COMPLETE REV

for
NCLEX-RN®

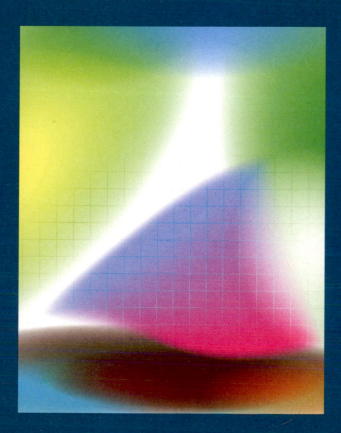

Donna F. Gauwitz, RN, MS

Nursing Consultant
Medical Legal Expert
Former Senior Teaching Specialist
School of Nursing—University of Minnesota, Twin Cities
Minneapolis, Minnesota

Former Nursing Education Specialist
Mayo Clinic
Rochester, Minnesota

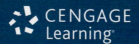

CENGAGE
Learning®

Australia • Brazil • Japan • Korea • Mexico • Singapore • Spain • United Kingdom • United States

**Complete Review for NCLEX-RN®,
Second Edition**
Donna F. Gauwitz

VP/General Manager, Skills & Product Planning:
Dawn Gerrain

Product Director, Health Care Skills:
Stephen Helba

Senior Director, Development:
Marah Bellegarde

Product Development Manager, Health Care
Skills: Juliet Steiner

Senior Content Developer, Health Care Skills:
Patricia A. Gaworecki

Product Assistant: Jenn Wheaton

Marketing Director: Michele McTighe

Marketing Manager: Scott Chrysler

Senior Production Director: Wendy Troeger

Production Manager: Andrew Crouth

Content Project Management: S4Carlisle

Art Direction: S4Carlisle

For product information and technology assistance, contact us at
Cengage Learning Customer & Sales Support, 1-800-354-9706

For permission to use material from this text or product,
submit all requests online at **www.cengage.com/permissions.**
Further permissions questions can be e-mailed to
permissionrequest@cengage.com

Library of Congress Control Number: 2013943064

ISBN-13: 978-1-133-28241-9

ISBN-10: 1-133-28241-5

Cengage Learning
200 First Stamford Place, 4th Floor
Stamford, CT 06902
USA

Cengage Learning is a leading provider of customized learning solutions with
office locations around the globe, including Singapore, the United Kingdom,
Australia, Mexico, Brazil, and Japan. Locate your local office at:
www.cengage.com/global

Cengage Learning products are represented in Canada by Nelson Education, Ltd.

To learn more about Cengage Learning, visit **www.cengage.com**
Purchase any of our products at your local college store or at our preferred
online store **www.cengagebrain.com**

Notice to the Reader

Printed in the United States of America
1 2 3 4 5 6 7 17 16 15 14 13

DEDICATION

This book is dedicated to my loving husband, William J. Gauwitz Jr., who is my best friend and always there encouraging me, supporting me, and cheering me on.

BRIEF CONTENTS

CONTENTS

CONTRIBUTORS

Mary Mescher Benbenek, RN, MS, CPNP, CFNP
Teaching Specialist
School of Nursing
University of Minnesota
Twin Cities, Minnesota
Chapter 30: Eyes, Ears, Nose, and Throat Disorders
Chapter 31: Respiratory Disorders

Margaret Brogan, RN, BSN
Registered Nurse/Expert
Children's Memorial Hospital
Chicago, Illinois
Chapter 36: Integumentary Disorders

Mary Lynn Burnett, RN, PhD
Assistant Professor of Nursing
Wichita State University
Wichita, Kansas
Chapter 3: Respiratory Disorders

Corine K. Carlson, RN, MS
Assistant Professor
Department of Nursing
Luther College
Decorah, Iowa
Chapter 16: Measurement and Drug Calculations
Chapter 32: Cardiovascular Disorders

Gretchen Reising Cornell, RN, PhD, CNE
Professor of Nursing
Utah Valley State College
Orem, Utah
Chapter 58: Health Issues of the Older Adult
Chapter 59: Delirium and Dementia
Chapter 67: Legal Issues for Older Adults

Vera V. Cull, RN, DSN
Former Assistant Professor of Nursing
University of Alabama
Birmingham, Alabama
Chapter 37: Musculoskeletal Disorders

Laura DeHelian, RN, PhD, APRN, BC
Advanced Practice Nurse
Neighboring Mental Health Services
Mentor, Ohio
Lecturer
Case Western Reserve University
Cleveland, Ohio
Chapter 47: Anxiety Disorders

Della J. Derscheid, RN, MS, CNS
Psychiatric Clinical Nurse Specialist
Department of Nursing
Mayo Clinic
Rochester, Minnesota
Chapter 52: Schizophrenia and Psychotic Disorders
Chapter 53: Paranoid Disorders

Ann Garey, MSN, APRN, BC, FNP
Nurse Practitioner
OB Services
Carle Foundation Hospital
Urbana, Illinois
Chapter 42: The Antepartal Period
Chapter 44: The Postpartal Period

Beth Good, RN, MSN, BSN
Teaching Specialist
University of Minnesota
Minneapolis, Minnesota
Chapter 51: Mood Disorders
Chapter 55: Substance Disorders

Samantha Grover, RN, BSN, CNS
Psychiatric Mental Health Clinical Specialist
MeritCare Health System
Moorhead, Minnesota
Chapter 50: Personality Disorders

Jeanne M. Harkness, RN, BA, MSN, BSN, AOCN
Clinical Practice Specialist
Jane Brattain Breast Center
Park Nicollet Clinic
St. Louis Park, Minnesota
Chapter 12: Hematological Disorders

Linda Irle, RN, MSN, APN, CNP
Coordinator, Maternal-Child Nursing
University of Illinois, Chicago
Urbana, Illinois
Family Nurse Practitioner, Acute Care
Carle Clinic
Champaign, Illinois
Chapter 44: The Postpartal Period

Amy Jacobson, RN, BA
Staff Nurse
United Hospital
St. Paul, Minnesota
Chapter 19: Drugs for the Cardiovascular System

Nadine James, RN, PhD
Assistant Professor of Nursing
University of Southern Mississippi
Hattiesburg, Mississippi
Chapter 9: Musculoskeletal Disorders

Lisa Jensen, CS, MS, APRN
Associate Chief Nurse/Mental Health
George E. Whalen VA Medical Center
Salt Lake City, Utah
Chapter 28: Psychotropic Drugs

Ellen Joswiak, RN, MA
Assistant Professor of Nursing
Luther College
Decorah, IA
Staff Nurse
Mayo Medical Center
Rochester, Minnesota
Chapter 64: Cultural Diversity

Betsy Ann Skrha Kennedy, RN, MS, CS, LCCE
Nursing Instructor
Rochester Community and Technical College
Rochester, Minnesota
Chapter 54: Post-Traumatic Stress Disorders

Robin M. Lally, PhD, RN, BA, AOCN, CNS
Teaching Specialist
School of Nursing
University of Minnesota
Minneapolis, Minnesota
Chapter 11: Oncology Disorders
Chapter 27: Antineoplastic Drugs
Chapter 66: Ethical Issues

Penny Leake, RN, PhD
Associate Professor
Luther College
Decorah, Iowa
Chapter 60: Case Management
Chapter 62: Home Health Care

Barbara Mandleco, RN, PhD
Associate Professor & Undergraduate Program
  Coordinator
College of Nursing
Brigham Young University
Provo, Utah
Chapter 29: Growth and Development
Chapter 35: Neurological Disorders

Gerry Matsumura, RN, PhD, MSN, BSN
Former Associate Professor of Nursing
Brigham Young University
Provo, Utah
Chapter 48: Somatoform Disorders
Chapter 49: Dissociative Disorders
Chapter 56: Sexual and Gender Identity Disorders

Alberta McCaleb, RN, DSN
Associate Professor
Chair, Undergraduate Studies
University of Alabama School of Nursing
University of Alabama at Birmingham
Birmingham, Alabama
Chapter 37: Musculoskeletal Disorders

Deana Moinari, RN, PhD
Associate Professor
Idaho State University
Pocatello, Idaho
Director of Rural Internship
Washington University
Spokane, Washington
Chapter 63: Hospice

JoAnn Mulready-Shick, RN, MS
Dean, Nursing and Allied Health
Roxbury Community College
Boston, Massachusetts
Chapter 20: Drugs for the Gastrointestinal System

Patricia Murdoch, RN, MS
Nurse Practitioner
University of Illinois, Chicago
Urbana, Illinois
Chapter 43: The Intrapartal Period
Chapter 45: Newborn Care

Jayme S. Nelson, RN, MS, ARNP-C
Adult Nurse Practitioner
Assistant Professor of Nursing
Luther College
Decorah, Iowa
Chapter 7: Neurological Disorders
Chapter 14: Perioperative Nursing
Chapter 22: Drugs for the Neurological System

Janice Nuuhiwa, MSN, CPON, APN/CNS
Staff Development Specialist
Hematology/Oncology/Stem Cell Transplant Division
Children's Memorial Hospital
Chicago, Illinois
Chapter 39: Oncology Disorders

Kristen L. Osborn, MSN, CRNP
Pediatric Nurse Specialist
UAB School of Nursing
UAB Pediatric Hematology/Oncology
Birmingham, Alabama
Chapter 40: Hematological Disorders

Karen D. Peterson, RN, MSN, BSN, PNP
Pediatric Nurse Practitioner
Division of Endocrinology
Children's Memorial Hospital
Chicago, Illinois
Chapter 34: Metabolic and Endocrine Disorders

Kristin Sandau, RN, PhD
Critical Care Education Coordinator
Abbott Northwest Hospital
Minneapolis, Minnesota
Chapter 4: Cardiovascular Disorders

Elizabeth Sawyer, RN, BSN, CCRN
Registered Nurse
United Hospital
St. Paul, Minnesota
*Chapter 13: Fluid, Electrolyte, and Acid-Base
  Disorders*

Lisa A. Seldomridge, RN, PhD
Associate Professor of Nursing
Salisbury University
Salisbury, Maryland
Chapter 8: Integumentary Disorders
Chapter 23: Drugs for the Integumentary System

Janice L. Vincent, RN, DSN
Assistant Professor
University of Alabama School of Nursing
University of Alabama at Birmingham
Birmingham, Alabama
Chapter 33: Gastrointestinal Disorders

Margaret Vogel, RN, MSN, BSN
Former Nursing Instructor
Rochester Community & Technical College
Rochester, Minnesota
Wound, Ostomy, and Continence Nurse
Enterstomal Therapy
Mayo Clinic
Rochester, Minnesota
Chapter 2: Eye, Ear, Nose, and Throat Disorders
*Chapter 17: Drugs for the Eyes, Ears, Nose,
  and Throat*

Mary Shannon Ward, RN, MSN
Director
Clinic Infectious Disease
Children's Memorial Hospital
Chicago, Illinois
Chapter 41: Infectious and Communicable Disorders

REVIEWERS

Dr. Geri Beers, RN, EdD
Associate Professor of Nursing
Samford University
Birmingham, Alabama

Nancy D. Bingaman, RN, MS
Nursing Instructor
Maurine Church Coburn School of Nursing
Monterey Peninsula College
Monterey, California

Carol Boswell, EdD, RN
Associate Professor
College of Nursing
Texas Tech University Health Sciences Center
Odessa, Texas

Judy A. Bourrand, RN, MSN
Assistant Professor
Ida V. Moffett School of Nursing, Samford University
Birmingham, Alabama

Clara Willard Boyle, RN, BS, MS, EdD
Associate Professor
Salem State College
Salem, Massachusetts

Rebecca Gesler, MSN, RN
Assistant Professor
Spalding University
Louisville, Kentucky

Loretta J. Heuer, PhD, RN, FAAN
Associate Professor
College of Nursing
University of North Dakota
Grand Forks, North Dakota

Susan Hinck, PhD, RN, CS
Associate Professor
Department of Nursing
Missouri State University
Springfield, Missouri

Mary M. Hoke, PhD, APRN-BC
Academic Department Head
New Mexico State University
Las Cruces, New Mexico

Ann Putnam Johnson, EdD, RN
Professor of Nursing
Associate Dean, College of Applied Sciences
Western Carolina University
Cullowhee, North Carolina

Brenda P. Johnson, PhD, RN
Associate Professor, Department of Nursing
Southeast Missouri State University
Cape Girardeau, Missouri

Pat S. Kupina, RN, MSN
Professor of Nursing
Joliet Junior College
Joliet, Illinois

Mary Lashley, RN, PhD, APRN, BC
Associate Professor
Department of Nursing
Towson University
Towson, Maryland

Melissa Lickteig, EdD, RN
Assistant Professor
School of Nursing
Georgia Southern University
Statesboro, Georgia

Caron Martin, MSN, RN
Associate Professor
School of Nursing and Health Professions
Northern Kentucky University
Highland Heights, Kentucky

Darlene Mathis, MSN, RN, APRN, BC, NP-C, CNE, CRNP
Assistant Professor and Certified Nurse Educator
Ida V. Moffett School of Nursing, Samford University
Family Nurse Practitioner
Birmingham Health Care
Birmingham, Alabama

Carol E. Meadows, MNSc, RNP, APN
Instructor
Eleanor Mann School of Nursing
University of Arkansas
Fayetteville, Arkansas

Margaret A. Miklancie, PhD, RN
Assistant Professor
College of Nursing & Health Science
George Mason University
Fairfax, Virginia

Frances D. Monahan, PhD, RN
Professor of Nursing
SUNY Rockland Community College
Consultant, Excelsior College

Deb Poling, MSN, APRN, BC, FNP, ANP
Assistant Professor
Regis University
Denver, Colorado
Case Manager
The Children's Hospital
Denver, Colorado

Abby Selby, MNSc, RN
Faculty
Mental Health and Illness
Eleanor Mann School of Nursing
College of Education and Health Professions
University of Arkansas
Fayetteville, Arkansas
PRN Educator
Mental Health Topics
Northwest Health System
Springdale, Arkansas

Sarah E. Shannon, PhD, RN
Associate Professor, Biobehavioral Nursing
and Health Systems
Adjunct Associate Professor, Medical History
and Ethics
University of Washington
Seattle, Washington

Susan Sienkiewicz, MA, RN
Professor
Community College of Rhode Island
Warwick, Rhode Island

Maria A. Smith, DSN, RN, CCRN
Professor
School of Nursing
Middle Tennessee State University
Murfreesboro, Tennessee

Ellen Stuart, MSN, RN
Professor
Mental Health Nursing
Grand Rapids Community College
Grand Rapids, Michigan

Karen Gahan Tarnow, RN, PhD
Faculty
School of Nursing
University of Kansas
Kansas City, Kansas

Janice Tazbir, RN, MS, CCRN
Associate Professor of Nursing
School of Nursing
Purdue University Calumet
Hammond, Indiana

Patricia C. Wagner, MSN, RNC
Clinical Assistant Professor
MCN Department, College of Nursing
University of South Alabama
Mobile, Alabama

PREFACE

Nursing is rapidly changing to meet the needs and demands of the health care environment. Clients are sicker, but due to the influx of technology, hospital stays are shorter. To meet these needs, nurses must not only be more skilled practitioners, but they also must be proficient in the areas of prioritization and delegation, as well as strengthen their roles as critical thinkers, decision makers, and leaders. As a result of the changing image of and demands on the nursing profession, the National Council of State Boards of Nursing has revised the National Council of Licensure Examination for registered nurses (NCLEX-RN®) to meet the challenges of health care in the twenty-first century. In order to be successful at passing the NCLEX-RN®, Cengage Learning has identified the need for a complete and comprehensive NCLEX-RN® review book that addresses all facets of nursing in this exciting and rapidly changing health care environment. *Complete Review for NCLEX-RN®* was developed to meet these challenges and prepare the graduates of nursing schools to be successful on the NCLEX-RN® and be the best prepared registered nurses that they can be.

CONCEPTUAL APPROACH

The concept for *Complete Review for NCLEX-RN®* resulted from the publisher's recognition of an identified need for a well-organized, readable, readily applicable, and comprehensive NCLEX-RN® review book. The text was developed to include a comprehensive content review of the subject matter covered in nursing school and practice questions that stimulate critical thinking skills and are representative of the types of questions found on the actual examination.

ORGANIZATION

Complete Review for NCLEX-RN® consists of 9 units, 67 chapters, and 1600 test questions primarily written at the application and analysis levels. After an introduction on preparing the graduate nurse to take the NCLEX-RN®, the units review all of the major topic areas covered in nursing school and tested on the NCLEX exam. Each chapter features a comprehensive content review followed by review questions with answers and rationales.

Unit I: Introduction

Chapter 1, Preparing for the NCLEX Examination, contains information on the development of the NCLEX-RN® and addresses the multitude of questions an NCLEX candidate may expect, ranging from applying and taking the exam to how the exam is scored and receiving the results.

Unit II: Medical-Surgical Nursing

Unit II covers all of the nursing content in medical-surgical nursing that is reflective of the NCLEX-RN®. Chapters are organized using a body-systems approach, with specialty chapters on perioperative nursing; oncology; and fluids, electrolytes, and acid-base disorders.

Each chapter begins with a brief overview of the anatomy and physiology necessary to develop an understanding of the disorders affecting that body system. This is followed by an overall assessment, including a health history and a physical examination. Diagnostic studies are next identified and include a description of the procedure followed by pre- and post-procedure care as applicable. Nursing diagnoses are also identified. Each chapter concludes with a review of the most frequently seen nursing disorders affecting the body system presented in the chapter. Each disorder begins with a description of the disorder, including pertinent incidence, etiological factors, and complications. The description is followed by an assessment of each disorder and includes clinical manifestations.

Diagnostic tests are identified for all disorders and cross-referenced to those procedures presented earlier in the chapter. Medical or surgical management is presented, if appropriate, and the review of each disorder concludes with nursing interventions.

Unit III: Pharmacology

This important unit of study addresses pharmacologic nursing from every aspect. Chapter 15, Medication Therapy, is a comprehensive overview of safe drug administration, drug uses, drug names, drug laws, and rights of medication administration. A drug assessment is presented, addressing the phases of the nursing process. The principles of drug administration are covered for oral, nasogastric, topical, and parenteral administrations. Intravenous administration—including vascular access devices, selection of the various types of veins, preparing and administering intravenous fluids and intravenous drugs, and complications and discontinuing therapy—is covered. The chapter concludes with a comprehensive review of blood therapy, including the types of blood, principles of blood therapy, blood therapy administration, and complications. Chapter 16, Measurement and Drug Calculations, begins with the system of measurements, including the metric, apothecary, and household measurement systems. Measurement conversion reviews ratio-proportion, formulas, and calculation methods, and includes pediatric dosage calculations. The content of the remainder of the chapters correlates with the content from the medical-surgical and pediatric units: Chapter 17, Drugs for the Eyes, Ears, Nose, and Throat; Chapter 18, Drugs for the Respiratory System; Chapter 19, Drugs for the Cardiovascular System; Chapter 20, Drugs for the Gastrointestinal System; Chapter 21, Drugs for the Endocrine System; Chapter 22, Drugs for the Neurological System; Chapter 23, Drugs for the Integumentary System; Chapter 24, Drugs for the Musculoskeletal System; Chapter 25, Drugs for the Genitourinary System; Chapter 26, Drugs for the Reproductive System; Chapter 27, Antineoplastic Drugs; and Chapter 28, Psychotropic Drugs. Each chapter is organized to reflect a category of drugs followed by the uses, adverse reactions, contraindications and precautions, drug interactions, nursing interventions, and types of drugs listed for each category.

Unit IV: Pediatric Nursing

Unit IV begins with Chapter 29, Growth and Development. This chapter covers growth and development principles, issues and theories of human development, as well as the growth and develop-

ment periods for the newborn, infant, toddler, preschooler, school-age, and adolescent child. The subsequent chapters are Chapter 30, Eyes, Ears, Nose, and Throat Disorders; Chapter 31, Respiratory Disorders; Chapter 32, Cardiovascular Disorders; Chapter 33, Gastrointestinal Disorders; Chapter 34, Metabolic and Endocrine Disorders; Chapter 35, Neurological Disorders; Chapter 36, Integumentary Disorders; Chapter 37, Musculoskeletal Disorders; Chapter 38, Genitourinary Disorders; Chapter 39, Oncology Disorders; Chapter 40, Hematological Disorders; and Chapter 41, Infectious and Communicable Disorders. These chapters have the same organization as the medical-surgical chapters in Unit II with one key exception: a category addressing the differences in the anatomy and physiology between the child and adult.

Unit V: Maternity and Women's Health Nursing

The maternity and women's health unit is composed of Chapter 42, The Antepartal Period, covering normal pregnancy and high-risk pregnancy conditions; Chapter 43, The Intrapartal Period, addressing the mechanisms and stages of labor and special intrapartal situations; Chapter 44, The Postpartal Period, covering the normal postpartum recovery period and postpartal complications; Chapter 45, Newborn Care, covering both anticipated and high-risk newborn conditions; and Chapter 46, Reproductive Disorders, which completes the unit. Each chapter is organized to be consistent with Unit II (Medical-Surgical Nursing) and Unit IV (Pediatric Nursing). These chapters begin with anatomy and physiology, assessment, diagnostic studies, nursing diagnoses, medical management, and nursing interventions.

Unit VI: Psychiatric Nursing

Unit VI reviews all of the psychiatric concepts covered on the NCLEX-RN® and includes Chapter 47, Anxiety Disorders; Chapter 48, Somatoform Disorders; Chapter 49, Dissociative Disorders; Chapter 50, Personality Disorders; Chapter 51, Mood Disorders; Chapter 52, Schizophrenia and Psychotic Disorders; Chapter 53, Paranoid Disorders; Chapter 54, Post-Traumatic Stress Disorders; Chapter 55, Substance Disorders; Chapter 56, Sexual and Gender Identity Disorders; and Chapter 57, Eating Disorders. Each chapter covers the unique features pertinent to the area of psychiatric nursing and applicable theories. Consistent with the previous units, each disorder begins with a description of the area of psychiatric nursing followed by assessment, diagnostic tests, medical management, and nursing interventions.

Unit VII: Gerontologic Nursing

There are two chapters in Unit VII: Chapter 58, Health Issues of the Older Adult, and Chapter 59, Delirium and Dementia. Topics addressed in Chapter 58 include theories of aging, effects of aging on individual body systems, and related issues such as sleep, immunity, pain, and polypharmacy. Delirium, dementia, and Alzheimer's disease are covered in Chapter 59.

Unit VIII: Community Health Nursing

Unit VIII reviews all aspects of community health nursing that may be covered on the NCLEX-RN®. The content includes Chapter 60, Case Management; Chapter 61, Long-Term Care; Chapter 62, Home Health Care; and Chapter 63, Hospice.

Unit IX: Legal and Ethical Issues in Nursing

Unit IX covers legal and ethical issues that are included on the NCLEX-RN®: Chapter 64, Cultural Diversity; Chapter 65, Leadership and Management; Chapter 66, Ethical Issues; and Chapter 67, Legal Issues for Older Adults.

FEATURES

Unique to *Complete Review for NCLEX-RN®* is the endorsement by the National Student Nurse Association. Also unique are the gerontologic, community health, and legal and ethical issues units. Additionally, this text is designed around the most up-to-date test plan and provides a comprehensive review of NCLEX-style questions. Every chapter and comprehensive test has priority and delegation questions that are heavily stressed in the current NCLEX-RN® test plan. This book has approximately 30% to 40% of the innovative-style questions to provide students with a well-rounded sampling of the alternate-item-format questions that they may encounter on the exam. It is through answering so many alternate-item-format questions in *Complete Review for NCLEX-RN®* that candidates will have increased confidence and be better prepared to pass the NCLEX-RN®.

Each answer to a review question includes the correct answer as well as the accompanying rationale for both the right and wrong options. The areas of client need, nursing process, cognitive level, and subject area were carefully planned and addressed to provide the student with a balanced and comprehensive sampling of the type of test questions that appear on the exam.

HOW TO USE THIS BOOK

The nursing school graduate should begin preparing for the test by reading Unit I, Chapter 1, Preparing for the NCLEX Examination. It is through reading this chapter that the student will develop an understanding of the preparation, testing experience, and post-testing procedures. Developing an understanding of what to expect will decrease the graduate's anxiety and better prepare him or her for the NCLEX-RN®.

After developing an understanding of the actual testing experience, the student should begin a review of the nursing content. It is recommended to begin with Unit II (Medical-Surgical Nursing) and go through each unit in sequence. After reading and reviewing the nursing content in each chapter, the student should take the chapter exam at the end of the chapter. The student may choose to take the whole chapter test before going through the rationales or choose to answer one question followed by reviewing the rationale for that question. Either way, it is through the rationales for the right and wrong options that a further review of nursing content is provided. Finally, it is important to have enough time to complete the actual exam. Take the entire chapter test for timing purposes. As a frame of reference, an estimated time allowance of 1 minute should be given per question. Some questions—regardless of whether multiple-choice or one of the alternate-format questions—may take more than a minute, whereas other questions will take less.

The concept, scope, and design of this text represent a commitment to help the graduate RN reach his or her full professional potential. Good luck on your NCLEX-RN® examination!

Donna Faye Gauwitz, RN, MS

ACKNOWLEDGMENTS

A very special thank you goes to Patty Gaworecki, Senior Content Developer, whom I worked with closely over the course of revising this book for her consultations and guidance.

I wish to thank all of the people behind the scenes at Cengage Learning who contributed in the publication process for this valuable book.

All of the contributors are thanked for their expertise in providing chapter content relevant to a thorough review of the nursing literature. The reviewers are thanked for their valuable comments about the manuscript.

I want to thank all of my nursing students at Methodist Hospital School of Nursing in Peoria, Illinois; Barry University in Miami Shores, Florida; Broward Community College in Pembroke Pines, Florida; and the University of Minnesota in Minneapolis, Minnesota, for their enthusiasm for my NCLEX-style test questions on their exams and their faith in my ability to prepare them to take the NCLEX-RN®. I want to thank all of the nursing graduates at Mayo Clinic in Rochester who took my NCLEX-RN® review course in their preparation to take the NCLEX-RN® and their positive feedback.

Last and most important, I want to thank my husband and best friend, William J. Gauwitz, for his continual support of my commitment to this book.

Donna Faye Gauwitz, RN, MS

ABOUT THE AUTHOR

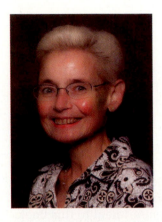

Donna Faye Gauwitz, RN, MS, received her diploma in nursing from St. Francis School of Nursing in Peoria, Illinois. After graduation, she worked on medical-surgical nursing units, specifically neurology, and on the psychiatric unit at St. Francis Hospital, a major acute care facility and trauma center in central Illinois. She immediately began work on her Bachelor of Science degree at Bradley University in Peoria, Illinois. After graduating with a BSN, Donna began her career in nursing education as a staff development coordinator at St. Francis Medical Center, orienting new graduate nurses to a large medical-surgical unit. She was also adjunct faculty at Illinois Central College in East Peoria, and at Illinois Wesleyan University in Bloomington, teaching medical-surgical and pediatric nursing. While at Illinois Central College, she developed and taught a new college course, "Introduction to Eating Disorders."

Donna further developed her research and publishing interests as a research assistant at the University of Illinois Department of Psychiatry and Behavioral Medicine in Peoria, and at Northwestern University College of Nursing in Chicago, Illinois. She did the research and wrote the proposal for an eating disorder clinic and became the director of the clinic at St. Francis Medical Center in Peoria, Illinois.

Her pursuit of advanced education took her to Northwestern University College of Nursing in Evanston, Illinois, to obtain her master's degree. After graduation from Northwestern University, Donna began her full-time teaching career at Methodist Medical Center in Peoria, Illinois, followed by teaching medical-surgical, orthopedics, rehabilitative, women's health, and neurology nursing at Barry University in Miami Shores, Florida, and Broward Community College in Pembroke Pines, Florida.

After relocating to Minnesota, she became a nursing education specialist for an acute care surgical unit at the Mayo Clinic in Rochester, Minnesota. Because of her unique expertise as an NCLEX-RN® item writer, while at the Mayo Clinic she was asked to teach NCLEX review courses for new registered nurse graduates to prepare them to take the NCLEX-RN®. Her love of nursing education then took her to the University of Minnesota as a senior teaching specialist and the coordinator of the Nursing Skills Laboratory in Minneapolis, Minnesota.

During her tenure in education, she had the opportunity to serve as an item writer eight times for the National Council of State Boards of Nursing in the development of the NCLEX-RN®. She was also asked to publish an article in *Insight,* a publication of the National Council of State Boards of Nursing. She further pursued her interest in publishing with three articles in the journal *Nursing* and one article in the *American Journal of Nursing.* She is also the author of *Administering Medications: Pharmacology for Health Careers.* Donna has also served as a medical expert in several malpractice cases.

Donna is a member of Sigma Theta Tau and has been listed in *Who's Who in American Nursing.*

INTRODUCTION

1 | Preparing for the NCLEX Examination

CHAPTER 1

PREPARING FOR THE NCLEX EXAMINATION

NATIONAL COUNCIL TEST PLAN FOR REGISTERED NURSES

The National Council of State Boards of Nursing (NCSBN) develops a licensure examination that is responsible for regulating entrance into nursing practice in the United States.

Development of the Test Plan

Before presenting the actual test plan for the NCLEX-RN®, it is essential to understand the NCLEX-RN® test development procedure. It takes 18 months for each item to be taken through every step of the test development procedure to ensure a completely valid and reliable exam that measures the knowledge, skill, and ability to be a safe entry-level registered nurse. The development of the NCLEX-RN® test plan goes through several steps.

First, a job analysis is performed every 3 years by surveying new graduates of schools of nursing for what skills and procedures they are most frequently performing. Hand washing and medication administration are two skills that new graduates respond are frequently performed. This job analysis serves as a guide in the development of the test plan from which the items are developed according to client need and the phase of the nursing process.

Second is the test plan, which guides the development of the NCLEX-RN®. Although every candidate's exam is different, each exam is developed to equally assess each candidate's knowledge; skill; and ability to promote, maintain, or restore a client's health and be a safe entry-level registered nurse.

After performing a job analysis and developing the test plan, the actual development of the exam begins. This process begins with the item writing workshop.

These workshops bring practicing registered nurses from across the country who work with new graduates to a designated site. Generally, item writers are nursing faculty from across the United States who teach in undergraduate schools of nursing or clinical preceptors working with new graduate nurses within their first 6 months of practice. An additional requirement an item writer must have is a master's or higher degree. Next, item reviewers are brought to the item review workshops in the same designated workshop sites. Item reviewers are registered nurses who are working directly with new graduates in clinical settings. "New graduates" are defined as those who have entered nursing practice in the past 6 to 12 months. These item reviewers review the items written by the item writers to determine if these items are a good representation of actual beginning nursing practice. After the items circulate through the item reviewers, the items go to an item sensitivity review workshop. The reviewers evaluate items for cultural diversity in the United States. The reviewers come from various ethnic and minority groups, representing a diversified background, cultural traditions, and viewpoints found in the United States and international test-taking populations.

The fourth step the items go through is an editorial review. These reviewers are made up of non-nurse individuals experienced in the editorial process. After the items have been reviewed for grammar and punctuation, the items are entered into the computer and followed by a member board item review process. The member board reviewers are registered nurses who work in a jurisdiction that is responsible for graduating registered nurses. Each nursing jurisdiction has a member board that reviews items. These reviewers review the items for accuracy of current nursing practice and level of difficulty.

After the member board review, the items are field tested. Fifteen of every 75 items are piloted on the NCLEX-RN®. After the member board review, the items go to the NCSBN for review and approval. The last step to complete the item development process is placing the items in the computerized adaptive test (CAT) pool. In addition to the actual item development process, a panel of judges directly impacts the total NCLEX-RN®. The panel of judges consists of registered nurse members elected every 3 years. These members are currently employed in clinical nursing practice and work with graduates within the first 6 to 12 months of practice.

COGNITIVE LEVELS

Each NCLEX-RN® item is written to the cognitive level based on Bloom's taxonomy and both the client needs category and subcategory. Although remembering and understanding, applying, analyzing, evaluating, and creating are the cognitive levels, the majority of the items on the NCLEX-RN® are written to applying, analyzing, evaluating, and creating. Items written at the applying, analyzing, evaluating, and creating levels are more difficult and require critical thinking to answer.

Remembering

The lowest cognitive level is remembering, which tests only simple recall. For example:

The normal range for the serum potassium level is _____.
Answer: 3.5 to 5.5 mEq/L

Rationale:
In this item, no more is required than memorization of a normal serum potassium level.

Understanding

The next cognitive level is understanding, which requires an understanding of written communication or information. It is simply ideas or concepts. For example:

Which of the following foods should the nurse include in the dietary instructions for a client on a low-residue diet for Crohn's disease?

1. Baked chicken and mashed potatoes
2. Lettuce salad and apple
3. Tacos and taco chips
4. Whole-grain toast and cornflakes cereal
Answer: 1

Rationale:
In this item, the stem tells you a low-residue diet is prescribed for Crohn's disease instead of requiring you to know what Crohn's disease is and what kind of diet is given in the treatment. For example, raw fruits (except bananas) and vegetables, seeds, and whole grains are to be avoided. Lettuce salad and apples are raw vegetables and fruit, respectively. Tacos and taco chips include both raw vegetables and whole grains. Whole-grain bread and cornflakes cereal are whole grains. Baked chicken is a meat that is permitted, and the mashed potatoes are a cooked vegetable.

Applying

As with many of the items, the level of difficulty can be increased by incorporating critical thinking skills. The third cognitive level is applying, which requires applying an idea or theory to a job-related situation. Information is used in a new way. Two examples will be given to better illustrate this cognitive level.

Example 1:
Which of the following foods should the nurse include in the dietary instructions for a client with Crohn's disease?
1. Baked chicken and mashed potatoes
2. Lettuce salad and apple
3. Tacos and taco chips
4. Whole-grain toast and cornflakes cereal
Answer: 1

Rationale:
The level of difficulty has been increased in this item, and the cognitive level has also been elevated from understanding to applying. In this item, you need to know that Crohn's disease is an inflammation of the bowel most commonly affecting the terminal ileum, jejunum, or colon and resulting in skip lesions (normal bowel followed by diseased bowel) characterized by abdominal pain, diarrhea, weight loss, fever, and fatigue. You also need to know what the diet of choice is for Crohn's disease (low residue) and what foods are permitted and what foods are to be avoided. A low-residue diet should avoid raw fruits, vegetables, and whole grains.

Example 2:
The nurse is collecting a nursing history from a client with acute pyelonephritis. Which of the following questions should the nurse ask?
1. "Have you noticed any blood in your urine?"
2. "Have you experienced a decrease in your urinary output?"
3. "Do you have pain when urinating?"
4. "Do you find you are experiencing dribbling at the end of urinating?"
Answer: 3

Rationale:
In this item, you must know that dysuria, or pain when urinating, is present in pyelonephritis. Asking about dysuria when collecting a nursing history supports the diagnosis.

Analyzing

The fourth cognitive level is analyzing, in which material or information is broken down into parts, detecting the relationship of the parts and the way they are organized. For example:

The nurse is caring for a client experiencing renal colic associated with nephrolithiasis. Which of the following nursing measures should receive priority in the client's plan of care?
1. Strain the urine.
2. Administer morphine sulfate.
3. Monitor intake and output.
4. Encourage ambulation.
Answer: 2

Rationale:
In this item you need to first understand what nephrolithiasis (kidney stone disease) is and the relationship to renal colic (severe and colicky pain in the flank area). After establishing that renal colic occurs from the nerves being stimulated during the passage of a kidney stone or clot, you must be able to prioritize the client's care. Although straining the urine, monitoring the intake and output, and encouraging ambulation are all appropriate nursing interventions, administering morphine sulfate is the priority.

Evaluating

The fifth cognitive level is evaluating, in which a stand or decision is justified. For example:

The nurse evaluates a client with hypernatremia to be at risk for cerebral edema when receiving which of the following intravenous solutions?
1. D5% water
2. 0.9% NS
3. D5% 0.9% NaCl
4. Lactated Ringer's solution
Answer: 1

Rationale:
D5% is given in the treatment of hypernatremia. The nurse must monitor the client for cerebral edema. 0.9% NS is an intravascular volume expander. D5% 0.9% NaCl is given for hypotonic dehydration and must be used cautiously in clients with heart failure or renal failure. Lactated Ringer's solution is used for burns and gastrointestinal fluid losses.

Creating

Creating is the sixth and final cognitive level. The focus is on creating new product or point of view. For example:

The nurse includes which of the following foods in formulating a low-residue diet for ulcerative colitis?
1. Strained green beans
2. Ham and bean soup
3. Fried scrambled eggs
4. Coconut pie
Answer: 1

Rationale:
A low-residue diet is the treatment of choice for ulcerative colitis. Strained vegetables such as strained green beans are permitted on a low-residue diet. Ham and bean soup, fried scrambled eggs, and coconut pie are to be avoided on a low-residue diet.

Client Needs and Client Needs Subcategories

In addition to each NCLEX-RN® item being written to a cognitive level, each item is written to client needs and client needs subcategories. The client needs category explains nursing tasks and competencies across the life span and in all client settings. There are four major categories of client needs (Table 1-1).

The first, Safe and Effective Care Environment, ensures client outcomes by directly delivering or indirectly supervising nursing care while maintaining the safety of clients, their families, or health care individuals. The second, Health Promotion and

Table 1-1 Categories of Client Needs

Client needs I	Safe and Effective Care Environment
Client needs II	Health Promotion and Maintenance
Client needs III	Psychosocial Integrity
Client needs IV	Physiological Integrity

Source: Used with permission from the National Council of State Boards of Nursing, 2013 Test Plan for the NCLEX-RN® Examination

Table 1-2 Client Needs Subcategories

Client Needs Category	Client Needs Subcategory
I. Safe and Effective Care Environment	Management of Care
	Safety and Infection Control
IV. Physiological Integrity	Basic Care and Comfort
	Pharmacological and Parenteral Therapies
	Reduction of Risk Potential
	Physiological Adaptation

Source: Used with permission from the National Council of State Boards of Nursing, 2013 Test Plan for the NCLEX-RN® Examination

Table 1-3 Management of Care Subcategory Content Areas

Advanced directives and living wills
Case management
Collaboration
Confidentiality
Delegation
Ethical issues
Informed consent
Management of care
Priorities
Rights of clients
Staff development

Source: Used with permission from the National Council of State Boards of Nursing, 2013 Test Plan for the NCLEX-RN® Examination

Table 1-4 Safety and Infection Control Subcategory Content Areas

Asepsis (medical and surgical)
Bioterrorism and planning for disasters
Equipment safety
Prevention of accidents and injuries
Prevention of errors
Safety in the home
Precaution procedures (airborne, contact, droplet, and standard)
Restraints

Source: Used with permission from the National Council of State Boards of Nursing, 2013 Test Plan for the NCLEX-RN® Examination

Maintenance, provides care directly to or indirectly to clients and their families, considering principles of growth and development while preventing health problems and promoting an optimal health status. Psychosocial Integrity is the third client needs category, and it provides care to clients with chronic mental illness or facilitates emotional support to families of clients with varying degrees of physical or mental illness. The fourth and last client needs category is Physiological Integrity, in which basic and advanced nursing care, including medications and parenteral therapies, are provided and the potential for risks is decreased.

Two of the four client needs categories have subcategories (Table 1-2).

The percent of items under each client needs category and subcategory on each candidate's examination is constantly being evaluated through research. The total percent of items on any candidate's examination for the client needs Safe and Effective Care Environment falls between 24% and 36%. There are two subcategories under Safe and Effective Care Environment. The first is Management of Care with 16% to 22% of the total items, and the second is Safety and Infection Control with 8% to 14% of the total items. These subcategory percentages are very reflective of health care in the twenty-first century, with delegation and the advent of new diseases such as severe acute respiratory syndrome (SARS), West Nile virus, and the possibility of diseases such as anthrax and smallpox. Items coming from the Management of Care (Table 1-3) and Safety and Infection Control (Table 1-4) come from many content areas.

The second client needs category is Health Promotion and Maintenance, which does not have a subcategory. The possibility of items on any candidate's examination ranges from 6% to 12%. Health Promotion and Maintenance provides direct and indirect care to clients and their families. This category considers principles of growth and development while preventing health problems and promoting an optimal health status, including development, obstetrics, health prevention, and promotion behaviors (Table 1-5).

Similar to Health Promotion and Maintenance, Psychosocial Integrity does not have subcategories under the client needs category. Psychosocial Integrity provides care to clients with chronic mental illness and facilitates emotional support to families of clients with varying degrees

Table 1-5 Health Promotion and Maintenance Client Needs Content Areas

Aging
Body image changes (anticipated)
Concepts of growth and development
Concepts of health and wellness
Education of clients and families
Family planning high-risk behaviors
Newborn care (antepartum, intrapartum, and postpartum)
Physical assessment skills
Prevention of disease
Self-care
Screening for health problems
Vaccinations and immunizations

Source: Used with permission from the National Council of State Boards of Nursing, 2013 Test Plan for the NCLEX-RN® Examination

Table 1-6 Psychosocial Integrity Client Needs Content Areas

Body image changes (unanticipated)
Changes in family or significant other roles
Chemical dependency
Concepts of death and dying
Coping strategies
Crisis management
Cultural issues
End-of-life issues
Family dynamics
Management of behavioral issues
Neglect and abuse
Spiritual issues
Stress
Therapeutic communication

Source: Used with permission from the National Council of State Boards of Nursing, 2013 Test Plan for the NCLEX-RN® Examination

Table 1-7 Physiological Integrity Client Needs Content Areas

Subcategory 1—Basic Care and Comfort
Alternative and complementary therapies
Comfort interventions that are not pharmaceutical
Devices considered assistive
Elimination issues
Hygienic issues
Mobility and immobility issues
Nutritional issues
Palliative care
Rest and sleep issues

Subcategory 2—Pharmacological and Parenteral Therapies
Adverse effects, contraindications, nursing implications, interventions
Blood and blood products
Calculations
Central venous access devices
Intravenous therapy
Medication administration
Parenteral nutrition

Subcategory 3—Reduction of Risk Potential
Complications of health deviations and surgical procedures
Conscious sedation
Diagnostic procedures
Interpretation of diagnostic and laboratory tests
Laboratory test procedures
Vital signs

Subcategory 4—Physiological Adaptation
Body systems alterations
Emergencies
Imbalances of fluid and electrolytes
Hemodynamics
Pathophysiology
Radiation therapy

Source: Used with permission from the National Council of State Boards of Nursing, 2013 Test Plan for the NCLEX-RN® Examination

of physical or mental illness. There are many content areas from which items are asked (Table 1-6).

The fourth and final client needs category is Physiological Integrity and encompasses the majority of items on the NCLEX-RN®, or 40% to 64%. As previously defined, Physiological Integrity deals with the most basic care to advanced nursing care, including medication and parenteral therapies, while decreasing potential risks. Because this client needs category makes up the largest percent of any candidate's examination, the content areas are broken down into each subcategory to give you an overview of study items (see Table 1-7).

SUCCESSFUL TEST PREPARATION

Being a successful test taker begins with the development of good study habits and techniques. Not only will developing these techniques help you in your own professional goal of becoming a safe and effective registered nurse, but they will also help you in your career when you teach clients.

Positive Attitude

The most important element to doing well on the NCLEX examination is a positive attitude. You may think this is easier said than done, but test-taking techniques will place you in a position of success and put you on the road to developing an "I can do it" attitude.

Perform mental exercises to help you develop a positive attitude. Use facts to help you think positively. Tell yourself that you did your work to the best of your ability in school, graduated from school, and now are ready to take the NCLEX-RN®. So again, look at the concrete facts. Set short-term, measurable goals.

Setting Goals

Short-term goals generally occur over a short period of time. *Measurable* means you can evaluate whether you were able to accomplish a goal. A short-term goal may be studying for the NCLEX-RN®. Set a realistic goal, such as studying a chapter a night from this NCLEX review book until you complete this book and accompanying questions both in the book and on the CD.

Long-term goals are goals that will occur over many months to years. For example, your long-term goal is to pass the NCLEX-RN®, making you the best possible nurse you can be.

Taking Care of Yourself

A basic criterion to being successful on a test is to take care of yourself. You should not alter your normal schedule as long as you are getting enough sleep and eating well. It is a proven fact that people function at their best when they get enough sleep. Sleep research has demonstrated a decrease in cognitive skills and reaction time when a person is suffering from sleep deprivation. In addition to adequate sleep, appropriate nutrition must be maintained. Think of yourself as an automobile. Much like a car without fuel, your body will not run without food and certainly not at its best. Eat three well-balanced meals a day to maintain a constant mental and physical alertness. It is important that you do not alter any of your normal routines. Do not drink more coffee or increase your intake for other caffeinated beverages or food such as cola products, tea, or chocolate. Taking more caffeine-containing products than usual may make you anxious and unable to concentrate.

TEST-TAKING STRATEGIES

Always begin by reading the entire question and all of the answers carefully before selecting a response. If the answer is not immediately known, using test-taking strategies can help to maximize your success.

Analyze the Stem

There are important points to learn about how stems are written that will make test taking easier. A good stem will not have a lot of extraneous information in it that is not necessary to answering the item. For example, names are never used on the NCLEX exam. They have no bearing on the item. Other biographical data such as age, gender, race, and occupation are never used unless they are necessary to answering the item. For example, some conditions occur more frequently in women or men, certain races or ages, or people with certain types of occupations, so this information is essential to present to correctly answer the item. For example, sickle cell anemia occurs in African Americans.

When starting to answer each question, carefully look at the stem. The stem is the part of the question asking the question. It may be stated as a question with a question mark or it may be a statement in which the answer completes the statement. There are other terms that may appear in a stem that also ask for you to prioritize and perform the most important intervention first. If "most appropriate," "most important," "essential," "most likely," "initial," or "best" appears in the stem, you are being asked to prioritize and decide which intervention should be first because it is more important than all of the other choices.

There are no negative stems in the actual NCLEX examination. You will never find an item that asks for the exception such as: "Which of the following would be the exception?" The NCLEX examination is not concerned with what the nurse would never do; rather, the NCLEX focuses on what the nurse should do in order to be a safe practitioner.

The following examples illustrate the different types of stems.

Age often affects the answer to the question. For example:

Which of the following should the nurse consider before starting an IV on a 4-year-old child?
1. Place the child in a supine position and apply bilateral wrist restraints.
2. Take the child to the hospital playroom to provide a comfortable and "safe" environment.

3. Assist the child to sit on the mother's lap with the child's leg between the mother's leg and the unused arm behind the mother.
4. Select the antecubital fossa for the insertion site to restrict the child's movement as little as possible.

Answer: 3

Rationale:
The most appropriate intervention for a 4-year-old child is to have the child sit on the mother's lap with the child's leg between the mother's leg and the unused arm behind the mother.

The stem can be stated as a question with a question mark. For example:

The nurse assesses a client's potassium level to be normal when it falls between what range of mEq/L?
Answer: 3.5 to 5.5

Another type of stem is a statement in which the answer completes the statement. For example:

The nurse is weighing a client in kilograms; the client weighs 65 kg. The client wants to know how many pounds that is. The most appropriate response by the nurse is _____.
Answer: 143

There are several versions of a stem asking a question with a question mark that are important for you to be familiar with. It is essential that you read the stem carefully and never read into what is being asked. First, you must identify all of the information presented in the stem.

Sometimes there is a sentence in addition to the actual stem asking the question. This information is intended to give you more background necessary to understanding the question and being able to answer it.

Example 1:
A stem can be presented with background information presented in two additional sentences. For example:

The nurse must weigh all clients and convert the weight in pounds to kilograms.

The nurse is assessing a client to weigh 189 pounds and converts this to how many kilograms?
Answer: 86

Often a stem presents the background information in the same stem sentence asking the question. For example:

A client with ulcerative colitis is experiencing abdominal pain, weight loss, and bloody diarrhea. The nurse assesses this client to have how many bloody diarrhea stools a day?
Answer: 15 to 20

Some stems may ask you to give the only correct answer. Other stems may ask for you to prioritize or ask what should be performed first. These are questions of higher difficulty, such as applying or analyzing, which are common on the NCLEX exam, so it is essential that you get comfortable with answering these questions.

Example 1:
The nurse correctly assists a client after a hip arthroplasty to get out of bed into which of the following chairs?
1. Wheelchair with footrest
2. Recliner chair with both legs elevated
3. Low soft lounge chair
4. Straight-back arm chair

Answer: 4

Rationale:
The only correct answer in this situation is to have the client sit in a chair with a straight back. The other choices of chairs would all be inappropriate and could result in harm or discomfort to the client.

Example 2:
After cataract surgery, a client complains of feeling nauseated. The priority nursing intervention for this client is to:
1. Offer dry cracker to eat.
2. Administer an antiemetic drug.
3. Instruct the client to deep breathe until the nausea subsides.
4. Explain that this is a normal occurrence after surgery.

Answer: 2

Rationale:
Although all of the interventions may be appropriate, the priority nursing intervention is to administer an antiemetic drug after surgery. Asking the priority is synonymous with asking what should be performed first.

Another version of prioritization is to ask what will be performed first. For example:

A client with a history of status epilepticus and diabetes is brought into the emergency department in the midst of a seizure. Which of the following should the nurse perform first?
1. Establish an airway.
2. Administer IV phenytoin (Dilantin).
3. Check the blood glucose level.
4. Start an IV line.
Answer: 1

Rationale:
Again, although the other interventions may be appropriate, the first intervention in any situation is to have a patent airway. Always remember that the ABCs (airway, breathing, and circulation) of care are the most important.

What you might see on the NCLEX exam is stems that use the word "avoid." These are frequently used in correlation to diet or nursing intervention questions. For example:

The nurse assists a client experiencing diarrhea to avoid which of the following foods when marking a menu?
Select all that apply.
[ ] 1. Steamed rice
[ ] 2. Bran cereal
[ ] 3. Orange juice
[ ] 4. Bananas
[ ] 5. Applesauce
[ ] 6. Fried eggs
Answer: 2, 3, 6

Rationale:
Bran cereal, orange juice, and fried eggs would all promote diarrhea and should be avoided on a diet for a client experiencing diarrhea. Steamed rice, bananas, and applesauce are all foods permitted in the diet of a client having diarrhea.

A stem asking for an abnormal finding so that an intervention may be performed does appear on the NCLEX exam. Reporting an abnormal finding is doing something essential to providing safe care. Remember, the most important point in any item is that the nurse is always doing something. For example:

The nurse is caring for a group of clients and reports which of the following clients as having an abnormal daily output?

1. A 2-day-old newborn with a daily urinary output of 60 mL
2. A 2-month-old infant with a daily urinary output of 400 mL
3. A 5-year-old child with a daily urinary output of 700 mL
4. A 35-year-old client with a daily urinary output of 1000 mL
Answer: 4

Rationale:
All of the choices are correct assessment findings except a 35-year-old client who has a daily urinary output of 1000 mL. The minimum daily output for an adult client should be 1500 mL.

Another type of stem requiring additional investigation is a type of item asking the nurse to seek more information. For example:

The nurse is reviewing the normal limits of a hearing assessment for a client who complains of decreased hearing. Which of the following findings would indicate the need for additional investigation?
1. Sound heard equally in both ears with the Weber test
2. 25 dB on the audiogram
3. Bone conduction greater than air conduction with the Rinne test
4. Pearly, shiny, and semitransparent tympanic membrane with an otoscope
Answer: 3

Rationale:
All of the choices are normal assessment findings except bone conduction greater than air conduction with the Rinne test. This necessitates that the nurse reports this finding so that further investigation may be done.

Alternative Style Items

The NCSBN introduced alternative format questions that include fill-in-the-blank, multiple-response, picture or graph "hot-spot," drag-and-drop or ordered-response, exhibit, and audio and video items.

Fill-in-the-Blank Questions

A fill-in-the-blank question may be a short phrase requiring one or two numbers to complete the sentence or a few descriptive sentences requiring an answer that generally includes one or two numbers. Additionally, the NCLEX frequently uses this format for calculation questions. Just enough information is given in a fill-in-the-blank question to answer the question. The information is specific, so it leads the test taker to only one possible answer. Fill-in-the-blank questions may be written at any of the cognitive levels (remembering, understanding, applying, analyzing, evaluating, and creating).

A remembering-level fill-in-the-blank question requires no more than a simple recall of a fact, such as a memorization of a word. It may be written as a question or as a statement with a missing word to complete the sentence. For example:

The nurse assesses a client's therapeutic digoxin level to be between what range ng/mL? _____.

Answer: 0.5 and 2

Rationale:
The therapeutic digoxin level is 0.5 to 2 ng/mL. Digoxin (Lanoxin) is an inotropic drug that acts as an antidysrhythmic.

Another version of the fill-in-the-blank question includes questions written at the understanding level or requiring an understanding of the material. For example:

The nurse should hang what percent of normal saline intravenous solution before starting a blood transfusion?
Answer: 0.9%

Rationale:
0.9% normal saline is the appropriate intravenous solution to hang when a client is going to receive blood to prevent hemolysis of red blood cells that may occur with a dextrose solution.

Questions written to the applying level apply understood material to a job-related situation. For example:

After initiating a blood transfusion, the nurse determines the client is experiencing an acute hemolytic reaction. When intervening in this situation, the priority is to stop the blood transfusion within how many minutes?
Answer: 15

Rationale:
An acute hemolytic reaction may occur within 15 minutes of a transfusion. The immediate intervention is to stop the blood followed by maintaining IV access with normal saline, sending the blood bag and tubing back to the blood bank, and obtaining a urine and blood sample.

Questions written to the analyzing level break down the material into parts and evaluate the relationship of the parts. For example:

The nurse compares a client who is 23 years old with a 70-year-old client for a spinal cord injury after a motor vehicle accident. The nurse appraises which age of the client to be at greatest risk for a spinal cord injury?
Answer: 23

Rationale:
Spinal cord injuries are most common in clients who are 16 to 30 years old after activities such as motor vehicle accidents.

A calculation question provides just enough information for the test taker to provide only one possible correct answer. For example:

The physician ordered methocarbamol (Robaxin) 1.5 g PO. Available are 750-mg tablets. How many tablets would you give?
Answer: 2

Rationale:
$$\frac{D}{H} = \frac{X}{V}$$

$1\ g = 1000\ mg$

$1.5\ g = 1500$

$$\frac{1500}{750} = \frac{x}{1}$$

$75x = 150$

$150 \div 75 = 2\ tabs$

The Multiple-Response Question

The multiple-response question has several correct options. The multiple-response question may be stated as a complete sentence ending with a question mark or an incomplete sentence requiring one of the options to complete the stem. Instead of having four options, you will have six options from which to choose the correct keys. Each option will have a little square box to the left of the number.

After reading each option, you will choose those options that relate to the stem as true statements and place an "x" in the boxes. Three examples are given to illustrate the possible options for a multiple-response question.

Example 1:
A nurse is caring for a client with diverticulitis. Which of the following measures would be essential to include in the client's plan of care?
[   ] 1. Increased fiber diet
[   ] 2. Bed rest
[   ] 3. Antihistamines
[   ] 4. Bulk-forming laxatives
[   ] 5. Relaxation techniques
[   ] 6. Antibiotics
Answer: 1, 4, 5

Rationale:
An increased fiber diet, bulk-forming laxative, and relaxation techniques are nursing measures for diverticulitis.

Example 2:
The nurse is caring for a 2-month-old child with an inguinal hernia. Which of the following would indicate to the nurse that the infant's hernia has strangulated?
[   ] 1. Reddened scrotum
[   ] 2. Bradycardia
[   ] 3. Inconsolable crying
[   ] 4. Abdominal distention
[   ] 5. Pain
[   ] 6. Lethargy
Answer: 1, 3, 5

Rationale:
Indications of a strangulated inguinal hernia in a newborn include a reddened scrotum, crying that is inconsolable, and pain.

Example 3:
When providing care for a child who is on oxybutynin chloride (Ditropan) for enuresis, the nurse should monitor the child for:
[   ] 1. Facial flushing
[   ] 2. Nasal congestion
[   ] 3. Diarrhea
[   ] 4. Blurred vision
[   ] 5. Dry mouth
[   ] 6. Nosebleeds
Answer: 1, 4, 5

Rationale:
Oxybutynin chloride (Ditropan) is an anticholinergic that may be used in the treatment of enuresis. Common adverse reactions include facial flushing, blurred vision, dry mouth, and constipation.

Picture or Graph Question

A picture or graph question is the third type of innovative question that the NCLEX-RN® has implemented. It asks you to identify something on a picture or graph as asked in the stem. Choosing the location on a picture, supplying some data on a graph, or filling in some information on a graph as asked in the stem is called identifying the hot spot and is considered the key. When you study, think about questions that could be asked about anatomy, tables, or graphs. For example:

The nurse selects which of the following IV site locations when starting an IV in the medial antebrachial vein?

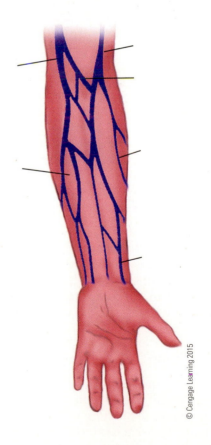

© Cengage Learning 2015

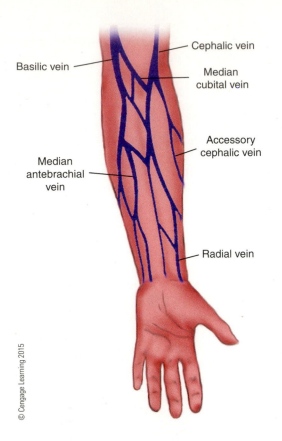

Cephalic vein

Basilic vein

Median cubital vein

Accessory cephalic vein

Median antebrachial vein

Radial vein

© Cengage Learning 2015

The test taker then chooses from the six unlabeled choices in the first figure. The choices represent the basilic, cephalic, median cubital, medial antebrachial, radial, and accessory veins, as shown in the second figure. The test taker would then write the appropriate name, medial antebrachial vein, on the correct spot in the figure.

Drag-and-Drop or Ordered-Response Item

The fourth style of item is drag and drop, in which a problem is presented and a list of items. The listed responses must be placed in a specified order. The unordered choices are presented on the left side of the computer screen. Placement of the new options is clicked on and dragged into the ordered box.

Exhibit Question

In this type of question, the student is presented with a problem and a chart-style exhibit. The Exhibit button at the bottom of the screen has to be clicked on to access the information behind each of three tabs. The chart-style exhibit is followed by a multiple-choice question based on the information found within each tab.

Audio and Video Questions

These question types are new to the exam and require you to either listen to an audio sound clip or view a short video in order to answer the question correctly.

EXAMINATION APPLICATION PROCESS

Shortly before or after graduation from your school of nursing, you will need to apply for licensure from the board of nursing in the state or territory in which you wish to practice. A frequently asked question is: "If I am graduating from nursing school in one state but am moving to another state, where should I take the NCLEX-RN®?" You should always apply for licensure in the state in which you want to practice. Although licensure may be transferred from one state to another, taking the NCLEX in the state in which you wish to practice saves you the time of applying for licensure in another state and saves you the additional cost of the reciprocity.

After applying to the state board of nursing, you will receive an NCLEX-RN® Examination Candidate Bulletin, which contains your application and provides detailed directions on how to apply for the NCLEX-RN®. It is a good idea to keep the candidate bulletin until you take the test and receive your results in case you have questions that the bulletin can answer for you. After completing the application, you should submit it with a certified check, cashier's check, or money order to the Pearson VUE group (the NCSBN's contracted testing service) or register by phone for an additional fee. After receiving your application, Pearson VUE will notify you by mail that your application has been received. Before submitting your application, if you have a disability, you should notify your state board of nursing that special accommodations are needed at the testing center.

Your state board of nursing will let Pearson VUE know of your eligibility to take the NCLEX-RN®. Pearson VUE will send you an Authorization to Test (ATT) and information on how to schedule and take the NCLEX-RN® as well as testing centers for your area, generally within 4 weeks of receipt of your ATT. The NCLEX-RN® is administered at Pearson VUE.

DAY OF THE TEST

After arranging a testing date and time, you should go to the testing center at least 30 minutes before your scheduled time to ensure you have all your allotted time for the test. If you arrive more than 30 minutes late for your scheduled test, you may have to forfeit your examination registration fee.

You will need to take your ATT form, current picture identification with your signature such as a driver's license, and a secondary form of identification such as a school ID or social security card with you the day of the test. After displaying your identification, your picture and thumbprint will be taken, and you will be asked to sign your name. You will also get a vein pattern test. A scanner reads your palm vein and the information is stored on a digital template. These requirements add an additional level of security to the process and the verification of the applicant.

You will not be allowed to take personal belongings such as papers, books, scratch paper, school materials, purse, pens, pencils, beepers, cell phones, or handheld calculators into your testing cubicle. There is no eating, drinking, or smoking in the testing area. Taking a nursing textbook or any NCLEX materials into the testing area is strictly prohibited and may result in your being asked to leave the testing center and your examination cancelled.

You will be given a note board and writing utensil to use during the test that can be replaced as often as necessary but at no time are to be removed from the facility.

You will be escorted to your testing cubicle for the first time for a brief orientation. There is fluorescent lighting used in the testing room, but if you would like a desk light, one will be provided for you.

You will have 6 hours to take the test, including a short tutorial before you begin the examination, two scheduled breaks, and unscheduled breaks as necessary. There is a 10-minute break that is mandatory after 2 hours of testing. After 3½ hours, there is another 10-minute break that is scheduled but is optional. You will be notified on the computer screen when it is time for all scheduled breaks. You will be required to leave your testing site during the scheduled breaks. You are also required to show your picture ID and sign your name before leaving and reentering the testing room. During your examination, you must raise your hand if you need anything or want to leave your testing cubicle for any reason.

Included in the computer tutorial before you begin your examination is a brief summary of the functions needed to use the computer to answer the items and three sample items. A frequently asked question is: "Do I have to be an expert at operating the computer to take the test?" The

answer is no. The tutorial will take you through step by step on how to highlight and record your answers. Also reviewed in the tutorial is the use of the on-screen calculator. Its use is optional when you have a calculation item. Even after starting your examination, you may raise your hand if you have a question about any function of the computer. At the end of your test, you will be given a brief questionnaire asking about your experience with the computerized NCLEX-RN®. After you have finished the questionnaire, you must raise your hand to be dismissed from the testing area. Your note board and writing utensil will be collected, and you will be dismissed.

The actual NCLEX-RN® exam may contain up to 265 items, including 15 new "tryout" items. This means that you may take up to 250 real items that will be scored and 15 tryout items. A tryout item is a first-time item that is being piloted to evaluate the level of difficulty of the item. It is not scored and does not affect your passing or failing the examination. It is very important that you understand that in no way is the test length indicative of passing or failing. You should plan on allowing yourself 1 minute per item, assuming you will need the 6-hour time limit to take the maximum number of items, or 265, but you can track your progress by referring to the timer in the upper-left corner of the screen and the item number in the upper-right corner. The minimum number of questions to pass the NCLEX is 75. The purpose behind displaying the test length and item number is to keep you informed of your progress so you can pace yourself.

TEST SCORING

Using the CAT, each candidate begins the NCLEX-RN® exam with an item of the same easy level of difficulty. If a candidate answers this item correctly, the next item will be slightly more difficult. If this item is answered correctly, the following item will be slightly more difficult, and the process will continue with more difficult items until an item is missed. If an item is missed, then the next item will be slightly easier. If that item is also missed, then the next item will be easier than the last one, and this process of administering an easier item will be continued until an item is answered correctly. Only answering an item correctly will result in the subsequent item's being more difficult. Putting this into perspective is that each item is individualized to fairly and completely evaluate your knowledge, skill, and ability to be a safe registered nurse. After each item, your competency level is computed by the computer and analyzed as to the area of the test plan and level of difficulty of that item. When you have answered 50% of your items correctly or incorrectly, the area of error is very small, and the indication is clear that you have either passed or failed. The goal of every candidate's examination is to answer 50% of all items correctly. This is why some candidates' examinations are short and may end after 75 items, meaning 50% or more of the 60 real or scored items were answered either correctly or incorrectly and the candidates either pass or fail. Every candidate's score is computer analyzed after the minimum number of items has been answered. After your items have been analyzed, one of three situations will occur. You will pass, fail, or continue to get more items. A candidate who answers all 265 items has simply taken more time and items to establish the margin of error.

Pearson VUE will transmit your NCLEX test results to your board of nursing. You may have heard a rumor that at the end of the test, the computer displays the word "pass" or "fail" on the screen. This is not true. Your board of nursing will send you your results. It generally takes 2 to 4 weeks to obtain results. After completing the examination, you will be given information on obtaining quick results after 48 hours of the scheduled exam. There is a small fee to obtain results by the Internet and phone.

RESULTS ANALYSES

A diagnostic profile is generated for all candidates who fail the NCLEX-RN®. The diagnostic profile will come in the mail with the results of your examination, which generally take 2 to 4 weeks to receive. If you opt to obtain your results 48 hours after your examination either by phone or the Internet and you happened to fail, you will have to wait for your mailed results to receive your diagnostic profile. The diagnostic profile will provide several pieces of information to help you in preparing for your retake examination. The first piece of information the diagnostic profile will provide you with is how close you were to the passing standard. It will also let you know how many total items you answered. Generally, candidates who answer all 265 items are either very close to the passing or failing standard.

On the back page of the diagnostic profile is an analysis of how well you did on each of the NCLEX-RN® Test Plan content areas designed to inform you on how to be successful on your future examination. The improvement needed in each of the content areas is outlined in this profile. The report gives the information that your performance was "Above the Passing Standard," "Near the Passing Standard," or "Below the Passing Standard" in the various test plan areas. These recommendations can only be used to identify *overall* weaknesses and strengths and can be used to further guide you in future preparation to retake the examination.

REFERENCES

National Council of State Boards of Nursing, Inc. (2013a). Frequently asked questions: Innovative NCLEX item formats. Retrieved from http://www.ncsbn.org

National Council of State Boards of Nursing Inc. (2013b). NCLEX Examination Candidate Bulletin. Retrieved from http://www.ncsbn.org

National Council of State Boards of Nursing, Inc. (2013c). NCLEX-RN Test Plan. Retrieved from http://www.ncsbn.org

Wendt, A., & Worcester, R. (2000). The National Council Licensure Examinations/differential item functioning process. *Journal of Nursing Education*, *39*(4), 185–187.

UNIT II

MEDICAL-SURGICAL NURSING

EYE, EAR, NOSE, AND THROAT DISORDERS

I. ANATOMY AND PHYSIOLOGY

A. FUNCTIONS OF THE VISUAL AND AUDITORY SYSTEMS

  1. EYES PROVIDE A PATHWAY FOR VISUAL STIMULI.

  2. EARS PROVIDE A PATHWAY FOR AUDITORY STIMULI.

  3. SPECIALIZED STRUCTURES IN THE EAR MAINTAIN A SENSE OF POSITION/EQUILIBRIUM (BALANCE).

B. EXTERNAL STRUCTURES OF THE EYE (SEE FIGURE 2-1)

  1. EYEBROWS, EYELIDS, AND EYELASHES

    a. Provide a physical barrier and protection from dust and foreign particles

    b. Distribute tears via the lacrimal glands and ducts

    c. Control the amount of light entering

Figure 2-1 External structures of the eye

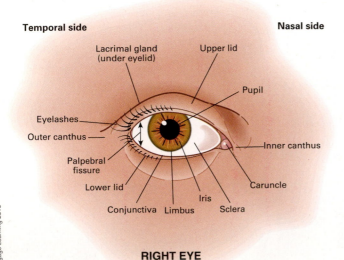

Temporal side   Nasal side

Lacrimal gland (under eyelid)   Upper lid

Pupil

Eyelashes

Outer canthus

Inner canthus

Palpebral fissure

Lower lid   Caruncle

Iris

Conjunctiva Limbus   Sclera

RIGHT EYE

© Cengage Learning 2015

  2. CONJUNCTIVA

    a. Transparent mucous membrane

    b. Covers the inner surfaces of the eyelid

    c. Underlying tissue that is pink in color

  3. SCLERA

    a. "White" of the eye

    b. Forms a tough shell and protects the intraocular structures

  4. CORNEA

    a. Transparent anterior portion of the globe

    b. Allows light to enter the eyeball

    c. Refracts (bends) light rays to focus on the retina

  5. LACRIMAL (TEAR) APPARATUS

    a. Glands and ducts that are located in the upper eyelid

    b. Provides secretions to moisten the eye and provides oxygen to the cornea

    c. Tears are drained into the nose.

  6. EXTRAOCULAR MUSCLES

    a. Each eye is moved by three pairs.

    b. Coordination of the simultaneous movement of the eyes in the same direction

C. INTERNAL STRUCTURES (SEE FIGURE 2-2)

  1. IRIS

    a. Provides the color of the eye

    b. The pupil is a round opening at the center of the eye allowing light to enter.

    c. Sympathetic stimulation causes dilation of the pupil.

    d. Parasympathetic stimulation causes constriction of the pupil.

  2. CRYSTALLINE LENS

    a. Transparent structure behind the iris

    b. Composed of a thick gel enclosed in a clear capsule

    c. Primary function is to bend light rays onto the retina

Figure 2-2 Lateral cross section of the interior eye

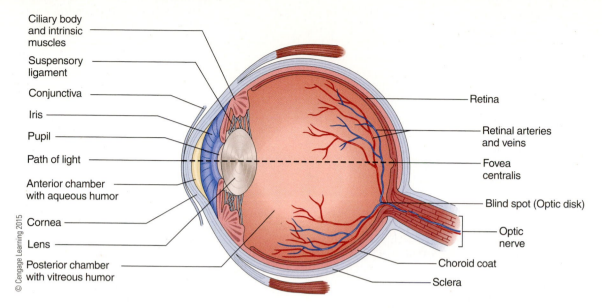

Ciliary body and intrinsic muscles
Suspensory ligament
Conjunctiva
Iris
Pupil
Path of light
Anterior chamber with aqueous humor
Cornea
Lens
Posterior chamber with vitreous humor

Retina
Retinal arteries and veins
Fovea centralis
Blind spot (Optic disk)
Optic nerve
Choroid coat
Sclera

© Cengage Learning 2015

3. CILIARY BODY
   a. Muscles attached to the lens capsule
   b. Facilitates focusing by change in shape
   c. Secretes aqueous humor
4. CHOROID
   a. Vascular structure that nourishes the ciliary body, iris, and outer retina
   b. Lies inside and parallel to the sclera
5. RETINA
   a. Lines the inside of the eye
   b. Rods are stimulated in a dark environment.
   c. Cones are stimulated to see colors in a bright environment.
   d. The center of visual acuity is the *fovea centralis*.
   e. The optic nerve area is a blind spot.
   f. Arteries and veins provide information about the vascular system.
   g. Responsible for converting images into form that the brain can understand

II. **ASSESSMENT**
   A. HEALTH HISTORY
      1. PAST HEALTH HISTORY
      2. MEDICATIONS (PAST, PRESENT, OVER THE COUNTER, HERBS)
      3. SURGERIES
   B. PHYSICAL EXAMINATION
      1. INSPECTION
         a. Eye—symmetry, color, pupil size
         b. PERRLA (pupils equally round and reactive to light accommodation)
         c. Lacrimal apparatus nontender
         d. Visual acuity 20/20 OU (both eyes); no diplopia (double vision)
         e. Conjunctiva clear; sclera white
         f. EOMI (extraocular movements intact)

         g. Disc margins sharp
         h. Retinal vessels normal; no hemorrhages, spots, or patches
         i. Note whether eyelids meet completely.
      2. PALPATION
         a. Check the eyelids for nodules.
         b. Palpate the eye by gently pushing into the orbit without discomfort.

III. **DIAGNOSTIC STUDIES**
   A. VISUAL ACUITY TEST
      1. DESCRIPTION: CLIENT READS FROM AN EYE CHART—FROM THE SNELLEN CHART AT 20 FEET (DISTANCE VISION TEST) OR FROM JAEGER'S CHART AT 14 INCHES (NEAR VISION TEST).
      2. PREPROCEDURE
         a. Instruct the client to cover one eye.
         b. Ask the client to identify all of the letters, beginning at any line on the chart.
         c. Repeat the instructions for the second eye exam.
      3. POSTPROCEDURE
         a. Determine the smallest line in which the client can identify all of the letters.
         b. Record the visual acuity designated by that line on the chart.
   B. SIX CARDINAL POSITIONS OF GAZE
      1. DESCRIPTION: MEASURES THE CRANIAL NERVES (III OCULOMOTOR, IV TROCHLEAR, VI ABDUCENS) AND THE EXTRAOCULAR MUSCLES
      2. PREPROCEDURE
         a. Hold the client's chin to prevent movement of the head and ask the client to watch your finger as it moves through the six cardinal fields of gaze.

      b. Ask the client to look to the extreme lateral (temporal) positions.

      c. Have the client follow your finger in the vertical plane, going from ceiling to floor.

      d. While the client stares straight ahead at a near fixed point, cover one eye and observe the uncovered eye for movement as it focuses on the designated point; repeat with the second eye.

  3. POSTPROCEDURE

      a. May observe a few horizontal nystagmic beats.

      b. If the eye moves rapidly to the right then slowly drifts to the left, it is called nystagmus to the right.

      c. Observe the coordinated movement of the globes and the upper lid.

C. CONFRONTATIONAL VISUAL FIELD TEST

  1. DESCRIPTION: MEASURES THE PERIPHERAL FIELD OF VISION OF THE CLIENT

  2. PREPROCEDURE

      a. At eye level with the client, ask her to look with both eyes into your eyes.

      b. While returning the client's gaze, place the hands about 2 feet apart, lateral to the client's ears.

      c. Instruct the client to identify when she sees your fingers move.

      d. Slowly move wiggling fingers of both hands along the imaginary bowl toward the client's line of gaze until she identifies them.

      e. Repeat this pattern for the upper and lower temporal quadrants for both eyes.

      f. Normally, a client sees both sets of fingers at the same time.

  3. POSTPROCEDURE

      a. If a defect is found, try to establish its boundaries.

      b. Diagram the location of the boundaries.

D. PUPIL FUNCTION TEST

  1. DESCRIPTION: MEASURES NORMAL PUPIL RESPONSE TO LIGHT

  2. PREPROCEDURE

      a. Ask the client to look into the distance, and shine a bright light obliquely into each pupil in turn.

      b. Always darken the room and use a bright light that focuses on one pupil only.

  3. POSTPROCEDURE

      a. Look for direct reactions to the light in the same eye.

      b. Observe for consensual reaction (constriction) in the opposite eye tested.

E. TONOMETRY

  1. DESCRIPTION: MEASURES INTRAOCULAR PRESSURE

  2. PREPROCEDURE

      a. Instill anesthetizing ophthalmic drops prior to applying the tonometer.

      b. Apply the tonometer to the corneal surface for pressure reading.

  3. POSTPROCEDURE

      a. Document the intraocular pressure.

      b. Normal intraocular pressure is 10–21 mm Hg.

F. SLIT LAMP MICROSCOPY

  1. DESCRIPTION: SLIT BEAM MAGNIFIES THE OCULAR STRUCTURES FOR EXAMINATION

  2. PREPROCEDURE

      a. Instruct the client to place her chin in the chin rest.

      b. Instruct the client that a powerful magnifier that is very bright will be used.

  3. POSTPROCEDURE

      a. Document the data from the magnification assessment.

G. OPHTHALMOSCOPE

  1. DESCRIPTION: PROVIDES A MAGNIFIED VIEW OF THE RETINA AND OPTIC NERVE WITH THE USE OF A LIGHT

  2. PREPROCEDURE

      a. Dilating eyedrops are contraindicated in head injury, coma, and narrow-angle glaucoma.

      b. Instill mydriatic (dilating) drops into both eyes, if not contraindicated.

      c. Glasses should be removed unless there is a marked nearsightedness or severe astigmatism.

      d. Darken the room, turn on the ophthalmoscope, and adjust the beam.

      e. Turn the lens disc to 0 diopters.

      f. The nurse should keep the index finger on the lens disc so that the scope can be focused during the exam.

      g. Use your right hand and eye to examine the client's right eye (avoid nose to nose).

      h. Hold the scope firmly braced under the medial aspect of the bony orbit.

      i. Keep the handle tilted laterally at about 20 degrees slant from vertical.

      j. Ask the client to look slightly up and over your shoulder and gaze at a point on the wall.

      k. From 15 inches away from the client, shine the light beam on the pupil; note the orange glow in the pupil—the red reflex; note any opacities.

      l. Find the retina in the vicinity of the optic disc; note the clarity of the disc outline, color of the disc (yellowish orange to creamy pink), size of the central physiologic cup, and symmetry.

m. Identify the arteries and veins; follow the vessels peripherally in four directions, noting the size and character of the arteriovenous crossings.

n. Inspect the fovea and macula by directing the light beam laterally.

o. Look for opacities in the vitreous or lens by rotating the lens disc progressively to diopters +10–12.

   3. POSTPROCEDURE

    a. Document the data from the exam regarding the red reflex, optic disc, retina, vessels, fovea, macula, vitreous, and lens.

    b. Review the last exam for comparison.

H. COLOR VISION TEST

   1. DESCRIPTION: DETERMINES THE CLIENT'S ABILITY TO DISTINGUISH COLORS

   2. PREPROCEDURE

    a. Ask the client to identify numbers or objects formed by a pattern of dots in a series of color plates.

   3. POSTPROCEDURE

    a. Document the exam findings on the client's color discrimination.

    b. Review the previous exam for comparison.

I. STEREOPSIS

   1. DESCRIPTION: EVALUATES THE CLIENT'S ABILITY TO SEE OBJECTS IN THREE DIMENSIONS; EXAMINES DEPTH PERCEPTION

   2. PREPROCEDURE

    a. Instruct the client to identify geometric patterns or figures that appear closer to her when viewed through special spectacles that provide a three-dimensional view.

   3. POSTPROCEDURE

    a. Document the client's depth perception.

    b. Review the previous exam for comparison.

J. KERATOMETRY

   1. DESCRIPTION: MEASURES THE CURVATURE OF THE CORNEA; OFTEN DONE PRIOR TO FITTING CONTACT LENSES, REFRACTIVE SURGERY, OR AFTER CORNEAL TRANSPLANT

   2. PREPROCEDURE

    a. Instruct the client on the reason for testing the cornea curvature.

   3. POSTPROCEDURE

    a. Inform the client on the findings and how that may impact the reason for the test.

IV. NURSING DIAGNOSIS

A. READINESS FOR ENHANCED SELF-CARE DEFICIT

B. ANXIETY

C. ACUTE PAIN

D. DISTURBED SENSORY PERCEPTION (VISUAL)

Nursing Diagnoses: Definitions and Classification 2012–2014. Copyright © 2012, 1994–2012 by NANDA International. Used by arrangement with John Wiley & Sons Limited.

V. CORRECTABLE REFRACTIVE ERRORS

A. MYOPIA

   1. DESCRIPTION

    a. Nearsightedness

    b. Blurred distance vision

    c. Abnormally elongated eyeball related to genetics

    d. Lens swelling with uncontrolled diabetes mellitus

   2. ASSESSMENT

    a. Client is able to see objects close to her.

    b. Client is unable to see objects clearly at an increasing distance.

   3. DIAGNOSTIC TESTS

    a. Refraction

    b. Snellen eye chart

   4. NURSING INTERVENTIONS

    a. Evaluate which lenses are used, the pattern of wear, and care practices.

    b. Must remove daily wear lenses each night or with sleep

    c. Identify whether contact lenses are present in an emergency situation (shining a light obliquely can assist to visualize a contact lens).

    d. After hand washing, you can remove a rigid contact lens (stand at the side of the lens that requires removal; hold a hand under the client's eye, and ask the client to blink, gently pulling on the upper and lower lids to cause the lens to fall into your hands or complete manual removal). After hand washing, you can remove a soft contact lens (stand at the side of your dominant hand, placing the middle finger on the lower eyelid against the cheekbone; gently pull the eyelid down against the cheek, with the thumb and index finger, and slide the lens down and off the cornea onto the sclera; bring your fingers together and gently pinch the lens off the eye).

    e. Store or cleanse the lens with appropriate cleansing solution.

    f. Instruct the client on the clinical manifestations of problems (redness, sensitivity, visual problems or pain) that must be managed by professionals.

   5. SURGICAL MANAGEMENT

    a. Keratorefractive surgery to alter corneal curvature

    b. Photorefractive keratectomy uses a laser to reshape the central cornea.

B. HYPEROPIA
   1. DESCRIPTION
      a. Farsightedness (blurred near vision)
      b. Eyeball is short; light focuses behind the retina.
   2. ASSESSMENT
      a. Able to see objects from a distance
      b. Unable to see objects at decreasing distances
   3. DIAGNOSTIC TESTS
      a. Refraction
      b. Snellen eye chart
   4. NURSING INTERVENTIONS
      a. Evaluate which lenses are used, the pattern of wear, and care practices.
      b. Must remove daily wear lenses each night or with sleep
      c. Identify whether contact lenses are present in an emergency situation (shining a light obliquely can assist to visualize a contact lens).
      d. Teach clinical manifestations of problems (redness, sensitivity, visual problems, or pain) that must be managed by professionals.
      e. If injury to the eye, do not remove lens.
   5. MEDICAL MANAGEMENT
      a. Corrective lens (glasses or contacts)
C. PRESBYOPIA
   1. DESCRIPTION
      a. Farsightedness with aging, due to decreased accommodation of the ciliary body
      b. Lens can no longer accommodate.
   2. ASSESSMENT
      a. Blurred near vision
      b. The client attempts to hold objects further from her eyes but her arms are not long enough.
   3. DIAGNOSTIC TESTS
      a. Refraction
      b. Reading normal page print
   4. NURSING INTERVENTIONS
      a. Teach the proper use and care of glasses or contacts, as above.
      b. Instruct the client to recheck vision every 1 to 2 years.
   5. MEDICAL MANAGEMENT
      a. Corrective lens (glasses or contacts)
D. ASTIGMATISM
   1. DESCRIPTION
      a. Uneven curvature of the cornea
      b. Unable to focus light at a clear point on the retina
   2. ASSESSMENT
      a. Refraction error
      b. Cylinder lens aligns to focus point
   3. DIAGNOSTIC TESTS
      a. Refraction

   4. NURSING INTERVENTIONS
      a. Instruct the client on the care of glasses or contact lens.

VI. UNCORRECTABLE VISUAL IMPAIRMENT
A. TOTAL BLINDNESS
   1. DESCRIPTION: NO LIGHT PERCEPTION AND NO USABLE VISION
B. FUNCTIONAL BLINDNESS
   1. DESCRIPTION: SOME LIGHT PERCEPTION BUT NO USABLE VISION
C. LEGALLY BLIND
   1. DESCRIPTION
      a. Meets criteria developed by the federal government for assistance and tax benefits
      b. Some usable vision
D. PARTIALLY SIGHTED
   1. DESCRIPTION: HAS CORRECTED VISUAL ACUITY GREATER THAN 20/200 IN THE BETTER EYE; GREATER THAN 20 DEGREES VISUAL FIELD
   2. ASSESSMENT FOR ALL THOSE WITH VISUAL IMPAIRMENT
      a. Interview the client regarding:
         1) Length of time with visual impairment
         2) Level of difficulty when doing certain tasks
         3) Personal meaning attached to visual impairment
         4) Coping strategies, emotional reactions, support systems
   3. DIAGNOSTIC TESTS
      a. Visual acuity
      b. Visual fields
   4. NURSING INTERVENTIONS
      a. Provide emotional support.
      b. Actively listen to the client.
      c. Involve the family, as appropriate.
      d. Introduce yourself to the client when entering or leaving.
      e. Utilize a normal tone of voice.
      f. Allow the client to hold onto your arm for guidance when walking.
      g. Describe the environment to help orient the client to movement and change.
      h. Describe the location of the food on the plate in terms of numbers on a clock.
E. EYE TRAUMA
   1. DESCRIPTION: BLUNT, PENETRATING, OR CHEMICAL INJURY TO THE EYE
   2. ASSESSMENT OF EYE EMERGENCY
      a. Pain
      b. Photophobia
      c. Redness
      d. Swelling
      e. Ecchymosis
      f. Tearing
      g. Blood in anterior chamber

h. Absent eye movements
i. Fluid drainage from the eye
j. Abnormal or decreased vision
k. Prolapsed globe
l. Abnormal intraocular pressure
3. DIAGNOSTIC TESTS
   a. Visual acuity
   b. Visual function
4. NURSING INTERVENTIONS
   a. Determine the mechanism of injury.
   b. Begin immediate irrigation for chemical exposure.
   c. Assess visual acuity after irrigation for chemical exposure.
   d. Stabilize foreign objects but do not remove.
   e. Elevate the head of the bed to decrease swelling.
   f. Keep the client NPO pending surgical intervention.
   g. Administer drugs and analgesia as ordered.
5. SURGICAL MANAGEMENT
   a. Repair for penetrating injury, globe rupture or globe avulsion (separation)

VII. **INFLAMMATION AND INFECTION OF THE EXTERNAL EYE (SEE TABLE 2-1)**
   A. DRY EYE DISORDERS
      1. DESCRIPTION: DRY EYES DUE TO DECREASED TEARING OR INCREASED TEAR EVAPORATION
      2. ASSESSMENT
         a. Sandy or gritty sensation in the eye
         b. Worsens during the day
         c. Improves after eye closure and sleep
      3. DIAGNOSTIC TESTS
         a. Physical examination

4. NURSING INTERVENTIONS
   a. Apply hot compresses and massage lid to help tear film expression.
   b. Instruct the client on the proper use of artificial tears to prevent contamination.
B. STRABISMUS (DOUBLE VISION)
   1. DESCRIPTION: INABILITY TO FOCUS TWO EYES SIMULTANEOUSLY ON AN OBJECT
   2. ASSESSMENT
      a. Sixth or third nerve damage
      b. Abnormal ocular muscles
   3. DIAGNOSTIC TESTS
      a. Cover-uncover test
      b. Corneal light reflex test
   4. MEDICAL MANAGEMENT
      a. Use of eye patch to strengthen weak muscles
      b. Surgical intervention on eye muscles to assist convergence

VIII. **CORNEAL DISORDERS**
   A. CORNEAL SCARS AND OPACITIES
      1. DESCRIPTION: DECREASE IN TRANSPARENCY OF LIGHT RAYS INTO THE EYE DUE TO INJURY OR DISEASE
      2. ASSESSMENT
         a. Impaired vision
         b. Altered appearance of the cornea (cloudy)
      3. DIAGNOSTIC TESTS
         a. Visual examination
         b. Visual acuity test
      4. SURGICAL MANAGEMENT
         a. Removal of full thickness of the cornea
         b. Replace with a donor cornea

Table 2-1 Inflammation and Infection of the External Eye

Infection	Location	Symptoms	Treatment
Hordeolum "sty"	Sebaceous glands lid margin	Red, swollen, acutely tender	Warm, moist compresses Antibiotics if indicated
Chalazion	Sebaceous glands lid margin	Swollen, nonpainful, reddened area	Warm, moist compresses Corticosteroids
Blepharitis	Eyelids	Reddened, crusts, burning, irritation, photophobia	Antibiotic ointment Antiseptic shampoo for scalp and eyebrows
Conjunctivitis "pink eye"	Conjunctiva	Redness, irritation, tearing, purulent drainage	Antibiotic drops Hand washing to prevent spread Allergy: artificial tears
Keratitis	Cornea	Ulceration, purulent drainage, pain, photophobia	Bacterial: topical antibiotics Viral: topical antivirals Chlamydial: systemic antibiotics Transplant if severe

B. KERATOCONUS
1. DESCRIPTION: BILATERAL GENERATIVE DISEASE OF THE RETINA, SOMETIMES FAMILIAL
2. ASSESSMENT
   a. Cornea has an altered shape (cone shaped).
   b. Blurred vision
3. DIAGNOSTIC TESTS
   a. Physical examination
   b. Visual acuity test
4. MEDICAL MANAGEMENT
   a. Astigmatism corrected with glasses or rigid contact lens
   b. Corneal transplant
C. CATARACT
1. DESCRIPTION: OPACITY WITHIN THE CRYSTALLINE LENS
2. ASSESSMENT
   a. Cloudy appearance in the affected eye developing gradually
   b. Decreased vision, abnormal color perception, and glare that is worse at night when the pupil dilates
3. DIAGNOSTIC TESTS
   a. Visual acuity test
   b. Ophthalmoscopy
   c. Slit lamp
4. NURSING INTERVENTIONS
   a. Instruct the client that topical drugs before surgery can produce stinging and burning (see Table 2-2).
   b. Postoperatively the client will not have depth perception until patch removal.
   c. May need special assistance until vision improves
   d. Client and family need instructions for eye techniques to prevent infection.
   e. Postoperative instructions to avoid bending, sneezing, and coughing
5. MEDICAL MANAGEMENT
   a. Nonsurgical
      1) Change prescription of glasses.
      2) Use magnifiers.
      3) Increase lighting.
      4) Administer topical drugs for pupil dilation (see Table 2-2).
6. SURGICAL MANAGEMENT (CONSIDERED AN ELECTIVE PROCEDURE)
   a. Lens removal
   b. Implantation of intraocular lens

Table 2-2 Topical Drugs for Pupil Dilation

Mydriatics	Phenylephrine HCl (Neo-Synephrine, Mydfrin)
Cycloplegics	Tropicamide (Mydriacyl, Tropicacyl)
	Scopolamine (Isopto Hyoscine)
	Atropine (Atropisol, Atropair)
	Contraindicated if glaucoma

D. RETINAL DETACHMENT
1. DESCRIPTION: A TEAR, OR HOLE IN THE RETINA, THAT SEPARATES IT FROM ITS BLOOD SUPPLY, RESULTING IN BLINDNESS
2. ASSESSMENT
   a. Light flashes, photophobia
   b. Ring in the field of vision
   c. Described as like a "curtain being drawn"
3. DIAGNOSTIC TESTS
   a. Visual acuity
   b. Slit lamp
   c. Ophthalmoscopy
4. NURSING INTERVENTIONS
   a. Prepare the client for surgery; this is an emergency situation.
   b. Administer antibiotics and corticosteroids as ordered.
   c. Administer analgesia as needed.
   d. Instruct the client to avoid positioning and activity that could increase intraocular pressure, such as lifting and bending, and protect the eye with glasses or an eye shield.
   e. Administer and educate the client about topical ophthalmic drugs.
5. SURGICAL MANAGEMENT
   a. Photocoagulation
   b. Cryoretinopexy
   c. Scleral buckling procedure
   d. Vitrectomy
   e. Intravitreal bubble
E. MACULAR DEGENERATION (AGE RELATED)
1. DESCRIPTION
   a. Degenerative process of the retina and macula resulting in the loss of central vision
   b. Most common in adults over 52 years of age
2. ASSESSMENT
   a. Appearance of *drusen* (yellowish exudate) in the fundus
   b. Blurred vision
   c. Presence of scotomas (shimmering island in the field of vision)
3. DIAGNOSTIC TESTS
   a. Visual acuity test
   b. Ophthalmoscopy
4. NURSING INTERVENTIONS
   a. Provide emotional support and direct services as needed.
   b. Engage in active listening and grief work facilitation.
   c. Identify successful coping strategies; involve the family.
   d. Discuss environmental concerns to promote safety.
   e. Inform the client on devices that may provide some vision enhancement.

F. GLAUCOMA
1. DESCRIPTION
   a. Increased intraocular pressure (IOP) with peripheral vision field loss and optic nerve atrophy
   b. When the rate of production of aqueous fluid is greater than the outflow, IOP can rise above normal limits.
   c. If IOP remains elevated, permanent visual damage may begin.
   d. Two types:
      1) Primary open-angle glaucoma (POAG)
      2) Primary closed-angle glaucoma (PACG)
   e. The third leading cause of blindness
2. ASSESSMENT
   a. Primary open-angle glaucoma (90%) develops slowly without clinical manifestations but individual gradually notices a gradual loss of peripheral vision; may be described as "tunnel vision."
   b. Chronic open-angle glaucoma (10%) has sudden severe pain in and around the eye, nausea and vomiting, and "colored halos around lights."
3. DIAGNOSTIC TESTS
   a. Slit lamp
   b. Tonometry
   c. Visual field test
   d. Ophthalmoscopic exam
4. NURSING INTERVENTIONS
   a. Instruct the client regarding the type of glaucoma and treatment plan.
   b. Emphasize the importance of monitoring vision.
   c. Instruct the client regarding the daily use, timing, and purpose of eyedrop administration.
   d. Darken the environment.
   e. Apply cool compresses to the forehead.
   f. Provide quiet space.
   g. If surgery is performed, instruct the client to avoid sudden head movements, coughing, and bending down because these can increase IOP; wear an eye shield at night to protect the operative eye; take stool softeners and increase fluids to avoid straining at stool.
5. MEDICAL MANAGEMENT
   a. Acute angle-closure glaucoma
      1) Cholinergic and hyperosmotic topical agents
      2) Laser peripheral iridotomy (new opening in the iris)
      3) Surgical iridectomy (new opening in the iris)
   b. Chronic open-angle glaucoma
      1) Drug therapy such as beta blockers, adrenergic antagonists, and miotics

6. SURGICAL MANAGEMENT
   a. Argon laser trabeculoplasty (open outflow of fluid channel)
   b. Trabeculectomy, with or without filtering implant (removal of a portion of the iris)
   c. Cryotherapy destruction of ciliary body (decreases production of aqueous humor)
G. ENUCLEATION
1. DESCRIPTION
   a. Removal of the eye
   b. Usually done for pain, infection, malignancy, or trauma
2. ASSESSMENT
   a. Primary indication is a blind and painful eye
   b. Glaucoma unresponsive to therapy, infection, or trauma
   c. Ocular malignancy not managed by chemotherapy, radiation, or cryotherapy
   d. Sympathetic ophthalmia (healthy eye develops an inflammatory response to primary eye trauma)
3. DIAGNOSTIC TESTS
   a. Ophthalmoscopic exam
   b. Tonometry
4. NURSING INTERVENTIONS
   a. Postoperatively, observe for indications of excessive bleeding or swelling, increased pain, displacement of implant, or elevated temperature.
   b. Instruct the client on instillation of topical ointments or drops.
   c. Instruct the client on wound cleansing and care.
   d. Instruct the client on conformer insertion into the socket if it falls out.
   e. Recognize and validate the client's emotional response.
   f. Provide support to the client and family because this can be a devastating loss.
   g. Six weeks after surgery, an ocularist may fit a prosthesis.
H. STRUCTURES OF THE EAR (SEE FIGURE 2-3)
1. EXTERNAL EAR
   a. Pinna or auricle external portion visible
   b. External auditory canal S-shaped with hair and sebaceous (wax) glands
   c. Functions to collect sound waves and transmit to the tympanic membrane (eardrum)
   d. Tympanic membrane partition between the external and middle ear
2. MIDDLE EAR
   a. Contains three tiny ossicles (bones: malleus, incus, and stapes)
   b. Vibrations cause ossicles to move and transmit sound to oval window.

Figure 2-3 Cross section of the ear

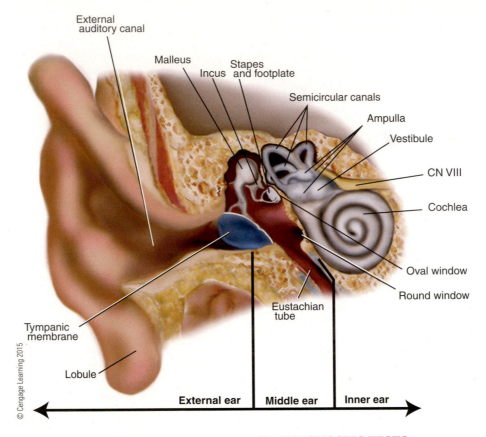

External
auditory canal

Malleus
Incus   Stapes
and footplate

Semicircular canals

Ampulla

Vestibule

CN VIII

Cochlea

Oval window

Round window

Eustachian
tube

Tympanic
membrane

Lobule

© Cengage Learning 2015

External ear   **Middle ear**   **Inner ear**

c. Eustachian tube equalizes pressure with a yawn or swallow.
d. Functions to conduct and amplify sound waves from the environment
3. INNER EAR
a. Composed of functional organs for hearing and balance
b. Cochlea contains the organ of Corti, the receptor for hearing.
c. Stimuli converted and transmitted to the brain via the vestibulocochlear nerve (CN VIII)
d. Three semicircular canals make up the organ of balance.

IX. ASSESSMENT
A. HEALTH HISTORY
1. PAST HEALTH HISTORY
2. MEDICATIONS (PAST, PRESENT, OVER THE COUNTER, HERBS)
3. SURGERIES
B. PHYSICAL EXAMINATION
1. INSPECTION
a. Ear—symmetry, canal
b. Presence of cerumen (wax) in the canal
c. Tympanic membrane (eardrum) intact
1) Pearly gray in color
2) Light reflex and landmarks intact
2. PALPATION
a. Denies pain or tenderness at auricles, tragus, or mastoid process

X. DIAGNOSTIC TESTS
A. RINNE TEST
1. DESCRIPTION:
a. Tuning fork test to distinguish between conductive and sensorineural hearing loss
2. PREPROCEDURE
a. Instruct the client that the activated tuning fork will be first held against the mastoid bone and, second, in front of the ear.
b. The client reports whether the sound is louder behind the ear (mastoid) or next to the ear. When the sound is no longer perceived behind the ear, move the fork next to the ear canal until the client indicates that the sound is no longer heard.
3. POSTPROCEDURE
a. The test is positive when the client reports that air conduction (AC) is heard longer than bone conduction (BC).
b. The test is negative if the client hears the tuning fork better by bone conduction.
B. WEBER TEST
1. DESCRIPTION: AN ACTIVATED TUNING FORK TEST FOR LATERALIZATION OF SOUND

2. PREPROCEDURE

   a. Instruct the client that a vibrating tuning fork will be placed on the midline skull and the forehead or teeth.

   b. Ask the client to indicate where the sound is heard best.

3. POSTPROCEDURE

   a. With a conductive loss in one ear, the sound is heard louder in that ear (lateralizes).

   b. With a sensorineural loss in one ear, the sound is louder in the unaffected ear.

C. AUDIOMETRY

   1. DESCRIPTION: TEST THAT PRESENTS A SERIES OF TONES AT VARYING INTENSITIES TO SCREEN FOR HEARING ACUITY AND DIAGNOSTIC FOR DEGREE AND TYPE OF HEARING LOSS

   2. PREPROCEDURE

      a. Instruct the client that the sounds will be presented through earphones.

      b. Instruct the client to respond verbally when a sound is heard.

      c. The response is recorded on an audiogram.

   3. POSTPROCEDURE

      a. A client with loss primarily in the higher frequencies has difficulty distinguishing high-pitched consonants such as in *cat*, *hat*, and *fat*, and the consonants are not heard.

      b. This type of hearing loss causes moderate difficulty in hearing normal speech.

      c. A hearing aid may be helpful to amplify sound but will not make sound clearer.

      d. An aid may not be helpful to the client who has problems with discrimination of sounds.

D. CALORIC TEST STIMULATION

   1. DESCRIPTION: USED TO DIAGNOSE DISEASE OF THE LABYRINTH. THIS IS DONE BY AN EAR IRRIGATION OF COLD OR WARM WATER AND MAY EVOKE NAUSEA AND VOMITING.

   2. PREPROCEDURE

      a. Instruct the client about the test procedure.

      b. Observe for nystagmus, nausea, and vomiting.

      c. Ensure client safety.

   3. POSTPROCEDURE

      a. Observe for the type of nystagmus, nausea and vomiting, falling, or vertigo.

      b. Decreased function is indicated by decreased response and indicates disease.

   c. The other ear is tested and the results are compared.

   d. Provide for client safety after the procedure.

E. POSTUROGRAPHY

   1. DESCRIPTION: TEST TO ASSESS THE BALANCE SYSTEM THAT IS ABLE TO ISOLATE ONE SEMICIRCULAR CANAL FROM OTHERS TO DETERMINE THE SITE OF A LESION CAUSING VESTIBULAR DISTURBANCE AND DEGREE OF DISABILITY

   2. PREPROCEDURE

      a. Give pretest instructions regarding intake of substances that can affect test results.

      b. Instruct the client that these tests are time consuming.

      c. If the vestibular is compromised, the client can experience distress, discomfort, and nausea and vomiting.

      d. Reassure that the test can be discontinued if not tolerated by the client.

   3. POSTPROCEDURE

      a. Assess for vertigo, nausea, and vomiting.

      b. Provide for client safety following the exam.

XI. **NURSING DIAGNOSIS**

   A. ANXIETY

   B. DISTURBED SENSORY PERCEPTION (AUDITORY)

   C. RISK FOR TRAUMA

   Nursing Diagnoses: Definitions and Classification 2012–2014. Copyright © 2012, 1994–2012 by NANDA International. Used by arrangement with John Wiley & Sons Limited.

XII. **EXTERNAL EAR AND CANAL DISORDERS**

   A. EXTERNAL OTITIS

      1. DESCRIPTION: INFLAMMATION OR INFECTION OF THE AURICLE AND EAR CANAL; MAY BE CALLED "SWIMMER'S EAR"

      2. ASSESSMENT

         a. Otalgia (pain) is due to swelling of the ear canal.

         b. Drainage may be serosanguineous (blood and serum) or purulent (pus).

         c. Swelling can block hearing and cause dizziness.

      3. DIAGNOSTIC TESTS

         a. Otoscope light exam

         b. Culture and sensitivity, if drainage is present

      4. NURSING INTERVENTIONS

         a. Cleanse the ear canal.

         b. Place a wick into the canal to deliver antibiotic otic drops.

         c. Administer topical antibiotic drops such as corticosteroids for inflammation.

   d. Administer Nystatin for fungal infections; corticosteroids are contraindicated.
   e. Apply warm moist compresses for surrounding tissue involvement.
   f. Carefully handle and dispose of drainage material.
   g. Administer otic drops at room temperature to prevent dizziness.
   h. Avoid touching the ear with the tip of the dropper to prevent contamination.
   i. Position ear so drops can run down the canal.
   j. Instruct the client to maintain the position for 2 minutes to allow dispersal of the drops.

B. CERUMEN AND FOREIGN BODIES IN THE EXTERNAL EAR CANAL
   1. DESCRIPTION: EARWAX (CERUMEN) CAN BECOME IMPACTED OR A FOREIGN BODY OBSTRUCTS EAR CANAL.
   2. ASSESSMENT
      a. Client complains of discomfort and decreased hearing.
      b. Earwax of an older adult client becomes thicker and drier due to canal hairs.
      c. Tinnitus (ringing in the ears)
      d. Vertigo
      e. Cough
      f. Cardiac depression (vagal stimulation)
   3. DIAGNOSTIC TESTS
      a. Otoscopic exam
      b. Audiogram
   4. NURSING INTERVENTIONS
      a. Irrigate the canal with body-temperature solution.
      b. A special or bulb syringe may be used to irrigate.
      c. Pull the auricle up and back while the client is in a sitting position.
      d. Avoid completely occluding the canal with the syringe tip.
      e. Use a cerumen spoon if the irrigation is not successful.
      f. Mild lubricant drops may be administered to soften the cerumen.
      g. Mineral oil may be used to drown an insect.
   5. MEDICAL MANAGEMENT
      a. Animate, inanimate, vegetable, or mineral objects must be removed by an audiologist.
      b. Deer ticks must be removed by microscope guidance via forceps.

C. MALIGNANCY OF THE EXTERNAL EAR
   1. DESCRIPTION
      a. Skin cancer involving the external ear

      b. Usually seen in fair-skinned persons with long-term exposure to the sun
   2. ASSESSMENT
      a. Chronic ulcer of the auricle
      b. Persistent drainage from the canal like otitis externa or blood tinged
   3. DIAGNOSTIC TESTS
      a. Biopsy of the involved area
      b. Computerized tomography (CT) scan
   4. NURSING INTERVENTIONS
      a. Prepare the client for biopsy and surgery to remove tissue.
      b. Instruct the client on the appearance of the carcinoma in the external ear.
   5. SURGICAL MANAGEMENT
      a. Removal of cancerous tissue
      b. Reconstruction of cosmetic deformities, if needed

XIII. MIDDLE EAR INVOLVEMENT
   A. ACUTE OTITIS MEDIA
      1. DESCRIPTION: INFLAMMATION OF THE MIDDLE EAR ASSOCIATED WITH UPPER RESPIRATORY INFECTIONS SUCH AS COLDS, SORE THROATS
      2. ASSESSMENT
         a. Pain, fever, malaise
         b. Headache and reduced hearing
      3. DIAGNOSTIC TESTS
         a. Otoscopic examination
         b. Visual examination
      4. NURSING INTERVENTIONS
         a. Administer analgesics to control pain.
         b. Instruct the client on prescribed systemic antibiotic use.
         c. Instruct the client on monitoring of pain and ear drainage.
         d. If surgery, avoid increased pressure such as blowing the nose or coughing.
         e. Instruct the client that if she must cough or sneeze she should leave her mouth open.
         f. Instruct the client to use care when getting up to prevent falls due to dizziness and loss of balance.
         g. Change dressings as needed.
      5. MEDICAL MANAGEMENT
         a. Amoxicillin for 10 days is the treatment of choice in the United States.
         b. Adults may also require antihistamine drugs
      6. SURGICAL MANAGEMENT
         a. Myringotomy is an incision into the eardrum to relieve pressure.
         b. Tympanostomy tube may be used for short- or long-term use.
   B. CHRONIC OTITIS MEDIA
      1. DESCRIPTION: CHRONIC INFECTION OF THE MIDDLE EAR DUE TO UNTREATED/REPEATED INFECTIONS

2. ASSESSMENT
   a. Purulent, mucus or serous discharge from the ear canal
   b. Hearing loss and sometimes ear pain, nausea, and dizziness
3. DIAGNOSTIC TESTS
   a. Otoscopic examination
   b. Culture and sensitivity, if drainage is present
   c. Mastoid x-ray
4. NURSING INTERVENTIONS
   a. Administer ear irrigations, such as ascetic acid (equal parts white vinegar and water).
   b. Administer otic drops as prescribed.
   c. Administer analgesics and antiemetics.
   d. Administer systemic antibiotics.
5. SURGICAL MANAGEMENT
   a. Tympanoplasty in reconstructing the eardrum
   b. Mastoidectomy to remove diseased tissue and source of infection
   c. Decongestants if fluid collection is due to allergy

C. OTOSCLEROSIS
1. DESCRIPTION: FIXATION OF THE STAPES, WHICH PREVENTS CONDUCTION OF SOUND TO THE INNER EAR
2. ASSESSMENT
   a. Hearing loss is asymmetric.
   b. May have difficulty hearing a phone conversation
   c. Tinnitus (ringing sensation)
3. DIAGNOSTIC TESTS
   a. Otoscopic examination
   b. Rinne test
   c. Weber test
   d. Audiogram
   e. Tympanometry
4. NURSING INTERVENTIONS
   a. Postoperatively, protect the client from injury to dizziness, nausea, and vomiting.
   b. Decrease sudden movements that may increase dizziness.
   c. Instruct the client to avoid coughing, sneezing, lifting, bending, or straining with bowel movements.

XIV. **INNER EAR PROBLEMS**
A. MÉNIÈRE'S DISEASE
1. DESCRIPTION: EPISODIC VERTIGO, TINNITUS, FLUCTUATING HEARING LOSS, AND EAR FULLNESS
2. ASSESSMENT
   a. Sudden, severe attacks of vertigo with nausea and vomiting
   b. Clinical manifestations begin between 30 and 60 years.
   c. 40% have bilateral involvement.

3. DIAGNOSTIC TESTS
   a. Audiometric studies
   b. Vestibular tests
   c. Electronystagmography
   d. Neurologic examination
4. NURSING INTERVENTIONS
   a. Provide for client safety to minimize vertigo.
   b. During Ménière's attack, keep the room darkened and the bed with the side rails up.
   c. Instruct the client to avoid sudden movements.
   d. Provide the client with a basin for emesis.
   e. Instruct the client to avoid fluorescent light or watching television, which may increase clinical manifestations.
   f. Assist the client with ambulation to prevent risk of fall.
   g. Administer drugs and fluid.
   h. Monitor intake and output.
   i. Postoperatively, the client may experience vertigo for weeks until adjusted.
5. MEDICAL MANAGEMENT
   a. Conservative therapy
      1) Sedative use of Valium or neuroleptics
      2) Anticholinergic (atropine)
      3) Management between attacks includes vasodilators, diuretics, antihistamines, a low-sodium diet, and avoidance of caffeine and nicotine.
6. SURGICAL MANAGEMENT
   a. Conservative surgical interventions
      1) Endolymphatic shunt
      2) Vestibular nerve section
   b. Destructive surgical interventions
      1) Labyrinthotomy
      2) Labyrinthectomy

B. PRESBYCUSIS
1. DESCRIPTION
   a. Hearing loss that may be common in the older adult
   b. There is a decline in word recognition ability and auditory sensitivity.
2. ASSESSMENT
   a. Difficulty understanding the spoken word due to loss of consonants
   b. Gradual decline in hearing sensitivity
   c. Vowels are heard but some consonants cannot be differentiated.
   d. Confusion and embarrassment between what is heard and spoken
3. DIAGNOSTIC TESTS
   a. Audiogram
   b. Otoscopic exam
   c. Rinne test

4. NURSING INTERVENTIONS
  a. Inform the client that noise exposure will intensify difficulty.
  b. Discuss with the client what the loss of hearing may mean.
  c. Encourage the client to use a hearing aid.
  d. Instruct the client on the care of a hearing aid.
5. MEDICAL MANAGEMENT
  a. Hearing aid
  b. Prognosis depends on the cause of the presbycusis.

C. LABYRINTHITIS
  1. DESCRIPTION: INFLAMMATION OF THE INNER EAR AFFECTING THE COCHLEAR OR VESTIBULAR PORTION
  2. ASSESSMENT
    a. Vertigo with nausea and vomiting
    b. Tinnitus and sensorineural hearing loss on the affected side
    c. Nystagmus (abnormal rhythmic jerking movement of the eyes)
  3. DIAGNOSTIC TESTS
    a. Nystagmus exam
    b. Calorie test stimulus
  4. NURSING INTERVENTIONS
    a. Discuss with the client safety concerns due to extreme unsteadiness.
    b. Implement physical therapy to help recondition the brain to reinterpret vestibular input.
  5. MEDICAL MANAGEMENT
    a. Antibiotics
    b. Antiemetics
    c. May need hearing aid if hearing loss occurs

D. ACOUSTIC NEUROMA
  1. DESCRIPTION: BENIGN TUMOR THAT OCCURS WHERE THE VESTIBULOCOCHLEAR NERVE (CN VIII) ENTERS THE AUDITORY CANAL OR TEMPORAL BONE FROM THE BRAIN
  2. ASSESSMENT
    a. Unilateral, progressive, sensorineural hearing loss
    b. Unilateral tinnitus
    c. Mild intermittent vertigo
    d. Reduced touch sensation in the posterior ear canal
  3. DIAGNOSTIC TESTS
    a. Neurologic tests
    b. Audiometric tests
    c. Vestibular tests
    d. CT scan
    e. Magnetic resonance imaging (MRI) scan
  4. NURSING INTERVENTIONS
    a. Protect the client from injury due to vertigo.
    b. Caution the client regarding hearing loss after surgery.

  c. Advise the client on equipment and support services available for hearing impairment.
  5. SURGICAL MANAGEMENT
    a. Surgical removal of the tumor
    b. Difficult to preserve hearing if medium- to large-size tumor (2–3 cm)

E. HEARING IMPAIRMENT AND DEAFNESS
  1. DESCRIPTION: DIFFICULTY HEARING OR COMPLETE LOSS OF SENSE OF HEARING
  2. ASSESSMENT
    a. Conductive hearing loss
      1) Hearing loss that involves the outer and middle ear sound conduction to inner ear
      2) Check for impacted earwax, middle ear disease, otosclerosis, stenosis.
    b. Sensorineural hearing loss
      1) Hearing loss that is caused by impairment of the inner ear or its central connections
      2) Congenital for hereditary factors
      3) Noise trauma over a period of time
      4) Aging (presbycusis)
      5) Ménière's disease
      6) Ototoxicity
      7) Systemic or immune disease
      8) Loss of ability to hear sound but not to understand speech
      9) Diminished ability to hear high-pitched sounds
      10) Words become difficult to distinguish; sound becomes muffled.
    c. Mixed hearing loss
      1) Caused by combination of conductive and sensorineural losses
    d. Central hearing loss
      1) Caused by problems in the central nervous system
      2) Unable to understand or put meaning to incoming sound
    e. Functional hearing loss
      1) May be caused by an emotional or psychologic factor
      2) Does not seem to hear or respond to pure tone hearing tests
      3) No organic cause can be identified.
  3. DIAGNOSTIC TESTS
    a. Test the young child for significant speech and language problems.
  4. NURSING INTERVENTIONS (SEE TABLE 2-3)
    a. Instruct the client about the type of hearing loss.
    b. Instruct the client regarding equipment and services that can aid audio communication.

Table 2-3 Communication with the Hearing-Impaired Client

Nonverbal Aids	Verbal Aids
Attend to hand movements.	Speak normally and slowly.
Shine good light on the speaker's face.	Use appropriate facial expressions.
Keep hands away from the face or mouth.	Enunciate clearly.
Avoid chewing, eating, smoking, or careless expressions while talking.	Use simple sentences.
Maintain eye contact.	Rephrase as needed, in different words.
Avoid distracting environments.	Write difficult names or words.
Use touch.	Avoid shouting.
Position self closer to the better ear.	Speak into the better ear with a normal voice.

© Cengage Learning 2015

c. Clients who are motivated and optimistic will be more successful with a hearing aid if the hearing impairment would benefit from it.

d. Instruct the client on the maintenance of the hearing aid.

e. Support the client during period of adjustment.

f. Instruct the client that, initially, she may need to adjust to voices such as her own or those of her family and friends or household sounds.

g. Instruct the client that she may need to experiment with increases and decreases in volume.

h. Instruct the client to expand environmental situations and sounds to prepare for differences.

i. Instruct the client to store the hearing aid in a cool, safe place.

j. Advise the client to purchase a 1-month supply at a time of the hearing aid batteries because the average battery life averages 1 week.

k. Instruct the client to cleanse ear molds weekly or as needed.

l. Encourage the client to learn speech or lip reading, which may be helpful in increasing communication.

m. Use verbal cues and gestures and facial expressions to help clarify messages.

n. Inform the client that many words may look alike when spoken, such as *rabbit* and *woman*.

o. Inform the client that cochlear implants may be used for acquired or congenital hearing loss.

5. SURGICAL MANAGEMENT

a. Cochlear implant, which stimulates auditory nerve fibers by electric current

b. Extensive training and rehabilitation are essential for maximum benefit.

XV. **ANATOMY AND PHYSIOLOGY OF THE NOSE AND THROAT (SEE FIGURE 2-4)**

A. FUNCTIONS OF THE NOSE AND THROAT

1. THE NOSE AND THROAT FORM THE UPPER PORTION OF THE AIRWAY.

2. THE NOSE FACILITATES THE SENSE OF SMELL.

3. THE NOSE AND THROAT ASSIST IN THE PRODUCTION OF THE VOICE.

B. NOSE

1. AIR ENTERS THE RESPIRATORY TRACT THROUGH THE NOSE.

2. HUMIDIFIES, WARMS, AND FILTERS INSPIRED AIR

3. NORMALLY, A LITER OF MOISTURE IS SECRETED BY THIS MUCOUS MEMBRANE DAILY.

4. CONTAINS TWO OPENINGS CALLED NARES

5. THIS ENTIRE AREA IS VERY VASCULAR.

C. SINUSES

1. AIR-FILLED CAVITIES WITHIN THE HOLLOW BONES THAT SURROUND NASAL PASSAGES

2. PROVIDE RESONANCE TO VOICE DURING SPEECH

D. PHARYNX

1. LOCATED BEHIND THE ORAL AND NASAL CAVITIES

2. DIVIDED INTO THREE SECTIONS: NASO-, ORO-, AND LARYNGOPHARYNX

3. PASSAGEWAY FOR BOTH RESPIRATORY AND DIGESTIVE TRACTS

E. LARYNX

1. LOCATED ABOVE THE TRACHEA AND JUST BELOW THE PHARYNX AT THE ROOT OF THE TONGUE

2. COMMONLY CALLED THE "VOICE BOX"

3. CONTAINS TWO PAIRS OF VOCAL CORDS, FALSE AND TRUE CORDS

Figure 2-4 Cross section of the nose and throat

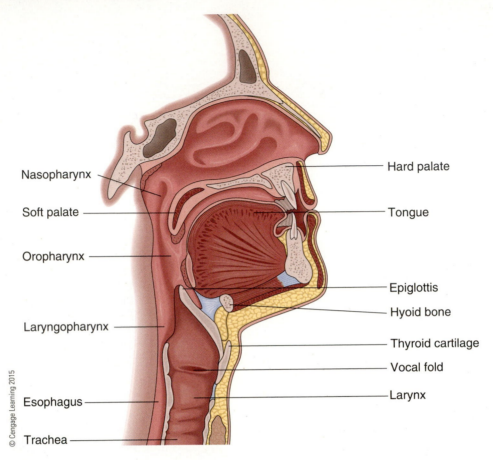

Nasopharynx

Soft palate

Oropharynx

Laryngopharynx

Esophagus

Trachea

Hard palate

Tongue

Epiglottis

Hyoid bone

Thyroid cartilage

Vocal fold

Larynx

© Cengage Learning 2015

4. THE OPENING BETWEEN THE TRUE CORDS IS THE GLOTTIS.
5. THE GLOTTIS PLAYS AN IMPORTANT ROLE IN COUGHING, A DEFENSE MECHANISM OF THE LUNGS.

F. EPIGLOTTIS
   1. LEAF-SHAPED STRUCTURE THAT IS ATTACHED TO THE TOP OF THE LARYNX
   2. PREVENTS FOOD FROM ENTERING THE TRACHEOBRONCHIAL TREE BY CLOSING DURING SWALLOWING

G. TRACHEA
   1. LOCATED IN THE FRONT OF THE ESOPHAGUS
   2. BRANCHES INTO THE RIGHT AND LEFT MAINSTEM BRONCHI

XVI. ASSESSMENT
   A. HEALTH HISTORY
      1. PAST HEALTH HISTORY
      2. MEDICATIONS (PAST, PRESENT, OVER THE COUNTER, HERBS)
      3. SURGERIES
   B. PHYSICAL EXAMINATION
      1. INSPECTION
         a. Nose—symmetry, color, shape, discharge, flaring, or narrowing
         b. Sinuses—tenderness, swelling, pain
         c. Throat—color, swelling, discharge
      2. PALPATION
         a. Nose—tenderness, swelling, drainage
         b. Sinuses—pain, tenderness, postnasal drip, color of exudate

XVII. DIAGNOSTIC STUDIES
   A. CULTURE: THROAT OR AREA OF INFECTION OR EXUDATE
      1. DESCRIPTION: USING A DACRON SWAB, VIGOROUSLY RUB THE PHARYNX, TONSILLAR PILLARS, AND AREAS OF PURULENCE, EXUDATE, OR ULCERATION.
      2. PREPROCEDURE
         a. Instruct the client to hold the mouth open for specimen collection.
         b. Throat collection may elicit gagging from the client.
         c. Assemble tongue blade, culture swab, kit.
      3. POSTPROCEDURE
         a. Send the appropriately labeled specimen to the lab for results.
         b. Notify the client of the results and prescribed treatment, if needed.

XVIII. NURSING DIAGNOSIS
   A. DISTURBED SENSORY PERCEPTION (NASAL)
   B. ACUTE PAIN
   C. RISK FOR INFECTION

   Nursing Diagnoses: Definitions and Classification 2012–2014. Copyright © 2012, 1994–2012 by NANDA International. Used by arrangement with John Wiley & Sons Limited.

XIX. NASAL-PHARYNGEAL DISEASES
   A. DEVIATED SEPTUM
      1. DESCRIPTION: DEFLECTION OF THE NORMALLY STRAIGHT NASAL SEPTUM
      2. ASSESSMENT
         a. Septum bent to one side
         b. Most commonly caused by trauma
         c. Obstruction to nasal breathing
         d. Nasal edema or dryness of the mucosa, with crusting and bleeding
         e. Mucus may be blocked, causing a sinus infection.
      3. DIAGNOSTIC STUDIES
         a. Culture of exudate
      4. NURSING INTERVENTIONS
         a. Instruct the client that swab may tickle the membrane or cause brief discomfort.
         b. Instruct the client on the proper handling of tissues and drainage to prevent infection of others.
         c. Instruct the client on the proper use of nasal decongestants or steroid sprays.
      5. SURGICAL MANAGEMENT
         a. Nasal septoplasty may be performed with or without rhinoplasty.
   B. NASAL FRACTURE
      1. DESCRIPTION: FRACTURE OF THE NASAL BONES MOST OFTEN CAUSED BY TRAUMA OF SUBSTANTIAL FORCE TO THE MIDDLE OF THE FACE
      2. ASSESSMENT
         a. Fracture types: unilateral, bilateral or complex
         b. Flattened appearance to the face
         c. Inability to breathe through the nostrils
         d. Presence of edema, bleeding, or hematoma
         e. Ecchymosis may be under one or both eyes
      3. DIAGNOSTIC TESTS
         a. Culture for cerebrospinal fluid (CSF) (indicative of a skull fracture)
      4. NURSING INTERVENTIONS
         a. Apply ice to the face and nose to reduce edema and bleeding.
         b. Monitor intranasal packing or external splints.
         c. Instruct the client not to take aspirin-containing drugs for 2 weeks to reduce bleeding risk.
         d. Assess respirations, pain management, bleeding, and edema.
         e. Instruct the client to detect early and late complications.
      5. SURGICAL MANAGEMENT
         a. Septoplasty
         b. Rhinoplasty
   C. EPISTAXIS
      1. DESCRIPTION
         a. Nosebleed occurs in all age groups, especially children and older adults.
         b. Caused by trauma, foreign bodies, abuse of nasal spray, illicit drug use, malformations, allergic rhinitis, or tumors
      2. ASSESSMENT
         a. Any condition that may prolong bleeding time or alters platelet count
         b. Ask the client if she is currently taking aspirin or nonsteroidal anti-inflammatory drugs (NSAIDs).
         c. Check blood pressure because hypertension may increase risk.
      3. DIAGNOSTIC TESTS
         a. Bleeding time
         b. Platelet count
      4. NURSING INTERVENTIONS
         a. Keep the client quiet.
         b. Place the client in a sitting position or leaning forward if possible.
         c. If reclining, elevate the head and shoulders.
         d. Apply direct pressure by pinching the entire soft lower portion of the nose for 10–15 minutes.
         e. Apply ice compresses to the nose and have the client suck on ice.
         f. Partially insert a small gauze pad into the bleeding nostril and continue pressure application.
         g. Obtain medical assistance if bleeding does not stop.
         h. Instruct the client to avoid vigorous nose blowing, strenuous activity, lifting, and straining for 4–6 weeks.
         i. Instruct the client to sneeze with the mouth open.
         j. Instruct the client to avoid the use of aspirin-containing products or NSAIDs.
      5. SURGICAL MANAGEMENT
         a. Anterior or posterior packing
         b. Cauterization
   D. ALLERGIC RHINITIS
      1. DESCRIPTION
         a. Reaction of the nasal mucosa to a specific antigen (allergen)

b. Attacks of seasonal rhinitis usually occur in the spring and fall caused by pollens from trees, flowers, or grasses.

2. ASSESSMENT
   a. Typical attacks last several weeks when pollen counts are high and disappears and recurs at the same time each year.
   b. Perennial rhinitis is present intermittently or constantly.
   c. Specific environmental triggers include pet dander, dust mites, molds, or foods.
   d. Perennial rhinitis resembles the common cold and the client may believe it is a cold.

3. DIAGNOSTIC TESTS
   a. Intradermal (skin) test of allergens
   b. Review the client's diary of reactions and activities precipitating the allergic event.

4. NURSING INTERVENTIONS
   a. Instruct the client to keep a diary of reactions and activities that precipitate reactions.
   b. Instruct the client to avoid triggers because this is the best therapy.
   c. Instruct the client to avoid house dust, dust mites, mold spores, pollens, pets, and smoke.
   d. Instruct the client regarding proper drug use (see Table 2-4).
      1) Antihistamines: monitor for sedative adverse reactions. Instruct the client to avoid driving or operating machinery, report palpitations, and avoid taking with alcohol or MAO inhibitors.
      2) Decongestants: contraindicated with cardiovascular disease, hypertension, diabetes mellitus, glaucoma, enlarged prostate, hepatic or renal disease. Instruct the client not to use decongestants for more than 3 days or more than 3–4 times per day.
      3) Corticosteroids: use on a regular basis, not p.r.n. Effect is delayed but decreases inflammation.

Discontinue use if nasal infection develops.
      4) Mast cell stabilizer: instruct the client of the correct use. The spray prevents clinical manifestation. Begin 2 weeks prior to pollen season or 10–15 minutes prior to exposure.
      5) Anticholinergics: instruct the client of the correct use. Spray prevents clinical manifestations with onset within 1 hour of use; may reduce the need for other drugs.

5. MEDICAL MANAGEMENT
   a. Antihistamines to block histamine binding
   b. Decongestants to promote vasoconstriction and reduce edema
   c. Corticosteroids to inhibit inflammation
   d. Mast cell stabilizers to inhibit degranulation of sensitized mast cells
   e. Anticholinergics to block hypersecretory effects, reduce drainage

E. ACUTE RHINITIS
   1. DESCRIPTION
      a. Common cold or acute coryza caused by viruses that invade the upper respiratory tract
      b. Most commonly spread by airborne droplet from an infected person while breathing, talking, sneezing, or coughing or by direct hand contact. Other factors such as chilling, fatigue, physical and emotional stress, compromised immune system may increase susceptibility.
   2. ASSESSMENT
      a. Tickling, irritation, sneezing, or dryness of nose or nasopharynx
      b. Copious thin nasal secretions initially, thicker discharge later
      c. Some nasal obstruction
      d. Watery eyes
      e. Elevated temperature
      f. General malaise
      g. Headache

Table 2-4 Method for Using an Intranasal Inhaler

Prior to using inhaler, gently blow nose to clear nostrils and follow these steps:
1. Remove the protective cap from the nasal inhaler.
2. Shake the canister well.
3. Hold the inhaler between the thumb and forefingers.
4. Tilt the head back slightly and insert the tip of the inhaler into one nostril, pointing it slightly toward the outside of the nostril. Hold the other nostril closed with one finger.
5. Press down on the canister to release one dose and at the same time gently inhale.
6. Hold your breath for a few seconds, then breathe out slowly through your mouth.
7. Remove the inhaler from one nostril and repeat the process with the other nostril. If more than one puff is prescribed, repeat actions 4–6.
8. Replace the protective cap on the inhaler.

3. NURSING INTERVENTIONS
   a. Instruct the client on how to contain secretions to prevent spread of infection to others.
   b. Encourage the client to rest, and instruct client on fluids and proper diet.
   c. Administer antipyretics and analgesics.
   d. Instruct the client that infection may spread to the throat, sinuses, middle ear, tonsils, and chest.
   e. Generally, antibiotics are not indicated unless bacterial invasion is evident or occurs.
   f. If the client's immune system is compromised, instruct the client to avoid crowded areas and others with cold clinical manifestations.
   g. Encourage frequent hand washing and avoiding hand-to-face contact.
   h. Instruct the client to report temperatures above 38°C (100.4°F), exudate on tonsils, tender lymph nodes, and sore, red throat.
   i. If pulmonary disease is present, instruct the client to report changes in consistency, color, and amount of sputum.

F. INFLUENZA
   1. DESCRIPTION
      a. Systemic viral infection of the body that has a remarkable ability to change over time; resolves in 7 days
      b. Each year flu causes significant morbidity and mortality.
   2. ASSESSMENT
      a. Headache
      b. Fever, chills
      c. Myalgia (aching muscles)
      d. Cough and sore throat
      e. Dyspnea and diffuse crackles indicate pulmonary complications.
   3. DIAGNOSTIC TESTS
      a. Clinical findings
   4. NURSING INTERVENTIONS
      a. Treatment is largely supportive.
      b. If a secondary infection develops, antibiotics will need to be given early. Secondary infection has some improvement for 2–3 days, then cough and purulent sputum develop.
      c. Administer influenza vaccination in clients at high risk (mid-October).

G. SINUSITIS
   1. DEFINITION
      a. Inflammation of the sinuses develops when the sinuses are narrowed or blocked by inflammation or swelling of the mucosa. Secretions that accumulate provide a medium for bacterial growth such as *Streptococcus pneumoniae*, *Haemophilus influenzae*, or *Moraxella catarrhalis*.
   2. ASSESSMENT
      a. Significant pain over the affected sinus
      b. Purulent nasal drainage
      c. Nasal obstruction, congestion, and swelling
      d. Fever and malaise
   3. DIAGNOSTIC TESTS
      a. Sinus x-rays
      b. Sinus computed tomogram (CT)
      c. Sinus cultures
   4. NURSING INTERVENTIONS
      a. Instruct the client to keep well hydrated by drinking six to eight glasses of water daily.
      b. Instruct the client to take hot showers or use humidification to promote secretion drainage.
      c. Instruct the client to report temperatures of 38°C (100.4°F) or higher.
      d. Administer analgesics to relieve pain.
      e. Instruct the client to take decongestants or expectorants to relieve swelling and improve breathing.
      f. Administer prescribed antibiotics, instructing the client to take the entire prescription and report continued clinical manifestations or change.
      g. Instruct the client to avoid smoking and exposure to smoke and environmental irritants that may worsen clinical manifestations.
      h. If allergies precipitate, follow directions regarding environment, drug therapy, and immunotherapy to reduce inflammation and prevent sinus infection.

H. POLYPS
   1. DEFINITION
      a. Benign projections of edematous mucous membrane that form in the sinus or nasal cavity
      b. These form slowly in response to repeated inflammation and may protrude into the airway.
   2. ASSESSMENT
      a. Nasal obstruction
      b. Nasal drainage (usually clear mucus)
      c. Speech distortion
   3. DIAGNOSTIC TESTS
      a. Clinical findings
   4. NURSING INTERVENTIONS
      a. Instruct the client regarding polyp formation.
      b. Inform the client of the effect of polyps by restriction of breathing.
      c. Promote a calming environment.
   5. SURGICAL MANAGEMENT
      a. Polypectomy

I. FOREIGN BODIES
   1. DESCRIPTION: FOREIGN BODIES LODGE IN THE UPPER AIRWAY; FOR EXAMPLE,

INORGANIC: BUTTONS OR BEADS;
ORGANIC: WOOD, PEAS, BEANS, PAPER

2. ASSESSMENT
   a. Asymptomatic
   b. Local inflammation and clear nasal discharge
   c. Discharge may become purulent and foul smelling.

3. NURSING INTERVENTIONS
   a. The foreign body may be removed by sneezing with the opposite nostril closed, or blowing the nose.
   b. Avoid irrigating or pushing the object backward because there is a danger of aspiration and airway obstruction.

4. MEDICAL MANAGEMENT
   a. Manual removal if other noninvasive methods fail

J. ACUTE PHARYNGITIS
1. DESCRIPTION
   a. Acute inflammation of the pharyngeal walls and may include the tonsils, palate, and uvula
   b. Can be caused by viral, bacterial, or fungal infection; 70% of cases are viral, 15–20% of cases are caused by strep.

2. ASSESSMENT
   a. "Scratchy throat" to pain so severe that swallowing is difficult
   b. Fungal, white irregular patches suggest *Candida albicans.*
   c. Viral: throat may appear mildly red with some congestion; about 70% of cases.
   d. Bacterial: "strep throat" from beta-hemolytic invasion accounts for 15–20% of cases.

3. DIAGNOSTIC TESTS
   a. Clinical findings
   b. Throat culture

4. NURSING INTERVENTIONS
   a. Encourage the client to increase fluid intake.
   b. Encourage the client to take cool, bland liquids, which will not irritate the throat.
   c. Avoid citrus juices because they irritate the membranes.
   d. Instruct the client to cover the mouth when coughing and to contain secretions in disposable tissues.
   e. Encourage hand washing and antibacterial wash to help prevent spread of infection.
   f. Administer analgesics 30 minutes prior to eating to enhance the ability to swallow.
   g. Administer prescribed antibiotics for suspected strep throat.
   h. Administer Nystatin to treat a fungal infection; swish and hold in the mouth before swallowing.

K. PERITONSILLAR ABSCESS
1. DESCRIPTION
   a. Complication of acute pharyngitis or tonsillitis if bacterial infection invades the tonsil
   b. Poses a threat to airway patency due to tonsil enlargement

2. ASSESSMENT
   a. High fever
   b. Leukocytosis
   c. Chills

3. DIAGNOSTIC TESTS
   a. Clinical findings
   b. Throat culture

4. NURSING INTERVENTIONS
   a. Protect and maintain the airway.
   b. Protect from secondary infection.
   c. Maintain intravenous antibiotic therapy.

5. SURGICAL MANAGEMENT
   a. Emergency tonsillectomy
   b. Elective tonsillectomy after the infection subsides

L. OBSTRUCTIVE SLEEP APNEA
1. DESCRIPTION
   a. Airway obstruction occurs when the tongue and soft palate fall backward and partially or completely obstruct the pharynx; characterized by repetitive cessation of airflow during sleep
   b. Cause may be involved with a small airway, altered respiratory control of muscles, and hormonal imbalance

2. ASSESSMENT
   a. Client has a generalized startle response, snorts and gasps during sleep.
   b. Apnea and arousal cycles occur repeatedly as many as 200–400 times in 6–8 hours of sleep.
   c. Frequent awakening at night
   d. Insomnia
   e. Excessive daytime sleepiness
   f. Morning headaches
   g. Personality changes and irritability
   h. Diminished ability to concentrate
   i. Impaired memory
   j. Disorientation occurs if awakened during periods of apnea.
   k. Failure to accomplish daily tasks
   l. Interpersonal difficulties
   m. May experience impotence
   n. Driving accidents
   o. May experience severe depression

3. DIAGNOSTIC TESTS
   a. Polysomnography
   b. Sleep studies

4. NURSING INTERVENTIONS
   a. Instruct the client to avoid sedatives and alcohol beverages for 3–4 hours prior to sleep.

   b. Referral to a weight-loss program may
      be beneficial.
   c. Apply an oral appliance that advances
      the mandible; may diminish clinical
      manifestations.
   d. Nasal continuous positive airway
      pressure (nCPAP) may be used.

   e. Bilevel positive airway pressure (BiPAP)
      delivers pressure during inspiration.
5. SURGICAL MANAGEMENT
   a. Uvulopalatopharyngoplasty (UPPP
      or UP3)
   b. Genioglossal advancement and hyoid
      myotomy (GAHM)

PRACTICE QUESTIONS

1. Which of the following should the nurse
   include in the discharge instructions for a client
   after cataract surgery?

   Select all that apply:
   [ ] 1. Use aseptic technique to apply eye
          medication
   [ ] 2. Expect an increase in pain after surgery
   [ ] 3. Avoid coughing, bending, or lifting
   [ ] 4. There are no eyedrops to use after surgery
   [ ] 5. The eye patch will cover the operative
          eye for 24 hours
   [ ] 6. A decrease in visual acuity is a
          complication

2. Which of the following should the nurse
   include in the assessment of the client's cranial
   nerves and extraocular eye muscles?
   1. Red reflex
   2. Six cardinal fields of gaze
   3. Disc characteristics
   4. Macular characteristics

3. When completing a measurement of the client's
   visual acuity, which of the following would be
   appropriate?
   1. Ophthalmoscope
   2. Penlight
   3. Visual field
   4. Snellen chart

4. The nurse collects a history from a client
   suspected of a sensorineural hearing loss.
   Which of the following findings supports the
   diagnosis and should be reported?
   1. The ability to hear high-pitched sounds
   2. Frequent ear irrigations for dry, hard cerumen
   3. A history of exposure to excessive noise
      over a period of time
   4. The client speaks softly

5. Which of the following nursing measures
   should receive priority in the client's plan of
   care after eye surgery?
   1. Prevent increased intraocular pressure and
      infection

2. Instruct on the importance of follow-up
3. Instruct on how to perform the Valsalva
   maneuver
4. Pain management

6. The nurse should consider which of the
   following drugs taken by a client with
   glaucoma?

   Drugs that
   1. increase intraocular pressure
   2. decrease intraocular pressure
   3. decrease vitreous humor
   4. cause anesthesia

7. The nurse implements which of the following
   interventions to reduce intraocular pressure
   following eye surgery?
   1. Applies hot compresses
   2. Provides bright lighting in the room
   3. Applies gentle pressure on the affected eye
   4. Keeps the head of the bed elevated

8. The nurse assesses which of the following to
   cause a conductive hearing loss?

   Select all that apply:
   [ ] 1. Cerumen
   [ ] 2. Loud noise
   [ ] 3. Otosclerosis
   [ ] 4. Ménière's disease
   [ ] 5. Ototoxicity
   [ ] 6. Middle ear disease

9. The client who just had cataract removal
   complains of nausea and severe pain in the
   operative eye. Which of the following nursing
   actions is the priority in this client's plan of
   care?
   1. Administer drugs for the pain and nausea
   2. Notify the physician immediately
   3. Assure the client that this is normal after
      surgery
   4. Turn the client to the operative side every
      2 hours

10. The client received instruction following cataract surgery. Which of the following statements by the client indicates the client understood the instruction?
    1. "Aspirin is all I need for the soreness."
    2. "I will sleep on the operative side."
    3. "I will wear an eye shield at night and glasses during the day."
    4. "I will not lift anything over 15 pounds."

11. Because a client has glaucoma, plans for nursing interventions should include
    1. a decrease in fluid intake.
    2. avoiding reading and watching television.
    3. a decrease in the amount of salt in the diet.
    4. eye medications must be taken for life.

12. Which of the following assessments indicate a client has sustained a retinal detachment?
    Select all that apply:
    [ ] 1. Floaters
    [ ] 2. A sharp, sudden pain in the eye
    [ ] 3. Photopsia
    [ ] 4. A reddened conjunctiva
    [ ] 5. Glare that is worse at night
    [ ] 6. Ring in the visual field

13. In planning the pre-op care for a client with a retinal detachment, the nurse should include which of the following in the plan of care?
    1. Restrict ambulation
    2. Maintain flat bed rest
    3. Place a patch over the affected eye
    4. Have client wear dark glasses for reading and television

14. For a client who sustained a chemical burn from battery acid, the nurse should include which of the following in the emergency procedures?
    1. Assess the visual acuity
    2. Irrigate the eye with sterile normal saline
    3. Swab the eye with antibiotic ointment
    4. Cover the affected eye with an eye patch

15. During the initial assessment the nurse observes the presence of bright red drainage on the eye dressing. Which of the following should be the nurse's first action?
    1. Report the findings to the physician
    2. Continue to monitor the vital signs and pain
    3. Note the amount of drainage on the client's record
    4. Mark the drainage on the dressing and monitor the amount and color

16. The nurse should instruct a client to buy how much of a supply of hearing aid batteries?

    _____

17. The nurse implements which of the following in the plan of care for a client who is hearing impaired?
    1. Speaks in a raised voice
    2. Speaks slowly
    3. Uses exaggerated facial expressions
    4. Has the light behind the nurse

18. The nurse is admitting a client in the emergency room with a foreign body in the ear identified as an insect. Which of the following interventions is a priority for the nurse to perform?
    1. Irrigate the affected ear
    2. Instill diluted alcohol in the affected ear
    3. Instill an antibiotic ointment into the affected ear
    4. Instill a cortisone ointment into the affected ear

19. The nurse correctly tells a client that the priority goal in the treatment for Ménière's disease is to
    1. maintain a sodium-free diet.
    2. eliminate environmental noise.
    3. preserve the remaining hearing.
    4. promote a quiet environment.

20. The nurse is collecting a history from a client suspected of having Ménière's disease. Which of the following assessment findings support the diagnosis?

    Select all that apply:
    [ ] 1. Purulent, foul-smelling drainage
    [ ] 2. Fever
    [ ] 3. Vertigo
    [ ] 4. Tinnitus
    [ ] 5. Increased discrimination in understanding of spoken words
    [ ] 6. Sensorineural hearing loss

21. A client has been receiving streptomycin and develops tinnitus, a disturbance in equilibrium, and hearing loss. The nurse reports this as a result of damage to which cranial nerve? ____

22. A client asks the nurse to explain what glaucoma is. Which of the following is the appropriate response by the nurse?
    1. "An opacity of the crystalline lens or its capsule."
    2. "A curvature of the cornea that becomes unequal."
    3. "A separation of the neural retina from the pigment retina."
    4. "An increase in the pressure within the eyeball."

23. Which of the following is the priority for the nurse to include in the teaching plan for a client with acute bacterial conjunctivitis?
    1. Instruct the client to avoid rubbing the eyes
    2. Apply hot moist compresses to the adherent crust on the eye
    3. Stress the importance of hand washing
    4. Instruct the client to avoid sharing towels

24. The nurse assesses a normal intraocular pressure to be _____.

25. A client who has a retinal detachment asks the nurse if a retinal detachment in the good eye is likely to occur. Which of the following responses by the nurse is most appropriate?
    1. "Chances are very high that you will experience another retinal detachment as you get older."
    2. "You should prevent trauma to your good eye because trauma can cause retinal detachment."
    3. "Clinical manifestations of retinal detachment are pain behind the eye, nausea, and dizziness and are to be reported immediately."
    4. "A retinal detachment can be prevented by having yearly ophthalmic examinations."

26. The registered nurse is making out assignments for the day. Which of the following nursing care activities may be delegated to certified assistive personnel?
    1. Instruct a client how to instill artificial tears
    2. Inform the client with cataracts of the post-op care
    3. Assess a client for a hearing loss
    4. Reinforce to a client with bacterial conjunctivitis the importance of hand washing

27. The nurse evaluates which of the following assessment findings to be normal in an older adult client?
    1. Hordeolum
    2. Exophthalmos
    3. Presbyopia
    4. Tinnitus

28. The nurse is reviewing the normal limits of a hearing assessment for a client who presents with decreased hearing. Which of the following findings would indicate the need for additional investigation?
    1. Sound heard equally in both ears with the Weber test
    2. Whispered words are repeated at 2 feet
    3. Bone conduction is heard twice as long as air conduction with the Rinne test
    4. Pearly gray tympanic membrane with otoscope

29. A client asks the nurse what a hordeolum is. Which of the following is the appropriate response by the nurse?
    1. "It is an inflammation of the cornea."
    2. "It is a chronic bacterial inflammation of the lid margin."
    3. "It is an infection of the conjunctiva."
    4. "It is an infection of the sebaceous glands on an eyelid follicle."

30. The registered nurse is preparing to delegate clinical assignments on a medical-surgical nursing unit. Which of the following assignments would be appropriate for the nurse to delegate to a licensed practical nurse?
    1. Instruct a client on the postoperative care following surgery for a cataract
    2. Develop an activity schedule for a client with glaucoma
    3. Perform an assessment of the ears for a client complaining of tinnitus
    4. Administer a drug intranasally to a client who has allergic rhinitis

ANSWERS AND RATIONALES

1. 1. 3. 5. Following cataract surgery, it is appropriate to use aseptic technique to apply eye medications; to instruct the client to avoid coughing, bending, or lifting; and to keep the operative eye patched for 24 hours. Using aseptic technique during the application of eye medications prevents an eye infection. Instructing the client to avoid coughing, bending, or lifting prevents increased intraocular pressure. The client should be instructed that although the eye patch covers the operative eye for only 24 hours, 1 to 2 weeks may be necessary to meet visual needs. A decreased visual acuity is not a complication. There should not be an increase in pain after surgery. All pain not relieved by medications should be reported.

2. 2. When assessing the cranial nerves (III, IV, and VI) and the six extraocular muscles, the six cardinal fields of gaze are utilized. The red reflex, disc characteristics, and macular characteristics are used to inspect the internal eye.

3. 4. The measurement of visual acuity includes the Snellen or E chart to test cranial nerve II. The ophthalmoscope and penlight illuminate inner eye structures, while the visual field evaluates cranial nerves and movement in the extraocular eye muscles.

4. 3. Sensorineural hearing loss is a permanent loss that is not correctable. It is a problem with the inner ear caused by excessive noise over a period of time, the aging process, Ménière's disease, ototoxicity, or congenital or other diseases.

5. 1. Increased intraocular pressure and infection can cause serious vision complications. Postoperative restrictions on head positioning, bending, coughing, and Valsalva maneuver will protect the eye from increased intraocular pressure and prevent injury. Follow-up care will be a concern later in the recovery process.

6. 1. Glaucoma causes increased intraocular pressure, which can damage the optic nerve. The drugs used to treat glaucoma would decrease intraocular pressure by decreasing aqueous humor in the anterior chamber. An anesthetic would not reduce the intraocular pressure.

7. 4. Elevating the head of the bed reduces intraocular pressure, as do applying cold compresses and dimming the lights in the room. Applying hot compresses or providing bright lights both would increase intraocular pressure. Pressure on the eye would also increase intraocular pressure.

8. 1. 3. 6. Conductive hearing loss is a correctable hearing loss that occurs in the middle and outer ear. It affects sound transmitted from the outer to inner ear. Causes include cerumen (earwax), otosclerosis, and middle ear disease. Sustained loud noise, Ménière's disease, and ototoxicity are causes of sensorineural loss.

9. 2. Severe pain and pain accompanied by complaints of nausea indicate an increase in intraocular pressure. These complaints need to be reported immediately to prevent damage to the eye. The physician may order drugs or take the client back to surgery. Turning on the operative side is to be avoided because it increases intraocular pressure.

10. 3. The client should wear an eye shield or glasses to protect the eye from injury or from rubbing the eye. Tylenol would be ordered for discomfort. Aspirin or drugs containing aspirin would not be used. The client should sleep on the unoperated side. The lifting restriction after surgery is 5 pounds or less. Lifting any more than 5 pounds would increase intraocular pressure.

11. 4. Eye medications are critical in the effective treatment of glaucoma. The client needs instruction that these are needed for the rest of his or her life. Decreasing salt and fluids will not decrease intraocular fluids. Normal reading or watching television will not affect glaucoma.

12. 1. 3. 6. Retinal detachment is the separation of the retina from the choroid layer, which is the blood supply. Clinical manifestations include photopsia (light flashes); floaters, "cobweb," "hairnet," or ring in the visual field; and loss of peripheral and central vision, all of which are painless.

13. 3. Placing an eye patch over the affected eye reduces eye movement. Occasionally bilateral patching may be needed. The size and the location of the retinal break may limit other activities, such as bending, coughing, and the Valsalva maneuver, to prevent further detachment and to promote drainage of fluid. Elevating the head of the bed prevents intraocular pressure.

14. 2. Emergency care following a chemical burn to the eye includes irrigating the eye immediately with a sterile saline or ocular solution. The irrigation should be continued for at least 10 minutes. After the irrigation, visual acuity will be assessed. Ointment or patching would retain the burn solution on the eye and cause further damage.

15. 1. Bright red drainage on the dressing may indicate hemorrhage and must be reported to the physician immediately. Although monitoring vital signs and the client's pain and recording the amount and color of the drainage are all important interventions, reporting the finding is the priority so emergency measures can be instituted.

16. 1 week

17. 2. Speak in a normal tone of voice to the client with impaired hearing. Avoid raising the voice because this does not improve communication. Face the client directly to facilitate lip reading. Moving closer to the better ear may be helpful, but avoid speaking into the impaired ear.

18. 2. Insects are killed before they can be removed unless a flashlight can coax them out. Mineral oil or diluted alcohol will suffocate the insect so that removal by forceps is possible. If the foreign object is vegetable matter it is not irrigated, because this would cause the object to expand and cause a worse impaction. Instilling an antibiotic or cortisone ointment into the affected ear may be done if an infection or inflammation is present.

19. 3. Ménière's disease is an inner ear disease with an unknown etiology that results in vertigo, tinnitus, and a sensorineural hearing loss. The goal of treatment is to preserve the remaining hearing. Nursing interventions include eliminating environmental noise, promoting a quiet environment, and restricting caffeine, nicotine, and alcohol. Prescribing a low-sodium diet has also been proven helpful in some clients.

20. 3. 4. 6. Clinical manifestations of Ménière's disease include sensorineural hearing loss, vertigo, and tinnitus.

21. 8th cranial nerve, VIII. The eighth cranial nerve is the acoustic nerve that is responsible for hearing. Damage to this cranial nerve results in a hearing loss. Streptomycin is an aminoglycoside anti-infective that may be ototoxic to the eighth cranial nerve.

22. 4. Glaucoma causes an increase in the intraocular pressure inside the eyeball. A cataract is the result of an opacity within the crystalline lens. A curvature of the cornea is an astigmatism. A separation of the retina is a detachment of the retina from its blood supply.

23. 3. Acute bacterial conjunctivitis ("pink eye") is very contagious. The priority nursing intervention is strict hand washing to prevent the spread of the infection to others. Then the client would be instructed not to share towels with others and not to rub or touch the eyes. Hot moist compresses may be used to soften adherent eye crusts.

24. 10–21 mm Hg

25. 2. There is only a 10% chance of a retinal detachment occurring in the good eye. Risk factors for retinal detachment include high myopia, aphakia, proliferative diabetic retinopathy, retinal lattice degeneration, and ocular trauma.

26. 4. Only a nurse can instruct, inform, and assess. Certified assistive personnel can reinforce teaching previously taught if it is within the scope of practice, such as hand washing.

27. 3. Presbyopia is a condition that causes farsightedness in the older adult client and leads to needing bifocals. A hordeolum is an infection of the sebaceous gland of the eyelid. Exophthalmos is an abnormal protrusion of the globe of the eye frequently seen in hyperthyroidism. Tinnitus is ringing in the ears and can be indicative of various medical conditions.

28. 3. In the Rinne test, the client should hear air conduction twice as long as bone conduction. It is normal for sound to be heard equally in both ears with the Weber test. The tympanic membrane should have a pearly gray appearance with the otoscope. It is also normal to be able to hear whispered words at 2 feet.

29. 4. A hordeolum is an infection of the sebaceous glands on an eyelid follicle. A chronic bacterial inflammation of the lid margin is a chalazion. Conjunctivitis is an infection of the conjunctiva.

30. 4. A licensed practical nurse may administer a drug intranasally. Assignments involving delegating, developing an activity plan, and performing an ear assessment should all be performed by a registered nurse.

REFERENCES

Daniels, R. (2010). *Delmar's manual of laboratory and diagnostic tests* (2nd ed.). Clifton Park, NY: Delmar Cengage Learning.

Daniels, R., & Nicoll, L. (2012). *Contemporary medical-surgical nursing.* Clifton Park, NY: Delmar Cengage Learning.

DeLaune, S.C., & Ladner, P. K. (2011). *Fundamentals of nursing: Standard and practice* (4th ed.). Clifton Park, NY: Delmar Cengage Learning.

Estes, M. (2010). *Health assessment and physical examination* (4th ed.). Clifton Park, NY: Delmar Cengage Learning.

Spratto, G. R., & Woods, A. L. (2012). *PDR nurse's drug handbook 2012.* Clifton Park, NY: Delmar Cengage Learning.

CHAPTER 3

RESPIRATORY DISORDERS

I. **ANATOMY AND PHYSIOLOGY**
  A. FUNCTIONS OF THE RESPIRATORY SYSTEM
    1. ENABLES OXYGEN TO DIFFUSE INTO THE BLOOD AND CARBON DIOXIDE TO DIFFUSE OUT OF THE BLOOD (RESPIRATION)
    2. PROVIDES FOR THE MECHANICAL MOVEMENT OF AIRFLOW BETWEEN THE ATMOSPHERE AND THE ALVEOLI (VENTILATION)
    3. INVOLVES THE MOVEMENT OF BLOOD INTO AND OUT OF THE CAPILLARY BEDS OF THE LUNGS TO ORGANS AND TISSUES (PERFUSION), DRIVEN BY THE CARDIOVASCULAR SYSTEM
  B. MAIN STRUCTURES
    1. UPPER AIRWAYS
    2. LOWER AIRWAYS
    3. ALVEOLI
    4. LUNGS
    5. DIAPHRAGM
    6. PULMONARY AND BRONCHIAL CIRCULATION (SEE FIGURE 3-1)
  C. UPPER RESPIRATORY TRACT
    1. NOSE AND SINUSES
      a. The nose is composed of bone (upper third) and cartilage (lower two-thirds).
      b. The nose contains two passages separated by a septum.
      c. Nasal passages (nostrils) contain hair follicles (vibrissae), a first defense to keep foreign particles or organisms from entering the lungs.
      d. Three major bony projections called turbinates, or conchae, are on the lateral walls of the nare.
      e. Turbinates increase the total surface area for filtering, heating, and humidifying inspired air before passing into the nasopharynx.
      f. The nose is the organ of smell (cranial nerve I: olfactory).

      g. Four air-filled paranasal sinuses provide resonance during speech.
    2. PHARYNX (THROAT)
      a. Serves as passageway for both respiratory and digestive tracts
      b. Located behind the oral and nasal cavities
      c. Divided into the nasopharynx, the oropharynx, and the laryngopharynx
      d. Nasopharynx lies above the soft palate and contains the adenoids and the distal opening of the eustachian tube.
      e. Oropharynx is located behind the mouth and below the nasopharynx and contains the tonsils.
      f. Laryngopharynx is located behind the larynx, or voice box, and above the trachea and contains the thyroid cartilage and the cricoid cartilage. It is the dividing point between the larynx and the esophagus.
    3. LARYNX
      a. The larynx contains the vocal cords.
      b. The opening between the vocal cords is the glottis.
      c. The glottis is important in coughing, the most fundamental defense mechanism of the lungs.
      d. The epiglottis is a leaf-shaped elastic structure attached to the top of the larynx and prevents food from entering the tracheobronchial tree.
      e. The epiglottis is the most important defense against aspiration.
  D. LOWER RESPIRATORY TRACT
    1. TRACHEA (WINDPIPE)
      a. Located anterior to the esophagus
      b. Extends from the lower border of the cricoid cartilage to the fourth or fifth thoracic vertebra
      c. Branches into the right and left mainstem bronchi at the carina

Figure 3-1 Structures of the respiratory tract

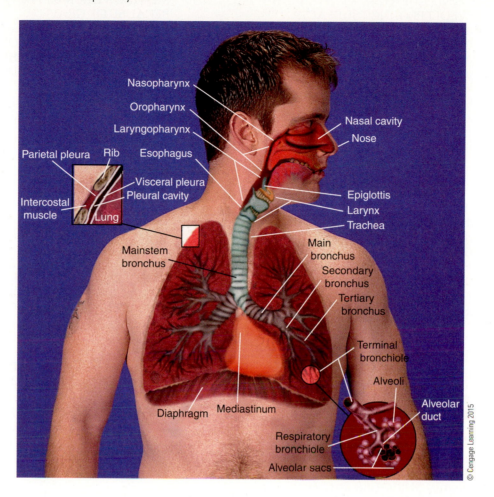

Nasopharynx
Oropharynx
Laryngopharynx
Parietal pleura Rib Esophagus
Visceral pleura
Pleural cavity
Intercostal muscle Lung
Mainstem bronchus
Diaphragm Mediastinum
Respiratory bronchiole
Alveolar sacs

Nasal cavity
Nose
Epiglottis
Larynx
Trachea
Main bronchus
Secondary bronchus
Tertiary bronchus
Terminal bronchiole
Alveoli
Alveolar duct

© Cengage Learning 2015

d. The carina is located at the sternal angle where the manubrium joins the sternum.

e. The trachea is composed of 6 to 10 C-shaped rings that are open in the back to not cause erosion or pressure on the esophagus.

2. MAINSTEM BRONCHI

a. The mainstem bronchi begins at the carina and resembles the trachea. The right bronchus is slightly wider, shorter, and more vertical than the left bronchus.

b. The right mainstem bronchus is more likely to be accidentally intubated and is where aspirated foreign objects are more likely to enter.

3. BRONCHI

a. The mainstem bronchi further divides into five secondary, or lobar, bronchi that enter each of the five lobes of the lung.

b. Each of the five lobar bronchi then branch into segmental and subsegmental divisions for each lobe.

4. BRONCHIOLES

a. The bronchioles, branching from the secondary bronchi, subdivide into smaller and smaller tubes as terminal and respiratory bronchioles.

b. Terminal and respiratory bronchioles are less than 1 mm in diameter, have no cartilage, and depend entirely on the elastic recoil of the lung for patency.

c. Terminal bronchioles contain no cilia and do not participate in gas exchange.

E. ALVEOLAR DUCTS AND ALVEOLI

1. ALVEOLAR DUCTS, WHICH LOOK LIKE A BUNCH OF GRAPES, BRANCH FROM THE RESPIRATORY BRONCHIOLES.

2. ALVEOLAR SACS ARISE FROM THESE DUCTS.

3. THE ALVEOLAR SACS CONTAIN CLUSTERS OF ALVEOLI, WHICH ARE THE MAIN UNITS OF GAS EXCHANGE.

4. THE LUNGS CONTAIN ABOUT 300 MILLION ALVEOLI, SURROUNDED BY PULMONARY CAPILLARIES.

5. IN A HEALTHY ADULT, THE SURFACE AREA FOR GAS EXCHANGE IN THE

LUNGS IS APPROXIMATE TO THE SIZE OF A TENNIS COURT.

6. THE ALVEOLI PRODUCE SURFACTANT, A LIPOPROTEIN THAT LINES THE ALVEOLI.

7. SURFACTANT REDUCES ALVEOLAR SURFACE TENSION AND PERMITS THE ALVEOLI TO EXPAND AS AIR FLOWS IN.

8. GAS EXCHANGE OCCURS IN THE RESPIRATORY BRONCHIOLES, ALVEOLAR DUCTS, AND THE ALVEOLI. THESE THREE STRUCTURES COMPOSE THE ACINUS.

F. LUNGS

1. THE LUNGS ARE SPONGE-LIKE, ELASTIC, CONE-SHAPED ORGANS LOCATED IN THE PLEURAL CAVITY IN THE THORAX.

2. THE APEX OF EACH LUNG EXTENDS ABOVE THE CLAVICLE; THE BASE OF EACH LUNG LIES JUST ABOVE THE DIAPHRAGM.

3. THREE LOBES AND 10 SEGMENTS ON THE RIGHT; 2 LOBES AND 8 SEGMENTS ON THE LEFT

4. THE PLEURA IS A CONTINUOUS SMOOTH MEMBRANE THAT TOTALLY ENCLOSES THE LUNG.

5. THE PARIETAL PLEURA LINES THE INSIDE OF THE THORACIC CAVITY AND THE UPPER SURFACE OF THE DIAPHRAGM.

6. THE VISCERAL PLEURA COVERS THE PULMONARY SURFACES, INCLUDING THE MAJOR FISSURES BETWEEN THE LOBES.

7. THE PLEURAL SPACE IS WHERE THE VISCERAL AND PARIETAL PLEURAE COME INTO CONTACT AND SLIDE OVER ONE ANOTHER.

8. A THIN FLUID (SURFACTANT) PRODUCED BY THE CELLS LINING THE PLEURA LUBRICATES THESE TWO SURFACES, ALLOWING THEM TO GLIDE SMOOTHLY AND PAINLESSLY DURING RESPIRATIONS.

9. THE CHEST WALL PROTECTS THE THORACIC CAVITY AND CONSISTS OF THE SKIN, RIBS, AND INTERCOSTAL MUSCLES (*INTERCOSTAL* MEANS "BETWEEN THE RIBS").

10. COMPLIANCE IS THE ABILITY OF THE LUNGS AND CHEST WALL TO EXPAND DURING INSPIRATION.

11. LUNG COMPLIANCE IS ENSURED BY ADEQUATE PRODUCTION OF SURFACTANT.

12. BOTH VENTILATION AND PERFUSION ARE GREATEST IN THE BASES OF THE LUNGS BECAUSE THE ALVEOLI IN THE BASES ARE MORE COMPLIANT (THEIR RESTING VOLUME IS LOW) AND BECAUSE OF GRAVITY.

13. THE GREATEST VOLUME OF PULMONARY BLOOD FLOW WILL NORMALLY OCCUR IN THE GRAVITY-DEPENDENT AREAS OF THE LUNG.

14. ELASTIC RECOIL ALLOWS THE LUNGS AND CHEST WALL TO RETURN TO THEIR RESTING STATE AFTER INSPIRATION.

15. THE PLEURAL SPACE NORMALLY HAS NEGATIVE PRESSURE.

G. DIAPHRAGM

1. THE DIAPHRAGM IS THE MAJOR MUSCLE OF INSPIRATION.

2. THE ACCESSORY MUSCLES OF RESPIRATION ARE THE SCALENE MUSCLES (ELEVATE THE FIRST TWO RIBS), STERNOCLEIDOMASTOID MUSCLES (RAISE THE STERNUM), TRAPEZIUS AND PECTORALIS MUSCLES (FIX THE SHOULDERS), AND VARIOUS BACK AND ABDOMINAL MUSCLES.

3. WHEN THE DIAPHRAGM CONTRACTS, IT MOVES DOWNWARD IN THE THORACIC CAVITY, CREATING A VACUUM THAT CAUSES AIR TO FLOW INTO THE LUNGS.

H. PULMONARY AND BRONCHIAL CIRCULATION

1. THERE ARE TWO SEPARATE SYSTEMS OF BLOOD FLOW THROUGH THE LUNGS.

2. BRONCHIAL ARTERIES ARISE FROM THE THORACIC AORTA AND ARE PART OF THE SYSTEMIC CIRCULATION. THEY CARRY BLOOD TO MEET THE METABOLIC DEMANDS OF THE LUNGS.

3. THE PULMONARY CIRCULATION IS COMPOSED OF A HIGHLY VASCULAR CAPILLARY NETWORK.

4. OXYGEN-DEPLETED BLOOD TRAVELS FROM THE RIGHT VENTRICLE OF THE HEART INTO THE PULMONARY ARTERY, WHICH BRANCHES INTO ARTERIOLES THAT FORM THE CAPILLARY NETWORKS.

5. THE CAPILLARIES ARE ENMESHED AROUND THE ALVEOLI WHERE GAS IS EXCHANGED.

6. EXTERNAL RESPIRATION INVOLVES PULMONARY CAPILLARIES (GAS EXCHANGE BETWEEN THE AIR IN THE ALVEOLI AND BLOOD IN THE PULMONARY CAPILLARIES).

7. FRESHLY OXYGENATED BLOOD TRAVELS THROUGH THE VENULES TO THE PULMONARY VEIN AND ON TO THE LEFT ATRIUM, WHERE IT IS

PUMPED THROUGHOUT THE SYSTEMIC CIRCULATION.

8. INTERNAL RESPIRATION INVOLVES SYSTEMIC CAPILLARIES (GAS EXCHANGE BETWEEN TISSUE CELLS AND BLOOD IN THE SYSTEMIC CAPILLARIES).

9. BODY POSITION HAS A SIGNIFICANT EFFECT ON THE DISTRIBUTION OF PULMONARY BLOOD FLOW.

II. **ASSESSMENT**
 A. HEALTH HISTORY
 1. MEDICAL AND FAMILY HISTORY
 2. AGE (RELATED TO CHANGES IN LUNG CAPACITY AND RESPIRATORY FUNCTION)
 3. SMOKING HISTORY (THE MOST SIGNIFICANT CONTRIBUTING FACTOR IN LUNG DISEASE; PACK-YEARS = NUMBER OF PACKS PER DAY TIMES NUMBER OF YEARS SMOKED)
 4. MEDICATION USE
 5. ALLERGIES
 6. TRAVEL AND AREA OF RESIDENCE
 7. DIET HISTORY
 8. HISTORY OF PREVIOUS UPPER RESPIRATORY INFECTIONS
 9. OCCUPATIONS HISTORY AND SOCIOECONOMIC STATUS
 10. CURRENT HEALTH PROBLEMS
 11. COUGH
 12. SPUTUM PRODUCTION (COLOR, CONSISTENCY, ODOR, AND AMOUNT OF SPUTUM VARY WITH DIFFERENT PULMONARY DISORDERS)
 13. CHEST PAIN
 14. DYSPNEA
 15. RESTLESSNESS
 16. IRRITABILITY
 17. CONFUSION
 18. HOARSENESS
 19. DYSRHYTHMIAS
 B. PHYSICAL EXAMINATION
 1. INSPECTION
 a. Note the anterior and posterior thorax with the client sitting.
 b. Symmetry of movement of the thorax
 c. Rate, depth, regularity, and effort of breathing
 d. Cyanosis or pallor
 e. Use of accessory muscles
 f. Presence of cough (nature and character of sputum)
 g. Duration of inspiratory and expiratory phases (inspiratory/expiratory ratio is normally 1:2)
 h. Clubbing of fingers (angle of nail bed greater than 160 degrees; distal phalangeal depth greater than interphalangeal depth; softening of nail beds)
 2. PALPATION
 a. Symmetry of respiratory movement (excursion)
 b. Tactile fremitus (vibration)
 c. Tenderness
 d. Detect painful areas or masses.
 e. Crepitus (subcutaneous emphysema)
 3. PERCUSSION
 a. Determines density of underlying structures
 b. Performed over the intercostals spaces
 c. Percussion penetrates only 2–3 inches. Deeper lesions are not detected by this technique.
 d. Diaphragmatic excursion—normal 1–2 inches (3–5 cm)
 e. Diaphragm is normally higher on the right because of the liver.
 f. Percuss the anterior and posterior chest wall (see Table 3-1).

Table 3-1 Percussion Sounds

Note	Pitch	Intensity	Quality	Duration	Comments
Resonance	Low	Moderate to loud	Hollow	Long	Normal lung tissue
Hyperresonance	Higher than resonance	Very loud	Booming	Longer than resonance	Trapped air; common findings over the lung in the presence of emphysema or asthma
Flat	High	Soft	Extreme dullness	Short	Normal finding over the sternum. Flatness percussed over the lung fields may indicate pleural effusion.
Dull	Medium	Medium	Thud-like	Medium	Common finding over the liver and kidneys. Dullness can be found over an atelectatic lung or consolidation.
Tympany	High	Loud	Musical, drum like	Short	Common findings over air pockets, such as the abdomen. May be found over a large pneumothorax

Table 3-2 Characteristics of Adventitious Breath Sounds

Breath Sound	Respiratory Phase	Timing	Description	Clear with Cough	Etiology	Conditions
Fine crackle	Predominantly inspiration	Discontinuous	Dry, high-pitched crackling and popping of short duration: sounds like hair rolled between fingers when held near ears	Possibly	Air passing through moisture in small airways that suddenly reinflate	Chronic obstructive pulmonary disease (COPD), congestive heart failure (CHF), pneumonia, pulmonary fibrosis, atelectasis
Coarse crackle	Predominantly inspiration	Discontinuous	Moist, low-pitched crackling and gurgling of long duration	Possibly	Air passing through moisture in large airways that suddenly reinflate	Pneumonia, pulmonary edema, bronchitis, atelectasis
Sonorous wheeze	Predominantly expiration	Continuous	Low-pitched snoring	Possibly	Narrowing of large airways or obstruction of bronchus	Asthma, bronchitis, airway edema, tumor, bronchiolar spasm, foreign body obstruction
Sibilant wheeze	Predominantly expiration	Continuous	High-pitched and musical	Possibly	Narrowing of large airways or obstruction of bronchus	Asthma, chronic bronchitis, emphysema, tumor, foreign body obstruction
Pleural friction rub	Inspiration and expiration	Continuous	Creaking, grating	Possibly	Inflamed parietal and visceral pleura; can occasionally be felt on thoracic wall as two pieces of dry leather rubbing against each other	Pleurisy, tuberculosis, pulmonary infarction, pneumonia, lung abscess
Stridor	Predominantly inspiration	Continuous	Crowing	Never	Partial obstruction of the larynx, trachea	Croup, foreign body obstruction, large airway tumor

© Cengage Learning 2015

4. AUSCULTATION
   a. Listen for normal breath sounds, adventitious sounds, and voice sounds.
   b. Instruct the client to breathe slowly and deeply through an open mouth.
   c. Listen to full respiratory cycle and compare bilaterally.
   d. Assess the client for possible hyperventilation during the assessment process (see Table 3-2).
5. AGING
   a. Affects the mechanical aspects of ventilation by decreasing chest wall compliance and elastic recoil of the lungs
   b. Changes in these elastic properties reduce ventilatory reserve.
   c. Aging causes the PaO_2 to decrease but does not affect the $PaCO_2$.

III. RADIOGRAPHIC AND SCANNING STUDIES
   A. CHEST X-RAY
      1. DESCRIPTION
         a. Gives information about the pulmonary and cardiac systems
         b. Evaluates the lung fields, clavicle and ribs, cardiac border, mediastinum, diaphragm, and the thoracic spine
         c. Also evaluates air trapping, consolidation, cavity formation, or presence of tumors
      2. PREPROCEDURE
         a. Instruct the client on the purpose of the procedure.
         b. Location of where the x-ray will be taken
         c. Procedure takes approximately 15 minutes.
         d. No restrictions on food, fluid, or medication prior to the procedure
         e. No sedation or anesthetic
         f. Views may be taken from several positions.
         g. Remove metal objects from the area of x-ray.
         h. Lead apron for men and women of childbearing age
         i. Instruct the client to take and hold his breath during the moment of x-ray.

3. PROCEDURE POSITIONS
   a. Anterior posterior (AP): x-ray beam passes the front to the back.
   b. Posterior anterior (PA): x-ray beam passes the back to the front.
   c. Lateral: position the client on the side, usually the left side against the film and arms raised over the head.
   d. Oblique: angle of the x-ray is directed between the PA and lateral views; used to evaluate pulmonary masses and infiltrates, especially of the mediastinum.
   e. Lateral decubitus: directs x-ray beam parallel to the floor with the client in a side-lying, supine, or prone position; used to identify small amounts of pleural effusion or subpulmonic effusion.
   f. Lordotic: the client leans backward against the x-ray film with the abdomen protruding; provides better visualization of the apices of the lungs, the area most commonly involved in pulmonary tuberculosis.
   g. Portable chest x-ray: performed at the client's bedside in more acute or critical situations; useful to detect atelectasis, effusions, pneumonia, and edema and to verify line or tube placement.
4. POSTPROCEDURE
   a. Return personal belongings and help the client dress if needed.
   b. For portable x-rays, assist the client back to a comfortable position and check any tubes, intravenous lines, or wires for proper placement and functioning if they were disturbed during the x-ray.
B. CHEST TOMOGRAPHY
   1. DESCRIPTION
      a. Tomography provides a two-dimensional view of tissue a few millimeters thick.
      b. Chest tomography provides more clarity in viewing lesions identified by plain x-ray.
      c. This procedure exposes the client to greater radiation than plain radiographs and is used only when absolutely necessary.
      d. Techniques such as computerized tomography (CT) of the chest have largely replaced this technique.
   2. PREPROCEDURE
      a. Instruct the client in positioning and that he needs to remain still during the study.
      b. Metal objects such as jewelry or clothing fasteners must be removed.
   3. PROCEDURE
      a. Client is positioned on the x-ray table in supine, side-lying, or prone position.

   b. X-ray machine moves above in circular or figure-eight motion.
   c. Client must remain very still but breathe in a normal pattern.
4. POSTPROCEDURE
   a. Same as chest x-ray.
C. COMPUTERIZED TOMOGRAPHY (CT) OR COMPUTERIZED AXIAL TOMOGRAPHY (CAT) SCAN
   1. DESCRIPTION
      a. A noninvasive procedure that uses tomographic roentgenography (x-ray) combined with a special scanning machine
      b. Can detect pulmonary densities, tumors, and lesions
      c. Provides consecutive cross-sectional "slices" or views of the thorax and produces a three-dimensional assessment of the lungs and the thorax
   2. PREPROCEDURE
      a. Inform the client about the procedure and its purpose.
      b. Determine sensitivity to the contrast medium.
      c. Client must be able to remain still during the procedure.
      d. Metallic objects must be removed.
      e. Inform the client that the contrast media (IV) may cause flushing, nausea, or sweating.
      f. Foods and fluids are withheld 4 hours prior to the procedure because of possible nausea.
      g. Procedure may take up to 2 hours.
      h. Have the client empty the bladder before the procedure.
   3. PROCEDURE
      a. Client is placed supine on a flat table within the scanning machine.
      b. Intravenous (IV) access is started, if not already available.
      c. Client is instructed to remain very still.
   4. POSTPROCEDURE
      a. Return the client's clothing and personal items.
      b. Encourage fluid intake to facilitate elimination of contrast medium.
      c. Client may resume diet.
D. LUNG SCAN (VENTILATION/PERFUSION; VQ SCAN)
   1. DESCRIPTION
      a. Identifies areas of the lung being ventilated and the distribution of pulmonary blood
      b. Used primarily to diagnose a pulmonary embolism
   2. PREPROCEDURE
      a. Inform the client about the procedure.
   3. PROCEDURE
      a. Involves injection of a radionuclide and several position changes

b. May also include inhalation of a radioactive gas or a radioaerosol with additional lung scans

4. POSTPROCEDURE

a. Inform the client that the radioactive substance will clear from the body in approximately 8 hours.

E. POSITRON-EMISSION TOMOGRAPHY (PET) SCAN

1. DESCRIPTION

a. Positron emission tomography (PET) is a nuclear study.

b. Scanning is done over time to allow for repeated or sequencing of three-dimensional images.

c. Useful for studying ventilation-perfusion relationships in the lung

2. PREPROCEDURE

a. Client must be able to remain still during the procedure.

b. Client must abstain from alcohol, tobacco, or caffeine for at least 24 hours prior to the test.

c. Client must avoid tranquilizers that alter mentation or insulin that alters glucose metabolism.

d. Inform client that the test takes 60–120 minutes to complete.

3. PROCEDURE

a. Client is placed on the examining table in supine position.

b. Chest is scanned 45 minutes after intravenous administration of the radionuclide.

c. Scanning is done for 1 hour.

4. POSTPROCEDURE

a. Assume standing position slowly to avoid postural hypotension.

b. Advise that radioactive substance is eliminated from the body within 6–24 hours.

c. Increase fluid intake to encourage elimination from the body.

F. FLUOROSCOPY

1. DESCRIPTION

a. These studies are done to evaluate movement of the chest and diaphragm during breathing and coughing.

b. They provide information about bronchiolar obstruction, loss of elasticity, or paralysis of the diaphragm.

c. May also be used in guidance of needle insertion for biopsy or removal of fluid during thoracentesis

2. PREPROCEDURE

a. Inform the client about the procedure.

b. If used in combination with contrasts or dyes, check for allergies.

3. PROCEDURE

a. Process is similar to conventional x-ray but fluoroscopy delivers much larger doses of radiation.

b. Newer equipment uses image intensifiers and reduces the amount of radiation exposure.

c. Provide tissues to the client for coughing.

4. POSTPROCEDURE

a. Same as conventional x-ray

IV. **ENDOSCOPIC STUDIES**

A. PURPOSE: INVASIVE TECHNIQUES PERFORMED TO VISUALIZE PULMONARY STRUCTURES AND OBTAIN TISSUE SPECIMENS

B. BRONCHOSCOPY

1. DESCRIPTION

a. Examination of tracheobronchial tree using a bronchoscope

b. May be performed in an operating room, a procedure room, radiology, or intensive care

c. To assess airway anatomy for tumors, obstruction, and atelectasis

d. To assist in diagnosis of infection or cancer and obtain a biopsy (diagnostic bronchoscopy)

e. To remove thick secretions, mucus plugs, or foreign bodies (therapeutic bronchoscopy)

2. PREPROCEDURE

a. Assess client stability.

b. Nothing by mouth (NPO) for several hours before the procedure (stop enteral feedings)

c. Assess for allergies to iodine, local anesthetics, or premedication.

d. Topical anesthetic administration into the oropharynx if no endotracheal tube or trach available

e. Remove dentures or bridges/plates.

3. PROCEDURE

a. A flexible fiberoptic bronchoscope is inserted through the mouth, nose, endotracheal tube, or tracheostomy tube.

b. Client is to be monitored by pulse oximetry.

4. POSTPROCEDURE

a. Monitor vital signs.

b. Monitor for hemoptysis.

c. Nothing by mouth (NPO) until gag reflex returns

d. Discourage smoking, coughing, or talking for several hours.

C. LARYNGOSCOPY

1. DESCRIPTION

a. Direct: to detect and remove lesions or foreign bodies in the larynx or to diagnose cancer with tissue biopsy. A fiberoptic laryngoscope is used.

b. Indirect: to assess the function of the vocal cords and obtain tissue biopsy. Observations are made of the other structures using a laryngeal mirror and light source.

2. PREPROCEDURE
   a. Written consent is required.
   b. Nothing by mouth for several hours before the test
   c. Assess for allergies to iodine, contrast media, or local anesthetics.
   d. Pretest drugs such as atropine and diazepam (Valium) are used to reduce secretions and anxiety.
   e. For indirect procedure, position the client in sitting position.
3. PROCEDURE
   a. Monitor for respirator problems and provide client reassurance.
   b. Local anesthetic is used in the mouth and throat.
   c. Monitor for vomiting and aspiration.
4. POSTPROCEDURE
   a. Monitor and assess vital signs and monitor for bleeding.
   b. Nothing by mouth until gag reflex returns
   c. Encourage coughing and fluid intake after gag reflex returns.
   d. Throat lozenges or gargles may help relieve sore throat.

D. MEDIASTINOSCOPY
   1. DESCRIPTION
      a. Purpose is to inspect and remove samples for biopsy of lymph nodes that drain the lung.
      b. Detects metastasis of lung cancer
      c. Used to obtain tissue for biopsy for diagnosis of tuberculosis or sarcoidosis
   2. PREPROCEDURE
      a. Written consent is required
      b. Inform the client on the reason for the procedure and purpose.
   3. PROCEDURE
      a. Procedure is done in the operating room with the client given local or general anesthetic.
      b. A suprasternal incision is used.
   4. POSTPROCEDURE
      a. Assess the client for bleeding, pneumothorax, and vocal cord paralysis.
      b. Assess the client for pain, and administer analgesics as ordered.

V. **INVASIVE PROCEDURES**
   A. THORACENTESIS
      1. DESCRIPTION: INVOLVES NEEDLE ASPIRATION OF PLEURAL FLUID OR AIR FROM THE PLEURAL SPACE FOR DIAGNOSTIC AND THERAPEUTIC PURPOSES
      2. PREPROCEDURE
         a. Requires written consent
         b. Position the client sitting on the side of the bed with the feet on a stool, leaning over the bedside table.
         c. Procure all of the supplies and equipment, including collections bottles.
      3. PROCEDURE
         a. Needle aspiration is performed by the physician using sterile technique.
         b. Assist with equipment.
         c. Stabilize and support the client.
         d. No more than 1200 ml should be removed at one time.
      4. POSTPROCEDURE
         a. Apply pressure to the puncture site.
         b. Use semi-Fowler's position or puncture site up.
         c. Monitor for shock, pneumothorax, respiratory arrest, subcutaneous emphysema.
         d. Assess breath sounds.
         e. Determine if the physician wants a follow-up chest x-ray.

   B. LUNG BIOPSY
      1. DESCRIPTION
         a. An invasive technique involving entering the lung or pleura to obtain tissue for analysis
         b. Used to make a definite diagnosis regarding the type of malignancy, infection, inflammation, or other type of lung disease
      2. PREPROCEDURE
         a. Written consent is required.
         b. Inform the client on the type of procedure.
         c. Anxiety is increased with use of word "biopsy" because of its association with cancer.
      3. PROCEDURE
         a. Transbronchial biopsy (TBB) and transbronchial needle aspiration (TBNA) are both performed in conjunction with bronchoscopy.
         b. Transthoracic needle aspiration (percutaneous approach for areas not accessible by bronchoscopy) using local anesthetic
         c. Open lung biopsy (in the operating room)
      4. POSTPROCEDURE
         a. Assessment of lung sounds, oxygenation status, and signs of respiratory distress
         b. Report clinical manifestations promptly.
         c. Monitor for hemoptysis or frank bleeding from vascular or lung trauma during the procedure.
         d. Postoperative care for open lung biopsy
         e. May need aspiration; assess the site for bleeding, apply pressure dressing.
         f. Chest tube management for open lung biopsy

C. THORACOTOMY
1. DESCRIPTION
   a. A surgical intervention that disrupts the negative pressure of the chest, requiring controlled ventilation throughout the procedure to maintain ventilation and pulmonary circulation
   b. Generally done for tumor resection, organ repair, or transplant
2. PREPROCEDURE
   a. Baseline labs (hematologic studies and arterial blood gas analysis)
   b. Chest x-ray, electrocardiogram, pulmonary function studies, lung scan
   c. Written surgical consent is required.
3. PROCEDURE
   a. General anesthesia
   b. Operating room procedure
4. POSTPROCEDURE
   a. Most common complications
      1) Hemorrhage
      2) Respiratory failure
      3) Wound infection
      4) Cardiac abnormalities
   b. Nursing interventions
      1) Instruct the client on what to expect postoperatively.
      2) Ventilator support
      3) Suctioning
      4) Drugs for pain and anxiety
      5) Chest tubes
   c. After extubation
      1) Coughing and deep breathing with splinting
      2) Fowler's position

3) Analgesics for comfort
4) Fluids (intravenous and oral)
5) Monitor labs (arterial blood gas)
6) Vital signs
7) Ambulation

VI. NONINVASIVE PROCEDURES
A. PULSE OXIMETRY
1. DESCRIPTION
   a. Indicates hemoglobin saturation using an infrared light and a sensor
   b. Recorded as SaO_2 or SpO_2, the expected reading for a healthy client is 95–100%. Pulse oximetry has poor accuracy at lower readings.
   c. It is meant to help alert the nurse to desaturation before clinical signs occur.
   d. Readings less than 91% require immediate assessment and action.
   e. Arterial blood gas analysis is required for accurate clinical determination of oxygenation status.
2. PREPROCEDURE
   a. Inform the client about the procedure.
3. PROCEDURE
   a. Affected by movement, hypothermia, decreased hemoglobin, edema, peripheral blood flow, and positioning of the device
4. POSTPROCEDURE
   a. Reassure the client that he is stable and that continuous monitoring is no longer necessary.
B. PULMONARY FUNCTION TESTING (SPIROMETRY) (SEE TABLE 3-3)

Table 3-3 Pulmonary Functions Tests

Test	Purpose
Forced vital capacity (FVC) Records the maximal amount of air that can be exhaled as quickly as possible after maximal inspiration	Gives indication of respiratory muscle strength and ventilatory reserve Often reduced in obstructive disease because of air trapping Often reduced in restrictive disease
Forced expiratory volume in 1 second (FEV_1) Records the maximal amount of air that can be exhaled in the first second of expiration	Effort dependent Declines normally with age Reduced in certain obstructive and restrictive disorders
FEV_1/FVC The ratio of expiratory volume in 1 second to FVC	Ratio provides a more sensitive indication of obstruction to airflow. Ratio is normal or increased in restrictive disease. Ratio is decreased in obstructive pulmonary disease (a hallmark).
Functional residual capacity (FRC) The amount of air remaining in the lungs after normal expiration Requires use of the helium dilution technique	Increased FRC indicates hyperinflation of air trapping (e.g., COPD). FRC is normal or decreased in restrictive pulmonary diseases.
Total lung capacity (TLC) The amount of air in the lungs at the end of maximal inhalation	Increased with air trapping associated with obstructive pulmonary disease Decreased in restrictive disease
Residual volume (RV) The amount of air remaining in the lungs at the end of a full, forced exhalation	Increased in obstructive pulmonary disease such as emphysema

1. DESCRIPTION
   a. Noninvasive technique used to determine lung volumes, ventilatory function, airway resistance, and distribution of gases
   b. Spirometry measures both volume and flow rate during forced expiration.
   c. May be useful in screening for pulmonary disease, guiding treatment changes, preoperative evaluation of pulmonary status, and determining breathlessness to differentiate pulmonary from cardiac dysfunction
2. PREPROCEDURE
   a. Inform the client on the purpose and value of the test.
   b. Usually withhold bronchodilators for 6 to 8 hours before the test.
3. PROCEDURE
   a. Can be done in the office or at the bedside
   b. Requires the client to breathe through the mouth (a nose clip is sometimes used to prevent air from escaping)
4. POSTPROCEDURE
   a. Note if any drugs were used during the test (e.g., bronchodilators) and alter the medication schedule as indicated.
   b. Observe the client for increased dyspnea or bronchospasm after the testing.

VII. LABORATORY TESTS
A. SPUTUM CULTURE
1. DESCRIPTION
   a. Identification of pathogenic organisms or abnormal cells
   b. First morning specimen preferred
2. PREPROCEDURE
   a. Provide sputum container (sterile) and teach use.
3. PROCEDURE
   a. Sputum is produced from a cough (from the lungs).
   b. May be obtained by expectoration or tracheal suctioning
   c. Approximately 15 ml is required.
   d. Always obtain a specimen before initiating antibiotic therapy.
   e. If suctioning is used to obtain a specimen, do not use saline during suctioning.
4. POSTPROCEDURE
   a. Label the container.
   b. Send to the lab.
B. ARTERIAL BLOOD GASES (ABGS) (SEE TABLE 3-4)
1. DESCRIPTION
   a. Arterial blood gas (ABG) analysis is used to determine pH and oxygen and carbon dioxide concentrations.

Table 3-4 Arterial Blood Gases: Normal Values

Parameter	ABGs
pH	7.35–7.45
PaO_2	80–100 mm Hg
$PaCO_2$	35–45 mm Hg
HCO_3	22–26 mEq/L
BE (base excess)	−2 to +2 mEq/L
SaO_2 (saturation of hgb)	> 95%

© Cengage Learning 2015

2. PREPROCEDURE
   a. Inform the client on the procedure.
   b. Assess the circulation of radial arterial flow using Allen's test.
   c. Ask the client to make a fist.
   d. Compress the ulnar and radial arteries.
   e. Ask the client to open the hand.
   f. Release the ulnar artery.
   g. Assess return of arterial blood flow.
   h. Repeat with release on the radial artery.
3. PROCEDURE
   a. If arterial line, assess patency, use sterile technique, aspirate and discard, withdraw the specimen, flush the line.
   b. If arterial artery puncture, use sterile technique.
4. POSTPROCEDURE
   a. Hold pressure over the radial arterial puncture for 5–15 minutes (depends on coagulation status).
   b. Be sure there are no air bubbles in the specimen and air is cleared.
   c. Label.
   d. Transport on ice and send immediately to the lab.
C. MANTOUX TEST
1. DESCRIPTION
   a. A skin test for tuberculosis (TB)
   b. A positive result only indicates the client was exposed to TB; it is not diagnostic for active TB.
2. PREPROCEDURE
   a. Ask about previous sensitivity to the test.
3. PROCEDURE
   a. Subdermal injection on the upper 1/3 inner surface of the forearm
   b. 0.1 ml of purified protein derivative (PPD) given subdermal, needle bevel up
4. POSTPROCEDURE
   a. Mark the spot with an ink pen.
   b. Read in 48–72 hours.
   c. Measure induration: if 10 mm or greater, it is a positive reading.

VIII. NURSING DIAGNOSIS
A. IMPAIRED GAS EXCHANGE
B. INEFFECTIVE BREATHING PATTERN

C. INEFFECTIVE AIRWAY CLEARANCE
D. ANXIETY
E. IMBALANCED NUTRITION: LESS THAN BODY REQUIREMENTS
F. ACTIVITY INTOLERANCE

Nursing Diagnoses: Definitions and Classification 2012–2014. Copyright © 2012, 1994–2012 by NANDA International. Used by arrangement with John Wiley & Sons Limited.

IX. PULMONARY THERAPIES/INTERVENTIONS
A. POSITIONING
   1. DESCRIPTION: EFFECTIVE POSITIONING PROMOTES BETTER VENTILATION AND MAY RELIEVE DYSPNEA.
   2. PREPROCEDURE
     a. Instruct the client on effective positioning.
   3. PROCEDURE
     a. If on bed rest, maintain in semi-Fowler's or high semi-Fowler's.
     b. Ambulatory clients should sit on the edge of the bed with their feet on the floor and two to three pillows on the overbed table or with clients resting elbows on the overbed table.
     c. If in a chair, the client should sit with feet on the floor shoulder-width apart and elbows supported on the knees to relax the upper body. Relax arms and hands.
     d. If standing, the client should position the back and hips against the wall with feet 12 inches from the wall, lean back, relax the shoulders, and bend slightly forward.
   4. POSTPROCEDURE
     a. Monitor for improvement in dyspnea.
B. INCENTIVE SPIROMETRY
   1. DESCRIPTION
     a. Device that provides assistive deep breathing exercises
     b. Should not replace other deep breathing and coughing interventions
     c. Generally used postoperatively
   2. PREPROCEDURE
     a. Obtain the device.
     b. Instruct the client on the proper use of the spirometry.
     c. Set the target volume as appropriate to the client and condition.
   3. PROCEDURE
     a. Client must seal the mouth around the mouthpiece.
     b. Inhale slowly and deeply to raise the cylinder in the column and ball in the chamber.
     c. Exhale slowly through pursed lips.
     d. Repeat the process, 10 repetitions, every 3–4 hours.

   4. POSTPROCEDURE
     a. Evaluate respiratory status.
     b. Document effort and response.
C. BREATHING TECHNIQUES
   1. DESCRIPTION
     a. Techniques to assist the client with better ventilation
     b. Pursed-lip breathing is recommended during any physical activity.
   2. PREPROCEDURE
     a. Inform the client on the techniques.
     b. Remind the client to always inhale before beginning the activity and exhale while performing the activity.
     c. Remind the client to not hold his breath during the activity.
     d. Provide tissues for coughing.
   3. PROCEDURE
     a. Pursed-lip breathing: breathe in through the nose and out through pursed lips (as if to whistle). Do not allow cheeks to puff. Spend at least twice the amount of time with exhalation as it takes to inhale. Use abdominal muscles to squeeze out as much air as possible with expiration.
     b. Diaphragmatic or abdominal breathing: the client consciously attempts to increase diaphragmatic movement by using the diaphragm and abdominal muscles. Most effective position is having the client sitting on the edge of the bed or chair with the feet on the floor. The client should bend slightly forward with the head tilted forward or take in gentle breath through the nose and mouth, then a deep breath, and hold to count of 5 and exhale. To learn the technique the client can:
       1) Lie on the back with the knees bent.
       2) Place the hands or a book on the abdomen.
       3) Begin breathing from the abdomen, keeping the chest still.
       4) Correct breathing technique allows hands or book on the abdomen to rise and fall with breaths.
     c. Controlled cough techniques: use diaphragmatic breathing position and technique. After three to five deep breaths, with pursed-lip technique, the client is to bend forward slowly while producing two or three strong coughs from the same breath. Pillow may be hugged tightly against the chest to provide chest support and reduce pain. Repeat the coughing procedure at least twice. Use controlled cough on arising early in the morning, before meals, and

before bedtime to expectorate accumulated mucus.

   4. POSTPROCEDURE
      a. Assess respiratory status.
      b. Reinforce proper use of technique.
      c. Provide for rest.

D. CHEST TUBES
   1. DESCRIPTION
      a. Closed drainage system to remove fluid or air, or both, from the pleural space
      b. Reestablish normal negative pressure in the pleural space.
      c. Promote reexpansion of the lungs.
      d. There are three possible chambers:
         1) Suction control
         2) Water seal chamber
         3) Drainage collection
      e. Commercial one-piece devices are available and are used more commonly than the two-bottle or three-bottle systems.
   2. PREPROCEDURE
      a. Written consent is required.
      b. Inform the client about the procedure.
   3. PROCEDURE
      a. May be done at the bedside or in the operating room
      b. Aseptic procedure
      c. Local anesthetic used for stab wound insertion sites
      d. Chest tube placed high for evacuation of air
      e. Chest tube placed low for evacuation of fluid or blood
   4. POSTPROCEDURE
      a. Check for bubbling and fluctuation.
      b. Turn the client, ask to cough and deep breathe.
      c. Note and document the initial amount and character of the drainage.
      d. Assess the tubing; should be coiled on the bed with no kinks or dependent loops.
      e. Keep collection chamber below the level of the heart.
      f. Maintain the water seal.
      g. Do not strip tubes; avoid milking tubes.
      h. X-ray confirmation of placement
      i. Attach to closed system for collection.
      j. Cover the site with occlusive dressing.
      k. Mark the collection container with the date and time to monitor drainage.
      l. Assess for subcutaneous emphysema around the insertion site.
      m. Monitor arterial blood gases.
      n. Monitor for shock.
      o. Respiratory assessment
      p. Do not clamp tubing (except briefly if the collection container is to be changed).
      q. Tape all connections.
      r. Be prepared for emergencies.
         1) If chest tube is accidentally pulled out, immediately cover the site with occlusive (Vaseline gauze) dressing.
         2) If collection chamber is damaged, immediately insert the end of the chest tube into sterile water until the system can be replaced.
         3) If there is continuous bubbling, assess for leaks in the system.

E. MECHANICAL VENTILATION (SEE TABLE 3-5)
   1. DESCRIPTION
      a. There are three types of ventilators used to deliver oxygen and artificial ventilation.
      b. A client who has been intubated will be attached to a ventilator using an endotracheal tube inserted through the nose or mouth or a tracheostomy tube.
      c. There are several modes of mechanical ventilation. These will be prescribed by the physician based on the client's situation (see Table 3-6).
   2. PREPROCEDURE
      a. Respiratory distress or failure is determined.
      b. Sedation is provided.
      c. Client is informed of the need for ventilator support.
      d. Client is intubated.

Table 3-5 Types of Ventilators

Volume cycled	Delivers preset tidal volume, independent of airway resistance or lung compliance Safety valve is set to terminate breath when peak inspiratory pressures are dangerous.
Pressure cycled	Delivers inspiratory volume until a preset pressure is reached This allows for varying tidal volumes to be delivered based on airway resistance. Normal lung compliance is required to use this mode.
Negative pressure	These ventilators generate subatmospheric pressure to the thorax and trunk to initiate respiration and do not require intubation. The "iron lung" is an example. Current resurgence of this model has potential for long-term home use. Other examples are the chest cuirass shell and poncho chest shell.

Table 3-6 Modes of Mechanical Ventilation

Mode	Delivery	Use	Considerations
Controlled mechanical ventilation (CMV)	Preset tidal volume Preset rate Ignores the client's own drive	Central nervous system (CNS) dysfunction Drug-induced paralysis or sedation Severe chest trauma (cannot use negative-pressure-driven effort)	Simple Least frequently used
Assist-control ventilation (ACV)	Preset tidal volume for every breath. Client initiates breath. Minimum rate preset (triggered if the client does not initiate)	Sensitivity is set to avoid hyperventilation if the client increases respiratory rate.	Risk of hyperventilation
Synchronized intermittent mandatory ventilation (SIMV)	Preset tidal volume. Client initiates breath. Machine assists for minimal preset rate.	Client can breathe spontaneously above the preset rate (own tidal volume).	Frequently used mode Used during weaning
Positive-end expiratory pressure (PEEP)	Pressures range from 2.5–10 cm H_2O pressure.	Frequently used in conjunction with mechanical ventilation to help keep alveoli and small airways open	Causes increased intrathoracic pressure, which may decrease venous return and cardiac output May potentiate hypotension and shock May cause pneumothorax if > 10 cm H_2O or decreased lung compliance
Pressure support ventilation (PSV)	Supports or augments the client's spontaneous inspiration at a preselected pressure level	Client controls inspiratory time and flow rate, expiratory time, frequency, tidal volume, and minute ventilation	May be used in combination with SIMV to improve tolerance and decrease work of breathing May be used alone for clients ready to attempt weaning
High-frequency ventilation	Delivers small tidal volumes at high rates using jet ventilation and high-frequency oscillation modes Delivers low tidal volume and high minute ventilation	Most frequently used in burn intensive care units and for clients with major airway disruption	Results in lower airway and intrathoracic pressures and may reduce barotraumas and circulatory depression
Inverse ratio ventilation (IRV)	Inspiratory phase prolonged Expiratory phase shortened	Client usually requires sedation to tolerate unusual breathing pattern.	Normal I/E = 1: 2–4 Improves alveolar function at lower levels of PEEP

© Cengage Learning 2015

3. PROCEDURE
   a. Endotracheal tube is passed.
   b. Placement is checked using auscultation, CO_2 detector, and chest x-ray.
4. POSTPROCEDURE
   a. Tape the endotracheal tube in place.
   b. Assess for irritation to oral cavity, teeth, lips.
   c. Assess respiratory status.
   d. Respiratory therapy to maintain settings and evaluate function of ventilator
   e. Nurse to note orders for ventilator settings and monitor client tolerance and response.
   f. Assess for complications.
      1) Barotrauma, which is major vessel or organ damage from ventilatory pressure with referring damage to the abdomen
      2) Tension pneumothorax
      3) Gastrointestinal because of the potential for gastric ulcers and hemorrhage from air swallowed with artificial airway
      4) Hypotension from decreased cardiac output
      5) Increased intracranial pressure
      6) Fluid imbalance from increased pressure on the baroreceptors in the thoracic aorta may cause increased production of antidiuretic hormone.
   g. Chest x-ray generally ordered to verify placement
   h. Ongoing care includes assessing weaning parameters (see Table 3-7).

Table 3-7 Ventilator Weaning

Weaning Process	Goals of Weaning
Can involve adjustments in:	Respiratory rate, < 25 breaths/min Tidal volume (V_T) at least 3–5 ml/kg
Oxygen	Heart rate and blood pressure within 15% of baseline
PEEP	Arterial pH ≥ 7.35
Ventilator modes	PaO_2 ≥ 60 mm Hg and stable
Ventilator settings	$PaCO_2$ ≤ 45 mm Hg and stable O_2 saturation ≥ 90% No cardiac dysrhythmias No use of accessory muscles for breathing

© Cengage Learning 2015

F. CHEST PHYSIOTHERAPY (CPT)
  1. DESCRIPTION: PERCUSSION AND VIBRATION OVER THE THORAX TO LOOSEN SECRETIONS IN THE AFFECTED AREAS OF THE LUNG
  2. PREPROCEDURE
      a. Inform the client about the procedure.
      b. Contraindicated if the procedure increases bronchospasm
      c. Contraindicated if history of pathological fractures, rib fractures, or osteoporosis
      d. Contraindicated in obesity
      e. Contraindicated if new incisions in the chest area or upper abdominal area
      f. Contraindicated if experiences pain in the chest
  3. PROCEDURE
      a. Can use cupped hands or percussion device
      b. Keep a thin layer of material between the hand or device and the skin.
      c. Stop if painful.
      d. Most effective first thing in the morning or 1 hour before or 2–3 hours after meals
      e. Instruct the client to take deep breaths and cough during the procedure.
  4. POSTPROCEDURE
      a. Assess oxygenation status.
      b. Offer oral hygiene.
G. POSTURAL DRAINAGE
  1. DESCRIPTION
      a. Use of gravity to drain secretions from segments of the lungs
      b. May be combined with chest physiotherapy (CPT)
  2. PREPROCEDURE
      a. Inform the client about the procedure.
      b. Determine any limitations in positioning.
      c. Contraindicated if increased intracranial pressure or unstable vital signs

  3. PROCEDURE
      a. Position the client with the lung segment to be drained in the uppermost position.
      b. Maintain position for 5–20 minutes or as tolerated.
      c. Stop if cyanosis or exhaustion increases.
      d. Optimum time is early in morning, 1 hour before meals, or 2–3 hours after meals
  4. POSTPROCEDURE
      a. Assess oxygenation status.
      b. Offer oral care.
H. PULMONARY CARE
  1. DESCRIPTION: A SERIES OF INTERVENTIONS TO PROMOTE THE PRODUCTION OF SPUTUM AND THE OPENING OF AIRWAYS
  2. PREPROCEDURE
      a. Inform the client about the process.
  3. PROCEDURE
      a. Cough
      b. Deep breathe
      c. Chest physiotherapy
      d. Turn and reposition
  4. POSTPROCEDURE
      a. Assess response.
      b. Assess oxygenation status.
I. INTERMITTENT POSITIVE PRESSURE BREATHING (IPPB)
  1. DESCRIPTION: DELIVERY OF AEROSOLIZED MEDICATIONS TO THE BRONCHIAL TREE BY POSITIVE PRESSURE BREATHING
  2. PREPROCEDURE
      a. Prepare equipment and medication.
      b. Inform the client about the procedure.
  3. PROCEDURE
      a. Client will breathe through a tube placed in the mouth until all medication is administered.
  4. POSTPROCEDURE
      a. Assess respiratory status.
      b. Assess for adverse reactions: dizziness, headache, anxiety.
      c. Monitor for cardiac dysrhythmias.
      d. Monitor for pneumothorax.
      e. Assess sputum production (amount and characteristics).
J. SUCTIONING
  1. DESCRIPTION
      a. Suctioning is indicated for clients who are unable to raise secretions after coughing or chest physiotherapy, to obtain a sputum sample, or to clear the airway of secretions or other substances (e.g., emesis, blood).
      b. Suctioning can be done via oral access (not sterile) or through an endotracheal tube or tracheostomy (sterile).

   2. PREPROCEDURE
      a. Assess the client's oxygenation status and need for suctioning.
      b. If suctioning for sterile sputum sample, do not use normal saline to obtain the specimen.
      c. Obtain a sterile suction kit.
      d. Set wall suction to 80–120 mm Hg.
   3. PROCEDURE
      a. Hyperoxygenate before suctioning.
      b. Use sterile technique.
      c. Adhere to standard precautions (mask, goggles, and gloves).
      d. Lubricate the suction catheter with sterile saline.
      e. Advance the catheter during inspiration without suction.
      f. After reaching the bronchial bifurcation, pull the catheter back 2–3 cm.
      g. Apply suction (intermittent) and remove the catheter with rotating motion.
      h. Suction a maximum of 10–15 seconds.
      i. Oxygenate the client.
      j. Assess for hypoxia and dysrhythmias.
      k. Assess need to suction again, rinse the catheter, and repeat the procedure if necessary.
   4. POSTPROCEDURE
      a. Rinse the catheter and discard with gloves.
      b. Document client response and character and amount of the sputum.
      c. Assess breath sounds and oxygenation status.
      d. Assess for adverse affects such as hypoxia, dysrhythmias, bronchospasm, and infection.

X. RESPIRATORY TERMS AND CONDITIONS

   A. DYSPNEA
      1. THE SUBJECTIVE SENSATION OF UNCOMFORTABLE BREATHING, THE FEELING OF INABILITY TO GET ENOUGH AIR
      2. IT IS OFTEN DESCRIBED AS BREATHLESSNESS, AIR HUNGER, SHORTNESS OF BREATH, LABORED BREATHING, AND PREOCCUPATION WITH BREATHING.
      3. PAROXYSMAL NOCTURNAL DYSPNEA (PND) IS A FORM OF DYSPNEA EXPERIENCED AT NIGHT, AFTER BEING ASLEEP FOR SEVERAL HOURS, DUE TO INCREASED VENOUS RETURN TO THE HEART WITH THE RECUMBENT POSITION.
      4. THE CLIENT AWAKENS WITH DYSPNEA. THIS IS ASSOCIATED WITH CARDIAC DISEASE.
   B. COUGH
      1. A PROTECTIVE REFLEX THAT CLEANSES THE LOWER AIRWAYS BY AN EXPLOSIVE EXPIRATION

      2. INHALED PARTICLES, ACCUMULATED MUCUS, INFLAMMATION, OR PRESENCE OF A FOREIGN BODY INITIATES THE COUGH REFLEX BY STIMULATING THE IRRITANT RECEPTORS IN THE AIRWAY.
   C. HEMOPTYSIS
      1. THE COUGHING UP OF BLOOD OR BLOODY SECRETIONS
      2. HEMOPTYSIS IS SOMETIMES CONFUSED WITH HEMATEMESIS, WHICH IS THE VOMITING OF BLOOD.
      3. BLOOD THAT IS COUGHED UP IS USUALLY BRIGHT RED, HAS AN ALKALINE pH, AND IS MIXED WITH FROTHY SPUTUM, WHEREAS BLOOD THAT IS VOMITED IS DARK, HAS AN ACIDIC pH, AND IS MIXED WITH FOOD PARTICLES.
   D. CYANOSIS
      1. A BLUISH DISCOLORATION OF THE SKIN AND MUCOUS MEMBRANES CAUSED BY INCREASING AMOUNTS OF DESATURATED OR REDUCED HEMOGLOBIN IN THE BLOOD
      2. GENERALLY DEVELOPS WHEN 5 g OF HEMOGLOBIN IS DESATURATED, REGARDLESS OF HEMOGLOBIN CONCENTRATION
      3. IT CAN RESULT FROM DECREASED ARTERIAL OXYGENATION (LOW PaO_2), PULMONARY OR CARDIAC RIGHT-TO-LEFT SHUNT, DECREASED CARDIAC OUTPUT, OR VASOCONSTRICTION.
      4. DOES NOT ALWAYS OCCUR WHEN THERE IS HYPOXIA. FOR EXAMPLE, SOMETIMES IMPAIRED CELLULAR OXYGENATION, SUCH AS SEVERE ANEMIA (FROM INADEQUATE HEMOGLOBIN CONCENTRATION) OR CARBON MONOXIDE POISONING (HEMOGLOBIN BOUND TO CARBON MONOXIDE INSTEAD OF OXYGEN), CAN CAUSE INADEQUATE OXYGENATION OF TISSUES WITHOUT CYANOSIS.
      5. INDIVIDUALS WITH POLYCYTHEMIA (AN ABNORMAL INCREASE IN NUMBER OF RED BLOOD CELLS) MAY HAVE CYANOSIS WHEN OXYGENATION IS ADEQUATE.
      6. THE CLINICAL FINDING OF CYANOSIS MUST BE INTERPRETED IN RELATION TO THE UNDERLYING PATHOPHYSIOLOGY.
      7. IF CYANOSIS IS SUGGESTED, THE PaO_2 SHOULD BE MEASURED.
      8. CENTRAL CYANOSIS, DECREASED OXYGEN SATURATION OF HEMOGLOBIN IN ARTERIAL BLOOD, IS BEST SEEN IN BUCCAL MUCOUS MEMBRANES AND LIPS.
      9. PERIPHERAL CYANOSIS, SLOW BLOOD CIRCULATION IN FINGERS AND TOES, IS BEST SEEN IN NAIL BEDS.

E. CLUBBING
   1. THE SELECTIVE BULBOUS ENLARGEMENT OF THE END (DISTAL SEGMENT) OF A DIGIT (FINGER OR TOE)
   2. USUALLY PAINLESS
   3. COMMONLY ASSOCIATED WITH DISEASES THAT INTERFERE WITH OXYGENATION, SUCH AS LUNG CANCER, BRONCHIECTASIS, CYSTIC FIBROSIS, PULMONARY FIBROSIS, LUNG ABSCESS, AND CONGENITAL HEART DISEASE

F. PULMONARY CHEST PAIN
   1. GENERALLY ORIGINATES FROM DISORDERS IN THE PLEURAE, AIRWAYS, OR THE CHEST WALL
   2. PLEURAL PAIN IS THE MOST COMMON PAIN CAUSED BY PULMONARY DISEASE.
   3. INFECTION AND INFLAMMATION OF THE PARIETAL PLEURA CAUSE PAIN WHEN THE PLEURA STRETCHES DURING INSPIRATION.
   4. THE PAIN IS USUALLY LOCALIZED TO A PORTION OF THE CHEST WALL, WHERE A UNIQUE BREATH SOUND CALLED A PLEURAL FRICTION RUB CAN BE HEARD OVER THE PAINFUL AREA.
   5. LAUGHING OR COUGHING MAKES PLEURAL PAIN WORSE.
   6. PLEURAL PAIN IS ALSO COMMON WITH PULMONARY INFARCTION (TISSUE DEATH) CAUSED BY PULMONARY EMBOLISM.
   7. PAIN CAUSED BY INFLAMMATION OF THE PARIETAL PLEURA IS CALLED PLEURISY OR PLEURITIS.
   8. IT CAN BE DIFFERENTIATED FROM CARDIAC PAIN, WHICH IS UNAFFECTED BY BREATHING.

G. ATELECTASIS
   1. COLLAPSE OF AFFECTED ALVEOLI AND ASSOCIATED LOBES OF THE LUNG

H. FLAIL CHEST
   1. USUALLY INVOLVES ONE SIDE OF THE CHEST (HEMITHORAX) RESULTING FROM MULTIPLE RIB FRACTURES ASSOCIATED WITH BLUNT CHEST TRAUMA
   2. MORE COMMON IN OLDER CLIENTS AND CAN HAVE A 40% MORTALITY RATE
   3. PARADOXIC RESPIRATION OF THE LOOSE SEGMENT OF CHEST WALL IS THE INWARD MOVEMENT OF THE THORAX DURING INSPIRATION, WITH OUTWARD MOVEMENT DURING EXPIRATION.
   4. GAS EXCHANGE IS SIGNIFICANTLY IMPAIRED.

XI. **RESPIRATORY DISORDERS**
A. PULMONARY EDEMA
   1. DESCRIPTION
      a. Cardiogenic
         1) Increased left ventricular filling pressures lead to increased pulmonary capillary hydrostatic pressure.
         2) Fluid fills the interstitial spaces and alveoli, decreasing gas exchange.
      b. Noncardiogenic
         1) Increased pulmonary capillary permeability as a result of injury that damages the alveolar capillary membrane
         2) Fluid shifts into the interstitial spaces and alveoli, decreasing gas exchange.
      c. Decrease in colloid oncotic pressure (COP)
         1) Protein fraction normally exerts pressure that opposes capillary hydrostatic pressure and helps keep fluid within the vessels.
         2) Clinical manifestations similar to cardiogenic pulmonary edema except that the heart is functioning normally
   2. ASSESSMENT
      a. Predisposing factors: heart disease (the most common cause), adult respiratory distress syndrome, inhalation of toxic gases, capillary injury and increases in capillary permeability
      b. Dyspnea
      c. Paroxysmal nocturnal dyspnea (PND)
      d. Crackles on auscultation
   3. DIAGNOSTIC TESTS
      a. Arterial blood gases
      b. Hemodynamic measurements from a pulmonary artery catheter
      c. Chest x-ray
   4. NURSING INTERVENTIONS
      a. Rotating tourniquets (rarely used): apply pressure cuffs to three limbs at a time, cuff inflation slightly above the client's diastolic blood pressure, cuff inflated for 45 minutes and released 15 minutes.
      b. Monitor daily weights.
      c. Assess respiratory status.
      d. Position the client in a semi-Fowler's position.
      e. Monitor intake and output.
      f. Monitor pulmonary artery pressures.
      g. Monitor hematocrit and hemoglobin.
      h. Assess for neck vein distention.
      i. Assess skin turgor.
      j. Administer drugs such as diuretics, analgesics, and bronchodilators.

B. **CHRONIC OBSTRUCTIVE PULMONARY DISEASE (COPD) OR CHRONIC AIRFLOW LIMITATION (CAL)**
1. DESCRIPTION
    a. A group of disorders associated with persistent or recurrent obstruction of airflow; includes chronic bronchitis, pulmonary emphysema, and bronchial asthma
    b. Pulmonary emphysema
        1) Destruction of alveoli, narrowing of small airways (bronchioles), and the trapping of air results in loss of lung elasticity.
        2) Primary contributing factor is smoking cigarettes
        3) Develop a deficiency of alpha antitrypsin (enzyme that blocks the action of proteolytic enzymes that are destructive to elastin and other substances in the alveolar walls)
    c. Chronic bronchitis
        1) Excessive mucus secretions within the airways and recurrent cough
        2) Contributing factors include heavy cigarette smoking, pollution, and infection.
        3) Copious sputum production
        4) Hypoxemia resulting in polycythemic: ruddy look to the skin, compensation
        5) Pulmonary hypertension leading to cor pulmonale
    d. Bronchial asthma
        1) Abnormal bronchial hyperreactivity to certain substances
        2) Extrinsic: antigen-antibody reaction triggered by food, drugs, or inhaled particles
        3) Intrinsic: pathophysiological conditions within the respiratory tract
        4) Status asthmaticus
            a) An asthma attack lasting more than 24 hours
            b) A medical emergency
            c) Usually responds to epinephrine hydrochloride (adrenalin) s.q. and aminophylline, theophylline, and ethylenediamine (Phyllocontin) IV and bronchodilator therapy (see Table 3-8)

Table 3-8 Comparison of Chronic Airflow Limitation Conditions/COPD

Chronic Bronchitis	Pulmonary Emphysema	Bronchial Asthma
Exposure to infectious or noninfectious irritants, especially tobacco smoke A chronic inflammation of the airways	Walls of individual air sacs torn; repair not possible Bronchioles collapse, trapping air	Swollen mucous membranes of bronchial tubes and surrounding tissue
Bronchial tubes narrowed as a result of thickened mucous membrane (often to twice the normal thickness), surrounding tissue inflammation	Lung tissue becomes inelastic; lungs enlarge, classic barrel-chest appearance	Muscles of bronchial tubes become spastic, causing narrowing. Thick mucus fills bronchial tubes and sacs.
Affects the small and large airways rather than the alveoli Excessive mucus production	Hyperinflation of the lung Enlarged alveoli prevent lung from returning to resting state.	Reversible airflow obstruction, airway inflammation, and airway hyperresponsiveness
Mucus and pus impede action of respiratory cilia.	Formation of bullae (air-filled spaces) that can be seen on x-ray examination	Breathing labored, expiration difficult Wheezing
Characterized by productive cough, mucus plugs, and recurrent respiratory infections	Small airway collapse and air trapping from positive intrathoracic pressures Exhalation difficult and prolonged	
History of smoking, air pollution, occupational exposure	History of chronic bronchitis	Commonly triggered by emotional stress, exercise, change in weather or allergen
ABGs: increased $PaCO_2$, decreased PaO_2 Respiratory acidosis	ABGs: increased $PaCO_2$, decreased PaO_2 Respiratory acidosis	Decreased pulmonary function tests with decreased peak flow (PEFR) that improve after treatment
Teach: proper use of medications, control of bronchospasms, methods to reduce exposure to pulmonary irritants, low-flow oxygen, proper use of inhalers and nebulizers, prevention of complications and infections, breathing exercises, energy conservation	Teach: proper use of medications, control of bronchospasms, methods to reduce exposure to pulmonary irritants, low-flow oxygen, proper use of inhalers and nebulizers, prevention of complications and infections, breathing exercises, energy conservation	Teach: proper use of medications, control of bronchospasms, methods to reduce exposure to pulmonary irritants, proper use of inhalers and nebulizers, prevention of complications and infections, breathing exercises, energy conservation, identify and eliminate exposure to pulmonary irritants, receive influenza immunization

2. ASSESSMENT
   a. Oxygenation status and level of consciousness
   b. Pulse oximetry
   c. Breathing pattern, rate, depth
   d. Chest expansion, dyspnea, nasal flaring
   e. Use of breathing techniques (e.g., pursed lip)
   f. Prolonged expiratory phase
   g. Use of accessory muscles
   h. Orthopnea
   i. Clubbing of fingers (classic with emphysema)
   j. Flattened diaphragm
   k. Barrel chest (classic with emphysema)
   l. Anorexia, weight loss
   m. Wheezing (classic with asthma)
   n. Anxiety
3. DIAGNOSTIC TESTS
   a. Arterial blood gas
   b. Chest x-ray
   c. Pulmonary function tests
   d. Sputum culture
4. NURSING INTERVENTIONS
   a. Instruct the client on the proper use and monitoring of oxygen.
   b. Instruct the client on energy conservation techniques.
   c. Encourage the client to sit for activities when possible.
   d. Inform the client not to hold the breath while performing activities.
   e. Be aware that activities involving the arms may increase dyspnea.
   f. Plan rest periods between activities.
   g. Instruct the client on breathing techniques.
   h. Instruct the client on pursed-lip breathing.
   i. Instruct the client on diaphragmatic breathing.
   j. Instruct the client on relaxation therapy.
   k. Instruct the client on pulmonary care.
   l. Instruct the client on controlled cough techniques.
   m. Plan to pace activities.
   n. Assess the quality and quantity of sputum, color, consistency, amount, and odor.
   o. Instruct the client on the medications and proper use of equipment.
   p. Instruct the client on the proper sequence of respiratory treatments.
   q. Instruct the client on the judicious use of bronchodilators and steroids.
   r. Instruct the client on the clinical manifestations of hypercapnia:
      1) Headache
      2) Drowsiness and fatigue

C. RESPIRATORY TRACT INFECTIONS (PNEUMONIA)
   1. DESCRIPTION
      a. An acute infection that causes inflammation of the parenchyma (alveolar spaces and interstitial tissue) of the lung
      b. The involved lung tissue becomes swollen and the air spaces fill with liquid.
      c. Pneumonia is caused primarily by specific organisms (bacteria, viruses, fungi, parasites, mycoplasma, or chemical irritants) and can be classified as community acquired and hospital associated (nosocomial) and those associated with immunocompromised status such as *Pneumocystis carinii* and *Aspergillus fumigatus*.
   2. ASSESSMENT
      a. Dullness on percussion due to consolidation
      b. Bronchial breath sounds auscultated over consolidated lung fields
      c. Crackles
      d. Tachypnea (respiratory rate > 20 breaths/min)
      e. Tachycardia (heart rate > 100 beats/min)
      f. Fever; sudden onset over 37.7°C (100°F)
      g. Shaking chills (with bacterial pneumonia)
      h. Chest pain
      i. Dyspnea
      j. Hacking cough
      k. Anxiety and confusion
   3. DIAGNOSTIC TESTS
      a. Arterial blood gases and pulse oximetry to determine need for oxygen
      b. Chest x-ray
      c. Sputum for culture and sensitivity testing
      d. Complete blood count (elevated WBC; depressed in mycoplasmal or viral pneumonia)
      e. Blood culture and sensitivity
   4. NURSING INTERVENTIONS
      a. Monitor vital signs (especially temperature); treat temperature as necessary.
      b. Provide for adequate hydration (oral) or administer IV fluids as ordered.
      c. Humidify inspired air.
      d. Encourage effective coughing.
      e. Relieve pain with analgesics.
      f. Monitor for dyspnea.
      g. Administer antibiotics for specific causative organism as ordered.
      h. Provide client and family teaching related to the disease process and

treatments, deep breathing and coughing techniques, importance of hand washing and need for adequate rest.

D. SEVERE ACUTE RESPIRATORY SYNDROME (SARS)
1. DESCRIPTION
   a. Respiratory illness of unknown cause that has recently been reported in a number of countries
   b. Believed to be spread by close contact when someone infected with the disease coughs droplets into the air and someone else breathes them in
   c. It may also be spread from touching objects that have become contaminated.
   d. The organism associated with SARS is coronavirus (SARS-CoV)
2. ASSESSMENT
   a. Fever greater than 38°C (100.4°F)
   b. Headache
   c. Overall feeling of discomfort
   d. Body aches
   e. Trouble breathing
   f. Dry cough
   g. Travel within 10 days on onset of symptoms to an area with documented or suspected community transmission of SARS
   h. Close contact within 10 days of onset of symptoms with a person known or suspected to have SARS
3. DIAGNOSTIC TESTS
   a. Laboratory detection of antibody to SARS-CoV
4. NURSING INTERVENTIONS
   a. Clinical manifestation management
   b. A combination of airborne, droplet, and contact precautions is recommended by the Centers for Disease Control and Prevention (CDC) until more is understood about transmission.

E. PULMONARY EMBOLISM
1. DESCRIPTION
   a. Obstruction of one or more pulmonary arteries by a thrombus or thrombi, originating somewhere in the venous system or in the right side of the heart
   b. May result from venous stasis, vessel wall injury, or hypercoagulability of the blood
   c. Predisposing factors
      1) Prolonged immobility
      2) Chronic lung disease
      3) Congestive heart failure
      4) Thrombophlebitis
      5) Hematologic disorders
      6) Lower extremity fractures or surgery
      7) Pregnancy or oral contraceptive use

2. ASSESSMENT
   a. Chest pain
   b. Tachycardia
   c. Dyspnea
   d. Petechiae
   e. Anxiety and restlessness
   f. Decreased breath sounds on auscultation, usually with pleural friction rub
   g. Signs of circulatory collapse (weak, rapid pulse; hypotension)
3. DIAGNOSTIC TESTS
   a. Arterial blood gases ($PaO_2 < 60$ mm Hg)
   b. Elevated LDH, bilirubin, and fibrin split products
   c. Deficient perfusion and ventilation lung scan (V/Q scan)
   d. Pulmonary angiogram indicates intra-arterial filling defect.
4. NURSING INTERVENTIONS
   a. Elevate the head of the bed to the semi-Fowler's position.
   b. Administer oxygen therapy as needed.
   c. Administer anticoagulants and thrombolytic therapy.
   d. Monitor for bleeding.
   e. Administer pain medication as prescribed to relieve chest pain.
   f. Prevent further emboli by reducing venous stasis.

F. PULMONARY HYPERTENSION
1. DESCRIPTION
   a. A complication of disorders in pulmonary circulation
   b. Causative factors include:
      1) Congenital heart disease with left-to-right shunt
      2) Congenital heart disease with diminished pulmonary blood flow
      3) Obstruction to pulmonary venous outflow
      4) Pulmonary embolism
      5) Chronic alveolar hypoxia
      6) Diffuse pulmonary fibrosis
2. ASSESSMENT
   a. Early:
      1) Hyperventilation
      2) Ague chest discomfort
   b. Late:
      1) Tachypnea, dyspnea, orthopnea, chest congestion
      2) Cyanosis of the lips and nail beds
      3) Edema of the hands and feet
      4) Anasarca (generalized, massive edema)
      5) Distended jugular veins
      6) Right ventricular heave (visible left parasternal systolic lift)
      7) Accentuated pulmonary component of the second heart sound

8) Right ventricular diastolic gallop
9) Pulmonary ejection click
10) Distant breath sounds
11) Basilar crackles
12) Mean pulmonary artery pressure (MAP) > 20 mm Hg (norm 8–15 mm Hg)

3. DIAGNOSTIC TESTS
   a. ABGs
   b. Chest x-ray
   c. Electrocardiography
   d. Pulmonary function tests
   e. Pulmonary angiography and perfusion scans
   f. Red blood cell and hematocrit levels may be increased.

4. NURSING INTERVENTIONS
   a. Administer oxygen therapy.
   b. Implement hemodynamic monitoring.
   c. Administer drugs to increase myocardial contractility and reduce right ventricular afterload such as diuretics, digitalis, bronchodilators, and vasodilators.

G. COR PULMONALE
   1. DESCRIPTION
      a. Right ventricular hypertrophy or failure, secondary to disease of the lungs, pulmonary vessels, or chest wall
      b. Occurs when there is increased pressure and pulmonary hypertension
      c. There is destruction of the pulmonary capillaries, increased resistance of the pulmonary capillary bed, and shunting of unaerated blood across the collapsed alveoli.
      d. Initially, the right heart fails, then the left heart fails because of decreased cardiac output.

   2. ASSESSMENT
      a. Right heart failure
      b. Peripheral edema (dependent)
      c. Jugular vein distension
      d. Left heart failure
      e. Dyspnea
      f. Cyanosis
      g. Cough
      h. Substernal pain
      i. Syncope on exertion
      j. Paroxysmal nocturnal dyspnea (PND) and orthopnea

   3. DIAGNOSTIC TESTS
      a. Chest x-ray
      b. Cardiac catheterization

   4. NURSING INTERVENTIONS
      a. Promote rest.
      b. Monitor oxygen status.
      c. Maintain a low-sodium diet.
      d. Administer drugs such as digoxin and diuretics.

H. CARBON DIOXIDE NARCOSIS (CO_2 NARCOSIS) (OXYGEN TOXICITY)
   1. DESCRIPTION
      a. Increased carbon dioxide due to chronic retention
      b. Secondary to excessive oxygen delivery
      c. With chronic respiratory disease and $PaCO_2$ retention, the hypoxic drive is triggered by low O_2 rather than high pCO_2.
      d. For these clients, a high O_2 concentration will suppress their drive to breathe.

   2. ASSESSMENT
      a. Signs of hypoxia
      b. Drowsy
      c. Irritable
      d. Hallucinations
      e. Convulsions
      f. Tachycardia
      g. Arrhythmias
      h. Poor ventilation

   3. DIAGNOSTIC TESTS
      a. Arterial blood gases
      b. Pulse oximetry

   4. NURSING INTERVENTIONS
      a. Avoid high concentrations of oxygen— keep below 3 L/min; no more than 70% oxygen delivered.
      b. Monitor oxygen levels and client response.

I. ACUTE RESPIRATORY FAILURE
   1. DESCRIPTION
      a. The exchange of O_2 for CO_2 in normal lungs cannot match the rate of O_2 consumption and CO_2 production in body cells, causing alveolar hypoventilation.
      b. PaO_2 < 60 mm Hg with or without hypercapnia ($PaCO_2$ > 50 mm Hg)
      c. Possible causes
         1) Airway obstruction
         2) Restrictive lung disease
         3) Central nervous system disorders, (e.g., head trauma or stroke [CVA])
         4) Drug overdose
         5) Anesthesia and surgical procedures

   2. ASSESSMENT
      a. Dyspnea
      b. Tachypnea
      c. Tachycardia
      d. Headache
      e. Cyanosis
      f. Anxiety, confusion, restlessness
      g. Decreased or absent breath sounds
      h. Adventitious breath sounds: crackles, wheezes

   3. DIAGNOSTIC TESTS
      a. ABGs with PaO_2 < 60 mm Hg, $PaCO_2$ > 50 mm Hg, and pH < 7.35
      b. ECG with cardiac dysrhythmias

    c. Chest x-ray with various lung field changes, depending on causative factors

    d. Assessment indicating compromise and hypoxia

  4. NURSING INTERVENTIONS

    a. Evaluate for the precipitating event and correct, if possible.

    b. Restore and maintain a patent airway by suctioning or endotracheal intubation.

    c. Provide oxygen therapy.

    d. Provide mechanical ventilation as required.

    e. Maintain effective tracheobronchial hygiene.

    f. Monitor vital signs and overall status.

    g. Monitor ABGs.

    h. Provide emotional support.

J. ADULT RESPIRATORY DISTRESS SYNDROME (ARDS)

  1. DESCRIPTION

    a. A form of acute respiratory failure caused by diffuse injury to the alveolar-capillary membrane characterized by:

      1) Refractory hypoxemia (responds poorly to high concentrations of oxygen)

      2) Decreased pulmonary compliance

      3) Dyspnea

      4) Noncardiogenic bilateral pulmonary edema

      5) Dense pulmonary infiltrates (ground-glass or "whited-out" appearance on x-ray)

    b. Usually follows an acute catastrophic event in clients with no previous pulmonary disease (within 24–48 hours)

    c. Oxygenation failure, with a $PaO_2 < 50$ mm Hg at oxygen concentrations of $> 50\%$

    d. Also called noncardiogenic pulmonary edema (older term is *shock lung*)

  2. ASSESSMENT

    a. Increasing dyspnea and use of accessory muscles

    b. Cyanosis

    c. Tachycardia

    d. Cough (blood-tinged, frothy sputum)

    e. Increasing hypoxemia

  3. DIAGNOSTIC TESTS

    a. Chest x-ray may be clear initially, later shows diffuse haziness or "whited-out" (ground-glass) appearance

    b. ABGs

    c. Sputum for culture and sensitivity

    d. Hemodynamic measures from pulmonary artery catheter (Swan-Ganz) show pulmonary capillary wedge pressure (PCWP) low to normal

  4. NURSING INTERVENTIONS

    a. Prepare for endotracheal intubation and mechanical ventilation.

    b. Administer sedation, if prescribed, to reduce O_2 consumption.

    c. Monitor for tension pneumothorax because high peak end expiratory pressure or PEEP is often used.

    d. Assess respiratory status and lung sounds.

    e. Suction as necessary.

    f. Monitor oxygenation: pulse oximetry, vital signs, ECG.

K. PLEURAL EFFUSION

  1. DESCRIPTION

    a. Excess nonpurulent fluid in the pleural space between the visceral and parietal pleurae

    b. Generally occurs as a secondary complication of another process

  2. ASSESSMENT

    a. Dullness to percussion over fluid

    b. Decreased or absent breath sounds over fluid

    c. Dyspnea

    d. Changes in vital signs (depending on size of effusion and amount of distress)

    e. Possible fever, tachypnea, tachycardia, hypotension

    f. Fear or anxiety

  3. DIAGNOSTIC TESTS

    a. Chest x-ray

    b. ABGs

    c. Thoracentesis

    d. Pleural fluid studies (culture, sensitivity, cytology)

  4. NURSING INTERVENTIONS

    a. Perform a respiratory assessment.

    b. Place the client in a Fowler's position.

    c. Prepare for thoracentesis.

    d. Monitor the client after the procedure.

    e. Monitor the vital signs.

    f. Administer drugs such as antibiotics and analgesics.

    g. Interventions depend on the etiology of the effusion.

L. EMPYEMA

  1. DESCRIPTION

    a. Collection of pus in the pleural space

    b. Commonly associated with pulmonary infection, lung abscess, or infected pleural effusion

    c. Predisposing factors are thoracic surgery and chest trauma.

  2. ASSESSMENT

    a. History of recent pneumonia or trauma

    b. Chest pain

    c. Dyspnea

     d. Cough
     e. Fever or chills
     f. Night sweats
     g. Weight loss
  3. DIAGNOSTIC TESTS
     a. Chest x-ray
     b. Sputum sample
     c. Pleural fluid analysis (thoracentesis)
     d. Ineffective thermoregulation
  4. NURSING INTERVENTIONS
     a. Prepare the client for chest tube insertion.
     b. Administer antibiotics.
     c. Perform a respiratory assessment.
     d. Prepare the client for a possible thoracotomy and decortication (removal) of a portion of the pleura.

M. CHEST TRAUMA
  1. DESCRIPTION
     a. Injury to the chest wall or lungs that interferes with inspiration, gas exchange, or expiration
     b. Collection of air, fluid, or blood in the pleural space; can come from outside the chest wall or inside the lung
     c. Hemothorax is blood in the pleural space.
     d. Pneumothorax is air in the pleural space.
     e. Open pneumothorax is a sucking chest wound.
     f. Causes:
       1) Trauma
       2) Gunshot, stabbing, motor vehicle accident
       3) Thoracic surgery
       4) Open thoracotomy
       5) Positive pressure ventilation
       6) Caused by positive pressure damage to a segment of the lung and exposure to the pleural space (mechanical ventilation)
       7) Iatrogenic
       8) Complication of thoracentesis or central venous line insertion
       9) Unknown
     g. Types
       1) Spontaneous: sudden and without warning
       2) Tension: due to buildup of pressure and results in shifting of internal organs and structures
       3) Open: from trauma
  2. ASSESSMENT
     a. Chest pain
     b. Shortness of breath, dyspnea
     c. Tachypnea
     d. Hypotension (may progress to shock)
     e. Tachycardia
     f. Hyperresonance and decreased breath sounds over the affected lung
     g. Asymmetric chest movement
     h. Anxiety, restlessness
     i. Diaphoresis
     j. Subcutaneous emphysema (crepitus) (especially with tension pneumothorax)
     k. Cyanosis
     l. Cardiovascular compromise
     m. Cardiac dysrhythmias
     n. Mediastinal shift (mediastinum pushed to the unaffected side)
     o. Tracheal deviation (deviation away from the injured side)
  3. DIAGNOSTIC TESTS
     a. ABGs
     b. Chest x-ray
  4. NURSING INTERVENTIONS
     a. Place the client in a high-Fowler's position.
     b. Assess vital signs and breath sounds.
     c. Provide oxygen therapy.
     d. Prepare the client for chest x-ray.
     e. Prepare the client for insertion of chest tubes.
     f. Provide comfort and reassurance to the client.

N. OCCUPATIONAL LUNG DISEASE (PNEUMOCONIOSES)
  1. DESCRIPTION
     a. Lung disorders resulting from occupational exposure to organic or inorganic dusts and noxious gases (see Table 3-9)
     b. Most common are:
       1) Silicosis
       2) Asbestosis
       3) Coal workers' pneumoconiosis (CWP, "black lung")
  2. ASSESSMENT
     a. History of exposure
     b. Asymptomatic in early stages
     c. Chronic cough
     d. Nonproductive in silicosis and asbestosis
     e. Productive of black fluid in CWP
     f. Dyspnea—progressive
     g. Recurrent upper respiratory infections
     h. Impaired diaphragmatic excursion
     i. Decreased chest expansion and diminished breath sounds
     j. Tachypnea
     k. Clubbing of digits (fingers and toes)
  3. DIAGNOSTIC TESTS
     a. Chest x-ray with findings of nodular formation, fibrosis, and interstitial densities
     b. Decreased pulmonary function tests
     c. ABGs with decreasing PaO_2 and increasing $PaCO_2$ as disease progresses

Table 3-9 Inhalation Disorders

Agents	Examples	Effects	Initial Symptoms	Treatment
Toxic gases	Smoke, ammonia, hydrogen chloride, sulfur dioxide, chlorine, phosgene, and nitrogen dioxide	Severe inflammation of the airways, alveolar and capillary damage, pulmonary edema	Burning of the eyes, nose, and throat; coughing; chest tightness; and dyspnea. Hypoxemia is common	Supplemental oxygen, mechanical ventilation with PEEP, support of the cardiovascular system. Steroids are sometimes used.
Oxygen	Oxygen toxicity	Oxygen concentrations of 50–75% for greater than 24–48 hours is associated with injury to cells of the lungs. Related to severe inflammatory response mediated primarily by oxygen radicals	Damage to alveolocapillary membranes, disruption of surfactant production, interstitial and alveolar edema, and decrease in compliance. Toxicity often cannot be differentiated from ARDS.	Ventilator support and reduction of inspired oxygen concentration to less than 60% as soon as tolerated by the individual
Pneumoconiosis silicosis (silica)	Inhaled particles, generally from the workplace	Permanent deposits; therefore, want to prevent further exposure and improve working conditions	Silicosis: fibrous nodules on x-ray; may be asymptomatic. Clinical manifestations include cough and dyspnea.	Silicosis: treat symptoms of frequent lower respiratory tract infections. Steroids may help.
Coal worker pneumoconiosis (coal) (black lung)			Coal: mild form is asymptomatic. Possible chronic bronchitis. Advanced form leads to severe pulmonary fibrosis. Productive cough and wheezing	Coal: no specific treatment. Those with severe complications often have associated cardiopulmonary dysfunction
Asbestosis (asbestos)			Asbestos: can cause fibrosis or tumor formation.	Asbestos: Supportive
Other less common inhalants: talc, fiberglass, clays, mica, slate, cement, cadmium, beryllium, tungsten, cobalt, aluminum, and iron			Can produce dyspnea on exertion, a nonproductive cough, hypoxemia, and decreased lung volume. May lead to respiratory failure and cardiac complications. Smoking markedly increases risk of developing bronchogenic cancer.	

4. NURSING INTERVENTIONS
   a. Teaching and care similar to those for clients with COPD

O. PULMONARY FIBROSIS
   1. DESCRIPTION
      a. A highly lethal interstitial lung disease
      b. Damage to lung tissue as a result of excessive wound healing
      c. Lung injury occurs, then inflammatory process, neutrophilic response, lymphocyte and macrophage response. Followed by exudation of serum proteins into alveolar space, collapse of alveolar units, and healing by fibrosis
   2. ASSESSMENT
      a. History of exposure to cigarette smoking, metal dust, organic dust, or wood fire
      b. Respiratory assessment
      c. Initially, clinical manifestations are slow and insidious, dyspnea.
      d. Progressive and severe dyspnea and hypoxemia
   3. DIAGNOSTIC TESTS
      a. Pulmonary function tests: shows decreased forced vital capacity
      b. Chest x-ray
      c. ABGS
   4. NURSING INTERVENTIONS
      a. Administer oxygen therapy.
      b. Perform a respiratory assessment.
      c. Position the client to assist breathing.
      d. Provide emotional support.
      e. Administer drugs such as corticosteroids or cytotoxic drugs.
      f. Administer morphine to minimize sensation of shortness of breath in later stages.

P. SARCOIDOSIS
1. DESCRIPTION
   a. Classified as an interstitial lung disease (also called "fibrotic lung disease")
   b. Hallmark of disease is noncaseating granulomas, which can occur in almost any organ or tissue of the body.
   c. Most commonly affecting the lung, but also affecting the liver, spleen, lymph nodes, eyes, small bones of the hands and feet, and skin
   d. Peak ages for sarcoidosis are 20–30 years and 45–65 years of age.
   e. For most clients, the illness resolves spontaneously. Others (10–15%) may develop pulmonary fibrosis and severe systemic disease.
   f. Thought to be activated by T lymphocytes
2. ASSESSMENT
   a. Nonproductive cough
   b. Dyspnea
   c. Chest discomfort
   d. Severe disease results in loss of lung compliance and functional ability to exchange gases
   e. Cor pulmonale (right-sided cardiac failure) often results from pumping against the noncompliant, fibrotic lung.
3. DIAGNOSTIC TESTS
   a. Chest x-ray (presence of granulomas)
   b. Computed tomographic (CT) scan
   c. Pulmonary function tests (PFT)
   d. Fiberoptic bronchoscopy
4. NURSING INTERVENTIONS
   a. Monitor the client for clinical manifestations.
   b. Instruct the client about medication regimen (corticosteroids 6–12 months) and adverse reactions.
   c. Implement physical care depending on clinical manifestations.

Q. TUBERCULOSIS
1. DESCRIPTION
   a. A reportable, communicable, infectious disease that can occur in any part of the body
   b. Organism is *Mycobacterium tuberculosis* (nonmotile, slow growing, nonsporulating, acid-fast rod).
   c. Spread by droplet nuclei (aerosolization) from laughing, sneezing, coughing
   d. Pulmonary TB involves the lungs. Causes caseation (tissue turned into a granular mass) in the lungs and Ghon tubercles, which can lie dormant for years, then become active and infect the client
   e. Miliary (hematogenous) TB is nonpulmonary and can affect any other part of the body.

   f. More likely to occur in overcrowded populations such as long-term care facilities and prisons
   g. Affects populations where their nutritional status is poor, the immune system is weak (older adults, HIV), substance abuse
   h. Inadequate treatment of primary infection leads to multidrug-resistant organisms.
2. ASSESSMENT
   a. Productive cough
   b. Hemoptysis
   c. Low-grade fever/chills
   d. Night sweats
   e. Dyspnea
   f. Progressive fatigue, malaise, lethargy
   g. Weight loss
   h. Anorexia, vomiting, indigestion
   i. Irregular menses
3. DIAGNOSTIC TESTS
   a. Mantoux test: positive if induration of 10 mm or more, read 48–72 hours after the test. For HIV-positive clients, a 5-mm induration or greater is considered positive.
   b. Sputum for acid-fast bacillus, x3
   c. Chest x-ray
   d. History and physical exam
5. NURSING INTERVENTIONS
   a. If hospitalized, the client is placed in airborne precautions.
   b. Administer drugs at night to minimize nausea.
   c. Instruct the client regarding the need for adequate nutrition, especially iron, protein, and vitamins.
   d. Instruct the client on the importance of adhering to the drug regimen, not missing doses, and continuing through the entire 6 to 12 months prescribed.
   e. Instruct the client to cover the mouth and nose with disposable tissues when sneezing, coughing, or laughing. Dispose of tissues in plastic bags. Wear a mask when in contact with crowds until the medication is effective in suppressing the infection.
   f. Return for monitoring of infectious status with sputum cultures every 2–4 weeks until cultures are negative (generally after 3 months of treatment).
   g. Instruct the client that others in the household will also require TB testing.

R. CARBON MONOXIDE POISONING
1. DESCRIPTION
   a. Carbon monoxide (CO) is a colorless, odorless, tasteless gas.
   b. Carbon monoxide binds to the hemoglobin molecule 200–250 times more tightly than oxygen.

Table 3-10 Carbon Monoxide Poisoning

Carbon Monoxide Level	Effects
1–10%	Low levels cause vasodilation and increase blood supply to major organs.
11–20%	Mild poisoning causes symptoms such as headache, visual changes, and slight dyspnea.
21–40%	Moderate poisoning causes symptoms such as headache, dizziness, tinnitus, drowsiness, decreased mental status, confusion, and pale or red-colored skin.
41–60%	Severe poisoning leads to convulsions, coma, or cardiopulmonary complications.
61–80%	Lethal poisoning leads to death.

© Cengage Learning 2015

   c. Carbon monoxide bound to hemoglobin forms carboxyhemoglobin (CoHb).
   d. Even when hemoglobin is bound by CO, the arterial blood (PaO_2) is normal.
   e. Vasodilation caused by carbon monoxide causes a "cherry-red" skin color.
   f. Normal levels of carbon monoxide are 1–10% (see Table 3-10).

2. ASSESSMENT
   a. Respiratory assessment
   b. Pulse oximetry may read high but reflect binding of carbon monoxide to hemoglobin, not oxygen.
   c. Carbon monoxide level is required to determine poisoning.
   d. Arterial blood gas analysis for $PaCO_2$ may reflect normal levels when hemoglobin is bound by carbon monoxide.
   e. Obtain history of circumstances of injury to determine possibility of carbon monoxide poisoning.
   f. Assess skin color.

3. DIAGNOSTIC TESTS
   a. Arterial blood gas analysis
   b. Carbon monoxide level

4. NURSING INTERVENTION
   a. Administer high-flow oxygen.
   b. Provide supportive care.

S. PLEURODESIS
  1. DESCRIPTION
   a. With chronic pulmonary effusions, the goal is to remove pleural fluid and prevent further accumulation.
   b. This procedure reduces or eliminates the need for repeated thoracentesis with malignant pulmonary disease.
   c. Sclerosing agents or talc are inserted into the intrapleural space via the chest tube.
   d. This causes adherence of the pleura to the chest wall (creates pleuritis between the visceral and parietal pleurae).

  2. ASSESSMENT
   a. Inform the client about the procedure and obtain informed consent.
   b. Obtain a cardiovascular and respiratory baseline assessment prior to the procedure.
   c. Monitor vital signs every 4 hours for 24 hours after the procedure. Client may experience fever and discomfort from pleuritis.

  3. DIAGNOSTIC TESTS
   a. Pleurodesis is conducted following thoracentesis.

  4. NURSING INTERVENTIONS
   a. Medicate the client with analgesics or sedative as ordered.
   b. Ensure that the chest tube is clamped immediately after instillation of the agent and remains clamped for the prescribed time.
   c. Assist the client with position changes if rotation is prescribed (limited research does not demonstrate that dispersion of the sclerosing agent is enhanced by rotation).
   d. When the chest tube is unclamped, note the amount and character of drainage.
   e. Perform a respiratory assessment every 8 hours and observe for respiratory distress and signs of pneumothorax.
   f. Administer analgesics as needed.

PRACTICE QUESTIONS

1. A client was admitted to the intensive care unit 36 hours ago following extensive pulmonary trauma. Which clinical manifestation would first alert the nurse that the client is experiencing adult respiratory distress syndrome (ARDS)?
   1. Blood-tinged, frothy sputum
   2. Dense pulmonary infiltrates with a "whited-out" appearance
   3. An increase in respiratory rate
   4. Increasing hypoxemia

2. A client with a history of asthma presents in the physician's office with complaints of difficulty breathing. While performing the initial assessment, the nurse becomes concerned that the client's respiratory status has worsened based on which of the following?
   1. Wheezing throughout the lung fields
   2. Noticeably diminished breath sounds
   3. Loud wheezing only on expiration
   4. Mild wheezing on inspiration

3. A home health nurse is visiting a client with severe chronic obstructive pulmonary disease (COPD) who is complaining of increased shortness of air. The client is on home oxygen at 2 L/min via an oxygen concentrator with a respiratory rate of 23 breaths/min. The most appropriate nursing action is to
   1. call emergency services to come to the home.
   2. reassure the client of being unnecessarily anxious.
   3. conduct further assessment of the client's respiratory status.
   4. consider increasing the oxygen to 4 L/min during the home visit.

4. The nurse is admitting a client with suspected tuberculosis (TB) to the acute care unit. The nurse places the client in airborne precautions until a confirmed diagnosis of active TB can be made. Which of the following tests is a priority to confirm the diagnosis?
   1. Chest x-ray that is positive for lung lesions
   2. Positive purified protein derivative (PPD) test
   3. Sputum positive for blood (hemoptysis)
   4. Sputum culture positive for *Mycobacterium tuberculosis*

5. A student health nurse is conducting tuberculosis (TB) testing. Students who had the purified protein derivative (PPD) test 48 hours ago have returned to have the results read and documented. The nurse determines that the test is positive if which of the following is present?
   1. The client complains of itching at the site
   2. There is a large area of erythema
   3. There is an induration of 10 mm or greater
   4. A bruise is present at the site of injection

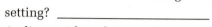
6. The nurse is aware that the optimal tidal volume for ventilator weaning is what setting? _____

7. A client with no history of respiratory disease has a sudden onset of dyspnea, chest pain, and tachycardia. A pulmonary embolism is suspected. The nurse anticipates which set of therapeutic orders to be prescribed for this client?

   Select all that apply:
   [ ] 1. Semi-Fowler's position
   [ ] 2. Oxygen at 2 L/min
   [ ] 3. High-Fowler's position
   [ ] 4. Morphine sulfate 2 mg intravenously
   [ ] 5. Oxygen at 4 L/min
   [ ] 6. Hydromorphine hydrochloride (Dilaudid) 2 mg intramuscular

8. A client with pulmonary edema is currently receiving 6 L/min of oxygen per nasal cannula. The most recent arterial blood gas (ABG) results indicate the following: pH = 7.30, pCO_2 = 50 mm Hg, pO_2 = 56 mm Hg, HCO_3 = 24 mm Hg. The nurse anticipates that the physician will order which of the following?
   1. Change nasal cannula to face mask at 6 L/min oxygen
   2. Add one ampule of sodium bicarbonate to the client's current intravenous fluids
   3. Change nasal cannula to partial rebreather mask at 8 L/min oxygen
   4. Intubate the client and place on mechanical ventilation

9. A registered nurse is planning the schedule for the day. Which of the following nursing tasks may the nurse delegate to a licensed practical nurse?
   1. Develop instructions for the client on pursed-lip breathing
   2. Clarify an order with the physician
   3. Instruct a client on a bronchoscopy
   4. Administer a purified protein derivative (PPD) to a client

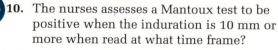
10. The nurses assesses a Mantoux test to be positive when the induration is 10 mm or more when read at what time frame?

    _____

11. The nurse has just received orders to provide chest physiotherapy for a client two times per day. The nurse evaluates which schedule to be most therapeutic?
    1. 7:00 a.m. and 1:00 p.m.
    2. 6:00 a.m. and 4:00 p.m.
    3. 9:00 a.m. and 5:00 p.m.
    4. 8:00 a.m. and 8:00 p.m.

12. The nurse assesses fluctuations in the water seal chamber of a client's closed chest drainage system. The nurse evaluates this finding as indicating
    1. the system is functioning properly.
    2. an air leak is present.
    3. the tubing is kinked.
    4. the lung has reexpanded.

13. The nurse assesses a college-age client complaining of shortness of breath after jogging and tightness in his chest. Upon further questioning, the client denies a sore throat, fever, or productive cough. The nurse notifies the physician that this client's clinical manifestations are most likely related to
    1. pneumonia.
    2. bronchitis.
    3. pneumoconiosis.
    4. asthma.

14. Which of the following is a priority to include in the instructions given to a client who has bronchitis?
    1. Avoid cigarette smoking
    2. Decrease overweight status
    3. Increase activity
    4. Avoid malnutrition

15. The nurse is assessing the respiratory status of a client following a thoracentesis. Which finding would indicate further assessment is needed?
    1. Equal bilateral chest expansion
    2. Scattered crackles, unchanged from baseline
    3. Diminished breath sounds on the affected side
    4. Respiratory rate of 22 breaths/minute

16. The nurse is admitting a client who complains of fever, chills, chest pain, and dyspnea. The client has a heart rate of 110, respiratory rate of 28, and a nonproductive hacking cough. A chest x-ray confirms a diagnosis of left lower lobe pneumonia. Upon auscultation of the left lower lobe, the nurse documents which of the following breath sounds?
    1. Bronchial
    2. Bronchovesicular
    3. Vesicular
    4. Absent breath sounds

17. The nurse is preparing a client with empyema for a thoracentesis. Which of the following should the nurse have available in the event that the procedure is ineffective?
    1. A ventilator
    2. A chest tube insertion kit
    3. An intubation tray
    4. A crash cart

18. A client is admitted to a burn unit with second- and third-degree burns over 18% of the body. An inhalation injury is also suspected. The nurse should monitor which of the following to determine the extent of carbon monoxide poisoning?
    1. Pulse oximetry
    2. Urine myoglobin
    3. Arterial blood gases
    4. Serum carboxyhemoglobin levels

19. Which of the following should the nurse include when suctioning a client's tracheostomy?
    1. Instill sterile saline down the trachea to stimulate a cough, then suction with continuous suctioning
    2. Insert the catheter until a cough reflex is obtained or until resistance is felt
    3. Adjust the wall suction to 150 mm Hg for the procedure
    4. Suction the client's mouth before entering the trachea

20. The nurse is evaluating the respiratory system of a client who admits to smoking a half pack per day for the last 5 years and 1 pack per day for 10 years prior to that. When evaluating the client's risk of developing a respiratory disease, the nurse calculates that the client has a smoking history of how many packs over the years?
    1. 2.5 pack-years
    2. 10 pack-years
    3. 12.5 pack-years
    4. 15 pack-years

21. A client with pneumonia has a poor appetite, is dyspneic and complains of decreased taste sensation, and is receiving chest physiotherapy treatments and breathing treatments. Which of the following actions should the nurse include to improve the client's appetite?
    1. Provide mouth care before meals
    2. Provide juice and fluids at the bedside
    3. Provide three balanced meals each day
    4. Increase fluid intake to 3 L a day

22. A client with left-sided heart failure is progressing to pulmonary edema. The nurse assesses the client and reports which of the following manifestations?
    1. Dry, hacking cough
    2. Bilateral crackles

3. Fever above 36.8°C or 101.5°F
4. Peripheral pitting edema

23. The nurse is performing a respiratory assessment of a client with pleurisy and compares the assessment findings with the previous day's assessment. Currently there is no friction rub, but one was auscultated the previous day. The nurse evaluates this finding as the result of
    1. the client taking more shallow breaths.
    2. a decreased inflammatory response.
    3. the effectiveness of the antibiotics.
    4. an accumulation of pleural fluid in the inflamed area.

24. The nurse is caring for a client following a cardiac bypass surgery. The nurse notes that in the first hour the chest tube drainage measured 90 ml. During the second hour the drainage dropped to 5 ml. The nurse suspects which of the following?
    1. The chest tube may be clotted
    2. The lungs have fully inflated
    3. The client is recovering normally
    4. The physician should be notified

25. The nurse should monitor a client admitted with a suspected diagnosis of pulmonary emphysema for which of the following clinical manifestations?

    Select all that apply:
    [ ] 1. Copious sputum production
    [ ] 2. Bilateral wheezing
    [ ] 3. Marked weight loss
    [ ] 4. Prolonged inspiratory phase
    [ ] 5. Barrel chest appearance
    [ ] 6. Severe dyspnea

26. The nurse is preparing to delegate which of the following nursing tasks to a licensed practical nurse?
    1. Administer morphine IV to a client experiencing a pulmonary embolism
    2. Monitor a client's chest tube for bubbling
    3. Assess a client for tactile fremitus
    4. Perform a sputum culture for a client

27. The nurse is reviewing the normal limits for a head and neck assessment. Which of the following findings would indicate the need for additional investigation?
    1. A small, discrete, movable lymph node
    2. The trachea is to the right of the suprasternal notch
    3. A thyroid gland that is not visible or palpable
    4. The muscles of the neck are symmetrical

28. The nurse is performing an assessment of the thorax and lungs on a 30-year-old client. Which of the following assessments does the nurse evaluate to be a normal adult finding?
    1. The thorax is barrel shaped
    2. The costal margin is greater than 90°
    3. The accessory muscles are used during inspiration and expiration
    4. The ribs articulate at a 45° angle with the sternum

29. The nurse correctly documents moist, low-pitched, gurgling breath sounds as
    1. sonorous wheezes.
    2. coarse crackles.
    3. sibilant wheezes.
    4. pleural friction rub.

30. When preparing a client to collect a sputum specimen, it would be essential for the nurse to explain which of the following aspects of the procedure?
    1. Avoid mouth care prior to collecting the specimen
    2. Breathe deeply followed by coughing up sputum
    3. Collect the specimen before bedtime
    4. Restrict fluids prior to expectorating sputum

ANSWERS AND RATIONALES

1. 3. Adult respiratory distress syndrome usually develops within 24 to 48 hours following an acute catastrophic event in clients with no previous pulmonary disease. In most cases, tachypnea and dyspnea are the first clinical manifestations. Blood-tinged, frothy sputum occurs later, after the development of pulmonary edema. The diffuse pulmonary infiltrates, resembling a ground-glass or "whited-out" appearance on a chest x-ray, will appear as ARDS progresses, whereas early chest x-rays are often normal. Hypoxemia will occur as ARDS progresses and the client becomes refractory to oxygen therapy.

2. 2. The severity of wheezing is not a reliable way to determine severity of an asthma attack. Some clients with minor attacks may have loud wheezing, whereas others may have severe attacks with mild wheezing. The client with severe asthma attacks may have no audible wheezing because of the decrease in airflow. For wheezing to occur, the client must be able to move air to produce sound. Wheezing usually occurs first on exhalation, and as the

asthma attack progresses, the client may wheeze during both inspiration and expiration. The significant finding with this assessment is that there are noticeably diminished breath sounds, which means reduced or absence of moving air. This may indicate severe obstruction and respiratory failure.

3. 3.   Further assessment is the most appropriate nursing action. Remember the nursing process; assessment is the first step. Calling for emergency services would be premature. Oxygen is not increased without the approval of the physician, and remember that with COPD the client's drive to breathe is triggered by low oxygen because of the carbon dioxide retention. For clients with COPD, oxygen should not generally be greater than 2 to 3 L/min. Reassurance that the client is unnecessarily anxious is inappropriate.

4. 4.   The most accurate way to diagnose TB is by sputum culture. Identifying the presence of tubercle bacilli is essential for a definitive diagnosis. Although hemoptysis is associated with more advanced cases of TB, it is not a confirmatory clinical manifestation. A positive PPD indicates exposure to TB, but gives no information about active disease. A chest x-ray with lesions may be present in a number of other diseases, not just TB.

5. 3.   An induration of 10 mm or greater is usually considered a positive result. For immunocompromised and HIV-positive clients, an induration of 5 mm or greater may be considered a positive result. Erythema is not a positive reaction. Itching or bruising is not indicative of a positive result. Remember, PPD skin tests are read 48 to 72 hours after administration.

6.   3–5 ml/kg.

7. 1. 4. 5.   Standard therapeutic interventions for a client with a pulmonary embolism include proper positioning, oxygen, and intravenous analgesics. Semi-Fowler's position is most appropriate because high-Fowler's position creates extreme flexion of the hips and slows venous return from the legs, which increases the risk of new thrombi. This client has no history of respiratory disease and is not limited to 2 to 3 L/min. Therefore, 4 L/min would be appropriate to help relieve dyspnea. Intravenous analgesics are prescribed to relieve chest pain. Morphine sulfate is the drug of choice and 2 mg is the appropriate intravenous dose. Morphine helps reduce pain and anxiety and can diminish congestion of blood in the pulmonary vessels because it causes peripheral venous dilation.

8. 4.   The client is exhibiting respiratory acidosis with severe hypoxemia. Intubation and mechanical ventilation are warranted in this situation. Changing the oxygen delivery system to a mask would not correct the hypoxemia. Changing the oxygen delivery system to partial rebreather mask, even with a slight increase in oxygen, would not correct the significant hypoxia, and the rebreather mask would increase the pCO_2 retention. Adding sodium bicarbonate to the IV fluids treats a clinical manifestation, not the underlying condition of respiratory distress, and sodium bicarbonate will not correct the hypoxemia.

9. 4.   It is not appropriate to assign a licensed practical nurse to develop a teaching plan, teach, or clarify an order with the physician. These are tasks reserved for the registered nurse. An LPN may administer a purified protein derivative to a client.

10.   48–72 hours

11. 2.   Chest physiotherapy and postural drainage are most effective upon first awakening and during the day 1 hour before or 2 to 3 hours after meals. This treatment should always be followed by oral hygiene. All of the other options are most effective either at or shortly after meal times.

12. 1.   In a closed drainage chest tube system, fluctuations in the water seal chamber during inhalation and exhalation (called tidaling) is a normal finding until the lung reexpands. If the fluctuations are absent, it may mean that there is an air leak, that the tubing is kinked, or that the lung has reexpanded and the client no longer requires chest drainage.

13. 4.   The exercise may have induced bronchospasms. Lack of fever or productive cough would reduce the possibility of the clinical manifestations representing pneumonia or bronchitis. The occupation as a college student decreases the likelihood of an occupationally related lung disease.

14. 1.   Cigarette smoking is one of the most significant risk factors for developing bronchitis. Bronchitis involves the major bronchi and is classified as acute or chronic. Acute bronchitis is bronchial airway inflammation related to smoke, irritants, or infection. Chronic bronchitis is a component of chronic obstructive pulmonary disease (COPD). It usually follows an upper respiratory infection such as rhinitis or sore throat. Malnutrition is considered a possible risk factor. Obesity or being active in sports is not correlated with bronchitis.

15. 3.   Following a thoracentesis, the nurse assesses breath sounds and vital signs. The nurse particularly looks for signs that may indicate a pneumothorax as a complication from the procedure. Signs that may indicate a pneumothorax include increased respiratory rate, dyspnea, retractions, diminished breath sounds, or cyanosis. Any of these signs should be reported to the physician immediately. Equal bilateral breath sounds are normal findings and a respiratory rate of 22 is slightly elevated and may be due to pain or anxiety. Scattered crackles, although not normal, have not changed from baseline and would not represent a complication as a result of the procedure.

16. 1. In the presence of pneumonia there will be bronchial breath sounds over the area of consolidation. The client may also have crackles in the affected side as a result of fluid in the interstitium and alveoli. Absence of breath sounds is not a usual finding and would not likely occur unless there was a serious complication.

17. 2. With empyema, the fluid to be removed from the pleural space is thick and "puslike." The physician may not be able to withdraw the fluid through needle aspiration and the client may require placement of a chest tube to adequately drain the purulent effusion. A ventilator, intubation tray, or crash cart is not likely to be necessary because there was no indication that the client was unstable.

18. 4. Carbon monoxide binds tightly to hemoglobin to form carboxyhemoglobin. Because carbon monoxide binds 200 times greater to hemoglobin than oxygen, there is decreased availability of oxygen to the cells. Clients are treated with 100% oxygen. Pulse oximetry will read falsely high, as it is a reading of how well the hemoglobin is bound, but not with oxygen. Urine myoglobin is indicative of by-products of muscle damage being excreted through the kidneys. Arterial blood gas pCO_2 may falsely represent the client's oxygenation status and is not a measure of carbon monoxide levels.

19. 2. Proper suctioning involves inserting the catheter gently until a cough reflex is stimulated or resistance is felt. It is then withdrawn with intermittent suction and a rotating motion using moderate suction pressure (80 to 120 mm Hg). Nursing research does not support the instillation of saline and the client's risk of aspiration and contamination are increased with this procedure. Airway suctioning is a sterile technique. If the client's mouth is to be suctioned it would be the last thing done, after airway suctioning and before discarding.

20. 3. The standard method for determining pack-year smoking history is to take the number of packs per day times the number of years. The number is recorded as the number of pack-years. $(0.50 \times 5) + (1.0 \times 10) = 2.5 + 10 = 12.5$ packs over the years.

21. 1. Because of the sputum production and expectoration, particularly during and after

treatments, the client will have decreased taste sensation. Providing oral care after pulmonary treatments and before meals will improve taste and appetite. Fatigue from breathing, activity, and treatments will also decrease energy. Providing more frequent small meals (not three large ones), increasing fluid intake, and offering fluids that appeal to the client are appropriate interventions for the client but will not impact appetite.

22. 2. A client with left-sided heart failure and pulmonary edema presents primarily with respiratory symptoms. Because of the fluid accumulation in the pulmonary vascular bed, there may be a productive cough with pink, frothy sputum. There is no fever associated with pulmonary edema, and peripheral pitting edema is more associated with right-sided heart failure.

23. 4. Initially a pleural friction rub is auscultated when there is inflammation between the pleural space and visceral pleura. With increasing inflammation, fluid accumulates between the two layers at the inflamed site and reduces the friction. The inflammatory process is still there and would be treated by anti-inflammatory drugs, not necessarily antibiotics (unless there were an infectious process involved). The client should be instructed to take adequately deep breaths for a good assessment of breath sounds and that should be consistent between assessments.

24. 1. The first hour after surgery, chest tube draining may be as high as 100 ml/hour but should taper off over the next several hours. There should not be a sudden significant increase or drop in the amount of drainage. In this case, a sudden drop may indicate that a clot has formed in the tube and the nurse will need to gently work the clot out of the tubing to prevent cardiac tamponade. Further assessment would need to be made before notifying the physician. A chest tube is not "milked" but can be gently manipulated. Chest tube drainage is not an indication of lung inflation. Chest drainage may taper off to minimal amounts before the tube is withdrawn, but that is based on the fluctuations in the water seal chamber being minimal and an evaluation by chest x-ray.

25. 3. 5. 6. Clients with pulmonary emphysema typically manifest symptoms of marked weight loss, barrel chest appearance, prolonged expiratory effort, marked dyspnea, and a cough late in the progression of the disease. There is scant mucus production. Copious sputum production is characteristic of chronic bronchitis. Bilateral wheezing is characteristic of bronchial asthma.

26. 4. A licensed practical nurse has the knowledge and skill to perform a sputum culture for a

client. Administering morphine IV to a client, monitoring a chest tube, or assessing a client for tactile fremitus are nursing tasks reserved for a registered nurse.

27. 2. The trachea should be midline in the suprasternal notch. It may be normal to feel a small, discrete, movable lymph node. It is clinically insignificant. The thyroid gland should not be visible or palpable and the muscles of the neck should be symmetrical.

28. 4. The thorax is generally slightly elliptical in shape, although the barrel-shaped chest may be normal in the infant and older adult. The costal angle should be less than 90° during exhalation and at rest. No accessory muscles should be used

during normal respirations. The ribs should also articulate at a 45° angle with the sternum.

29. 2. Low-pitched gurgling breath sounds are coarse crackles. Sonorous wheezes are low-pitched breath sounds. Sibilant wheezes are high-pitched musical breath sounds. A pleural friction rub is a creaking sound.

30. 2. Breathing deeply should be followed by coughing up sputum in the collection process of a sputum specimen. Mouth care should be offered prior to collecting a sputum specimen. The specimen should be collected in the morning and fluids encouraged before coughing up the specimen.

REFERENCES

Daniels, R. (2010). *Delmar's manual of laboratory and diagnostic tests* (2nd ed.). Clifton Park, NY: Delmar Cengage Learning.

Daniels, R., & Nicoll, L. (2012). *Contemporary medical-surgical nursing.* Clifton Park, NY: Delmar Cengage Learning.

DeLaune, S. C., & Ladner, P. K. (2011). *Fundamentals of nursing: Standard and practice* (4th ed.). Clifton Park, NY: Delmar Cengage Learning.

Estes, M. (2010). *Health assessment and physical examination* (4th ed.). Clifton Park, NY: Delmar Cengage Learning.

Spratto, G. R., & Woods, A. L. (2012). *PDR nurse's drug handbook 2012.* Clifton Park, NY: Delmar Cengage Learning.

CHAPTER 4

CARDIOVASCULAR DISORDERS

I. **ANATOMY AND PHYSIOLOGY**
   A. FUNCTIONS AND STRUCTURES OF THE CARDIOVASCULAR SYSTEM
      1. TRANSPORT OXYGEN AND NUTRIENTS TO CELLS
      2. REMOVE METABOLIC WASTES
      3. TRANSPORT HORMONES THROUGHOUT THE BODY
   B. HEART
      1. FOUR-CHAMBERED, MUSCULAR ORGAN LOCATED WITHIN THE MEDIASTINAL SPACE BETWEEN THE LUNGS, PALPABLE AT THE FIFTH INTERCOSTAL SPACE, SLIGHTLY LEFT OF MIDCLAVICULAR LINE
      2. HEART IS ENCASED IN THE PERICARDIUM (PERICARDIAL SAC) MADE UP OF A VISCERAL (INNER) LAYER AND A PARIETAL (OUTER) LAYER.
      3. PERICARDIAL SPACE IS LOCATED BETWEEN LAYERS OF PERICARDIAC SAC, PROVIDING LUBRICATION AND THEREFORE DECREASING FRICTION WITH EACH CONTRACTION.
   C. HEART LAYERS
      1. ENDOCARDIUM (INNER LAYER)
      2. MYOCARDIUM (MIDDLE, MUSCULAR LAYER)
      3. EPICARDIUM (OUTER LAYER)
   D. HEART CHAMBERS
      1. FOUR CHAMBERS SEPARATED BY A SEPTUM
         a. Right atrium receives deoxygenated blood from the body through the superior and inferior vena cava
         b. Right ventricle receives blood from the right atrium through the tricuspid valve
         c. Left atrium receives oxygenated blood from the lung through the pulmonary veins
         d. Left ventricle receives blood from the left atrium through the mitral valve
   E. CARDIAC VALVES
      1. ATRIOVENTRICULAR (AV) VALVES
         a. The tricuspid and mitral valves prevent blood from flowing back into the atria during ventricular diastole.
         b. Chordae tendineae attached to the papillary muscles in the wall of the ventricles prevent the valve leaflets from collapsing backward into the atria.
      2. SEMILUNAR VALVES
         a. The pulmonic and aortic valves prevent blood from flowing back into the ventricles during ventricular diastole.
   F. BLOOD FLOW TO THE MYOCARDIUM
      1. THE CORONARY SINUSES (JUST ABOVE THE AORTIC VALVES) ARE OPENINGS TO THE CORONARY ARTERIES (THEY FILL DURING DIASTOLE).
      2. LEFT MAIN CORONARY ARTERY DIVIDES INTO THE LEFT ANTERIOR DESCENDING (LAD) ARTERY AND ITS BRANCHES AND THE CIRCUMFLEX ARTERY AND ITS BRANCHES, WHICH SUPPLY BLOOD TO THE LEFT ATRIUM AND LEFT VENTRICLE
      3. THE RIGHT CORONARY ARTERY AND ITS BRANCHES SUPPLY BLOOD TO THE RIGHT ATRIUM, RIGHT VENTRICLE, AND INFERIOR AND POSTERIOR WALL OF THE LEFT VENTRICLE. IT SUPPLIES BLOOD TO A-V NODE IN 90% OF THE POPULATION.
   G. ELECTRICAL DEPOLARIZATION
      1. SODIUM IONS SHIFT RAPIDLY INTO THE CARDIAC CELLS WHILE POTASSIUM IONS SHIFT OUT.
      2. CELL MEMBRANES BECOME DEPOLARIZED, WITH THE CHANGE TO POSITIVE CHARGE OCCURRING INSIDE THE CELLS.
      3. ELECTRICAL IMPULSES PASS THROUGH THE ELECTRICAL CONDUCTION SYSTEM AND THE CELLS THEMSELVES.

Figure 4-1 Electrical conduction system

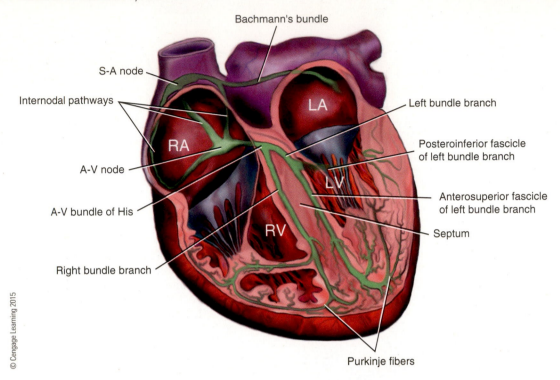

Bachmann's bundle

S-A node

Internodal pathways

RA

A-V node

A-V bundle of His

Right bundle branch

LA

Left bundle branch

Posteroinferior fascicle
of left bundle branch

LV

Anterosuperior fascicle
of left bundle branch

Septum

RV

Purkinje fibers

© Cengage Learning 2015

H. ELECTRICAL CONDUCTION SYSTEM (SEE FIGURE 4-1)
  1. SINOATRIAL (S-A) NODE IS THE NATURAL PACEMAKER OF THE HEART
    a. Located in right atrium
    b. Proper origin of electrical impulses
    c. Beats at 60–100 times per minute
  2. ATRIOVENTRICULAR (A-V) NODE
    a. Located at the base of the right atrium
    b. Allows for brief pause of impulse so atrial contraction and emptying can be completed
    c. If origin of impulse, beats at 40–60 times per minute
  3. BUNDLE OF HIS
    a. Located along the septum
    b. Delivers impulse via the left bundle branch (dividing into anterior and posterior fascicles) to the left ventricles and to the right bundle branch in the right ventricle
  4. PURKINJE FIBERS
    a. Located along the wall of both ventricles
    b. Should result in simultaneous ventricular contractions
    c. If origin of impulse, beats at 20–40 times a minute
I. MECHANICAL SYSTEM OF HEART (ELECTRICALLY TRIGGERED)
  1. SYSTOLE (CONTRACTION) OCCURS WHEN BLOOD IS EJECTED FROM THE VENTRICLES.

  2. DIASTOLE (RELAXATION) OCCURS WHEN VENTRICLES ARE AT REST.
J. CARDIAC OUTPUT (MECHANICAL EFFICIENCY)
  1. CARDIAC OUTPUT (CO) MEASURES THE EFFICIENCY OF THE HEART: THE AMOUNT OF BLOOD EJECTED FROM EACH VENTRICLE IN 1 MINUTE (AVERAGE ADULT CO = 4–8 L/MIN)
  2. CARDIAC OUTPUT (CO) = STROKE VOLUME (SV) × HEART RATE (HR). STROKE VOLUME (SV) MEASURES THE AMOUNT OF BLOOD EJECTED FROM THE VENTRICLE WITH EACH HEARTBEAT.
  3. FACTORS THAT AFFECT CARDIAC OUTPUT:
    a. Heart rate (regulated by the autonomic nervous system)
    b. Stroke volume, which is affected by:
      1) Preload: the volume of blood in the ventricle (stretch placed on myocardial muscle fibers) before contraction
      2) Afterload: the resistance against which the left ventricle must pump
      3) Contractility: force of contraction, which can increase SV by improving ventricular emptying

K. ANATOMY AND PHYSIOLOGY OF THE VASCULAR SYSTEM

   1. BLOOD VESSELS THROUGH WHICH BLOOD CIRCULATES FROM THE HEART INCLUDE: ARTERIES, ARTERIOLES, CAPILLARIES, VENULES, AND VEINS.

     a. Arteries have thick, elastic walls to accept the pulsatile systolic flow of oxygenated blood away from the heart (with the exception of the pulmonary artery, which carries deoxygenated blood from the right ventricle to the lungs).

     b. Arterioles have thin, less elastic walls that are sensitive to changes in O_2 and wastes, and constrict or dilate correspondingly (a main determinate of blood pressure).

     c. Capillaries have very thin walls through which the exchange of cellular wastes and nutrients take place.

     d. Venules obtain blood from capillaries and deposit it into veins.

     e. Veins have thin, valvular walls through which deoxygenated blood returns (with the exception of the pulmonary veins, which carry oxygenated blood to the left atrium from the lungs) to the heart.

L. REGULATION OF THE CARDIOVASCULAR SYSTEM

   1. AUTONOMIC NERVOUS SYSTEM

     a. Sympathetic

       1) Increases heart rate and force of contractility

       2) Stimulates the heart's beta-adrenergic receptors for epinephrine and norepinephrine

     b. Parasympathetic

       1) Decreases heart rate

       2) Stimulates the vagus nerve

   2. BARORECEPTORS (LOCATED IN THE AORTIC ARCH AND CAROTID SINUS)

     a. Perceive pressure changes in the arterial system, responding with messages to the brainstem

     b. Results in appropriate increased or decreased heart rate, and constriction or vasodilation via the autonomic nervous system in order to compensate

   3. CHEMORECEPTORS (LOCATED IN THE AORTIC ARCH AND CAROTID BODY)

     a. Perceive chemical changes in the blood (e.g., decreased pO_2 and increased pCO_2)

     b. Results in vasoconstriction

   4. RENAL SYSTEM SENSES WHEN BLOOD FLOW TO THE KIDNEYS DECREASES, RESULTING IN SODIUM AND WATER BEING RETAINED AND RELEASE OF HORMONES TO FURTHER RETAIN FLUIDS

   5. OTHER FACTORS MAY ALSO AFFECT THE CARDIOVASCULAR SYSTEM (E.G., EXERCISE, EMOTION, TEMPERATURE).

M. BLOOD PRESSURE

   1. SYSTOLIC BLOOD PRESSURE (SBP)

     a. Highest pressure caused by blood forced against the wall of the arteries during each ventricular contraction

     b. Normal SBP for adults is 90–135.

   2. DIASTOLIC BLOOD PRESSURE (DBP)

     a. Lowest pressure of blood against the walls of the arteries while the ventricles are at rest

     b. Normal DBP for adults is 60–85.

II. ASSESSMENT

A. HEALTH HISTORY

   1. PAST HEALTH HISTORY

   2. MEDICATIONS (PAST, PRESENT, OVER THE COUNTER, HERBAL)

   3. SURGERIES/PROCEDURES

   4. SUBJECTIVE EXAMINATION (DETAILED DESCRIPTION OF ANY SYMPTOMS FROM THE CLIENT: ONSET, DESCRIPTION, ACTIVITY INTOLERANCE, DYSPNEA, ORTHOPNEA)

B. PHYSICAL EXAMINATION

   1. INSPECTION

     a. General: activity level, color, alertness, pain, dyspnea, vital signs, presence of distended neck veins

     b. Thorax:

       1) Visible scars from previous surgery; normal skin color

       2) Thorax symmetrical with no visible pulsation (pulsation of the aortic arch or innominate arteries may be observed as normal)

       3) Angle of Louis (raised notch where the manubrium and body of the sternum are joined at the second intercostal) may be used as a marker to count intercostal spaces

     c. Peripheral: edema, cyanosis, wounds, uneven hair distribution, pain

   2. PALPATION

     a. Skin should be warm, dry.

     b. Point of maximum impulse (PMI) may be palpated at the fifth ICS at the midclavicular line (abdominal aorta may be visibly and palpably pulsing as normal)

     c. Unless the client has a very thin chest wall, pulsations are not normally felt in the heart's auscultatory areas because these thrills ("purring" or abnormal pulsation) may reflect valvular disorder and turbulent blood flow.

Figure 4-2 Auscultatory areas of the heart

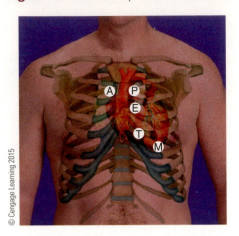

© Cengage Learning 2015

d. Peripheral
　1) Feet normally have pedal pulses present (scale: 0 is absent pulse; 11 is weak; 21 is normal; 31 is bounding).
　2) Capillary refill time should be less than 3 seconds.

3. PERCUSSION
　a. Right-sided heart border should not be distinguishable.

4. AUSCULTATION
　a. Auscultatory areas: (see Figure 4-2)
　　1) Aortic valve: second ICS to the right of the sternum
　　2) Pulmonic valve: second ICS to the left of the sternum
　　3) Tricuspid valve: fourth ICS left of the sternum
　　4) Mitral valve (apex): fifth ICS at the left midclavicular line
　b. Normal heart tones include S1 (systole) and S2 (diastole).
　c. Extra heart sounds are abnormal, with the exception of a splitting of S2, which may be heard at the pulmonic area during inspiration (see Table 4-1).
　d. Murmurs are heard when there is a turbulent blood flow through normal or abnormal valves (see Table 4-2).
　　1) Are described according to loudness on a 6-point scale
　　2) Are described according to timing in the cardiac cycle: systolic occurs between S1 and S2 such as in aortic stenosis or mitral regurgitation, whereas diastolic occurs between S2 and S1 (late in cycle) such as in mitral stenosis or aortic regurgitation.
　　3) Are described by location where the murmur is best heard
　e. Peripheral: a bruit is an abnormal buzzing heard through the stethoscope placed over a vessel, and indicates a narrowed or bulging wall of the vessel (e.g., femoral artery, carotid artery).

Table 4-1 Abnormal Heart Sounds: Gallops and Rubs

Sound	Description	Possible Cause
Paradoxical Splitting of S2	"Extra" sound heard between S1 and S2 during expiration	Severe myocardial depression (myocardial infarction, aortic stenosis or regurgitation of the pulmonic valve)
S3 (Ventricular Gallop) (Note: May be normal for those < 40 years old)	Low-intensity vibration of ventricular walls, usually occurs immediately after S2	Ventricular filling defects (left ventricular failure, mitral valve regurgitation, ventricular septal defect)
S4 (Atrial Gallop)	Low-frequency vibration of the atrial walls, usually occurs immediately before S1 of the next cycle	Abnormal atrial contraction (hypertension, anemia, left ventricle hypertrophy, aortic stenosis, old age)
Summation Gallop (Quadruple Gallop)	Combination of S3 and S4; sounds like a horse galloping	Severe heart failure
Pericardial Friction Rub	Often transient, short, high-pitched grating sound; often best heard while the client is sitting forward and exhaling	Inflammation, infection, or infiltration (pericarditis, cardiac tamponade)

© Cengage Learning 2015

Table 4-2 Abnormal Heart Sounds: Murmurs

Severity	Description
Grade I	Very faint
Grade II	Faint, but consistently audible
Grade III	Loud, but of moderate intensity
Grade IV	Loud, with palpable thrill
Grade V	Very loud, thrill present, audible with a stethoscope partially off the client's chest
Grade VI	Extremely loud, audible even without a stethoscope

© Cengage Learning 2015

C. CARDIAC WAVEFORMS EXAMINATION
　1. INITIAL EVALUATION IS USUALLY DONE BY STANDARD 12-LEAD ELECTROCARDIOGRAM (ECG); MAY BE MONITORED CONTINUOUSLY USING TELEMETRY.
　2. BASELINE
　　a. Represents resting phase; "isoelectric line"
　　b. Should be flat and straight
　　c. Any positive deflections are those that occur above baseline.
　　d. Any negative deflections are those that occur below baseline.

Figure 4-3 Normal sinus rhythm

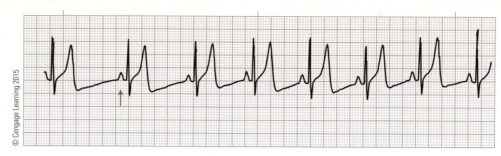

Figure 4-4 Sinus bradycardia

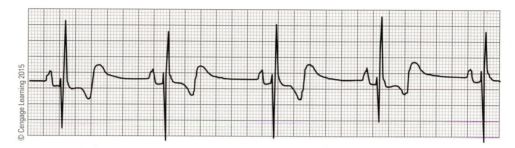

3. P WAVE
   a. Represents atrial depolarization (contraction)
   b. Should be positive deflection, rounded
4. QRS WAVE
   a. Represents ventricular depolarization
   b. The shape depends on viewing direction (which lead is used).
   c. Q is the first negative deflection (but not present in all leads).
   d. R is the first positive deflection.
   e. S is a negative deflection following the R (but not present in all leads).
5. PR INTERVAL
   a. Represents electrical impulse traveling through the AV node where it pauses briefly, then to the Purkinje fibers of the ventricles
   b. Measures from 0.12 to 0.20 second
6. T WAVE
   a. Represents repolarization of ventricles
   b. Usually positive deflection, rounded
   c. If an ectopic beat (extra) occurs on the T wave, the ventricles are irritable and may cause a dangerous R-on-T ventricular tachycardia.
7. QT INTERVAL
   a. Represents total time for ventricular depolarization and repolarization
   b. Measurement varies with gender and heart rate.

8. ST SEGMENT
   a. Represents early ventricular repolarization
   b. Should be isoelectric
   c. Elevation above baseline may indicate myocardial infarction (MI).
9. U WAVE
   a. Represents slowed repolarization of ventricular Purkinje fibers (often hypokalemia)
   b. Not normally present; may follow T wave but be smaller
D. CARDIAC RHYTHMS
   1. NORMAL SINUS RHYTHM (SEE FIGURE 4-3)
      a. Rate: 60–100 beats/minute and regular; SA node origin
      b. P wave: normal
      c. PR interval: normal
      d. QRS complex: normal
   2. SINUS BRADYCARDIA (SEE FIGURE 4-4)
      a. Rate: 60 beats/minute and regular
      b. P wave: normal
      c. PR interval: normal
      d. QRS complex: normal
      e. Possible causes: parasympathomimetic drugs, intracranial pressure, inferior MI, may be normal in trained athletes
      f. Significance: may cause decreased cardiac output (CO), which may result in low BP, dizziness, angina, change in level of consciousness
      g. Treatment: if symptomatic, give atropine and hold all parasympathomimetic drugs.

Figure 4-5 Sinus tachycardia

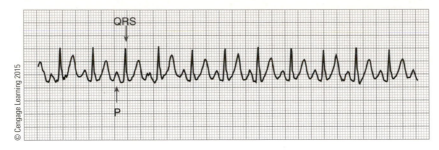

Figure 4-6 Premature atrial contractions

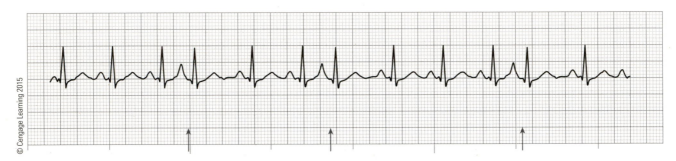

Figure 4-7 Paroxysmal supraventricular tachycardia

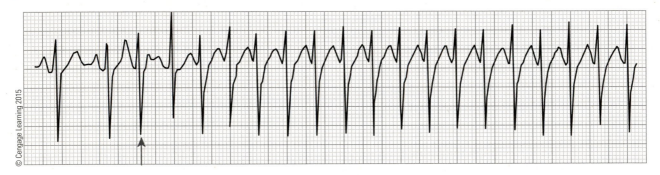

3. SINUS TACHYCARDIA (SEE FIGURE 4-5)
   a. Rate: > 100 beats/minute and regular (S-A node origin)
   b. P wave: normal
   c. PR interval: normal
   d. QRS complex: normal
   e. Possible causes: exercise, pain, fever, hypotension, myocardial ischemia, congestive heart failure, anemia, hyperthyroidism; also drugs such as theophylline, epinephrine, caffeine
   f. Significance: may decrease CO
   g. Treatment: treat underlying cause. Some clients may be prescribed beta blockers.

4. PREMATURE ATRIAL CONTRACTIONS (SEE FIGURE 4-6)
   a. Rate: usually 60–100 beats/minute and irregular (origin is different foci in either atrium)
   b. P wave: abnormal shape; P wave comes early

   c. PR interval: normal or varied
   d. QRS complex: usually normal
   e. Possible causes: emotional stress, stimulants such as caffeine, tobacco, alcohol, or diseases such as infection, inflammation, hyperthyroidism, chronic obstructive pulmonary disease (COPD), heart disease, or enlarged atrium
   f. Significance: may increase in frequency and become supraventricular tachycardia (SVT)
   g. Treatment: depends on clinical manifestations. Withdraw stimulants. Some clients may be prescribed digoxin (Lanoxin), quinidine (quinidine gluconate or quinidine sulfate), procainamide (Pronestyl), or beta blockers.

5. PAROXYSMAL SUPRAVENTRICULAR TACHYCARDIA (PSVT) (SEE FIGURE 4-7)

Figure 4-8 Atrial flutter

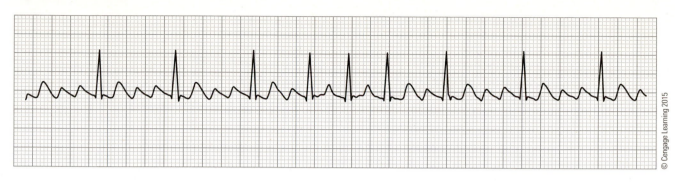

© Cengage Learning 2015

a. Rate: 100–300 beats/minute and regular (origin is above the bundle of His) ("paroxysmal" refers to sudden onset)

b. P wave: abnormal shape (may be difficult to view due to fast rate)

c. PR interval: variable

d. QRS complex: usually normal

e. Possible causes: overexertion, stress, stimulants, rheumatic heart disease, digitalis toxicity, coronary artery disease, or cor pulmonale

f. Significance: depends on heart rate and symptoms (> 180 beats/minute may result in decreased CO with hypotension and ischemia)

g. Treatment: may include vagal stimulation by the physician only (carotid massage or Valsalva's maneuver); drugs (IV adenosine [Adenocard], verapamil [Calan], diltiazem [Cardizem], digoxin [Lanoxin]; or [especially in those with Wolff-Parkinson-White syndrome or recurrent SVT]), radiofrequency catheter ablation (destroying of an accessory pathway) may be performed.

6. ATRIAL FLUTTER (SEE FIGURE 4-8)

a. Rate: atrial: 350–600 beats/minute; ventricular at < 100 beats/minute is considered "controlled" but > 100 beats/minute is "uncontrolled" (both are often irregular).

b. P wave: sawtooth, and more P waves than QRS complexes

c. PR interval: not measurable

d. QRS complex: usually normal

e. Possible causes: coronary artery disease, hypertension, mitral valve disorders, cardiomyopathy, pulmonary embolus, cor pulmonale, and use of drugs such as digoxin (Lanoxin)

f. Significance: if ventricular rate is consistently high, may result in decreased cardiac output, including hypotension, angina, heart failure. The client is at increased risk for

embolized clot from the heart to the brain, causing a stroke.

g. Treatment: depends on heart rate and clinical manifestations. Cardioversion may be attempted to convert the client to normal sinus rhythm using synchronized electrical cardioversion, chemical cardioversion with IV ibutilide (Corvert), or radiofrequency catheter ablation. Drugs such as verapamil (Calan), diltiazem (Cardizem), and digoxin (Lanoxin) may be used on a long-term basis. Blood thinners such as warfarin (Coumadin) may be indicated to prevent clots.

7. ATRIAL FIBRILLATION (SEE FIGURE 4-9)

a. Rate: atrial 350–600 beats/minute and irregular; ventricular > 100 beats/minute is considered "controlled" but > 100 beats/minute is "uncontrolled" (both are often irregular).

b. P wave: chaotic, atrial activity with no distinguishable P wave

c. PR interval: not measurable

d. QRS complex: usually normal

e. Possible causes: usually underlying heart disease, also in alcoholism, infection, stress

f. Significance: if the ventricular rate is consistently high, may result in decreased cardiac output, hypotension, angina, heart failure. Client has increased risk for embolized clot from the heart to the brain, causing a stroke.

g. Treatment: depends on heart rate and clinical manifestations. Cardioversion may be attempted to convert the client to normal sinus rhythm using synchronized electrical cardioversion, chemical cardioversion with IV ibutilide (Corvert), or radiofrequency catheter ablation. Drugs such as verapamil (Calan), diltiazem (Cardizem), amiodarone (Cordarone), and digoxin (Lanoxin) may be used on a long-term basis. Blood thinners such as warfarin

Figure 4-9 Atrial fibrillation

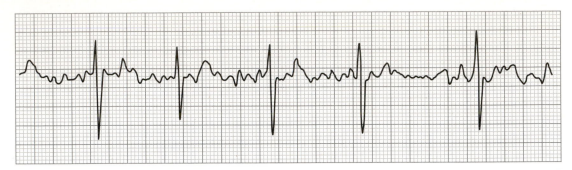

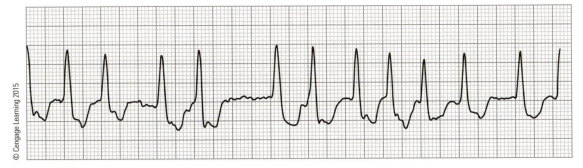

© Cengage Learning 2015

(Coumadin) may be indicated to prevent clots. Dabigatran etexilate (Pradaxa) anticoagulant given to reduce the risk of stroke and systemic embolism in nonvascular atrial fibrillation.

8. JUNCTIONAL RHYTHMS (JUNCTIONAL ESCAPE, ACCELERATED JUNCTIONAL, AND JUNCTIONAL TACHYCARDIA) (SEE FIGURE 4-10)
   a. Rate: 40–140 beats/minute and regular (originates in the A-V node)
   b. P wave: abnormal (may be before QRS or hidden)
   c. PR interval: variable
   d. QRS complex: usually normal
   e. Possible causes: may be normal in athletes with sinus bradycardia, or occur with acute MI or dysfunctional S-A node. Accelerated junctional rhythm may be seen in inferior MI, digoxin toxicity, acute rheumatic fever, and during open heart surgery.
   f. Significance: depends on heart rate and clinical manifestations
   g. Treatment: junctional escape rhythms should not be suppressed (atropine may be given in symptomatic clients to stimulate the S-A node); if digoxin (Lanoxin) toxicity is suspect, level should be drawn and digoxin held.

9. FIRST-DEGREE HEART BLOCK (SEE FIGURE 4-11)
   a. Rate: 60–100 and regular (but impulse is delayed in the A-V node)
   b. P wave: normal
   c. PR interval: > 0.20 second
   d. QRS complex: normal
   e. Possible causes: MI, ischemic heart disease, rheumatic fever, hyperthyroidism, drugs such as digoxin and beta blockers
   f. Significance: may lead to higher degrees of blocks
   g. Treatment: digoxin (Lanoxin) serum level

10. SECOND-DEGREE HEART BLOCK, TYPE I (WENCKEBACH) (SEE FIGURE 4-12)
    a. Rate: atrial is normal and regular but ventricular is slower and irregular.
    b. P wave: normal
    c. PR interval: progressively lengthens
    d. QRS complex: normal, except after the longest PR interval, a single QRS is dropped
    e. Possible causes: MI, ischemic heart disease, or drugs that slow the heart
    f. Significance: often transient after an MI but may be a warning sign of worsening block
    g. Treatment: usually none. If the client is symptomatic, atropine may be given; a temporary or permanent pacemaker may be placed.

11. SECOND-DEGREE HEART BLOCK, TYPE II (MOBITZ) (SEE FIGURE 4-13)
    a. Rate: usually normal (may be irregular)
    b. P wave: occurs in multiples

Figure 4-10 (A) Junctional escape rhythms; (B) accelerated junctional rhythm; (C) junctional tachycardia

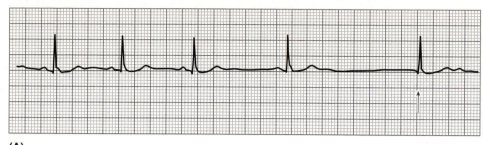

(A)

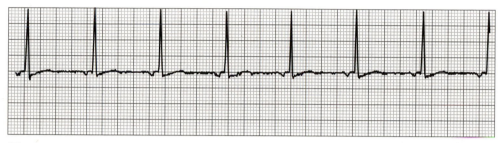

(B)

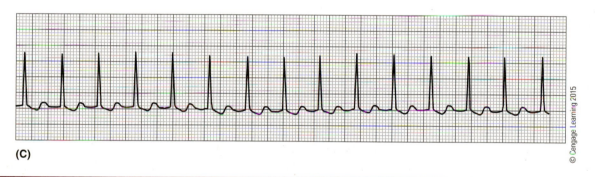

(C)

Figure 4-11 First-degree heart block

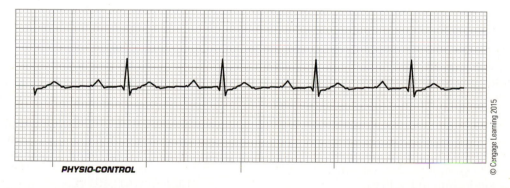

PHYSIO-CONTROL

c. PR interval: normal or prolonged
d. QRS complex: widened, preceded by
> 1 P wave
e. Possible causes: MI, rheumatic and
atherosclerotic heart disease, digoxin
toxicity
f. Significance: may lower cardiac output
and may progress to third-degree block

g. Treatment: permanent pacemaker
(temporary pacemaker in emergencies);
drugs to increase heart rate may
be tried until the pacemaker is
placed, including atropine,
epinephrine (Adrenalin Chloride),
or dopamine (dopamine
hydrochloride).

Figure 4-12 Second-degree heart block, type I Wenckebach

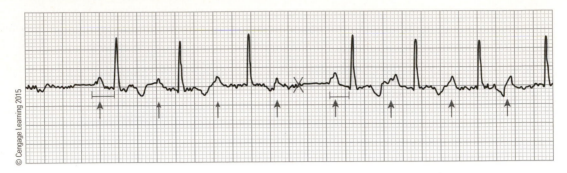

Figure 4-13 Second-degree heart block, type II Mobitz

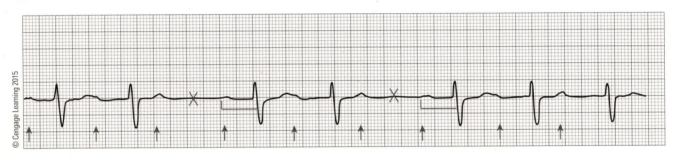

Figure 4-14 Third-degree heart block

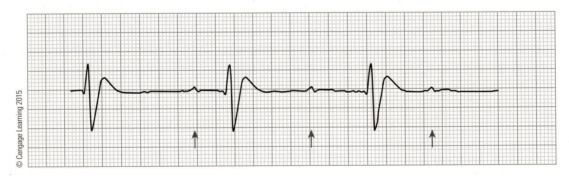

12. THIRD-DEGREE HEART BLOCK (SEE FIGURE 4-14)
    a. Rate: ventricular rate is 20–40 beats/minute and regular (originates in ventricles).
    b. P wave: normal, but not connected with QRS complex
    c. PR interval: varies
    d. QRS complex: often widened, no connection to P waves
    e. Possible causes: calcification of cardiac conduction system, heart disease, cardiomyopathy, myocarditis, open heart surgery
    f. Significance: decreased cardiac output (hypotension, syncope, angina, and decreased level of consciousness possible)
    g. Treatment: emergency temporary or permanent pacemaker drugs to increase heart rate (epinephrine [Adrenaline Chloride], and dopamine [dopamine hydrochloride]), may be tried while waiting for a pacemaker; cardiopulmonary resuscitation (CPR) may be required for very low rates and poor cardiac output.

13. PREMATURE VENTRICULAR CONTRACTIONS (PVCS) (SEE FIGURE 4-15)
    a. Rate: varies; irregular, due to premature beats
    b. P wave: may occur any time relative to a PVC
    c. PR interval: not measurable
    d. QRS: wide and abnormal (>0.12)

Figure 4-15 Premature ventricular contractions

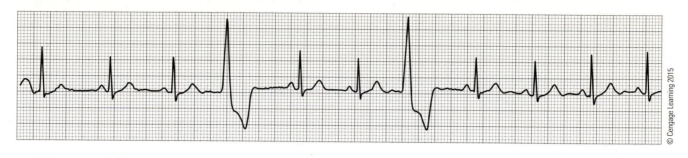

© Cengage Learning 2015

Figure 4-16 Ventricular tachycardia

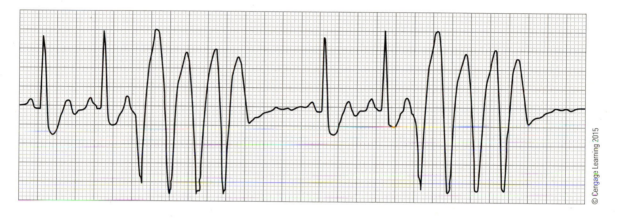

© Cengage Learning 2015

e. Possible causes: age, hypokalemia, hypoxia, fever, exercise, stress, MI, congestive heart failure (CHF), as well as stimulants (caffeine, alcohol, nicotine)

f. Significance: depends on frequency or number of PVCs. Frequent PVCs may proceed ventricular tachycardia or fibrillation. Isolated PVCs are usually asymptomatic.

g. Treatment: address possible cause (remove stimulants or treat hypokalemia or fever); drugs may include IV or PO amiodarone (Cordarone) or lidocaine (Xylocaine HCl).

14. VENTRICULAR TACHYCARDIA (GREATER THAN OR EQUAL TO THREE PVCS IN A ROW) (SEE FIGURE 4-16)

a. Rate: 120–180 beats/minute and usually quite regular

b. P wave: not usually visible due to being hidden in QRS complex; dissociation with A-V node

c. PR interval: not measurable

d. QRS complex: wide and distorted

e. Possible causes: acute MI, coronary artery disease, potassium imbalance, cardiomyopathy, mitral valve prolapse, prolonged QT (from medications)

f. Significance: may be asymptomatic if unsustained (< 30 seconds). If

sustained, decreased cardiac output will eventually occur (possible hypotension, dyspnea, angina, decreased level of consciousness). May proceed to ventricular fibrillation

g. Treatment: amiodarone or lidocaine IV if the client has a pulse with this rhythm. If the client has no pulse, CPR should be initiated and immediate synchronized electrical cardioversion is indicated. Drugs for pulseless ventricular tachycardia also include epinephrine (Adrenalin Chloride).

15. VENTRICULAR FIBRILLATION (SEE FIGURE 4-17)

a. Rate: not measurable, irregular

b. P wave: not present

c. PR interval: not present

d. QRS interval: not measurable

e. Possible causes: acute MI, ischemia, cardiomyopathy, catheter stimulation of ventricle, electrical shock, hyperkalemia, hypoxemia

f. Significance: absolute loss of any cardiac output (so no pulse), resulting in apnea and seizures

g. Treatment: immediate CPR, nonsynchronized defibrillation, epinephrine (Adrenalin Chloride), and amiodarone

Figure 4-17 Ventricular fibrillation

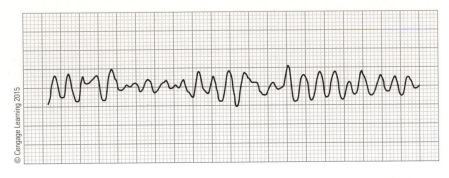

© Cengage Learning 2015

Figure 4-18 Asystole

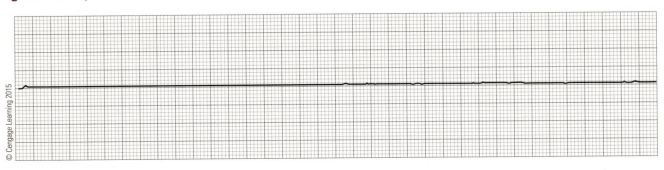

© Cengage Learning 2015

16. ASYSTOLE (SEE FIGURE 4-18)
   a. Rate: no ventricular beats
   b. P wave: if present, not followed by QRS
   c. PR interval: if present, not measurable due to no QRS
   d. QRS interval: absent
   e. Possible causes: hypoxia, hyperkalemia, hypokalemia, preexisting acidosis, drug overdose, hypothermia
   f. Significance: no cardiac output with this lethal rhythm
   g. Treatment: confirm unresponsiveness and verify asystole in more than one lead to confirm that "flatline" is not merely due to a lead being pulled off the client's chest, CPR, intubation, IV access, epinephrine (Adrenalin Chloride) and atropine.

III. DIAGNOSTIC STUDIES AND TREATMENT PROCEDURES
   A. LABORATORY TESTS (SEE TABLE 4-3)
   B. CARDIAC MONITORING: ELECTROCARDIOGRAM (ECG)
      1. DESCRIPTION
         a. Tracing of the electrical activity of the heart detected on the body surface
         b. Helpful in detecting cardiac dysrhythmias, cardiac ischemia, MI, and many other conditions
      2. PREPROCEDURE
         a. Inform the client that no discomfort is experienced.
         b. Apply patches to clean, dry skin (avoid hair if possible) with careful placement to ensure accuracy.
         c. Instruct the client to remain motionless (muscle activity may cause interference referred to as artifact).
      3. POSTPROCEDURE
         a. Remove patches gently from the client's skin.
   C. HOLTER MONITOR
      1. DESCRIPTION: RECORDING OF ECG RHYTHM FOR 24–48 HOURS ON AN OUTPATIENT BASIS
      2. PREPROCEDURE
         a. Prepare clean, dry skin and apply electrodes.
         b. Inform the client that the skin may be irritated by electrodes.
         c. Instruct the client to avoid bath or shower during monitoring.
         d. Stress the importance of keeping an accurate diary of clinical manifestations and activities (which can be correlated with any abnormal rhythms upon review of monitor's memory).

Table 4-3 Common Cardiac Laboratory Tests

Test	Significance
Creatinine Kinase (CK) CK-MB (Myocardial Bands) Troponin	CK: elevated after any striated muscle damage CK-MB and troponin: elevated after cardiac muscle damage (used for ruling out myocardial infarction)
Cholesterol	Blood lipid Elevation is a cardiovascular (CV) risk factor.
Triglycerides	Fatty acids Elevation is a CV risk factor.
Lipoproteins (HDL, LDL)	Specific breakdown helpful for determining CV risk factor
Potassium, Magnesium	Electrolytes; high or low levels may interfere with cardiac rhythm.
Heparin level (currently more commonly used)	Evaluates coagulation sequence
Partial Thromboplastin Time (PTT)	Heparin level guides appropriate IV dosing for heparin.
International Normalized Ratio (INR) (currently more commonly used)	Evaluates coagulation sequence
Prothrombin Time (PT)	Elevated level desired to prevent clots for those at risk Normal level required before the client has invasive procedure (to prevent bleeding)
Hemoglobin (Hgb)	Needed to transport oxygen to cells and remove carbon dioxide Decreased level may exacerbate angina
C-reactive Protein	(Inflammatory marker) elevation may indicate increased risk for plaque rupture
Homocysteine	Elevation may be a CV risk factor.
Sodium (Na^+)	Decrease may indicate fluid overload in heart failure.
Hemoglobin A1C	Evaluates average of blood glucose level from the past several weeks Elevations may indicate poor diabetes control, which is a risk factor for CV.
White Blood Count (WBC)	Elevation may indicate infection (bacterial endocarditis); commonly elevated after an MI
Medication Levels (digoxin, quinidine)	Evaluates therapeutic drug levels Subtherapeutic or excessive levels may necessitate change of dosing.
Calcium (Ca^+)	Elevation may shorten QT interval and cause cardiac dysrhythmias.

© Cengage Learning 2015

D. CHEST X-RAY
  1. DESCRIPTION: X-RAY VISUALIZATION TO EXAMINE LUNG FIELDS, SIZE OF THE HEART, AND ANY FLUID AROUND THE HEART
  2. PREPROCEDURE
    a. Inquire about frequency of recent x-rays and possibility of being pregnant.
    b. Provide lead shield for the part of the body not being viewed.
    c. Remove any obstructing metal or jewelry.
E. EXERCISE TREADMILL TEST (GRADED EXERCISE TEST OR GXT)
  1. DESCRIPTION: CLIENT WALKS ON A TREADMILL OR RIDES AN EXERCISE BIKE WHILE BEING MONITORED FOR ECG RHYTHMS AND VITAL SIGNS IN ORDER TO ASSESS FOR CORONARY ARTERY DISEASE (CAD) OR LEFT VENTRICULAR FUNCTION (LVF).
  2. PREPROCEDURE
    a. Instruct the client to wear walking shoes.
    b. Place electrode patches in an accurate position on clean, dry skin.
  3. POSTPROCEDURE
    a. Assess that the client's vital signs and ECG rhythm have returned to normal and that no symptoms of dyspnea, angina, or dizziness remain.
F. ECHOCARDIOGRAM
  1. DESCRIPTION: ULTRASOUND WAVES PICKED UP BY A TRANSDUCER PLACED ON DIFFERENT POSITIONS OVER THE CHEST WALL TO ASSESS FLOW OF BLOOD, CONGENITAL HEART DEFECTS; ESTIMATES LEFT VENTRICULAR FUNCTION
  2. PREPROCEDURE
    a. No contraindications
    b. Place the client on the left side, facing the equipment.

G. STRESS ECHOCARDIOGRAM
1. DESCRIPTION: COMBINATION EXERCISE TREADMILL AND ECHOCARDIOGRAM TO COMPARE RESTING IMAGES WITH IMMEDIATE POSTEXERCISE TO ASSESS FOR CHANGE IN LEFT VENTRICULAR WALL MOTION AND THICKENING
2. PREPROCEDURE
   a. Assess that the client is able to reach peak exercise (e.g., no foot ulcers).
   b. Inform the client of the importance of returning quickly to the exam table for immediate imaging after exercise.
3. POSTPROCEDURE
   a. Assess that the client has returned to baseline vitals signs, with no dyspnea or angina.

H. TRANSESOPHAGEAL ECHOCARDIOGRAM (TEE)
1. DESCRIPTION
   a. A probe with a transducer tip is swallowed by the client.
   b. Visualization for valvular abnormalities, possible thrombus, bacterial endocarditis, congenital heart defects
2. PREPROCEDURE
   a. NPO at least 6 hours before the test
   b. Local anesthetic, but IV sedation is used so a designated driver needs to take the client home.
   c. Instruct the client that the procedure lasts about 15 minutes.
3. POSTPROCEDURE
   a. Suction may be needed for oral secretions.
   b. Monitor the vital signs and oxygen saturation (client may need O_2 due to sedation).
   c. Observe for esophageal perforation, dysrhythmias, vasovagal reactions.
   d. Verify that the client's gag reflex is intact before offering lukewarm fluid/foods.

I. NUCLEAR CARDIOLOGY: THALLIUM
1. DESCRIPTION:
   a. Thallium (a radioactive isotope) is injected IV so that the scintillation camera can count radioactive uptake (areas of poor uptake indicate infarction).
   b. Useful for assessing the extent of disease in a coronary artery and predict the effectiveness of bypass surgery or angioplasty
2. PREPROCEDURE
   a. Start the IV line.
   b. Inform the client that an isotope is used only in a small diagnostic amount and will lose radioactivity in a few hours.
   c. For stress tests, thallium is injected 1 hour before the client exercises, 5–10 minutes after, and then after 2–4 hours.

d. Client should eat only a light meal during injection and testing period.
   e. Inform the client that the arms will be extended behind the head in a supine position.
3. POSTPROCEDURE
   a. Monitor vital signs.
   b. Assess for dyspnea or angina.

J. NUCLEAR CARDIOLOGY: DIPYRIDAMOLE THALLIUM
1. DESCRIPTION
   a. Dipyridamole (Persantine) is injected to vasodilate coronary arteries so increased blood flow will make scanning with thallium more effective.
   b. Used when the client is unable to tolerate exercise such as with severe peripheral vascular disease
2. PREPROCEDURE
   a. Instruct the client to hold all caffeine products for 12 hours in advance.
   b. Instruct the client on the purpose of dipyridamole (Persantine).
3. POSTPROCEDURE
   a. Monitor the vital signs.
   b. Assess for dyspnea or angina.

K. NUCLEAR CARDIOLOGY: TECHNETIUM OR SESTAMBI SCAN
1. DESCRIPTION
   a. IV injection of this isotope
   b. High uptake will be visualized in areas of MI (even 1–6 days post-MI).
2. PREPROCEDURE (SEE THALLIUM.)

L. CARDIAC CATHETERIZATION, CORONARY ANGIOGRAM, AND PERCUTANEOUS CORONARY INTERVENTION (PCI)
1. DESCRIPTION
   a. Insertion of a catheter into the heart via a vein (for the right side of the heart) or femoral or brachial artery (for the left side of the heart)
   b. Useful for obtaining measurement of ventricular function and diagnoses of coronary artery disease
   c. In a coronary angiogram, dye can be injected to provide further assessment of structure and motion of the heart.
   d. In a percutaneous coronary intervention (PCI), an attempt to correct the blockage in the artery can be made.
      1) Angioplasty: blocked area of an artery is "ballooned" open, with plaque left pressed around the walls of the artery
      2) Angioplasty with stent: after blockage is "ballooned," a mesh stent is left in place to help support the walls of the vessel to stay open.
      3) Atherectomy: plaque is "shaved" off by rotating blade.

2. PREPROCEDURE
   a. NPO 6–18 hours
   b. Verify written consent.
   c. Assess that laboratory values are within range.
   d. Review the client's allergies and creatinine (dye allergy is possible for those allergic to shellfish; dye may be harmful to the kidneys for those with elevated creatinine or diabetes mellitus).
   e. Inform the client that sedation will be given and a local anesthetic will be administered at the catheter entry site, and a feeling of warmth and fluttering of the heart may be experienced as the catheter is passed.
   f. Instruct the client to inhale when the catheter is inserted.
   g. Attach the ECG leads and monitor the client during the 1- to 2-hour procedure.

3. POSTPROCEDURE
   a. Observe the insertion site for overt bleeding or hematoma (bleeding beneath skin).
   b. Instruct the client to call immediately if there are signs of bleeding from the insertion site.
   c. If bleeding or hematoma occurs, hold firm pressure with three fingers just above the insertion site.
   d. Monitor ECG and vital signs.
   e. Assess the extremities for peripheral pulses, color, temperature, sensation every 15 minutes times 4, then with decreased frequency.
   f. Instruct the client on duration of bed rest (from 2–6 hours, depending on if the vein or artery was used, and if a closure device was used after sheath pull).
   g. Encourage fluids to promote excretion of the dye.
   h. After angioplasty with stent, ask the client to take clopidogrel (Plavix) temporarily to reduce platelet aggregation around the new stent.
   i. Complications may include: breakage of the tip of the catheter; blood loss; allergic reaction to dye; air or blood embolism; dysrhythmia; MI; cerebrovascular accident (CVA); punctured ventricle, septum, or lung tissue; and, rarely, death.

M. INTRACORONARY ULTRASOUND
   1. DESCRIPTION
   a. Tiny ultrasound probe inserted into the coronary artery
   b. Provides evaluation for plaque size and consistency, artery walls, and effectiveness of treatment
   2. PREPROCEDURE
   a. Same as for Cardiac Catheterization, Coronary Angiogram, and Percutaneous Coronary Intervention (PCI)
   3. POSTPROCEDURE
   a. Same as for Cardiac Catheterization, Coronary Angiogram, and Percutaneous Coronary Intervention (PCI)

N. ELECTROPHYSIOLOGY STUDY (EPS)
   1. DESCRIPTION: INVASIVE STUDY TO ASSESS THE ELECTRICAL ACTIVITY OF THE HEART USING CATHETERS INSERTED VIA THE VEINS TO THE RIGHT SIDE OF THE HEART
   2. PREPROCEDURE
   a. Verify written consent.
   b. Assess that laboratory values are within normal range.
   c. Antidysrhythmic medications may be stopped by the physician several days before the procedure.
   d. NPO 6–8 hours before
   e. Sedation as ordered
   f. Continuous ECG monitoring
   3. POSTPROCEDURE
   a. Same as for Cardiac Catheterization, Coronary Angiogram, and Percutaneous Coronary Intervention (PCI), except no dye is used

O. HEMODYNAMIC MONITORING
   1. DESCRIPTION:
   a. Invasive monitoring done at the hospital bedside to assess pressures of CV system using intra-arterial and pulmonary artery catheters
   b. Central venous pressure (CVP) measures right atrium pressure (preload) and can be used as a guide for overhydration or underhydration.
   c. Provides information about arterial blood pressure, intracardiac pressures, cardiac output

P. PACEMAKER
   1. DESCRIPTION:
   a. Medical device that takes over the function of a client's nonfunctioning S-A node or A-V node
      1) Indications include treatment for bradycardias, heart blocks.
      2) New use includes treatment for tachycardic rhythms, with overdrive pacing capabilities to pace faster than tachycardic rhythm, in order to reset and slow it.
      3) Newest uses include treatment for vasovagal syncope, hypertrophic cardiomyopathy, and heart failure.
      4) Automatic implantable cardioverter defibrillator
   b. May be temporary (placed during an emergency or during open heart surgery) with the energy source outside the body. Wires are threaded

transvenously to stimulate the muscle of the right ventricle.

  c. May be permanent, with the battery surgically implanted under a pocket of skin in the chest wall. Battery is attached to pacer electrodes, threaded transvenously to the endocardium of the right ventricle or atrium.

2. PREPROCEDURE

  a. NPO for several hours prior to the procedure

  b. Fit the client for a sling to be worn immediately after surgery on the side of the pacemaker to prevent the client from abducting the arm away from the body and possibly dislodging the position of electrodes on the myocardium.

  c. Assess that preoperative laboratory values are within parameters.

3. POSTPROCEDURE

  a. Continuous ECG monitoring to make sure the pacemaker is functioning appropriately

    1) Parameters and low limit of the pacemaker should be known by the nurse, who then ascertains that it is functioning within limits ("failure to sense" occurs if the pacemaker fires inappropriately while the client's own rhythm is functioning within limits).

    2) Each spike on the ECG strip represents an electrical charge to the myocardium from the pacemaker and should be followed by the appropriate atrial or ventricular contraction ("failure to capture" occurs if spike is not followed by contraction).

    3) Premature ventricular contractions (PVCs) may occur if the electrode has moved from the original surgical placement.

  b. IV antibiotics are often given prophylactically before and after the procedure.

  c. Chest x-ray is obtained after placement to verify lead placement and rule out pneumothorax.

  d. Insertion site is checked for swelling or bleeding, discharge, or redness.

  e. Instruct the client before discharge regarding the following:

    1) Monitor for signs of infection (temperature, discharge, redness).

    2) Encourage compliance with ordered activity restrictions, including avoiding abduction of the operative side above the shoulder level until the electrode

adheres to the heart (up to 3–4 weeks).

    3) Encourage avoiding close proximity to high-output electrical generators, running engines, or magnets such as magnetic resonance imaging (MRI); no need to avoid microwave ovens.

    4) Instruct the client on how to take her pulse, and call the physician if it is not within a specified range.

    5) Encourage the client to keep the pacemaker identification card in the wallet.

    6) Instruct the client on the importance of follow-up checks with the clinic, some of which may be done over the telephone with a borrowed transmitter device.

Q. CORONARY ARTERY BYPASS GRAFT SURGERY (CABG)

1. DESCRIPTION

  a. Surgical placement of new conduits to provide coronary artery blood flow when existing coronary arteries are not patent (not open)

  b. Often the saphenous vein and left internal mammary artery are used.

  c. May be done with or without cardiopulmonary bypass pump and stopping of the heart

2. PREPROCEDURE

  a. Tour the client and family through the intensive care unit (ICU) and waiting room.

  b. Inform the client that memories from preanesthesia and the operating room preanesthesia may occur after surgery.

  c. Inform the client that the alarms may be noisy in the ICU.

  d. Discuss the purpose of the ECG leads and arterial lines for blood pressure monitoring, urinary catheter for drainage, and chest tubes with bloody drainage for preventing fluid buildup in the chest.

  e. A pen and paper may be used to communicate while endotracheal tube does not permit speech. The tube may be removed within hours after surgery.

  f. Have the client practice using the incentive spirometer.

  g. Instruct the client to ask for pain medication, and to splint the chest incision while coughing and moving.

  h. Inform the client that anorexia may be experienced for a few weeks.

  i. Discuss how depression is common among those recovering from CABG surgery and when to seek help for this.

j. Introduce cardiac rehabilitation activities and support groups.

k. Assess baseline data.

  1) Echocardiogram, angiography, chest x-ray, ECG

  2) Laboratory work, including coagulation times (clients on warfarin [Coumadin] need to discontinue this medication prior to surgery to avoid bleeding complications)

  3) Availability of cross-matched blood for transfusions, if needed, in addition to blood cell savers that recycle the client's own blood during surgery

3. POSTPROCEDURE (SEE TABLE 4-4)

  a. Transport by at least two nurses and an anesthesiologist to assist in bringing the client from surgery directly to the ICU on the bed

  b. Monitor ECG, hemodynamic and oxygen saturation readings, and chest tube output (sudden increase in chest tube drainage greater than 150 ml an hour may indicate abnormal bleeding), nasogastric tube may be used.

  c. Suction the client while on ventilator, obtain ABGs, and attempt to wean off the ventilator.

d. Obtain frequent vital signs for the first 4 hours.

e. Check peripheral pulses and extremity warmth every 1–2 hours.

f. Assist the client to turn from side to side, splint chest incision, use incentive spirometer, and to ambulate early to prevent complications of prolonged bed rest.

g. Assess the chest and any donor site incisions.

h. Discuss discharge plans with the client and family (hospital stay 4–6 days).

R. PERIPHERAL ARTERIOGRAPHY AND VENOGRAPHY

  1. DESCRIPTION

    a. Injection of radiopaque dye to check the patency of arteries or veins in the extremities (usually the legs)

    b. Serial x-rays done to assess for occlusion, atherosclerotic plaques, aneurysms, or traumatic injury

  2. PREPROCEDURE

    a. Assess for allergy to dye or shellfish, or elevated creatinine (which may allow damage to kidneys from the dye).

    b. Assess baseline peripheral pulses.

  3. POSTPROCEDURE

    a. Observe the insertion site for bleeding, hematoma.

Table 4-4 Nursing Care: Complications After Open Heart Surgery

Complication	Assessment	Intervention
Low cardiac output	Hypotension, low urine output, cool extremities, larger-than-normal blood loss	IV crystalloids or colloids, RBCs (for fluid deficit) Diuretics, inotropic drugs, vasopressor drugs
Cardiac tamponade	Decreased chest tube output and muffled heart sounds, pulsus paradoxus	Clot may need to be removed from the chest tube or the chest tube may need to be changed. If no chest tube, pericardiocentesis (removal of fluid by aspiration) Client may need to return to surgery.
Dysrhythmias	Frequent PVCs Atrial fibrillation Bradycardic rhythms	Treat serum potassium imbalance. Verify catheter placement is correct in the heart. Antidysrhythmic drugs Use of temporary pacer wires placed during surgery to pace low heart rate and overdrive pace tachycardic rhythms
Emboli	Dyspnea, faintness, positive lung scans Most common on the third day post-op, especially with those who used saphenous (leg) vein graft	Anticoagulant therapy Observe for neurologic changes (cerebral emboli).
Fever	Elevated temperature	Blood, urine cultures Antibiotic therapy
Intraoperative myocardial infarction	ECG changes post-op Unusually elevated cardiac markers	Monitor oxygen saturation. (See myocardial infarction section.)

b. Hold firm pressure with three fingers directly above the site if bleeding or hematoma occurs.

c. Monitor ECG and vital signs.

d. Assess the extremities for peripheral pulses, color, temperature, sensation every 15 minutes times 4, then with decreased frequency.

e. Instruct the client on bed rest.

f. Encourage fluids to dilute the dye and promote excretion.

g. Complications can include: breakage of the tip of the catheter; blood loss; allergic reaction to dye; air or blood embolism; dysrhythmias; MI; CVA; punctured ventricle, septum, or lung tissue; and, rarely, death.

IV. NURSING DIAGNOSES

A. INEFFECTIVE TISSUE PERFUSION: CARDIOPULMONARY

B. DECREASED CARDIAC OUTPUT

C. RISK FOR ACTIVITY INTOLERANCE

D. ACUTE PAIN

E. ANXIETY

Nursing Diagnoses: Definitions and Classification 2012–2014. Copyright © 2012, 1994–2012 by NANDA International. Used by arrangement with John Wiley & Sons Limited.

V. CARDIOVASCULAR DISEASES

A. VENTRICULAR SEPTAL DEFECT (VSD)

1. DESCRIPTION

a. Congenital opening in the septum that allows blood to flow between the right and left ventricles

b. Associated with Down's syndrome, renal anomalies, prematurity, fetal alcohol syndrome

c. May result from myocardial infarction

2. ASSESSMENT

a. Early clinical manifestations: failure to thrive, loud systolic murmur and palpable thrill, tachycardia, grunting respirations

b. Some adults may be undiagnosed and asymptomatic but are at increased risk for CVA.

3. DIAGNOSTIC TESTS

a. Chest x-ray, ECG, echocardiogram, cardiac catheterization, laboratory tests

4. NURSING INTERVENTIONS

a. Administer oxygen.

b. Administer drugs.

c. Promote good nutrition.

d. Encourage rest.

e. Treat presenting clinical manifestations.

5. SURGICAL MANAGEMENT

a. Open heart repair of the septum

b. Recent angiogram procedure allows for balloon closure of opening

B. RHEUMATIC FEVER AND HEART DISEASE

1. DESCRIPTION

a. Rheumatic fever is a systemic inflammatory disease occurring primarily in young adults.

b. For some, it may lead to heart, joint, central nervous system (CNS), or skin involvement.

c. Caused by group A streptococcal upper airway infection

d. Infection usually occurs 2–3 weeks before cardiac symptoms.

2. ASSESSMENT

a. Carditis: murmurs, enlargement and heart failure, pericarditis

b. Polyarthritis: temporary inflammation of the joints

c. Chorea: weakness, ataxia

3. DIAGNOSTIC TESTS

a. Lab tests include: throat culture, serum antistreptolysin titer, as well as erythrocyte sedimentation rate and C-reactive protein for nonspecific systemic inflammatory response.

b. Echocardiogram may show valvular insufficiency and pericardial fluid or thickening.

c. Chest x-ray may show heart failure.

4. NURSING INTERVENTIONS

a. Bed rest during acute clinical manifestations

b. Administer antibiotics (usually penicillin).

c. Administer salicylates and corticosteroids as anti-inflammatory agents for fever and joint pain.

d. Encourage the client to seek prompt medical attention for sore throat, which could be streptococcal.

e. Encourage good nutrition, hygienic practices, and rest to reduce rheumatic fever outbreaks.

f. Provide additional prophylaxis for dental or surgical procedures to prevent recurrence of rheumatic fever.

g. Instruct the client to seek medical attention if clinical manifestations such as excessive fatigue, dizziness, palpitations, or dyspnea with activity develop (signs of valvular heart disease).

5. SURGICAL MANAGEMENT (FOR CLIENTS WHO DEVELOP VALVULAR HEART DISEASE)

a. Valvuloplasty: balloon is passed through the femoral vein or artery to dilate the stenotic mitral or aortic valve.

b. Commisurotomy: during open heart surgery, the surgeon cuts out calcium from the commissures (leaflets) to widen valve opening.

c. Valve replacement: prosthetic (synthetic) or biologic (from a pig or cow) valves are used to surgically replace the defective valve.

C. VALVULAR HEART DISEASE
1. DESCRIPTION
   a. Mechanical disruption of blood flow due to either:
      1) Stenosis: narrowing of valve opening, which does not allow for sufficient opening and leads to decrease ventricular filling (AV valves) and decreased ventricular ejection (semilunar valves)
      2) Regurgitation (also called valvular insufficiency): incomplete closure of the valve leaflets, resulting in the backward flow of blood
   b. Contributing factors include: rheumatic heart disease, congenital causes, Marfan syndrome, hypertension, endocarditis, myocardial infarction, and gender (e.g., mitral valve prolapse is more common among women).
2. ASSESSMENT
   a. Clinical manifestations vary according to the type and severity of defect (some clients may be without clinical manifestations) (Table 4-5)
   b. Commonly occurring clinical manifestations are dyspnea, weakness, and fatigue.
3. DIAGNOSTIC TESTS
   a. Echocardiogram to evaluate valvular structure and function
   b. ECG
   c. Cardiac catheterization
   d. Chest x-ray
4. NURSING INTERVENTIONS
   a. Administer oxygen

b. Administer and instruct the client on the purpose of prescribed digoxin, anticoagulants, nitroglycerin, beta blockers, diuretics, vasodilators, and ACE inhibitors and possible side effects to report.
   c. Instruct the client on a low-sodium diet.
   d. Instruct the client on the need for prophylactic antibiotics prior to dental or surgical procedures to prevent bacterial endocarditis.
   e. Assist with cardioversion if needed.
5. SURGICAL MANAGEMENT
   a. Valvuloplasty
   b. Commisurotomy
   c. Valve replacement (for severe mitral or aortic valvular disease)
D. ENDOCARDITIS (INFECTIVE OR BACTERIAL)
1. DESCRIPTION
   a. Bacterial or fungal infection of the myocardium, heart valves, or prosthetic valves
   b. May result in vegetative growths on valves, endocardial lining, or blood vessels, which may interfere with valvular functioning
   c. Infectious vegetation may embolize to the kidneys, spleen, central nervous system, or lungs.
   d. Associated with IV drug used, prosthetic valves, mitral valve prolapse, rheumatic heart disease, congenital defects, or syphilis
2. ASSESSMENT
   a. Weakness, fatigue
   b. Weight loss
   c. Joint pain (arthralgia)
   d. Intermittent night sweats
   e. Loud murmur, possibly new murmur with fever

Table 4-5 Clinical Findings for Valvular Heart Disease

Valvular Disease	Clinical Finding
Mitral stenosis	Dyspnea, fatigue, atrial fibrillation, heart failure, loud S1, diastolic murmur
Mitral valve regurgitation (insufficiency)	Chronic: fatigue, weakness, dyspnea with activity, systolic murmur or thrill, or both Acute: pulmonary edema and shock
Mitral valve prolapse	Palpitations, dyspnea, angina, syncope (some clients are asymptomatic; occurs more often in women)
Aortic regurgitation (insufficiency)	Palpitations, angina, syncope, left-sided heart failure, visible apical pulse, soft S1 or presence of S3, possible systolic murmur at the left sternal border (some clients are chronic but asymptomatic for years, then present with dyspnea)
Aortic stenosis	Palpitations, angina, syncope, left-sided heart failure, decreased cardiac output, S4 (often discovered in youth)
Pulmonary stenosis	Syncope, angina, right-sided heart failure, systolic murmur at the left sternal border, split S2 (congenital; rare)

3. DIAGNOSTIC TESTS
   a. Positive blood cultures
   b. White blood cell count (WBC) may be normal or elevated.
   c. Echocardiogram (transesophageal is especially helpful)
4. NURSING INTERVENTIONS
   a. Administer antibiotics (penicillin, gentamycin [Garamycin]).
   b. Support bed rest during acute stage.
   c. Administer analgesics for aches.
   d. Monitor for adequate fluid intake.
5. SURGICAL MANAGEMENT
   a. Replacement of defective or vegetative heart valve may be needed.

E. MYOCARDITIS
   1. DESCRIPTION
      a. Inflammation of the myocardium (heart muscle)
      b. Often asymptomatic with a spontaneous recovery
      c. May occasionally result in cardiomyopathy and heart failure
      d. Causes include infection, immune reactions (rheumatic fever), radiation therapy, toxins, alcoholism.
   2. ASSESSMENT
      a. Fatigue, dyspnea
      b. Fever, mild chest soreness
      c. Tachycardia, palpitations (S3, S4 gallops)
      d. Mitral murmur and pericardial friction rub (scratchy sound over the intercostal space on the left chest)
      e. Heart failure (left or right)
   3. DIAGNOSTIC TESTS
      a. Elevated CK-MB, WBC, eosinophil sedimentation rate (ESR)
      b. Positive blood culture
      c. ECG
      d. Chest x-ray
      e. Echocardiogram
      f. Endomyocardial biopsy
   4. NURSING INTERVENTIONS
      a. Administer antibiotics and diuretics.
      b. Administer antipyretics and possibly antidysrhythmics and anticoagulants.
      c. Administer corticosteroids and immunosuppressants.
      d. Administer oxygen.
      e. Provide for rest.
   5. SURGICAL MANAGEMENT
      a. Often not necessary
      b. May include temporary pacemaker, cardiac assist devices, or transplantation

F. HYPERTENSION (HTN)
   1. DESCRIPTION
      a. An elevation of systolic or diastolic blood pressure of 140/90 mm Hg or greater is considered high (between 120/80 mm Hg and 139/89 mm Hg is considered prehypertension).
      b. Primary hypertension (essential HTN) is the most common.
      c. Secondary hypertension results from another source (such as renal failure).
      d. *Malignant hypertension* is the term for either primary or secondary hypertension that is severe.
      e. Major contributor to coronary artery disease (CAD), cerebrovascular accidents (CVAs), and renal failure
      f. Caused by increased blood viscosity or reduced lumen size of the vessels
         1) Arterial bed thickens
         2) Sympathetic nervous system increases
         3) Circulating blood volume increases due to renal or hormonal dysfunction
         4) Angiotensin II rises, resulting in constriction of vessels and increased circulating volume
      g. Hypertrophy results as the left ventricle attempts to keep up with increased workload and oxygen demands.
      h. End result of chronic hypertension is cardiac dilation; heart failure may develop when hypertrophy cannot maintain cardiac output.
      i. Promotes atherosclerosis, leading to angina and MI
      j. Contributes to peripheral vascular disease and kidney damage
   2. ASSESSMENT
      a. Diagnosis is based on at least two consecutive readings after initial screening.
      b. Occipital headache, blurred vision
      c. Fatigue
      d. Edema, nocturia
      e. Many clients are asymptomatic.
   3. DIAGNOSTIC TESTS
      a. Serial BP measurements
      b. Creatinine, BUN, K^+ (potassium) to check for kidney damage from untreated HTN
      c. Urinalysis to check for protein in the urine
      d. Complete blood count
   4. NURSING INTERVENTIONS
      a. Administer diuretics.
      b. Administer calcium-channel blockers.
      c. Administer angiotensin-converting enzyme (ACE) inhibitors.
      d. Administer alpha-receptor blockers and agonists.
      e. Administer beta blockers.
      f. Treat underlying cause such as secondary hypertension.

g. Instruct the client on lifestyle modification to decrease risk factors (weight, diet, stress).

h. Instruct the client that possible laboratory tests may be ordered to assess if potassium or magnesium supplements are needed due to a loss in the urine from diuretics.

G. AORTIC ANEURYSM

1. DESCRIPTION

a. Degenerative changes in the tunica media (muscular layer of the aorta) cause the aorta to stretch outward and "bulge."

b. Blood pulsating against the aneurysm weakens it further, potentially contributing to a hemorrhagic separation in the aortic wall.

c. A saccular aneurysm occurs when there is an outpouching of the arterial wall.

d. A fusiform aneurysm occurs when a spindle-shaped enlargement encompasses the entire aortic circumference.

e. A false aneurysm occurs when the entire wall is injured, with blood contained in surrounding tissue (a sac eventually forms and communicates with an artery or the heart).

2. ASSESSMENT

a. Ascending thoracic aneurysm: pain, difference in blood pressure between the left and right arms

b. Descending thoracic aneurysm: sudden pain between the shoulder blades radiating to the chest, dyspnea, hoarseness, dry cough

c. Abdominal aneurysm: pulsating mass in periumbilical area, systolic bruit over the aorta, lumbar pain radiating to the flank and groin (although clients may be asymptomatic)

d. Dissecting aneurysm: sudden "ripping" pain that may radiate to the chest, back, neck, or abdomen (may lead to blood loss, shock, and even death)

3. DIAGNOSTIC TESTS

a. Aortography

b. Echocardiogram (possibly transesophageal)

c. CT or MRI

d. ECG

e. Hemoglobin

f. X-rays

4. NURSING INTERVENTIONS

a. Administer antihypertensives.

b. Administer negative inotropic agents to reduce the contractile force of pressure on the arteries.

1) Administer oxygen.

2) Administer narcotics for pain.

3) Administer IV fluids and blood transfusions, if dissecting the aneurysm results in hypovolemic shock.

5. SURGICAL MANAGEMENT

a. Elective or emergency repair of the aneurysm may be necessary.

H. CORONARY ARTERY DISEASE (CAD)

1. DESCRIPTION

a. Accumulation of atherosclerotic (fatty, fibrous) plaque in the lumen of the coronary arteries results in decreased blood flow of oxygen and nutrients to the myocardial tissue.

b. Occurs more commonly among males and postmenopausal females and those with diabetes mellitus

c. Diseased arteries are altered so they cannot dilate and compensate for the blockage (lesion).

d. Ischemia develops (reversible change in the artery at the cellular and tissue levels), which indicates a lack of oxygen.

e. If untreated, myocardial infarction (MI) may result (irreversible damage to the myocardial tissue due to the myocardium switching from aerobic to anaerobic metabolism).

2. ASSESSMENT

a. Angina

b. Nausea and vomiting

c. Cool extremities

d. Older adults and clients with diabetes mellitus may be asymptomatic or experience only fatigue and exertional dyspnea.

3. DIAGNOSTIC TESTS

a. ECG

b. Exercise tests or nuclear imaging

c. Coronary angiography

d. Lipid profile

4. NURSING INTERVENTIONS

a. Administer nitrates, beta-adrenergic or calcium-channel blockers, antiplatelet, antilipemic, or antihypertensive drugs.

b. Instruct the client on lifestyle modification that may alter the effects of CAD (weight control, no smoking, consistent exercise, and a diet low in fat and sodium).

5. SURGICAL MANAGEMENT

a. Angioplasty ("ballooning" open of clogged artery)

b. Angioplasty with stent placement to keep newly opened artery patent

c. Atherectomy ("shaving" of plaque by a rotating blade)

d. Coronary artery bypass surgery (for those with left main coronary artery blockage, or > 2 vessel disease unresponsive to medical or angioplasty treatment), which uses the client's own saphenous vein from the leg, radial artery, or internal mammary artery as a graft to bypass blood supply from the aorta

I.   MYOCARDIAL INFARCTION (MI)
1. DESCRIPTION
   a. Irreversible cell damage (necrosis) of muscle tissue due to prolonged ischemia (20 minutes) of the coronary artery
   b. MI is defined by the location of the damage.
      1) Right coronary artery (RCA) occlusion results in inferior MI or right ventricular infarction.
      2) Left circumflex artery (CX) occlusion results in lateral wall infarction.
      3) Left anterior descending artery (LAD) results in anterior wall infarction.
   c. MI is defined by the extent of the damage.
      1) Q-wave (transmural) damage occurs when all layers of the myocardium are affected.
      2) Non-Q-wave (subendocardial) damage occurs only in the inner or middle layers of the myocardium.
   d. Result of damage
      1) Infarcted myocardial cells release cardiac enzymes into the bloodstream (CK-MB, troponin).
      2) Within 24 hours, the infarcted area becomes edematous and cyanotic.
      3) Within several days, leukocytes arrive and remove dead cells.
      4) By week 3, scar formation may inhibit contractility.
      5) Compensatory mechanisms (increased heart rate [HR], vascular constriction, renal retention of sodium and water) may be enabled by the body in an attempt to increase cardiac output.
   e. Ventricular dilation may occur due to the heart's remodeling process after MI.
2. ASSESSMENT
   a. Crushing substernal chest pain that may radiate to the left arm, jaw, neck, or shoulder blades
   b. Nausea and vomiting
   c. Cool extremities, diaphoresis, anxiety (due to release of catecholamines)
   d. Blood pressure and pulse elevated in early stage (due to activation of the sympathetic nervous system)
   e. Jugular vein distension
   f. Many older adults do not have common signs of chest pain, but rather dyspnea, fatigue, and syncope. Women and those with diabetes mellitus may experience dyspnea, back pain, or be asymptomatic.
3. DIAGNOSTIC TESTS
   a. Serial 12-lead ECGs: have previous ECG available to compare for changes (e.g., > 2 mm ST elevation in the chest leads)
   b. Serial cardiac enzymes (CK-MB, troponin)
   c. Echocardiogram
   d. Nuclear imaging
   e. Cardiac catheterization
4. NURSING INTERVENTIONS
   a. Immediate action within 10 minutes of the onset of clinical manifestations, as prompted by the acronym: "MONA greets every client" (morphine, oxygen, nitroglycerin, aspirin).
      1) Administer oxygen 2–3 L/minute.
      2) Administer nitroglycerin (if BP > 90 systolic and no use of sildenafil [Viagra] in the past 24 hours).
      3) Administer one aspirin (for antiplatelet effect, if no allergy or active bleeding or recent surgical intervention).
      4) Administer IV morphine.
   b. Continuous cardiac monitoring, as well as ECGs
   c. IV fibrinolytic (thrombolytic) therapy within 6 hours from the onset of clinical manifestations (if the client meets criteria)
   d. Administer IV or SQ heparin.
   e. Limit the client's physical activity for the first 12 hours upon gradual increase of activity; verify that the client is not exceeding the target rate.
   f. Administer beta blockers (to slow heart rate, reducing myocardial demand).
   g. Apply patches, if needed, for transcutaneous pacing or defibrillation as needed according to the rhythm.
   h. Administer appropriate drugs as needed according to the rhythm (atropine for slow, symptomatic rates; antidysrhythmics for symptomatic dysrhythmias).
   i. In the recovery stage of MI, the client may need cardiac rehabilitation, as well as education about drugs, taking own pulse, daily weights, reasons to call the physician. If clinical manifestations reoccur, the client should take one nitroglycerin tablet and if no relief, call 911.
   j. Offer the family availability of CPR classes, social and spiritual support.

k. Refer to the dietician for assistance in managing weight, lipids, diabetes, carbohydrates, and salt.

l. Refer to tobacco or other chemical substance intervention if needed.

5. SURGICAL MANAGEMENT

a. Immediate cardiac catheterization may be needed, with possible percutaneous intervention (e.g., percutaneous transluminal coronary angioplasty, or PTCA), possible stent placement, or other intervention.

b. CABG may be needed for multiple lesions (blockages) or left main coronary artery disease.

J. CARDIOMYOPATHY

1. DESCRIPTION

a. Decreased cardiac output due to damaged heart muscle is classified by type:

1) Dilated cardiomyopathy occurs when all four chambers are dilated due to loss of muscle tone from damaged fibers, such as from post-MI.

2) Hypertrophic cardiomyopathy occurs when there is asymmetrical thickening of the septum and left ventricular hypertrophy.

3) Restrictive cardiomyopathy occurs when ventricular filling is restricted due to left ventricular hypertrophy and endocardial thickening (end stage is irreversible).

b. Although often idiopathic, possible causes include: infection, hypertension, postpartum, heart disease (ischemic or valvular), drugs, alcohol, genetic trait, thyroid disease, amyloidosis, or sarcoidosis.

2. ASSESSMENT

a. Dyspnea, orthopnea

b. Peripheral edema, peripheral cyanosis

c. Fatigue, elevated liver enzymes

d. Murmurs, gallops

3. DIAGNOSTIC TESTS

a. ECG

b. Chest x-ray

c. Echocardiogram

d. Nuclear cardiology scans

4. NURSING INTERVENTIONS

a. Treat the underlying cause.

b. Administer ACE inhibitors, diuretics, digoxin, isorbide, beta blockers, antidysrhythmics, anticoagulants as indicated.

c. Instruct the client on lifestyle modification and management of clinical manifestations.

5. SURGICAL MANAGEMENT

a. Cardioversion if uncontrolled atrial fibrillation

b. Pacemaker

c. Revascularization (angioplasty, CABG)

d. Ablation (purposeful damaging) of the A-V node and implant of a dual-chamber pacemaker

e. Mitral valve replacement

f. Heart transplant

K. HEART FAILURE

1. DESCRIPTION

a. Ineffective pumping by the heart, resulting in intravascular and interstitial volume overload, as well as poor tissue perfusion

b. Compensatory mechanisms are triggered (increased heart rate, contractility, peripheral vascular resistance, venous return, as well as fluid retention due to angiotensin).

c. After long-term compensatory mechanisms, ventricular hypertrophy occurs due to the heart muscle's increased attempts to force blood out into the systemic circulation.

d. Possible causes: hypertension, left ventricular hypertrophy or infarction, aortic or mitral valve stenosis (right-sided heart failure eventually results from left-sided heart failure)

2. ASSESSMENT

a. Left-sided heart failure

1) Dyspnea, orthopnea

2) Fatigue

3) Crackles in the lung fields

4) Tachycardia, possible S3 and S4 heart sounds

5) Point of maximum impulse deviated to the left, away from the sternum (due to enlarged heart)

b. Right-sided heart failure

1) Weight gain, peripheral edema

2) Right upper quadrant pain, feeling of fullness (due to eventual liver engorgement)

3) Jugular venous distension

3. DIAGNOSTIC TESTS

a. Chest x-ray

b. Echocardiogram

c. Abnormal liver enzymes and elevated BUN and creatinine

d. Hemodynamic monitoring (using a Swan-Ganz catheter to measure pressures in the heart)

4. NURSING INTERVENTIONS

a. Treat the underlying cause (if known).

b. Administer oxygen if low saturations on room air.

c. Administer ACE inhibitor daily for clients with left ventricle dysfunction.

   d. Administer diuretics, nitrates, morphine.
   e. Assist the client to sit up comfortably to breathe.
   f. Instruct the client on a low-sodium diet, and to call the physician if increased daily weights or dyspnea are experienced at home.
   g. Inform the client that potassium or magnesium values will be checked regularly and that supplements may be used if daily diuretics are administered, due to the client's increased risk for electrolyte imbalance.
   h. Outpatient IV dobutamine, milrinone (Primacor), or nesiritide (Natrecor) may be of benefit for end-stage heart failure.
5. SURGICAL INTERVENTION
   a. CABG surgery or angioplasty in some cases
   b. Heart transplant in severe cases
   c. Recent left-ventricular assist devices may be of benefit.

L. PERICARDIAL EFFUSION AND CARDIAC TAMPONADE
1. DESCRIPTION: SUDDEN INCREASE IN FLUID (USUALLY BLOOD) IN THE PERICARDIAL SAC, CAUSING THE HEART TO BE COMPRESSED, LIMITING DIASTOLIC FILLING AND CARDIAC OUTPUT
2. ASSESSMENT
   a. Neck vein distension (elevated central venous pressure)
   b. Muffled heart sounds
   c. Pulsus paradoxus. Assessment is:
      1) Inflate the cuff above the systolic pressure.
      2) Deflate the cuff gradually, noting when sounds are first audible on expiration.
      3) Repeat step 2, this time identifying when sounds are also audible on inspiration
      4) Subtract the inspiratory systolic pressure from the expiratory systolic pressure (>10 mm Hg difference is suspicious for tamponade).
   d. Diaphoretic, cool skin
   e. Dyspnea, tachycardia
3. DIAGNOSTIC TESTS
   a. Chest x-ray
   b. ECG
   c. Echocardiogram
   d. Pulmonary artery catheterization
4. NURSING INTERVENTIONS
   a. Administer oxygen.
   b. Continuous ECG and hemodynamic monitoring

   c. Assist with emergent pericardiocentesis.
   d. Administer inotropic drugs, and possibly heparin antagonist or vitamin K if the client has been on heparin or coumadin that may have increased bleeding into the pericardial sac.
5. SURGICAL MANAGEMENT
   a. Pericardiocectomy
   b. If tamponade was sustained from trauma, assist with blood transfusion as the client is readied for sternotomy or pericardial tap to drain the fluid.

M. SHOCK
1. DESCRIPTION
   a. Clinical syndrome of reduced perfusion to organs and tissues
   b. Hypovolemic shock: rapid fluid loss (hemorrhage, severe burns, ascites, peritonitis)
   c. Cardiogenic shock: MI, cardiomyopathy and heart failure, pericardial tamponade, tension pneumothorax, pulmonary embolism
   d. Anaphylactic shock: severe allergy to medicine, food, or contrast media; reaction to incompatible blood transfusion, or venom
   e. Septic shock: gram-negative and gram-positive bacteria, or other systemic infections
   f. Neurogenic shock: spinal cord injury, spinal anesthesia, severe pain, medication, hypoglycemia
2. ASSESSMENT
   a. Tachycardia (may not be present if the client is on beta blockers)
   b. Restlessness, tachypnea
   c. Diminishing urine output
   d. Hypotension, cold clammy skin develops
   e. Loss of consciousness, shallow Cheyne-Stokes respirations, and anuria develop at late stages.
3. DIAGNOSTIC TESTS
   a. Blood, urine, or sputum cultures (to identify the organism if septic)
   b. WBC and ESR rates
   c. Hematocrit and coagulation studies
   d. Arterial blood gases
   e. Chest x-ray
   f. Echocardiogram
   g. ECG
4. NURSING INTERVENTIONS
   a. Treat the underlying cause (e.g., infection, allergic response).
   b. Maintain airway, breathing, respirations.
   c. Infuse intravenous fluids to help maintain blood pressure.

d. Continuous hemodynamic monitoring

e. For cardiogenic shock: inotropic drugs, vasodilators, intra-aortic balloon pump therapy, thrombolytic therapy

f. For anaphylactic shock, administer epinephrine, oxygen, IV fluids.

g. For septic shock, administer antibiotic therapy, inotropic and vasopressor drugs.

h. For neurogenic shock, administer vasopressor drugs.

5. SURGICAL MANAGEMENT

a. For cardiogenic shock, ventricular assist device or heart transplant may be needed.

N. CHRONIC PERIPHERAL ARTERIAL DISEASE (PAD)

1. DESCRIPTION

a. Chronic peripheral arterial disease progressive narrowing and eventual obstruction of lower extremity arteries (e.g., aortoiliac, femoral, popliteal, tibial) with no cure, only palliative treatment

2. ASSESSMENT

a. Chronic peripheral arterial disease occurs most often with clients who smoke and those who have diabetes mellitus, hyperlipidemia, or hypertension.

b. Pain often occurs in the legs during exercise.

c. Decreased pulses, ulcers over pressure points of lower extremities, thin and hairless skin, cool temperature

d. Foot is pale when elevated, and usually less painful as well as reddish (dependent rubor) when hanging off the bed.

3. DIAGNOSTIC TESTS

a. Ultrasound

b. Segmental blood pressures of the thigh, below the knee, and at the ankles (extremity blood pressure drops in arteries as disease progresses)

c. Peripheral arterial angiography

4. NURSING INTERVENTIONS

a. Identify the risk factors and support the client through progression of disease such as hypertension, lipid, and diabetes management, as well as exercise to develop collateral circulation.

b. Instruct the client on how to care for the feet (daily visual inspection, keeping the skin clean and dry, proper shoes, avoidance of chemicals, cold, or heat).

c. Administration of pentoxifylline (Trental) to reduce blood viscosity; antiplatelet agents or anticoagulants may be recommended.

5. SURGICAL MANAGEMENT

a. Arterial bypass using the client's own donor vein or synthetic graft material to deliver blood around the affected area of the artery

b. Endarterectomy may be performed to open the artery and remove plaque.

c. Amputation is least desired but necessary if gangrene has developed.

O. ACUTE ARTERIAL OCCLUSIVE DISORDERS

1. DESCRIPTION

a. Sudden occlusion of an artery, resulting from localized thrombus in a diseased vessel, embolization from the heart (infective endocarditis, MI, atrial fibrillation, valvular disease), or trauma to a vessel

b. Arterial thrombus in the right side of the heart may embolize to the lungs, causing a pulmonary embolus.

c. Arterial thrombus in the left side of the heart may embolize anywhere in the systemic circulation.

2. ASSESSMENT

a. Abrupt onset

b. Pain, pulselessness, pallor, paresthesia

c. Potential paralysis and inability to adapt to temperature changes

d. If unresolved, may develop into tissue necrosis and gangrene within hours, resulting in loss of extremity

3. DIAGNOSTIC TESTS

a. Ultrasound of extremity

b. Angiogram of extremity

4. NURSING INTERVENTION

a. Initiate heparin therapy immediately.

b. Infuse catheter-directed thrombolytic therapy (tPA, retaplase) if the client is a candidate and the radiologist has inserted a peripheral catheter into the femoral artery.

c. Frequent assessment of extremity: color, motion, sensitivity, pulses by handheld Doppler

d. Management of pain is very important: painful ischemia may need IV narcotic administration.

e. Instruct the client that long-term anticoagulation may be needed.

5. SURGICAL MANAGEMENT

a. Recently formed thrombus may be lysed ("broken up") by catheter-directed thrombolytic therapy.

b. Peripheral angioplasty

c. Surgical embolectomy or thrombectomy (removal of blocking plaque)

d. Amputation is least desired but necessary if gangrene has developed.

P. THROMBOPHLEBITIS
1. DESCRIPTION
    a. Acute deep vein thrombophlebitis: inflammations and thrombus formation, commonly in the deep leg veins (femoral, popliteal)
    b. Venous stasis is a risk factor that occurs most often in people who are overweight, have heart failure or atrial fibrillation, or have just undergone prolonged sitting such as in a car or airplane trip. Pregnant and postpartum women are also at risk.
    c. Endothelial damage is a risk factor that occurs when a client is receiving IV agents that may be irritating, as well as having an IV catheter in the same site for a prolonged period.
    d. Hypercoagulability of blood is a risk factor that occurs in hematologic disorders, such as cancer, or those who smoke or use oral contraceptives.
2. ASSESSMENT
    a. Superficial thrombophlebitis may present with a hard, cord-like vein, surrounded by warm, red, tender skin.
    b. Deep vein thrombophlebitis may present with edema of one leg only, pain, warm skin, and a fever, or the client may be asymptomatic.
    c. Involvement of the vena cavae may result in the client's extremities becoming cyanotic.
    d. Homan's sign (pain upon dorsiflexion of the foot) is not reliable, because it may be present under other conditions.
3. DIAGNOSTIC TESTS
    a. Anticoagulation studies
    b. Venous Doppler or duplex scanning of the lower extremities
    c. Lung scan or pulmonary arteriogram may be done to rule out pulmonary embolus if the client is at high risk or displays hypoxia and chest pain.
4. NURSING INTERVENTIONS
    a. Administer continuous IV heparin or subcutaneous injections of low-molecular-weight heparin (e.g., Lovenox).
    b. Support bed rest with bathroom privileges.
    c. Elevate the extremity above the heart.
    d. Inform the client on the need for elastic compression stockings and anticoagulation therapy.
    e. Measure the size of the affected and unaffected extremity daily to measure progress.
5. SURGICAL MANAGEMENT
    a. Intracaval filter insertion to prevent clots from embolizing through the circulatory system

PRACTICE QUESTIONS

1. During a routine physical examination, a client reports recent occipital headaches, blurred vision, fatigue, and increasing edema. The nurse reports these findings as indicative of
    1. endocarditis.
    2. hypovolemic shock.
    3. hypertension.
    4. ventricular tachycardia.

2. A client's parents ask the nurse, "What is the prognosis of myocarditis?" The most appropriate response by the nurse is
    1. "A heart transplant would be very promising."
    2. "Most often, a person will do well with coronary artery bypass surgery."
    3. "A coronary angioplasty would only involve a 1- to 3-day hospitalization."
    4. "Recovery usually happens without any special treatment."

3. The nurse is planning the care for a client in the acute stage of bacterial endocarditis. Which of the following interventions should the nurse include?

    Select all that apply:
    [ ] 1. Rest
    [ ] 2. Fluid restriction
    [ ] 3. Vitamin K (Aquamephyton)
    [ ] 4. Analgesics
    [ ] 5. Antibiotics
    [ ] 6. Physical therapy

4. A client who has hypertension asks the nurse why a urine sample is needed. The nurse informs the client it is to check for
    1. protein, which may indicate the kidneys are affected.
    2. illegal drugs, which may have caused the hypertension.

3. infection, which may cause the blood pressure to rise.
4. the appropriate drug level of the antihypertensive medication.

5. Which of the following orders should the nurse question in a client who has been admitted with a possible myocardial infarction and active peptic ulcer disease?
   1. Nitroglycerin SL
   2. Oxygen by nasal cannula
   3. Morphine IV
   4. Aspirin PO

6. The nurse's client asks, "How did I get rheumatic heart disease?" The most appropriate response by the nurse is that rheumatic heart disease is frequently a result of
   1. hypertension.
   2. streptococcal infection.
   3. genetic tendency.
   4. pregnancy.

7. Which of the following interventions are a priority during exacerbation of left-sided heart failure?

   Select all that apply:
   [ ] 1. Metered dose inhaler of albuterol
   [ ] 2. High-Fowler's position
   [ ] 3. Oxygen
   [ ] 4. IV fluids
   [ ] 5. Incentive inspirometer
   [ ] 6. Diuretics

8. The nurse is preparing a client to be discharged after a new diagnosis of heart failure. Which of the following statements by the client shows an appropriate understanding of the nurse's teaching?
   1. "I will do weekly finger-stick monitoring of my sodium levels."
   2. "I will call my doctor if I gain more than 2 pounds in a day."
   3. "I will take my angiotensin-converting enzyme (ACE) inhibitor as needed for shortness of breath."
   4. "I will not take my diuretic pill on weekends when I am traveling, in order to avoid incontinence."

9. The nurse should monitor a client after a coronary angioplasty for which of the following clinical manifestations indicating cardiac tamponade?

   Select all that apply:
   [ ] 1. Muffled heart sounds
   [ ] 2. Headache
   [ ] 3. Hypotension
   [ ] 4. Vision changes
   [ ] 5. Cool, diaphoretic skin
   [ ] 6. Tachycardia

10. The nurse is caring for a client who has an allergy to penicillin. Immediately after receiving cefazolin (Ancef) IV for prophylaxis for a pacemaker insertion, the client becomes restless, tachycardic, and hypotensive. Which of the following interventions should the nurse implement as the priority?
    1. Administer epinephrine (adrenaline)
    2. Obtain stat blood culture
    3. Administer thrombolytic therapy
    4. Administer atropine

11. After a myocardial infarction, a client has concerns about when it is safe to resume sexual activity. The most appropriate response by the nurse is
    1. "You should really talk to your doctor about that."
    2. "Continue with the sexual practice with which you are most comfortable."
    3. "You need to first undergo a cardiac stress test."
    4. "When you're able to climb two flights of stairs comfortably."

12. In preparing a client for a transesophageal echocardiogram (TEE), the nurse should include which of the following in the client education?
    1. "You will be able to eat only soft foods for the first day after the procedure."
    2. "You will need a designated driver to take you home."
    3. "The procedure involves a series of x-rays that may require you to come back."
    4. "The procedure involves a balloon that will press plaque against the blocked walls of your coronary artery."

13. After receiving a permanent pacemaker, the client asks the nurse if there are any activities to avoid during a vacation scheduled for 4 months after discharge. Which of the following is the most appropriate response by the nurse?
    1. "There are no restrictions on your activity."
    2. "You should avoid working over a running engine."
    3. "Avoid standing in front of microwave ovens."
    4. "Swimming in the ocean should be avoided."

14. After a client with coronary artery disease develops heavy, substernal chest pain, which of the following interventions should the nurse do first?
    1. Administer 2 puffs of albuterol (Proventil) by mouth
    2. Administer 1 tablet of nitroglycerin under the tongue every 5 minutes; call 911 if no relief after 15 minutes

3. Administer 0.04-mg IV push nitroglycerin slowly over 1 to 2 minutes
4. Administer immediate synchronized cardioversion

15. The nurse assists the client with coronary artery disease to select which of the following menu choices?

Select all that apply:
[ ] 1. Mozzarella cheese
[ ] 2. Grilled cheddar cheese sandwich
[ ] 3. Tomato juice
[ ] 4. Peanut-butter sandwich
[ ] 5. 2% milk
[ ] 6. Tortilla

16. In caring for a client with a cardiac history, the client has a temperature of 39.4°C or 103°F, becomes tachycardic, hypotensive, and short of breath while exhibiting cool, clammy skin and a decreased urine output. The client also has positive blood cultures. The nurse should include which of the following in the plan of care for this client?
1. Assistance with pericardiocentesis
2. Administration of antihypertensives
3. Administration of vasopressors
4. Assistance with defibrillation

17. Which of the following should the nurse include in the preoperative teaching for a client scheduled for coronary artery bypass graft (CABG) surgery?
1. A liquid diet will be ordered for the first 4 to 5 days postoperatively
2. Coughing is to be avoided in order to protect the sternal incision
3. The hospital stay is generally about 10 days
4. High-calorie supplements are encouraged in the first few weeks postoperative

18. The nurse observes the ECG rhythm of a client who has received a new permanent pacemaker for third-degree heart block. Several spikes are noted on the rhythm, but are not followed by any other waveforms. The nurse recognizes this as
1. an indication that the pacemaker is adhering to the heart.
2. a normal finding because spikes should never be seen on a pacemaker ECG rhythm strip.
3. the sinoatrial (S-A) node is beating appropriately but may not show up on the rhythm strip.
4. an abnormal finding because every spike on the ECG strip should be followed by a waveform.

19. The nurse assesses the left foot of a client with known coronary artery disease that has become suddenly cold, painful, and pulseless. Which of the following would be the priority intervention for this client?
1. Notify the physician
2. Provide education to the client about probable bypass surgery for the client's leg the following week
3. Instruct the client on importance of daily doses of warfarin (Coumadin)
4. Instruct the client to restrict activity, keeping it warm and elevated until it heals

20. Plans for nursing interventions for a client in the acute stage of bacterial endocarditis should include which of the following interventions?
1. Daily ECGs
2. Administration of analgesics as needed
3. Strict fluid restriction
4. Aggressive physical therapy

21. Which of the following is a priority for the nurse to report when obtaining a history from a client scheduled for a coronary angiogram?
1. A history of rheumatic heart disease
2. A history of allergy to shellfish
3. A recent diagnosis of hyperlipidemia
4. A previous coronary angioplasty to the right coronary artery

22. Which of the following should the nurse include in the plan of care for a client following a coronary angiogram?
1. Vigorous leg exercises
2. Immediate cardiac stress test
3. Encourage fluids
4. Activity restriction for 4 to 6 weeks

23. The nurse is teaching a class to student nurses on rheumatic fever. Which of the following should the nurse include in the class? Rheumatic fever
1. occurs mainly in the elderly.
2. is more likely to develop after a varicella zoster infection.
3. is diagnosed easily with a throat culture and serum antistreptolysin titer.
4. may be diagnosed by a series of two-step blood cultures.

24. Which of the following should the nurse include in the plan of care for the client experiencing pain from a deep vein thrombosis (DVT) of the leg who is receiving heparin and warfarin (Coumadin)? Administration of
1. aspirin 325 mg p.o. every 4 hours.
2. patient-controlled analgesic of IV morphine.

3. hydromorphine hydrochloride (Dilaudid) 2 mg intramuscular every 4 hours.
4. ibuprofen (Motrin) 400 mg p.o. every 6 hours p.r.n.

25. The client with a recent diagnosis of cardiomyopathy asks the nurse, "What contributed to my getting this illness?" The most appropriate response is to say that the majority of clients with cardiomyopathy also have
    1. hypertension.
    2. a viral infection.
    3. a genetic trait.
    4. an unknown cause.

26. The nurse is teaching the client what to expect after coronary artery bypass graft surgery (CABG). Which of the following client statements demonstrates that the client correctly understood the teaching?
    1. "I will be given a pen and paper to communicate, because I will still have a breathing tube in my throat."
    2. "I will be fed with a tube into my stomach until I can eat again."
    3. "Pain medicine is generally not needed after this surgery."
    4. "The nurses will be checking on me every 4 hours."

27. The nurse evaluates the PR interval to have what measurement? _____

28. The nurse reports the following ECG strip to be indicative of which of the following dysrhythmias?
    1. Ventricular fibrillation
    2. Atrial flutter
    3. Atrial fibrillation
    4. Ventricular tachycardia

29. The nurse assesses the rate of ventricular tachycardia to be at what rate?

    _____

30. A client is brought to the emergency room with a third-degree heart block after experiencing an acute anterior myocardial infarction. Which of the following interventions is the priority on an emergency basis?
    1. Temporary pacemaker
    2. Administer lidocaine
    3. Cardioversion
    4. Administer atropine

31. The nurse should include which of the following in the plan of care of a client after a pacemaker is inserted?
    1. Instruct the client to avoid lifting the arm on the pacemaker side above shoulder height

2. Encourage the client to exercise the shoulder and arm on the side of the pacemaker four times a day
3. Encourage the client to wash the pacemaker incision with warm soapy water twice a day
4. Instruct the client to avoid the use of microwave ovens

32. Following morning assessments, the registered nurse may delegate which of the following clients with a dysrhythmia to a licensed practical nurse to care for? A client with
    1. ventricular tachycardia.
    2. sinus bradycardia.
    3. ventricular fibrillation.
    4. sinus rhythm with a second-degree A-V block type II (Mobitz II).

33. The nurse is monitoring the ECG tracing on the central monitors on a cardiac unit. Which of the following dysrhythmias is a priority for the nurse to report first?
    1. Sinus rhythm with a first-degree A-V block
    2. Supraventricular tachycardia (SVT)
    3. Atrial fibrillation
    4. Idioventricular rhythm (ventricular escape rhythm)

34. The nurse prioritizes the following clients with dysrhythmias in order of their care. Prioritize the following clients, from highest to lowest priority, in the order in which care should be performed.
    ___ 1. A client with sinus bradycardia
    ___ 2. A client with atrial flutter
    ___ 3. A client with ventricular fibrillation
    ___ 4. A client with sinus tachycardia

35. In caring for a client with atrial flutter, which of the following goals would have priority?
    1. Reduce the ventricular rate to below 100 beats per minute
    2. Identify and treat the underlying cause
    3. Control the heart rate and maintain cardiac output
    4. Increase the heart rate

36. Which of the following should the nurse include in the plan of care for a client with sinus tachycardia?
    1. Administer lidocaine
    2. Assess the client
    3. Administer atropine
    4. Cardioversion

ANSWERS AND RATIONALES

1. 3. Clinical manifestations of hypertension include blurred vision, fatigue, occipital headaches, and increased edema.

2. 4. A heart transplant is a late-stage intervention for cardiomyopathy, which rarely results from myocarditis. Coronary artery bypass surgery is indicated for people with > 2 vessel disease not responsive to medical treatment. Coronary angioplasty is indicated for people with coronary artery lesions causing angina-related symptoms. Myocarditis is often asymptomatic and most often resolves spontaneously.

3. 1. 4. 5. Rest is indicated during the acute stage of bacterial endocarditis, along with acetaminophen (Tylenol) or salicylic acid (aspirin) for aches and antibiotics to fight the infectious organism. Steroids are not indicated and fluids should be encouraged rather than restricted. Vitamin K is used for reversal of warfarin (Coumadin) that would cause the blood to be too thin.

4. 1. Hypertension is not normally caused by illegal drugs nor by infection. Drug levels are more frequently done by serum analysis rather than urine, and appropriate levels of antihypertensives are judged by the serial blood pressure readings of the client. A urine test that showed high levels of microalbuminuria and proteinuria may indicate that the client's hypertension has caused poor blood supply to the kidneys, resulting in renal dysfunction.

5. 4. Nitroglycerin, oxygen, morphine, and aspirin are all appropriate interventions for a client suspected of having a myocardial infarction. However, a client with an active peptic ulcer should not be considered a candidate for aspirin, due to its antiplatelet effects possibly promoting more gastrointestinal (GI) bleeding.

6. 2. Rheumatic heart disease commonly occurs in children after an infection of group A beta-hemolytic streptococcal pharyngitis.

7. 2. 3. 6. Nursing interventions that are a priority for a client with an acute exacerbation of left-sided heart failure include having the client assume a high-Fowler's position, oxygen, and diuretics to reduce the fluid volume. Albuterol is used for a client with asthma. IV fluid flush would be harmful for a client experiencing respiratory distress from left-sided heart failure.

8. 2. While finger-stick glucose levels are done by clients to monitor their diabetes, sodium finger-stick levels are not done. ACE inhibitors need to be taken daily, as prescribed (not p.r.n.). Diuretic pills may be delayed a few hours before a big event, but not skipped or the client may end up with a heart failure exacerbation. A client who calls about a sudden weight gain may receive instructions from the health care provider to come in to be evaluated or may be instructed to take an extra diuretic pill at home.

9. 1. 3. 5. 6. Clinical manifestations of cardiac tamponade include muffled heart sounds, tachycardia, low blood pressure, and cool, diaphoretic skin. These clinical manifestations indicate shock, possibly caused by a dissection (cutting) of a coronary artery, a ventricle, or the septum during the coronary angioplasty.

10. 1. Blood cultures and IV antibiotics are appropriate for a client in septic shock. Thrombolytic therapy is indicated for some clients experiencing an acute MI or peripheral clot. Atropine would be appropriate for an individual who has symptomatic bradycardia or heart block. The client has a known allergy to penicillin, and cefazolin (Ancef) is a related cephalosporin, so the client is likely experiencing a severe allergic reaction. The priority intervention for anaphylactic shock would be to monitor the airway and give epinephrine, while infusing rapid IV fluids for hypotension.

11. 4. Discussing timing for the client to resume sexual activity should be handled matter-of-factly by the nurse while discussing other activities. The client may not be physically ready to continue with comfortable sexual practices immediately after the myocardial infarction. The client needs an objective indicator. A cardiac stress test is not necessary prior to resuming sexual activity, while the ability to climb two flights of stairs comfortably is a good guideline.

12. 2. After a transesophageal echocardiogram (TEE), the client should be able to eat lukewarm food as soon as the gag reflex returns, usually just a few hours after receiving anesthetizing spray in the back of the throat. X-rays are not involved, nor is the client undergoing a balloon procedure such as the coronary angioplasty. Having a designated driver will be needed after a transesophageal echocardiogram because the client has received IV sedation.

13. 2. Early microwave ovens required avoidance by persons with pacemakers, but not current models. Swimming would be contraindicated for the first few weeks due to abduction of the arm while the leads were still adhering to the muscle of the heart. However, 4 months postoperatively, the client should be able to abduct arms for swimming. Working over a running engine, as well as being near high-frequency power waves, is contraindicated for anyone with a permanent pacemaker.

14. 2. Administering albuterol (Proventil) in a situation where a client had exercise-induced asthma and experienced shortness of breath would be appropriate. However, for a client with known cardiac disease who is experiencing chest pain, the inhaler would not be appropriate. Nitroglycerin is not given IV push. Immediate synchronized cardioversion is appropriate for the client in pulseless ventricular tachycardia or ventricular fibrillation. Correct administration of nitroglycerin for a client who has coronary artery disease involves 1 nitroglycerin tablet every 5 minutes (if blood pressure is above 90 systolic) for up to 3 tablets, then calling 911 if no relief.

15. 1. 6. Cheddar cheese has higher fat content than mozzarella cheese, and a canned vegetable drink often has high sodium content. Peanut-butter is a high-fat item. Skim milk is preferred to 2%. Tortilla is a low-fat item.

16. 3. A client who is exhibiting a temperature of 39.4°C, or 103°F, becomes tachycardic, hypotensive, and has shortness of breath with cold, clammy skin and a decreased urine output has signs of septic shock (systemic infection) with known positive blood cultures. A pericardiocentesis is an intervention for cardiac tamponade, a condition that may also result in shock, but is also generally accompanied by muffled heart sounds and pulsus paradoxus, neither of which are presented in this client. Antihypertensive drugs would cause the client's blood pressure to drop even further. If the client were in a pulseless ventricular tachycardia or fibrillation, emergency defibrillation would be indicated, but no dysrhythmia is present in the scenario. Vasopressors are indicated to raise the blood pressure. Rapid IV fluid administration and inotropic drugs may be used as well.

17. 4. The first meal after coronary artery bypass graft surgery may be clear liquids, but the client quickly progresses to a low-fat and low-salt diet as soon as it can be tolerated. Coughing is important to clear the airways, and is done by splinting the sternum with a pillow. Hospital stays are generally 4 to 5 days. A poor appetite may be present for the first few weeks and clients are encouraged to try high-calorie supplements.

18. 4. Although it is true that the pacemaker leads need time to adhere to the heart muscle after implantation, the correct precaution is to keep the affected side's arm near the body for about 1 to 3 weeks. It does not mean that the device won't function properly as soon as it is implanted. Spikes are seen on an ECG waveform strip when the pacemaker discharges an electrical stimulus to the heart and should be followed by a P wave (for atrial depolarization) or a QRS wave (ventricular depolarization) as indicated by pacemaker programming.

19. 1. Scheduling bypass surgery for a week after the left foot of a client has suddenly become cold, painful, and pulseless is not an aggressive enough treatment, as ischemia, tissue necrosis, and gangrene may happen within several hours from an acute arterial occlusion. Warfarin (Coumadin) anticoagulant therapy would be likely after the intervention for this occlusion, but is not the nurse's immediate priority. Keeping the limb elevated may actually cause more pain, and is indicated for someone with venous stasis or venous phlebitis. The nurse needs to notify the physician immediately so this client can be seen and arrangements can be made for immediate transport to a hospital where the client can be evaluated for possible catheter-directed thrombolytic therapy, emergency embolectomy, or bypass surgery.

20. 2. Antibiotics to combat the bacterial infection and analgesics for aches that may occur are appropriate interventions for acute-stage bacterial endocarditis. Adequate fluid intake is important also. However, aggressive physical therapy is contraindicated in the acute stage because the client needs to reserve some physical resources for recovery. Daily ECGs are not necessary for acute bacterial endocarditis.

21. 2. Although obtaining a clear record of the client's cardiac history is important prior to a coronary angiogram, it is a priority to notify the physician of an allergy to shellfish. The client with a shellfish allergy is more likely to be allergic to the contrast dye used in the procedure. An order may be given to give diphenhydramine (Benadryl), steroids, or extra IV fluids before the procedure. The chart should be marked for an allergy to shellfish.

22. 3. The client's leg on the side where the cardiologist entered the femoral artery needs to remain still for a period of time after the procedure (usually 2 to 4 hours) in order to allow the arterial site to seal. A cardiac stress test would not be indicated because the angiogram provides a more definitive diagnostic work-up. A 4- to 6-week activity restriction may be indicated after a large myocardial infarction, but not for a simple coronary angiogram, after which the client can begin walking hours later. The client should be encouraged to drink fluids to protect the kidneys from the contrast dye.

23. 3. Rheumatic fever occurs primarily in young adults and is mostly likely to develop after a group A beta-hemolytic streptococcal upper respiratory infection. Diagnosis is not done by a series of blood cultures, but rather with a throat culture and serum antistreptolysin titer.

24. 2. A daily dose of aspirin would be ordered for antiplatelet effect, not for pain control. A client with a deep vein thrombosis would be receiving heparin therapy, so intramuscular injections should be avoided (due to possible hematoma formation at injection sites). Ibuprofen (Motrin) is also contraindicated for a client receiving oral anticoagulants due to possible drug interaction. The best solution to this client's pain would be patient-controlled IV analgesic.

25. 4. Although hypertension, viral infection, or a genetic trait may all be possible reasons for developing cardiomyopathy, the majority of cases are idiopathic (unknown reason).

26. 1. A nasogastric tube may be used to decompress the stomach after coronary artery bypass graft surgery, but is not immediately used for feeding unless the client cannot eat in the days following surgery. Pain medication is offered regularly because the client will most likely experience pain in the sternal incision as well as leg, if a graft was taken from there. Immediately after CABG surgery the nurses will be assessing the client every 15 minutes and more frequently as needed until the client becomes stable. It is correct that the client should expect to use hand signals and writing to communicate in the first few hours after surgery while on the ventilator.

27.   0.12 to 0.20 second

28. 2. Atrial flutter is a dysrhythmia characterized by a very irritable atrium. The atria fire at a rate of 250 to 350 beats per minute. The waveforms produced resemble the teeth of a saw. Ventricular fibrillation is a lethal rhythm characterized by a chaotic rhythm that originates in the ventricles. It is an unorganized and uncoordinated series of rapid impulses that cause the heart to fibrillate rather than contract. Atrial fibrillation is an extremely irritable rhythm originating in the atrium. There is a constant generalized quivering with no sign of organized atrial activity. Ventricular tachycardia is a lethal rhythm that exists when three or more premature ventricular contractions (PVCs) occur in a row at a rate greater than 100 beats per minute.

29.   120–180 beats per minute

30. 1. A third-degree heart block is a lethal rhythm. It is the complete blockage of the atrial impulses into the ventricles. The block may be at the A-V node, bundle of His, or bundle branches, resulting in the atria and ventricles beating independently of each other. The atrial rate is usually normal while the ventricular rate is very slow and below 55 beats per minute. The causes may be an anterior myocardial infarction, coronary artery disease, surgery, aging, or drug toxicity such as digoxin, procainamide (Procanbid), or verapamil (Calan).

31. 1. A client who had a pacemaker inserted should be instructed to stay on bed rest for 12 hours with minimal activity of the affected arm and shoulder to prevent dislodging the leads of the pacemaker. The client should also be instructed to keep the insertion area dry for 1 week postinsertion. It is not necessary to avoid microwave ovens because they do not threaten the function of the pacemaker.

32. 2. Ventricular tachycardia and ventricular fibrillation are lethal dysrhythmias that require immediate intervention to maintain life. Sinus rhythm with a second-degree A-V block type II (Mobitz II) requires pacemaker placement. Sinus bradycardia is a dysrhythmia that generally goes unnoticed because the client can compensate for the decreased cardiac output. Treatment is not necessary unless the client becomes symptomatic.

33. 4. Idioventricular rhythm (ventricular escape rhythm) is a lethal rhythm in which there is a high pacemaker failure. No impulses are conducted to the ventricles from above the bundle of His. Supraventricular tachycardia (SVT) is a term used to describe tachydysrhythmias that cannot be classified more accurately. Treatment depends on the severity of the client's clinical manifestations. A sinus rhythm with a first-degree A-V block is a consistent delay in the A-V conduction. Generally no intervention is recommended. Atrial fibrillation is a constant quivering of the heart caused by extreme atrial irritability. The atrial rate is controlled with calcium-channel blockers and beta blockers. Cardioversion may be necessary and is most successful if performed within 3 days of treatment.

34. 3. 2. 4. 1. A client with sinus bradycardia is generally symptomatic with treatment not being necessary. A client with sinus tachycardia should be assessed for the cause and treated as needed. The most common drugs used are beta blockers. The ventricular response is controlled in a client with atrial flutter through the administration of calcium-channel blockers. Ventricular fibrillation is a lethal rhythm in which the heart fibrillates. A code and CPR must be performed immediately or the client will die.

35. 3. The goal for a client with atrial fibrillation is to reduce the ventricular response rate to below 100 beats per minute. An appropriate goal for a client with sinus tachycardia is to identify and treat the underlying cause. It is a priority to control the heart rate and maintain cardiac output in a client with atrial flutter. A goal of increasing the heart rate would be an appropriate goal for a client with a junctional rhythm.

36. 2. Sinus tachycardia is a dysrhythmia in which the S-A node discharges at more than 100 beats per minute. The nursing interventions include assessing the client for the cause and treat as needed. The most commonly used drugs are beta blockers.

REFERENCES

Anatomical Chart Company. (2011). *Atlas of pathophysiology* (3rd ed.). Springhouse, PA: Springhouse.

Daniels, R. (2010). *Delmar's manual of laboratory and diagnostic tests* (2nd ed.). Clifton Park, NY: Delmar Cengage Learning.

Daniels, R., & Nicoll, L. (2012). *Contemporary medical-surgical nursing*. Clifton Park, NY: Delmar Cengage Learning.

Estes, M. (2010). *Health assessment and physical examination* (4th ed.). Clifton Park, NY: Delmar Cengage Learning.

Hazinnski, M. F., Cummins, R. O., & Field, J. M. (Eds.). (2010). *2010 handbook of emergency cardiovascular care for health providers*. Dallas, TX: American Heart Association.

Lewis, K. M., & Handal, K. (2000a). *Sensible analysis of the 12-lead ECG*. Clifton Park, NY: Delmar Cengage Learning.

Lewis, K. M., & Handal, K. (2000b). *Sensible ECG analysis*. Clifton Park, NY: Delmar Cengage Learning.

Miller, E., III, & Jehn, M. L. (2004). New high blood pressure guidelines create new at-risk classification. *Journal of Cardiovascular Nursing, 19*(6), 367–371.

Spratto, G. R., & Woods, A. L. (2012). *PDR nurse's drug handbook 2012*. Clifton Park, NY: Delmar Cengage Learning.

CHAPTER 5

GASTROINTESTINAL DISORDERS

I. ANATOMY AND PHYSIOLOGY

A. FUNCTIONS OF THE GASTROINTESTINAL SYSTEM
   1. SUPPLY NUTRIENTS TO THE CELLS OF THE BODY
   2. INGESTION OF FOOD
   3. DIGESTION (BREAKDOWN) OF FOOD
   4. ELIMINATION OF THE WASTE PRODUCTS OF DIGESTION

B. MOUTH AND ORAL CAVITY
   1. LIPS AND BUCCAL (ORAL) CAVITY
   2. TEETH USED IN MASTICATION (CHEWING)
   3. TONGUE USED IN TASTE, DEGLUTITION (SWALLOWING), AND SPEECH
   4. PAROTID, SUBMAXILLARY, AND SUBLINGUAL SALIVARY GLANDS PRODUCE SALIVA CONTAINING MUCUS FOR LUBRICATION AND PTYALIN (AMYLASE) TO BEGIN DIGESTION.

C. ESOPHAGUS
   1. HOLLOW, MUSCULAR TUBE APPROXIMATELY 10 INCHES LONG
   2. RECEIVES FOOD FROM THE PHARYNX, WHICH IS PROPELLED INTO THE STOMACH THROUGH PERISTALSIS (CONTRACTION OF MUSCULAR LAYERS)
   3. CONTAINS THE LOWER ESOPHAGEAL SPHINCTER (LES), WHICH IS IMPORTANT IN PREVENTING THE REFLUX OF GASTRIC ACID

D. STOMACH (SEE FIGURE 5-1)
   1. LIES IN THE LEFT UPPER QUADRANT OF THE ABDOMEN
   2. CONTAINS THE FUNDUS, THE BODY, AND THE ANTRUM
   3. SITE FOR COMPLEX AND MECHANICAL PROCESSES FOR DIGESTION
      a. Gastric juices secreted by small glands within the rugae
      b. Pepsinogen secreted by chief cells, which converts to pepsin to begin the breakdown of protein
      c. Hydrochloric acid secreted by parietal cells, resulting in acidity of gastric juices and aids in the protection against ingested organism
      d. Intrinsic factor secreted for the absorption of vitamin B_{12}
      e. Chyme, a semisolid substance, results from the partial digestion of food by the salivary enzyme mylase, the gastric enzyme pepsin, and hydrochloric acid.
   4. USUAL CAPACITY IS 1 TO 1.5 L
   5. SERVES AS RESERVOIR FOR FOOD—3 TO 4 HOURS AVERAGE LENGTH OF TIME FOOD REMAINS IN THE STOMACH

E. SMALL INTESTINE (SEE FIGURE 5-1)
   1. LIES IN ALL FOUR ABDOMINAL QUADRANTS
   2. MEASURES 10 TO 30 FEET
   3. CONSISTS OF THE DUODENUM, JEJUNUM, AND ILEUM
      a. Duodenum
         1) Shortest section
         2) Significant role in digestion
         3) Hormonal secretions
         4) Contains openings of pancreatic and common bile ducts
      b. Jejunum
         1) Second section composed of circular folds
         2) Provides surface area for digestion and absorption
      c. Ileum
         1) Terminates with ileocecal valve separating the small intestine from the large intestine
         2) Prevents the reflux of contents of the large intestine into the small intestine

Figure 5-1 Structures of the abdomen

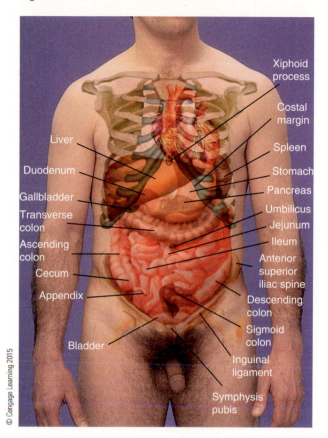

© Cengage Learning 2015

F. LARGE INTESTINE (SEE FIGURE 5-1)
 1. MEASURES 5 TO 6 FEET LONG
 2. EXTENDS FROM THE ILEOCECAL VALVE TO THE ANUS
 3. CONSISTS OF THE ASCENDING, TRANSVERSE, DESCENDING, AND SIGMOID COLON
 4. LIMITED DIGESTION FUNCTIONS
  a. Absorbs water and electrolytes
  b. Forms feces (75% water and 25% solid wastes)
  c. Secretes mucus
  d. Synthesizes vitamins B and K
G. LIVER (SEE FIGURE 5-1)
 1. LARGEST SOLID ORGAN IN THE BODY
 2. LIES IN THE RIGHT HYPOCHONDRIAC AND EPIGASTRIC REGIONS
 3. FOUR MAJOR FUNCTIONS
  a. Storage of carbohydrates, amino acids, vitamins, minerals, and blood
  b. Detoxification of drugs, hormones, and bacteria
  c. Metabolism of carbohydrates, proteins, fats, and ammonia to urea
  d. Synthesis and secretion of 600 to 1000 ml of bile every day

H. GALLBLADDER (SEE FIGURE 5-1)
 1. LIES IN THE RIGHT UPPER QUADRANT
 2. STORES AND CONCENTRATES BILE
 3. DURING THE DIGESTION OF FATS, CONTRACTS, FORCING BILE INTO THE DUODENUM
 4. SPHINCTER OF ODDI KEEPS THE AMPULA OF VATER CLOSED EXCEPT WHEN STIMULATED BY FOOD
 5. BILE RELEASED IN THE PRESENCE OF CHOLECYSTOKIN, PANCREOZYMIN, AND PARASYMPATHETIC STIMULATION THROUGH THE CYSTIC AND COMMON BILE DUCTS INTO THE DUODENUM
 6. STORES 30 TO 50 ML
I. PANCREAS (SEE FIGURE 5-1)
 1. LARGE ELONGATED ACCESSORY ORGAN OF DIGESTION
 2. LIES IN A TRANSVERSE POSITION IN BOTH THE RIGHT AND LEFT UPPER QUADRANTS
 3. EXOCRINE GLAND SECRETING BICARBONATE AND PANCREATIC ENZYMES AIDING IN THE PROCESS OF DIGESTION
 4. ENDOCRINE GLAND CONSISTING OF ISLETS OF LANGERHANS COMPOSED OF BETA CELLS SECRETING INSULIN AND ALPHA CELLS SECRETING GLUCAGON

II. **ASSESSMENT**
A. HEALTH HISTORY
 1. PAST HEALTH HISTORY
 2. MEDICATIONS (PAST, PRESENT, OVER THE COUNTER, HERBS)
 3. SURGERIES
B. PHYSICAL EXAMINATION
 1. INSPECTION
  a. Mouth—symmetry, color, size, odor, teeth
  b. Abdomen—skin changes, symmetry, contour, masses, movement
   1) Peristalsis is only visible in a thin adult.
   2) Aortic pulsation may be seen in the epigastric region.
  c. Rectum and anus—color, lumps, tissues, external hemorrhoids
 2. AUSCULTATION
  a. Bowel sounds
   1) Perform prior to percussion and palpation.
   2) Auscultate all four quadrants.
   3) High-pitched gurgling occurring every 5 to 15 seconds
   4) Listen 5 minutes to all four quadrants before determining absence.
  b. Aortic bruit indicates turbulent blood flow.

3. PERCUSSION
   a. Determines presence of fluid, distention, and masses
   b. Liver 2.4 to 5 inches (6–12 cm) dullness at the right midclavicular line
   c. Tympany predominant sound of the abdomen
4. PALPATION
   a. Mouth—ulcers, indurations, tenderness
   b. Abdomen
      1) Light palpation (1 cm)—detects tenderness, masses, swelling, muscular resistance, cutaneous hypersensitivity
      2) Deep palpation (4–8 cm)—outlines abdominal organs and masses
      3) Round tenderness—indicates peritoneal inflammation
      4) Liver—may be felt 0.4 to 0.8 inch (1 to 2 cm) below the right costal margin
      5) Spleen—felt only if enlarged, rupture can occur if continued

III. DIAGNOSTIC STUDIES
A. UPPER GI OR BARIUM SWALLOW
   1. DESCRIPTION: X-RAY STUDY WITH FLUOROSCOPY AND CONTRAST MEDIUM (BARIUM)
   2. PREPROCEDURE
      a. NPO for 8 to 12 hours
      b. No smoking
   3. POSTPROCEDURE
      a. Encourage 6 to 8 glasses of water daily.
      b. Offer laxative—stools may be white for 72 hours.
B. LOWER GI OR BARIUM ENEMA
   1. DESCRIPTION: X-RAY STUDY VISUALIZING THE COLON
   2. PREPROCEDURE
      a. Day before the test:
         1) Clear liquid for lunch and dinner
         2) 8 ounces of fluid every hour for 8 to 10 hours
         3) 10 ounces of magnesium citrate or x-prep in mid to late afternoon
         4) Prescribed number of 5 mg bisacodyl (Dulcolax) tablets—usually 3 or 4
         5) Maybe NPO after midnight
      b. Day of the test:
         1) Bisacodyl (Dulcolax) suppository early morning or tap water enema
         2) Continue NPO or clear liquid diet up to the procedure
         3) Contrast medium (barium) administered rectally with the client on a tilt table

3. POSTPROCEDURE
   a. Increase fluids.
   b. Offer laxative—stools may be white for 72 hours.
C. ORAL CHOLECYSTOGRAM (GB SERIES)
   1. DESCRIPTION: X-RAY VISUALIZATION OF THE GALLBLADDER TO DETERMINE THE PATENCY OF THE BILIARY DUCT SYSTEM WHILE ASSESSING THE ABILITY OF THE GALLBLADDER TO CONCENTRATE, CONTRACT, AND EMPTY
   2. PREPROCEDURE
      a. Day before the test:
         1) Assess for allergy to iodine or seafood.
         2) Evaluate the bilirubin level—if greater than 2 mg/dl, will not visualize the gallbladder.
         3) Low-fat or fat-free meal for dinner
         4) Six radiopaque iopanoic acid (Telepaque) tablets are administered 5 minutes apart beginning 2 hours after dinner.
         5) Inform the radiologist if vomiting or diarrhea occurs after ingestion of the dye.
         6) NPO after ingestion of the dye
   3. POSTPROCEDURE
      a. May be given fatty meal to enhance excretion of the dye
      b. Assess for slight dysuria as the dye is excreted.
D. CHOLANGIOGRAM
   1. DESCRIPTION: X-RAY VISUALIZATION OF THE HEPATIC AND COMMON BILE DUCTS
   2. PREPROCEDURE
      a. Day before the test:
         1) Assess for allergy to iodine or seafood.
         2) Evaluate the bilirubin level—contraindicated if greater than 3.5 mg/dl.
      b. Day of the test:
         1) NPO after midnight
         2) Radiographic dye is administered intravenously.
   3. POSTPROCEDURE
      a. Two to 6 hours after the test, assess for delayed reaction to the dye (dyspnea, rashes, tachycardia, hives).
      b. Assess for slight dysuria as the dye is excreted.
E. PERCUTANEOUS TRANSHEPATIC CHOLANGIOGRAM
   1. DESCRIPTION
      a. X-ray visualization of the intrahepatic, extrahepatic biliary ducts and, occasionally, the gallbladder after

direct administration of the radiopaque dye into the intrahepatic duct

  b. Useful in clients who are jaundiced

  2. PREPROCEDURE

  a. Assess for allergy to iodine or seafood.

  b. Evaluate coagulation studies.

  c. Type and cross match blood.

  d. NPO after midnight

  3. POSTPROCEDURE

  a. Maintain bed rest for several hours.

  b. Assess for bleeding and sepsis.

  c. Monitor vital signs.

  d. Avoid analgesics to prevent covering up abdominal signs associated with hemorrhage or bile leakage.

F. UPPER GI ENDOSCOPY (ESOPHAGOGASTRODUODENOSCOPY [EGD])

  1. DESCRIPTION: DIRECT VISUALIZATION OF THE UPPER GASTROINTESTINAL TRACT USING A LONG, FLEXIBLE, FIBEROPTIC-LIGHTED SCOPE

  2. PROCEDURE

  a. Day before the test:

  1) NPO after midnight

  2) Remove the client's dentures and other oral devices.

  3) Inform the client that speaking during the procedure is not possible because of the fiberscope.

  b. Day of the test:

  1) Client is placed in the left lateral decubitus position to facilitate easier insertion of the endoscope.

  2) Topical anesthetic spray naloxone (Xylocaine) is applied to the throat to inactivate the gag reflex.

  3) Atropine may be given to reduce secretions.

  4) Glucagon may be given as a smooth muscle relaxant.

  5) Biopsies may be taken if indicated.

  3. POSTPROCEDURE

  a. Maintain NPO until gag reflex returns, usually 2 to 4 hours.

  b. Assess the gag reflex by tickling the back of the throat.

  c. Monitor for signs of perforation (bleeding, abdominal pain, elevated temperature, dyspnea, or dysphagia).

  d. Offer warm saline gargles or throat lozenges for relief of sore throat.

  e. Maintain bed rest with the side rails elevated until sedation wears off.

G. ENDOSCOPIC RETROGRADE CHOLANGIOPANCREATOGRAPHY (ERCP)

  1. DESCRIPTION: RADIOGRAPHIC VISUALIZATION OF THE COMMON BILE AND PANCREATIC DUCTS WITH THE USE OF A FIBEROPTIC ENDOSCOPE

  2. PREPROCEDURE

  a. Day before the test:

  1) NPO after midnight

  2) Inform the client that breathing will not be compromised with the endoscope.

  3) Instruct the client that lying very still is essential to allow for good visualization of the ducts.

  b. Day of the test:

  1) Remove the client's dentures.

  2) Sedative with a narcotic is administered for relaxation.

  3) Client is placed in supine left lateral position to facilitate insertion of the endoscope.

  4) Topical anesthetic spray naloxone (Xylocaine) is applied to the pharynx to inactivate the gag reflex.

  5) Place the client in several positions throughout the procedure to permit passage of a small catheter into the ductal system for the injection of radiographic dye so x-ray films may be taken.

  6) Glucagon is often administered to minimize spasms and improve visualization of the ampulla of Vater.

  3. POSTPROCEDURE

  a. Maintain NPO until gag reflex returns.

  b. Monitor for the signs of ERCP-induced pancreatitis (abdominal pain, nausea, and vomiting).

  c. Monitor for signs of ERCP-induced cholangitis (septicemia).

  d. Offer warm saline gargles or throat lozenges for relief of sore throat.

  e. Maintain bed rest with the side rails elevated until sedation wears off.

H. COLONOSCOPY

  1. DESCRIPTION: DIRECT VISUALIZATION OF THE ENTIRE COLON FROM THE ANUS TO THE CECUM WITH A FLEXIBLE FIBEROPTIC SCOPE

  2. PREPROCEDURE

  a. Day before the test:

  1) 1 gallon of GoLYTELY or Colace administered the evening before the procedure (1 glass every 10 minutes until gone)

  2) Bisacodyl (Dulcolax) tablets and enemas may be given.

  3) Clear liquid diet beginning at noon and up to 8 hours before the procedure, then NPO

  b. Day of the test:

  1) Client is placed in left lateral decubitus position to insert the colonoscope.

         2) Administer ordered sedative medication—usually midazolam (Versed).

         3) Atropine may be given to decrease colonic secretions.

         4) Client's position will be changed to facilitate the colonoscope as it is directed toward the cecum.

    3. POSTPROCEDURE

      a. Maintain bed rest with the side rails up until sedation wears off.

      b. Inform the client that abdominal cramping may be experienced because air was injected into the colon during the procedure.

      c. Monitor for signs of colon perforation (abdominal distention and tenderness).

      d. Monitor vital signs for signs of hemorrhage (increased pulse and decreased blood pressure).

      e. Offer food after assessing for evidence of bowel perforation.

      f. Instruct the client to push fluids to compensate for dehydration from bowel preparation.

I. PROCTOSIGMOIDOSCOPY

    1. DESCRIPTION: DIRECT VISUALIZATION OF THE ANUS, RECTUM, AND SIGMOID COLON WITH THE USE OF A FIBERSCOPE

    2. PREPROCEDURE

      a. Day before the test:

         1) Administer an enema the evening before the procedure.

      b. Day of the test:

         1) Clear liquid breakfast

         2) Administer the enema the morning of the procedure.

         3) Client is placed in the lateral decubitus position and assisted into the knee-chest position during the procedure.

    3. POSTPROCEDURE

      a. Inform the client that abdominal discomfort and flatulence may be experienced because air was injected into the bowel during the procedure.

      b. Monitor for signs of rectal bleeding.

J. LIVER BIOPSY

    1. DESCRIPTION: INSERTION OF A NEEDLE BETWEEN THE SIXTH AND SEVENTH OR EIGHTH AND NINTH INTERCOSTAL SPACE ON THE RIGHT SIDE TO OBTAIN A SPECIMEN OF HEPATIC TISSUE

    2. PREPROCEDURE

      a. Day before the test:

         1) Obtain the client's coagulation study (PT, clotting or bleeding time).

         2) Type and cross match.

         3) Obtain baseline vital signs.

         4) Obtain informed consent.

      b. Day of the test:

         1) Administer the prescribed sedative.

         2) Place the client in the supine or left lateral position.

         3) Instruct the client to exhale and hold the exhalation, allowing the liver to descend, decreasing the risk of a pneumothorax.

    3. POSTPROCEDURE

      a. Place the client on the right side for 1 to 2 hours, pressing a liver capsule against the chest wall to decrease risk of hemorrhage.

      b. Monitor vital signs for evidence of hemorrhage (increased pulse, decreased blood pressure) and peritonitis (increased temperature).

K. GASTRIC ANALYSIS

    1. DESCRIPTION: CONTENTS OF THE STOMACH ARE ASPIRATED TO DETERMINE THE AMOUNT OF ACID PRODUCED DURING THE RESTING OR BASAL STATE (BASAL ACID OUTPUT [BAO]) AND DURING THE STIMULATED STATE (MAXIMAL ACID OUTPUT [MAO]).

    2. PREPROCEDURE

      a. Day before the test:

         1) Instruct the client not to smoke, chew gum, or take anticholinergic medications before the procedure.

         2) NPO after midnight

      b. Day of the test:

         1) Nasogastric tube is inserted with a syringe attached to aspirate gastric contents and discard first specimen.

         2) Four subsequent samples are taken and analyzed every 15 minutes apart (these are the BAO).

         3) Histamine is administered subcutaneously and eight samples are taken and analyzed every 15 minutes apart (these are the MAO).

         4) Inform the client that histamine may produce a flushing sensation.

    3. POSTPROCEDURE

      a. Monitor the client for histamine side effects such as intestinal, bronchial, and uterine spasms.

L. GASTRIC EMPTYING STUDIES

    1. DESCRIPTION: RADIONUCLIDE STUDY IN WHICH THE STOMACH IS SCANNED UNTIL GASTRIC EMPTYING IS COMPLETE AFTER THE INGESTION OF A "TEST MEAL," EITHER SOLID OR LIQUID CONTAINING TECHNETIUM (TC)

2. PREPROCEDURE
   a. Day before the test:
      1) NPO after midnight
      2) No laxatives
      3) No sleeping pills
   b. Day of the test:
      1) Client ingests a solid "test meal" consisting of a cooked egg white containing Tc or a liquid "test meal" consisting of a glass of orange juice containing Tc.
      2) Inform the client that only a small dose of radionuclear material is ingested and is safe.
      3) Place the client in a supine position and images are taken under a gamma camera every 2 minutes every hour depending on emptying time.
3. POSTPROCEDURE
   a. Instruct the client that no radiation precautions need to be taken in the disposal of bodily secretions.
   b. Reinforce safety of the dose of the radioactive material.

M. STOOL SPECIMEN
1. FECAL FAT
   a. Description: stool is collected continuously over 3 days and fecal fat is measured to evaluate presence of malabsorption.
   b. Preprocedure
      1) 3-day collection
         a) 100 g of fat ingested per day for 3 days
         b) Instruct the client to defecate in a clean dry container and to avoid urinating or placing toilet paper in the container.
         c) Instruct the client to avoid laxatives or enemas during the test.
         d) Send each stool specimen to the lab immediately in an acute care setting, or instruct the client to keep all stool in a large stool container in the freezer at home until completion of the test.
   c. Postprocedure
      1) Instruct the client to resume a normal diet.
2. STOOL FOR OCCULT BLOOD
   a. Description: stool sample is obtained to determine presence of gastrointestinal bleeding.
   b. Preprocedure
      1) Instruct the client to avoid red meats, raw vegetables, fruits, and vitamin C for 3 days before the test.
      2) Instruct the client to avoid taking nonsteroidal anti-inflammatory drugs, anticoagulants, and steroids for 7 days before the test.
      3) Instruct the client to defecate in an appropriate container, keeping the stool specimen free from urine or toilet paper.
3. TYPES OF TESTS FOR OCCULT BLOOD
   a. Hemoccult test
      1) Open the front cover of the Hemoccult slide and apply a thin smear of stool.
      2) Open the back cover of the Hemoccult slide and apply two drops of developer on the slide.
      3) Bluish discoloration indicates presence of occult blood.
   b. Hematest
      1) Place a small smear of stool on the guaiac filter paper.
      2) Put a Hematest tablet in the middle of the stool sample.
      3) Place 2 or 3 drops of water on the tablet.
      4) Bluish discoloration indicates presence of occult blood.
4. POSTPROCEDURE
   a. Resume normal diet and medications.
   b. Stool culture
      1) Description: stool sample is obtained to determine presence of a bowel infection.
      2) Procedure
         a) Instruct the client not to void urine with the stool sample.
         b) Dip a sterile swab into the purulent fecal matter and place the swab in a sterile test tube.
         c) Send the specimen immediately to the lab.

N. UREA BREATH TEST
1. DESCRIPTION: BREATH SAMPLE TAKEN AFTER INGESTION OF CARBON-LABELED UREA CAPSULE TO DETERMINE PRESENCE OF *HELICOBACTER PYLORI*
2. PREPROCEDURE
   a. Instruct the client to avoid loperamide (Pepto-Bismol) and antibiotics for 1 month prior to the test.
   b. Instruct the client to avoid omeprazole (Prilosec), lansoprazole (Prevacid), or esomeprazole (Nexium) for 1 week prior to the test.
   c. Instruct the client to avoid nizatidine (Axid), ranitidine (Zantac), famotidine (Pepcid), or cimetidine (Tagamet) for 24 hours prior to the test.
3. PROCEDURE
   a. Client ingests a carbon-labeled urea capsule.
   b. Breath sample is taken 10 to 20 minutes later.

O. PARACENTESIS
1. DESCRIPTION: INSERTION OF A NEEDLE INTO THE PERITONEAL CAVITY TO REMOVE ASCITIC FLUID
2. PREPROCEDURE
   a. Instruct the client to empty the bladder (prevents accidental trauma from the needle during the procedure).
   b. Measure abdominal girth.
   c. Obtain the client's weight.
   d. Obtain baseline vital signs.
   e. Place the client in a high-Fowler's position in the bed or in a chair with the back supported and feet flat on a stool.
3. POSTPROCEDURE
   a. Monitor vital signs.
   b. Measure and compare preprocedure weight and abdominal girth.
   c. Monitor serum protein and electrolyte levels because of high albumin and electrolytes, especially sodium.

d. Monitor the dressing over the needle puncture site for bleeding.

IV. BLOOD CHEMISTRIES (SEE TABLE 5-1)

V. GASTROINTESTINAL TUBES
A. NASOGASTRIC (NG) TUBES
1. DESCRIPTION: POLYURETHANE OR SILICONE TUBE PASSED THROUGH THE NARE INTO THE STOMACH FOR PURPOSES OF FEEDING, INTERMITTENT SUCTION, OR GASTRIC DECOMPENSATION WITH CONTINUOUS SUCTION
2. TYPES OF TUBES
   a. Levin: single lumen tube used for tube feeding or to provide intermittent gastric suction
   b. Salem sump: double-lumen air-vented tube used for gastric decompensation with continuous suction
3. INSERTION
   a. Place client in a high-Fowler's position.

Table 5-1 Blood Chemistries

Test	Significance
Albumin	Decreased in chronic liver disease or malabsorption
Ammonia	Elevated in severe liver disease
Amylase	Elevated in acute pancreatitis
Bilirubin	Elevated in biliary obstruction or impaired liver function
Calcium	Decreased in acute pancreatitis or malabsorption syndrome
Cholesterol	Elevated in biliary obstruction or extensive liver disease
Glucose (fasting)	Elevated in pancreatic insufficiency Decreased in pancreatitic hypofunction, tumor, or dumping syndrome
Lactic Dehydrogenase (LDH)	Elevated in metastatic cancer of the liver
Lipase	Elevated in acute pancreatitis, liver disease, or perforated peptic ulcer
Phosphatase, Alkaline	Elevated in biliary obstruction
Potassium	Decreased in severe diarrhea, vomiting, starvation, fistula along gastrointestinal (GI) tract, or pyloric obstruction
Protein	Elevated in cirrhosis Decreased in other liver diseases or malabsorption
Sodium	Decreased in severe diarrhea or vomiting
Serum Glutamicoxaloacetic (SGOT) or Asparate Aminotransferase (AST)	Elevated in acute hepatitis
Serum Glutamate Pyruvate (SGPT) or Alanine Aminotransferase (ALT)	Elevated in liver disease
Triglycerides	Elevated in liver disease Decreased in malnutrition
Urea Nitrogen (BUN)	Decreased in malnutrition or severe liver damage
Vitamin B$_{12}$	Decreased in pernicious anemia or after a gastrectomy

b. Measure the tube from the tip of the nose to the tip of the earlobe to the tip of the sternum and mark with tape.

c. Lubricate the tip of the tube only with a water-soluble lubricant that can be easily dissolved if the tube accidentally enters the lung.

d. Ask the client to hyperextend the neck, advancing the tube toward the nasopharynx.

e. Instruct the client to tilt the head forward when the tube is felt in the oropharynx (throat).

f. Offer the client small sips of water from a glass with a straw and encourage to swallow.

g. Stop passing the tube if the client gags, and wait a few minutes before proceeding.

h. Withdraw the tube slightly if gagging continues and inspect throat for coiling.

i. Assess correct placement of tube by:
  1) Checking the pH of the aspirated contents (pH of 4 or less indicates gastric secretions)
  2) Inserting 5–10 ml of air into a stethoscope placed over the stomach and listen for a swish of air
  3) Taking an x-ray, leaving the stylet or guidewire in place (most reliable method for checking placement of tube)

j. Secure the tube to the bridge of the nose with tape and to the gown.

B. INTESTINAL TUBES
  1. DESCRIPTION: POLYURETHANE OR SILICONE TUBE PASSED THROUGH THE NOSE INTO THE SMALL INTESTINE FOR PURPOSES OF REMOVING INTESTINAL CONTENTS OR DECOMPRESSING THE BOWEL
  2. TYPES OF TUBES
    a. Cantor and Harris tubes: single-lumen tubes with mercury at the tip of the tube
    b. Miller Abbott tube: double-lumen tube using one lumen for mercury and the other for drainage
  3. INSERTION
    a. Same as nasogastric tube but add 3 to 4 cm (8 to 10 in.) to the measurement for correct tube placement.
    b. After inserting the nasogastric tube into the stomach with the client in high-Fowler's position, turn the client on the right side to allow for advancement of the tube through the pylorus of the stomach and into the small intestine (may take up to 24 hours to reach the small intestine).

c. Confirm placement by testing the pH of aspirate followed by x-ray before taping in place.

C. NURSING CARE OF NASOGASTRIC AND INTESTINAL TUBES
  1. FREQUENT ORAL CARE, OFFERING HARD CANDY OR ICE CHIPS TO PREVENT DRYNESS
  2. ASSESS NARE FOR IRRITATION OR DRAINAGE, APPLYING WATER-SOLUBLE LUBRICANT TO THE ENCRUSTED NARE.
  3. ACCURATE INTAKE AND OUTPUT

VI. NURSING DIAGNOSES
  A. IMBALANCED NUTRITION: LESS THAN BODY REQUIREMENTS
  B. ACUTE PAIN
  C. INEFFECTIVE THERAPEUTIC REGIMEN MANAGEMENT
  D. DIARRHEA
  E. CONSTIPATION
  F. DEFICIENT FLUID VOLUME

Nursing Diagnoses: Definitions and Classification 2012–2014. Copyright © 2012, 1994–2012 by NANDA International. Used by arrangement with John Wiley & Sons Limited.

VII. GASTROINTESTINAL DISEASES
  A. GASTROESOPHAGEAL REFLUX DISEASE (GERD)
    1. DESCRIPTION
      a. Reflux of gastric or duodenal contents, or both, into the esophagus
      b. Result of incompetent lower esophageal sphincter (LES)
    2. ASSESSMENT
      a. Heartburn (pyrosis)
      b. Regurgitation
      c. Dysphagia
    3. DIAGNOSTIC TESTS
      a. Barium swallow
      b. Esophagoscopy
      c. Esophageal manometry
      d. Esophageal acid monitoring
    4. NURSING INTERVENTIONS
      a. Instruct the client to eat a high-protein, low-fat diet, avoiding alcohol, carbonated beverages, milk products, acidic fruits, and chocolate.
      b. Instruct the client to avoid late-night eating, lying down for 2 to 3 hours after eating, or wearing tight clothes around the waist and bending over.
      c. Instruct the client to sleep with the head of the bed elevated on 4- to 6-inch blocks.
      d. Teach the client regarding the safe administration of prescribed histamine H_2-receptor blockers, proton pump inhibitors, and antisecretory, anticholinergic, or cholinergic drugs.

    e. Instruct the client to avoid the use of anticholinergic drugs, which decrease gastric emptying.

    f. Instruct the client to take an antacid 1 to 3 hours after meals and at bedtime.

    g. Encourage the client to stop smoking.

  5. SURGICAL MANAGEMENT

    a. Antireflux surgery may be necessary if conservative treatment fails.

B. HIATAL HERNIA

  1. DESCRIPTION

    a. Herniation of a portion of the stomach through an opening into the diaphragm

    b. Commonly asymptomatic and found on a routine upper GI tract x-ray

    c. Occurs more frequently in older women

    d. Two types:

      1) Sliding hernia results when a portion of the stomach and the gastroesophageal junction slip into the thoracic cavity.

      2) Paraesophageal or rolling hernia results when the fundus and greater curvature of the stomach rolls through the diaphragmatic defect and forms a pocket on the side of the esophagus.

    e. Contributing factors include obesity, pregnancy, ascites, tumors, trauma, advanced age, constant recumbent position, and heavy lifting.

    f. Complications include hemorrhage, ulceration, stenosis, and strangulation of the hernia.

  2. ASSESSMENT

    a. Pyrosis

    b. Retrosternal or substernal pain

    c. Dysphagia

  3. DIAGNOSTIC TESTS

    a. Barium swallow

    b. Esophagoscopy

  4. NURSING INTERVENTIONS

    a. Instruct the client to avoid alcohol and smoking.

    b. Instruct the client to sleep with the head of the bed elevated on 4- to 6-inch blocks.

    c. Instruct the client to avoid activities that increase intra-abdominal pressure such as coughing, straining, and bending forward.

    d. Instruct the client on diet modifications, including small, frequent bland meals, weight loss, and not eating 2 hours before bedtime.

  5. SURGICAL MANAGEMENT

    a. Goal is to reinforce the LES and reduce gastric reflux.

    b. Valvuloplasties or antireflux procedures include Nissen fundoplication, Hill gastropexy, and Belsey's fundoplication, involving wrapping of the fundus of the stomach around the lower esophagus.

    c. Success of surgery depends on the correct tightness of the wrap (too tight results in dysphagia and gas-bloat syndrome; too loose results in continual reflux).

C. ESOPHAGITIS

  1. DESCRIPTION

    a. Inflammation of the esophagus

    b. Causes include chemical irritants, physical irritants such as smoking, alcohol, and temperature extremes of food and fluids.

  2. ASSESSMENT

    a. Achalasia (cardiospasm)

    b. Pyrosis

  3. DIAGNOSTIC TESTS

    a. Esophagoscopy

  4. COMPLICATIONS

    a. Barrett's esophagus

      1. The result of an incompetent lower esophageal sphincter

      2. May occur after years of esophagitis and heartburn

      3. The lining of the esophagus is damaged by the acid of the stomach.

  5. NURSING INTERVENTIONS

    a. Instruct the client to eliminate the cause and prevent reflux of gastric acid.

    b. Instruct the client to take medication as ordered even after clinical manifestations subside.

D. GASTRITIS

  1. DESCRIPTION

    a. Inflammation of the gastric mucosa

    b. May be acute or chronic

    c. Causes include corticosteroids, nonsteroidal anti-inflammatory drugs, digitalis, aspirin, alcohol, smoking, spicy foods, prolonged vomiting, reflux of bile salts post-gastroduodenostomy and post-gastrojejunostomy, central nervous system lesions, and *Helicobacter pylori* (*H. pylori*).

  2. ASSESSMENT

    a. Anorexia

    b. Nausea

    c. Vomiting

    d. Epigastric distress

    e. Feeling of fullness

  3. DIAGNOSTIC TESTS

    a. Gastroscopy with biopsy for definitive diagnosis

    b. Breath, serum, urine, gastric tissue biopsy for diagnosis of *H. pylori*

    c. Complete blood count and stool tests diagnostic for anemia and occult blood

4. NURSING INTERVENTIONS
a. In acute phase, bed rest, NPO, nasogastric (NG) tube, and replacement of fluids and electrolytes lost through vomiting and diarrhea
b. Blood transfusions for hemorrhagic gastritis
c. Administer antacids or H_2 antagonists as prescribed; administer antibiotics if *H. pylori* is diagnosed.
d. Gradual reintroduction of clear liquids and bland foods when symptoms subside
e. Instruct the client to eliminate the cause.

E. ATROPHIC GASTRITIS
1. DESCRIPTION: CHRONIC INFLAMMATION OF THE STOMACH RESULTING FROM DEGENERATION OF GASTRIC MUCOSA, RESULTING IN PERNICIOUS ANEMIA
2. ASSESSMENT
a. Vitamin B_{12} deficiency
b. Hypochlorhydria (decreased acid production)
c. Achlorhydria (lack of acid production)
3. DIAGNOSTIC TESTS
a. Parietal cell antibody and intrinsic factor serum tests
4. NURSING INTERVENTIONS
a. Vitamin B_{12} injections may be necessary for life.
b. Stress the importance of close medical supervision because of the higher incidence of gastric cancer.

F. UPPER GASTROINTESTINAL BLEEDING
1. DESCRIPTION
a. Sudden or insidious occult bleeding from the upper gastrointestinal tract
b. May be capillary, arterial, or venous in origin
c. 1500 ml of blood or loss of 25% of intravascular blood volume is a massive upper GI bleed.
d. Has a 10% mortality rate
2. ASSESSMENT
a. Hematemesis (bright red or "coffee ground" emesis)
b. Melena (black tarry, foul-smelling stools occurring from the digestion of blood in the GI tract and the presence of iron, indicating a slow GI bleed)
c. Occult blood (small amount of blood appearing in gastric secretions detectable only by guaiac test)
3. DIAGNOSTIC TESTS
a. Fiberoptic panendoscopy
b. Angiography
4. NURSING INTERVENTIONS
a. Blood and fluid replacement
b. Oxygen therapy

c. Monitor vital signs every 15 to 30 minutes.
d. Assess for shock.
e. Hourly urine output
f. NG tube and possible cool water, ice, or saline lavages (except in esophageal varices)
g. Identify and eliminate the cause after the client stabilizes.
h. Frequent mouth care
5. MEDICAL MANAGEMENT
a. Vasopressin (Pitressin) to produce vasoconstriction in a client who is a poor surgical risk
b. Somatostatin (Sandostatin) administered early when bleeding is related to esophageal varices
c. Magnesium trisilicates and aluminum hydroxide antacids most useful because they are nonabsorbable
6. SURGICAL MANAGEMENT
a. Surgical intervention aimed at the site of bleeding when medical treatment fails

G. PEPTIC ULCER DISEASE
1. DESCRIPTION
a. Erosion of the GI mucosal membrane and classified as acute or chronic depending on the degree of mucosal involvement
b. May develop in the lower esophagus, stomach, duodenum, or jejunum
c. Acute ulcer associated with mild inflammation, superficial erosion of short duration resolving quickly when eliminating the cause
d. Chronic ulcer extends through the muscular wall with the formation of fibrous tissue of long duration
2. TYPES
a. Gastric ulcer
1) Superficial lesion predominantly occurring in the antrum of the stomach as a result of normal to decreased gastric acid production with a high recurrence rate
2) More common in 50–60 years of age, women, unskilled laborers, and people of lower socioeconomic status
3) Causes include smoking, drug, alcohol, NSAIDs, aspirin, corticosteroids, caffeine, incompetent pyloric sphincter, and after severe burns, head trauma, or major surgery.
4) Clinical manifestations include burning or gaseous pressure in the left upper epigastrium, back, and upper abdomen occurring 1–2 hours after eating, nausea, vomiting, and weight loss.

b. Duodenal ulcer
1) Penetrating lesion occurring in the first 2 cm of the duodenum as a result of increased gastric acid with a high recurrence rate
2) More common in the 35- to 45-year-old age group, men, and postmenopausal women
3) Causes include smoking, drug, alcohol, chronic obstructive pulmonary disease (COPD), Zollinger-Ellison syndrome, pancreatic disease, hyperparathyroidism, and chronic renal failure.
4) Clinical manifestations include burning, cramping, and pressure-like pain across the midepigastrium and back occurring 2–4 hours after eating that is relieved with antacids.

3. THREE MAJOR COMPLICATIONS INCLUDE:
a. Hemorrhage occurs most commonly and with a higher frequency in duodenal ulcers.
b. Perforation is the most lethal complication, frequently occurring in large penetrating posterior duodenal ulcers that have not healed and invade the pancreas, manifesting as severe upper abdominal pain.
c. Gastric outlet obstruction most commonly occurs after a long history of ulcer pain that becomes worse at the end of the day and may be relieved with self-induced vomiting.

4. DIAGNOSTIC TESTS
a. Fiberoptic endoscopy with biopsy to diagnose the site of the ulcer and presence of *H. pylori*
b. Urea breath tests

5. NURSING INTERVENTIONS DURING ACUTE EPISODE
a. NPO and NG tube to low intermittent suction
b. IV fluid replacement
c. Bed rest
d. Monitor vital signs.
e. Administer antacids, H$_2$-receptor antagonists, proton pump inhibitors, anticholinergics, and sedatives as prescribed.

6. NURSING INTERVENTIONS WITH A COMPLICATION
a. Hemorrhage
1) NPO and NG tube for gastric decompensation and possible ice or cool water lavage
2) IV fluid and blood replacement
3) Monitor vital signs.

b. Perforation
1) NPO and NG tube for gastric decompensation
2) IV fluid replacement
3) Administer broad-spectrum antibiotics as prescribed to treat peritonitis.
4) Insert an indwelling urinary catheter and monitor output hourly.
5) Monitor vital signs.
c. Gastric outlet obstruction
1) NPO and NG tube to continuous suction to remove food and fluids and to facilitate the process of healing
2) Clamp NG tube for 8 to 12 hours followed by measurement of gastric residue.
3) Gradually begin oral fluids when gastric aspirate is less than 200 ml, followed by gradual introduction of solid foods as gastric aspirate continues to decrease and with absence of vomiting.
4) IV fluids and electrolyte replacement
5) Administer antacids, H$_2$-receptor antagonist, and proton pump inhibitors as prescribed.

7. MEDICAL MANAGEMENT WITH A COMPLICATION
a. Recommended operative procedure for perforation is reinforcement of the area with an omentum graft.
b. Endoscopic balloon dilation may be performed to remove pyloric obstruction.

8. SURGICAL MANAGEMENT FOR PEPTIC ULCERS
a. Criteria for surgical intervention include inability of the ulcer to heal; repeated recurrence, especially prepyloric and pyloric ulcers; multiple ulcer sites; malignant ulcer; drug-induced ulcer; or the presence of trauma, burns, or sepsis.
b. Types
1) Gastroduodenostomy or Billroth I involves the removal of the distal two-thirds of the stomach with anastomosis to the duodenum.
2) Gastrojejunostomy or Billroth II involves the removal of the distal two-thirds of the stomach with anastomosis to the jejunum and is the preferred surgical procedure to prevent recurrent duodenal ulcers.

3) Vagotomy involves the severing of the vagus nerve to eliminate HCl acid stimulus.

4) Pyloroplasty involves creating an enlarged pyloric sphincter to facilitate passage of gastric contents.

5) Billroth I or II with a vagotomy may be the preferred procedure to eliminate HCl acid secretion.

9. POSTOPERATIVE COMPLICATIONS
   a. Dumping syndrome
      1) Most commonly occurs after a Billroth II, resulting in abdominal cramps, urge to defecate, borborygmi, generalized weakness, sweating, palpitations, and dizziness within 30 minutes of meals and lasting no longer than an hour
      2) Usually self-limiting within months
      3) Small, dry, low-carbohydrate meals and refined sugar with moderate protein and fat recommended
      4) Fluids are permitted between meals but not with meals.
   b. Postprandial hypoglycemia
      1) Results from ingestion of concentrated carbohydrate causing release of excessive insulin followed by hypoglycemia
      2) Clinical manifestations include weakness, diaphoresis, mental confusion, palpitations, tachycardia, and anxiety.
      3) Candy or high-sugar fluid given to relieve hypoglycemia, followed by limiting sugar consumption with meals
   c. Bile reflux gastritis
      1) Results after gastric surgery involving the pylorus due to chronic exposure to bile
      2) Symptoms include increasing epigastric distress after meals that may be relieved by vomiting.
      3) Cholestyramine (Questran) administered before or with meals binding with bile salts and eliminating the source of irritation
      4) Aluminum hydroxide antacids may be given.

10. POSTOPERATIVE MANAGEMENT
    a. NPO and NG tube to decompress the remaining stomach and to decrease pressure on the suture line to facilitate healing
    b. Monitor the gastric aspirate, expecting bright red for the first 24 hours, followed by yellowish green within 36 to 48 hours.
    c. Monitor vital signs.
    d. Strict intake and output
    e. Monitor the dressing for bleeding or infection.
    f. Instruct the client on how to splint the abdomen during coughing and deep breathing.
    g. IV fluid and electrolyte replacement
    h. Gradual reintroduction of clear liquids and measurement of residual aspirate 1 to 2 hours prior to removing the NG tube
    i. Monitor for pernicious anemia—a long-term complication after partial gastrectomy requiring lifetime injections of vitamin B_{12} (see Table 5-2).

H. APPENDICITIS
   1. DESCRIPTION
      a. Inflammation of the appendix frequently occurring between 11 and 30 years of age
      b. Causes include obstruction of the lumen of the appendix by a fecalith (accumulation of feces), foreign body, tumor, or intramucal thickening as a result of lymphoid hyperplasia.
   2. ASSESSMENT
      a. Periumbilical pain that is continuous, persistent, and shifts to the right lower quadrant, localizing at McBurney's point (between the umbilicus and right iliac crest—signs of peritoneal irritation)
      b. Anorexia
      c. Nausea
      d. Vomiting
      e. Rebound tenderness
      f. Muscle guarding
   3. DIAGNOSTIC TESTS
      a. History and physical
      b. White blood cell (WBC) count

Table 5-2 Peptic Ulcer

Preventive Measures
• Identify and eliminate the cause.
• Get adequate physical and emotional rest.
• Avoid alcohol, smoking, and spicy irritating foods.
• Eat small frequent meals.
• Avoid NSAIDs, aspirin, and gastric-irritating medications unless prescribed by a physician (take with food).
• Avoid lying down after eating.
• Take antacids and H_2-antagonist as prescribed, avoiding interchanging over-the-counter brands, which may result in harmful side effects.

4. SURGICAL MANAGEMENT
   a. Immediate appendectomy unless appendix has ruptured; if appendix has ruptured, but no peritonitis, IV fluids and antibiotics for 6 to 8 hours before surgery.

I. PERITONITIS
   1. DESCRIPTION
      a. Acute or chronic inflammation of the peritoneum
      b. Bacterial causes include ruptured appendix, pancreatitis, peritoneal dialysis, obstruction in the GI tract, and gunshot or stab wound.
      c. Chemical causes include perforated peptic ulcer and rupture of a fallopian tube from an ectopic pregnancy.
      d. Complications include hypovolemic shock, septicemia, paralytic ileus, intra-abdominal abscess, and organ failure.
   2. ASSESSMENT
      a. Abdominal pain
      b. Tenderness over the involved site
      c. Rebound tenderness
      d. Muscle rigidity and spasm
      e. Abdominal distention and ascites
      f. Fever, tachycardia, and tachypnea
      g. Nausea and vomiting
   3. DIAGNOSTIC TESTS
      a. Complete blood count
      b. Abdominal paracentesis with culture
      c. Laparotomy
   4. NURSING INTERVENTIONS
      a. NPO and NG suction
      b. Antibiotic therapy
      c. IV fluid and electrolyte replacement
      d. Analgesics
      e. Assist the client to flex the knees for increased comfort.
      f. Accurate intake and output
   5. SURGICAL MANAGEMENT
      a. Emergency surgery may be necessary to eliminate the source of infection.
      b. Evacuate the abdominal cavity and insert drains if a perforation has occurred.

J. GASTROENTERITIS
   1. DESCRIPTION
      a. Inflammation of the stomach and small intestine
      b. Causes may be viral, bacterial, or parasitic.
      c. Generally self-limiting and does not require hospitalization
      d. Older adults may require hospitalization because of the inability to compensate for dehydration.
   2. ASSESSMENT
      a. Frequent watery diarrhea
      b. Nausea and vomiting
      c. Abdominal cramps

3. NURSING INTERVENTIONS
      a. Instruct the client to increase fluids rich in glucose and electrolytes (Pedialyte, Gatorade).
      b. NPO if vomiting is present
      c. Older adults may require hospitalization and IV fluid replacement.
      d. Administer antibiotics as prescribed.
      e. Identify and eliminate the cause.

K. INFLAMMATORY BOWEL SYNDROME
   1. DESCRIPTION
      a. Chronic, recurrent inflammation of the intestinal tract characterized by periods of exacerbations and remissions
      b. Cause is unknown but possible theories include infectious agent, autoimmune reaction, food allergies, and heredity.
      c. Types
         1) Crohn's disease
         2) Ulcerative colitis

L. CROHN'S DISEASE
   1. DESCRIPTION
      a. Chronic, nonspecific inflammatory bowel disorder that may occur in any part of the GI tract but frequently seen in the terminal ileum, jejunum, and colon with an insidious onset
      b. Commonly occurs between the ages of 15 and 30 years, with a slightly higher incidence in women, Jewish population, and upper-middle-class urban populations
      c. Complications include strictures, obstruction, fistulas, fat malabsorption, and gluten intolerance.
   2. ASSESSMENT
      a. Diarrhea
      b. Fatigue
      c. Abdominal pain
      d. Weight loss
      e. Fever
   3. DIAGNOSTIC TESTS
      a. Barium enema (skip lesions)
      b. Sigmoidoscopy and colonoscopy with biopsy
      c. Complete blood count
      d. Serum chemistries
   4. NURSING INTERVENTIONS
      a. Monitor frequency and character of stools.
      b. Daily weights
      c. Assess for signs of malnutrition.
      d. Administer IV fluids and TPN as ordered.
      e. Administer good skin care, cleaning the perianal area and providing sitz baths.
      f. Increase fluids.
      g. Provide a diet high in protein, calories, and vitamins; low in roughage, residue, and fat; and milk free.
      h. Administer sulfasalazine (Azulfidine) and corticosteroids as prescribed.

i. Administer immunosuppressive drugs as ordered if corticosteroids are unsuccessful.
   5. SURGICAL MANAGEMENT
      a. Intestinal resection may be necessary when medical management fails.
M. ULCERATIVE COLITIS
   1. DESCRIPTION
      a. Continuous inflammation beginning in the rectum and sigmoid colon extending upward into the colon but rarely affecting the small intestine
      b. Most commonly occurs between the ages of 15 and 25 years and less frequently between 50 and 80 years of age with a slightly higher incidence in women, Jewish population, and upper-middle class urban populations
      c. Complications include hemorrhage, strictures, perforation, toxic megacolon, colonic dilation, malabsorption, and a significant increased risk of active colitis present for more than 10 years.
      d. Ranges from mild localized disorder to an acute fulminating crisis that may result in a perforated colon, fatal peritonitis, and toxemia
   2. ASSESSMENT
      a. Bloody diarrhea ranging from 2 to 20 stools per day depending on the extent of the disease

      b. Abdominal cramping
      c. Weight loss
      d. Fever
      e. Anemia
      f. Tachycardia
      g. Dehydration
   3. DIAGNOSTIC TESTS
      a. Blood studies including a complete blood count, serum electrolyte panel, and serum protein
      b. Sigmoidoscopy
      c. Colonoscopy
      d. Barium enema
   4. NURSING INTERVENTIONS
      a. Provide for both physical and mental rest.
      b. Monitor and record the characteristics of the stools.
      c. Increase fluids and maintain a strict intake and output.
      d. Meticulous skin care, avoiding harsh soaps, and providing sitz baths
      e. NPO during acute exacerbation followed by a diet high in protein and calories, low in residue (see Table 5-3), and milk free
      f. Instruct the client to avoid smoking.
      g. Administer vitamin and iron supplements as ordered.
      h. Administer sulfasalazine (Azulfidine) and corticosteroids orally as prescribed (forms of each may be given as retention enema depending on the severity of the disease).

Table 5-3 Low-Residue Diet

Goal: To reduce the frequency of bowel movement by providing a diet that does not stimulate the intestinal tract and is low in fiber

Food	Permitted	Avoided
Beverages	Coffee, tea, carbonated strained fruit juices without pulp	Fruit juices with pulp, alcohol
Milk	Up to 2 cups/day including cooking (avoid completely for more restricted diet)	Yogurt with fruit
Meat	Bake or broiled meats without skin, creamy peanut butter	Fried, smoked, or pickled cured meats, ham
Egg	All except fried	Fried
Cheese	Cottage cheese, American, cheddar	All others
Soup	All made with permitted foods	Pea, ham and bean
Vegetables	Strained vegetables and without skins	Raw vegetables, vegetables with skins, peas, dried beans, legumes
Fruits	Strained fruits and without skins	Raw fruits, fruits with skins or seeds
Bread	White bread, crackers, melba toast	Whole-grain or bran breads, all hot breads (pancakes, muffins, biscuit)
Cereal	Cooked, refined, or strained such as cream of wheat or rice, grits, dry cereals without bran, noodles	Whole-grain or bran and those with nuts and raisins
Fats	Butter, cream, oil, mayonnaise, plain gravy	Spicy gravy
Desserts	Plain desserts including cakes, cookies, and puddings	Desserts with nuts, raisins, or coconut; pies, rich cakes; cobblers
Condiments	Salt, sugar, cinnamon, allspice, paprika, vinegar, lemon juice	All others

i. Administer immunosuppressive drugs in severe cases when other drug regimens fail.

5. SURGICAL MANAGEMENT
   a. Indicated if the client fails to respond to treatment with frequent debilitating exacerbations, massive bleeding, perforation, strictures, obstruction, dysplasia, or carcinoma
   b. Types
      1) Total proctocolectomy with permanent ileostomy
         a) One-stage procedure that removes the colon, rectum, and anus with closure of the anus creating a stoma in the right lower quadrant with the end of the terminal ileum
         b) Curative procedure
      2) Total proctocolectomy with continent ileostomy
         a) Creates an internal pouch (Kock's pouch) with a one-way nipple valve that is emptied at intervals with the insertion of a catheter
         b) Curative but has a high complication rate
      3) Total colectomy and ileal reservoir
         a) Consists of two procedures 8 to 12 weeks apart
         b) First procedure includes a colectomy, rectal mucosectomy, construction of ileal reservoir, and anastomosis with temporary ileostomy.
         c) Second procedure involves closure of the ileostomy when the capacity of the reservoir is increased.
         d) Goal is to gain control and decrease the number of stools daily.
   c. Postoperative management
      1) Measure drainage daily from ileostomy (1500 to 2000 ml) and from abdominal drain (100 to 150 ml).
      2) Reassure the client that incontinence of mucus is a temporary result of the surgery.
      3) Instruct the client to begin Kegel exercises several weeks postoperatively.
      4) Make a referral to an enterostomal therapy nurse.

N. DIVERTICULOSIS AND DIVERTICULITIS
   1. DESCRIPTION
      a. Diverticular disease has two clinical forms (diverticulosis and diverticulitis) consisting of outpouches of the mucosa (diverticula) that push through the surrounding muscle, most commonly in the sigmoid colon.
      b. Diverticulosis consists of multiple noninflamed diverticula with the client generally asymptomatic.
      c. Diverticulitis consists of multiple inflamed diverticula with retention of hardened stool (fecalith), resulting in a symptomatic client.
      d. More common in older adults and slightly more prevalent in men
      e. Cause unknown but research suggests diet low in fiber and high in refined carbohydrates reduces fecal residue, narrows the bowel lumen, and leads to high intra-abdominal pressure during defecation.
      f. Complications of diverticulitis include perforation with peritonitis, bowel obstruction, and hemorrhage.
   2. ASSESSMENT
      a. Abdominal pain and tenderness generally in the left lower quadrant
      b. Fever and chills
      c. Nausea and vomiting
      d. Leukocytosis
   3. DIAGNOSTIC TESTS
      a. Barium enema and colonoscopy (except in acute diverticulitis because of the risk of perforation and peritonitis)
      b. Complete blood count
      c. Urinalysis
   4. NURSING INTERVENTIONS
      a. Instruct the client to select high-fiber foods.
      b. Encourage the client to increase fluids.
      c. Administer bulk laxatives and anticholinergics as prescribed.
      d. Encourage the client to lose weight and avoid activities that increase intra-abdominal pressure such as straining at stool, vomiting, bending, lifting, or tight clothing.
      e. Bed rest, NPO, IV fluids and broad-spectrum antibiotics in acute diverticulitis
   5. SURGICAL MANAGEMENT
      a. Colon resection with temporary colostomy may be necessary to drain an abscess or resect an inflammatory obstructing mass.

O. INTESTINAL OBSTRUCTION
   1. DESCRIPTION
      a. Intestinal contents cease to flow through the GI tract, requiring emergency treatment.
      b. Two types:
         1) Mechanical obstruction is the most common and the result of an occlusion of the intestinal tract by adhesions, hernias, or neoplasms.

2) Nonmechanical obstruction is the result of a neuromuscular (paralytic ileus, pseudobstruction) or vascular (emboli, atherosclerosis of the mesenteric arteries) condition.
c. Complications include strangulation and gangrene.

2. ASSESSMENT
   a. Obstruction high in the small intestine has a rapid onset resulting in frequent copious bile containing vomitus that may be projectile, intermittent crampy abdominal pain, and minimal or the absence of abdominal distention.
   b. Obstruction in the large intestine has a gradual onset resulting in infrequent vomitus that may be foul smelling and orangish brown, crampy abdominal pain with severe abdominal distention, and lack of all stool.
   c. Borborygmi (high-pitched bowel sounds above the obstruction)
   d. Low-grade fever unless strangulation

3. DIAGNOSTIC TESTS
   a. Abdominal x-rays
   b. Barium enema (except when perforation is suspected)
   c. Sigmoidoscopy and colonoscopy
   d. Complete blood count, serum electrolyte, amylase, and BUN

4. NURSING INTERVENTIONS
   a. NPO and NG or intestinal tube to decompress the intestine
   b. IV fluid and electrolyte replacement
   c. Administer analgesics as ordered.
   d. Monitor vital signs and bowel sounds.

5. SURGICAL MANAGEMENT
   a. Mechanical obstructions commonly require resection of the obstructed intestine.

P. HERNIA
1. DESCRIPTION
   a. Part of an internal organ protrudes through an abdominal opening causing abdominal, inguinal, or femoral bulge.
   b. Types:
      1) Inguinal hernia is most common and frequently occurs in men.
      2) Femoral hernia is more common in women and can easily strangulate.
      3) Ventral or incisional hernia results from a weakness in an old abdominal incision.
      4) Umbilical hernia is more common in children, resulting when the umbilical opening fails to close after birth, and frequently resolves as the child grows.

   c. Hernias may be reducible (can be manipulated back into the abdominal cavity), irreducible or incarcerated (cannot be manipulated back into the abdominal cavity because of an obstruction to the intestinal flow, usually by adhesions), or strangulated (intestinal flow and blood supply is obstructed, resulting in acute intestinal obstruction).

2. ASSESSMENT
   a. Palpable bulge over the affected site when the client stands or bears down
   b. Pain when tension is applied to the herniated area
   c. Vomiting, abdominal distention, and persistent pain with strangulation

3. DIAGNOSTIC TESTS
   a. History and physical (detects palpable mass)
   b. Abdominal x-ray (detects obstruction)

4. NURSING INTERVENTIONS
   a. Instruct the client how to apply a truss (pad with a belt) over the hernia to reduce it.
   b. Postoperatively:
      1) Maintain accurate intake and output (difficulty voiding frequently requires catheterization).
      2) Apply an ice bag to the scrotal area after inguinal hernia repair (scrotal edema).
      3) Discourage coughing but instruct the client how to deep breathe and turn.
      4) Instruct the client how to splint the incision for support and to sneeze with the mouth open.
      5) Instruct the client to avoid heavy lifting 6 to 8 weeks postoperatively.
         a) Surgery depends on the size of the hernia and risk of strangulation.
         b) Surgery may be either herniorrhaphy (simple reduction) or hernioplasty (reduction with reinforcement of weakened area with wire, fascia, or mesh).

Q. HEMORRHOIDS
1. DESCRIPTION
   a. Dilated hemorrhoidal veins classified as internal or external
   b. Causes include straining at stool, prolonged standing or sitting, pregnancy, obesity, and portal hypertension.

2. ASSESSMENT
   a. Bleeding with defecation and pain occurs with internal hemorrhoids.

b. Generally, pain and bleeding are rare with external hemorrhoids unless thrombosis occurs.

3. DIAGNOSTIC TESTS
   a. Inspection
   b. Digital examination
   c. Sigmoidoscopy

4. NURSING INTERVENTIONS
   a. Instruct the client on the importance of a high-fiber diet and increased fluid intake.
   b. Instruct the client to take stool softeners and use ointments such as dibucaine (Nupercanial), anti-inflammatories, or astringents.
   c. Apply ice packs for several hours followed by warm packs.
   d. Postoperatively:
      1) Administer prescribed analgesics because pain is severe (also before defecation).
      2) Offer warm sitz baths.
      3) Educate on the importance of diet, fluids, and drugs as ordered.

5. MEDICAL MANAGEMENT
   a. Injection of sclerosing solution into the tissue surrounding the hemorrhoids (shrinks supporting tissue causing fibrosis)
   b. Rubber band ligation with internal hemorrhoids
   c. Photocoagulation, diathermy, or cryotherapy

6. SURGICAL MANAGEMENT
   a. Hemorrhoidectomy is excision of hemorrhoids performed when excessive bleeding, pain, or prolapse is present.

R. HEPATITIS
   1. DESCRIPTION
      a. Inflammation of the liver
      b. Classified as viral (most common and includes hepatitis A, B, C, D, E, and G), nonviral (also called noninfectious and caused by drugs or chemicals), and bacterial (rare)
      c. Types of hepatitis (see Table 5-4)
      d. Complications

Table 5-4 Types of Hepatitis

Type	Incubation	Causes/Transmission	Period of Infection
Hepatitis A	2 to 7 weeks (average 4 weeks)	Fecal-oral Crowded and poor sanitary conditions Fecal contamination of food, including undercooked shellfish from contamination by food handler, and fecal-contaminated water	Present in feces 2 weeks before onset of symptoms and 2 weeks after onset of symptoms No carrier state
Hepatitis B	7 to 24 weeks (average 8 to 10 weeks)	IV drug users Accidental needle sticks Contaminated blood products Sexual activity (vaginal, seminal secretions) Saliva (urine, feces, tears, sweat, and breast milk not infectious unless contaminated with blood) Perinatal	Before and after onset of symptoms Small percent develop chronic lifetime carrier state
Hepatitis C	2 to 24 weeks (average 8 weeks)	IV drug users Contaminated blood products Hemodialysis Tattooing Sexual activity Organ donation Perinatal	1 to 2 weeks before onset of symptoms and throughout clinical course May be lifetime with chronic carrier
Hepatitis D	2 to 26 weeks	Same as Hepatitis B	Same as Hepatitis B Occurs as primary infection along with hepatitis B or in a carrier state of hepatitis B Contributing factor to fulminant hepatitis B
Hepatitis E	2 to 8 weeks (average 3 to 4 weeks)	Fecal-oral Most frequently contaminated drinking water and in underdeveloped countries (rare in the United States)	Unknown—may be similar to hepatitis A
Hepatitis G	Coincides with other forms of hepatitis	Blood transfusion	Frequently exists with other forms of hepatitis

1) Chronic persistent hepatitis is most common, generally benign, characterized by hepatomegaly and fatigue, requiring no special treatment, liver function test may be abnormal for years, and convalescence may be delayed.

2) Chronic active hepatitis is the continuation of symptoms associated with hepatitis B and C and differential diagnosis made with liver biopsy (demonstrates necrosis that may progress to cirrhosis).

3) Fulminant hepatitis is a rare, severe, life-threatening form of hepatitis resulting in necrosis or liver failure.

2. ASSESSMENT: CLINICAL MANIFESTATIONS ARE CLASSIFIED IN THREE PHASES:

  a. Preicteric phase

    1) Lasts 1 to 21 days

    2) Precedes jaundice

    3) Anorexia, nausea, vomiting

    4) Right upper quadrant abdominal pain

    5) Decreased smell and taste

    6) Weight loss

    7) Malaise, headache, arthralgia

    8) Low-grade fever

    9) Hepatomegaly and lymphadenopathy

  b. Icteric phase

    1) Lasts 2 to 4 weeks

    2) Jaundice

    3) Dark urine

    4) Pruritus

    5) Fever subsides.

    6) Clay-colored stools

    7) Fatigue

    8) Hepatomegaly

  c. Posticteric phase (convalescent phase)

    1) Jaundice disappears but does not mean recovery.

    2) Lasts an average of 2 to 4 months

    3) Significant malaise and fatigue

3. DIAGNOSTIC TESTS

  a. Liver function tests

  b. Hepatitis serology

  c. Physical examination reveals hepatomegaly.

4. NURSING INTERVENTIONS

  a. Bed rest

  b. Diet high in calories, carbohydrates, and protein, and low in fat

  c. Meticulous skin and mouth care

  d. Daily weights

  e. Administer antiemetics as prescribed (avoid phenothiazines because of hepatotoxic effects).

  f. Administer interferon in hepatitis B, C, and chronic hepatitis.

  g. Instruct the client to scratch with the knuckles, not the nails.

  h. Instruct the client to avoid alcohol (cough syrups and mouthwashes with high alcohol content) and any over-the-counter medications such as acetaminophen (Tylenol) because they are hepatotoxic.

5. PREVENTIVE MEASURES

  a. Hepatitis A:

    1) Instruct the client on the importance of hand washing after bowel movements and before eating.

    2) Immune globulin may be given preventively and also up to 2 weeks after exposure (day care center, traveling to underdeveloped countries).

    3) Instruct the client on the proper preparation of food.

  b. Hepatitis B:

    1) Hepatitis B vaccine (routine vaccine for all newborns and adolescents, high-risk individuals such as health care workers, IV drug users, persons with multiple sexual partners, sexual partners of hepatitis B carriers, and prison inmates)

    2) Instruct the client on the importance of hand washing and gloves when exposure to blood is anticipated.

    3) Instruct the client to use a condom for sexual intercourse.

    4) Instruct the client to avoid sharing razors and toothbrushes.

    5) Dispose of needles and syringes in puncture-resistant containers.

  c. Hepatitis C:

    1) Screen all blood, organ, and tissue donors.

    2) Hepatitis B preventive control measures

S. CIRRHOSIS

1. DESCRIPTION

  a. Chronic disease with an insidious onset characterized by diffuse destruction and fibrotic regeneration of hepatic cells

  b. Highest incidence in men over the age of 50 years with a history of alcoholism

  c. High mortality rate

  d. Most common cause is alcoholism.

  e. Four types:

    1) Alcoholic cirrhosis, also called portal or nutritional cirrhosis, previously called Laënnec's, is

caused by alcohol abuse, resulting in fatty changes and widespread scar tissue in the liver.

   2) Postnecrosis cirrhosis is a complication of viral, toxic, or autoimmune hepatitis and results in scar tissue.
   3) Biliary cirrhosis results from biliary obstruction and infection.
   4) Cardiac cirrhosis results from severe right-sided heart failure.

   f. Complications include portal hypertension, jaundice, esophageal varices, peripheral edema, ascites, renal failure, hepatic encephalopathy, and coma.

2. ASSESSMENT
   a. Early manifestations:
      1) Anorexia, nausea, vomiting, and dyspepsia
      2) Flatulence, change in bowel habits (diarrhea or constipation)
      3) Dull, heavy right upper abdominal or epigastric pain
      4) Fever, weight loss, and fatigue
      5) Hepatomegaly and splenomegaly
   b. Late manifestations:
      1) Jaundice
      2) Peripheral edema and ascites
      3) Skin lesions such as spider angiomas and palmar erythema
      4) Hematologic conditions including bleeding tendencies, anemia, thrombocytopenia, and leukopenia
      5) Endocrine conditions including testicular atrophy, menstrual irregularities, gynecomastia, loss of axillary and pubic hair
      6) Peripheral neuropathy
      7) Asterixis (liver flap characterized by the inability of the client to hold the arms and hands extended forward and to make rapid flexion and extension movements)
      8) Fector hepaticus (musty, sweet breath odor)

3. DIAGNOSTIC TESTS
   a. Liver profile
   b. Liver biopsy
   c. Complete blood count
   d. Prothrombin time

4. NURSING INTERVENTIONS
   a. Bed rest
   b. Meticulous skin care and teach the client to scratch with the knuckles, not the nails.
   c. Administer cholestyramine (Questran) for pruritus.
   d. Strict intake and output
   e. Monitor daily weights and offer between-meal snacks.

   f. Assist the client to a semi-Fowler's or Fowler's position for dyspnea.
   g. Provide good oral hygiene.
   h. Instruct the client to avoid aspirin and hepatoxic over-the-counter drugs.
   i. Offer high-calorie (3000 kcal per day), high-carbohydrate, and low-fat diet.
   j. Restrict protein in the diet when hepatic encephalopathy is present.
   k. Restrict sodium in the diet when edema and ascites are present.

T. PANCREATITIS
   1. DESCRIPTION
      a. Inflammation of the pancreas
      b. May be acute or chronic
      c. Ranges from mild edema to severe hemorrhagic necrosis
      d. Common in middle-aged men
      e. Causes include biliary tract disease, alcoholism, surgical trauma, penetrating duodenal ulcer, hyperparathyroidism, hyperlipidemia, renal failure, certain drugs such as thiazide diuretics, oral contraceptives, corticosteroids, NSAIDs, and sulfonamides and following endoscopic retrograde cholangiopancreatography (ERCP).
      f. Two most common local complications are pseudocyst (cavity surrounding the pancreas filled with necrotic products and liquid secretions) and an abscess (large fluid-filled cavity within the pancreas).
      g. Most common systemic complications are pleural effusion, atelectasis, pneumonia, and tetany.

   2. ASSESSMENT
      a. Acute pancreatitis
         1) Severe, continuous left upper quadrant pain that radiates to the back, aggravated by eating, and not relieved by vomiting
         2) Flexion of the spine is an attempt to relieve the pain.
         3) Flushing, cyanosis, and dyspnea
         4) Nausea and vomiting
         5) Low-grade fever and leukocytosis
         6) Hypotension and tachycardia
         7) Decreased or absent bowel sounds
      b. Chronic pancreatitis
         1) Heavy, gnawing, occasional burning or crampy left upper quadrant abdominal pain
         2) Malabsorption and weight loss
         3) Mild jaundice with dark urine and steatorrhea
         4) Diabetes mellitus

   3. DIAGNOSTIC TESTS
      a. Serum and urinary amylase, serum lipase (most specific), serum bilirubin,

alkaline phosphatase, and sedimentation rate
   b. White blood cell count
   c. Fecal fat determinations
   d. Blood and urine glucose
   e. Endoscopic retrograde cholangiopancreatography
4. NURSING INTERVENTIONS
   a. Acute pancreatitis
      1) Meperidine (Demerol) was once thought to be the drug of choice because it doesn't cause spasms of the sphincter of Oddi. All opioids cause some degree of spasms. Also, because normepridine (toxic metabolite) can result in seizures, it is no longer the preferred drug to be used in acute pancreatitis.
      2) Assist the client to assume pain relief positions (flex the trunk and draw the knees up or side-lying with the head elevated 45 degrees).
      3) NPO and jejunostomy tube to decrease gastric and pancreatic secretions
      4) IV fluid (lactated Ringer's) and electrolyte replacement
      5) Monitor the client for fever and other signs of an infection.
      6) Monitor serum glucose to assess the development of diabetes mellitus from damage to the B-cells islets of Langerhans.
      7) Blood volume replacement if shock is present
      8) Administer H_2 antagonists and antacids as ordered.
      9) Restart food with small, frequent high-carbohydrate, high-protein, and low-fat diet.
     10) Instruct the client to avoid alcohol.
   b. Chronic pancreatitis
      1) All nursing interventions listed for acute pancreatitis
      2) Administer pancreatin (Viokase) and pancrelipase (Cotazym), which contain amylase, lipase, and trypsin, given to replace pancreatic enzymes.
      3) May give bile salts to facilitate absorption of fat-soluble vitamins
      4) Surgery may be necessary to divert bile flow or relieve ductal obstruction.
U. CHOLECYSTITIS AND CHOLELITHIASIS
   1. DESCRIPTION
      a. Cholecystitis
         1) Inflammation of the gallbladder
         2) Usually associated with cholelithiasis

         3) Generally caused by *Escherichia coli* in the absence of gallstones
         4) Incidence higher in multiparous women over 40 years of age, postmenopausal women, sedentary lifestyle, obesity, a familial tendency, and Native American or Caucasian populations
         5) Complications include cholangitis, pancreatitis, biliary cirrhosis, carcinoma, and peritonitis.
      b. Cholelithiasis
         1) Actual cause is unknown but theories include infection and disturbances in the metabolism of cholesterol.
         2) Gallstones made up of precipitates of cholesterol, bile salts, bilirubin, calcium, and protein (mixed cholesterol stones most common)
   2. ASSESSMENT
      a. Cholecystitis
         1) Mild indigestion to severe pain and tenderness in the right upper quadrant that may radiate to the right shoulder and scapula
         2) Nausea, vomiting, dyspepsia, heartburn, fat intolerance, and flatulence
      b. Cholelithiasis
         1) May be asymptomatic (symptoms dependent on whether gallstone is mobile or lodged in a duct)
         2) Biliary colic occurs when the stone attempts to move forward, causing spasms, tachycardia, diaphoresis, and prostration.
         3) Jaundice, dark amber foamy urine, clay-colored stools, steatorrhea, and pruritus when obstruction of bile flow is present
   3. DIAGNOSTIC TESTS
      a. Ultrasonography
      b. Oral cholecystogram
      c. IV cholangiogram
      d. Percutaneous transhepatic cholangiography
      e. Liver function tests
      f. White blood cell count
      g. Serum enzymes
   4. NURSING INTERVENTIONS
      a. NPO and NG tube to decompress stimulation of the gallbladder
      b. Administer prescribed analgesic
      c. Administer prescribed anticholinergics to decrease secretions, biliary contractions, and spasms.
      d. Use baking soda, Alpha Keri lotion, and lotions containing calamine, and administer cholestyramine (Questran) if ordered for pruritus.

e. Instruct the client on a low-fat and low-calorie diet if weight reduction is needed.
5. MEDICAL MANAGEMENT
   a. Methyl tertiary terbutyl ether (MTBE) is instilled via a percutaneous catheter into the gallbladder to dissolve the stones.
   b. Extracorporeal shock-wave lithotripsy (ESWL) involves locating the stones with an ultrasound followed by high-energy shock waves to dissolve the stones (usually occurs within 2 hours).
   c. Hydrocholeretic drugs such as dehydrocholic acid (Decholin) may be administered postoperatively if there is no obstruction to stimulate the production of bile with a low specific gravity.

6. SURGICAL MANAGEMENT
   a. Endoscopic sphincterotomy (papillotomy) involves passing the endoscope into the duodenum with an electrodiathermy knife attached to the endoscope to widen the sphincter of Oddi, removing the stone or allowing it to pass.
   b. Laparoscopic cholecystectomy involves removing the gallbladder through one of four small punctures in the abdomen through the use of a laparoscope allowing the client to return to normal activities within 2 to 3 days.
   c. Cholecystectomy involves removing the gallbladder through a right subcostal incision with the insertion of a T-tube to drain excess bile and ensure patency of the common bile duct.

PRACTICE QUESTIONS

1. The nurse is assessing a client's gastrointestinal tract. Which of the following subjective assessments should be included?
   1. Rebound tenderness
   2. Diarrhea
   3. Generalized red abdominal rash
   4. Hematuria

2. In planning the postprocedure care for a client who has a barium enema, the nurse should include which of the following?

   Select all that apply:
   [ ] 1. Position the client on the right side
   [ ] 2. Observe and record the amount of rectal drainage
   [ ] 3. Encourage fluids
   [ ] 4. Maintain bed rest for 12 hours
   [ ] 5. Monitor the client for a rise in body temperature and abdominal pain
   [ ] 6. Administer a laxative

3. When providing care for a client who has had an upper gastrointestinal endoscopy, the nurse should include which of the following interventions?
   1. Assist the client to maintain a right-side lying position
   2. Provide the client with a fatty "test meal"
   3. Keep the client NPO until the gag reflex returns
   4. Administer the prescribed bulk-forming laxative

4. The nurse is caring for a client with gastroesophageal reflux disease. Which of the following measures would be essential to include in the client's discharge instructions?

   Select all that apply:
   [ ] 1. Small, frequent meals
   [ ] 2. Avoid fluids at mealtime
   [ ] 3. High-calorie and high-protein diet
   [ ] 4. Bulk-forming laxatives
   [ ] 5. Sleep with the head of the bed elevated
   [ ] 6. Avoid caffeine in the diet

5. The nurse is caring for a client with gastroenteritis. Which of the following nursing measures should receive priority in the client's plan of care?
   1. Maintain a clean environment free from odors
   2. Assist the client to wash hands and face before meals
   3. Encourage fluids and monitor intake and output
   4. Provide foods the client likes and allow plenty of time for meals

6. The nurse is caring for a client with diverticulitis. Which of the following diets would be essential to include in the client's plan of care?
   1. High-fiber diet
   2. Low-fat, high-carbohydrate, and high-protein diet, avoiding alcohol

3. High-calorie, high-carbohydrate, and low-fat diet
4. Diet high in protein and calories, low in residue, and milk free

7. The registered nurse is making out the clinical assignments for the day. Which of the following nursing tasks is appropriate to delegate to a licensed practical nurse?
   1. Plan an activity schedule for a client following a Billroth I
   2. Develop a plan of care for a client following a total proctocolectomy
   3. Assess the client's understanding of the care following an ileostomy
   4. Assist the client to select a low-fat diet following a cholecystectomy

8. The nurse is collecting a nursing history from a client suspected of having an obstruction of the alimentary canal. Which of the following questions should the nurse ask first to elicit the most accurate assessment?
   1. "Are you frequently awakened during the middle of the night because of pain?"
   2. "Have you recently lost a lot of weight?"
   3. "Do you have difficulty swallowing food or liquids?"
   4. "Have you experienced any bleeding?"

9. The nurse is caring for a client with peptic ulcer disease. Which of the following observations should the nurse report immediately?

   Select all that apply:
   [ ] 1. Hypotension
   [ ] 2. Thirst
   [ ] 3. Headache
   [ ] 4. Tachycardia
   [ ] 5. Restlessness
   [ ] 6. Diarrhea

10. When preparing a client for insertion of a nasogastric tube, it is essential for the nurse to include which of the following aspects of the procedure?
    1. Instruct the client to avoid swallowing when the tube is felt in the back of the throat
    2. Assist the client to assume a left-side-lying or recumbent position
    3. Tilt the client's head back when the tube is being inserted
    4. Measure the tube from the tip of the nose to the earlobe to the xiphoid process

11. The nurse monitors a client for signs of dumping syndrome. Which of the following does the nurse evaluate as early clinical manifestations?

    Select all that apply:
    [ ] 1. Hematemesis

[ ] 2. Abdominal muscle rigidity
[ ] 3. Tachycardia
[ ] 4. Vertigo
[ ] 5. Sweating
[ ] 6. Diarrhea

12. A client scheduled for a vagotomy asks the nurse what a vagotomy is. Which of the following statements by the nurse best describes the purpose of the vagotomy?
    1. "It decreases food transit time in the stomach."
    2. "It regenerates the gastric mucosa."
    3. "It reduces the stimulus to acid secretion."
    4. "It stops stress-related reactions."

13. The nurse is caring for a client who is jaundiced. The nurse should implement which of the following in the plan for this client's pruritus?
    1. Monitor the client's temperature and assess the client's color
    2. Instruct the client to scratch with knuckles instead of nails
    3. Administer prescribed analgesic and assist the client to bathe frequently
    4. Encourage the client to eat a high-protein, low-cholesterol diet

14. The nurse assesses a client to be experiencing dumping syndrome within what time frame of a meal after a Billroth II?

    _____

15. The nurse is admitting a client with a diagnosis of preicteric (prodromal phase) hepatitis. Which of the following would the nurse expect to be the priority assessment finding?
    1. Clay-colored stools
    2. Anorexia
    3. Jaundice
    4. Pruritus

16. A client is diagnosed with hepatitis A and asks the nurse how to avoid infecting other family members. The nurse's response would be based on the understanding that the spread of hepatitis A is primarily
    1. through sexual contact with an infected person who does not show symptoms of the disease.
    2. by contaminated needles from a person who has some form of hepatitis.
    3. through blood transfusions of improperly prepared blood.
    4. from person to person through fecal contamination or contaminated food and water.

17. The nurse assesses a client with ulcerative colitis to experience how many bloody diarrhea stools per day?

    _____

18. The nurse is discharging a client with chronic pancreatitis. Which of the following measures would be essential to include in the client's discharge instruction?
    1. Weight reduction and exercise program
    2. Bowel retraining program including daily laxative administration
    3. Diet modifications avoiding high-fat foods, caffeine, and alcohol
    4. Relaxation techniques and stress management

19. A nurse evaluates a client to experience a burning or gaseous pressure in the left epigastrum, back, and upper abdomen occurring how may hours after eating?

    _____

20. In preparing the client for an endoscopic cholecystectomy, the nurse should include which of the following post-op information?

    Select all that apply:
    [ ] 1. "There is a small midline abdominal incision."
    [ ] 2. "You will be NPO for 2 days followed by a low-fat diet."
    [ ] 3. "Your activity will be restricted."
    [ ] 4. "Generally the pain is minimal."
    [ ] 5. "There is a low incidence of wound infection."
    [ ] 6. "The hospital stay is generally 1 to 2 days."

21. The nurse performs which part of the gastrointestinal assessment first?
    1. Auscultation
    2. Palpation
    3. Inspection
    4. Percussion

22. When preparing a client for a colonoscopy, it would be essential for the nurse to explain which of the following aspects of the procedure?
    1. Stools will be white until all the barium is expelled
    2. Bowel sounds will be monitored hourly for 12 hours
    3. The client will be positioned on the right side with the legs straight
    4. The client must begin a clear liquid diet beginning at noon the day before

23. A client experiences regurgitation and dyspepsia. The nurse assists the client to assume an upright position. Which of the following statements by the nurse would best describe the purpose of this measure?
    1. "It prevents the flow of gastric contents into the esophagus."
    2. "It decreases the inflammatory changes in the esophagus."
    3. "It enhances and strengthens esophageal peristalsis."
    4. "It increases the lower esophageal pressure."

24. Because a client has Crohn's disease, plans for nursing intervention should include
    1. weight-reduction measures and low-calorie diet.
    2. frequent application of lubricant lotion and discouraging scratching.
    3. teaching the importance of follow-up liver function test after discharge.
    4. perianal care and restoration of fluids and electrolytes.

25. During an acute exacerbation of Crohn's disease, which of the following nursing diagnoses should have priority?
    1. Imbalanced nutrition: less than body requirements related to anorexia and diarrhea
    2. Anxiety related to altered self-concept and health status
    3. Fatigue related to decreased nutrient intake and anemia
    4. Knowledge deficiency related to lack of information about disease process

26. The nurse is evaluating the pain complaints of four clients. Which client does the nurse report to the physician as having symptoms indicative of peptic ulcer disease?
    1. Low, colicky abdominal pain
    2. A gnawing epigastric pain relieved by food
    3. Left upper quadrant pain that radiates to the back
    4. Right upper quadrant pain radiating to the right shoulder

27. The nurse observes a staff member caring for a client after a vagotomy and partial gastrectomy. Which of the following indicates that the staff member is irrigating the nasogastric tube correctly?
    1. Inject 10 ml distilled water, clamp tube for 30 minutes, then disconnect suction for 30 minutes
    2. Insert 20 ml of air and clamp off suction for 1 hour
    3. Administer 20 ml of prescribed antibiotic and increase pressure of suction
    4. Fill syringe with 30 ml of normal saline, inject into tube, and withdraw slowly

28. In planning the postoperative care for a client with an ileostomy, the nurse would select which of the following as the priority nursing diagnosis?
    1. Disturbed body image related to the ostomy
    2. Risk for deficient fluid volume related to excess fluid loss

3. Ineffective sexuality patterns related to loss of sexual desire
4. Risk for impaired skin integrity related to fecal drainage

29. The nurse is caring for a client receiving continuous nasogastric feedings. The nurse observes the client for aspiration that could be the result of
    1. use of unclean equipment and reflux into the esophagus.
    2. administering tube feedings at either a cold or warm temperature.
    3. too rapid administration and incomplete stomach emptying.
    4. allergic reaction to feeding administered.

30. The nurse is caring for a client receiving medications through a nasogastric tube. Which of the following is the appropriate method for the nurse to administer these medications?
    1. Mix all medications together and administer as a bolus and flush with 20 to 30 ml normal saline or water at the end
    2. Administer those medications that are compatible and flush with 60 ml normal saline or water at the end
    3. Administer each medication individually and flush with 100 ml normal saline or water at the end
    4. Administer each medication individually, flush with 5 to 10 ml normal saline or water between each medication, and flush with 20 ml at the end

31. The nurse is assessing a client postoperatively following a hemorrhoidectomy. Which of the following assessments would be most important for the nurse to include?
    1. The client's ability to assume a sitting position
    2. The degree of embarrassment the client expresses
    3. Inspection of the rectal area for bleeding
    4. Presence of nausea and vomiting

32. The nurse is caring for a client 2 hours after a hemorrhoidectomy. The client asks the nurse, "Should I be having severe pain?" The most appropriate response by the nurse would be:
    1. "Yes and I'll get you a pain medication."
    2. "This is a minor surgery and the pain is also minor."
    3. "I'll call your physician because I don't know why you are having so much pain."
    4. "Try changing your position and take some deep breaths to relax you."

33. The nurse is caring for a client 1 week postoperatively following a colostomy. Which of the following assessment findings would be a priority for the nurse to report?
    1. The client is experiencing flatulence

2. The color of the stoma is dusky blue
3. The skin under the colostomy bag is red
4. The client appears depressed

34. The nurse is discharging a client with an ileostomy. Which of the following would the nurse include in the discharge instructions?
    1. A drainage appliance only needs to be worn in public
    2. Bowel regularity will be established within 2 weeks
    3. Report any signs of bleeding from the stoma
    4. Increase fluids rich in electrolytes, such as Gatorade

35. A client with a colostomy is experiencing an increased odor and asks the nurse what is contributing to this. The most appropriate response by the nurse is
    1. "There are no foods that affect odor."
    2. "Food such as eggs, asparagus, fish, and broccoli will increase the odor."
    3. "The odor is normal but a pouch deodorant will help."
    4. "Changing the pouch and washing the stoma daily will eliminate the odor."

36. The nurse evaluates which of the following clients to be at greatest risk for developing alcoholic cirrhosis (Laënnec's)?
    1. A 55-year-old male who has chronic alcoholism
    2. A 28-year-old male who had a recent exposure to a hepatotoxic drug
    3. A 70-year-old male who has a history of right-sided heart failure
    4. A 40-year-old female who has a biliary obstruction

37. The nurse should assess a client suspected of having peritonitis for which of the following clinical manifestations?

    Select all that apply:
    [ ] 1. Pyrosis
    [ ] 2. Abdominal tenderness
    [ ] 3. Diarrhea
    [ ] 4. Muscle rigidity
    [ ] 5. Abdominal pain
    [ ] 6. Tachycardia

38. The nurse assesses which of the following clients to most likely develop a problem with constipation?
    1. A client who consumes a high-fiber diet
    2. A client who is receiving trimethoprim-sulfamethoxazole (Bactrim)
    3. A client who is receiving dicyclomine hydrochloride (Bentyl)
    4. A client who has a 1500-ml fluid intake per day

39. The nurse assesses a client for the presence of a gastric outlet obstruction. Which of the following findings should be reported?

    Select all that apply:
    [ ] 1. Large abdominal peristaltic waves
    [ ] 2. Sudden severe upper abdominal pain
    [ ] 3. Shoulder pain
    [ ] 4. Projectile vomiting
    [ ] 5. Rigid, boardlike abdomen
    [ ] 6. Weight loss

40. The nurse assesses a client with hepatic encephalopathy for asterixis by
    1. asking the client to extend an arm, dorsiflex the wrist, and extend the finger.
    2. assessing the client for azotemia, oliguria, and intractable ascites.
    3. assessing the client for a musty, sweet breath odor.
    4. asking the client to draw a cross and noting any deterioration in the figure construction.

41. Which of the following should the nurse include when performing a Hematest?
    1. Open the front flap on the cover of the slide, apply a thin smear of stool in the first box only
    2. Open the flap on the back of the slide and apply a drop of developing solution
    3. Place test tablet on top of the stool specimen on guaiac paper and follow with 2 drops of water
    4. Document results after waiting five minutes to observe color changes

42. The nurse obtains a pH of 8.0 when aspirating for gastric contents when assessing correct tube placement. The nurse evaluates a pH of 8.0 to be

    1. alkaline, which indicates respiratory secretions.
    2. a neutral pH.
    3. acidic, confirming gastric secretions.
    4. indicative of intestinal secretions.

43. Based on an understanding of the adverse reactions to drugs, which of the following drugs does the nurse evaluate from the medication history to cause constipation?
    1. Fluoxetine (Prozac)
    2. Digoxin (Lanoxin)
    3. Amoxycillin (Polymox)
    4. Amitriptyline (Elavil)

44. When assessing a client with a nasogastric tube, the nurse discovers it is set on continuous high suction. Which of the following nursing actions should the nurse implement?
    1. Clamp the tube for 30 minutes, then reconnect it to continuous high suction
    2. Call the physician and remove the tube
    3. Irrigate the tube with 30 ml of normal saline and record the characteristics of the drainage
    4. Change the suction to low intermittent suction

45. During an inspection of the abdomen, which of the abdominal findings should the nurse report as abnormal?
    1. Bilateral symmetrical abdomen
    2. Flat abdominal contour
    3. Strong abdominal pulsations
    4. Depressed umbilicus beneath the abdominal surface

ANSWERS AND RATIONALES

1. 1. Assessment includes both subjective and objective data. Rebound tenderness is sudden pain when the examiner palpating the abdomen removes the examining fingers and the client complains of pain. Diarrhea, generalized red abdominal rash, and hematuria are all observable and therefore objective, not subjective, data.

2. 3. 6. As a result of the barium being administered rectally for a barium enema, increasing fluids and administering a laxative are encouraged to resume normal defecation and prevent an impaction. Positioning the client on the right side and maintaining bed rest for 12 hours is postprocedure care for a liver biopsy. Rectal bleeding would be assessed after a colonoscopy. A rise in body temperature and abdominal pain

would indicate a possible perforation following an endoscopy.

3. 3. Because a topical anesthesia spray, usually lidocaine, is administered during an upper gastrointestinal endoscopy to facilitate passage of the endoscopy, assessing the return of the gag reflex is crucial postprocedure prior to administering food and fluids to prevent aspiration. Positioning the client on the right side is postprocedure care following a liver biopsy. Providing the client a fatty "test meal" may be ordered following an oral cholecystogram to check for gallbladder emptying. Administering a laxative is not necessary because no barium is used during an upper endoscopy to cause constipation.

4. 1. 5. 6. Small, frequent meals, avoiding caffeine, and sleeping with the head of the bed elevated prevent the gastric secretions from going backward through an incompetent lower esophageal sphincter (LES) that occurs in gastroesophageal reflux disease. Avoiding fluids at mealtime and providing for rest after meals is the treatment for dumping syndrome. A high-calorie, high-protein diet with 2000 ml of fluid daily is recommended in malnutrition after certain gastrointestinal diseases or surgery. Low-roughage, high-fiber diet and bulk-forming laxatives are recommended to treat diverticulitis.

5. 3. Although maintaining a clean environment free from odors, assisting the client to wash the hands and face before meals, and offering foods the client likes are appropriate nursing interventions for a client with gastroenteritis, encouraging fluids and monitoring the intake and output are the priority interventions.

6. 1. Diverticulitis is treated with a high-fiber diet and bulk-forming laxatives. If a diet is low in fiber and with the decreased bulk of the stool, the bowel lumen narrows, leading to high intra-abdominal pressure during defecation. This contributes to the formation of the diverticula. A low-fat, high-carbohydrate, and high-protein diet avoiding alcohol is the diet of choice for pancreatitis. A high-calorie, high-carbohydrate, and low-fat diet is the diet for cirrhosis. A diet high in protein and calories, low in residue, and milk free is the diet for ulcerative colitis.

7. 4. A licensed practical nurse may assist a client in selecting the specific foods on a selected diet. Only a registered nurse may develop, assess, and plan interventions.

8. 3. Difficulty swallowing food or liquids is the most appropriate assessment to determine the presence of an obstruction of the alimentary canal. Pain and weight loss may also occur with an obstruction but would not be the first clinical manifestation that the client would present with. Bleeding would be diagnostic with cancer, not an obstruction.

9. 1. 4. 5. Hypotension, tachycardia, and restlessness are all indicative of hemorrhage in a client with a peptic ulcer and must be reported immediately. Thirst, headache, and diarrhea are all clinical manifestations a client may experience with or without peptic ulcer disease but do not indicate an emergency situation.

10. 4. It is correct to measure from the tip of the nose to the tip of the earlobe to the xiphoid process prior to inserting a nasogastric tube to determine correct placement. Instructing the client not to swallow when the tube is felt in the back of the throat is incorrect, because the nurse would encourage a client to swallow as the tube is being passed. The client should be in a high-Fowler's position for insertion of the tube. The head should be tilted forward when the tube is felt in the throat.

11. 3. 4. 5. 6. Vertigo, tachycardia, sweating, and diarrhea are early manifestations that occur in a client with dumping syndrome. Hematemesis, melena, and hypotension occur with a gastrointestinal bleed. Abdominal pain, muscle rigidity, nausea, and vomiting occur in peritonitis. Epigastric distress after meals relieved by vomiting occurs in bile reflux gastritis, another postoperative complication of peptic ulcer surgery.

12. 3. A vagotomy severs the vagus nerve and eliminates the hydrochloric acid stimulus.

13. 2. Pruritus occurs as a result of an accumulation of bile salts under the skin. Scratching with the knuckles instead of the nails maintains the skin's integrity and prevents tearing.

14.   30 minutes

15. 2. Anorexia is a clinical manifestation that occurs in the preicteric phase of hepatitis. Clay-colored stools, jaundice, and pruritus are all clinical manifestations that occur in the icteric phase of hepatitis.

16. 4. Hepatitis A is transmitted by the fecal-oral route and by contaminated food and water. Sexual contact with an infected person, contaminated needles, and contaminated blood are modes of transmission for hepatitis B and C.

17.   2–20

18. 3. A diet low in fat and avoiding caffeine and alcohol are recommended for chronic pancreatitis. Weight reduction, exercise program, bowel retraining program, relaxation techniques, and stress management are not interventions pertinent to pancreatitis.

19.   1–2

20. 4. 5. 6. The laparoscopic cholecystectomy is a minor procedure with few complications. There is decreased wound infection, minimal pain, and a 1- to 2-day hospital stay. An abdominal incision, nasogastric tube, NPO, low-fat diet, pain, Jackson-Pratt drain, and restricted activity would occur in an open cholecystectomy.

21. 3. Inspection should be the first phase of the gastrointestinal assessment, followed by auscultation, percussion, and palpation. Inspection should be performed first, before there is any stimulation of the intestinal organs and contents.

22. 4. The client will be on clear liquids beginning at noon and for up to 8 hours before the procedure, then NPO. The client will be placed in the left lateral decubitus position to facilitate the insertion of the colonoscope. There is no barium administered and the vital signs, not the bowel sounds, will be monitored postprocedure for signs of hemorrhage.

23. 1. An upright position is the best position for a client experiencing regurgitation and dyspepsia. It prevents the flow of gastric contents into the esophagus.

24. 4. A client with Crohn's disease experiences frequent loose stools. The client may have as many as 20 stools per day, so nursing interventions for perianal care and restoration of fluids and electrolytes are important. Weight-reduction measures and a low-calorie diet are appropriate interventions for cholecystitis. Teaching the importance of follow-up liver function tests after discharge would be an intervention for hepatitis. Frequent application of a lubricant lotion and discouraging scratching are appropriate interventions for a client experiencing jaundice.

25. 1. The priority nursing diagnosis for a client with Crohn's disease is imbalanced nutrition: less than body requirements related to anorexia and diarrhea. Other less important nursing diagnoses include fatigue related to decreased nutrient intake and anemia, knowledge deficiency related to lack of information about the disease process, and anxiety related to altered self-concept and health status.

26. 2. A gnawing epigastric pain relieved by food is indicative of peptic ulcer disease. Low, colicky abdominal pain is a clinical manifestation of diverticulitis. Upper left quadrant pain that radiates to the back is classic in pancreatitis. Right upper quadrant pain that radiates to the right shoulder is characteristic of cholecystitis.

27. 4. The correct procedure for irrigating a nasogastric tube is to fill a syringe with 30 ml normal saline followed by injecting it into the tube and withdrawing slowly.

28. 2. The priority nursing diagnosis for a client with an ileostomy is risk for deficient fluid volume related to excess fluid loss. The client with an ileostomy has continuous liquid stools, which can result in a fluid volume deficit unless the client takes in an adequate amount of fluids. Other less important nursing diagnoses include disturbed body image related to the ostomy, ineffective sexuality patterns related to loss of sexual desire, and risk for impaired skin integrity related to fecal drainage.

29. 3. Administering a continuous nasogastric feeding too fast places the client at risk for aspiration. Aspiration could also be the result of incomplete stomach emptying. Use of unclean equipment and reflux into the esophagus places the client at risk for infection manifested by

diarrhea. Administering a tube feeding at either too cold or too warm a temperature may result in spasms. An allergic reaction to the feeding administered is the result of an intolerance to the feeding.

30. 4. The appropriate procedure for administering medications through a nasogastric tube is to administer each medication separately. After each medication is administered individually, 5 to 10 ml of normal saline or water should be administered between medications followed by a 20-ml flush at the end.

31. 3. Post-op care following a hemorrhoidectomy includes a high-fiber diet, increased fluid intake, stool softeners, and inspecting the area for bleeding.

32. 1. The pain following a hemorrhoidectomy can be persistent and severe. It is important that the nurse understands this and does not disregard the client's complaints.

33. 2. It is a priority that the nurse reports the stoma of a colostomy that becomes dusky blue. This indicates ischemia. A client who has a colostomy may experience flatulence after eating gas-forming foods. The skin under the colostomy bag that becomes red may be a sign of irritation. A client who is depressed may be having a difficult time adjusting to the colostomy.

34. 4. Because a client with an ileostomy has continuous liquid stools, the potential for losing electrolytes exists. The client should be encouraged to drink fluids rich in electrolytes, such as Gatorade. Regularity is not established with an ileostomy, so an appliance must be worn at all times.

35. 2. Although changing the colostomy pouch and a pouch deodorant may help the odor of a colostomy, the most appropriate intervention is to instruct the client to avoid odor-forming foods such as eggs, asparagus, fish, and broccoli.

36. 1. Alcoholic (Laënnec's) cirrhosis is associated with alcohol abuse. Postnecrotic cirrhosis is the result of a toxic substance. Chronic biliary obstruction may cause biliary cirrhosis. Cardiac cirrhosis may result from a long-standing right-sided heart failure.

37. 2. 4. 5. 6. Clinical manifestations of peritonitis include abdominal pain, tenderness, and distention. Other clinical manifestations include muscle rigidity, fever, nausea, vomiting, tachycardia, and tachypnea. Diarrhea is a characteristic of many gastrointestinal disorders, such as gastroenteritis. Pyrosis may also be included in many other gastrointestinal disorders.

38. 3. Dicyclomine hydrochloride (Bentyl) is a cholinergic blocking drug generally given for

hypermotility and spasms of the gastrointestinal tract associated with an irritable colon, spastic colon, or mucous colitis. Constipation is a common adverse reaction to Bentyl. Other gastrointestinal adverse reactions include nausea, vomiting, and dry mouth. A high-fiber diet would be given to prevent constipation. Trimethoprim-sulfamethoxazole (Bactrim) is an antibiotic frequently given for a urinary tract infection. A common adverse reaction is diarrhea. A client with a fluid intake of 1500 ml could develop constipation but Bentyl is a more likely cause of constipation.

39. 1. 4. 6.   Clinical manifestations of a gastric outlet obstruction include loud peristalsis, large and visible peristaltic abdominal waves, vomiting that relieves the pain, and accompanying weight loss. Sudden severe upper abdominal pain, shoulder pain, and a rigid, boardlike abdomen are classic in perforation of a peptic ulcer.

40. 1.   Asking the client to extend the arm, dorsiflex the wrist, and extend the finger is asterixis, or liver flap, which is a clinical manifestation that occurs as coma approaches in hepatic encephalopathy. Asking the client to draw a cross and noting any deterioration in the figure construction is also a clinical manifestation of hepatic encephalopathy. A musty, sweet breath odor occurs in some clients with hepatic encephalopathy. Azotemia, oliguria, and intractable ascites are manifestations of hepatorenal syndrome, a serious complication of cirrhosis.

41. 3.   The correct way to perform a Hematest is to place a test tablet on top of the stool on guaiac paper followed by 2 drops of water. Two minutes should elapse before assessing the results. A Hemoccult slide test is performed by opening the flap of the slide and applying a thin smear of stool in the first box only. The slide cover is then closed and the slide turned over. The flap on the back is open and 2 drops of Hemoccult developing solution is applied in each box.

42. 1.   When checking for correct nasogastric tube place, a pH of 8.0 indicates the presence of alkaline and respiratory secretion. Fluid aspirated with a pH higher than 6.0 indicates pleural fluid from the tracheobronchial tree. A range of 1.0 to 4.0 indicates proper tube placement. Fluid aspirated with a pH higher than 6.0 may also indicate the tube is placed in the intestine because the intestinal secretions are less acidic than the stomach.

43. 4.   Fluoxetine (Prozac) is a selective serotonin reuptake inhibitor that causes diarrhea. Digoxin (Lanoxin) is a cardiac glycoside that may cause diarrhea. Amoxycillin (Polymox) is an antibiotic that causes diarrhea. Amitriptyline (Elavil) is a tricyclic antidepressant that may cause constipation.

44. 4.   A nasogastric tube should be set on low intermittent suction to prevent trauma to the stomach. A tube set on continuous high suction may cause trauma to the gastric tissue and may actually suck out the stomach wall.

45. 3.   A strong abdominal pulsation may indicate a widened pulse pressure and an aortic aneurysm. A bilateral symmetrical abdomen, flat abdominal contour, and a depressed umbilicus beneath the abdominal surface are all normal findings.

REFERENCES

Daniels, R. (2010). *Delmar's manual of laboratory and diagnostic tests* (2nd ed.). Clifton Park, NY: Delmar Cengage Learning.

Daniels, R., & Nicoll, L. (2012). *Contemporary medical-surgical nursing*. Clifton Park, NY: Delmar Cengage Learning.

DeLaune, S. C., & Ladner, P. K. (2011). *Fundamentals of nursing: Standard and practice* (4th ed.). Clifton Park, NY: Delmar Cengage Learning.

Estes, M. (2010). *Health assessment and physical examination* (4th ed.). Clifton Park, NY: Delmar Cengage Learning.

Spratto, G. R., & Woods, A. L. (2012). *PDR nurse's drug handbook 2012*. Clifton Park, NY: Delmar Cengage Learning.

CHAPTER 6

ENDOCRINE DISORDERS

I. ANATOMY AND PHYSIOLOGY

A. FUNCTIONS OF ENDOCRINE GLANDS

1. MAJOR ENDOCRINE GLANDS INCLUDE PITUITARY, THYROID, PARATHYROID, ADRENALS, PANCREAS, AND GONADS.
2. ENDOCRINE GLANDS SECRETE CHEMICALS (HORMONES) DIRECTLY INTO THE BLOODSTREAM AND HAVE A DIRECT OR INDIRECT EFFECT ON THE METABOLISM OF WATER AND ELECTROLYTES.
3. HORMONES REGULATE THE INTERNAL ENVIRONMENT IN THE BODY.
4. SOME HORMONES TARGET SPECIFIC TISSUES, AND OTHERS AFFECT A VARIETY OF TISSUES AND CELLS OF THE BODY.
5. HORMONE CONCENTRATION IN THE BLOOD IS REGULATED BY NEGATIVE FEEDBACK MECHANISMS.
6. HORMONES ARE CLASSIFIED AS STEROID HORMONES (CORTISONE), PEPTIDES (INSULIN), AND AMINE HORMONES (EPINEPHRINE).
7. FUNCTIONS AND STRUCTURE ARE AFFECTED BY LACK OF BLOOD SUPPLY, INFECTION, TUMOR GROWTH, OVERSTIMULATION, AND OVERGROWTH.

B. PITUITARY GLAND (SEE FIGURE 6-1)

1. ROUND STRUCTURE LOCATED ON THE INFERIOR ASPECT OF THE BRAIN
2. THE ANTERIOR LOBE REGULATES PRODUCTION OF SEVERAL HORMONES, INCLUDING THE GROWTH HORMONE, THYROID-STIMULATING HORMONE (TSH), AND ADRENOCORICOTROPIC HORMONE.
   a. Growth hormone plays a role in growth of bones, muscles, and cells and affects carbohydrate, protein, and fat metabolism.
   b. Thyroid-stimulating hormone is necessary for growth and function of the thyroid gland and controls release of thyroid hormones.
   c. Adrenocorticotropic hormone (ACTH) controls release of glucocorticoids and adrenal androgens from the adrenal cortex.
3. THE POSTERIOR LOBE RELEASES ANTIDIURETIC HORMONE (ADH), WHICH CONSERVES WATER, THEREBY MAINTAINING BLOOD VOLUME.

C. THYROID GLAND (SEE FIGURE 6-1)

1. BUTTERFLY-SHAPED ORGAN IN THE LOWER NECK ANTERIOR TO THE TRACHEA
2. RELEASES HORMONES T_4 (THYROXINE), T_3 (TRIIODOTHYRONINE), AND CALCITONIN
3. T_4 PLUS T_3 MAKE UP THE THYROID HORMONE.
4. T_4 AND T_3 CONTAIN IODINE MOLECULES BOUND TO AMINO ACIDS.
5. T_4 AND T_3 SYNTHESIZED AND STORED IN THE THYROID ARE BOUND TO PROTEINS UNTIL RELEASED INTO THE BLOOD.
6. IODINE INGESTED ORALLY IS ABSORBED INTO THE BLOOD IN THE GASTROINTESTINAL (GI) TRACT, WHERE IT IS PICKED UP BY THE THYROID GLAND, CONCENTRATED IN THE GLAND, AND REACTS WITH TYROSINE TO FORM THYROID HORMONES.
7. THE MAJOR ROLE OF THYROXINE IS TO REGULATE METABOLISM SO THAT O_2 CONSUMPTION AND HEAT PRODUCTION KEEP PACE WITH THE BODY'S NEEDS AND ACTIVITIES.
8. BY CONTROLLING METABOLISM, THYROXINE HAS A ROLE IN REGULATING:
   a. Growth and development
   b. Carbohydrate, fat, and protein metabolism

c. Reproduction
d. Vitamin requirements
e. Resistance to infection

9. PRODUCTION OF THYROXINE IS DEPENDENT ON INGESTION OF SUFFICIENT PROTEIN AND IODINE AND ON RELEASE OF THE THYROID-STIMULATING HORMONE FROM THE ANTERIOR PITUITARY GLAND.

10. CALCITONIN IS RELEASED WHEN THERE ARE HIGH LEVELS OF PLASMA CALCIUM, CAUSING CALCIUM TO BE DEPOSITED IN BONES.

D. PARATHYROID GLAND (SEE FIGURE 6-1)

1. FOUR SMALL GLANDS EITHER ATTACHED TO OR EMBEDDED IN THE POSTERIOR ASPECT OF THE THYROID GLAND

2. SECRETES THE HORMONE PARATHORMONE

3. PARATHORMONE CAUSES AN INCREASE IN PLASMA CALCIUM IONS AND DECREASE IN PLASMA PHOSPHATE ION CONCENTRATION (INVERSE RELATIONSHIP).

E. ADRENAL GLANDS (SEE FIGURE 6-1)

1. TWO SMALL STRUCTURES THAT CAP THE TOP OF THE KIDNEYS

2. INNER PORTION IS THE MEDULLA; OUTER PORTION IS THE CORTEX

3. MEDULLA FUNCTIONS AS PART OF THE AUTONOMIC NERVOUS SYSTEM AND SECRETES THE CATECHOLAMINE HORMONES EPINEPHRINE (ADRENALIN) AND NOREPINEPHRINE.

4. ACTION OF EPINEPHRINE IS TO RESPOND TO "FIGHT OR FLIGHT" BY CONVERTING LIVER GLYCOGEN TO GLUCOSE FOR ENERGY, BOOSTING THE O_2 CARRYING CAPACITY OF THE BLOOD, AND INCREASING CARDIAC OUTPUT.

5. ACTION OF NOREPINEPHRINE IS TO PRODUCE EXTENSIVE VASCULAR CONSTRICTION, CAUSING MARKED INCREASE IN BLOOD PRESSURE (BP)

6. ADRENAL CORTEX SECRETES:

a. Mineralocorticoids (aldosterone—main one)
b. Glucocorticoids (cortisol—most important one)
c. Androgenic adrenocorticoids (17 ketosteroids)
d. Aldosterone has a major role in concentration of Na^+ in the body, acting on renal tubules to cause increased sodium retention, secondary H_2O retention, and K^1 excretion. These actions sustain normal BP and cardiac output.

e. Cortisol promotes gluconeogenesis (converts amino acids and fats to glycogen) and influences protein catabolism, and is used extensively for inflammation and allergic reactions.
f. Androgens oppose the catabolic effects of glucocorticoids and have sexual effects of masculinization.

F. PANCREAS (SEE FIGURE 6-1)

1. HAS AN EXOCRINE FUNCTION AND AN ENDOCRINE FUNCTION

2. ENDOCRINE FUNCTION IS CONTROLLED BY THE ALPHA AND BETA CELLS OF THE ISLETS OF LANGERHANS.

3. ALPHA CELLS SYNTHESIZE GLUCAGON, WHICH RAISES BLOOD SUGAR BY PROMOTING CONVERSION OF GLYCOGEN TO GLUCOSE IN THE LIVER.

4. BETA CELLS SYNTHESIZE INSULIN, WHICH LOWERS BLOOD SUGAR BY PROMOTING TRANSPORT OF GLUCOSE INTO THE CELLS.

5. INSULIN PLAYS A KEY ROLE IN THE METABOLISM OF CARBOHYDRATES, FATS, AND PROTEIN BY:

a. Stimulating active transport of glucose into the muscle and adipose tissue cells.
b. Regulating the rate at which carbohydrates are burned by the cell for energy.
c. Promoting conversion of glucose to glycogen for storage in the liver.
d. Promoting conversion of fatty acids into fat, which can be stored as adipose tissue.
e. Stimulating protein synthesis within the tissues.

6. THE RATE OF INSULIN SECRETION IS REGULATED BY BLOOD SUGAR LEVELS.

7. CARBOHYDRATES ARE THE BODY'S PREFERRED FUEL AS WELL AS ITS MOST IMMEDIATE SOURCE OF ENERGY.

8. IF THE BODY CANNOT BURN CARBOHYDRATES, IT WILL CONVERT FAT FIRST AND THEN PROTEIN.

9. BODY WILL BURN CARBOHYDRATES RATHER THAN FATS AND PROTEIN IF:

a. Carbohydrate intake is adequate.
b. Sufficient insulin is present to get glucose into the cells.
c. Reserve stores of glycogen are present.

10. CARBOHYDRATE METABOLISM INVOLVES:

a. Active transport of glucose into the cells and the release of energy.
b. Storage of glucose not immediately needed for energy as glycogen and fat.

Figure 6-1 Structures of the endocrine system

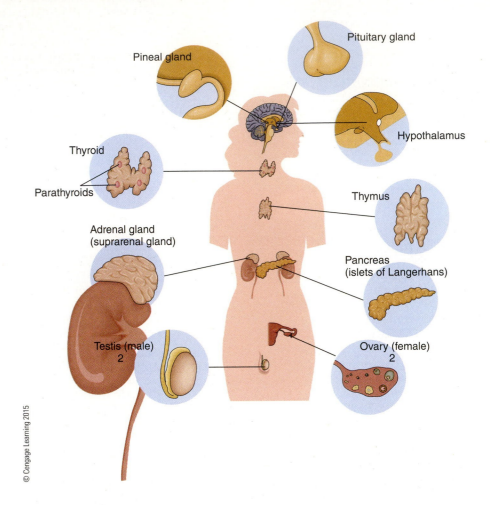

Pineal gland

Pituitary gland

Thyroid

Parathyroids

Hypothalamus

Thymus

Adrenal gland
(suprarenal gland)

Pancreas
(islets of Langerhans)

Testis (male)
2

Ovary (female)
2

© Cengage Learning 2015

c. Conversion of glycogen back to glucose whenever blood glucose level drops.

d. Conversion of fats and proteins to glucose or glycogen whenever these two carbohydrate substances are depleted and energy is needed.

II. ASSESSMENT

A. HEALTH HISTORY
   1. INCREASED OR LESSENED ENERGY LEVELS AND PRESENCE OF FATIGUE
   2. CHANGES IN HEAT AND COLD INTOLERANCE
   3. WEIGHT CHANGES
   4. CHANGES IN SEXUAL FUNCTION AND SECONDARY SEX CHARACTERISTICS
   5. CHANGES IN MENTAL STATUS
   6. EXCESSIVE THIRST (DIABETES MELLITUS OR DIABETES INSIPIDUS)
   7. FREQUENT URINATION (DIABETES MELLITUS OR DIABETES INSIPIDUS)
   8. FAMILIAL TENDENCY
   9. MULTIPLE ENDOCRINE DISORDERS ARE COMMON.

B. PHYSICAL EXAMINATION
   1. EXOPHTHALMUS (HYPERTHYROIDISM)
   2. HYPERPIGMENTATION OF THE SKIN (ADDISON'S DISEASE)
   3. HARD, NONPITTING EDEMA (MYXEDEMA)
   4. DELAYED HEALING (DIABETES MELLITUS)
   5. ENLARGED PHYSICAL FEATURES (ACROMEGALY OR CUSHING'S SYNDROME)
   6. EXCESSIVE GROWTH (GIGANTISM)
   7. ALTERATIONS IN HAIR TEXTURE (THYROID) OR AMOUNT (OVARIAN OR ADRENAL CONDITIONS)
   8. VITAL SIGN CHANGES—INCREASED TEMPERATURE AND HEART RATE (HYPERTHYROIDISM), INCREASED HEART RATE AND BLOOD PRESSURE (PHEOCHROMOCYTOMA)

III. DIAGNOSTIC STUDIES

A. STIMULATION AND SUPPRESSION TESTS FOR PITUITARY, THYROID, AND ADRENAL GLANDS
   1. DESCRIPTION
      a. Stimulating hormones (TSH, ACTH, follicle-stimulating hormone [FSH], or luteinizing hormone [LH]) given and response of target gland evaluated
      b. If target gland responds, dysfunction of hypothalamus or pituitary gland is suspected.
      c. Suppression tests are helpful in determining if negative feedback mechanism is operational.

B. FLUID DEPRIVATION TEST
   1. DESCRIPTION
      a. Test is performed by withholding fluids to determine response of the posterior pituitary gland in releasing antidiuretic hormone (ADH).
         1) Inability to increase specific gravity and urine osmolality with weight loss, increased serum osmolality, and elevated serum sodium are characteristics of diabetes insipidus.
   2. PROCEDURE
      a. Day of the test:
         1) Fluids withheld for 8–12 hours or until 3% to 5% of body weight is lost
         2) Patient weighed frequently throughout the test
         3) Plasma and urine osmolality studies performed at the beginning and end of the test
         4) Monitor closely for tachycardia, excessive weight loss, and hypotension.
   3. POSTPROCEDURE
      a. Continue to monitor closely for signs of vasomotor collapse. Client continues to excrete large volume of urine and may develop vascular collapse because of massive output of H_2O.
      b. Fluids resumed slowly to avoid water intoxication

C. THYROID-STIMULATING HORMONE TEST
   1. DESCRIPTION
      a. A serum immunoassay test for measuring serum TSH concentrations.
      b. Useful for monitoring thyroid hormone replacement therapy and for determining whether disorder is in the thyroid gland, pituitary gland, or hypothalamus
      c. Elevated levels indicate primary hypothyroidism.
      d. Low levels indicate hyperthyroidism.

   2. PREPROCEDURE
      a. Prior to the test:
         1) Question the client as to the use of products that contain iodine, such as medications, food supplements, and topical antiseptics, which will alter results.
   3. POSTPROCEDURE: NONE

D. SERUM FREE THYROXINE (FT_4)
   1. DESCRIPTION
      a. Directly measures free (unbound) thyroxine
      b. Useful in confirming an abnormal TSH
   2. PREPROCEDURE
      a. Prior to the test:
         1) Question the client as to the use of products that contain iodine, such as medications, food supplements, and topical antiseptics, which will alter results.
   3. POSTPROCEDURE: NONE

E. RADIOACTIVE IODINE (RAI) UPTAKE
   1. DESCRIPTION
      a. Measurement of the rate of absorption of a tracer dose of ^{123}I in the thyroid gland
      b. Thyroid gland normally takes up 5% to 35% of tracer dose in 24 hours.
      c. High uptake in hyperthyroidism; low uptake in hypothyroidism
      d. Drugs may increase or decrease results.
   2. PREPROCEDURE
      a. Prior to the test:
         1) Question the client as to the use of products that contain iodine, such as medications, food supplements, and topical antiseptics, which will alter results.
         2) Instruct the client in the 24-hour urine collection procedure.
         3) Client needs to know that the tracer dose is small and harmless.
      b. Day of the test:
         1) Client is given ^{123}I capsule.
         2) 24-hour urine collection is started after the tracer dose is given.
         3) Thyroid is scanned at intervals of 2, 6, and 24 hours after the tracer dose is given.
      c. Postprocedure
         1) Client reassurance

F. FINE-NEEDLE ASPIRATION BIOPSY
   1. DESCRIPTION: EXAMINATION OF A SAMPLE OF THYROID TISSUE OBTAINED THROUGH A SMALL-GAUGE NEEDLE TO DETERMINE IF THE CELLS FROM A THYROID MASS ARE BENIGN OR MALIGNANT
   2. PREPROCEDURE
      a. Obtain written consent.
      b. Explain the procedure.

3. POSTPROCEDURE
   a. Light pressure applied to the site
   b. Client reassurance due to fear of malignancy (cancer)
G. THYROID SCAN
   1. DESCRIPTION
      a. Use of a radioisotope and scintillation detector or other device to provide an image of the thyroid gland that identifies the location, size, shape, and function of the thyroid gland
      b. ^{123}I most common isotope used
   2. PREPROCEDURE
      a. Prior to the test:
         1) Question the client as to the use of products that contain iodine, such as medications, food supplements, and topical antiseptics, which will alter test results.
         2) Question the client regarding radiographic studies using contrast media within the previous 3 months because they may alter test results.
      b. Day before the test:
         1) NPO after midnight
      c. Day of the test:
         1) Radioisotope administered by the radiologist
   3. POSTPROCEDURE
      a. Client may resume food and fluids.
H. 24-HOUR URINE FOR FREE CATECHOLAMINES
   1. DESCRIPTION
      a. Collection of a 24-hour urine for the evaluation of the free catecholamines, metanephrines (MN), and vanillylmandelic acid (VMA)—the metabolic end products of epinephrine and norepinephrine.
      b. Useful in diagnosing pheochromocytoma, a tumor of the adrenal medulla
   2. PREPROCEDURE
      a. Prior to the test:
         1) Question the client as to prior ingestion of foods such as coffee, tea, bananas, chocolate, vanilla, and aspirin, which will alter test results.
         2) Obtain special bottles from the laboratory for the 24-hour urine collection.
         3) Instruct the client in the procedure for 24-hour urine collection.
   3. POSTPROCEDURE
      a. Transport urine to the laboratory in a properly labeled container.
I. FASTING BLOOD SUGAR
   1. DESCRIPTION
      a. Plasma glucose test to determine the presence of excessive glucose when the client has symptoms of diabetes mellitus
      b. A fasting plasma glucose of 126 mg/dl or higher on two consecutive tests is significant for a diagnosis of diabetes mellitus.
   2. PREPROCEDURE
      a. Day before the test:
         1) No caloric intake for at least 8 hours prior to the procedure
   3. POSTPROCEDURE
      a. Client may resume food and fluids.
J. ORAL GLUCOSE TOLERANCE TEST
   1. DESCRIPTION
      a. A test in which the client drinks a concentrated glucose solution followed by a blood glucose determination 2 hours later
      b. A blood glucose level of 200 mg/dl or higher 2 hours after the glucose ingestion is significant for a diagnosis of diabetes mellitus.
   2. PREPROCEDURE
      a. Three days before the test:
         1) A diet high in carbohydrates (200–300 g) is eaten each day for 3 days.
      b. Day before the test:
         1) NPO for 10 hours before the test except for water
      c. Day of the test:
         1) Client is given a specified amount of glucose (75 g or 100 g) as a lemon-flavored or glucola solution after fasting blood and urine samples are obtained.
         2) Blood and urine samples obtained at 30 minutes, 1 hour, and 2 hours
         3) Test may take up to 5 hours to complete.
   3. POSTPROCEDURE
      a. Monitor the client for clinical manifestations of hyperglycemia and hypoglycemia.

IV. **NURSING DIAGNOSES**
   A. ACTIVITY INTOLERANCE
   B. IMBALANCED NUTRITION: LESS THAN BODY REQUIREMENTS (HYPERTHYROIDISM)
   C. IMBALANCED NUTRITION: MORE THAN BODY REQUIREMENTS (HYPOTHYROIDISM, CUSHING'S SYNDROME)
   D. HYPOTHERMIA (HYPOTHYROIDISM)
   E. CONSTIPATION (HYPOTHYROIDISM)
   F. INEFFECTIVE THERAPEUTIC REGIMEN MANAGEMENT
   G. RISK FOR INFECTION (DIABETES MELLITUS, CUSHING'S SYNDROME)
   H. FATIGUE

V. ENDOCRINE DISORDERS

A. ANTERIOR PITUITARY DISORDERS

1. DESCRIPTION
   a. Secretion of anterior pituitary hormones under control of releasing factors secreted by the hypothalamus
   b. Major hormones secreted from the anterior pituitary are adrenocorticotropic hormone (ACTH), thyroid-stimulating hormone (TSH), growth hormone, follicle-stimulating hormone (FSH), luteinizing hormone (LH), and prolactin.
   c. ACTH, TSH, FSH, and LH have specific target glands that normally respond to the specific hormone secreted.
   d. Prolactin stimulates milk production.
   e. Growth hormone has widespread effects on the body.
   f. Acromegaly—hypersecretion of growth hormone after puberty (epiphyseal plates closed) due to hyperpituitary function, may be caused by a tumor.
      1) Bones enlarge transversely, not vertically.
      2) Features are coarse and heavy.
      3) Frontal sinuses are pronounced.
      4) Hands and feet are conspicuously wider.
      5) Lips are heavy and tongue is enlarged.
      6) Elongated forehead and lantern jaw
   g. Most common conditions resulting from hypersecretion of anterior pituitary hormones are Cushing's syndrome (increased ACTH) and acromegaly (increased growth hormone).
   h. Hyposecretion of anterior pituitary hormones (panhypopituitarism) is usually caused by tumors, trauma, or hemorrhage.
      1) All hormones secreted by the anterior pituitary usually affected
      2) Clinical manifestations according to which hormone is not secreted in adequate amounts
      3) Tumors manifested by visual problems (pressure on the optic nerve) and headaches (increased intracranial pressure)
      4) Tumors treated by surgical removal (hypophysectomy), stereotactic or conventional radiation therapy, and drugs (bromocriptine or octreotide)
      5) Hypophysectomy partially or totally removes the pituitary gland through transfrontal, subcranial, or oronasal transsphenoidal surgical approaches.
      6) Hormone replacement necessary depending on the extent of gland tissue removed

i. Nursing interventions
   1) Nursing interventions following hypophysectomy via the transphenoid approach:
      a) Observe closely for leakage of cerebrospinal fluid from the nose or constant swallowing.
      b) Assess nasal drip (clear nasal drip that tests positive for protein content may indicate cerebrospinal fluid leak).
      c) Monitor vital signs closely for changes.
      d) Nasal packing to remain in place for at least 24 hours. Client should not blow the nose, strain, or bend over.
      e) Assess visual acuity at regular intervals (decreased acuity may indicate hematoma development).
      f) Observe mental alertness for clinical manifestations of impending thyroid crisis or Addisonian crisis.
      g) Corticosteroid drugs are started immediately post-op because of lack of ACTH, which is necessary for functioning of the adrenal cortex.
      h) Administer thyroid replacement if prescribed. (Thyroid replacement is not given until the client begins to show clinical manifestations of hypothyroidism. Stored thyroid hormone may serve the client for several weeks.)
      i) Measure and record output every 2 hours for several days and measure urinary specific gravity after each voiding because fluid and electrolyte changes may occur early due to lack of ADH (diabetes insipidus).
      j) Vasopressin (ADH) of the posterior pituitary is started early when signs of fluid imbalance appear.
      k) Administer water carefully. Client may be thirsty. Water intoxication may occur if H_2O replacement is excessive.

l) Administer testosterone for impotence in males (lack of gonadotropic hormone).

m) Estrogen-progestin is given to stimulate ovarian function in females.

n) Instruct the client that lifetime hormonal replacement therapy is necessary, with frequent medical follow-up.

o) If the client is receiving steroids, be aware that stress may increase the need for increased dose and stress may seriously upset hormonal balance.

B. POSTERIOR PITUITARY DISORDERS
   1. DIABETES INSIPIDUS
      a. Description
         1) Disorder of the posterior lobe of the pituitary gland involving absence of vasopressin (ADH)
         2) ADH increases reabsorption of H_2O from the renal tubules, and, when absent, large amounts of urine are excreted, leading to fluid and electrolyte imbalance.
         3) If fluids are withheld, client continues to excrete large volumes of urine, leading to severe dehydration.
      b. Assessment
         1) Insatiable thirst (polydipsia)
         2) Large volume of dilute urinary output (polyuria)
         3) Urine specific gravity between 1.001 and 1.005
      c. Diagnostic tests
         1) Fluid deprivation test
         2) Plasma osmolality
         3) Urine osmolality
         4) Plasma levels of vasopressin
         5) Stimulating test with administration of desmopressin (synthetic vasopressin) to monitor response
      d. Nursing interventions
         1) Instruct the client regarding long-term ADH replacement therapy with desmopressin or lypressin intranasally, or vasopressin tannate in oil intramuscularly (IM).
   2. SYNDROME OF INAPPROPRIATE SECRETION OF ANTIDIURETIC HORMONE (SIADH)
      a. Description: excessive ADH secretion from the posterior pituitary resulting in low urinary output and high urine osmolality, hyponatremia, and high urine Na^+ concentration

b. Assessment
   1) Abrupt weight gain without edema
   2) Neurological clinical manifestations such as muscle twitching, headaches, and seizures
   3) Hyponatremia, causing muscle cramps and weakness
   4) Low urinary output
   5) Gastrointestinal manifestations such as abdominal cramps, anorexia, and vomiting
c. Diagnostic tests
   1) Serum sodium
   2) Urinary sodium
d. Nursing interventions
   1) Frequent neurological checks (observe for clinical manifestations of hyponatremia)
   2) Monitor daily weights.
   3) Accurate intake and output
   4) Restrict fluid intake to 1000 ml per day.
   5) Measure specific gravity.
   6) Monitor vital signs.
   7) Administer hypertonic saline.
   8) Administer furosemide (Lasix) if the serum sodium level is above 125 mEq/L.
e. Medical management
   1) Treat the underlying cause (central nervous system [CNS] disorders, cancer, body response to some drugs, such as those that stimulate the release of the antidiuretic hormone).

C. THYROID DISORDERS
   1. HYPERTHYROIDISM
      a. Description
         1) Graves' disease, most common type, caused by increase in secretion of thyroid hormones as a result of abnormal stimulation of the thyroid gland by circulating immunoglobulins
         2) Often precipitated by stressor
         3) Untreated hyperthyroidism progresses to myocardial hypertrophy with death due to heart failure.
      b. Assessment
         1) Hyperexcitability
         2) Nervous, jittery, and tense
         3) Overly alert
         4) Exaggerated reactions
         5) Heat intolerance
         6) Increased perspiration
         7) Fine tremors of hands
         8) Weight loss in spite of increased appetite
         9) Velvety skin texture

10) Palpitations and breathlessness
11) Exophthalmos
12) Increased pulse rate
13) Dysrhythmias
14) Increase in systolic blood pressure only

c. Diagnostic tests
1) TSH
2) T_3 and T_4
3) Serum T_4
4) Radioactive iodine uptake

d. Medical management
1) Treated by irradiation, pharmacotherapy, or surgery
2) Radioactive iodine destroys overactive thyroid cells and is treatment of choice for the older adult.
3) One oral dose of ^{123}I or ^{131}I is usually sufficient but the client must be observed closely for several years for clinical manifestations of hypothyroidism.
4) Synthroid used posttreatment to prevent hypothyroidism
5) Pharmacotherapy inhibits hormone synthesis or hormone release.
6) Drugs most frequently used include propylthiouracil (Propacil, PTU), or methimazole (Tapazole) with improvement noted in 1 to 2 weeks.
7) Once clinical manifestations subside, the client is placed on a maintenance dose, then gradually withdrawn.

e. Surgical management
1) Potassium iodide compounds (Lugol's solution and SSKI) given with antithyroid drugs and beta-adrenergic blockers (propranolol) to prepare the client for thyroidectomy.
2) Lugol's solution and SSKI (iodine preparations) decrease the release of thyroid hormones from the thyroid gland and decrease the vascularity of the thyroid gland before surgery.
3) Beta-adrenergic blockers given to control sympathetic nervous system effects (tachycardia, anxiety, tremors, etc.)
4) Thyroidectomy performed in select cases
5) Usually removing 5/6 of the thyroid gland (subtotal thyroidectomy) sufficient to cause remission
6) Surgery performed only after the client's thyroid function has returned to normal

f. Nursing interventions
1) Postoperative
a) Have tracheostomy set at the bedside.
b) Institute measures to prevent tension on the suture line.
c) Position for comfort in semi-Fowler's with the head elevated and supported by pillows.
d) Assess dressing for hemorrhage.
e) Assess for complaints of pressure or fullness at the incision site.
f) Monitor vital signs.
g) Assess for voice changes or respiratory difficulty.
h) Make certain that IV calcium gluconate is available for emergency use.

2. THYROID STORM (THYROTOXICOSIS)
a. Description
1) Life-threatening, uncontrolled hyperthyroidism with increased amounts of thyroid hormones released into the blood and markedly increased metabolism
2) Onset spontaneous but often after stressor
3) Temperature may rise to 41°C (106°F) because the body is unable to release heat from increased metabolism.

b. Assessment
1) Extreme temperature elevation
2) Marked respiratory distress
3) Tachycardia
4) Apprehension
5) Restlessness that progresses to delirium, coma, and death from heart failure

c. Nursing interventions
1) Implement aggressive and immediate interventions to prevent death.
2) Monitor for cardiac arrhythmias.
3) Change linen frequently if the client is diaphoretic.
4) Provide a cool room.

d. Medical management
1) Measures to decrease temperature and heart rate
2) Measures to prevent vascular collapse through the use of antithyroid drugs, humidified O_2, hypothermia blankets, ice packs, hydrocortisone, and Tylenol

3. HYPOTHYROIDISM
a. Description
1) General slowing of body activities caused by a reduction in secretion of thyroid hormones

2) Can range from mild to advanced form called myxedema
3) Most common cause in adults is autoimmune Hashimoto's thyroiditis
b. Assessment
   1) Slow development of fatigue, hair loss, brittle nails, numbness and tingling of the fingers, and menorrhagia or amenorrhea in young women
   2) Weight gain
   3) Dry and thickened skin
   4) Apathy and expressionless face
   5) Slurred speech and thickened tongue
   6) Puffy and watery eyes
   7) Sleepiness
   8) Constipation
   9) Intolerance to cold
   10) Slow pulse rate
   11) Subnormal temperature
   12) Increase in diastolic blood pressure
c. Diagnostic tests
   1) TSH
   2) FT_4
   3) Serum lipids (hyperlipidemia)
   4) Serum cholesterol (hypercholesterolemia)
d. Nursing interventions
   1) Instruct the client on the need for lifetime thyroid hormone replacement therapy (Synthroid or Levothroid).
   2) Monitor closely for myocardial ischemia or infarction.
   3) Instruct the client in a diet high in proteins and low in calories until weight returns to normal.
   4) Administer sedatives, opioids, and anesthetic agents to these clients because these clients are sensitive.
   5) Provide these clients with extra blankets because they tend to be cold.
   6) Offer a diet high in bulk and roughage and fluid content for constipation.
   7) Encourage a low-calorie diet for weight loss.

4. MYXEDEMA
   a. Description
      1) Severest form of hypothyroidism noted by nonpitting edema from accumulations of mucopolysaccharides in tissues
      2) Myxedema coma, often preceded by infection, progresses to decreased blood flow to brain, hypotension, hypoglycemia, bradycardia, hypothermia, hypoventilation, and death.

   b. Assessment
      1) Periorbital edema
      2) Puffy hands and feet
      3) Profound lethargy and apathy
      4) Slowed body metabolism

D. PARATHYROID DISORDERS
   1. HYPERPARATHYROIDISM
      a. Description
         1) Caused by overproduction of parathormone by the parathyroid gland
         2) Characterized by bone decalcification, elevated serum calcium levels, decreased serum phosphate levels, increased calcium and phosphorus in the urine, and decreased neuromuscular irritability
         3) Renal calculi, obstruction, pyelonephritis, and renal failure are complications due to increased renal calcium and phosphorus levels in the renal pelvis and parenchyma.
      b. Assessment
         1) Nausea and vomiting
         2) Weakness and fatigue
         3) Bone pain
         4) Polyuria
         5) Polydipsia
         6) Increased emotional irritability
         7) Neuromuscular irritability
      c. Diagnostic tests
         1) Serum calcium (elevated)
         2) Serum phosphates (low)
         3) Urinary calcium and phosphates (elevated)
         4) Radioimmunoassays for parathormone
      d. Nursing interventions
         1) Encourage fluids to prevent renal calculi.
         2) Encourage ambulation.
         3) Measures to prevent falls (osteoporosis can lead to pathologic fractures)
         4) Instruct the client on a diet low in calcium and high in phosphorus.
      e. Surgical management
         1) Surgery usually performed, with part or all of the gland removed
         2) Prior to surgery, electrolyte imbalance treated with oral phosphorus, fluids forced to 2000 ml per day, IV saline and Lasix to aid in the renal clearance of calcium, and cranberry and prune juice to prevent stone formation
         3) Postoperative goals related to prevention of complications of hemorrhage, airway obstruction, injury to recurrent laryngeal nerve, and tetany

2. HYPOPARATHYROIDISM
   a. Description
      1) Disorder in which there is insufficient secretion of parathormone caused by inadequate blood supply to the parathyroid gland, mechanical injury, or inadvertent removal of all or some of parathyroid glands during thyroid or neck surgery
      2) Clinical manifestations related to imbalance of calcium and phosphorus, increased calcification of bone, and increased neuromuscular activity that may progress to tetany
   b. Assessment
      1) Numbness and tingling in extremities and around the neck (mild tetany)
      2) Painful muscle spasms, seizures, carpal spasm, marked anxiety and apprehension, bronchospasm, laryngeal stridor, and cardiac dysrhythmias (severe tetany)
   c. Diagnostic tests
      1) Serum phosphate (elevated)
      2) Serum calcium (low)
      3) Bone density (increased)
      4) Urinary calcium and phosphorus (low)
   d. Nursing interventions
      1) Place the tracheostomy set at the bedside.
      2) Place calcium gluconate at the bedside.
      3) Perform Trousseau's sign (constrict blood flow to the wrist) or Chvostek's sign (tap facial muscle) to assess for tetany.
      4) Instruct the client on a diet high in calcium and low in phosphorus.
      5) Instruct the client to take large daily doses of vitamin D orally, calcium salts, and aluminum hydroxide gel or aluminum carbonate (Gelusil Ampojel) after meals.
   e. Medical management
      1) Treatment goals are to raise serum calcium levels, eliminate symptoms of hypoparathyroidism and hypocalcemia, and correct state of tetany if present.
      2) Calcium gluconate in saline is given parenterally to treat tetany (should be kept at bedside for emergency use).
      3) Parathormone is given in severe cases but many clients exhibit allergic response.

E. ADRENAL DISORDERS
   1. CUSHING'S SYNDROME
      a. Description
         1) Disorder characterized by excessive secretion of the glucocorticoid "cortisol" from the adrenal cortex; usually due to tumor
         2) Excessive glucocorticoids result in protein wasting, capillary fragility, and adipose tissue accumulations.
         3) Any client with autoimmune disorders, allergic reactions, and posttransplant procedures who is receiving large doses of glucocorticosteroids for extended periods of time may exhibit symptoms of Cushing's syndrome.
            a) Dosage must be tapered before discontinuance.
      b. Assessment
         1) Moon face and buffalo hump
         2) Purple striae on breasts, axilla, and legs
         3) Truncal obesity with slender limbs
         4) Reduced resistance to infection
         5) Hypertension
         6) Electrocardiogram (ECG) abnormalities
         7) Muscle weakness
         8) Hyperglycemia
         9) Changes in secondary sex characteristics
        10) Altered mental status (frank psychosis)
      c. Diagnostic tests
         1) Serum sodium (increased)
         2) Serum glucose (increased)
         3) Serum potassium (decreased)
         4) Plasma and urinary levels of cortisol
         5) Overnight dexamethasone suppression test
         6) 24-hour urinary free cortisol level
         7) High- or low-dose dexamethasone test
      d. Nursing interventions
         1) Measures to minimize risk for injury and infection
         2) Monitor for potential complications preoperative.
         3) Client teaching according to the type of scheduled surgery
         4) Provide mental and physical rest.
         5) Maintain skin integrity.
         6) Improve nutritional status (diet low in calories, carbohydrates, and sodium but ample protein and potassium content).
         7) Measures to improve body image
         8) Encourage healthy mental functioning.

9) Assess for postoperative complications (addisonian crisis).

e. Medical management

1) Interventions dependent on cause

f. Surgical management

1) If clinical manifestations are caused by a pituitary tumor, tumor is removed by hypophysectomy or ablated by irradiation.

2) If clinical manifestations are caused by adrenal cortex tumor, tumor is surgically resected (adrenalectomy).

3) If both adrenal glands are involved (bilateral total adrenalectomy), client will need lifetime adrenal cortex hormone replacement therapy.

2. PRIMARY ALDOSTERONISM

a. Description

1) Condition in which there is excessive secretion of aldosterone from the adrenal cortex; usually due to tumor

2) Client exhibits signs and symptoms of hypokalemia and alkalosis and has normal or elevated serum sodium levels

3) Adrenalectomy performed if caused by a tumor

4) Postoperative care includes temporary (unilateral) or permanent (bilateral) replacement of corticosteroids, fluid management, and insulin for hyperglycemia.

5) If not treated early, advances to hypertension, cardiovascular disease, and renal insufficiency

6) Spironolactone, an aldosterone antagonist, given if the client is unable to have surgery.

b. Assessment

1) Hypertension

2) Muscle weakness

3) Leg cramps

4) Generalized fatigue

5) Polyuria

6) Polydipsia

7) Tetany

8) Paresthesia

c. Diagnostic tests

1) Serum sodium (unchanged or high)

2) Serum potassium (low)

3) Aldosterone (high)

4) Renin (low)

5) Measurement of aldosterone levels after salt loading

d. Nursing interventions

1) Observe for changes in vital signs.

2) Assess for clinical manifestations of adrenal insufficiency, adrenal crisis, or hemorrhage.

3. ADDISON'S DISEASE

a. Description

1) Disorder in which there is hypofunction of the adrenal cortex, resulting in an insufficient secretion of both mineralocorticoids and glucocorticoids

2) Because these hormones are essential for life, client will die unless replacement therapy is initiated.

3) Usually caused by autoimmune response or atrophy of adrenal glands

4) Develops without warning and often precipitated by stress, for example, infection, trauma, or surgery

b. Assessment

1) Loss of strength

2) Nausea and vomiting

3) Abdominal pain

4) Diarrhea

5) Bronze-like pigmentation of the skin (hyperpigmentation)

6) Hyperpigmentation of pressure points of the knees, elbows, and along the belt line

7) Brownish gums

8) Hypoglycemia

9) Hypotension

10) Loss of some secondary sex characteristics in women (pubic and axillary hair)

c. Diagnostic tests

1) Serum glucose (low)

2) Serum sodium (low)

3) Serum potassium (high)

4) Serum cortisol levels (low)

5) White blood cell count (increased)

6) Adrenocorticosteroid hormones in the blood and urine (decreased)

d. Nursing interventions

1) Instruct the client in need to take lifelong replacement drug therapy.

2) Instruct the client to increase salt intake when ill, experiencing stress, or in hot weather.

3) Instruct the client that edema and weight gain may indicate the need to decrease the dosage of steroids, and symptoms of dizziness, lightheadedness, and weight loss may indicate the need to increase the dosage.

4) Instruct the client and family in administration of Solu-Cortef for emergency use.

5) Instruct the client to wear and carry medical alert information that advises of need for steroids at all times.

4. ADDISONIAN CRISIS
   a. Description
      1) Untreated Addison's disease progresses to addisonian crisis characterized by severe hypotension, shock, coma, vascular collapse, and death.
      2) Occurs when client fails to take prescribed replacement therapy or as a complication of surgery or other treatment of pituitary or adrenal glands
   b. Medical management
      1) Goals of emergency care are to reverse shock, restore blood circulation, and replace needed steroids.
      2) Client given hydrocortisone (Solu-Cortef) intravenously, fludrocortisone (mineralocorticoid), followed with 5% dextrose in saline (glucose and saline replacements), vasopressors, blood transfusions, and serum albumin.
      3) Essential that all forms of stimuli, for example, loud noises, bright lights, and movement, be eliminated.

5. PHEOCHROMOCYTOMA
   a. Description
      1) Disorder caused by a tumor (usually benign) in the adrenal medulla, resulting in increased secretion of epinephrine and norepinephrine
      2) Clinical manifestations depend on amount of epinephrine and norepinephrine secreted.
      3) Diagnosed by symptoms of the sympathetic nervous system (fight or flight), with increased metabolism, and increased blood glucose levels occurring with hypertension
   b. Assessment
      1) Headache
      2) Diaphoresis
      3) Palpitations
      4) Tachycardia
      5) Apprehension
      6) Hypertension (intermittent or persistent)
      7) Postural hypertension (frequent)
      8) Flushing
      9) Constipation
   c. Diagnostic tests
      1) 24-hour urine for catecholamines (MN and VMA)
      2) Total plasma catecholamine levels for epinephrine and norepinephrine
         a) Physical, mental, and chemical factors may affect results.
      3) Computerized tomography (CT) scans, magnetic resonance imaging (MRI), ultrasound, and MIBG scintigraphy helpful in identifying location of adrenal tumor
   d. Nursing interventions
      1) Monitor closely for shock and hemorrhage.
      2) Frequent assessment of ECG changes, arterial pressures, fluid and electrolyte balance, and blood glucose levels
      3) Instruct the client in use and precautions of corticosteroids if adrenalectomy is performed.
   e. Medical management
      1) During acute episodes, alpha-adrenergic blocking agents or smooth muscle relaxants are used to lower blood pressure.
      2) Once blood pressure is stable, client is prepared for surgery with phenoxybenzamine (Dibenzyline), a long-acting alpha blocker, or beta-adrenergic blocking agents (Inderal) if cardiac clinical manifestations unresponsive to alpha blockers.
   f. Surgical management
      1) Adrenalectomy is treatment of choice.
         a) During surgery, there is danger of excessive production of catecholamines as the tumor is manipulated, causing very high BP levels and cardiac arrhythmias.
         b) Fluids, plasma, and plasma substitutes are given to lessen the effect of hypotension.
         c) Hypotension occurs as soon as the tumor is removed—lasts for 24–48 hours post-op.
         d) Corticosteroid replacement is necessary if bilateral adrenalectomy, and frequently given in unilateral adrenalectomy for initial postoperative period.

F. PANCREATIC ENDOCRINE DISORDERS
   1. DIABETES MELLITUS
      a. Description
         1) A chronic metabolic disease of the pancreas resulting from insufficient secretion of insulin
         2) Insufficient insulin produces a disorder of carbohydrate metabolism with a subsequent derangement of protein and fat metabolism.

3) Diabetes mellitus is classified as type 1 (insulin dependent), type 2 (noninsulin dependent). Diabetes mellitus is associated with other diseases and gestational diabetes.

4) Type 1 is characterized by the inability to produce insulin as beta cells are destroyed.

5) Type 1 may be due to genetic susceptibility and autoimmune response.

6) Type 1 onset may be sudden with nausea, vomiting, and complaints of abdominal pain.

7) In Type 2, some insulin is produced but the amount is insufficient due to impaired insulin secretion or insulin resistance.

8) Client with type 2 is usually obese with slow onset of symptoms.

9) Type 2 is treated with weight reduction, oral antidiabetic agents, and exercise.

b. Assessment
   1) Polyuria
   2) Polydipsia
   3) Polyphagia
   4) Weakness and fatigue
   5) Numbness and tingling of extremities
   6) Frequent infections
   7) Vision changes
   8) Slow healing of injured tissue
   9) Weight loss

c. Diagnostic tests
   1) Serum glucose (diagnosed by laboratory findings of high blood glucose levels on more than one laboratory testing)

d. Complications
   1) Complications of insulin therapy include hypoglycemia, hyperglycemia, lipodystrophy, erratic insulin action, insulin allergy, and insulin resistance.
   2) Acute complications of diabetes include hypoglycemic reaction (insulin reaction) and diabetic ketoacidosis.
   3) Hypoglycemic reaction occurs when blood glucose falls to less than 50–60 mg/dl.
   4) Chronic complications of diabetes include vascular degenerative changes, neuropathy, ocular disturbances, kidney disease, and foot and leg problems.
   5) Vascular degenerative changes (macrovascular) occur because diabetics are more prone to atherosclerotic changes, for

example, coronary artery disease, cerebrovascular disease, and peripheral vascular disease.

6) Neuropathies occur because diabetes affects the peripheral, autonomic, and spinal nerves, leading to decreased sensation of pain and temperature, unsteady gait, cardiovascular changes, delayed gastric emptying, neurogenic bladder, and sexual dysfunction.

7) Ocular disturbances such as diabetic retinopathy may progress to blindness.

8) Microvascular changes in the kidneys due to diabetes may result in end-stage renal disease.

9) Foot and leg problems often leading to amputation develop as a result of neuropathy and peripheral vascular disease.

e. Nursing interventions
   1) Focus on assisting the client to learn about diabetes, promoting self-care, and teaching measures for control of the disease and prevention of complications.
   2) Client teaching includes role of nutrition, exercise, monitoring blood glucose levels, administration of antidiabetic medications or insulin, clinical manifestations of hyperglycemia and hypoglycemia, and prevention of complications.
   3) Dietary instructions should include:
      a) All carbohydrates—simple and complex—should be eaten in moderation.
      b) Meal plans may utilize exchange lists, MyPlate, and glycemic index.
      c) Important to stress consistency in eating, monitoring food intake in relation to insulin or oral hypoglycemic agents and exercise, and adhering to an individualized diet plan
   4) Instructions regarding exercise should include:
      a) Clients with diabetes need regular exercise.
      b) An increase in activity will decrease the need for insulin or oral antidiabetic agents. However, an unusual amount of exercise can precipitate a hypoglycemic reaction. Clients need to carry some form of

rapid-acting glucose with them to treat hypoglycemia.

c) If exercise is less than usual, client will require either a lighter diet or more insulin.

d) If exercise is more than usual, client will require either more food or less insulin.

5) Client teaching regarding blood glucose monitoring should include:

a) Frequency of monitoring depends on many variables.

b) If prone to frequent glycosuria or continual hyperglycemia, instruct the client to perform urine testing for ketonuria with dipsticks.

6) Client teaching regarding administration of antidiabetic medications and insulin

7) Client teaching regarding clinical manifestations of hyperglycemia and hypoglycemia should include:

a) Hyperglycemia occurs when there is not enough insulin or antidiabetic drug or too much food.

b) Clinical manifestations of hyperglycemia include polyuria, polydipsia, polyphagia, fatigue and weakness, numbness and tingling in the hands and feet, and slow wound healing.

c) Hypoglycemic reaction is caused by too large a dose of insulin or antidiabetic drug or too little food.

d) Vomiting, diarrhea, more exercise than usual, or emotional stress may precipitate a hypoglycemic reaction.

e) Hypoglycemic reaction is likely to occur at peak action time of the type of insulin or antidiabetic agent.

f) Early or moderate clinical manifestations of hypoglycemic reaction include weakness, shakiness, diaphoresis, hunger, nervousness, irritability, palpitations, tremors, headache, blurred or double vision, and numbness of the lips and tongue.

g) Sources of glucose such as fruit juice, hard candy, sugar, honey, or glucose tablets should be readily available to treat early

Table 6-1 Client Teaching Regarding Foot Care

- Wash feet daily and dry them carefully, especially between the toes
- Inspect feet and between toes for blisters, cuts, and infections
- Use a mirror to see the bottom of the feet
- Avoid activities that will restrict the blood flow to the feet, especially smoking and crossing the legs
- Wear comfortable, well-fitting, and closed-toed shoes
- Avoid going barefoot
- Wear new shoes for short intervals
- Always wear stockings
- Inspect inside of shoes for rough edges, nail points, or foreign objects
- Avoid temperature extremes (test water with hands before getting in)
- Avoid using water bottles or heating pads
- Have feet examined regularly by a physician
- Have toenails cut straight across
- See a podiatrist for treatment of corns or calluses

© Cengage Learning 2015

symptoms of early or moderate hypoglycemia.

h) In advanced hypoglycemic reaction, client becomes stuporous and unconscious.

i) Advanced stage treated with injection of glucagon, adrenalin, or dextrose 50% IV

8) Client teaching regarding foot care (see Table 6-1)

f. Medical management

1) Focus on controlling diabetes and preventing complications through diet, exercise, and pharmacological therapy.

2) Nutritional goals focus on controlling weight, maintaining a constant blood sugar level, and providing all the essential foods for healthy living.

3) The dietary plan includes caloric distribution of 50% to 60% carbohydrates, 20% to 30% fat, and 10% to 20% protein.

4) Pharmacologically, clients are treated with insulin or oral antidiabetic agents.

5) Insulin therapy may be given once or twice a day or given three to four times a day according to blood glucose monitoring results.

6) Clients with type 1 diabetes taking insulin who are NPO for diagnostic examinations or surgery will have the insulin dosage changed but not eliminated.

7) Oral antidiabetic agents include sulfonylureas, biguanides, alpha glucosidase inhibitors, thiazolidinediones, and meglitinides.

8) Clients with type 2 diabetes taking oral antidiabetic agents may need to take insulin during periods of stress, for example, surgery, infection, and emotional trauma.

2. DIABETIC KETOACIDOSIS
   a. Description
      1) Extreme hyperglycemia that occurs when there is an absence of insulin or markedly inadequate amount of insulin
      2) Hyperglycemia occurs when glucose is not transported across the cell membrane because of lack of insulin.
      3) Without available carbohydrate for cellular fuel, the liver converts glycogen store to glucose (gluconeogenesis).
      4) As the need for cellular fuel grows more critical, the body breaks down fats into free fatty acids and glycerol.
      5) Excessive amounts of free fatty acids are mobilized from adipose tissue cells and converted to ketone bodies in the liver.
      6) The liver accelerates the rate of production of ketone bodies.
      7) As fat metabolism increases, the liver produces too many ketone bodies, resulting in accumulation of ketone bodies in the blood (ketosis) and in the urine (ketonuria).
      8) The process of burning fats for fuel in the absence of carbohydrates results in four pathologic events: incomplete lipid metabolism, dehydration, lactic acidosis, and electrolyte imbalance.
      9) State of dehydration results in loss of sodium and potassium and increased creatinine, blood urea nitrogen, hemoglobin, and hematocrit.
      10) Precipitating causes include taking too little insulin; omitting doses of insulin; overeating; an increased need for insulin due to surgery, trauma, or pregnancy; and insulin resistance.
   b. Assessment
      1) Polyuria
      2) Polydipsia
      3) Nausea and vomiting
      4) Abdominal pain

5) Acetone breath (fruity odor)
6) Kussmaul's breathing (deep, rapid respirations)
7) Dehydration
   c. Diagnostic tests
      1) Serum glucose (levels vary greatly but may be elevated to 800–1000 mg/dl)
      2) Serum bicarbonate (low)
      3) pH (low)
      4) Serum ketones (high)
      5) Urinary ketones (present)
      6) Serum electrolytes (hypokalemia)
   d. Nursing interventions
      1) Frequently monitor vital signs.
      2) Assess for fluid overload during hydration process.
      3) Monitor ECG for signs of hyperkalemia.
      4) Monitor urine output to ensure adequate renal function.
      5) Monitor fluid and electrolyte balance.
      6) Monitor blood glucose levels.
      7) Administer fluids, insulin, and electrolytes as ordered.
      8) Provide client education to prevent further episodes of acidosis.
   e. Medical management
      1) Primary goal is to shift metabolism from fats to carbohydrates and thus restore carbohydrate utilization.
      2) Secondary goal is to reverse shock, correct fluid and electrolyte imbalance, and correct factors that led to acidosis.
      3) Dehydration due to polyuria, rapid breathing, diarrhea, and vomiting is treated initially with rapid administration of (0.9%) normal saline at 500–1000 ml over 2–3 hours, then 0.45% normal saline to continue rehydration.
      4) Plasma expanders may be needed to treat severe hypotension.
      5) Potassium balance restored with potassium added to IVs
      6) Acidosis treated with IV administration of rapid-acting insulin ordered as units per hour
      7) Hourly glucose measurements done when blood sugar levels reach 250–300 mg/dl. Dextrose is added to IV solution to prevent hypoglycemia.

3. HYPERGLYCEMIC HYPEROSMOLAR NONKETOTIC SYNDROME
   a. Description
      1) State of hyperglycemia and hyperosmolarity with a lack of effective insulin

2) Client has persistent hyperglycemia leading to osmotic diuresis, resulting in loss of water and electrolytes.

3) Water shifts from the intracellular to extracellular fluid space, resulting in dehydration, hypernatremia, and increased osmolarity.

4) Occurs in older adults after an illness or as a result of taking medications that cause insulin dependency.

b. Assessment

1) Hypotension

2) Polyuria

3) Polydipsia

4) Dehydration

5) Tachycardia

6) Neurological changes

c. Diagnostic tests

1) Serum glucose (levels from 600–1200 mg/dl)

2) Serum osmolality (above 350 mOsm/kg)

3) Serum sodium (low)

4) Serum potassium (low)

5) Blood urea nitrogen (BUN) (high) (levels 70–90 mg/dl)

d. Medical management

1) Treated the same as diabetic ketoacidosis (DKA), although insulin does not play as critical a role because client is not in acidosis

2) Neurologic clinical manifestations take 3–5 days to clear.

PRACTICE QUESTIONS

1. The nurse performs which of the following assessments in a client with severe anterior pituitary deficiency caused by the growth of a tumor?

   Select all that apply:
   [ ] 1. Intolerance to heat
   [ ] 2. Hyperglycemia
   [ ] 3. Polyuria
   [ ] 4. Bradycardia
   [ ] 5. Hypoglycemia
   [ ] 6. Dehydration

2. The nurse should include which of the following in preoperative instructions for a client with an anterior pituitary tumor who is scheduled for a total hypophysectomy using the transsphenoid approach?
   1. Avoid sneezing or blowing the nose after surgery
   2. Drink 10 glasses of fluids the day before surgery
   3. Do not rinse the mouth with any solutions until the packing is removed
   4. Support the neck when getting out of bed

3. The nurse is collecting a nursing history from a client admitted with diabetes insipidus. Which of the following questions should the nurse ask?
   1. "Have you experienced a change in temperature where you feel very hot or very cold?"
   2. "Have you noticed a change in how you react to people or situations?"

   3. "Have you experienced a change in urinary frequency or amount?"
   4. "Have you noticed a change in how you function sexually?"

4. The nurse should include which of the following in the discharge instructions of a client with diabetes insipidus?
   1. Follow-up appointments are not necessary with the physician unless there is an acute illness
   2. The prescribed hormone drugs will need to be taken for a lifetime
   3. Extra fluids should be taken cautiously when experiencing a major stressor
   4. Changes in diet and exercise may require changes in medication dosages

5. The nurse should report which of the following client assessments as consistent with a diagnosis of Graves' disease?

   Select all that apply:
   [ ] 1. Lethargy
   [ ] 2. Exophthalmus
   [ ] 3. Heat intolerance
   [ ] 4. Weight loss
   [ ] 5. Cold, clammy skin
   [ ] 6. Bradycardia

6. Which of the following client statements should the nurse report to the physician prior to scheduling a radioactive iodine uptake and excretion test?
   1. "I've been taking over-the-counter cough medicine for the past 2 weeks."

2. "My husband and I are vegetarians."

3. "We like to drink a glass of wine with our meals."

4. "I take a baby aspirin every day since my heart attack last year."

7. Which of the following should the nurse include in the teaching plan for a client who has hyperthyroidism and is treated with ^{123}I?
   1. A single dose of the radioactive iodine is sufficient
   2. Body excretions are considered radioactive for 1 week
   3. An increase in temperature and pulse rate should be reported
   4. Symptoms of hyperthyroidism should subside in 1 to 2 weeks

8. The nurse develops a plan of care for the immediate postoperative period for a client who had a thyroidectomy. The plan should include measures to
   1. correct fluid and electrolyte balance.
   2. administer medications to decrease vascularity of the thyroid glands.
   3. promote range-of-motion exercises of the neck.
   4. prevent complications of respiratory obstruction.

9. The nurse implements which of the following interventions in the plan of care for a client with hypothyroidism?
   1. Applying lotion for skin care
   2. Providing a cool temperature in the room
   3. Scheduling periods of rest
   4. Administering p.r.n. medications for diarrhea

10. The nurse is caring for a client with myxedema. Which of the following would indicate to the nurse that the client's condition is deteriorating?
    1. An increase in pulse rate and respirations
    2. Cold skin and episodes of chills
    3. Difficulty in arousing the client for medications
    4. Client complaints of palpitations

11. The nurse should include which of the following in the preoperative teaching plan for a client with hyperparathyroidism who is scheduled to have a portion of his parathyroid gland removed?
    1. Force fluids to at least 3000 ml per day
    2. Take over-the-counter supplements of vitamin D daily
    3. Maintain bed rest as much as possible
    4. Adhere strictly to the high-calcium diet

12. The postoperative orders for a client who has had the parathyroid gland removed include using Chvostek's sign to assess for signs of tetany. Which of the following is the appropriate assessment technique the nurse should implement?
    1. Occlude the blood flow in the wrist
    2. Observe respiratory rate and depth
    3. Listen for a crowing sound with inspirations
    4. Tap sharply over the facial nerves

13. The diet prescribed for a client with hypoparathyroidism should be high in calcium and low in phosphorus. The nurse instructs the client to include which of the following foods?
    1. Milk
    2. Green leafy vegetables
    3. Cauliflower
    4. Cheese

14. The nurse is admitting a client suspected of having Cushing's syndrome. Which of the following assessments supports the diagnosis of Cushing's syndrome?

    Select all that apply:
    [ ] 1. Slender trunk with enlarged arms and legs
    [ ] 2. Hypertension
    [ ] 3. Hyperglycemia
    [ ] 4. Decreased body and facial hair
    [ ] 5. Hyperpigmentation of the skin on the breasts and abdomen
    [ ] 6. Fat pad accumulations above the clavicles

15. The nurse evaluates which of the following nursing diagnoses to be most important for a client with Cushing's syndrome?
    1. Ineffective breathing patterns related to depressed respirations
    2. Risk for infection related to altered protein metabolism and inflammatory response
    3. Pain related to tissue and nerve injury and anxiety
    4. Ineffective therapeutic regimen management related to lack of knowledge about the need for lifelong replacement therapy

16. The nurse would report which of the following laboratory results as consistent with a diagnosis of primary aldosteronism?
    1. Serum potassium of 3 mEq/L
    2. Serum phosphorus of 3 mg/dL
    3. Serum sodium of 130 mEq/L
    4. Serum calcium of 12 mg/dL

17. Which of the following nursing interventions should be included in a plan of care for a client with Addison's disease?
    1. Administer the prescribed diuretics
    2. Give diet instructions for a low-carbohydrate, low-protein diet
    3. Monitor for signs of Na$^+$ and K$^+$ imbalances
    4. Encourage self-care activities

18. Which of the following questions should the nurse ask during an admission interview for a client admitted with a diagnosis of pheochromocytoma?
    1. "Do you ever notice or feel an increase in your heart beating?"
    2. "Do you suddenly feel warm and flushed when you get out of bed?"
    3. "Do your symptoms subside when you eat simple sugars?"
    4. "Do the attacks make you feel like you want to rest a while and sleep?"

19. The nurse conducts a health history for a client with type 1 diabetes mellitus. Which of the following client statements best describes the onset characteristics of this type of diabetes?
    1. "I was diagnosed during the fifth month of my pregnancy."
    2. "One day I passed out after I had terrible nausea, vomiting, and abdominal pain."
    3. "When I hit 40, I began to notice I was picking up weight and urinating more frequently."
    4. "My fasting blood sugars are always between 110 mg/dL and 126 mg/dL."

20. Which of the following should be included in the assessment of a client with diabetes mellitus who is experiencing a hypoglycemic reaction?

    Select all that apply:
    [ ] 1. Tremors
    [ ] 2. Nervousness
    [ ] 3. Extreme thirst
    [ ] 4. Flushed skin
    [ ] 5. Profuse perspiration
    [ ] 6. Constricted pupils

21. The client with diabetes mellitus asks the nurse which blood sugar test is most significant in determining that one is diabetic. The best response of the nurse would be which of the following?
    1. "When you have two consecutive fasting blood sugars of 126 or more in a short period of time."
    2. "Whenever you have a blood sugar taken and it is 150 or more."
    3. "When your blood sugar is in the range of 150 and 190 a couple of hours after you drink a special glucose solution."
    4. "When your blood sugar is 175 or more an hour after you have eaten a meal."

22. Which of the following nutritional goals would be most important in the teaching plan for a client with diabetes mellitus?
    1. Limit saturated fats to 20% of total calories
    2. Maintain body weight at 10 to 15 lbs above ideal body weight
    3. Avoid eating snacks between meals
    4. Include all essential food components in the diet plan

23. The nurse should instruct a client with diabetes mellitus and the client's family about the clinical manifestations of diabetic ketoacidosis before discharge. Which of the following should be included?

    Select all that apply:
    [ ] 1. Dehydration
    [ ] 2. Shallow, labored respirations
    [ ] 3. Acetone breath
    [ ] 4. Tremors
    [ ] 5. Cold, clammy skin
    [ ] 6. Abdominal pain

24. Which of the following should the nurse include in the instructions given to a client with diabetes mellitus on how to prevent hypoglycemia?
    1. Eat a meal or snack every 4 to 5 hours while awake
    2. Have a family member learn to inject insulin if symptoms appear
    3. Increase insulin if moderate exercise is planned
    4. Ingest complex carbohydrates if symptoms appear

25. The nurse instructs a client with diabetes mellitus that the priority self-care activity for preventing the complication of diabetes is which of the following?
    1. Learn to administer insulin properly and know the signs of hyperglycemia and hypoglycemia
    2. Follow the prescribed diabetic diet closely unless medical condition changes
    3. Keep the blood glucose levels controlled at or near normal levels
    4. Report to the physician immediately any kidney, vascular, or neurological changes

26. The nurse is observing a staff member preparing to give a client in diabetic ketoacidosis 40 units of NPH insulin IV bolus. Which of the following interventions by the nurse is appropriate?
    1. Assist the staff member preparing the injection by rotating the vial of NPH insulin prior to drawing up the insulin
    2. Instruct the staff member to follow the NPH IV bolus with 5 to 10 units per hour in normal saline
    3. Ask the staff member to give the client the NPH insulin IV bolus for the experience
    4. Tell the staff member that only regular insulin may be administered intravenously

27. The registered nurse is delegating tasks to be performed to a nursing unit. Which of the following tasks may be delegated to a licensed practical nurse?
    1. Develop the nutritional plan for a client with diabetes mellitus
    2. Assess ECG changes in a client with pheochromocytoma who had an adrenalectomy
    3. Implement the teaching plan for a client with Addison's disease
    4. Monitor the blood pressure in a client with primary aldosteronism

28. The nurse is caring for a client with diabetes mellitus who received 6 units of regular insulin at 0730. The nurse should monitor the client for clinical manifestations of hypoglycemia at which of the following times?
    1. 0930 to 1030
    2. 0800 to 0830
    3. 1200 to 1400
    4. 1500 to 1700

29. Which of the following is a priority for the nurse to monitor in a client with pheochromocytoma?
    1. Weight
    2. Serum glucose level
    3. Blood pressure
    4. Temperature

30. The nurse identifies which of the following clients to be at greatest risk for developing primary hyperaldosterism?
    1. A client with untreated lung cancer
    2. A client with a lesion of the hypothalamus
    3. A client with a history of meningitis and peripheral neuropathy
    4. A client with hypertension and hypokalemia not treated with diuretics

ANSWERS AND RATIONALES

1. **4. 5.** The anterior pituitary gland secretes several hormones, primarily ACTH, TSH, FSH, LH, and prolactin. A tumor in the anterior pituitary gland results in hyposecretion of one or more of the hormones secreted. Bradycardia would indicate a deficiency in thyroid hormones, and hypoglycemia would indicate a deficiency in adrenocorticotropic hormones. Intolerance to heat would be characteristic of hyperthyroidism, and hyperglycemia would indicate an increase in ACTH. Polyuria would be characteristic of excessive secretion of ADH from the posterior pituitary or excessive secretion of ACTH. Dehydration and polyuria are characteristics of diabetes insipidus, a posterior pituitary disorder.

2. **1.** A transsphenoid hypophysectomy is a surgical approach through the oral-nasal cavity. Any stress on the nasal cavity, such as sneezing or blowing one's nose, may precipitate the leakage of cerebrospinal fluid. These clients are not dehydrated prior to surgery, so they don't need increased fluids. Postoperatively, clients may rinse their mouths with warm saline. Because the surgery involves the upper lip and nose, supporting the neck is not necessary.

3. **3.** The client with diabetes insipidus has a deficiency in ADH secreted from the posterior pituitary gland. The client will experience voiding frequent large volumes of dilute urine. Questions regarding changes in heat and cold tolerance and mental status would be appropriate for thyroid disorders. Changes in sexual function are appropriate for anterior pituitary disorders and disorders with the sexual organs.

4. **2.** Clients with disorders involving a deficiency in hormone production will need to take replacement hormones for the rest of their lives. The client with diabetes insipidus is deficient in ADH and so will need to take the replacement vasopressin for a lifetime. These clients need periodic follow-up to monitor response to medication dose and route. Major stressors, such as illness or surgery, will affect hormone requirements, so a client with diabetes insipidus will need increased fluids for fluid replacement until vasopressin dosages can be regulated. Diet and exercise do not have an effect on medication dosages for diabetes insipidus but do have an effect for diabetes mellitus.

5. **2. 3. 4.** Hyperthyroidism, also known as Graves' disease (an increase in the production of thyroid hormones), is characterized by an increase in the metabolic rate, protruding eyeballs (exophthalmus), and an accumulation of fluid in the fat pads behind the eyes. The client also experiences hyperexcitability, nervousness, heat intolerance, and weight loss despite increased appetite. Lethargy and bradycardia are characteristics of decreased metabolism. An increased metabolic rate results in increased body warmth.

6. 1. Medications and foods containing iodine alter the results of radioactive iodine tests. Over-the-counter cough medicines may contain iodide. A vegetarian diet and wine are not food sources of iodine. Aspirin is not a medicinal source of iodine.

7. 3. Hyperthyroid clients treated with ^{123}I need to be observed closely for signs of hyperthyroidism indicating treatment was not successful. Hypothyroidism results indicate overresponse. Some clients need a second dose. Clients have a fear about radioactive substances, but clients are not considered to be radioactive and no radiation precautions are necessary. It takes approximately 3 to 4 weeks before the symptoms of hyperthyroidism subside.

8. 4. A thyroidectomy is removal of the thyroid gland through a neck incision. Immediately postoperatively there is the potential complication of airway obstruction by edema formation. Fluid and electrolyte balance would be monitored during the operative period and would not be imbalanced immediately post-op. Medications to decrease the vascularity of the thyroid glands would be done preoperatively. Range-of-motion exercises to the neck are not started until several days postoperatively.

9. 1. The client with hypothyroidism has decreased metabolism, which results in a slowing down of all body processes. Characteristically, the skin is very dry and thickened and requires lubrication. With a decrease in metabolic rate, the client will be cold and will be prone to constipation. These clients are very lethargic and sleep much of the time and therefore need to be encouraged to participate in activities to the greatest extent possible.

10. 3. The most life-threatening complication for the client with myxedema is myxedema coma. This client already has decreased metabolism, and as the condition worsens, cardiac, respiratory, and neurological systems slow down even more. The client then goes into a coma and may die from circulatory and respiratory collapse. If a client with myxedema becomes unable to be aroused, the client may be progressing into a coma. In myxedema the client experiences a decrease in pulse rate and respirations, has cold skin, and often has complaints of being chilled due to the decreased metabolic rate. Clients with increased metabolism complain of palpitations.

11. 1. Hyperparathyroidism is caused by an overproduction of the parathyroid hormone parathormone from the parathyroid glands. Parathormone takes calcium from the bone and concentrates it in the blood. As a result, these clients are prone to renal stones. Forcing fluids dilutes the urine and prevents precipitation of kidney stones. Remaining in bed contributes to stone formation. With an increased level of calcium in the blood, the client should be on a diet low in calcium. Vitamin D would not be necessary to enhance the absorption of calcium.

12. 4. Tetany is neuromuscular irritability characterized by tremors and spasms. Chvostek's sign is performed by tapping sharply over the facial nerves and is positive if that causes twitching or spasms in the region of the eyes, nose, and mouth. Occluding the blood flow in the wrist is Trousseau's sign. Respiratory obstruction and laryngeal spasm assessments are important measures to detect impending tetany but are not Chvostek's sign.

13. 2. Milk and cheese products are high in calcium but also high in phosphorus. Green leafy vegetables have a higher calcium and lower phosphorus ratio, but spinach should be avoided as it contains oxalate, which forms insoluble calcium substances. Cauliflower has a high phosphorus content in relation to calcium.

14. 2. 3. 6. Cushing's syndrome is an overproduction of glucocorticoids and androgens from the adrenal cortex. These hormones produce fat pad accumulations and a "buffalo hump" in the neck and supraclavicular areas. Hypertension and hyperglycemia are also clinical manifestations. The client has fat pad accumulations in the trunk. Protein wasting results in slender arms and legs. The excessive androgens cause virilization with increased body and facial hair. Hyperpigmentation of the skin is a result of insufficient adrenal cortex hormones.

15. 2. The anti-inflammatory effects of increased corticosteroids may mask the signs of inflammation and infection. These clients do not have changes in respiratory status or pain. Lifelong replacement therapy is not necessary unless the client had an adrenalectomy.

16. 1. Excessive production of aldosterone from the adrenal cortex (primary aldosteronism) is characterized by a severe decline in serum potassium levels, causing muscle weakness and fatigue, and decline in serum hydrogen ions, leading to alkalosis. Hypertension is the major sign of primary aldosteronism, with serum sodium levels that are normal or elevated. Serum calcium levels are low, as the hypokalemic alkalosis may decrease the ionized serum calcium levels, leading to tetany. A serum phosphorus level of 3 mg/dL is within the normal range.

17. 3.   Addison's disease is a deficiency of adrenal glucocorticoids and mineralocorticoids resulting in major disturbances in sodium (hyponatremia) and potassium (hyperkalemia). These clients need lifelong replacement therapy of glucocorticoids and mineralocorticoids. A high-carbohydrate, high-protein diet is ordered. With insufficient glucocorticoids and mineralocorticoids, the client is at risk for developing addisonian crisis when under any stress, including self-care activities.

18. 1.   Pheochromocytoma is a tumor in the adrenal medulla that secretes excessive amounts of epinephrine and norepinephrine. Palpitations are a major clinical manifestation. Postural hypotension occurs frequently and would be noted with dizziness and cold and clammy skin. Hyperglycemia is another classic manifestation. Clinical manifestations that subside when simple sugars are eaten are characteristic of hypoglycemia. The "attacks" that occur are a result of the release of the catecholamines and cause the client to be extremely anxious, tremulous, and weak.

19. 2.   Type 1 diabetes mellitus usually has an acute onset with nausea, vomiting, and abdominal pain and is often diagnosed after the client becomes comatose with ketoacidosis. Diabetes mellitus diagnosed during pregnancy is classified as gestational diabetes. Type 2 diabetes mellitus has a gradual onset and usually occurs in clients over 30. Clients with consistent fasting blood sugar levels that are slightly over normal are classified as borderline diabetics with impaired glucose intolerance.

20. 1. 2. 5.   In hypoglycemia, the blood glucose levels fall, resulting in sympathetic nervous system responses such as sweating, tremors, and nervousness. Extreme thirst and flushed skin are clinical manifestations present in hyperglycemia. Dilated pupils are a sympathetic response.

21. 1.   Fasting plasma glucose levels are abnormal if they are 126 mg/dL or more, and two consecutive fasting blood sugars of 126 mg/dL or more is indicative of diabetes mellitus. Random plasma glucose levels and 2-hour postload glucose are not abnormal until they are more than 200 mg/dL. A 1-hour postmeal plasma glucose level of 175 mg/dL is within the normal range.

22. 4.   The diabetic diet should be a well-balanced meal including all the essential food elements. Saturated fats should be limited to 10% of total calories. Achieving and maintaining ideal weight is necessary to gain control of blood sugar levels. Spacing meals throughout the day is less taxing on the pancreas.

23. 1. 3. 6.   In diabetic ketoacidosis (DKA), the body burns fats, which increases the amount of ketone bodies. An increase in ketone bodies causes acetone breath, which has a fruity odor. In DKA the respirations are deep but not labored. Other clinical manifestations of DKA include dehydration, abdominal pain, orthostatic hypotension, and tachycardia. DKA is a state of hyperglycemia. Tremulousness and cold, clammy skin are signs of hypoglycemia.

24. 1.   Meals or snacks every 4 to 5 hours while awake will maintain consistent blood sugar levels and should help to prevent hypoglycemia. Hypoglycemia is treated with injections of glucagon to raise the blood sugar level. Exercise burns calories so that less insulin is needed. Hypoglycemia is treated by ingesting simple carbohydrates.

25. 3.   The main goal in the management of the diabetic is to prevent the vascular and neuropathic complications from occurring by keeping the blood glucose levels at normal or near-normal levels through an interrelated mix of insulin, diet, and exercise. Proper administration of insulin and adherence to diet will not prevent complications. The renal, vascular, and neurological changes have already begun by the time the client notices changes.

26. 4.   Only regular insulin, which is clear, may be administered intravenously.

27. 4.   A licensed practical nurse cannot perform tasks that involve developing, assessing, or implementing. Those are tasks that only the registered nurse can perform. A licensed practical nurse may monitor the blood pressure in a client with aldosteronism.

28. 1.   Regular insulin is a short-acting insulin that has an onset of 30 minutes to 1 hour. The peak is between 2 and 3 hours and the duration is between 4 and 6 hours. A hypoglycemia reaction is most likely to occur during the peak, so if regular insulin was given at 0730, a hypoglycemic reaction would occur between 0930 and 1030.

29. 3.   Pheochromocytoma is a disorder caused by a tumor of the adrenal medulla characterized by intermittent or persistent hypertension. It is a priority to stabilize the blood pressure so surgery may be performed to remove the tumor.

30. 4.   Primary hyperaldosterism should be suspected in a client with hypertension and hypokalemia not treated with diuretics.

REFERENCES

Daniels, R. (2010). *Delmar's manual of laboratory and diagnostic tests* (2nd ed.). Clifton Park, NY: Delmar Cengage Learning.

Daniels, R., & Nicoll, L. (2012). *Contemporary medical-surgical nursing.* Clifton Park, NY: Delmar Cengage Learning.

Estes, M. (2010). *Health assessment and physical examination* (4th ed.). Clifton Park, NY: Delmar Cengage Learning.

Spratto, G. R., & Woods, A. L. (2012). *PDR nurse's drug handbook 2012.* Clifton Park, NY: Delmar Cengage Learning.

CHAPTER 7

NEUROLOGICAL DISORDERS

I. **ANATOMY AND PHYSIOLOGY OF THE NERVOUS SYSTEM (SEE FIGURE 7-1)**
   A. **FUNCTIONS OF THE NERVOUS SYSTEM (SEE FIGURE 7-2)**
   B. **DIVISIONS**
      1. CENTRAL NERVOUS SYSTEM
         a. Brain
         b. Spinal cord
      2. PERIPHERAL NERVOUS SYSTEM
         a. Cranial nerves
         b. Spinal nerves

      3. AUTONOMIC NERVOUS SYSTEM (SEE TABLE 7-1)
         a. Sympathetic nervous system
         b. Parasympathetic nervous system
   C. **CENTRAL NERVOUS SYSTEM**
      1. BRAIN
         a. Skull: hard bony covering for the brain
         b. Cerebrum
            1) Covered by a thin layer called the cerebral cortex
            2) Contains the gray and white matter

Figure 7-1 Structures of the brain

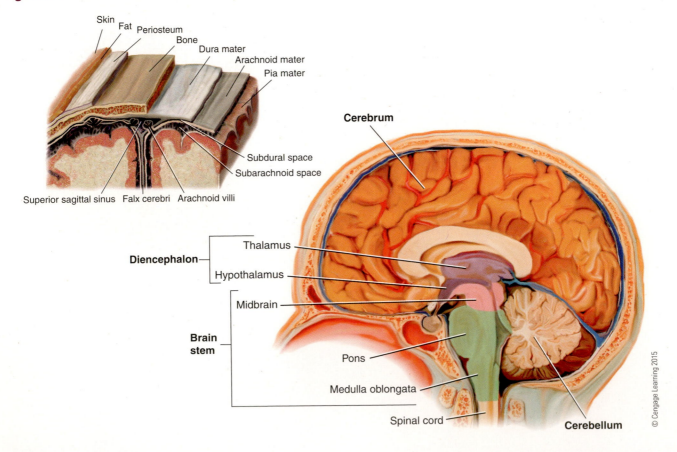

Skin
Fat
Periosteum
Bone
Dura mater
Arachnoid mater
Pia mater

Subdural space
Subarachnoid space

Superior sagittal sinus   Falx cerebri   Arachnoid villi

Cerebrum

Diencephalon
Thalamus
Hypothalamus

Midbrain

Brain stem

Pons

Medulla oblongata

Spinal cord

Cerebellum

© Cengage Learning 2015

Figure 7-2 Functional areas of the brain

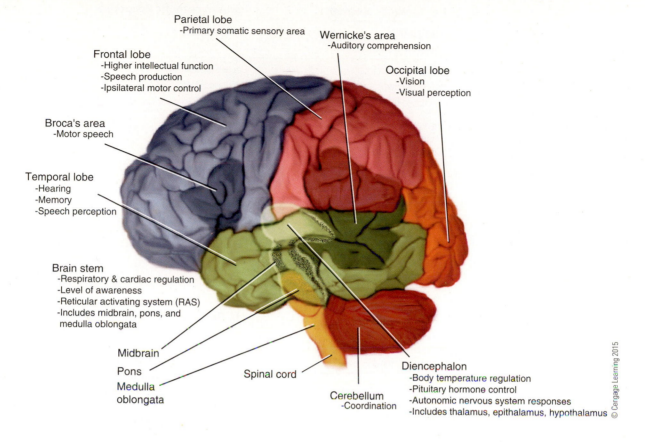

Parietal lobe
-Primary somatic sensory area

Wernicke's area
-Auditory comprehension

Frontal lobe
-Higher intellectual function
-Speech production
-Ipsilateral motor control

Occipital lobe
-Vision
-Visual perception

Broca's area
-Motor speech

Temporal lobe
-Hearing
-Memory
-Speech perception

Brain stem
-Respiratory & cardiac regulation
-Level of awareness
-Reticular activating system (RAS)
-Includes midbrain, pons, and
 medulla oblongata

Midbrain

Pons

Medulla
oblongata

Spinal cord

Cerebellum
-Coordination

Diencephalon
-Body temperature regulation
-Pituitary hormone control
-Autonomic nervous system responses
-Includes thalamus, epithalamus, hypothalamus

© Cengage Learning 2015

a) Gray matter: contains association and projection pathways that transmit impulses to communicate information to the various areas of the brain

b) White matter: contains neurons, the basic cells of the central nervous system composed of the body (controls function of neuron), axon (carries impulse away from cell body), and dendrite (carries impulse toward the cell body)

3) Divided into right and left hemispheres

a) Right hemisphere: receives and controls information from the left side of the body; controls perception of the physical environment, music, art, spirituality, and verbal communication (creative activity)

b) Left hemisphere: receives and controls information from the right side of the body; controls

problem solving, calculation, language, interpretation, analysis, reading, writing, and verbal communication (analytical activity)

c. Thalamus

1) Has a role in sensations such as pain, temperature, and touch

2) Controls emotions such as pleasantness and unpleasantness

3) Role in the arousal and alerting mechanism

4) Involved in mechanisms that produce complex reflex movements

d. Hypothalamus

1) Serves as a regulator and coordinator of autonomic activities

2) Plays a role in how the emotions express themselves in bodily sensations

3) Essential role in regulating the water balance, waking state, and appetite control

4) Assists in the control of the reproductive function

5) Critical role in temperature regulation

Table 7-1 Sympathetic and Parasympathetic Responses

System	Sympathetic Response	Parasympathetic Response
Neurological	Pupils dilated Heightened awareness	Pupils normal size
Cardiovascular	Increased heart rate Increased myocardial contractility Increased blood pressure	Decreased heart rate Decreased myocardial contractility Vasodilation
Respiratory	Increased respiratory rate Increased respiratory depth Bronchial relaxation	Bronchial constriction
Gastrointestinal	Decreased gastric motility Decreased gastric secretions Increased glycogenolysis Decreased insulin production Sphincter contraction	Increased gastric motility Increased gastric secretions Sphincter dilatation
Genitourinary	Decreased urine output Decreased renal blood flow	Normal urine output

© Cengage Learning 2015

e. Cerebellum
  1) Controls skeletal muscles to ensure smooth and coordinated muscle movements, equilibrium, and posture
f. Brainstem
  1) Medulla
    a) Critical control over vital functions such as cardiac, respiratory, and vasomotor
    b) Role in nonvital functions such as sneezing, coughing, vomiting, hiccoughing, and swallowing
  2) Pons
    a) Responsible for regulation of respirations
  3) Midbrain
    a) Functions as a reflex center for pupillary reflexes and eye movement
g. Meninges
  1) Composed of the dura, arachnoids, and pia matter, which are coverings of the brain that protect, support, and nourish
2. SPINAL CORD
  a. Continuation of the brain
  b. Supported by the vertebral column
  c. Covered by the meninges
  d. Controls body movement and visceral function, transmits information to and from the brain, and interprets sensory information from the trunk, extremities, and internal organs
  e. 31 pairs of spinal nerves
3. CEREBROSPINAL FLUID
  a. Produced in the choroid plexus

  b. Secreted by the lateral ventricles, circulated through the third and fourth ventricles and subarachnoid space
  c. Bathes the brain and spinal cord while providing shock absorption
  d. Clear, colorless appearance
  e. 0–5 cells/ml lymphocytes, 15–45 mg/dl protein, 45–100 mg/dl glucose
  f. Pressure is 70–180 mm H_2O
  g. Average daily amount in the adult is approximately 125 ml
  h. Approximately 550 ml secreted, circulated, and absorbed daily
D. PERIPHERAL NERVOUS SYSTEM
  1. CRANIAL NERVES (SEE TABLE 7-2)
    a. 12 pairs of cranial nerves that have sensory, motor, or mixed functions
  2. SPINAL NERVES (SEE TABLE 7-3)
    a. 31 pairs of spinal nerves that exit the spinal cord through the vertebral column containing afferent (sensory) and efferent (motor) nerves
E. AUTONOMIC NERVOUS SYSTEM
  1. TWO SUBDIVISIONS (SYMPATHETIC AND PARASYMPATHETIC) THAT WORK ANTAGONISTICALLY TO CONTROL THE INVOLUNTARY FUNCTIONS OF CARDIAC, SMOOTH MUSCLE, AND GLANDS
  2. PRIMARY FUNCTION IS TO MAINTAIN INTERNAL HOMEOSTASIS OF THE BODY
  3. SYMPATHETIC SYSTEM ACTIVATED BY "FIGHT-OR-FLIGHT" RESPONSE (SEE TABLE 7-1)
  4. PARASYMPATHETIC SYSTEM CONSERVES, RESTORES, AND FACILITATES ESSENTIAL BODY FUNCTIONS (SEE TABLE 7-1).

Table 7-2 Cranial Nerves

Cranial Nerve	Function	Assessment	Expected Findings
Olfactory (I)	Sensory: smell	Have client identify smells, such as coffee or alcohol, with one nostril occluded; repeat for opposite nostril.	Correct identification of smell or ability to choose smell from a list of choices.
Optic (II)	Sensory: vision	Ask client to read printed material, identify number of fingers held in front of client, or read from Snellen eye chart. Test visual fields by having client identify when the examiner's finger enters visual field.	Vision intact or correctable with lenses. Visual field intact.
Oculomotor (III)	Motor: pupil constriction	Cranial nerves III, IV, and VI are tested together. Inspect for ptosis, or drooping of eyelid. Assess extraocular eye muscles by having client follow the examiner's finger to each quadrant of the visual field. Assess for accommodation by asking the client to look at the examiner's finger held 4 to 6 inches from the client's nose, and then to follow the finger to 18 inches from the client's nose. Ask client about double vision.	Pupils are equal and round and react equally to light. No ptosis or double vision. Eyes move smoothly and consensually inward and downward. As the examiner's finger moves away from the client, the pupil will accommodate by dilating; as the finger moves closer, the pupil will normally constrict.
Trochlear (IV)	Motor: upper eyelid elevation, extraocular eye movement	See oculomotor (III).	Eyes should move smoothly and consensually upward and outward without nystagmus or diplopia.
Trigeminal (V)	Sensory: cornea, nose, and oral mucosa Motor: mastication	Test corneal reflex by lightly touching cornea with a small piece of cotton. Check sensation of face by touching lightly with a cotton ball while the client's eyes are closed and asking the client whether sensation is present. Check motor function by having client clench jaws shut while the examiner palpates the contraction of the termporalis and masseter muscles.	Corneal reflex as evidenced by rapid blinking when cotton swept across cornea. Feeling cotton ball on face indicates that facial sensation is intact. Jaw movement symmetrical and able to overcome resistance.
Abducens (VI)	Motor: extraocular eye movement	See oculomotor (III).	Eyes move outward.
Facial (VII)	Motor: facial muscles; Sensory: taste (anterior two-thirds of tongue)	Ask client to smile, show teeth, wrinkle forehead, or whistle. Have client close eyes lightly and keep them closed against the examiner's trying to open them. Have client identify salt and sugar when dabbed on tongue.	Facial movement symmetrical; sense of taste intact.
Acoustic (VIII)	Sensory: hearing, equilibrium	Assess ability to hear ticking watch or whispered voice. Observe gait for swaying. Perform Romberg test (refer to assessment of motor function).	Sense of hearing intact; no swaying or loss of balance.
Glossopharyngeal (IX)	Sensory: sensation to throat and taste (posterior one-third of tongue) Motor: swallowing	Have client identify taste of salt and sugar on back of tongue. Have client say "ah" and assess for symmetrical position of uvula. Test gag reflex by touching back of pharynx with tongue depressor. Observe swallowing ability and speech patterns.	Taste sensation intact; uvula raises symmetrically; gag reflex intact; swallowing and speech intact.
Vagus (X)	Motor and sensory	Test along with glossopharyngeal nerve.	
Spinal Accesssory (XI)	Motor: movement of uvula, soft palate, sternocleidomastoid muscle, trapezius muscle	Place examiner's hand on side of client's face and ask client to turn head against resistance; have client shrug shoulders against resistance of the examiner's hand.	Ability to move shoulder and head against resistance.
Hypoglossal (XII)	Motor: tongue movement	Ask client to stick out tongue and observe for symmetry, deviation to side; have client push tongue against tongue depressor and move tongue from side to side.	Tongue should be centrally aligned, able to push against resistance of tongue depressor; no fasciculations (involuntary twitching of muscle fibers) should be present.

Table 7-3 Spinal Nerves

Nerves	Number of Pairs
Cervical	8
Thoracic	12
Lumbar	5
Sacral	5
Coccyx	1

© Cengage Learning 2015

Table 7-4 Levels of Consciousness

Alert	Oriented, opens eyes spontaneously, responds appropriately.
Lethargic	Sleepy; slow to respond, but responds appropriately; oriented; opens eyes in response to verbal stimuli.
Stuporous	Aroused only in response to painful stimuli; never fully awake; conversation, if present, is confused or unclear; opens eyes to painful stimuli.
Semicomatose	May move in response to painful stimuli; does not converse; protective blink, swallowing, and pupil reflexes are present.
Comatose	Unresponsive except to severe pain; protective reflexes are absent; pupils are fixed; no voluntary movement.

© Cengage Learning 2015

Table 7-5 Glasgow Coma Scale

Behavior	Response	Score
Eye-Opening Response	Spontaneous	4
	To verbal command	3
	To pain	2
	No response	1
Best Verbal Response	Oriented, conversing	5
	Disoriented, conversing	4
	Use of inappropriate words	3
	Incomprehensible sounds	2
	No response	1
Best Motor Response	Obeys verbal commands	6
	Moves to localized pain	5
	Flexion withdrawal to pain	4
	Abnormal posturing—decorticate	3
	Abnormal posturing—decerebrate	2
	No response	1
Total		3 to 15

© Cengage Learning 2015

II. ASSESSMENT

A. HEALTH HISTORY
1. PAST MEDICAL HISTORY
2. SURGERIES
3. MEDICATIONS (CURRENT, PAST MEDICATIONS, OVER-THE-COUNTER MEDICATIONS, ALTERNATIVE THERAPIES)
4. ASSESS EXPOSURE TO PERINATAL TOXINS SUCH AS SMOKING, ALCOHOL, RADIATION, AND VIRUSES.
5. ASSESS DEVELOPMENTAL DELAYS IN WALKING, TALKING, ETC.
6. ASSESS THE CLIENT'S ABILITY TO PERFORM ACTIVITIES OF DAILY LIVING.
7. ASSESS WHETHER THE CLIENT IS LEFT- OR RIGHT-HANDED.
8. ASSESS IF THE CLIENT HAS EXPERIENCED A LOSS OF SENSATION, WEAKNESS, TINGLING, TREMORS, SYNCOPE, HEADACHES, SEIZURES, OR PARALYSIS.
9. ASSESS IF THE CLIENT HAS EXPERIENCED ANY CHANGES IN MEMORY, LANGUAGE, OR PROBLEM-SOLVING ABILITY.
10. ASSESS SLEEP, REST, ELIMINATION, SEXUAL PATTERNS.

B. PHYSICAL ASSESSMENT
1. ASSESS FOR ORIENTATION TO PERSON, PLACE, AND TIME.
2. ASSESS LEVEL OF CONSCIOUSNESS AND MENTAL STATUS (SEE TABLE 7-4).
3. PERFORM GLASGOW COMA SCALE (SEE TABLE 7-5).
4. ASSESS CRANIAL NERVES (SEE TABLE 7-2).
5. ASSESS VITAL SIGNS.
6. ASSESS CEREBELLAR FUNCTION BY OBSERVING THE CLIENT'S GAIT AND POSTURE.
7. ASSESS COORDINATION BY PERFORMING THE FINGER-TO-NOSE TEST, SHALLOW KNEE BEND, AND RAPID PRONATION AND SUPINATION OF THE HANDS.
8. PERFORM THE HEEL-TO-SHIN TEST.
9. PERFORM SENSORY EXAMINATION.
   a. Tactile sensation
      1) Stroke the client's arms and legs with the eyes closed and ask the client if the cotton ball is felt.
   b. Pain and temperature
      1) Touch the client with a cotton-tipped applicator or the rounded edge of a paperclip; ask the client whether the sensation is sharp or dull.
      2) Touch the client with an item that is cold or hot and ask the client if the item is hot or cold.
   c. Vibration
      1) After striking a tuning fork, place the end of the handle on the client's

wrists followed by the ankles and
ask if the vibrations are felt.

   d. Proprioception

      1) With the eyes closed, move the
client's joint of a finger or great toe
up and down in space and ask the
client how the joint is being moved.

      2) Romberg sign

         a) Client stands with the feet
together and arms at the side
with the eyes first open and then
closed; observe for swaying,
indicating a cerebellar problem
(minimal swaying acceptable).

   e. Stereognosis

      1) With the eyes of the client closed,
place an object such as a coin in
the client's hand and ask the client
to identify it.

   f. Graphesthesia

      1) With the eyes of the client closed,
hold the client's hand extended
and draw a letter or number and
ask the client to identify it.

   g. Integration of sensation

      1) With the eyes of the client closed,
simultaneously touch both sides of
the client's body with a sharp
object and ask the client to identify
the number of objects felt.

   h. Assess reflexes

      1) Biceps reflex: strike the antecubital
space with the elbow flexed.

      2) Triceps reflex: strike the triceps
tendon above the elbow with the
arm flexed.

      3) Brachioradialis reflex: strike the
radius 3 to 5 cm above the wrist on
a relaxed arm.

   i. Patellar reflex: strike the patellar
tendon below the patella with the legs
freely hanging.

   j. Achilles reflex: strike the Achilles
tendon in a leg flexed at the knee and
the foot dorsiflexed at the ankle.

10. ASSESS THE PUPILS.

11. ASSESS FOR MENINGEAL IRRITATION.

   a. Brudzinski's sign: flex the head and
neck onto the chest while observing for
flexion of the hip and knees, indicating
a positive response.

   b. Kernig's sign: flex the leg at the hip,
bring the knee to a 90-degree angle,
followed by attempting to extend the
leg while observing the client for pain
and spasms.

III. DIAGNOSTIC STUDIES

  A. X-RAY OF THE SKULL AND SPINE

    1. DESCRIPTION: X-RAY STUDY OF THE
SKULL AND SPINE USED TO RULE OUT
FRACTURES, DISLOCATIONS, AND
CURVATURES OF THE SPINE

    2. PREPROCEDURE

      a. Explain the purpose of the procedure.

      b. Instruct the client to lie still.

    3. POSTPROCEDURE

      a. No follow-up is needed.

  B. LUMBAR PUNCTURE

    1. DESCRIPTION: INSERTION OF A SPINAL
NEEDLE THROUGH THE L3–L4 INTO
THE SUBARACHNOID SPACE TO
OBTAIN CEREBROSPINAL FLUID FOR
LABORATORY ANALYSIS TO MEASURE
PRESSURE OR INSTILL MEDICATIONS

    2. PREPROCEDURE

      a. Obtain a written consent.

      b. Instruct the client to empty the bladder.

      c. Instruct the client to lie still during the
procedure.

    3. PROCEDURE

      a. Assist the client to assume a lateral
recumbent position with the knees
flexed.

    4. POSTPROCEDURE

      a. Instruct the client to lie flat, generally
4–8 hours, to prevent a spinal
headache.

      b. Encourage fluids.

      c. Monitor the puncture site for leakage
of cerebrospinal fluid (CSF) and
hematoma.

  C. CEREBRAL ANGIOGRAPHY

    1. DESCRIPTION: X-RAY STUDY OF THE
CEREBRAL VASCULAR SYSTEM
FOLLOWING AN INJECTION OF
CONTRAST MEDIUM, GENERALLY
INTO THE FEMORAL ARTERY

    2. PREPROCEDURE

      a. Explain the procedure.

      b. Obtain a written consent.

      c. Assess for allergies to iodine.

      d. NPO for 8–12 hours.

      e. Inform the client that a warm sensation
may be experienced with injection of
the dye.

      f. Instruct the client to lie still during the
procedure.

      g. Inform the client that groin discomfort
may be felt when the groin puncture is
made.

    3. PROCEDURE

      a. Administer sedation as prescribed.

    4. POSTPROCEDURE

      a. Maintain the client on bed rest,
generally for 8–12 hours.

      b. Monitor puncture dressing.

      c. Monitor vital signs.

      d. Apply pressure to the puncture site
with a sandbag.

      e. Encourage fluids.

      f. Assess the extremity for skin color, temperature, and capillary refill.

      g. Assess the area distal to the injection site.

D. MYELOGRAPHY

    1. DESCRIPTION: AIR CONTRAST OR WATER CONTRAST X-RAY STUDY INSERTED INTO THE SUBARACHNOID SPACE OF THE SPINE

    2. PREPROCEDURE

      a. Explain the procedure.

      b. Obtain a written consent.

      c. Assess allergies to iodine.

      d. NPO for 2–4 hours

      e. Instruct the client that a warm sensation may be felt with the injection of the dye.

      f. Instruct the client to void.

      g. Instruct the client to lie still during the procedure.

      h. Inform the client that during the procedure, the table will be tilted up and down to facilitate injection of the dye.

      i. Hold phenothiazine or tricyclic antidepressant, which may lower the seizure threshold.

    3. PROCEDURE

      a. Administer sedation as prescribed.

    4. POSTPROCEDURE

      a. Elevate the head of the bed 60° if a water-soluble agent was used, otherwise, 30–45°.

      b. Monitor the client for headaches, fever, stiff neck, or photophobia, which may indicate meningitis.

      c. Wait 48 hours before restarting phenothiazine or tricyclic antidepressant.

      d. Maintain the client on bed rest, generally for 8–12 hours.

      e. Encourage fluids.

      f. Monitor urine output.

E. POSITRON EMISSION TOMOGRAPHY (PET) SCAN

    1. DESCRIPTION: NUCLEAR SCAN THAT HAS AN ADVANTAGE OVER COMPUTERIZED TOMOGRAPHY (CT) OR MAGNETIC RESONANCE IMAGING (MRI) BECAUSE IT NOT ONLY PROVIDES INFORMATION ON THE BLOOD FLOW, OXYGEN UPTAKE, AND GLUCOSE TRANSPORT, BUT ALSO INFORMATION ON THE FUNCTION OF THE BRAIN

    2. PREPROCEDURE

      a. Explain the procedure.

      b. Instruct the client to void.

      c. Assess for allergy to iodine.

      d. Instruct the client to lie still during the procedure.

      e. Instruct the client to avoid caffeine, smoking, and alcohol for 24 hours.

      f. Obtain baseline vital signs and neurological assessment.

    3. PROCEDURE

      a. Administer sedation as prescribed.

      b. May offer relaxation tapes or mental relaxation exercises to facilitate lying still

    4. POSTPROCEDURE

      a. Instruct the client to wash hands after voiding and bowel movements because radionuclide is excreted in the urine and feces.

      b. Encourage fluids.

F. MAGNETIC RESONANCE IMAGING (MRI)

    1. DESCRIPTION: NONINVASIVE SCANNING TEST THAT HAS THE ADVANTAGE OVER CT SCANNING BECAUSE IT RELIES ON THE INTERACTION BETWEEN THE BODY'S CHEMISTRY AND A MAGNETIC FIELD

    2. PREPROCEDURE

      a. Explain the procedure.

      b. Obtain a written consent.

      c. Reassure the client that there is no radiation exposure.

      d. Remove any hairpins, glasses, jewelry, watch, and other metal objects.

      e. Offer the client earplugs for the loud knocking and thumping noises.

      f. Instruct the client to lie still during the procedure.

      g. Assess the client for a pacemaker, cerebral aneurysm clips, or other metal objects that would be affected by a magnetic field.

      h. Instruct the client to void.

    3. PROCEDURE

      a. Administer sedation as prescribed.

    4. POSTPROCEDURE

      a. No special postprocedural care

G. COMPUTERIZED TOMOGRAPHY (CT) SCAN

    1. DESCRIPTION: COMPUTERIZED ANALYSIS OF TOMOGRAPHIC X-RAYS PROVIDING THREE-DIMENSIONAL CROSS SECTIONS OF TISSUE STRUCTURES OF THE BRAIN

    2. PREPROCEDURE

      a. Explain the procedure.

      b. Obtain a written consent.

      c. NPO for 4 hours

      d. Remove hairpins, wigs, and all hair accessories.

      e. Assess for allergy to iodine.

      f. Instruct the client to lie still during the procedure.

    3. PROCEDURE

      a. Administer sedation as prescribed.

      b. Place the client's head in a holding device.

    c. Start an intravenous line.

    d. Xenon and oxygen mix may be administered by mask or endotracheal tube.

  4. POSTPROCEDURE

    a. Encourage fluids.

    b. Monitor the client for adverse reactions of xenon gas.

H. ELECTROENCEPHALOGRAPHY (EEG)

  1. DESCRIPTION: NONINVASIVE STUDY THAT EVALUATES THE ELECTRICAL ACTIVITY OF THE BRAIN

  2. PREPROCEDURE

    a. Explain the procedure.

    b. Inform the client to avoid fasting, which may result in hypoglycemia and adversely affect the results.

    c. Instruct the client to wash the hair the night before the procedure.

    d. Avoid hairsprays, oils, or hairpins the day of the procedure.

    e. Instruct the adult client to sleep no more than 5 hours the night before.

    f. Instruct a child client to sleep no more than 5–7 hours the night before.

    g. If prescribed, consult the physician before administering an anticonvulsant.

    h. Instruct the client to lie still during the procedure.

    i. Instruct the client to avoid caffeine-containing products, alcohol, and illegal drugs.

  3. PROCEDURE

    a. Assist the client to a reclining chair or bed.

    b. Attach the electrodes to the scalp with electrode gel.

    c. Reinforce lying still with the eyes closed.

    d. Monitor the client for seizure activity.

    e. If prescribed, instruct the client to deeply breathe 20 times in a 3-minute period to induce hyperventilation, producing cerebral vasoconstriction and alkalosis, which may result in seizure activity.

    f. If prescribed, place a bright light in front of client and perform 1 to 20 flashes of light per second with the eyes first open then closed (photic stimulation—seizures are light sensitive).

    g. If prescribed, sleep may be induced with oral or intravenous sedation that may induce brain waves, indicating certain types of epilepsy (frontal lobe epilepsy).

  4. POSTPROCEDURE

    a. Remove the electrode gel from the client's scalp.

    b. Offer the client shampoo to wash the hair.

    c. Inform the client who had a sleep EEG to have someone else drive him home.

    d. Monitor the client for seizure activity.

IV. NURSING DIAGNOSES

  A. RISK FOR ASPIRATION

  B. GRIEVING

  C. RISK FOR INEFFECTIVE CEREBRAL TISSUE PERFUSION

  D. INEFFECTIVE AIRWAY CLEARANCE

  E. IMPAIRED PHYSICAL MOBILITY

  F. IMPAIRED VERBAL COMMUNICATION

  G. RISK FOR INJURY

  H. INEFFECTIVE THERAPEUTIC REGIMEN MANAGEMENT

  I. RISK FOR IMPAIRED SKIN INTEGRITY

  J. IMPAIRED URINARY ELIMINATION PATTERN

  K. IMPAIRED NUTRITION: LESS THAN BODY REQUIREMENTS

Nursing Diagnoses: Definitions and Classification 2012–2014. Copyright © 2012, 1994–2012 by NANDA International. Used by arrangement with John Wiley & Sons Limited.

V. NEUROLOGICAL DISORDERS

  A. HEADACHES

    1. DESCRIPTION

      a. Headache or cephalalgia is a clinical manifestation rather than a disease.

      b. Head pain caused by stimulation of pain-sensitive structures in the head

      c. Affects more than 45 million individuals annually

      d. Classified as primary tension, migraine, or cluster

    2. TYPES

      a. Tension type

        1) Most common type

        2) Characterized by a steady pressure in the head

        3) Generally bilateral

        4) Referred to as a muscle contraction, psychogenic or rheumatic headache

        5) No aura

        6) May occur daily

      b. Migraine

        1) Characterized by unilateral or bilateral throbbing pain

        2) May be preceded by prodrome and aura (sensation of light or warmth)

        3) Aura may last for 30 minutes.

        4) Etiology unknown but may be neurological, vascular, or chemical

        5) May be triggered by chocolate, alcohol, bright lights, menstruation, or stress

        6) May last hours to days

        7) Generally occurs after awakening and improves with sleep

c. Cluster
  1) Episodic headaches peaking in 10 minutes and lasting 90 minutes occurring for weeks to months followed by remission
  2) Generally occurs unilaterally around or behind one eye and is severe
  3) More frequent in men between the ages of 20 and 50 years
  4) Characterized by an abrupt onset without a prodrome
3. ASSESSMENT
  a. Tension type
    1) Photophobia
    2) Phonophobia
    3) Pressure or tightness bilaterally
    4) Worse with activity
  b. Migraine
    1) Migraine with aura
      a) Unilateral numbness, tingling, or burning sensations in the lips, hands, or face
      b) Dizziness
      c) Confusion
      d) Weakness
      e) Scintillating scotomata (perceived flashing of light in one quadrant or visual field)
    2) Migraine without aura
      a) Unilateral, severe, pulsating head pain that is worse with activity
      b) Nausea and vomiting
      c) Photophobia
      d) Phonophobia
4. DIAGNOSTIC TESTS
  a. Complete history and physical
  b. CT scan or MRI may be done if there is a neurological abnormality on assessment.
5. NURSING INTERVENTIONS
  a. Tension type
    1) Nonnarcotic analgesics
    2) Butalbital and aspirin (Fiorinal)
    3) Butalbital and acetaminophen (Fioricet)
    4) Acetaminophen and isometheptene (Midrin)
    5) Muscle relaxants
    6) Tricyclic antidepressants
    7) Beta-adrenergic blocking agents
  b. Migraine
    1) Nonnarcotic analgesics
    2) Serotonin receptor agonists
      a) Eletriptan (Relpax)
    3) Ergotamine tartrate (Ergomar)
    4) Acetaminophen and isometheptene (Midrin)
    5) Corticosteroids
    6) Beta-adrenergic blocking agents

  7) Antidepressants
  8) Calcium-channel blockers
    a) Verapamil (Isoptin)
  9) Valproate (Depakene)
  10) Methysergide (Sansert)—reserved for clients with one or more headaches weekly
  c. Cluster
    1) Ergotamine tartrate (Ergomar)
    2) Methysergide (Sansert)
    3) Prednisone
    4) Verapamil (Isoptin)
    5) Lithium carbonate (Eskalith)
6. GENERAL NURSING INTERVENTIONS
  a. Biofeedback
  b. Relaxation therapy
  c. Stress management
  d. Provide the client medication instructions.
  e. Encourage the client to keep a diary of the characteristics of the headaches.
  f. Instruct the client to avoid trigger-producing foods such as caffeine, alcohol, cheese, chocolate, onions, ice cream, salt, vinegar-containing products, and nicotine.
B. EPILEPSY
  1. DESCRIPTION
    a. Paroxysmal abnormal electrical discharges of neurons in the brain
    b. Over half of causes are idiopathic.
    c. Variety of other possible causes include metabolic disturbances, electrolyte imbalances, acidosis, hypoglycemia, hypoxia, dehydration, water intoxication, alcohol or barbiturate withdrawal, hypertension, septicemia, systemic lupus erythematosus, brain injury, cerebrovascular accidents, diabetes mellitus, and heart, liver, or kidney diseases
    d. Most common causes in children under the age of 6 years are birth trauma, infectious agents, or inherited diseases such as phenylketonuria
  2. TYPES
    a. Tonic-clonic
      1) Formerly called grand mal
      2) Generally begins with a loss of consciousness followed by the tonic phase (stiffening of the body) for 10–20 seconds and concludes with a clonic phase lasting 30–40 seconds
      3) Tongue or cheek biting, incontinence of feces or urine, excessive salivation, cyanosis, and muscle aching may occur.
      4) Client may complain of not feeling normal for several hours or days postseizure and lacks all memory of the seizure.

b. Typical absence
   1) Formerly called petit mal
   2) More common in children but rare beyond adolescence
   3) May briefly lose consciousness—may appear as daydreaming
   4) May occur as many as 100 times
   5) May be induced by bright flashing lights or hyperventilation
c. Myoclonic
   1) Brief, sudden jerking of extremities
   2) May be severe enough to result in the client falling to the ground
d. Akinetic, atonic, astatic
   1) Terms used interchangeably—akinetic (cessation of movement), atonic (loss of muscle tone), or astatic (loss of balance)
   2) Formerly called drop attack—generally causes falling to the ground
   3) Characterized by a temporary loss of muscle tone followed by a sudden loss of consciousness that resolves by the time the client hits the ground
   4) Activities return immediately following the seizure.
e. Partial seizures (focal seizures)
   1) Simple type
      a) Generally retains consciousness
      b) May report an aura
      c) Clinical manifestations include unusual sensations, unilateral extremity movement, dream states, fear, anger, flushing, sweating, pupil dilation, change in heart rate, and epigastric discomfort.
   2) Complex type
      a) Generally loses consciousness for 1 to 3 minutes
      b) Characteristic clinical manifestations include automatisms (inappropriate behaviors such as lip smacking, reaching for real or imaginary items, picking at objects, or continuation of behaviors being performed prior to the seizure).
      c) Client has no memory of behavior postseizure.
f. Status epilepticus
   1) Serious complication requiring immediate medical intervention to prevent irreversible brain damage or death due to hypoxia
   2) Period of one continuous seizure lasting longer than 10 minutes or several seizures occurring during a 30-minute time frame

   3) Most common causes include a sudden withdrawal of anticonvulsant medication, head injury, cerebral edema, metabolic disturbances, or a sudden alcohol withdrawal.
   4) Emergency medical interventions include:
      a) Maintaining the client's airway, breathing, and circulation is the priority.
      b) Administer prescribed oxygen per nasal cannula or face mask.
      c) If possible, insert an airway, but never force the airway into the client's mouth.
      d) Establish an intravenous line of 0.9% normal saline and administer prescribed drugs such as diazepam (Valium), lorazepam (Ativan), valproate (Depacon), phenytoin (Dilantin), or fosphenytoin (Cerebyx).
3. ASSESSMENT
   a. Phases of possible seizure activity
      1) Prodromal: precedes seizure activity with a sign or activity
      2) Preictal or aura: period right before a seizure in which a sensory warning may be present
      3) Ictal: period of main seizure activity
      4) Postictal: recovery period following a seizure
4. DIAGNOSTIC TESTS
   a. Comprehensive history
   b. EEG—controversial because many clients have a normal EEG between seizures
   c. Laboratory tests such as complete blood count (CBC), serum chemistry, urinalysis (UA), and kidney and liver studies to rule out metabolic disorders
   d. CT scan
   e. MRI scan
   f. Cerebral angiography
   g. PET scan
5. NURSING INTERVENTIONS
   a. Document date, time, duration, and description of the seizure.
   b. Protect the client from injury during the seizure.
   c. Place the client in a lateral position.
   d. Maintain the airway.
   e. Suction as needed.
   f. Never restrain the client.
   g. Loosen restrictive clothing.

h. Administer prescribed drugs.
i. Instruct the client to wear a medical alert bracelet.
j. Instruct the client to avoid stress, fatigue, excessive alcohol intake, and hypoglycemia.
k. Instruct family members to assist the client to the ground at the onset of the seizure.
l. Provide a list of community resources.
m. Instruct the client to take all anticonvulsant medications and to consult the physician before taking over-the-counter medications.
n. Inform the client on state laws regarding driving or operating machinery.

C. MENINGITIS
1. DESCRIPTION: CEREBROVASCULAR INFECTION RESULTING IN AN INFECTION OF THE PIA MATER, ARACHNOID OF THE BRAIN, SPINE, AND CEREBROSPINAL FLUID
2. TYPES
   a. Bacterial meningitis
      1) Most common in fall and winter
      2) Causative organisms include *Streptococcus pneumoniae*, *Neisseria meningitidis*, and *Haemophilus influenzae*.
      3) Occurs in high-density populations such as college dormitories, prisons, and the military
      4) *H. influenzae* vaccine given to high-risk populations
   b. Viral meningitis
      1) Generally self-limiting
      2) Occurs as a sequela to several viral illnesses including herpes simplex, mumps, measles, and herpes zoster
   c. Fungal meningitis
      1) Occurs most commonly in clients with acquired immunodeficiency syndrome (AIDS)
3. ASSESSMENT
   a. Nuchal rigidity
   b. Kernig's sign—90° flexion of the hip followed by an attempt to extend the knee results in pain.
   c. Brudzinski reflex—flexion of the head and neck toward the chest results in flexion of the hip and knees.
   d. Increased intracranial pressure
   e. Vascular dysfunction
   f. Headaches
   g. Nausea and vomiting
4. DIAGNOSTIC TESTS
   a. Cerebrospinal fluid
   b. Complete blood count
   c. Serum electrolytes

d. Chest x-ray
e. Sinus x-ray
5. NURSING INTERVENTIONS
   a. Monitor vital signs and neurological status every 4 hours.
   b. Administer prescribed antipyretics.
   c. Maintain strict intake and output.
   d. Administer prescribed anticonvulsants.
   e. Administer prescribed antibiotics.
   f. Provide low lighting in the client's room.
   g. Administer prescribed analgesics.
   h. Maintain seizure precautions.
   i. Perform frequent vascular assessment to prevent vascular complication from septic emboli generally present in the hands and, if left untreated, leads to gangrene.
   j. Rifampin may be administered as prophylaxis for individuals who have had close contact with the client.

D. ENCEPHALITIS
1. DESCRIPTION
   a. Inflammation that causes edema and hemorrhage increases intracranial pressure, and may result in death.
   b. Most commonly caused by viral infection but may also be caused by bacterial, fungal, or parasitic infection
   c. Mosquitoes and ticks are the most common causes and are generally endemic.
2. ASSESSMENT
   a. Fever
   b. Nausea and vomiting
   c. Stiff neck
   d. Change on level of consciousness
   e. Increased intracranial pressure
   f. Mental and personality changes
   g. Headache
   h. Kernig's sign
   i. Brudzinski's sign
   j. Myoclonic jerks
   k. Seizure activity
3. DIAGNOSTIC TESTS
   a. Cerebrospinal fluid analysis
   b. EEG
   c. MRI
   d. PET
4. NURSING INTERVENTIONS
   a. Assess vital and neurologic signs every 2 hours.
   b. Elevate head of the bed 30° to 45°.
   c. Turn, cough, and deep breathe every 2 hours.
   d. Maintain patent airway.
   e. Administer prescribed diuretics such as Mannitol and corticosteroids such as Decadron to control edema.

f. Administer prescribed drugs such as acyclovir (Zovirax), which is the treatment of choice for herpes encephalitis.

E. BRAIN ABSCESS

1. DESCRIPTION
   a. Accumulation of pus within the brain
   b. Occurs as the result of a local or systemic infection
   c. Most common organisms are *Staphylococcus aureus* and *Streptococci*
   d. May spread by direct access such as from a tooth, mastoid, or sinus or by indirect access such as a skull fracture, brain trauma, pulmonary infection, or endocarditis

2. ASSESSMENT
   a. Headache
   b. Fever
   c. Nausea and vomiting
   d. Increased intracranial pressure

3. DIAGNOSTIC TESTS
   a. CT scan
   b. MRI scan

4. NURSING INTERVENTIONS
   a. Administer prescribed antimicrobials.
   b. Assist with drainage of the abscess if indicated.
   c. Monitor dressing after drainage of abscess.
   d. Monitor neurological function after drainage of abscess.

F. PARKINSON'S DISEASE

1. DESCRIPTION
   a. Disorder of the basal ganglia resulting in bradykinesia (slowing down in movement), rigidity (increased muscle tone), tremor at rest, and impaired postural reflexes
   b. More common in men after the age of 60 years
   c. Exact cause unknown but results from substantial degeneration of the substantia nigra, leading to a decrease in dopamine
   d. Most common complications include dysphagia, pneumonia, malnutrition, and aspiration.

2. ASSESSMENT
   a. Tremor
   b. Rigidity
   c. Bradykinesia
   d. Stooped posture
   e. Abducted fingers that flex at the metacarpophalangeal joints
   f. Slow and shuffling gait
   g. Short, cautiously taken steps
   h. "Pill-rolling" hand movement
   i. Masklike face
   j. Drooling
   k. Dysphagia
   l. Micrographia—handwriting gets smaller
   m. Arms swing when ambulating
   n. Dysarthria
   o. Soft-spoken speech
   p. Mood swings
   q. Difficulty sleeping
   r. Slow reaction time
   s. Dementia

3. DIAGNOSTIC TESTS
   a. Complete history and physical
   b. Positive diagnosis is made when at least two of the three classic manifestations are present (tremor, bradykinesia, or rigidity).

4. NURSING INTERVENTIONS
   a. Administer prescribed dopaminergics such as carbidopa/levodopa (Sinemet) to treat rigidity.
   b. Administer prescribed anticholinergic such as trihexyphenidyl (Artane) and benztropine (Cogentin) to treat tremor.
   c. Bromocriptine mesylate (Parlodel) may be administered to increase dopaminergic receptors.
   d. MAO inhibitors such as selegiline (Eldepryl) to inhibit the release of levodopa
   e. Catechol *O*-methyltransferase (COMT) inhibitors such as entacapone (Comtan) in conjunction with Sinemet
   f. Encourage the client to participate in physical, occupational, and speech therapies.
   g. Instruct the client to perform breathing exercises to prevent respiratory problems.
   h. Encourage the client to wear elastic stockings for orthostatic hypotension.
   i. Encourage the client to provide self-care activities.
   j. Monitor intake and output.
   k. Assess the client for dysphagia.
   l. Provide the client with an upright chair with arms and small blocks behind the legs when sitting.
   m. Place an elevated toilet seat on the toilet.

5. SURGICAL MANAGEMENT
   a. Stereostatic pallidotomy and thalamotomy ablate areas in the thalamus to reduce tremor and rigidity.
   b. Deep brain stimulation involves placement of an electrode unilaterally to control tremors.
   c. Fetal tissue transplantation is experimental for motor clinical manifestations.

G. MULTIPLE SCLEROSIS (MS)
1. DESCRIPTION
   a. Progressive autoimmune degenerative disorder of the spinal cord and brain
   b. Occurs in clients 20 to 40 years of age
   c. Characterized by periods of remissions and exacerbations
   d. Etiology unknown but viral, immunologic, and genetic theories exist
   e. Affects women slightly more than males
   f. More common in cold-weather climates
   g. Clinical manifestations aggravated by fatigue, overexertion, extreme temperatures, and stress
2. ASSESSMENT
   a. Fatigue
   b. Stiffness of legs
   c. Hyperactive deep tendon reflexes
   d. Unsteady gait
   e. Positive Babinski's reflex
   f. Clonus
   g. Absent abdominal reflexes
   h. Intention tremor (tremor occurring with activity)
   i. Dysmetria (immobility to direct or limit movement)
   j. Dysdiadochokinesia (inability to stop one motor movement and substitute another)
   k. Lack of coordination
   l. Tinnitus
   m. Vertigo
   n. Hearing loss
   o. Speech difficulties including dysarthria, ataxia, and slow speech
   p. Dysphagia
   q. Visual problems including blurred vision, diplopia, scotomas, and nystagmus
   r. Facial pain
   s. Paresthesia
   t. Decreased temperature perception
   u. Bowel and bladder problems
   v. Sexual difficulties
   w. Cognitive impairments such as decreased short-term memory and concentration
3. DIAGNOSTIC TESTS
   a. No specific diagnostic tests
   b. Complete history and physical
   c. Cerebrospinal fluid analysis
   d. MRI
4. NURSING INTERVENTIONS
   a. Bed rest during an acute episode
   b. Prevent complications of immobility
   c. Instruct the client on possible triggers and methods for avoidance.
   d. Instruct the client on health promotion to avoid illness, fatigue, and extreme temperatures.
   e. Encourage the client to eat a well-balanced diet, including high-fiber foods, and increase fluid intake to prevent constipation.
   f. Administer prescribed anticholinergics for bladder spasticity.
   g. Instruct the client on self-catheterization if appropriate.
   h. Provide emotional support.
   i. Administer prescribed corticosteroids during exacerbations.
   j. Administer prescribed immunosuppressive drugs during exacerbations.
   k. Administer prescribed anticholinergics for bladder spasticity.
   l. Administer prescribed cholinergics for urinary retention.
   m. Administer prescribed muscle relaxants for spasticity.
   n. Administer dalfampridine (Ampyra), which improves walking.
   o. Administer fingolimod (Gilenya), which is indicated to treat clients with relapsing forms of MS to decrease frequency of clinical exacerbation to delay the physical disability.

H. AMYOTROPHIC LATERAL SCLEROSIS
1. DESCRIPTION
   a. Rare progressive degenerative disorder involving the motor system characterized by atrophy of the hands, forearms, and legs that leads to paralysis and death
   b. Occurs between the ages of 40 and 70 years
   c. More common in males
   d. Death generally occurs within 2 to 5 years.
   e. Cause unknown
2. ASSESSMENT
   a. Fatigue
   b. Muscle atrophy
   c. Weakness
   d. Dysarthria
   e. Dysphagia
   f. Fasciculations of the face
3. DIAGNOSTIC TESTS
   a. No specific diagnostic test
   b. Complete history and physical
   c. Creatine kinase (CK) is elevated.
   d. Muscle biopsy
4. NURSING INTERVENTIONS
   a. Provide the client and family emotional support.
   b. Administer prescribed riluzole (Rilutek) to slow disease progression.
   c. Prevent complications of immobility.
   d. Implement aspiration precautions.
   e. Implement pain relief interventions.

I. HUNTINGTON'S DISEASE
  1. DESCRIPTION
     a. Hereditary autosomal dominant trait disorder of chromosome number 4
     b. Fifty percent of children with a parent with the disorder will likely inherit the disorder.
     c. No known cure—death generally occurs within 15 years after onset.
     d. Occurs between the ages of 3 and 50 years
  2. STAGES
     a. Stage I—onset of neurological or psychological clinical manifestations lasting approximately 5 years
     b. Stage II—increased dependence of others lasting approximately 5 years
     c. Stage III—loss of independence lasting approximately 5 years
  3. ASSESSMENT
     a. Progressive mental changes leading to dementia
     b. Choreiform movements (rapid jerky movements) in the extremities, trunk, and facial muscles
     c. Hesitant or explosive speech
     d. Bowel and bladder incontinence
     e. Respiratory difficulties
  4. DIAGNOSTIC TESTS
     a. No specific diagnostic test
     b. Family history
     c. Physical examination
  5. NURSING INTERVENTIONS
     a. Genetic counseling is the priority.
     b. Supportive treatment
     c. Administer prescribed haloperidol (Haldol) to suppress movement.
     d. Provide for client safety.
     e. Increase caloric intake.
J. MYASTHENIA GRAVIS (MG)
  1. DESCRIPTION
     a. Chronic autoimmune neuromuscular disorder involving a fluctuating weakness of the skeletal muscles in which the antibodies attack the number and effectiveness of acetylcholine (Ach) at the neuromuscular junction
     b. Characterized by periods of remissions and exacerbations
     c. Occurs between the ages of 10 and 65 years, with the peak age in the second and third decades of life
     d. More common in females
  2. ASSESSMENT
     a. Muscle weakness that increases with activity during the day but improves with rest
     b. Ptosis
     c. Diplopia
     d. Dysphagia
     e. Respiratory difficulty
     f. Speech difficulty

  3. DIAGNOSTIC TESTS
     a. Complete history and physical
     b. Thyroid functioning
     c. Serum protein electrophoresis
     d. Acetylcholine receptor antibody (AchR) test
     e. CT scan
     f. Positive client response to cholinergic drugs
     g. Tensilon test
        1) Tensilon retards the breakdown of acetylcholine, which, in turn, increases the availability of Ach, providing short-term improvement to clients with MG.
        2) Administration of tensilon to a client in cholinergic crisis will result in no change or a worsening of weakness.
        3) Administration of tensilon to a client in myasthenic crisis results in temporary improvement of muscle weakness.
        4) Carries a slight risk of ventricular fibrillation and cardiac arrest
        5) Antidote for tensilon is atropine sulfate.
     h. Electromyography (EMG)
  4. NURSING INTERVENTIONS
     a. Assess the client for respiratory difficulty.
     b. Maintain emergency equipment at bedside.
     c. Suction the client as needed.
     d. Provide chest physiotherapy as appropriate.
     e. Assess the client for dysphagia.
     f. Provide small frequent high-calorie meals.
     g. Encourage the client to remain upright for 30 to 60 minutes after eating.
     h. Encourage the client to participate in activities early in the day or following administration of drugs.
     i. Encourage frequent rest periods.
     j. Encourage the client to work with the speech and language pathologist.
     k. Ask "yes" or "no" questions.
     l. Instruct the client to use artificial tears to prevent corneal abrasions.
     m. Encourage the client to wear eye protection at bedtime.
     n. Inform the client about services provided through the Myasthenia Gravis Foundation.
     o. Administer prescribed cholinesterase inhibitors such as pyridostigmine (Mestinon).
        1) Monitor the client for cholinergic crisis (nausea, vomiting, diarrhea, abdominal pain, hypotension,

pallor, blurred vision, pupillary miosis, and facial twitching) caused by an acute worsening of the muscle weakness as a result of overmedication of anticholinesterase drugs.

    2) Monitor the client for myasthenia crisis (tachycardia, tachypnea, hypertension, cyanosis, anoxia, bowel and bladder incontinence, decreased urinary output, and absent cough or swallowing reflex) caused by increase in muscle weakness as a result of undermedication of anticholinesterase drugs.

  p. Administer prescribed immunosuppressive drugs such as prednisone (Deltasone), azathioprine (Imuran), or cyclophosphamide (Cytoxan).

  q. Assist with plasmapheresis—process that removes antibodies from the plasma, generally six exchanges in 14 days to decrease clinical manifestations.

  5. SURGICAL MANAGEMENT
    a. Thymectomy is most effective when performed within 2 years after the onset of the disorder.

K. GUILLAIN-BARRÉ SYNDROME
  1. DESCRIPTION
    a. Also known as acute idiopathic polyneuritis or polyradiculoneuropathy
    b. An uncommon, acute, rapidly progressing, and potentially fatal polyneuritis
    c. The immune system destroys the myelin sheath.
    d. Exact etiology unknown but research suggests cell-mediated immunologic reaction
    e. Often associated with history of acute respiratory or gastrointestinal illness, surgery, trauma, or immunization 1–8 weeks before the onset of the disorder
    f. Women between the ages of 30 and 50 years are more susceptible.
    g. Respiratory failure is a serious complication.
  2. ASSESSMENT
    a. Symmetrical ascending weakness of the lower extremities
    b. Paresthesia
    c. Paralysis
    d. Decrease in muscle tone
    e. Decreased or absent deep tendon reflexes
    f. Hypertension
    g. Bradycardia

    h. Orthostatic hypotension
    i. Absent bowel and bladder function
    j. Facial weakness
    k. Dysphagia
    l. Extraocular eye movements
    m. Pain—generally worse at night
    n. Difficulty communicating
  3. DIAGNOSTIC TESTS
    a. Complete history and physical
    b. Cerebrospinal fluid analysis
    c. Electromyography (EMG)
    d. Nerve conduction studies
    e. Respiratory function studies
  4. NURSING INTERVENTIONS
    a. Promote optimal airway exchange.
    b. Monitor arterial blood gases.
    c. Maintain emergency intubation equipment at the bedside.
    d. Provide oxygen, suctioning, and chest physiotherapy as needed.
    e. Monitor the client for dysphagia and implement dysphagia interventions as appropriate.
    f. Administer prescribed analgesics.
    g. Implement communication interventions.
    h. Provide emotional support.
    i. Prevent complications of physical immobility.
    j. Assist with plasmapheresis as appropriate.
    k. Administer prescribed immunoglobins.

L. TETANUS
  1. DESCRIPTION
    a. Also known as lockjaw
    b. Severe form of polyneuritis and polyradiculitis affecting the cranial and spinal nerves
    c. Etiology is anaerobic bacillus, *Clostridium tetani*.
    d. Generally enters the body from a traumatic wound such as a gunshot, compound fracture, dental infection, animal bite, or dirty needles during illegal drug use
    e. Incubation period ranges from 7 to 21 days with an average of 7 days.
    f. Milder form of the disorder and better prognosis experienced with a longer incubation period
  2. ASSESSMENT
    a. Trismus (stiff jaw)
    b. Stiff neck
    c. Opisthotonos (severe arching of the back)
    d. Retraction of the head
    e. Pain
    f. Laryngeal or respiratory spasms
    g. Diaphoresis
    h. Hypertension
    i. Tachycardia

3. DIAGNOSTIC TESTS
   a. No specific diagnostic test
   b. History and physical examination
4. NURSING INTERVENTIONS
   a. Monitor CBC, serum electrolytes, arterial blood gases (ABGs), glucose, clotting factors, and albumin.
   b. Place the client in a dark, quiet room away from noise.
   c. Administer prescribed sedation.
   d. Avoid unnecessary touching of the client.
   e. When touching the client is necessary, use a firm touch.
   f. Maintain a warmer-than-normal temperature.
   g. Avoid covering the client with bed linens.
   h. Priority is to ensure tetanus prophylaxis by antitoxin.
   i. Wash the wound with warm soapy water to decrease incidence of tetanus.

M. BOTULISM
   1. DESCRIPTION
      a. Serious and potentially fatal paralytic disease resulting from contaminated food with *Clostridium botulinum*
      b. *C. botulinum* is found in the soil and has spores that are difficult to destroy.
      c. Most common cause is improper home canning
      d. Incubation period is 18 to 36 hours.
   2. ASSESSMENT
      a. Diplopia
      b. Dysphagia
      c. Dysarthria
      d. Weakness
      e. Paralytic ileus
      f. Constipation
      g. Abdominal pain
      h. Respiratory failure
   3. DIAGNOSTIC TESTS
      a. Complete history
      b. Stool culture for *C. botulinum*
      c. CBC
   4. NURSING INTERVENTIONS
      a. Administer prescribed botulism antitoxin (ABE) after the client is tested for hypersensitivity and immediately after the diagnosis is made.
      b. Lavage the stomach or administer laxatives or high-colonic enemas to prevent absorption.
      c. Monitor the client for respiratory paralysis.
      d. Implement tracheostomy and mechanical ventilation interventions as appropriate.
      e. Report the disorder to the Centers for Disease Control and Prevention (CDC).

   f. Primary prevention should be the goal.
   g. Instruct clients on proper canning of home foods, particularly those with a low-acid content.
      1) Boil foods for 10 minutes.
      2) Remove bad spots from all fruits and vegetables before canning.
      3) Ensure canning jar is airtight.
      4) Store canned foods in a cool location.
      5) Discard any canned container that swells or looks bad when opened.

N. STROKE
   1. DESCRIPTION
      a. Ischemia or hemorrhage to a section of the brain leads to cell death.
      b. Serious medical emergency necessitating immediate interventions to prevent permanent disability
      c. Causes include thrombus, embolus, hemorrhage, ruptured aneurysm, and arteriovenous malformation (AVM).
      d. Modifiable risk factors include obesity, smoking, alcohol, substance abuse, sedentary lifestyle, oral contraceptives, diabetes mellitus, hyperlipidemia, and hypertension.
      e. Nonmodifiable risk factors include being of African American, Hispanic, or Asian American descent; male; older adult; and family history.
   2. TYPES
      a. Ischemic
         1) Results from an occlusion of a cerebral artery by a thrombus or embolus
         2) Further divided into thrombotic (accounts for half of all strokes generally associated with atherosclerosis) and embolic (accounts for a third of all strokes and results from a emboli breaking off and traveling to the cerebral or carotid arteries with the middle cerebral artery being the most common)
      b. Transient ischemic attacks (TIAs) or reversible ischemic neurologic deficit (RIND) are warning signs that precede ischemic strokes.
         1) Referred to as "silent stroke"
         2) TIA is a temporary loss of neurological function often lasting less than 15 minutes but no more than 24 hours.
         3) RIND is a temporary loss of neurological function lasting more than 24 hours but less than 1 week.
         4) Indication of progressing cerebrovascular disease

c. Hemorrhagic
  1) Interruption of vessel wall integrity accounting for a bleed into the brain tissue as a result of hypertension, an aneurysm (weakening or ballooning of an artery), subarachnoid hemorrhage, intracranial hemorrhage, or arteriovenous malformation (embryonic abnormality resulting in a conglomeration of spaghetti-like tangles and thin-walled dilated vessels prone to rupture)

3. ASSESSMENT (SEE TABLE 7-6)
  a. Altered level of consciousness
  b. Hemiparesis (weakness) or neglect (unawareness of weakness on one side of the body)
  c. Denial of disorder
  d. Proprioceptive or spatial difficulty (decreased awareness of the body in space)
  e. Failure to make appropriate decisions
  f. Inappropriate judgment
  g. Poor memory
  h. Aphasia (impaired communication)
    1) Expressive aphasia: difficulty in the ability to write or speak
    2) Receptive aphasia: difficulty with verbalization of sounds and words
    3) Global aphasia: impairment of all verbal and understanding of communication
  i. Dysarthria
  j. Alexia (difficulty reading)
  k. Agraphia (difficulty writing)
  l. Hemiplegia (one-sided paralysis)
  m. Agnosia (inability to read, write, or understand material)
  n. Hemianopsia (blindness in one side of visual field)
  o. Ptosis
  p. Amaurosis fugax (temporary period of blindness in one eye)
  q. Dysphagia
  r. Emotional stability

4. DIAGNOSTIC TESTS
  a. Complete history and physical
  b. Complete blood count
  c. Thrombin and prothrombin times
  d. Cerebrospinal fluid analysis
  e. CT scan
  f. MRI scan
  g. Angiography
  h. ECG

5. NURSING INTERVENTIONS
  a. Primary prevention
    1) Instruct clients and families on reducing modifiable risk factors as the priority.
  b. Acute stroke management
    1) Maintain airway, breathing, and circulation.
    2) Assess the client's level of consciousness.
    3) Perform cranial nerve assessment.
    4) Administer prescribed antihypertensives.
    5) Monitor fluid and electrolytes.
    6) Elevate the head of the bed 30°.

Table 7-6 Characteristic Findings in Left- and Right-Hemisphere Stroke

	Left-Hemisphere Stroke	**Right-Hemisphere Stroke**
Communication	Aphasia Alexia Agraphia	Altered sense of humor
Vision	Unable to distinguish words and letters Difficulty reading Decreased in right visual field	Left visual field neglect Absence of depth perception
Hearing	Normal	Decreased
Memory	May be affected	Disoriented to person, place, and time Confusion
Behavior	Cautious and slow Worthlessness Depression Anxiety Frustration Guilt	Impulsive Euphoria Denial of health state Failure of appropriate judgment Confabulation Smiles constantly Poor insight into physical limitations

© Cengage Learning 2015

7) Monitor for increased intracranial pressure.

8) Administer prescribed analgesics.

9) Administer prescribed diuretic such as mannitol (Osmitrol) and furosemide (Lasix) to decrease cerebral edema.

10) Insert a Foley catheter.

11) Administer prescribed anticoagulants such as heparin and warfarin (Coumadin).

12) Administer prescribed platelet inhibitors such as ticlopidine (Ticlid), clopidogrel (Plavix), and dipyridamole (Persantine).

c. Intermediate stroke management

1) Maintain patent airway.

2) Assess for dysphagia.

3) Maintain upright position for 30 minutes after eating.

4) Thicken fluids as appropriate.

5) Maintain hemostasis, preventing fluid overload.

6) Monitor vital signs frequently.

7) Administer prescribed low-molecular-weight heparin (Lovenox) to prevent deep vein thrombosis.

8) Prevent complications of immobility.

9) Perform active range of motion.

10) Administer good skin care.

11) Initiate a bladder retraining program.

12) Increase fiber and fluids in the diet to prevent constipation.

13) Offer emotional support.

14) Approach the client from the unaffected side.

15) Implement aphasia interventions.

a) Avoid environmental distractions.

b) Talk directly to the client.

c) Avoid letting family members answer for the client.

d) Allow plenty of time for the client to answer.

e) Ask simple "yes" and "no" questions.

f) Avoid unnecessary communication when the client is fatigued.

g) Encourage gestures or pointing at items to facilitate communication.

h) Honestly tell the client if he is not understood.

i) Speak to the client in a normal tone and volume.

j) Attempt to communicate one idea at a time.

d. Rehabilitative nursing interventions

1) Encourage participation in care.

2) Encourage the client to participate in occupational therapy.

3) Encourage the client to participate in speech therapy.

4) Assess the client for rehabilitative aids.

5) Instruct the client on medications.

6) Encourage importance of scheduled follow-up with health care provider.

7) Instruct the client on the importance of frequent blood pressure checks.

O. SPINAL CORD INJURY

   1. DESCRIPTION

a. Injury to the spinal cord as a result of an incomplete (some sensory and motor function remains below the site of the injury) or complete (total loss of all sensory and motor function below the site of the injury) loss of sensory and motor function

b. Caused by a variety of traumas, including motor vehicle accidents, sports injuries, falls, and violence

c. The greatest at risk population is the 16- to 30-year-old age category

d. Complications include:

1) Spinal shock

a) Occurs immediately following the injury

b) Characterized by decreased reflexes, loss of sensation, and flaccid paralysis below the site of injury

c) Lasts days to months

2) Neurogenic shock

a) The loss of vasomotor tone results from the injury.

b) Characterized by hypotension, bradycardia, and dry warm extremities

c) Generally occurs with a cervical or high thoracic injury

3) Autonomic dysreflexia (hyperflexion)

a) A response to visceral stimulation after resolution of spinal shock

b) Occurs in injury that occurs at T6 or above

c) Most common cause is an overdistended bladder or bowel

d) May be life threatening

e) Characterized by severe hypertension (systolic greater than 300 mm Hg), bradycardia (30–40 beats per minute), diaphoresis and flushing above the site of injury, throbbing headache, blurred vision, nausea, nasal congestion, and piloerection (body hair erection)

    f) Nursing interventions include elevation of the head of the bed 45°, insertion of a Foley catheter or perform a digital rectal examination as prescribed, and monitor the blood pressure and pulse.

2. TYPES OF INJURY
    a. Incomplete
        1) Central cord syndrome: occurs most commonly in older clients in the cervical cord area with weakness present predominantly in the upper extremities
        2) Anterior cord syndrome: most commonly results from a flexion injury with motor paralysis and loss of pain and temperature below the site of injury
        3) Posterior cord syndrome: rare condition with a loss of proprioception
        4) Brown-Séquard syndrome
            a) Loss of motor function, position, vibratory sense, and ipsilateral (same side) and vasomotor paralysis

            b) Contralateral (opposite side) pain and temperature remains intact below the level of injury.
        5) Conus medullaris syndrome and cauda equina syndrome: lower limb flaccid paralysis, bowel and bladder dysfunction in the lumbar and sacral areas

3. ASSESSMENT OF CLINICAL MANIFESTATIONS RELATED TO THE LOCATION OF THE INJURY (SEE TABLE 7-7)
    a. Altered level of consciousness, sensory function, and motor function
    b. Bradycardia
    c. Hypotension
    d. Poikilothermism (the body has a decreased ability to sweat and shiver below the level of injury)
    e. Hypoventilation
    f. Urinary retention
    g. Paralytic ileus
    h. Neurogenic bowel
    i. Skin breakdown
    j. Loss of body weight
    k. Deep vein thrombosis
    l. Gastric distention

4. DIAGNOSTIC TESTS
    a. Complete history and physical
    b. Complete spinal x-rays
    c. CT scan
    d. MRI scan

Table 7-7 Spinal Cord Level of Injury

Level of Injury	Characteristics	Potential Capabilities
C1–C3	Most likely incompatible with life Heart and respirations severely compromised	Ventilator dependent May be able to operate a wheelchair with a chin or mouth stick
C4–C5	Heart and respirations compromised Minimal neck sensation with C4 Total neck; minimal shoulder, back, biceps, and elbow movement exists	May breathe without ventilator May be able to operate wheelchair with mobile hand supports with C5, may be able to assist with feeding with assistive devices
C6–C8	Vagus nerve compromised below the site of injury, resulting in a decreased respiratory capacity	Upper back abduction, elbow flexion, wrist extension, and minimal thumb movement in C6 Movement extends to elbow extension with finger extension with C7–C8 injury
T1–T6	Compromised respiratory capacity	Full movement of back, upper extremities, and hands exists. Able to fully operate a wheelchair and operate a car with hand controls May be able to stand with body support
T7–T12	Lower level of vagus nerve involvement	Full innervation of thoracic and intercostal muscles May be able to stand with leg braces and ambulate with crutches
L1–L2	Minimal function of legs and pelvis Unable to stand independently	Able to sit independently May be able to ambulate with long leg braces
L3–L4	Some impairment of leg, genitourinary (GU), and gastrointestinal (GI) organs	Able to flex quadriceps and hips Support of hamstring muscles with short leg braces allows ambulation. May be able to ambulate with the use of a cane

5. NURSING INTERVENTIONS
  a. Priority is to maintain airway, breathing, and circulation.
  b. Monitor the client for cardiac dysrhythmias, autonomic dysreflexia, spinal and neurogenic shock.
  c. Assess the client for urinary retention and constipation.
  d. Implement interventions to prevent skin breakdown.
  e. Prevent complications of immobility.
  f. Offer the client and family psychological support.
  g. Immobilize cervical injury with skeletal traction.
      1) Skull tongs (Gardner-Wells, Barton, or Crutchfield tongs)
         a) Traction is applied with weights attached at the end.
         b) Displacement of skull pins and infection around insertion on tongs may occur.
         c) May be used with Stryker frame or kinetic treatment table
      2) Halo fixator
         a) Four pins inserted into the skull with a metal halo ring connected to a chest vest when a stable spine is present to allow for greater mobility of the client
         b) Avoid turning the client by the halo device.
         c) Assess the proper size of the chest vest by ensuring that one finger can be inserted and moves freely under the vest.
  h. Immobilize thoracic, lumbar, and sacral injury (Taylor splint).
      1) Bed rest
      2) Immobilize the site of injury with plastic or fiberglass body cast.
      3) A brace or corset must be worn when out of bed.
  i. Administer prescribed corticosteroids such as methylprednisolone (Solu-Medrol) in the first 8 hours after the injury.
  j. Administer prescribed atropine for bradycardia.
  k. Administer prescribed inotropic and sympathomimetic drugs such as dopamine hydrochloride (Intropin) and isoproterenol (Isuprel) for severe hypotension.
  l. Administer a prescribed plasma expander such as dextran in the prevention or treatment of hypotension by increasing capillary blood flow in the spinal cord.
  m. Administer prescribed dantrolene (Dantrium) and baclofen (Lioresal) for muscle spasticity.
  n. Assist with emergency surgery such as decompensation laminectomy and spinal fusion and insertion of rods such as Harrington rods.
  o. Encourage the client to participate in self-care as much as possible.
  p. Inform the client of the benefit for a 1- to 3-month stay in a rehabilitation hospital to regain as much independence as possible.

P. SPINAL CORD TUMORS
  1. DESCRIPTION
    a. Tumor originating or spreading to the spinal cord
    b. Primary spinal cord tumors are rare.
    c. Most occur as metastasis from the breast, lungs, thyroid, breasts, prostate, colon, and uterus.
  2. CLASSIFICATIONS
    a. Intramedullary tumors are rare tumors originating within the spinal cord.
    b. Extramedullary tumors account for most spinal cord tumors originating outside the spinal cord.
  3. ASSESSMENT OF CLINICAL MANIFESTATIONS DEPEND ON THE SITE OF ORIGIN OF THE TUMOR.
    a. Pain
       1) Most common
       2) Often radicular pain (nerve root) aggravated by coughing, straining, sneezing, or lying down
    b. Weakness
    c. Clumsiness
    d. Spasticity
    e. Hyperactive reflexes
    f. Numbness
    g. Tingling
    h. Decrease in temperature sensation
    i. Ataxia
    j. Tightness around the trunk
    k. Bladder incontinence
    l. Bowel incontinence
    m. Loss of sexual function
    n. Paralysis
  4. DIAGNOSTIC TESTS
    a. Spinal x-rays
    b. CT scan
    c. MRI scan
    d. EMG
  5. NURSING INTERVENTIONS
    a. Assess sensory and motor function.
    b. Assess vital signs every 4 hours.
    c. Administer prescribed corticosteroids to decrease tumor-induced edema.
    d. Administer prescribed analgesics.
    e. Prevent complications of immobility.

f. Implement bowel and bladder retraining programs.

g. Provide small, frequent, high-caloric meals to maintain metabolic needs.

h. Offer the client and family emotional support.

6. SURGICAL MANAGEMENT

 a. Laminectomy

 b. Decompression, partial or total resection of the tumor

 c. Radiation

   1) Low-grade malignant tumors such as meningioma, astrocytoma, and ependymoma

   2) Monitor the client for radiation myelopathy, which develops over a period of 6–12 months.

 d. Chemotherapy

   1) Proven use is very limited in primary tumors but may be used in conjunction with metastatic cancers such as breast cancer.

Q. TRAUMATIC BRAIN INJURY

1. DESCRIPTION

 a. Any injury to the brain or scalp as a result of trauma

 b. Occurs when a mechanical force comes in contact with a portion of the brain (generally the frontal or temporal lobes) directly or indirectly

 c. Most common causes include vehicle accidents often compounded by drug or alcohol use, acts of violence, falls, and sports-related injury.

 d. Occurs most frequently in males between the ages of 10 and 39 years

 e. Based on the degree of injury, may have a poor prognosis, with death often occurring immediately after the injury as a result of the actual trauma, hemorrhage, or shock

2. TYPES

 a. Minor

   1) Laceration of the scalp

     a) Tearing of the vessels of the scalp that may cause profuse bleeding

     b) Has a good prognosis

     c) Small incidence of infection may occur

   2) Contusion

     a) Brief loss of consciousness following an injury to the cerebral cortex, diencephalon, or brainstem

     b) The client may also experience amnesia and headaches.

     c) Generally resolves spontaneously but may experience continued headache, lethargy, decreased memory and concentration, and behavioral and personality changes

     d) Instruct the client to notify the physician if clinical manifestations persist.

 b. Major

   1) Contusion

     a) Bruising of the brain

     b) Frequently associated with a fracture

     c) Coup (injury at the site of impact) and contrecoup (injury opposite the site of impact)

     d) A common complication is seizures.

   2) Fractures

     a) Generally include linear, depressed, or comminuted fractures

     b) Clinical manifestations include Battle's sign (postauricular ecchymosis), raccoon eyes (periorbital edema and ecchymosis), rhinorrhea (leakage of cerebrospinal fluid from the nose), and otorrhea (fluid from the ear).

   3) Epidural hematoma

     a) Arterial bleed generally the result of a temporal bone fracture between the dura and the inner surface of the skull

     b) Clinical manifestations include periods of talkativeness followed by periods of unconsciousness, often within minutes of the injury.

     c) May lead to coma

   4) Subdural hematoma

     a) Venous bleed generally the result of a laceration of brain tissue

     b) Slow bleeding into the space beneath the dura and above the arachnoid

     c) Classified as acute (occurring in 48 hours), subacute (occurring from 48 hours to 2 weeks), or chronic (occurring from 2 weeks to months) after the injury

     d) Clinical manifestations include increased intracranial pressure, decreased level of consciousness, and headache.

     e) Has a high mortality rate

   5) Intracranial hematoma

     a) Intracranial hemorrhage often the result of a fracture or torsion of the brainstem

6) Herniation

    a) Shift of brain tissue and downward herniation of some portion of the brain tissue, generally the temporal lobe or the brainstem

    b) Clinical manifestations include ptosis, decreased level of consciousness, nonreactive pupils, and Cheyne-Stokes respirations.

    c) May be life threatening

3. ASSESSMENT

  a. Amnesia

  b. Increased intracranial pressure

  c. Systemic hypotension

  d. Hypoxia

  e. Hypercapnia

  f. Cushing reflex (severe hypertension and wide pulse pressure is a late sign)

  g. Tachycardia

  h. Hypovolemic shock

  i. Cardiac dysrhythmias

  j. Lethargy

  k. Behavioral changes

  l. Nonreactive and pinpoint pupils

  m. Ataxia

  n. Weakness

  o. Decreased muscle tone

  p. Headache

  q. Nausea and vomiting

  r. Papilledema

  s. Stiff neck

  t. Difficulty swallowing and speaking

4. DIAGNOSTIC TESTS

  a. CT scan

  b. MRI scan

  c. Arteriogram

  d. Cerebral blood flow studies

  e. Cervical spine x-ray

5. NURSING INTERVENTIONS

  a. Assess vital signs every 1 to 2 hours.

  b. Avoid extreme flexion or extension of the neck.

  c. Log roll the client.

  d. Elevate the head of the bed to 30 degrees.

  e. Assess using the Glascow Coma Scale.

  f. Administer lubricating eyedrops or tape the eyes shut to prevent corneal abrasions.

  g. Provide warm or cold compresses to the eyes to decrease periorbital ecchymosis.

  h. Place an eye patch over the eye for clinical manifestations of diplopia.

  i. Monitor the client for rhinorrhea or otorrhea.

  j. Avoid nasogastric or nasotracheal suctioning.

  k. Administer good skin care.

  l. Prevent complications of immobility.

  m. Implement bowel and bladder interventions if appropriate.

  n. Monitor the client for seizures.

  o. Instruct the client's family to notify the physician if increased drowsiness, nausea, vomiting, seizures, visual or sensory problems, behavior changes, bradycardia, or stiff neck occur because they indicate complications and generally occur within 3 days of discharge.

  p. Instruct the client to avoid alcohol, operating heavy machinery, playing contact sports, or taking warm baths.

  q. Monitor the client for increases in intracranial pressure.

  r. Instruct the client and family on methods to prevent head injury.

6. SURGICAL MANAGEMENT

  a. Craniotomy

    1) May be performed to decrease intracranial pressure to remove ischemic tissue

PRACTICE QUESTIONS

1. Which of the following would the nurse assess in a client who has a degeneration of the neurons that synthesize and release dopamine?

1. Bradycardia and hypotension
2. Insomnia and mania
3. Hand tremors and muscle rigidity
4. Pupil dilation and dysuria

2. As the nurse assesses a client undergoing diagnostic testing for myasthenia gravis, which of the following findings would be most supportive of the diagnosis of myasthenia gravis?

1. A history of a spinal cord injury
2. A history of a viral infection
3. A history of muscle weakness improved with rest
4. A history of an autoimmune disease

3. Which of the following clinical manifestations would the nurse expect to find in a client with meningitis?

   Select all that apply:
   [ ] 1. Headache
   [ ] 2. Dysphagia
   [ ] 3. Nuchal rigidity
   [ ] 4. Fever
   [ ] 5. Dysarthria
   [ ] 6. Vomiting

4. The nurse correctly explains to a client's family that the reason a stroke on the right side of the brain results in paralysis on the left side of the body is because the pyramidal pathways cross over at the end of which of the following?
   1. Medulla
   2. Thalamus
   3. Pons
   4. Midbrain

5. The nurse assists a client who had a stroke to make which of the following menu choices?

   Select all that apply:
   [ ] 1. Chicken sandwich
   [ ] 2. Taco salad
   [ ] 3. Sliced tomato
   [ ] 4. Angel food cake
   [ ] 5. Potato chips
   [ ] 6. Bacon, lettuce, and tomato sandwich

6. The nurse is teaching a class on the prevention of cerebrovascular accidents. Which of the following risk factors should the nurse identify as the most important factor contributing to a stroke?
   1. Sedentary lifestyle
   2. Hypertension
   3. Smoking
   4. Obesity

7. The nurse is caring for a client who has aphasia following a cerebrovascular accident. Which of the following nursing interventions should the nurse include in the plan of care?
   1. Assume that the client cannot understand what is said
   2. Establish long-term goals with the client
   3. Attempt repetition with phrases when speaking to the client
   4. Speak to the client in a louder-than-usual voice

8. The nurse evaluates a client to have an acute subdural hemotoma because it occurred within what time frame?

   _____

9. During an initial interview with a client who has had an anterior cord syndrome spinal cord injury, the nurse would expect to find which of the following assessment findings?

   Select all that apply:
   [ ] 1. Motor weakness that is greater in the upper extremities than in the lower ones
   [ ] 2. Impairment in the sensations of touch, position, vibration, and motion
   [ ] 3. Hypesthesia
   [ ] 4. Flaccid bowel and bladder function
   [ ] 5. Decreased pain
   [ ] 6. Loss of temperature below the level of the injury

10. Which of the following actions is a priority for the nurse to perform first in a client with a spinal cord injury who complains of a headache?
    1. Administer a beta-adrenergic blocker
    2. Take the blood pressure
    3. Assess the pupillary reaction
    4. Insert a Foley catheter

11. The nurse is caring for a client suspected of having botulism. The nurse should assess the client for which of the following?

    Select all that apply:
    [ ] 1. Headache
    [ ] 2. Muscle weakness
    [ ] 3. Drowsiness
    [ ] 4. Stiff jaw and neck
    [ ] 5. Respiratory and eye problems
    [ ] 6. Opisthotonos

12. Because a client with a spinal cord injury is at risk for pneumonia, atelectasis, and respiratory arrest, the nurse should plan to
    1. position the client in a prone position.
    2. monitor the hemoglobin and hematocrit levels.
    3. administer propoxyphene (Darvon) 65 mg p.o. every 4 hours.
    4. have the client count to 10 out loud without taking a breath.

13. The nurse is caring for a client with Parkinson's disease. Which of the following nursing interventions should the nurse include in the plan of care?
    1. Elevate the client's legs
    2. Offer the client the bedpan every 2 hours
    3. Encourage the client to sit in a reclining, soft chair without arms
    4. Instruct the client to eat a high-calcium diet

14. The physician tells a client with multiple sclerosis that it is a chronic progressive neurologic condition. The client asks the nurse, "Will I experience pain?" The most appropriate response by the nurse is which of the following?
    1. "Tell me about your fears regarding pain."
    2. "Analgesics will be ordered to control the pain."

3. "Pain is not a characteristic symptom of this disease process."
4. "Let's make a list of the things you need to ask your physician."

15. The nurse is caring for a client with amyotrophic lateral sclerosis. Which of the following nursing diagnoses should have priority?
   1. Impaired skin integrity related to disuse
   2. Anticipatory grieving related to inevitable death
   3. Acute pain related to inflammation
   4. Self-care deficit related to paralysis

16. The nurse is caring for a client with Guillain-Barré syndrome. Which of the following would indicate the client's condition is deteriorating?
   1. Weakness and paresthesia
   2. Pain and muscle aches
   3. Urinary retention
   4. Respiratory infection

17. A client's family asks the nurse what meningitis is. The nurse's response should be based on an understanding that meningitis is a
   1. fatal form of polyneuritis.
   2. cerebrospinal infection.
   3. collection of pus in the brain tissue.
   4. rare progressive loss of motor neurons.

18. The nurse is admitting a client diagnosed to have a cerebrovascular accident involving left-brain damage. The nurse evaluates which of the following to be clinical manifestations of a cerebrovascular accident involving left-brain damage?

   Select all that apply:
   [ ] 1. Paralyzed right side
   [ ] 2. Aphasia
   [ ] 3. Left-sided neglect
   [ ] 4. Paralyzed left side
   [ ] 5. Depression
   [ ] 6. Denial of deficits

19. Which of the following is a priority when suctioning a client with increased intracranial pressure?
   1. Limit the suction passes to 30 seconds
   2. Suction the client as needed
   3. Suction the client at least every hour
   4. Schedule the suctioning with other nursing tasks

20. The nurse is caring for a client with an arterioventricular malformation who is scheduled for surgery. Which of the following should be the priority in the care provided to this client?
   1. Offer psychologic support
   2. Encourage a high-protein and high-calorie diet

3. Avoid activities that will increase the blood pressure
4. Administer intravenous fluids to prevent dehydration

21. The nurse is caring for a client in the first 48 hours following a spinal cord trauma. Which of the following nursing interventions should the nurse include in the plan of care?
   1. Encourage a high-protein and high-roughage diet
   2. Insert a nasogastric tube
   3. Position the client in a prone position
   4. Administer a daily tap-water enema

22. Immediately following a spinal cord injury, a client's family asks the nurse, "Is the damage the client presents with in the emergency room as bad as it seems?" The most appropriate response by the nurse is which of the following?
   1. "Because of edema around the spinal cord, it is difficult to evaluate the extent of the injury for up to 1 week."
   2. "Unfortunately, yes, the injury is exactly as it appears."
   3. "Probably not, because the client will probably regain a lot of function."
   4. "The injury is so severe that death is imminent within days."

23. The nurse is admitting a client suspected of Parkinson's disease. Which of the following does the nurse observe that supports the diagnosis?

   Select all that apply:
   [ ] 1. Chorea movements
   [ ] 2. Tremor noticeable at rest
   [ ] 3. Paresthesia
   [ ] 4. Rigidity
   [ ] 5. Bradykinesia
   [ ] 6. Muscle wasting

24. The nurse should instruct a client with myasthenia gravis to remain upright for how long after eating?

   _____

25. The nurse is preparing a client with myasthenia gravis for a plasmapheresis. Which of the following laboratory tests must be obtained and assessed prior to this procedure?

   Select all that apply:
   [ ] 1. Creatine phosphokinase (CPK)
   [ ] 2. Complete blood count (CBC)
   [ ] 3. Blood urea nitrogen (BUN)
   [ ] 4. Platelets
   [ ] 5. Clotting studies
   [ ] 6. Urine for protein

26. The nurse is assessing a client with myasthenia gravis at 1600. Which of the following assessment findings should the nurse anticipate the client to report?
    1. Double vision and muffled, nasal-quality speech
    2. Tremors of the hands when attempting to lift objects
    3. Improvement of muscle strength with mild exercise
    4. Numbness and tingling of the extremities

27. The nurse's plan of care for a client with Guillain-Barré syndrome is based on an understanding of which of the following disease processes?
    1. Decreased secretion of acetylcholine and an increase of cholinesterase at the myoneural junction
    2. Segmental demyelination of the ventral and dorsal nerve roots in the spinal cord and medulla
    3. Chronic inflammation, demyelination, and scarring of the CNS
    4. Decreased secretion of the neurotransmitter dopamine with an anticholinergic effect

28. Which of the following should the nurse assess to provide the most accurate information regarding a client suspected of having a C4 injury?
    1. Ask the client to shrug the shoulders while applying downward pressure
    2. Ask the client to straighten the flexed arms while applying resistance
    3. Ask the client to grasp an object and make a fist
    4. Ask the client to lift the arms while applying resistance

29. A client has difficulty communicating because of expressive aphasia following a cerebrovascular accident. When the nurse asks how the client is feeling, the spouse answers for the client. The nurse should
    1. ask how the spouse knows how the client is feeling.
    2. acknowledge the spouse but look at the client for a response.
    3. instruct the spouse to let the client answer.
    4. return later to speak to the client after the spouse has gone home.

30. Which statement made by the spouse of a client with multiple sclerosis indicates to the nurse an understanding of the home-care needs for this client?
    1. "I'm going to feed my spouse from now on."
    2. "I've learned how to take care of a Foley catheter."
    3. "I will put up handrails in the shower."
    4. "I will make my spouse stay in bed as much as possible."

31. The nurse should consider which of the following when planning the care of a client with Lou Gehrig disease, or amyotrophic lateral sclerosis (ALS)?
    1. Death frequently occurs from decreased respiratory function
    2. Successful treatment consists of IV methylprednisolone (Solu-Medrol)
    3. Life expectancy after diagnosis is 25 years
    4. Higher incidence in females between the ages of 15 and 50

32. The nurse is caring for a client with a spinal cord trauma following a motorcycle accident. It is a priority for the nurse to monitor for and immediately report which of the following findings?

    Select all that apply:
    [ ] 1. Hypotension
    [ ] 2. Bradycardia
    [ ] 3. Pain
    [ ] 4. Inflammation at the site of the injury
    [ ] 5. Ecchymosis
    [ ] 6. Warm, dry extremities

33. Passive range of motion exercises have been prescribed for a recent cerebral vascular (CVA) client with left hemiplegia. Which of the following would be most important for the nurse to include in the exercise treatment plan?
    1. Begin the exercises on the first day of hospitalization during the acute phase
    2. Perform each movement slowly and smoothly, repeating five times during the exercise period
    3. Position each joint higher than the joint proximal to it
    4. Schedule the exercises once a shift along with another nursing activity

34. A new nurse caring for a client with glioblastoma asks a nurse the prognosis for this client. Based on an understanding of a glioblastoma, the nurse informs the new nurse that the prognosis is
    1. successful with chemotherapy.
    2. dependent on the client's overall condition.
    3. curable with surgery.
    4. extremely grave.

35. The nurse should implement which of the following methods of assisting during a seizure?

    Select all that apply:
    [ ] 1. Turn the client on the side
    [ ] 2. Restrain the client
    [ ] 3. Turn on the lights
    [ ] 4. Observe the seizure activity
    [ ] 5. Open the airway with a padded tongue blade
    [ ] 6. Provide for client privacy

36. The nurse should inform a client with a seizure disorder to avoid which of the following?

Select all that apply:
[ ] 1. Excess noise
[ ] 2. Stress
[ ] 3. Infections
[ ] 4. A high chocolate intake
[ ] 5. Alcohol
[ ] 6. Fatigue

37. In planning the post-op care after cranial surgery, the nurse should place the client in which of the following positions?
1. Flat bed rest
2. Side-lying position
3. Elevate the head of bed 30°
4. Trendelenburg

38. The nurse is preparing a plan of care for a client post-op following a craniotomy. The nurse formulates which of the following goals as the priority goal when caring for this client?
1. Prevent increased intracranial pressure
2. Maintain a safe environment
3. Prevent infection
4. Maintain skin integrity

39. The nurse reviews the report of a client's cerebrospinal fluid analysis. Which of the following findings should the nurse report?
1. Glucose 60 mg/dl
2. Total protein 30 mg/dl
3. Clear, colorless appearance
4. White blood cells 100/ml

40. When assessing cranial nerve X, the nurse will need which of the following?
1. A tongue blade
2. A tuning fork
3. An ophthalmoscope
4. Cotton and a safety pin

41. A student nurse asks the nurse what cranial nerve is responsible for smell. The most appropriate response by the nurse is what cranial nerve?

42. A mother asks the nurse if the seizures her child is experiencing will last a lifetime. The appropriate response by the nurse would be which of the following?
1. "The tonic-clonic seizures your child is experiencing will last a lifetime but can be successfully controlled with an antiepileptic drug."
2. "Your child is experiencing a type of seizure called typical absence seizure and it may or may not go away. Each child is different."
3. "The type of seizure your child has is called akinetic seizure and it may or may not go away. Each child is different."
4. "Psychomotor seizures are hard to predict and you should ask your doctor."

43. The nurse is caring for a client with increased intracranial pressure. Which of the following assessment findings should the nurse immediately report?
1. Nausea
2. Fever
3. Headache
4. Absence of papillary response

44. The nurse determines there are how many spinal nerves in the sacral area?

45. The registered nurse is delegating nursing tasks for the day. Which of the following tasks may be appropriately delegated to unlicensed assistive personnel?
1. Instruct a client with headaches to keep a diary of the characteristics of the headaches
2. Plan sample menu selections for a client who had a stroke
3. Monitor the temperature in a client who had a spinal cord injury
4. Assess cranial nerve VII in a client suspected of having trigeminal neuralgia

ANSWERS AND RATIONALES

1. 3. Dopamine is a neurotransmitter that inhibits the excitatory functions of acetylcholine-producing neurons. It is through dopamine's ability to inhibit and balance the excitatory functions that coordinated, refined movement can occur. Without the inhibiting effects of dopamine, the client experiences difficulty initiating voluntary movement and muscle

rigidity. A "pill-rolling" tremor is present. Bradycardia, hypotension, insomnia, mania, pupil dilation, and dysuria are not signs of the lack of dopamine.

2. 4. Myasthenia gravis is an autoimmune disease of the neuromuscular junction that is manifested by a fluctuating skeletal muscle weakness. Antibodies attack the acetylcholine at the

neuromuscular junction, preventing muscle contraction. There is no correlation to a spinal cord injury. Although there is no known cause of multiple sclerosis, there is research indicating a correlation to a viral infection. Muscle strength is generally increased after rest.

3. 1. 3. 4. 6.   Headache, nuchal rigidity or resistance to flexion of the neck, fever, nausea, and vomiting are the classic clinical manifestations of meningitis.

4. 1.   The crossover of the pyramidal pathways at the end of the medulla results in the opposite side of the body being affected when the cerebrovascular accident (CVA) occurs in the other side. For example, when the CVA is on the right side, the paralysis is on the left side of the body. The pons and midbrain, like the medulla, are parts of the midbrain. The thalamus is located in the cerebrum and lies above the brainstem.

5. 1. 3. 4.   A high-fat diet is a modifiable risk factor in clients at risk for a cerebrovascular accident. Chicken sandwich, sliced tomato, and angel-food cake is the menu with the lowest fat content. Bacon, potato chips, and taco salad are not only high in fat but also high in sodium, which would predispose a client to hypertension and risk for another stroke.

6. 2.   A sedentary lifestyle predisposes a client to obesity and cardiovascular disease, which increases the risk of a cerebrovascular accident. Smoking and obesity are modifiable risk factors that do increase the risk of a stroke, but hypertension is supported by research to put the client at the greatest risk for a stroke. Successful treatment of hypertension is the best prevention of a CVA.

7. 3.   When aphasia occurs with a cerebrovascular accident, repetition proves beneficial in enhancing the client's understanding of what is said. An assumption should never be made that the client understood what was said. The client may be experiencing expressive, receptive, or global aphasia. The client cannot focus to plan a long-term goal. Speaking louder to the client serves no purpose because the client is not hard of hearing. The client benefits most from presenting only one idea at a time, simple "yes" and "no" questions, repetition, and never rushing the client.

8.   48 hours

9. 3. 5. 6.   Motor weakness that is greater in the upper extremities than the lower ones is present in a central cord syndrome. Impairment in the sense of touch, position, vibration, and motion is present in Brown-Sequard's syndrome, in which a disruption in one half of the spinal cord has occurred, either from a lesion or a transection. Flaccid bowel and

bladder function and paralysis of the lower extremities represent damage to the lowest portion of the spinal cord. Hypesthesia, decreased pain, and loss of temperature below the level of injury represent the anterior cord syndrome because the posterior cord is still intact, and therefore the sensations of touch, vibration, motion, and position are unaffected.

10. 2.   The priority action in a client who has sustained a spinal cord injury and is complaining of a severe headache is to take the blood pressure. A severe headache and a systolic blood pressure of 300 mm Hg are suggestive of autonomic dysreflexia or hyperreflexia, which are life threatening if left untreated.

11. 2. 5.   General gastrointestinal symptoms (nausea, vomiting, and abdominal pain) occur 6 to 48 hours after ingestion of food suspected to be contaminated. However, involvement of the nervous system progresses very quickly over 2 to 4 days, with symptoms of eye problems, muscle weakness, and respiratory problems that can be life threatening. Headache, fever, nausea, and vomiting occur with meningitis. Drowsiness, confusion, and seizures are all findings that may occur with a head injury or brain abscess. Opisthotonos, stiff jaw, and stiff neck are clinical manifestations that are classic in tetanus.

12. 4.   A prone position is not desirable for a client who has sustained a spinal cord injury because it would further decrease the vital capacity and could even predispose the client to a cardiac arrest. Monitoring the hemoglobin and hematocrit levels would be important interventions when there is blood loss from other injuries. Administering Darvon is not an appropriate intervention for a client with a spinal cord injury.

13. 1.   Elevating the legs is an important intervention in the client with Parkinson's disease because ankle edema occurs. Offering the bedpan every 2 hours is an intervention for multiple sclerosis. Reclining in a soft chair without arms is incorrect because a client with Parkinson's disease needs an upright, firm chair with arms to facilitate getting out of the chair because of the decrease in mobility. A high-calcium diet is incorrect because a diet with foods that are easily chewed and high in roughage is recommended for the difficulties with chewing and also to prevent constipation.

14. 3.   The clinical manifestations of multiple sclerosis include weakness or paralysis of the extremities, numbness or tingling, visual disturbances, bowel or bladder disturbances, and gait and balance difficulties. Pain is not a clinical manifestation of multiple sclerosis. By providing this information, the nurse educates and reassures the client. Telling the client to make a list for the physician shifts responsibility from the nurse to the physician. Reflecting the client's fears about pain is not the most appropriate response. Providing accurate information is most appropriate.

15. 2.   The priority nursing diagnosis for a client with amyotrophic lateral sclerosis (ALS) is anticipatory grieving related to inevitable death. ALS is a fatal neurological disease in which there is a loss of motor neurons. Death generally results when the respiratory muscles are affected and respiratory function is compromised.

16. 4.   Guillain-Barré syndrome is a fatal disease that is characterized by an ascending paralysis affecting the peripheral nervous system. Respiratory infection and failure are the most common complications.

17. 2.   Meningitis is a cerebrospinal infection. Purulent exudate forms in bacterial meningitis, but does not form in viral meningitis. Meningitis is not associated with polyneuritis or a progressive loss of motor neurons.

18. 1. 2. 5.   Clients who have left-sided brain damage are aware of their deficits and often experience anxiety or depression. Aphasia and paralysis on the right side are also common clinical manifestations of left-side brain damage. Paralysis or neglect of the left side and a denial of any deficits are common in right-sided brain damage.

19. 1.   Suctioning can cause an increase in intracranial pressure and should be used cautiously. The client must be closely assessed during suctioning and suction passes should be limited to 30 seconds. The client should be allowed to rest for several minutes between suction passes, manually hyperventilated, and preoxygenated with 100% oxygen prior to suctioning.

20. 3.   Arterioventricular malformation is a congenital malformation that results in a tangled web of dilated and thin-walled vessels. The abnormality in the capillary network of these vessels causes the development of an impaired communication between the arterial and venous systems. Any increase in the pressure within the vessels may cause them to rupture. As a result, all activities should be avoided that increase the blood pressure.

21. 2.   A nasogastric tube connected to low intermittent suction may be inserted following a spinal cord trauma to relieve gastric distention. This is particularly necessary if the injury is above the T5 level. Hypomotility results with the possibility of a paralytic ileus or gastric distention.

22. 1.   It is difficult to ascertain the client's permanent level of disability until after the resolution of edema surrounding the spinal cord. It is edema that can cause compression of the spinal cord and increase ischemic damage to the spinal cord. The spinal cord damage caused by edema is typically evident within a week. Telling the family not to worry about the extent of the injury, as the injury is lethal, may be inaccurate and robs the family of any hope.

23. 2. 4. 5.   Parkinson's disease is a neurological disorder with three classic features: tremor, rigidity, and bradykinesia.

24.   30 minutes

25. 2. 4. 5.   Plasmapheresis is a procedure that removes anti-Ach receptor antibodies by way of a machine called a cell separator. This machine separates the plasma from the blood. Plasmapheresis may be useful in clients in crisis being prepared for surgery or when corticosteroids are to be avoided.

26. 1.   Myasthenia gravis is an autoimmune disease resulting in alterations of the skeletal muscles. The clinical manifestations are more prominent late in the day because the skeletal muscles are weakest then and strongest early in the day. The eye, breathing, speaking, chewing, and swallowing muscles are predominantly involved.

27. 2.   Guillain-Barré syndrome, often referred to as postinfectious polyneuropathy, is a segmental demyelination of the ventral and dorsal nerve roots in the spinal cord and medulla. A decrease in acetylcholine at the neuromuscular junction is myasthenia gravis. Parkinson's disease is a decrease in the secretion of dopamine. A chronic inflammation, demyelination, and scarring of the CNS is characteristic of multiple sclerosis.

28. 1.   Asking a client to shrug the shoulders while applying resistance will provide the most accurate information in a client suspected of having a C4 injury. Asking a client to straighten the flexed arms while applying resistance would assess for a C7 injury. Asking the client to grasp an object and make a fist would assess for a C8 injury. Asking the client to lift the arms while applying resistance would assess for a C5 injury.

29. 3.   Expressive aphasia is a difficulty in both writing and speech. It is important to allow a client with expressive aphasia sufficient time to speak. No one should speak for the client because this serves only to increase the client's frustration.

30. 3.   A goal in the nursing management of multiple sclerosis is to promote the client's independence while ensuring the client's comfort and safety. Assistive devices such as handrails in the shower encourage independence and safety. It is also essential to promote mobility and prevent complications.

31. 1. Death from amyotrophic lateral sclerosis (ALS), also known as Lou Gehrig disease, typically comes from a respiratory infection related to decreased respiratory function. There is no cure for ALS. Riluzole (Rilutek) may be given to retard the progression of the disease. Clients typically live for only 2 to 6 years after learning of their diagnosis. The disease affects twice as many men as women.

32. 1. 2. 6. Hypotension, bradycardia, and warm, dry extremities indicate the presence of neurogenic shock and occur as the result of a loss of vasomotor tone. Neurogenic shock most commonly occurs with a cervical or high-thoracic injury. Pain would indicate the preservation of sensation. Ecchymosis and inflammation at the site of the injury would be expected with the injury.

33. 1. Although positioning each joint of a CVA client higher than the joint proximal to it is worthy, the nursing goal is to maintain musculoskeletal function. This is accomplished by initiating passive range-of-motion exercises during the acute phase and on the first day of hospitalization. Muscle atrophy secondary to lack of innervation and to inactivity can develop in as little as a month.

34. 4. A glioblastoma is a highly malignant brain tumor with a very poor prognosis.

35. 1. 4. 6. When a client is having a seizure, it is a priority for the nurse to place the client on the side, observe all seizure activity, and protect the client from harm. The purpose of placing the client on the side is to prevent aspiration. Nothing should be given by mouth, nor should the client be restrained.

36. 2. 5. 6. It is important for the nurse to instruct a client who has had a seizure to avoid stress, fatigue, and alcohol. The nurse should instruct the client on stress control techniques and methods to promote sleep. A well-balanced diet is also recommended.

37. 3. Following a craniotomy, the best position to place the client in is to have the head of the bed elevated 30° to prevent increased intracranial pressure.

38. 1. The primary goal following a craniotomy is to prevent increased intracranial pressure. Fluid and electrolytes and body position are crucial to prevent an increased intracranial pressure. An elevated head position should be maintained and extreme neck flexion avoided. Maintaining a head-elevated position decreases sagittal sinus pressure, promotes venous drainage, and decreases vascular congestion.

39. 4. Normal cerebrospinal fluid should have a clear and colorless appearance. Protein should be 15 to 45 mg/dl. Protein levels higher than this may indicate a tumor or an infection. Normal glucose ranges between 45 to 75 mg/ml. Glucose levels higher than 75 mg/ml indicate the presence of an infection, leukemia, or cancer. The white blood cells range is 0.8/ml. Levels higher than this indicate an infection or a tumor.

40. 1. Cranial nerve (CN) X is the vagus nerve and is responsible for the gag reflex. Assessment of the gag reflex is done with a tongue blade inserted in the mouth and gently touched to the posterior pharynx or soft palate. It is essential to assess CN X in a client suspected of a decreased level of consciousness or after certain procedures where an anesthetic or an anesthetic spray was used.

41. I

42. 2. Typical absence (petit mal) seizures occur in children but rarely extend into adolescence. These seizures may completely cease or develop into another type of seizure.

43. 4. Absence of papillary response is an ominous sign and may indicate impending herniation and should be reported immediately to the physician. Fever is a common complication following an injury to the brain and should also be reported, but absence of papillary response is a priority. Headache and nausea are all clinical manifestations a client may experience but do not indicate an emergency.

44. 5

45. 3. Unlicensed assistive personnel cannot instruct or plan nursing activities. Performing assessment techniques is also not a function of unlicensed assistive personnel.

REFERENCES

Daniels, R. (2010). *Delmar's manual of laboratory and diagnostic tests* (2nd ed.). Clifton Park, NY: Delmar Cengage Learning.

Daniels, R., & Nicoll, L. (2012). *Contemporary medical-surgical nursing.* Clifton Park, NY: Delmar Cengage Learning.

Estes, M. (2010). *Health assessment and physical examination* (4th ed.). Clifton Park, NY: Delmar Cengage Learning.

Spratto, G. R., & Woods, A. L. (2012). *PDR nurse's drug handbook 2012.* Clifton Park, NY: Delmar Cengage Learning.

CHAPTER 8

INTEGUMENTARY DISORDERS

I. ANATOMY AND PHYSIOLOGY
A. FUNCTIONS OF THE SKIN
1. **PROTECTION AGAINST INVASION BY ORGANISMS**
   a. Intact epidermis is a mechanical barrier against mechanical, thermal, chemical, and radiant trauma.
   b. Oily and slightly acidic secretions from sebaceous glands limit growth of organisms.
   c. Thickness of epidermal layer on the palms and soles cushions against damage.
2. **REGULATION OF BODY TEMPERATURE**
   a. Skin adjusts heat loss to balance metabolic heat production.
   b. Heat loss depends on blood flow to the skin.
   c. Blood flow to the skin varies with changes in the body's core temperature and environmental temperature.
   d. Blood vessels dilate during warm temperatures and constrict during cold.
   e. With excessive heat, sweat is produced by eccrine glands and cooling is enhanced by evaporation from the skin.
3. **PREVENTION OF EXCESSIVE LOSS OF WATER AND ELECTROLYTES**
   a. Skin is a barrier to prevent loss of water and electrolytes.
   b. Prevents subcutaneous tissue from drying out
   c. Damage to the skin, for example, burns, causes extreme loss of both water and electrolytes.
4. **MANUFACTURES VITAMIN D**
   a. In presence of sunlight or ultraviolet radiation, vitamin D is synthesized.
   b. Vitamin D is critical in the absorption of calcium and phosphate in the diet.
5. **DETECTION OF SENSATION (TOUCH, PRESSURE, VIBRATION, PAIN)**
   a. Specialized receptors detect touch (Meissner's corpuscles), pressure

(Merkel cells and Rufini endings), vibration (Pacinian corpuscles), and hair movement (hair follicle endings).
   b. Temperature is sensed by thermoreceptors in the epidermis.
   c. Pain is detected by free nerve endings throughout the epidermis, dermis, and hypodermis.
   d. Density of receptors determines sensitivity of the skin. The fingers and face are very sensitive because they have the highest density of touch receptors.
6. **PROVISION OF EXTERNAL APPEARANCE**
   a. Integral to self-image and self-esteem
   b. Skin diseases were once perceived as punishment for being spiritually and physically "unclean."
7. **PROCESSING OF ANTIGENIC SUBSTANCES**
   a. Langerhans cells in the epidermis and dermis are important in cell-mediated immune response.
   b. Antigens entering immunologically competent skin induce an immune response of Langerhans and T cells.
   c. Immune response may be involved in inflammatory skin diseases.
B. MAIN STRUCTURES (SEE FIGURE 8-1)
1. **THREE LAYERS**
   a. Epidermis
   b. Dermis
   c. Hypodermis (subcutaneous)
2. **EPIDERMAL APPENDAGES**
   a. Eccrine (sweat) glands
   b. Apocrine glands
   c. Sebaceous (oil) glands
   d. Hair follicles
   e. Nails
C. EPIDERMIS
1. **THIN, OUTER SKIN LAYER MADE OF KERATINOCYTES**

Figure 8-1 Cross section of the skin

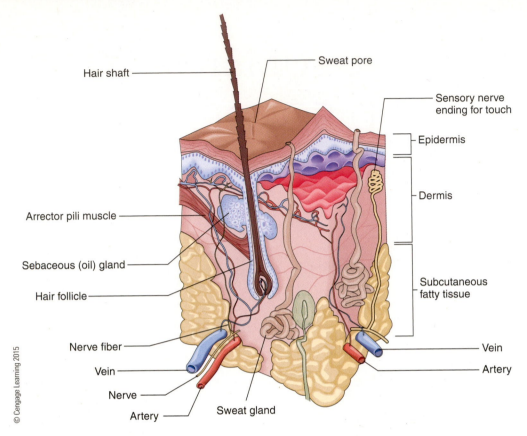

Hair shaft

Sweat pore

Sensory nerve ending for touch

Epidermis

Dermis

Arrector pili muscle

Subcutaneous fatty tissue

Sebaceous (oil) gland

Hair follicle

Nerve fiber

Vein

Vein

Artery

Nerve

Artery

Sweat gland

© Cengage Learning 2015

2. THICKNESS RANGES FROM 0.04–1.6 MM
3. THINNEST ON EYELIDS; THICKEST ON THE PALMS OF THE HANDS AND SOLES OF THE FEET
4. CONSTANTLY REGENERATES
5. PROVIDES SKIN COLOR FROM CAROTENOIDS (YELLOW), MELANIN (BROWN), OXYGENATED HEMOGLOBIN IN ARTERIOLES AND CAPILLARIES (RED), REDUCED HEMOGLOBIN IN VENULES (BLUE)

D. DERMIS
1. DENSE LAYER UNDER THE EPIDERMIS; 1–4 MM THICK
2. LYMPHATIC, VASCULAR, NERVE SUPPLIES AND SWEAT GLANDS ARE LOCATED HERE.
3. CONTAINS FIBROBLASTS, MACROPHAGES, MAST CELLS, AND LYMPHOCYTES FOR HEALING
4. ELASTICITY OF SKIN IS PROVIDED BY COLLAGEN AND ELASTIN IN THIS LAYER.

E. HYPODERMIS (SUBCUTANEOUS LAYER)
1. THICKNESS IS DETERMINED BY AGE AND HEREDITY.
2. PROVIDES INSULATION FROM HOT/ COLD, PROTECTS FROM TRAUMA,

SERVES AS A SOURCE OF ENERGY AND HORMONE METABOLISM
3. THICKEST ON THE BACK AND BUTTOCKS

F. ECCRINE (SWEAT) GLANDS
1. PRODUCE SWEAT FOR TEMPERATURE REGULATION
2. MOST NUMEROUS ON PALMS, SOLES, FOREHEAD, AND AXILLAE
3. STIMULATED BY HEAT, EXERCISE, EMOTIONS

G. APOCRINE GLANDS
1. ROLE IN HUMANS IS NOT WELL ESTABLISHED.
2. DO NOT FUNCTION UNTIL PUBERTY AND REQUIRE HIGH OUTPUT OF SEX HORMONE TO BE ACTIVE
3. LOCATED IN THE AXILLAE, BREAST AREOLAE, ANOGENITAL AREA, EAR CANALS, AND EYELIDS

H. SEBACEOUS (OIL) GLANDS
1. RELEASE SEBUM (OIL) TO THE FACE, SCALP, UPPER BACK, AND CHEST
2. ASSOCIATED WITH HAIR FOLLICLES

I. HAIR FOLLICLES
1. FOUND ON ALL SKIN SURFACES EXCEPT THE PALMS AND SOLES
2. EACH FOLLICLE IS AN INDEPENDENT UNIT.

3. TYPICAL LOSS IS 50–100 HAIRS/DAY
4. MELANOCYTES IN THE BULB OF THE HAIR FOLLICLE DETERMINE HAIR COLOR.
5. USUALLY FOUND WITH SEBACEOUS GLANDS
6. ARRECTOR PILI MUSCLES OF THE DERMIS ATTACH TO HAIR FOLLICLES AND ELEVATE HAIRS WHEN THE BODY TEMPERATURE FALLS (GOOSE BUMPS).

J. NAILS
1. HORNY SCALES OF THE EPIDERMIS
2. NAIL MATRIX, MADE OF KERATIN, IS LOCATED IN THE PROXIMAL NAIL BED.
3. GROWTH IS 0.1 MM/DAY. COLD WEATHER AND ILLNESS SLOW GROWTH.
4. TRAUMA TO THE NAIL MATRIX DISTORTS NAIL SHAPE.

II. **ASSESSMENT**
A. HEALTH HISTORY
1. PAST MEDICAL HISTORY
2. MEDICATIONS (PHOTOSENSITIZING, CORTICOSTEROIDS)
3. ALLERGIES TO FOODS, MEDICATIONS
4. FAMILY HISTORY (ALOPECIA, PSORIASIS, SCABIES, LUPUS)
5. OCCUPATION AND TRAVEL
6. HABITS
B. PHYSICAL EXAMINATION
1. INSPECTION
   a. Begin at the head and include the hair, scalp, nails, mucous membranes, skin (especially the axillae), skin folds, external genitalia, webs between the toes and fingers, palms of the hands, and soles of the feet.
   b. Identify primary lesions—how they looked when they first appeared (macule, papule, plaque, nodule, tumor, wheal, vesicle, bulla, cyst, pustule).
   c. Describe secondary lesions—changes over time or from irritation or infection (scale, crust, erosion, ulcer, scar, lichenification, excoriation, fissure, atrophy).
   d. Hair distribution, color, texture, and condition of the scalp
   e. Nail color, shape, texture, and thickness
   f. Skin color, moisture, temperature, texture, turgor, edema, tenderness, odor, and lesions
   g. Describe the location, distribution, size, arrangement, color, and configuration of lesions.
2. PALPATION
   a. Limited, except moisture, temperature (examiner uses the dorsum of the hand), texture, edema
   b. Turgor is palpated by pinching the skin over the forearm and letting go. If elevated for more than 3 seconds, turgor is decreased.
3. ESTABLISH SKIN ASSESSMENT PARAMETERS (SEE TABLE 8-1)
4. EVALUATE COMMON SKIN CHANGES ASSOCIATED WITH AGING (SEE TABLE 8-2).
5. ASSESS FOR PRIMARY LESIONS (SEE FIGURE 8-2).
6. ASSESS FOR SECONDARY LESIONS (SEE FIGURE 8-3).

Table 8-1 Skin Assessment Parameters

Parameter	Normal	Abnormal
Integrity	Skin intact; no diseased or injured tissue	Broken skin; open areas such as fissures, ulcers, excoriations. Rash or lesions such as papules, nodules, vesicles, pustules, wheals, scales.
Color	Varies with skin type and race: pink, tanned, olive, brown	Pallor—pale skin, especially in face, conjunctivae, nail beds, and oral mucous membranes. Cyanosis—bluish discoloration noticed in lips, earlobes, and nail beds. Jaundice—a yellowing of the skin, mucous membranes, and sclera. Erythema—reddish hue to the skin as in sunburn and inflammation.
Temperature and Moisture	Usually warm and dry, depending on environmental temperature	Cool, cold, moist, clammy, or warmer than normal
Texture	Smooth, soft. Thickness varies in different areas.	Loose, wrinkled, rough, thickened, thin, oily, flaking, scaling
Turgor and Mobility	An assessment of skin hydration. Normally skin moves freely. A pinched fold of skin returns immediately to normal position.	Taut with edema; slack with dehydration. Rigid in some diseases such as scleroderma
Sensation	Distinguishes hot and cold, sharp and dull	Numbness, tingling, insensitive to pressure and sharp objects
Vascularity	Clear; no discoloration	Telangiectasia—permanent dilation of groups of superficial capillaries and venules. Petechiae—pinpoint hemorrhagic spots. Ecchymosis—large, irregular, hemorrhagic areas.

Table 8-2 Common Skin Changes Associated with Aging

Skin Change	Description
Adolescence	
Folliculitis	Inflammation of the hair follicle
Acne	Inflammation of the pilosebaceous follicle
Increased Perspiration	Response to heat, emotional stress, exercise
Apocrine Secretion	Related to sex hormone activity
Pigmented Nevi	Benign cluster of melanocyte-like cells
Adulthood	
Melasma	Blotchy pigmentation
Alopecia	Baldness associated with genetic and hormonal factors; also associated with certain medications
Excessive Facial or Body Hair	Androgen-related problem in women
Actinic Keratosis	Slightly raised, red papules; premalignant
Sebaceous Cyst	Potentially infectious enclosed cyst in the dermis
Acrochordon	Small, flesh-colored papule
Older Adulthood	
Xerosis	Dry skin from decreased natural oils and sweat
Wrinkling	Natural change from loss of elasticity, subcutaneous fat, sun exposure, smoking, gravity
Skin Tears	Epidermal thinning; associated with corticosteroid use
Senile Lentigines	Black or brown flat lesions (liver spots)
Seborrheic Keratosis	Harmless raised black or brown spots or wart-like growths
Cherry Angiomas	Dilated blood vessels that form small loops

© Cengage Learning 2015

III. DIAGNOSTIC STUDIES

A. CULTURE AND SENSITIVITY
1. DESCRIPTION
   a. Specimen is obtained to confirm presence of microorganisms.
   b. Used to determine most appropriate antibiotic for treatment
2. PROCEDURE
   a. Obtain a culturette sterile swab and tube.
   b. Swab the lesion, collecting any exudate that is present.
   c. Place the swab in the tube. Crush the bottom of the tube to activate the preservative.
   d. Label the container and send it to the lab immediately.
3. POSTPROCEDURE
   a. Wash hands.
   b. Cover with dressing if necessary.
B. POTASSIUM HYDROXIDE EXAM AND FUNGAL CULTURE/WOOD'S LIGHT EXAM
1. DESCRIPTION
   a. Specimen obtained to confirm the presence of a fungal infection.
   b. Skin, hair, or nails can be tested.
2. PROCEDURE
   a. Fine scales from edge of site are scraped with a scalpel blade onto the glass slide.
   b. A drop of potassium hydroxide is placed on the specimen, which is examined under microscope.
   c. For culture, scraping or a portion of the dystrophic nail is implanted in the culture medium.
   d. Wood's light (black light) used in a dark room also detects superficial fungal infections.
3. POSTPROCEDURE
   a. Wash hands.
   b. Place a dressing over the lesion if necessary.
C. SCABIES SCRAPING
1. DESCRIPTION
   a. Specimen from unscratched lesion to confirm scabies
   b. Sample linear burrow, if present, to look for eggs or feces.
2. PROCEDURE
   a. Using a #15 scalpel blade, scrape off the top of the lesion or linear burrow, if present.
   b. Place shavings on a microscope slide, cover with immersion oil, and view.

Figure 8-2 Types of primary skin lesions

NONPALPABLE

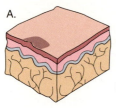

A.

Macule:
    Localized changes in skin
    color of less than 1 cm
    in diameter
Example:
    Freckle

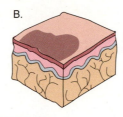

B.

Patch:
    Localized changes in skin
    color of greater than 1 cm
    in diameter
Example:
    Vitiligo, stage 1 of pressure
    ulcer

PALPABLE

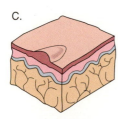

C.

Papule:
    Solid, elevated lesion less
    than 0.5 cm in diameter
Example:
    Warts, elevated nevi,
    seborrheic keratosis

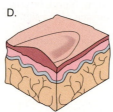

D.

Plaque:
    Solid, elevated lesion
    greater than 0.5 cm
    in diameter
Example:
    Psoriasis, eczema,
    pityriasis rosea

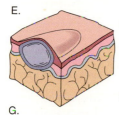

E.

Nodules:
    Solid and elevated; however,
    they extend deeper than
    papules into the dermis or
    subcutaneous tissues,
    0.5–2.0 cm
Example:
    Lipoma, erythema nodosum,
    cyst, melanoma, hemangioma

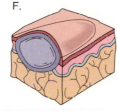

F.

Tumor:
    The same as a nodule only
    greater than 2 cm

Example:
    Carcinoma (such as advanced
    breast carcinoma); **not** basal ce
    or squamous cell of the skin

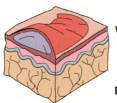

G.

Wheal:
    Localized edema in the
    epidermis causing irregular
    elevation that may be red
    or pale
Example:
    Insect bite, hive, angioedema

FLUID-FILLED CAVITIES WITHIN THE SKIN

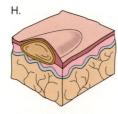

H.

Vesicle:
    Accumulation of fluid between
    the upper layers of the skin;
    elevated mass containing
    serous fluid; less than 0.5 cm
Example:
    Herpes simplex, herpes
    zoster, chickenpox, scabies

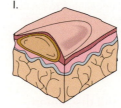

I.

Bullae:
    Same as a vesicle only
    greater than 0.5 cm
Example:
    Contact dermatitis, large
    second-degree burns,
    bullous impetigo, pemphigus

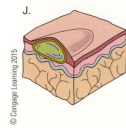

J.

Pustule:
    Vesicles or bullae that
    become filled with pus,
    usually described as less
    than 0.5 cm in diameter
Example:
    Acne, impetigo, furuncles,
    carbuncles, folliculitis

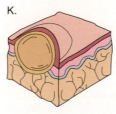

K.

Cyst:
    Encapsulated fluid-filled or
    a semi-solid mass in the
    subcutaneous tissue or
    dermis
Example:
    Sebaceous cyst, epidermoid
    cyst

Figure 8-3 Type of secondary lesions

ABOVE THE SKIN SURFACE

A.
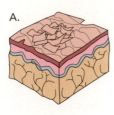
Scales:
Flaking of the skin's surface
Example:
Dandruff, psoriasis, xerosis

B.
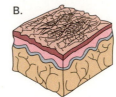
Lichenification:
Layers of skin become
thickened and rough as a
result of rubbing over a
prolonged period of time
Example:
Chronic contact dermatitis

C.
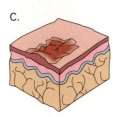
Crust:
Dried serum, blood, or pus
on the surface of the skin
Example:
Impetigo, acute eczematous
inflammation

D.
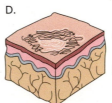
Atrophy:
Thinning of the skin surface
and loss of markings
Example:
Striae, aged skin

BELOW THE SKIN SURFACE

E.
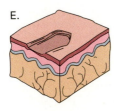
Erosion:
Loss of epidermis
Example:
Ruptured chickenpox vesicle

F.
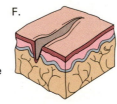
Fissure:
Linear crack in the epidermis
that can extend into the derm
Example:
Chapped hands or lips,
athlete's foot

G.
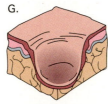
Ulcer:
A depressed lesion of
the epidermis and upper
papillary layer of the dermis
Example:
Stage 2 pressure ulcer

H.
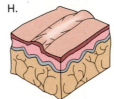
Scar:
Fibrous tissue that replaces
dermal tissue after injury
Example:
Surgical incision

I.
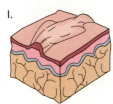
Keloid:
Enlarging of a scar past
wound edges due to excess
collagen formation (more
prevalent in dark-skinned
persons)
Example:
Burn scar

J.
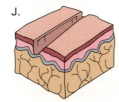
Excoriation:
Loss of epidermal layers
exposing the dermis
Example:
Abrasion

© Cengage Learning 2015

    c. Expect slight bleeding and discomfort
       when the lesion is opened.
  3. POSTPROCEDURE
    a. Wash hands.
    b. Place a dressing over the lesion if
       bleeding occurs.
D. PATCH TESTING
  1. DESCRIPTION
    a. Application of small amounts of
       substances to determine which produce
       allergic skin responses

    b. Differentiates irritant dermatitis from
       allergic dermatitis
  2. PROCEDURE
    a. Small amount of allergens are applied to
       the skin using specially prepared tape.
    b. Instruct the client about local inflammatory
       skin reactions and the importance of
       wearing the patch for 48 hours.
    c. Erythema, papules, or vesicles indicate
       positive reaction.
    d. Read at 48, 72, and 96 hours.

E. BIOPSY
   1. DESCRIPTION
      a. Removal of skin specimen for microscopic exam
      b. Types include shave, dermal punch, and surgical excision.
      c. All use local anesthetic.
   2. PROCEDURE
      a. If a large biopsy is anticipated, avoid aspirin and aspirin-containing products for 48 hours prior to the biopsy. Notify the physician if taking anticoagulants. Review history for clotting disorders. Remind the client of need for antibiotics if having valve or joint replacement. Eat a light meal prior to the procedure to avoid fainting.
      b. Local anesthetic is administered.
      c. Cleanse the skin with antibacterial solution.
      d. Shave biopsy—specimen of epidermis and upper dermis removed with #15 scalpel blade or curved scissors. Apply pressure to the site.
      e. Punch biopsy—stretch skin tight, punch pressed into dermal layer, rotated back and forth to free the specimen, base cut with scissors. Apply pressure to site. Sutures are applied if needed.
      f. Surgical excision—full-thickness specimen, larger area. Site is marked with gentian violet pen. Lesion is excised using a scalpel. Apply pressure for hemostasis. Incision is closed with sutures. Cover with sterile nonstick dressing.
   3. POSTPROCEDURE
      a. Instruct the client in wound care, using antibacterial ointment and nonadherent dressing.
      b. Instruct in signs of wound infection to report.
      c. Advise the client how and when biopsy results will be reported.

IV. **NURSING DIAGNOSES**
   A. RISK FOR INFECTION
   B. IMPAIRED SKIN INTEGRITY
   C. RISK FOR DEFICIENT FLUID VOLUME
   D. ACUTE PAIN
   E. INEFFECTIVE HEALTH MAINTENANCE
   F. SITUATIONAL LOW SELF-ESTEEM
   G. DISTURBED BODY IMAGE
   Nursing Diagnoses: Definitions and Classification 2012–2014. Copyright © 2012, 1994–2012 by NANDA International. Used by arrangement with John Wiley & Sons Limited.

V. **INTEGUMENTARY DISORDERS**
   A. PRURITUS
      1. DESCRIPTION
         a. Itching
         b. Clinical manifestations associated with many things, from dry skin to skin cancer

      2. ASSESSMENT
         a. Location, degree, and interference with activities of daily living
         b. Skin changes, including excoriation, length of fingernails
      3. DIAGNOSTIC TESTS
         a. Depends on the underlying problem
      4. NURSING INTERVENTIONS
         a. Maintain hydration.
         b. Bathe or shower daily for 15–20 minutes with warm water, mild soap, followed by application of emollient.
         c. Apply topical drugs such as menthol, camphor, urea, and lactic acid.
         d. Avoid use of topical anesthetics and antihistamines. Systemic antihistamines may be beneficial, including hydroxyzine (Atarax), diphenhydramine (Benadryl), and chlorpheniramine (Chlor-Trimeton), as may tricyclic antidepressants (doxepin HCl (Sinequan) and amitriptyline HCl (Elavil).
         e. Use topical steroids only as a last resort.
         f. Administer reduced doses of antihistamines to older adult clients because of drowsiness.
   B. ATOPIC DERMATITIS
      1. DESCRIPTION
         a. Common, relapsing pruritic eczema
         b. Often associated with asthma and allergic rhinitis (hay fever)
      2. ASSESSMENT
         a. Red, oozing, crusty rash in acute phase
         b. Dry, brownish-gray colored scales in chronic form
         c. Located on elbow bends, backs of knees, neck, eyelids, and backs of hands and feet
         d. Characterized by intense itching that may lead to viral, bacterial, or fungal infections and scarring
      3. DIAGNOSTIC TESTS
         a. Culture and sensitivity if infection is suspected
         b. Patch testing for allergies
      4. NURSING INTERVENTIONS
         a. Administer daily skin care with superfatted soap (Dove, Basis, Eucerin, Neutrogena, Aveeno, Cetaphil) to hydrate and lubricate the skin.
         b. Apply topical emollients (Aquaphor, Eucerin, Cetaphil creams) two to three times per day after bathing.
         c. Instruct the client to avoid extremely hot water, bubble baths.
         d. Instruct the client to wash all new clothes before wearing. Avoid using fabric softener.
         e. Encourage the client to wear loose-fitting, cotton-blend clothing and keep room temperature cool.

f. Instruct the client to take showers with mild soap and to apply an appropriate moisturizer immediately after swimming.

g. Instruct the client to keep fingernails short, smooth, and clean and avoid scratching.

h. Instruct the client to avoid known allergens. Encourage careful label reading.

i. Help the client understand that there is no "cure." If antibiotics are ordered, remind of the importance of finishing the entire prescription.

j. Instruct the client on the clinical manifestations of infection that should be reported.

C. STASIS DERMATITIS
1. DESCRIPTION
   a. Very dry skin, shallow ulcers on the lower legs
   b. Caused by venous insufficiency
2. ASSESSMENT
   a. Itching, brown-stained skin, open shallow ulcers that are slow to heal
   b. Feeling of heaviness in the legs
   c. Dilated veins
3. DIAGNOSTIC TESTS
   a. Culture and sensitivity, if infection is suspected
4. NURSING INTERVENTIONS
   a. Goal is to improve venous return.
   b. Elevate the legs above the level of the heart several times a day.
   c. Instruct the client to wear support hose or elastic bandages wrapped from the toes to the thighs.
   d. Instruct the client to avoid crossing the legs and standing for prolonged periods in one place.
   e. Encourage the client to perform calf exercises and walking.
   f. Elevate the foot of the bed.
   g. Apply moisture-retaining dressings or Unna boots for ulcers.
   h. Skin grafts may be required to heal large ulcers.

D. CONTACT DERMATITIS
1. DESCRIPTION
   a. Irritant contact dermatitis— inflammatory response to chemical or physical irritant (cleaning product, fragrance, skin care product)
   b. Allergic contact dermatitis—delayed hypersensitivity response to allergen (poison ivy, nickel in jewelry)
2. ASSESSMENT
   a. Irritant dermatitis—redness, vesicles, ulceration; usually localized
   b. Allergic dermatitis—itching, stinging, redness, swelling within an hour to 2 weeks after contact; may involve extensive areas of the body

3. DIAGNOSTIC TESTS
   a. Patch testing to identify allergens
4. NURSING INTERVENTIONS
   a. Instruct the client to avoid causative agent.
   b. Instruct the client to avoid allergens.
   c. Apply topical drugs such as menthol, camphor, urea, and lactic acid, and Aquaphor, Eucerin, and Cetaphil creams to control pain and itching.
   d. Administer systemic antihistamines such as hydroxyzine (Vistaril) and diphenhydramine (Benadryl) and topical or systemic steroids as prescribed.

E. INTERTRIGO
1. DESCRIPTION
   a. Superficial inflammatory dermatitis that occurs between two skin surfaces that are touching one another
   b. Heat, friction, and moisture (humidity, urinary incontinence) worsen the condition.
2. ASSESSMENT
   a. Redness, maceration, itching and burning between two skin surfaces, commonly the neck creases, axillae, antecubital fossae, perineum, finger and toe webs, abdominal skinfolds, and beneath the breasts
   b. Erosions, fissures, and infection with bacteria of *Candida albicans* may occur.
3. DIAGNOSTIC TESTS
   a. Culture and sensitivity if infection is suspected
4. NURSING INTERVENTIONS
   a. Goal is to promote drying and aeration of body skin folds.
   b. Instruct the client in proper hygiene with careful drying; may use a hair dryer on cool setting to get skin folds dry.
   c. Encourage the client to wear loose-fitting, cotton-blend clothing, and periodic removal or changing of clothing.
   d. Instruct the client to use talcor cellulose-containing powder (Zeasorb) if the skin is unbroken.
   e. Avoid cornstarch because it encourages *C. albicans* overgrowth.
   f. Low-potency topical corticosteroids (hydrocortisone 1.0% or 2.5% cream or lotion) or combination steroid and antifungal (Vytone 1%) may be used for short-term application if inflammation or fungal infection is present.
   g. Cool soaks with tap water or Burrow's solution three to four times a day are useful to remove exudates. Folded gauze or clean cotton handkerchiefs may be placed in skin folds to promote healing.

F. PSORIASIS VULGARIS
1. DESCRIPTION
   a. Chronic, recurrent inflammatory disorder involving keratin synthesis
   b. Genetic predisposition is suspected.
2. ASSESSMENT
   a. Itching; red, dry scaly patches of varying sizes with periods of remission and exacerbation
   b. Anxiety and stress precede flares.
   c. Commonly seen on the scalp, elbows, knees, and sacral region; usually symmetrical
3. DIAGNOSTIC TESTS
   a. No specific tests
4. NURSING INTERVENTIONS
   a. Mild conditions may be treated with natural sunlight or topical therapy (triamcinolone). Keratolytic agents (salicylic acid) may be used to remove scales to allow topical agents to penetrate.
   b. Apply anthralin, an effective topical for widespread psoriasis. It stains fabric, hair, skin, furniture, and bathroom fixtures. Careful application and hand washing are recommended.
   c. Administer scalp care, which includes the use of tar shampoos to remove scales followed by topical corticosteroids. Use of a shower cap enhances absorption of steroids.
   d. Apply all topical agents only to lesions, avoiding contact with normal skin.
   e. Apply oral methotrexate in small doses to inhibit DNA synthesis in lesions that are considered severe cases and are unresponsive to other topical agents.
   f. Monitor the client's electrolytes, complete blood count (CBC), and liver function studies if methotrexate is used. Because of chromosomal abnormalities associated with methotrexate, effective birth control for both men and women is imperative during treatment.
   g. Administer etretinate (Tegison) only as a last resort.
   h. Instruct the client about ultraviolet light treatments.
   i. Assist the client with coping because many clients feel "dirty" due to the appearance of their lesions.
   j. Prevent secondary infection by keeping the skin clean and dry.
   k. Assist the client with controlling factors that cause a flare-up such as stress, anxiety, poor diet, and lack of exercise.

G. ACNE VULGARIS
1. DESCRIPTION
   a. Common, self-limiting condition caused by excess production of oil, abnormal keratinization of epithelium of follicles, and proliferation of bacteria
   b. Exacerbations associated with menstrual cycles, heat, humidity, and excessive perspiration
2. ASSESSMENT
   a. Presence of comedones (blackheads), pustules, papules, and nodules
3. DIAGNOSTIC TESTS
   a. None
4. NURSING INTERVENTIONS
   a. Treatment depends on the severity of the outbreak.
   b. Instruct the client to use water-based, noncomedogenic products and cosmetics.
   c. Instruct the client to use products with benzoyl peroxide for antimicrobial effect (Desquam, Banzagel, Persa-Gel, Panoxyl).
   d. Administer topical antibiotics such as clindamycin (Cleocin) and erythromycin if prescribed.
   e. Administer topical retinoids such as tretinoin (Retin-A and Avita) or adapalene (Differin) alone or with benzoyl peroxide.
   f. Administer systemic antibiotics such as tetracycline or erythromycin for several months to suppress growth of acne and reduce inflammation if topical agents are ineffective. Instruct the client to report vaginitis or gastrointestinal upset.
   g. Administer prescribed hormone therapy with estrogens to suppress sebaceous gland activity for 3–4 menstrual cycles to determine effectiveness.
   h. Use isotretinoin (Accutane) for severe acne resistant to management. Because of teratogenicity, female clients must have a pregnancy test prior to beginning treatment and use an effective contraceptive for at least 1 month before starting treatment.
   i. Monitor a client on isotretinoin (Accutane) for elevated triglycerides.
   j. Instruct the client to avoid vitamin A while on isotretinoin (Accutane).
   k. Inform the client that all acne therapies require at least 4–8 weeks to see improvement.

H. ACNE ROSACEA
1. DESCRIPTION
   a. Chronic inflammatory skin eruptions of the face, cheeks, bridge of the nose
   b. Associated factors include fair skin, caffeine, alcohol (especially wine), sunlight, extremes of temperature, spicy foods, and emotional stress.

c. Onset between 30 and 50 years of age, with women more commonly affected than men

2. ASSESSMENT
   a. Redness, papules, pustules, telangiectases
   b. Sebaceous hyperplasia of the nose after many years of chronic inflammation
   c. Eyelid inflammation and conjunctivitis

3. DIAGNOSTIC TESTS
   a. None

4. NURSING INTERVENTIONS
   a. Instruct the client to avoid triggers that provoke facial vasodilation.
   b. Administer topical metronizadole (MetroGel), which is the drug of choice.
   c. Assist the client in dealing with body image changes related to the disease.

I. SKIN TEARS
   1. DESCRIPTION
      a. Wounds resulting from separation of the epidermis from underlying connective tissue, usually caused by trauma
      b. Most common on the forearm, hand, elbow, and upper arm
      c. Thinning of the epidermis and reduced adhesion of the dermis to the epidermis contribute to risk in older adults.

   2. ASSESSMENT
      a. Location, size, ability to replace flap over the wound

   3. DIAGNOSTIC TESTS
      a. None

   4. NURSING INTERVENTIONS
      a. Irrigate blood from the site with normal saline.
      b. Reaffix the flap to approximate wound edges if able.
      c. Close the wound with wound closure strips (Steri-strips) and cover with nonadherent, moisture-retaining dressing (petrolatum gauze).
      d. Apply rolled gauze dressing to protect from further injury.
      e. Prevent injuries by using protective gloves on the client's hands, soft armrests on wheelchairs.
      f. Avoid covering skin tear wound with a transparent dressing.
      g. Monitor for clinical manifestations of infection.
      h. Instruct the client on appropriate wound care.

J. PRESSURE ULCERS
   1. DESCRIPTION
      a. Lesion on the skin caused by unrelieved pressure (bedsores, decubitus ulcers) on the skin and can extend to the subcutaneous tissue and muscle
      b. High pressure on bony prominences contributes to development.

c. Immobility, age, moisture, poor nutrition, friction, and shear are risk factors that can be controlled.

2. ASSESSMENT
   a. Risk factors should be identified on a regular basis using a scale such as the Braden scale.
   b. Observe the skin over the sacrum, heel, greater trochanter, and ischial tuberosities.
   c. Review lab data—albumin, total protein, hemoglobin, hematocrit, and lymphocytes.
   d. If ulcer is present, note location, size, depth, stage of drainage, and condition of surrounding skin.

3. DIAGNOSTIC TESTS
   a. Culture and sensitivity if infection is suspected
   b. Bone scan to confirm osteomyelitis

4. NURSING INTERVENTIONS
   a. Redistribute pressure using a special bed, foam heel protectors, and pillows between the knees. Change position frequently, keeping pressure off any broken areas. Keep the head of the bed as low as possible.
   b. Use pressure-relieving seat cushions for clients who are out of bed. Instruct the client to reposition every 15 minutes. Avoid donut-type devices because they tend to cause pressure ulcers.
   c. Encourage a dietary intake high in protein and vitamin C to aid healing. Supplement as needed to maintain a positive nitrogen balance.
   d. Assess and manage pain associated with the ulcer and its care.
   e. Keep the client's skin dry. Change linen and clothing as frequently as necessary. Use warm water and mild soap and dry carefully. Use topical agents that act as barriers to moisture if the client is incontinent.
   f. Provide wound care with normal saline using a 35-ml piston syringe with a 19-gauge angiocatheter on the tip. Apply dressings that keep the wound moist and the surrounding skin dry.
   g. Use clean gloves and clean dressings.
   h. Minimize shearing and friction through proper positioning, getting assistance for transfers, and the use of draw sheets.
   i. Provide consistency in wound care to monitor progress.
   j. Inform the client that Stages III and IV ulcers and those over 2 cm in diameter may require surgical repair with musculocutaneous flap grafts.

k. Stages of pressure ulcers
  1) Stage 1: area is reddened, but skin is not broken.
  2) Stage 2: epidermal and dermal layers are involved.
  3) Stage 3: subcutaneous tissues are involved.
  4) Stage 4: muscle and bone may be involved.

K. **ACTINIC KERATOSES**
  1. DESCRIPTION
    a. Common, epithelial, precancerous lesion
    b. Caused by sun exposure, especially in older white adults
  2. ASSESSMENT
    a. Irregular shape, flat, or slightly red macule or papule with indistinct border
    b. Face, tops of ears, back of the neck, forearms, and back of the hand are the most common locations.
    c. Scale of lesions can be shed or peeled off but grows back.
    d. Varies in size, from pinhead to several centimeters; often appear in clusters; easier to palpate than see
  3. DIAGNOSTIC TESTS
    a. Shave or excisional biopsy to determine if squamous cell cancer is present
  4. NURSING INTERVENTIONS
    a. Administer topical application of 5-fluorouracil (5-FU, Efudex) for treating widespread disease, but it may cause inflammatory response.
    b. Apply 5-fluorouracil (5-FU) twice daily with a gloved hand. Skin may be covered with gauze. Instruct the client that erosion, ulceration, necrosis, and reepithelialization may occur.
    c. Discontinue 5-fluorouracil (5-FU) when the skin becomes ulcerated. Apply topical corticosteroids to reduce inflammation and pain. Complete healing takes 1–2 months after therapy is stopped.
    d. Instruct the client to minimize skin exposure, use sunscreen, and wear protective clothing.
  5. MEDICAL MANAGEMENT
    a. Cryotherapy with liquid nitrogen is used for single or small numbers of lesions. Minor discomfort is caused when nitrogen is applied. Causes a blister that should not be disturbed.
    b. Electrodesiccation and curettage, use of a hot spark to kill the lesion, is done under local anesthesia. Wound must be kept moist with topical antibiotic ointment (Bacitracin).
    c. Laser excision vaporizes lesions under local anesthesia.

L. SKIN CANCER (SEE CHAPTER 11, SECTION N)

M. **CELLULITIS**
  1. DESCRIPTION
    a. Skin infection that extends into the dermis and subcutaneous fat usually caused by *Staphylococcus pyogenes*
    b. If untreated, may lead to gangrene, abscesses, and sepsis
    c. Risk factors include age, diabetes, malnutrition, presence of wounds or ulcers, and use of systemic steroids.
  2. ASSESSMENT
    a. Deep red erythematous areas, tender and swollen
  3. DIAGNOSTIC TESTS
    a. Culture and sensitivity to isolate organism
  4. NURSING INTERVENTIONS
    a. Apply soaks to the affected area to reduce edema and inflammation.
    b. Monitor the client's vital signs for evidence of sepsis.
    c. Administer antibiotics as prescribed.
    d. Prevent cross-contamination by thorough hand washing.
    e. Use standard precautions as appropriate.

N. HERPES ZOSTER
  1. DESCRIPTION
    a. Infection caused by the reactivation of the varicella virus in clients who have had chickenpox
    b. Those who have not had chickenpox are at risk after exposure to a person with herpes zoster
  2. ASSESSMENT
    a. Presence of vesicles grouped on an erythematous base along a dermatome
    b. Vesicles appear 1–2 days after onset of pain and itching at the site.
    c. Eruption usually clears in 2 weeks.
    d. Postherpetic pain (residual pain) and itching are major complications.
  3. DIAGNOSTIC TESTS
    a. Viral culture
    b. Tzanck's smear to establish presence of herpes zoster
  4. NURSING INTERVENTIONS
    a. Assess pain for constant, intermittent, burning, location, and the presence of deep visceral pain.
    b. Administer antiviral drugs such as acyclovir (Zovirax) and Valtrex early in the disease to reduce pain and shorten the course of the disease.
    c. Administer analgesics as needed for pain relief.
    d. Use topical therapy for itching such as cool compresses, antipruritic medications like Caladryl.

e. Continue intervention and support as long as postherpetic pain is present, often for many months. Inform the client that tricyclic antidepressants, phenothiazines, or electrical stimulating units may be helpful for pain control.

O. INFECTIOUS DISORDERS OF THE SKIN (SEE TABLE 8-3)

P. BURNS

  1. DESCRIPTION

     a. Injury resulting from direct contact with or exposure to any thermal, chemical, electrical, or radiation source

     b. Energy from heat source is transferred through body tissues.

     c. Depth of injury is related to temperature and duration of exposure.

  2. TYPES

     a. Thermal

        1) Caused by exposure or contact with flame, hot liquids, semiliquids (steam), semisolids (tar), or hot objects

     b. Chemical

        1) Caused by contact with strong acids, bases, or organic compounds

        2) Chemicals used in household cleaning, industry, agriculture, and the military are capable of causing injury.

        3) Splash injuries to the eye and inhalation injuries are particularly serious.

     c. Electrical

        1) Caused by contact with exposed or faulty electrical wiring, high-voltage power lines, or lightning

        2) Extent of injury is influenced by duration of contact, voltage, type of current, pathway of the current, and tissue resistance to the current.

     d. Radiation

        1) Least common type of burn associated with nuclear radiation accidents, use of radiation in industry, and therapeutic irradiation

Table 8-3 Infectious Disorders of the Skin

Disease	Organism	Clinical Manifestations	Medical Management
Bacterial Infections			
Impetigo Contagious	*Staphylococcus aureus*	Begins as a small vesicle; becomes a weeping lesion; forms a light brown crust. Usually on the face and upper trunk. More common in children. More common in spring and fall. Poor hygiene coupled with warm weather facilitates the spread of the disease.	Cleanse the affected area at least 3 times a day. Apply an antibiotic ointment. Occasionally, systemic antibiotics are needed.
Carbuncle	*Staphylococcus aureus*	Begins as infected hair follicles in the dermis. Symptoms are redness, swelling, pain. Yellow cores of pus develop. Carbuncles usually occur on the nape of the neck and upper back. Obese or malnourished persons with poor hygiene as well as diabetics are most susceptible to carbuncles.	Warm, moist soaks may help "bring the boil to a head." Once the carbuncle ruptures or is incised and drained, pain subsides. Carbuncles tend to recur. The staphylococcus organism may be resistant to topical antibiotics. Systemic antibiotic may be needed.
Viral Infections			
Herpes Zoster (shingles)	V-Z (varicella-zoster)	Clusters of small vesicles over the course of a peripheral sensory nerve. Two-thirds of clients have lesions just in the thoracic region. Lesions can occur over the trigeminal nerve, affecting the face, scalp, and eyes. Crusts develop in several days. Symptoms are mild to severe pain, itching, fever, malaise. In older adults, pain can last for months or years. Persons who have not had chickenpox risk contracting the disease if they care for herpes zoster clients with open lesions. Persons who previously had chickenpox, but developed only partial immunity to it, may still be susceptible to herpes zoster.	Acyclovir (Zovirax) is given to clients in severe pain or to immunosuppressed clients. Analgesics help control the pain. Narcotic analgesics are prescribed for severe pain. Antipruritic topical medications decrease the itching.
Herpes Simplex, Type 1 and 2 (fever blisters, cold sores) Type 2 (genital)	*Herpes simplex virus*	Type 1—a cluster of vesicles on an erythematous base occurring most commonly at the corners of the mouth or at the edge of the nostrils. Type 2—lesions in the vagina or cervix of a woman or on the penis of a man. The lesions itch, burn, and frequently break open, forming a crust. Healing occurs in about 10 days.	Topical use of antiviral agents such as acyclovir decreases discomfort. Even with treatment, cold sores and fever blisters tend to recur, especially with fever, upper respiratory infections, and stress. Oral administration of acyclovir helps to prevent recurrence of genital herpes.

Disease	Organism	Clinical Manifestations	Medical Management
Warts	Human papillomavirus	Seen as small, painless round papules on hands, face, and neck. On the bottom of the feet, warts grow inward from the pressure and are painful (plantar warts). Warts in the anogenital region itch. Genital warts increase the risk of cervical cancer.	No treatment is indicated for painless warts; they tend to disappear eventually. Plantar warts may be removed by cryosurgery or with locally applied chemicals such as nitric acid. Warts are not highly contagious from person to person but may be spread on the person's own body by rubbing or scratching. Genital warts are spread by sexual intercourse.
Fungal Infections			
Tinea (ringworm) *Tinea capitis* (ringworm of the scalp) *Tinea corporis* (ringworm of the body) *Tinea cruris* ("jock itch") *Tinea pedis* (athlete's foot)	*Microscorim audouini*	Tinea is a superficial infection of the skin, called ringworm because of its circumscribed appearance, typically round, and reddened with slight scaling. Lesions of tinea corporis have a pale center. Itching is common with tinea cruris. Itching and burning occur with tinea pedis. Tinea is spread easily. Jock itch and athlete's foot are more common among men than women.	Treat mild infections with a topical antifungal drug such as miconazole nitrate (Micatin) or tolnaftate (Aftate). Severe infections are treated with oral administration of griseofulvin microsize (Grisactin).
Parasitic Infections			
Scabies	*Sarcoptes scabiei* (female itch mite)	The itch mite burrows under the skin, lays eggs, and deposits fecal material. Short, dark-red wavy lines may be seen on hands, wrists, elbows, axillary folds, nipples, waistline, and gluteal folds. Pruritus is severe and can persist for up to 3 months after treatment. Scratching leads to secondary infection. Scabies is spread by prolonged contact and is frequently seen in several members of a family.	Apply the scabicide, lindane (Kwell), topically to the entire body at bedtime so that the medication remains on the skin 8 to 12 hours. Treat all family members even if they do not have symptoms. Wash all underclothing and bed and bath linens in hot water. Change linens daily.
Pediculosis (lice)	*Pediculus* capitis (head lice) *Pediculus corporis* (body lice) *Phthirius pubis* (pubic lice)	Eggs, or nits, of *P. capitis* attach themselves firmly to a hair shaft on the head or in a beard. Nits have a gray, pearly appearance. The pubic louse resembles a tiny crab that attaches itself to pubic hair. Body lice live in the seams of clothing. The bite of the louse causes severe pruritus. Scratching leads to secondary infection.	Lindane (Kwell) is applied topically to the hair as a shampoo or to the body as a cream or lotion. Repeat the treatment again in 8 to 10 days. Wash or dry-clean clothing and linens. Disinfect combs and brushes. Vacuum carpets and furniture; then spray with a pediculicide.

2) The length of exposure, distance from the source of radiation, strength of the radiation source, and amount of shielding between the source and the person determine the extent of injury.

e. Inhalation injury
1) Caused by exposure to smoke and noxious gases such as carbon monoxide
2) Type of smoke, length of exposure to asphyxiants, and thermal injury to lung tissue are components of inhalation injuries.

3. ASSESSMENT
a. Burn severity assessed by depth, size, location, age, and general health of the client, mechanism of injury
b. Depth classified by layers of skin that are injured
1) Partial thickness—involvement of the epidermal layer only (first degree). Is red, blanches with pressure, is painful for 48–72 hours, and heals in 3–7 days.
2) Partial thickness—involvement of the dermal layer (second degree). Is wet, shiny, weeping, with blisters, and blanches with pressure. It is painful and sensitive to touch and air currents. Healing rates vary with depth and presence of infection.
3) Full thickness—involvement of the subcutaneous layer (third degree). Varies in color such as deep red, white, black, or brown; is dry, often with thrombosed blood vessels visible. Client has loss of sensation and requires grafting for healing.
4) Full thickness—involvement to the bone (fourth degree). Varies in color, with visible charring and limited movement. Client has loss

Figure 8-4 Rule of nines

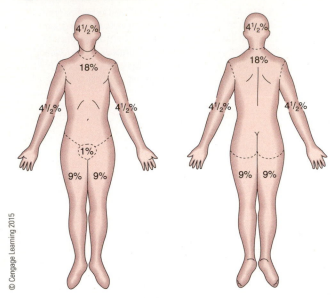

© Cengage Learning 2015

of sensation and requires grafting for healing. Amputation of extremities is likely.

c. Size of burn is determined by Rule of Nines or using an age-specific burn diagram.

  1) The Rule of Nines is a quick tool to estimate burn size based on anatomic sections of the body, with each representing 9% or a multiple of 9 (see Figure 8-4).

  2) A burn diagram charts the percentages for body segments according to age and is more accurate.

d. The location of the burn is important to anticipate other injuries.

  1) Burns of head, neck, and chest are typically associated with inhalation injuries.

  2) Burns of the face may involve the eyes and ears, both requiring special care.

  3) Perineal burns often become infected because of contact with urine and feces.

  4) Circumferential burns may compromise circulation or cause inadequate chest expansion.

e. Age affects severity and outcome of burn. Mortality is higher for children under age 4 and clients older than 65.

f. General health influences response to injury and treatment. Mortality rates increase for clients with cardiac, respiratory, and alcohol-related illnesses.

g. Mechanism of injury determines type of initial treatment and need for any special procedure.

h. Assess for airway and breathing while extent of burn injury is determined.

  1) Lips, tongue, oropharynx, and nares for redness, blisters, ulceration, soot

  2) Respiratory rate, effort, stridor, wheezing, cyanosis, and carboxyhemoglobin levels

  3) Check for circumferential burns of chest or trunk.

4. DIAGNOSTIC TESTS

a. Carboxyhemoglobin level: detects carbon monoxide in blood

b. Serum electrolytes, blood urea nitrogen (BUN), creatinine, hematocrit, blood glucose: determine electrolyte imbalances, kidney function, hydration status, body's response to stress

c. Chest x-ray: determines pulmonary status for clients with suspected inhalation injuries

d. Electrocardiograph: continuous monitoring for all clients with extensive burns, electrical burns, or history of cardiac disease

5. NURSING INTERVENTIONS—INITIAL/ EMERGENT CARE

a. Stop the burning process, which begins at the scene, and transport to the burn center as quickly as possible.

  1) Flames, scald injuries—wet down with cool water.

  2) Chemical burns—remove clothing and jewelry, brush off any chemical powder residual, wet down with cool water.

  3) Electrical burns—turn off the electrical source before touching the victim.

b. Monitor airway, breathing; administer 100% oxygen via a face mask.

  1) Carbon monoxide levels may be elevated, causing impaired vision, flushed face, headache, nausea, impaired dexterity, dizziness, tachycardia, and tachypnea.

  2) Keep $PaO_2 > 90$ mm Hg, $PaCO_2$ 35–45 mm Hg, and $SaO_2 > 95\%$, respiratory rate 16–24 breaths/ minute with normal pattern and depth, clear breath sounds.

  3) Instruct the client in the use of the incentive spirometry, deep breathing, and coughing, and perform at least every 2 hours. Keep the head of the bed elevated.

  4) Have suction equipment available.

c. Replace fluids and electrolytes.
   1) Monitor for hyponatremia, hyperkalemia, and elevated hematocrit in the first 36 hours.
   2) Fluid loss through injured skin is massive (blisters, generalized edema, open wounds), especially if the burn is greater than 15% of the total body surface area.
   3) Start two large-bore IVs in the nonburned area, if possible, with Ringer's lactate solution.
   4) Insert indwelling foley catheter and monitor urine output every hour to ensure there is at least 30 ml/hr or 0.5 ml/kg/hr. Observe for dark brown or red color, which indicates presence of myoglobin or hemoglobin.
   5) Keep heart rate < 120 beats/minute.

d. Prevent aspiration.
   1) Insert a nasogastric tube for an unconscious client or a client with 20% or greater burned areas.
   2) Restrict oral intake to prevent ileus.

e. Minimize pain.
   1) IV narcotics such as morphine sulfate are given in 5- to 10-minute intervals until pain is under control.
   2) Avoid intramuscular (IM) and subcutaneous (SC) injections because of erratic absorption from poorly perfused tissue.
   3) Avoid oral medications because of aspiration risk and possible ileus.

f. Prevent tissue ischemia.
   1) Remove any constricting jewelry, clothing. Limit use of blood pressure cuffs on injured extremities.
   2) Distal pulses are assessed using a Doppler stethoscope.
   3) Escharatomy (cutting open of dead, dry tissue) may be needed to restore circulation.
   4) Fasciotomy, deeper incision into fascia, may be needed in clients with electrical or crush injuries.

g. Provide initial wound care.
   1) Clean wounds with mild soap and warm water, trimming nonviable tissue and shaving hair within a 1-inch margin from wound edge.
   2) Administer tetanus toxoid.
   3) Use strict aseptic technique to avoid cross-contamination.
   4) Apply topical antimicrobial and cover with loose gauze dressing.

   5) Keep the client warm as hypothermia can be a problem— use sterile sheets; increase room temperature.

h. Assist with coping.
   1) Grieving process is common, beginning with shock, disbelief, and feelings of being completely overwhelmed.
   2) Reassure the client and family; provide information in small amounts about the extent of injuries, treatments under way, and client progress.

6. NURSING INTERVENTIONS—ACUTE PHASE
   a. Acute phase begins approximately 48–72 hours postburn when the client is hemodynamically stable and diuresis has begun. In addition to concerns above, emphasis is placed on restorative care.
   b. Monitor for development of pneumonia or atelectasis.
   c. Prevent hypothermia.
   d. Prevent infection.
      1) Instruct the family on isolation attire, including masks, caps, shoe covers, gowns, gloves.
      2) Advise the family not to visit if they have an infection of any kind.
      3) Observe all invasive lines for any swelling, redness, purulence. Check blood, urine, and sputum cultures for microorganisms.
      4) Monitor for clinical manifestations of sepsis, including headache, chills, anorexia, nausea, changes in vital signs, confusion, and restlessness.
   e. Provide nutritional support.
      1) Metabolic rates are 100% higher than normal, depending on the extent of the burn.
      2) Weigh the client daily.
      3) If the client is able to eat, offer small frequent meals that are high in calories and proteins. Encourage the family to bring favorite foods.
      4) Gastrointestinal complications may prohibit eating, and tube feeding or parenteral nutrition may be ordered.
   f. Minimize pain.
      1) Combination therapies are often used, including patient-controlled analgesia, inhalation analgesics such as nitrous oxide, oral analgesics, and narcotic

agonist-antagonists. Nonsteroidal anti-inflammatory drugs may be used cautiously due to risk of gastrointestinal irritation.

2) Hypnosis, guided imagery, art and play therapy, relaxation techniques, biofeedback, and music therapy are also beneficial.

3) Provide all interventions so the client will have maximum benefit during painful procedures.

g. Provide wound care.

1) Medicate prior to wound care.

2) Cleansing is done by showering, spraying, or "tubbing."

3) Debriding to remove eschar (dead tissue) is accomplished by mechanical, enzymatic, or surgical interventions.

a) Mechanical—use scissors or forceps to trim or loosen the tissue during or after hydrotherapy. Wet-to-dry dressings also mechanically remove necrotic tissue. Both of these processes are painful.

b) Enzymatic—use proteolytic and fibrinolytic enzyme ointments to remove dead tissue.

c) Surgical—may remove thin layers of eschar (tangential) or deep layers (fascial) to expose healthy tissue.

4) Topical antimicrobials

a) Used on partial- and full-thickness burns once or twice a day after cleaning and debriding

b) Wound may be covered with antimicrobial cream and left open to the air for greater freedom of movement and ease of inspection, or covered with gauze dressings wrapped from distal to proximal.

c) Commonly used agents include silver sulfadiazine (Silvadene), mafenide acetate (Sulfamylon), silver nitrate, bacitracin, polymyxin B, and neomycin sulfate.

5) Temporary wound coverings

a) Biologic—amniotic membrane, human cadaver skin or pig skin, may be used to cover, protect, or debride.

b) Biosynthetic—nylon fabric (Biobrane), dermal and epidermal analogs (Integra), alginates (Curasorb, Kalginate),

hypoallergenic films (Bioclusive, Op-site), and fine mesh gauze impregnated with ointment (Aquaphor) are used to promote healing or cover donor sites used for skin grafts.

h. Provide therapeutic positioning.

1) Pain, presence of dressings, and wound contractures limit mobility.

2) Burned areas must be maintained in anticontracture positions using splints and occupational and physical therapy for best return of function.

3) Encourage participation in activities of daily living and as much movement as possible every 2–4 hours.

i. Provide psychological support.

1) Changes in self-esteem related to changes in body image are common.

2) Provide accepting atmosphere and time for communication.

3) Instruct the client and family about the client's projected appearance to reduce misconceptions.

4) Encourage the client to interact with others, including burn support groups.

j. Instruct the client on self-care.

1) Wound care

a) Use of dressings, topical antimicrobials

b) Lubricate grafts, donor sites, and healed burn wounds using alcohol-free moisturizer at least three times a day.

c) Wear pressure garments 23 hours a day to reduce scarring.

d) Avoid direct sun for 1 year postinjury.

2) Medications—dosage, precautions, and adverse reactions

3) Nutritional maintenance

4) Support and peer groups

5) Importance of follow-up care

7. SURGICAL MANAGEMENT

a. Grafting procedures autografts

1) Use of the superficial layer of the client's own unburned skin

2) Epidermis is split in layers— "split-thickness" graft.

3) Sheet grafts are used to cover burns in a visible area.

4) Meshed grafts have many little slits that allow for expansion of the donor skin to cover larger or irregular areas. Meshed pattern is visible when healed.

5) Full-thickness grafts, consisting of epidermis and dermis, are used to cover deeper wounds.

6) Graft adherence depends on development of a fibrin and collagen network. Graft is not disturbed, and the area is immobilized. Small blebs of serum are removed from graft sites with a small needle and cotton-tip applicator.

7) Donor site is covered with dressing and observed for infection. Donor sites can be reused after it has healed.

8) Epithelial autografting uses small full-thickness skin specimen that is sent to the lab for culture and growth. It takes 3–4 weeks to have a large enough piece to use.

PRACTICE QUESTIONS

1. Which of the following nursing activities should the registered nurse delegate to a licensed practical nurse?
   1. Instruct a client with acne vulgaris on the use of tretinoin (Retin-A)
   2. Develop a plan of care on the irrigation of a skin ulcer with normal saline
   3. Obtain a health history from a client admitted with a pressure sore on the coccyx
   4. Monitor the vital signs of a client with cellulitis for evidence of sepsis

2. Which of the following is a priority to include when instructing a client to perform a skin assessment?
   1. "Evaluate the evenness of skin color, moisture, and temperature."
   2. "Look for any changes in moles, especially color and size."
   3. "Begin performing skin examinations after age 40."
   4. "Assess the entire body and look for changes in skin or moles."

3. The nurse assesses a client's skin and finds an elevated, solid lesion on the client's great toe. It is pink, nontender, and 0.5 cm in size. Which of the following is the most appropriate action by the nurse?
   1. Notify the physician immediately
   2. Gather more information about the lesion from the client
   3. Instruct the client to cover the lesion with an adhesive bandage
   4. Determine what the client has been doing to treat the lesion

4. The nurse instructs a client with pruritus to apply an emollient immediately after bathing. The nurse understands that the rationale for this intervention is to
   1. prevent evaporation of water from the epidermis.
   2. cause vasodilation that will reduce the symptoms of pruritus.
   3. provide extra fat to the subcutaneous tissue.
   4. protect the skin from further irritation.

5. The nurse is discharging a client who developed a skin tear while hospitalized for surgery. The nurse instructs the client in wound care for the skin tear. Which of the following would be essential to include in the wound care instructions for this client?
   1. Cover the skin tear with a transparent dressing
   2. Use a nonadherent dressing over the wound
   3. Eat a high-fat diet to help the wound heal more quickly
   4. Drink 3000 ml of water every day to keep the skin hydrated

6. The nurse is teaching a mother about caring for her 4-year-old with atopic dermatitis. Which of the following statements by the mother indicates that the teaching has been successful?
   1. "I prevent the spread of dermatitis by using separate towels for the children."
   2. "We will all switch to soy milk."
   3. "I will keep my child out of the sun."
   4. "I will avoid using fabric softeners in the laundry."

7. The nurse is teaching a class on the treatment of psoriasis with methotrexate. Which of the following should the nurse include in her teaching?
   1. Methotrexate is recommended only for those over the age of 50
   2. It is important to monitor serum albumin, total protein, and blood glucose
   3. An effective birth control for both men and women must be taken
   4. Topical steroids used with methotrexate provide the most effective therapy

8. The nurse is providing diet instructions for a client with acne rosacea. Which of the following describes the most appropriate dietary restrictions?

   Select all that apply:
   [ ] 1. Avoid spicy foods
   [ ] 2. Limit the intake of foods rich in omega-3 fatty acids
   [ ] 3. Avoid chocolate
   [ ] 4. Avoid caffeine
   [ ] 5. Restrict the use of products containing phenylalanine
   [ ] 6. Avoid fried foods

9. The nurse is evaluating the following four clients for the development of a pressure ulcer. Which of the following clients is at greatest risk for the development of a pressure ulcer?
   1. A 52-year-old obese female, 2 days post-op for a knee replacement, who has an indwelling urinary catheter
   2. A 74-year-old thin male, who is awaiting surgery for a fractured left hip
   3. A 91-year-old emaciated female with a blood sugar of 160 mg/dl, who is sitting in a wheelchair
   4. A 67-year-old obese male, who has cellulitis of his right lower leg

10. The nurse is instructing a client with herpes zoster on self-care. Which of the following statements by the client indicates the teaching has been successful?
    1. "I will stay away from my young grandchildren."
    2. "Frequent cool baths will help my herpes heal more quickly."
    3. "I will use topical diphenhydramine to dry up the lesions."
    4. "I will avoid using fabric softener in the laundry."

11. When assessing for changes in skin color in an African-American client, the nurse should assess which of the following first?
    1. Soles of the feet
    2. Palms of the hand
    3. Conjunctiva or sclera
    4. Nail beds or oral mucosa

12. The nurse is preparing to teach a class on the prevention of skin problems. Which of the following is a priority for the nurse to instruct clients to avoid?
    1. Sunlight
    2. Radiation
    3. Alkaline soaps
    4. Vitamin E

13. The nurse is caring for a client during the emergent phase of a burn injury. Which of the following assessments would provide the nurse

with the most accurate information regarding this client's full-thickness burns?
    1. Leathery, dry, hard skin
    2. Red, fluid-filled vesicles
    3. Massive edema at the injury site
    4. Serous exudates from a shiny, dark-brown wound

14. Prioritize the emergency management of a burn, from highest to lowest priority, with 1 as the highest priority.
    ____ 1. Establish and maintain an airway
    ____ 2. Assess for associated injuries
    ____ 3. Establish an IV line with a large-gauge needle
    ____ 4. Remove the client from the burn source

15. Using an open method of skin care, which of the following should the nurse include when caring for a client with deep partial-thickness burns of both legs?
    1. Ensure that sterile water is used in the debridement tank
    2. Apply topical silver sulfadiazine (Silvadene) with clean gloves
    3. Use clean gloves to remove the dressings and wash the wounds
    4. Wear a cap, mask, gown, and gloves when caring for the client

16. The nurse notifies the physician that a client who is 12 hours postburn has abdominal distention and faint, intermittent bowel sounds. Which of the following should the nurse perform?
    1. Withhold oral intake except water
    2. Insert a nasogastric tube
    3. Administer a histamine-blocking medication
    4. Reposition the client in preparation for an enema

17. The nurse is caring for a client with a burn injury who has a nursing diagnosis of impaired physical mobility related to limited range of motion secondary to pain. Which of the following is the priority nursing intervention for this client?
    1. Encourage the client to perform range-of-motion exercises in the absence of pain
    2. Instruct the client on the importance of exercise to prevent contractures
    3. Provide an analgesic medication before physical activity and exercise
    4. Arrange for the physical therapist to increase activity during hydrotherapy

18. Which of the following statements by a client who received instructions on pain control prior to a dressing change indicates the instructions were understood?
    1. "I will ask for my midazolam (Versed) 1 hour before the dressing change."

2. "I will ask for acetaminophen (Tylenol) 2 hours before my dressing change."
3. "I will put on my favorite music to take my mind off my pain."
4. "I will ask the nurse for IV morphine 5 minutes before my dressing change."

19. The client who has burns on the face, neck, and chest asks why a pressure garment must be worn so many hours a day prior to dressing changes. Which of the following statements by the nurse provides the most accurate explanation?
    1. "The pressure garment protects your skin from sunlight and further damage."
    2. "It provides support and splinting to keep your body in alignment."
    3. "It reduces the thickness of the scar tissue."
    4. "The pressure garment helps trap the oils in your skin."

20. The nurse is planning to debride and remove scales and crusts of skin lesions to the left leg of a client. Which of the following is a priority intervention for this client?
    1. Cool oatmeal bath
    2. Warm saline dressings
    3. Cool sodium bicarbonate bath
    4. Warm magnesium sulfate dressings

21. A client with chronic skin lesions on the face and arms admits to the nurse of being unable to look in the mirror. Based on this information, which of the following nursing diagnoses would the nurse identify?
    1. Anxiety related to personal appearance
    2. Disturbed body image related to perception of unsightly lesions
    3. Social isolation related to poor self-image
    4. Deficient knowledge related to lack of understanding of use of cover-up techniques

22. The nurse is caring for a client with full-thickness burns who is receiving fluid replacement. Which of the following would indicate to the nurse that the client's condition is deteriorating?
    1. Systolic blood pressure (BP) of 86
    2. 30 to 50 ml/hr urine output
    3. Respiratory rate of 18/minute
    4. Pulse rate of 85

23. During the acute phase of a burn injury, the nurse assists a client with deep partial-thickness burns of the left arm to make which of the following menu choices that are most appropriate?
    Select all that apply:
    [ ] 1. Fried chicken
    [ ] 2. Turkey sandwich with lettuce and tomato
    [ ] 3. Barbecued pork on a roll
    [ ] 4. Mashed potatoes
    [ ] 5. Milkshake
    [ ] 6. Cola beverage

24. A client with psoriasis is being treated with psoralen plus UVA light phototherapy. During the course of therapy, the client is instructed to wear protective eyewear to block all UV rays. Which of the following statements by the client indicates a correct understanding of the teaching?
    1. "I should wear sunglasses continuously for 6 hours after taking the medication."
    2. "I should wear sunglasses until my pupils can constrict when exposed to light."
    3. "I will wear sunglasses for 12 hours after treatment to prevent retinal damage."
    4. "I should wear sunglasses for 24 hours following treatment when indoors near a bright window."

25. Which of the following assessments would provide the nurse with the most accurate information regarding a client in the emergent phase of burn care?
    Select all that apply:
    [ ] 1. Extreme thirst
    [ ] 2. Decreased pulse
    [ ] 3. Warm and flushed feeling
    [ ] 4. Decreased bowel sounds
    [ ] 5. Dehydration
    [ ] 6. Decreased blood pressure

26. A client with burns over the face, arms, and trunk is requesting pain medication. When intervening in this situation, the nurse should administer which of the following drugs of choice for pain control in burn management?
    1. Meperidine (Demerol)
    2. Morphine
    3. Oxycodone/aspirin (Percodan)
    4. Propoxyphene/acetaminophen (Darvocet)

27. In planning the care for a severely burned client, the nurse should select which of the following as the priority nursing diagnosis?
    1. Pain related to burn injury and treatments
    2. Impaired physical mobility related to contractures
    3. Risk for deficient fluid volume related to a fluid shift, evaporation, and plasma loss
    4. Imbalanced nutrition: less than body requirements related to the body's need for an increased calorie intake

28. The nurse implements which of the following nursing measures as preventing dilutional hyponatremia in a client with burns?
    1. Instruct the client on the sodium content in foods

2. Administer a diuretic

3. Encourage the client to drink fluids other than water

4. Encourage the client to exercise vigorously

29. Which of the following nursing interventions should the nurse include in the rehabilitative phase of burn care?
   1. Establish and maintain a patent airway
   2. Insert two large-bore catheters percutaneously
   3. Administer range-of-motion exercises

4. Use Parkland formula to calculate fluid requirement

30. Which of the following nursing tasks should the nurse delegate to unlicensed assistive personnel?
   1. Remove a dressing on a skin tear of a client's leg
   2. Advise a client with acne to use water-based cosmetics
   3. Assist with bathing of a client with a burn
   4. Encourage a client with acne rosacea to verbalize feelings

ANSWERS AND RATIONALES

1. 4. A licensed practical nurse may not instruct, develop a teaching plan, or obtain a health history. Those are activities reserved for the registered nurse. A licensed practical nurse may monitor the vital signs of a client with cellulitis for evidence of sepsis. A licensed practical nurse is trained to monitor vital signs for deviations from normal and then report those changes to a registered nurse.

2. 4. Skin self-examination includes the entire body, looking for any changes in skin color as well as changes in moles. Although evaluating the evenness of skin color, moisture, and temperature is an appropriate intervention, it is limited in its focus to two insignificant characteristics of skin moisture and temperature. These do not change with development of skin cancer. Inspecting moles is also an important part of a skin examination, but limits the skin assessment to moles only and negates the rest of the assessment. Performing a skin examination is an ongoing assessment and not just something that begins after age 40.

3. 2. More information is needed about the lesion to help determine an appropriate course of action. The findings do not require immediate attention from the physician. It is inappropriate to determine a plan of action without completing a thorough assessment. Determining what the client has been doing to treat the lesion only gathers part of the data needed to determine a plan of action.

4. 1. Emollients seal in water and hydrate the skin. Emollients do not affect the blood vessels. The emollient is not in contact with the subcutaneous tissue. The primary function of an emollient is to rehydrate the skin. Intact skin is the best defense against irritation.

5. 2. Use of a nonadherent dressing is the most helpful in treatment of skin tears. A transparent dressing causes maceration of the skin and may cause further skin trauma with removal. A diet high in fat does not help with healing. A diet high in protein and vitamin C is more likely to help healing. The primary treatment of skin tears is protecting them from further trauma so they can heal.

6. 4. Fabric softeners often contain chemicals or components that are irritants for those with atopic dermatitis. Dermatitis is not a contagious condition, so using separate towels is not necessary. Avoidance of certain foods in treating atopic dermatitis is controversial. It is recommended that only known allergens be avoided. The sun is not a trigger for atopic dermatitis.

7. 3. Because methotrexate is associated with chromosomal abnormalities, both men and women must use highly effective birth control during therapy. Methotrexate may be used in clients with very severe disease who have been unresponsive to other therapies, regardless of age. The appropriate lab work to monitor when a client is taking methotrexate includes blood chemistry and liver and renal function studies. Methotrexate is only used when all other treatment options fail.

8. 1. 4. Spicy foods, hot and cold drinks with caffeine, and alcohol all worsen acne rosacea. Foods rich in omega-3 fatty acids, chocolate, fried foods, and products containing phenylalanine are unrelated to controlling rosacea.

9. 2. Risk factors for the development of pressure sores include bony prominences, inability to change position independently, and a bed-rest status. These factors pose the highest risk for the client.

10. 1. People who have not had chickenpox may get it from exposure to those with herpes zoster. Cool baths, although soothing, do not speed up the healing process. Topical diphenhydramine is useful for itching but will not accelerate the healing process. The use of fabric softener is unrelated to herpes zoster.

11. 4. Assessment of the skin of those with naturally darker pigmentation should be done in an area where the epidermis is thin or in areas of least pigmentation, such as the nail beds or oral mucosa. The soles of the feet and palms of the hands are the second best options. It would not be appropriate to inspect the conjunctiva or sclera of an African-American client for skin color because of the possibility of yellowing.

12. 1. Limiting exposure to the sun is the most important preventive measure in reducing the risk of developing skin cancer and premature aging. Radiation and alkaline soaps are less common causes of skin problems. Overexposure to vitamin E does not cause skin problems.

13. 1. A burn that has leathery, dry, and hard skin describes a full-thickness burn in the emergent phase. A burn that is a red, fluid-filled vesicle with massive edema at the injury site describes a deep partial-thickness burn during the emergent phase. Serous exudate from a shiny, dark-brown wound describes a partial-thickness burn in the acute phase.

14. 4. 1. 3. 2. It is a priority to remove a client from the burning source, followed by establishing and maintaining an airway. Establishing an IV line with a large-gauge needle and assessing for associated injuries would follow in priority.

15. 2. The open method requires cleansing the wounds, applying a topical antimicrobial, and leaving the wounds open to air. Either saline or an electrolyte solution is best to use in the debridement tank. It would be inappropriate to use the open method with a partial-thickness burn because there are no dressings in place.

16. 2. Paralytic ileus is common in the postburn phase and is best treated with a nasogastric tube to suction for decompression. All oral intake should be withheld. Administering a histamine-blocking medication will not improve peristalsis, although it may be given to reduce the possibility of aspirating acidic stomach contents. It would not be appropriate to prepare the client at this time for administration of an enema. Once there is evidence of peristalsis (bowel sounds are present, the client passes flatus), an enema may be administered.

17. 3. Control of pain is crucial before clients will participate in their prescribed exercise routine.

This is best facilitated by administering an analgesic medication before physical activity. Controlling the pain should be followed by encouraging range of motion and instructing the client on the importance of exercise to prevent contractures. Arranging for a client to see a physical therapist does not address pain control. In fact, most burn patients find hydrotherapy to be very painful because of the debridement that must occur at that time.

18. 4. Pain control in a burn injury includes administering IV morphine just prior to the dressing change. Midazolam (Versed) is a good drug for pain control but it must be administered too far in advance to be of maximal benefit. Acetaminophen (Tylenol) is not an adequate analgesic for pain associated with full-thickness burns. Listening to music may be a good adjunct therapy to medication to control pain prior to a dressing change for a burn, but it is usually not enough by itself to control a client's pain.

19. 3. Pressure garments flatten scar tissue, giving the client more mobility and resulting in a better cosmetic appearance. Wearing a pressure dressing does protect the site from further injury, but this is not the major reason for wearing a pressure garment. Wearing a pressure dressing does not support or splint the body part, nor does it trap the oils in the skin.

20. 2. Debridement is best accomplished using a warm solution. Saline is the best choice. A cool oatmeal or sodium bicarbonate bath is best used for pruritus. Magnesium sulfate will not be helpful for the person with scaly and crusty skin.

21. 2. Defining characteristics for disturbed body image include verbalization of self-disgust and inability to look at oneself in the mirror. Anxiety would be an appropriate nursing diagnosis only if the client verbalizes or demonstrates anxiety related to appearance. Social isolation or deficient knowledge would be an appropriate diagnosis only if the client verbalizes these as problems.

22. 1. A decrease in the systolic blood pressure to less than 90 mm Hg indicates evaporation, plasma loss, and a fluid shift into the interstitium secondary to the burn injury. A urinary output of between 30 and 50 ml per hour, respiration rate of 18, and a pulse rate of 85 are all considered normal.

23. 2. 4. 5. A turkey sandwich with lettuce and tomato, mashed potatoes, and a milkshake provide the highest-quality protein with the best representation of food groups for a client who has a partial-thickness burn of one arm. It is also manageable by a client who has only one hand that is usable. Fried chicken is high in fat,

and barbecued pork is spicy and may not be tolerated well. A cola beverage, although high in calories, is void of nutrients.

24. 4. Psoralen is absorbed by the lens of the eye, so protective eyewear must be used for 24 hours after taking the medication. Because UVA penetrates glass, the sunglasses must also be worn inside.

25. 1. 4. 6. The emergent phase of a burn injury is also called the resuscitative phase. It begins with the onset of the burn and generally lasts 1 to 2 days but may continue for approximately 5 days. Initially there is fluid loss and the presence of edema. It continues until diuresis begins. The client will exhibit thirst and chilling due to fluid and heat loss. Decreased bowel sounds or even absent bowel sounds may be present from an adynamic ileus resulting from trauma or a potassium shift. Signs of hypovolemic shock would include decreased blood pressure and increased pulse.

26. 2. Morphine sulfate is the drug of choice in the treatment of burns. Meperidine (Demerol) may also be used but is not the drug of choice. Oxycodone/aspirin (Percodan) and propoxyphene/acetaminophen (Darvocet) are not strong enough drugs to provide adequate pain relief.

27. 3. The priority nursing diagnosis for a client with burns is risk for deficient fluid volume related to a fluid shift, evaporation, and plasma loss.

28. 3. The client is encouraged to drink fluids other than water as a means of preventing dilutional hyponatremia, also known as water intoxication. Fluids rich in electrolytes and calories are offered.

29. 3. Administering range-of-motion exercises is an appropriate intervention for the rehabilitative phase of burn care. Establishing and maintaining a patent airway, inserting two large-bore catheters percutaneously, and using the Parkland formula to calculate fluid requirement are interventions reserved for the emergent and acute phase of burn management.

30. 3. Removing a dressing, providing client instruction, and encouraging a client to verbalize feelings are all activities that require the skills of a qualified nurse. Although socialization is a skill that unlicensed assistive personnel may perform, encouraging a client to verbalize feelings is a skill that requires the expertise of the nurse in assisting the client to deal with the expressed feelings. Unlicensed assistive personnel may assist with the bathing of a client who sustained a burn.

REFERENCES

Daniels, R. (2010). *Delmar's manual of laboratory and diagnostic tests* (2nd ed.). Clifton Park, NY: Delmar Cengage Learning.

Daniels, R., & Nicoll, L. (2012). *Contemporary medical-surgical nursing.* Clifton Park, NY: Delmar Cengage Learning.

DeLaune, S. C., & Ladner, P. K. (2011). *Fundamentals of nursing: Standard and practice* (4th ed.). Clifton Park, NY: Delmar Cengage Learning.

Estes, M. (2010). *Health assessment and physical examination* (4th ed.). Clifton Park, NY: Delmar Cengage Leaning.

Spratto, G. R., & Woods, A. L. (2012). *PDR nurse's drug handbook 2012.* Clifton Park, NY: Delmar Cengage Learning.

CHAPTER 9

MUSCULOSKELETAL DISORDERS

I. ANATOMY AND PHYSIOLOGY

A. FUNCTIONS OF THE MUSCULOSKELETAL SYSTEM
  1. HOLDS THE SKELETON TOGETHER
  2. GIVES THE BODY SHAPE
  3. ALLOWS THE BODY TO MOVE
  4. BREAKS DOWN CALCIUM
  5. ASSISTS IN THE METABOLISM PROCESS
  6. MAKES RED BLOOD CELLS

B. BONE (SEE FIGURE 9-1)
  1. THE HUMAN SKELETON HAS 206 BONES.
  2. WHEN SKELETON FIRST FORMS, IT IS MADE OF FLEXIBLE CARTILAGE.
  3. OSSIFICATION (THE PROCESS OF CHANGING FLEXIBLE CARTILAGE INTO CALCIUM AND COLLAGEN) TAKES ABOUT 20 YEARS TO COMPLETE.
  4. ABOUT 70% OF ADULT BONE IS COMPOSED OF MINERALS; REMAINING 30% IS ORGANIC MATTER (MAINLY COLLAGEN).
  5. IN ADULTS, THERE ARE TWO FORMS OF BONE: COMPACT AND CANCELLOUS.
    a. Compact bone (hard outside) is solid, looks like ivory, and is very strong, with holes and channels running through it carrying blood vessels and nerves.
    b. Cancellous bone (inside compact bone) looks like sponge and is made up of a meshlike network of tiny pieces of bone called trabeculae.
  6. SPACES IN TRABECULAE ARE FILLED WITH RED MARROW (FOUND MAINLY AT BONE ENDS) AND YELLOW MARROW (MOSTLY FAT).
  7. CHILD BONE IS SMALLER THAN ADULT BONE AND CONTAINS "GROWING ZONES" CALLED GROWTH PLATES.
  8. GROWTH PLATES ARE COLUMNS OF MULTIPLYING CARTILAGE CELLS THAT GROW IN LENGTH AND THEN CHANGE INTO BONE.
  9. BONE BUILDING CONTINUES THROUGHOUT LIFE AS THE BODY CONSTANTLY RENEWS THE BONES' LIVING TISSUE.
  10. IN CHILDREN, APPROXIMATELY 3% OF BONE IS BROKEN DOWN AND REBUILT EACH YEAR.
  11. ADULT BONE TURNOVER IS MUCH SLOWER THAN CHILDREN'S.
  12. BONE CONTAINS THREE TYPES OF CELLS: OSTEOBLASTS, OSTEOCYTES, AND OSTEOCLASTS.
    a. Osteoblasts make new bone and help repair damaged bone.
    b. Osteocytes carry nutrients and waste products from blood vessels in bone.
    c. Osteoclasts break down bone and help to "sculpt" and shape it.
      1) Very active in children
      2) Work on remodeling bone during growth and as fractures heal

C. MUSCLE (SEE FIGURE 9-2)
  1. THERE ARE MORE THAN 650 MUSCLES (COMPRISE HALF OF A PERSON'S BODY WEIGHT).
  2. MUSCLES ARE CONNECTED TO BONES BY TENDONS.
  3. THERE ARE THREE DIFFERENT KINDS OF MUSCLES: SKELETAL, SMOOTH, AND CARDIAC.
  4. SKELETAL MUSCLES ARE ATTACHED TO BONE, MOSTLY IN THE LEGS, ARMS, ABDOMEN, CHEST, NECK, AND FACE.
    a. Called striated because fibers have horizontal stripes
    b. Contract (shorten or tighten) quickly and powerfully
    c. Tire easily and have to rest between workouts
    d. Size varies greatly depending on the job they do.
    e. Known as voluntary muscles because the person can control their movement
    f. Controlled by the brainstem

205

Figure 9-1 Anterior and posterior views of the adult human skeleton

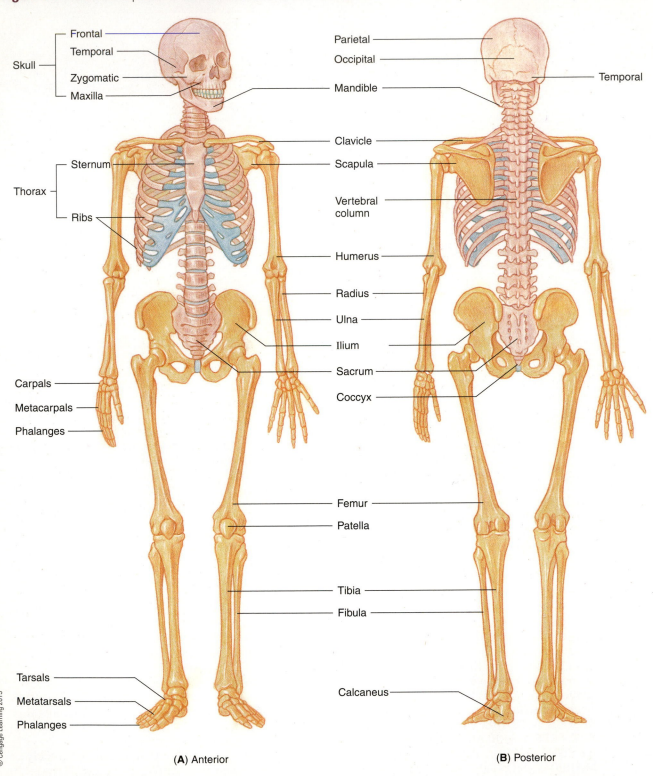

Skull
— Frontal
— Temporal
— Zygomatic
— Maxilla

Parietal
Occipital
Temporal

Mandible

Clavicle

Thorax
— Sternum
— Ribs

Scapula

Vertebral column

Humerus

Radius

Ulna

Ilium

Carpals

Sacrum

Metacarpals

Coccyx

Phalanges

Femur

Patella

Tibia

Fibula

Tarsals

Calcaneus

Metatarsals

Phalanges

© Cengage Learning 2015

(A) Anterior   **(B)** Posterior

g. Regulated by the cerebral motor cortex and cerebellum

5. SKELETAL MUSCLE FIBERS ARE DIFFERENT IN STRUCTURE OR FUNCTION.

6. DURING MOVEMENT, THE MOTOR CORTEX SENDS ELECTRICAL SIGNALS THROUGH THE SPINAL CORD AND PERIPHERAL NERVES TO THE MUSCLES (CONTRACTION OCCURS).

Figure 9-2 Muscular system: anterior and posterior views

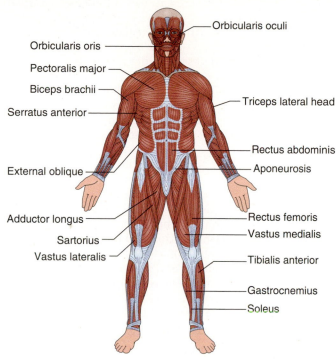

Orbicularis oculi
Orbicularis oris
Pectoralis major
Biceps brachii
Serratus anterior
Triceps lateral head
Rectus abdominis
Aponeurosis
External oblique
Adductor longus
Rectus femoris
Vastus medialis
Sartorius
Vastus lateralis
Tibialis anterior
Gastrocnemius
Soleus

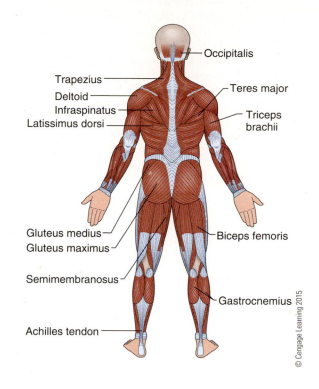

Occipitalis
Trapezius
Deltoid
Infraspinatus
Latissimus dorsi
Teres major
Triceps brachii
Gluteus medius
Gluteus maximus
Biceps femoris
Semimembranosus
Gastrocnemius
Achilles tendon

© Cengage Learning 2015

a. Motor cortex on the right side controls muscles on the left side of the body, and vice versa.
b. Cerebellum coordinates muscle movements ordered by the motor cortex.
c. Sensors in muscles and joints tell cerebellum and other parts of the brain where and how the arm or leg is moving and what position it is in (feedback results in smooth, coordinated motion).

7. MUSCLES MOVE BODY PARTS BY CONTRACTING AND THEN RELAXING.
8. MUSCLES PULL BONES BUT CANNOT PUSH THEM BACK TO THE ORIGINAL POSITION.
   a. Work in pairs of flexors and extensors.
   b. A flexor contracts to bend the limb at the joint (bring it closer to the body).
   c. When movement is completed, the flexor relaxes and the extensor contracts (extending or straightening the limb at the same joint).

D. TENDON
1. TOUGH, CORDLIKE TISSUES
2. ALLOW MUSCLES TO PULL ON BONES
3. NARROW BANDS ON TOP OF THE HANDS ARE TENDONS (PULLING ON FINGERS MAKE TENDONS MOVE).

E. LIGAMENT
1. LONG FIBROUS STRAPS THAT WRAP AROUND JOINTS
2. FASTEN BONES TO OTHER BONES

F. CONNECTIVE TISSUE
1. CARTILAGE: FLEXIBLE, RUBBERY SUBSTANCE THAT SUPPORTS BONES AND PROTECTS BONES WHEN RUBBING TOGETHER

G. JOINTS
1. JOINTS ARE CLASSIFIED BY HOW MUCH THE BONES THEY CONNECT WITH CAN MOVE AGAINST ONE ANOTHER AND IF THEY CONTAIN SYNOVIAL FLUID (LUBRICATES THE JOINT).
2. CARTILAGINOUS JOINTS ARE PARTIALLY MOVABLE (LINKED BY CARTILAGE, AS IN THE SPINE).
   a. Each vertebra in the spine moves in relation to the one above and below it.
   b. Together these movements give the spine flexibility.
3. THREE KINDS OF FREELY MOVABLE JOINTS THAT PLAY A BIG PART IN VOLUNTARY MOVEMENT ARE HINGE, PIVOT, AND BALL-AND-SOCKET JOINTS.
   a. Hinge joints allow movement in one direction, such as those in the knees and elbows.
   b. Pivot joints allow rotating motion, such as the side-to-side movement of the head.
   c. Ball-and-socket joints allow the greatest freedom of movement, such as those in the hips and shoulders, where the

spherical end of the long bone fits into the hollow of another bone.

4. SYNOVIAL JOINTS ARE FILLED WITH SYNOVIAL FLUID, WHICH ACTS AS A LUBRICANT FOR EASE OF JOINT MOVEMENT).

II. ASSESSMENT

A. HEALTH HISTORY
1. PAST HEALTH HISTORY (CHRONIC DISEASES, FRACTURES, GENETIC PROBLEMS, PSORIASIS)
2. MEDICATIONS (PAST, PRESENT, OVER THE COUNTER, HERBS, VITAMIN, MINERALS)
3. SURGERIES (NUMBER, TYPE, DATES, COMPLICATIONS)
4. USE OF ASSISTIVE DEVICES (TYPE OF DEVICE, WHEN PRESCRIBED, FOR WHAT REASON, WHO PRESCRIBED IT)
5. FAMILY HISTORY (SOME MUSCULOSKELETAL DISEASES ARE HEREDITARY)
6. PSYCHOSOCIAL AND LIFESTYLE HISTORY (OCCUPATION, RECREATION, ECONOMIC IMPACT, COPING MECHANISMS, LIVING ARRANGEMENTS)

B. PHYSICAL EXAMINATION
1. DISORDERS IN MUSCULOSKELETAL SYSTEM THAT AFFECT OTHER SYSTEMS
   a. Chest and vertebral fractures affect respiration.
   b. Infection of the bone may invade the bloodstream and spread systemically.
   c. Connective tissue disease may affect the heart.
   d. Fractures may injure adjacent organs.
2. DISORDERS IN OTHER SYSTEMS THAT AFFECT THE MUSCULOSKELETAL SYSTEM
   a. Psoriasis may be related to psoriatic arthritis.
   b. Nutrient deficits produced by disorders in gastrointestinal or hematologic systems may affect bone.
   c. Nervous system deficits in muscle control can lead to atrophy.
   d. Malignancies often metastasize to bone.
3. INSPECTION
   a. Bone and joints—inspect symmetry, size, movement, pain, swelling, and range of motion (ROM) of the extremities and the trunk.
      1) Assess newborns for developmental hip dysplasia (asymmetry of gluteal folds, abduction of legs, or shortening of femur).
      2) Assess children's:
         a) Ability to sit upright—normal to achieve this by 8 months in age
         b) Pronation of feet—common at ages 12–30 months
         c) Genu varun (bowleg)—normal for 1 year after learning to walk
         d) Lordosis (swayback)—common under 5 years old
      3) Assess older adults for:
         a) Speed and coordination—slower with decreased muscle tone and nerve conduction
         b) Fracture and compressed vertebrae—may be due to osteoporosis
         c) Osteoarthritis changes
         d) Surgical scars from joint replacement
   b. Muscles—inspect size, symmetry, contour, movement, contractures, fasciculations, tremors, color, and texture of overlying skin.
   c. Tendon and ligament—inspect movement and pain.
   d. Posture—inspect the front for symmetric shoulders, anterior iliac crests, trochanters, and knees for symmetry. From the back, inspect symmetry of scapulae, posterior iliac crests, and trochanters.
   e. Gait—inspect each phase of stance and swing, cadence (rhythm of gait), length of stride, posture during each phase, and swinging of arms.
4. AUSCULTATION—LISTEN FOR GRINDING OR RUBBING OF BONE ON BONE.
5. PALPATION
   a. Bone—assess for deformities, tenderness, or swelling, which may indicate fractures, neoplasms, or osteoporosis.
      1) Assess newborns'
         a) Clavicles for mass or crepitus, which may be the result of a fracture during delivery
         b) Arms and legs by holding the arms and legs out and letting go—normal if the newborn returns to the fetal position
         c) Muscle strength by holding the newborn lightly under the arms—normal if the newborn does not fall through your hands
      2) Assess older adults for:
         a) Muscle mass—may be decreased in older age
         b) Muscle strength, resistance to fatigue, reaction time—decreased in older age
         c) Tenderness of the joints, smoothness of movement, presence of nodules, active and

passive ROM, which may be measured with a goniometer to measure the angle of a joint in degrees

3) Assess muscle strength on a scale of 0% to 5%:

0 = 0% strength—complete paralysis

1 = 10% strength—no movement but contraction is palpable or visible

2 = 25% strength—full movement against gravity with support

3 = 50% strength—normal movement against gravity

4 = 75% strength—normal movement against gravity and against minimal resistance

5 = 100%—normal movement against gravity and against full resistance

4) Assess tonicity—tone of the muscle at rest should be firm, not atonic.

5) Assess flaccidity—weakness or laxness of the muscle

6) Assess spasticity—sudden involuntary muscle contraction

III. DIAGNOSTIC STUDIES

A. BONE X-RAY

1. DESCRIPTION: IDENTIFIES TEXTURE AND CONTOUR OF BONES. CLIENT STANDS ON THE FLOOR OR LIES ON A FLAT BED AND THE X-RAY IS TAKEN.

2. PREPROCEDURE

a. Remove any clothing with metallic devices from the area to be x-rayed.

3. POSTPROCEDURE

a. None

B. MAGNETIC RESONANCE IMAGING (MRI)

1. DESCRIPTION

a. Noninvasive technique using a magnetic field to view tissue

b. Clients with metal devices such as pacemakers and hip or knee prosthesis cannot have an MRI.

c. Contrast dye may be used in the procedure to view additional tissue.

d. Full body scan lasts 60 to 90 minutes.

2. PREPROCEDURE

a. Assess clothing for any metal devices.

b. Assess for allergy to dye if contrast is used.

c. Offer the client earplugs.

3. POSTPROCEDURE

a. None

C. BONE SCANS

1. DESCRIPTION: SCANNING OF DESIGNATED AREA AFTER RADIOACTIVE SUBSTANCE INJECTED TO IDENTIFY OSTEOLYTIC AND OSTEOBLAST ACTIVITY

2. PREPROCEDURE

a. Inject the radioactive substance 2–3 hours prior to the procedure so that the substance settles in the bone and is concentrated in areas where osteoblast activity is increased.

3. POSTPROCEDURE

a. Assess the client for allergic reaction.

D. ARTHROGRAPHY

1. DESCRIPTION: DYE IS INJECTED INTO A JOINT TO OUTLINE SOFT TISSUE DEFECTS, INTRA-ARTICULAR GROWTHS, AND ABNORMAL JOINT CONTOURS UNDER STRICT STERILE PROCEDURES.

2. PREPROCEDURE

a. Inform the client of the procedure.

3. POSTPROCEDURE

a. Assess the client for allergic reaction and signs of infection.

E. ARTHROSCOPY

1. DESCRIPTION: SURGICAL INSERTION OF ARTHROSCOPE INTO THE JOINT TO VISUALIZE JOINT SURFACES. ADDITIONAL SURGICAL PROCEDURES MAY BE PERFORMED, SUCH AS SHAVING BONE AND CARTILAGE, REPAIR OR REMOVE MENISCI, REPAIR LIGAMENT, REMOVE LOOSE BODIES, OR BIOPSY TISSUE.

2. PREPROCEDURE

a. Inform the client of the procedure such as performed in the operating room.

b. No eating or drinking 8 hours prior to the procedure

c. Instruct the client to have a responsible adult drive him home because local or general anesthesia is used.

3. POSTPROCEDURE

a. Activity level may be restricted.

b. Monitor for abnormal neurovascular changes such as paresthesia, muscle weakness, coolness, color changes, sluggish capillary refill, altered skin temperature, and clinical manifestation of infection.

c. If assistive device such as a crutch, cane, or walker is used, instruct the client on proper use and have the client return demonstrate.

d. Keep the sterile dressing dry.

e. Administer analgesic if prescribed.

f. Monitor the client for infection, bleeding, or nerve damage.

F. BLOOD TESTS (SEE TABLE 9-1)

G. URINE TESTS (SEE TABLE 9-2)

H. JOINT ASPIRATION

1. DESCRIPTION

a. Analysis of joint contents to find hemarthrosis (blood in the joint) or

Table 9-1 Blood Tests for the Musculoskeletal System

Serum Component	Normal Values	Reason for Test and Comments
Alkaline phosphate	30–85 IU/ml	• Liver and bone cancer • Elevated in fracture, osteomalacia, Paget's disease
Antinuclear antibodies (ANA) total (if positive types of ANA identified—anti-DNA, anti-Sm, etc.)	Less than 1:20	Elevated in lupus, rheumatoid arthritis, Sjogren's syndrome, liver disease, scleroderma, and other conditions
Antiphospholipid antibodies		
Aspartate aminotransferase (AST or SGOT) Alanine aminotransferase (ALT or SGPT)	5–40 units per liter 7–56 units per liter	• Liver function • Many medications are caustic to the liver.
Bleeding time	1–9 minutes	Anticoagulant therapy
Blood chemistry		
• Glucose • Blood urea nitrogen (BUN) • Creatinine • Sodium (Na) • Potassium (K) • Chloride (Cl)	• 65–110 mg/dl • 7–25 mg/dl • Less than 1.5 mg/dl • 135–147 mEq/L • 3.5–5.4 mEq/L • 96–109 mEq/L	• Steroids can increase glucose. • Kidney function; many medications are caustic to kidneys. • Kidney function; many medications are caustic to kidneys. • Gastrointestinal tract, kidney, and lung function • Calcium metabolism; medications may interfere with calcium metabolism.
Calcium	9–10.5 mg/dl	• Decreased in osteomalacia • Elevated in Paget's disease
Complement assay • C^3 • C^4	• Male: 80–180 mg/dl; female: 76–120 mg/dl • Male/female: 15–45 mg/dl	Decreased in rheumatoid arthritis, lupus
Complete blood count		
• Red blood cell (RBC) • White blood cell (WBC) • Hemoglobin (HgB) • Hematocrit (Hct) • Platelet (PLT)	• Male: 4.7–$6.1 \times 10^6/ml^3$; female: 4.2–$5.4 \times 10^6/ml^3$ • 4,000 to 10,000 cells per cubic milliliter • Male: 13–18 g/dl; female: 12–16 g/dl • Male: 45–52%; female: 37–48% • 150,000–400,000/UL	• Anemia, dietary deficiency • High WBC indicates infection; low may be due to medications. • Anemia, bleeding • Anemia, bleeding • High PLT indicates malignancy, blood diseases, or rheumatoid arthritis. Low PLT indicates blood diseases, infections, and as the result of certain medications.
C-reactive protein (CRP)	Less than 8 mg/ml	• Inflammation • Elevated in rheumatoid arthritis
Erythrocyte sedimentation rate (ESR)	• Male: up to 15 mm/hr • Female: up to 20 mm/hr • Children: up to 10 mm/hr • Older adults: up to 30 mm/hr	• Inflammation • Elevated in rheumatoid arthritis, osteoarthritis, lupus
HLA-B27	Genetic marker is present in the blood reported as either positive or negative.	• Distinguish spondyloarthropathies from other types of arthritis. • Positive in 90% of people with a spondylarthropathy diagnosis and 5–8% of the general population
Immunoglobulins (IgG)	13–23%	Elevated in rheumatoid arthritis, lupus
International normalized ratio (INR)	2–3 or 2.5–3.5 in clients on anticoagulant therapy	Coumadin anticoagulant therapy
Parathyroid hormone (PTH)	Less than 2000 pg/ml	Decreased in osteomalacia
Partial thromboplastin time (PTT)	60–70 seconds or 1.5 to 2.5 times control in clients on heparin	Heparin anticoagulant therapy
Phosphorus	3.0–4.5 ng/dl	• Medications can increase phosphorus levels (vitamin D) • Decreased in osteomalacia
Prothrombin time (PT)	11–12.5 seconds or 1.5 to 2.5 times control in clients on Coumadin	Coumadin anticoagulant therapy

Serum Component	Normal Values	Reason for Test and Comments
Rheumatoid factor	Less than 1:20	• Measurement of the reactive IgM antibodies • 80% of clients with rheumatoid arthritis have positive titers. • Lupus and Sjogren's syndrome may cause a low positive titer. • Heart disease, liver disease, mononucleosis, and other conditions may also cause a positive result.
Uric acid	Male: 4.5–6.5 mg/dl; female 2.5–5.5 mg/dl	Elevated in Paget's disease
25 Hydroxyvitamin	16–74 ng/ml	Elevated in osteomalacia

© Cengage Learning 2015

pyarthrosis (pus in joint) with examination of synovial fluid
    b. Also used to remove fluid within the joint
  2. PREPROCEDURE
    a. Inform the client of the procedure.
  3. POSTPROCEDURE
    a. Monitor the client for infection.

IV. NURSING DIAGNOSES
  A. RISK FOR PERIPHERAL NEUROVASCULAR DYSFUNCTION (FRACTURES)
  B. ACUTE PAIN
  C. RISK FOR IMPAIRED SKIN INTEGRITY
  D. IMPAIRED PHYSICAL MOBILITY
  E. INEFFECTIVE THERAPEUTIC REGIMEN MANAGEMENT

Nursing Diagnoses: Definitions and Classification 2012–2014. Copyright © 2012, 1994–2012 by NANDA International. Used by arrangement with John Wiley & Sons Limited.

V. MUSCULOSKELETAL EQUIPMENT
  A. CASTS AND SPLINTS
    1. DESCRIPTION
      a. Cast—made of synthetic material or plaster of paris, which circumferentially encases the affected body part
      b. Splint—made of synthetic material or plaster of paris, which supports one or both sides of the affected body part and is secured with straps or elastic bandage
    2. USES AND TYPES
      a. Used to immobilize or correct the affected part of the body
        1) Cast—absolute immobilization prescribed for deformity, trauma, or disorder
        2) Splint—immobilization

Table 9-2 Urine Tests for the Musculoskeletal System

Urine Component	Normal Values	Reason for Test
Calcium	2.5–7.5 mmol/day	Elevated in Paget's disease
Culture and sensitivity	Negative bacteria present	Assess musculoskeletal disease.
Hydroxyproline	120–470 mmol/24 hr	Elevated in Paget's disease
Uric acid	1.5–4.5 mmol/24 hr	Elevated in gout
Urinalysis	Negative	Assess musculoskeletal disease.
Acetone	Negative	
Albumin	Negative	
Bacteria	Negative	
Bilirubin	Rare	
Casts	Clear amber	
Color	Negative	
Glucose	Not strong	
Odor	4.6–8.0	
pH	2–3/HPF	
RBC	1.005–1.030	
Specific gravity	4–5/HPF	
WBC		

© Cengage Learning 2015

   b. Types
      1) Upper extremity—trimmed to permit thumb and index finger opposition such as a short arm, long arm cast or arm cylinder, or hanging arm splint
      2) Lower extremity—may be made ambulatory and includes short leg, long leg, leg cylinder, or hinge cast or splint
      3) Spica—incorporates part or all of the trunk and part or all of one or more extremities such as the shoulder, hip, or thumb
      4) Body—cover only the body trunk

3. CARE
   a. Instruct the client to avoid getting the cast wet, removing padding, inserting foreign objects, or covering with plastic for prolonged periods of time.
   b. Elevate the extremity above the level of the heart.
   c. Perform range-of-motion exercises above and below the cast as permitted.
   d. Inform the client to report any increased pain, burning, or tingling.
   e. Assess the surrounding skin for excoriated area or a foul odor.

4. COMPLICATIONS (SEE TABLE 9-3)

B. CRUTCHES
  1. DESCRIPTION: MECHANICAL AID USED TO ASSIST IN WALKING. CLIENT MUST BE MEASURED FOR ACCURATE FIT AND ASSESSED FOR STABILITY OF GAIT AND UPPER BODY STRENGTH TO ENSURE SAFETY.
  2. USES AND TYPES
   a. Axillary—used in a client with a stable gait with good upper body strength and balance; requires weight bearing with the hands
   b. Lofstrand—metal cuff around the forearm that stabilizes the wrist to make walking safer and easier; used when balance is decreased
   c. Platform—has a cuff for the upper arm and is used when balance is decreased; does not put weight on hands or wrists
  3. CARE
   a. Instruct the client that the weight of the body should be on the arms, not the axillae.
   b. Instruct the client to maintain an erect posture.
   c. Instruct the client to replace worn-out crutch tips and to avoid using crutch tips when wet.
   d. Instruct the client to wear shoes with a low heel.

4. COMPLICATIONS
   a. Injured radial nerve from pressure on the axillae
   b. Falls
   c. Hand blisters
   d. Fatigue
5. CRUTCH GAITS (SEE FIGURE 9-3)

C. CANES
  1. DESCRIPTION: MECHANICAL AID USED TO ASSIST WALKING.
  2. USES AND TYPES
   a. Standard straight leg—wooden is 36 inches long and aluminum is usually adjustable.
   b. Quad cane—has four legs and provides additional support when balance and/or upper body strength is decreased.
  3. CARE
   a. Instruct the client to hold the cane on the stronger side of the body.
   b. Position the tip of the cane 6 inches to the side and front of the foot then move the affected leg, or, if stronger, move the cane and affected leg at the same time. Move the unaffected leg last.
  4. COMPLICATIONS
   a. Falls

D. WALKERS
  1. DESCRIPTION: MECHANICAL AID TO ASSIST IN WALKING FOR CLIENTS WHO NEED MORE SUPPORT THAN A CANE
  2. USES AND TYPES
   a. Standard
     1) Most stable of all walkers—has four legs that are usually adjustable.
     2) Walker must be picked up to use.
   b. Four wheeled—least stable of all walkers; has four wheeled legs
   c. Two wheeled—more stable than a four-wheeled walker because it has only two wheeled legs
  3. CARE
   a. Instruct the client to move the walker and affected leg ahead 6 inches, then move the stronger leg ahead and repeat.
   b. Instruct the client that the arms should bear the weight in the second step after the affected leg is moved forward 6 inches.
  4. COMPLICATIONS
   a. Falls

E. TRACTION
  1. DESCRIPTION: APPLICATION OF A PULLING FORCE TO A PART OF THE BODY BY PULLEYS AND WEIGHTS TO CORRECT DEFORMITIES, IMPROVE JOINT CONTRACTURES, TREAT DISLOCATION, PROVIDE IMMOBILIZATION, TREAT DISEASE PROCESSES

Table 9-3 Complications of Casts

Complication	Type Cast/Splint/Traction	Signs/Symptoms	Treatment	Prevention
Peroneal nerve palsy	Lower extremity	Pain, tingling, paresthesia of the leg and foot Proper positioning Reapply cast/traction.	Passive dorsiflexion exercises and brace for ambulation Proper positioning during application	Observe for pressure on nerve.
Compartment syndrome	Upper and lower extremities	Pain with passive motion Pallor Pulselessness Paresthesia Pressure Paralysis	Relieve constriction with bivalve cast, cut padding/reapply cast/rewrap traction. Possible fasciotomy Detect early by reporting symptoms to the physician.	Proper positioning during application
Constrictive edema	All	Increased swelling Altered circulatory or neurologic status	Remove wrap and reapply loosely. Bivalve cast: cut padding and wrap. Elevate the extremity.	Proper positioning during cast application Do not wrap tightly. Assess for signs/symptoms. Elevate the extremity.
Constipation/impaction	All if on bed rest	Inconsistent/no bowel movements Alternating constipation and diarrhea (indicate impaction)	Alter/add to diet (e.g., juices, roughage) Laxative Enemas	Assess diet. Assess bowel movements. Individualized bowel program
Renal calculi (increased serum calcium due to resorption from bone)	All if on bed rest	Flank pain (constant or intermittent) Difficult urination Decreased urinary output	Notify the physician. X-ray Treatment by size/location	Increase fluids (3 L/day). Limit milk and milk products. Monitor intake and output.
Pressure area/ulcer	All	Reddened area Pain Irritability/restlessness Drainage through cast Temperature	Notify the physician. Bivalve cast Treatment depends on findings.	Proper application of cast/traction Maintain correct handling of cast/traction.
Pin infection	Casts/tractions with pins or wires	Erythema at the site Drainage or odor, or both Pin migration Temperature Pain	Antibiotics Pin removal in surgery if severe	Meticulous pin care Assess for infection.
Cranial nerve damage	Halo cast	Abnormal eye movements Pupil changes Blurred vision Diplopia Difficulty swallowing/control of tongue/speech	Depends on severity Continue to assess. Pin removal in surgery	Assess for signs/symptoms. Neurovascular checks
Superior mesenteric artery syndrome (cast syndrome)	Hip/spica cast	Nausea/vomiting Abdominal pain/fullness Shortness of breath	Nothing by mouth Intravenous fluids X-ray of abdomen	Assess symptoms. Document and notify the physician immediately.
Apprehension	Cast removal		Nasogastric suction Surgery to remove ischemic bowel	

© Cengage Learning 2015

Figure 9-3 Various crutch gaits

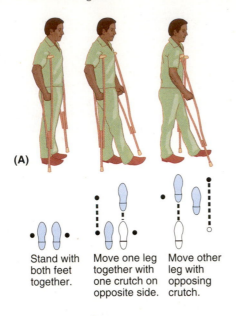

(A)

Stand with both feet together.

Move one leg together with one crutch on opposite side.

Move other leg with opposing crutch.

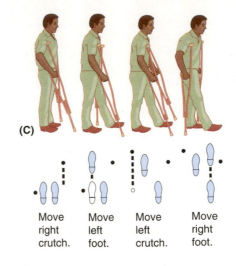

(C)

Move right crutch.

Move left foot.

Move left crutch.

Move right foot.

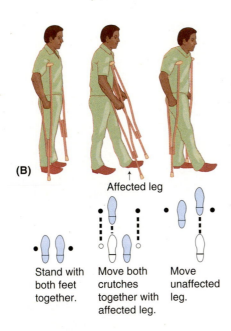

(B)

Affected leg

Stand with both feet together.

Move both crutches together with affected leg.

Move unaffected leg.

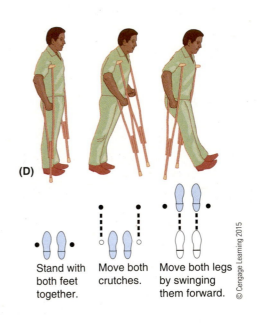

(D)

Stand with both feet together.

Move both crutches.

Move both legs by swinging them forward.

© Cengage Learning 2015

2. USES AND TYPES
   a. Skeletal
      1) Force applied directly to the bone by inserting pins, wires, or tongs into bone
      2) May have 40 lb of traction up to 8 weeks at a time
      3) Used to reduce fractures
   b. Manual
      1) Completed by the application of the hands of a health care worker
      2) Temporary form of traction until application of a cast to reduce a fracture

   c. Skin
      1) Usually 5 lb of traction is applied directly to the skin.
      2) May be used continuously or intermittently
   d. Traction type: upper extremity
      1) Dunlops (sidearm)
         a) Used to immobilize the arm to correct contractures or fractures
         b) Pull is outward.
         c) Elbow in flexion usually 90°
         d) May be skin or skeletal traction

2) Olecranon pin (overhead arm)
  a) Used to immobilize the arm to correct contractures or fractures
  b) Pull is upward.
  c) Elbow in flexion usually 90°
  d) May be skin or skeletal traction

e. Traction type: lower extremity
  1) Buck's (extension)
    a) Used to immobilize the leg to correct contractures of the knee and joint or a fracture of the hip or femoral shaft
    b) A form of skin traction
    c) Pull on the lower extremity with the knee and hip fully extended
  2) Russell
    a) Used to immobilize the leg, generally for a fracture of the femur or hip
    b) A form of skin traction
    c) Exerts pull on the lower extremity
  3) Balanced traction with Thomas ring splint and Pearson attachment
    a) Used to immobilize the leg to correct a fracture, generally of the femoral shaft of the femur, acetabulum, hip, or tibia
    b) Entire leg is supported with a ring placed at the groin of the affected leg to support the thigh off the bed.
    c) Skeletal type of traction

3. CARE
  a. Traction is attached to the bed frame.
  b. Trapeze should always be applied to the frame to assist the client with movement. This allows raising the buttocks off the bed for skin care.
  c. Ensure that ropes hang freely and there is no friction against the ropes.
  d. Maintain good body alignment—the client is positioned high in the bed so the feet do not press against the foot of the bed.
  e. Apply weights slowly to avoid jerking motion.
  f. Assess pressure points for skin breakdown and administer good skin care.
  g. Perform neurovascular checks.
  h. Avoid elevating the head of the bed greater than 25°—would promote migration of the client to the end of the bed.

4. COMPLICATIONS
  a. Major complications are listed in Table 9-3.

b. Additional complication of infection of the pin or wire with skeletal traction

F. FIXATORS
  1. DESCRIPTION: SURGICAL IMPLANTED DEVICES
  2. USES AND TYPES
    a. Internal fixation:
      1) To align and stabilize the fracture until healing occurs when closed techniques fail to reduce fracture
      2) Pins, wires, screws, screw and plate, rods are inserted into the bone.
    b. External fixation:
      1) At least two bars are placed horizontally under and above the fracture.
      2) Used for complex fractures with extensive soft tissue involvement, nonunion, bone grafting
      3) Midframes—used for hands and feet
      4) Large frames—used for tibia or pelvis
  3. CARE
    a. Instruct the client that meticulous pin care must be performed, usually with half-strength hydrogen peroxide and normal saline.
    b. Assess for infection, pin loosening, and proper alignment with x-ray.
  4. COMPLICATIONS
    a. Anesthesia risks
    b. Infection
    c. Disruption of blood supply
    d. Device failure

VI. MUSCULOSKELETAL PROBLEMS AND DISEASES
  A. SPRAINS
    1. DESCRIPTION
      a. Most common type of injury to the musculoskeletal system
      b. Injury to ligamentous structures surrounding a joint
      c. Etiology—wrenching or twisting motion; common areas—ankles and wrists
      d. Classification according to the number of ligament fibers torn:
        1) First degree—few torn
        2) Second degree—partial disruption
        3) Third degree—complete tearing of the ligament
      e. Complications from severe sprain:
        1) Avulsion fracture (the ligament pulls loose a fragment of the bone)
        2) Unstable joint structure, leading to subluxation or dislocation
        3) Hemarthrosis (bleeding in the joint space)
        4) Disruption of the synovial lining

2. ASSESSMENT
   a. First degree—there is mild tenderness and slight swelling.
   b. Second degree—there is more swelling and tenderness.
   c. Third degree—a gap in the muscle may be apparent or felt through the skin if the muscle is torn (extremely painful due to the exposed nerve endings).
3. DIAGNOSTIC TESTS
   a. X-ray to rule out fracture
4. NURSING INTERVENTIONS
   a. Encourage rest and limit movement.
   b. Apply ice to the affected area 20–30 minutes with breaks of 10–15 minutes during the acute phase, generally during the first 24–48 hours after injury.
      1) Cold therapy is used in the acute phase of most musculoskeletal injuries.
      2) Vasoconstriction and the reduction of nerve impulses occur with cold therapy, which provides analgesia and reduced muscle spasms, edema, inflammation, and local metabolic requirements.
   c. Apply warm, moist heat intermittently 20–30 minutes to reduce swelling and provide comfort after the acute phase has passed.
   d. Apply compression of the affected extremity for periods of 30 minutes followed by removing it for 15-minute intervals.
   e. Elevate the affected extremity.
   f. Administer analgesia and muscle relaxants as prescribed.
   g. Administer nonsteroidal anti-inflammatory drugs to decrease pain and edema.
5. SURGICAL MANAGEMENT
   a. May be necessary if disruption of the ligament or muscle structure, fracture, or dislocation occurs
B. STRAINS
   1. DESCRIPTION
      a. Stretching of the muscle and its fascial sheath
      b. Acute strain can result in partial or complete rupture of the muscle
      c. Minor strains are self-limiting and resolve in 3–6 weeks.
      d. Complications from severe strain: partial or complete rupture of the muscle
   2. ASSESSMENT
      a. Pain
      b. Edema
      c. Decreased function
      d. Bruising

3. DIAGNOSTIC TESTS
   a. X-ray to rule out fracture
4. NURSING INTERVENTIONS
   a. See the nursing interventions for sprains
5. SURGICAL MANAGEMENT
   a. See the surgical management for sprains
C. CARPAL TUNNEL SYNDROME
   1. DESCRIPTION
      a. Form of repetitive stress injury
      b. Characterized by progressive compression of median nerve caused by narrowing of the carpal tunnel in the wrist through overuse
      c. Normally seen in women aged 30 to 60; is a serious occupational health problem
      d. Complications—if untreated, partial paralysis, sensory disturbances, atrophy of the muscles of the palm and first three fingers
   2. ASSESSMENT
      a. Numbness
      b. Paresthesia
      c. Pain of the hand and fingers progressing up the arm in time
      d. Inability to clench the fist
      e. May be decreased strength and flexibility of the thumb
      f. Clinical manifestations generally increased at night and in the morning
      g. Temperature of the palm may be cold; palm may be discolored or chapped.
   3. DIAGNOSTIC TESTS
      a. X-ray to rule out fracture
      b. Electromyography
         1) Electrodes are placed at specific places along the median nerve to assess diminished nerve conduction of the electrical current.
         2) Delayed conduction of 5 milliseconds for positive diagnosis
      c. Phalen's wrist-flexion test
         1) Client places the elbow on the table, letting the wrist drop.
         2) Positive test is indicated when carpal tunnel syndrome occurs in the hand/fingers in 60 seconds or less.
      d. Tinel sign
         1) Percuss the median nerve at the wrist.
         2) Positive test is indicated when tingling occurs in the thumb/first three fingers.
      e. Compression test
         1) Blood pressure cuff is inflated above systolic pressure on the forearm for 1½ minutes.

2) Positive test is indicated when carpal tunnel syndrome is present after the 1½ minutes.

4. NURSING INTERVENTIONS
   a. Immobilize the affected area using a splint for 1–2 weeks.
   b. Apply compression of the affected wrist.
   c. Administer analgesia or muscle relaxants as prescribed.
   d. Administer nonsteroidal anti-inflammatory drugs to decrease pain.
   e. Instruct the client who has a surgical repair that no heavy lifting or direct pressure on the palm is permitted for 2–3 weeks.

5. SURGICAL MANAGEMENT
   a. Decompression is achieved by resecting the carpal ligament and may need synovectomy or removal of the synovium.

D. BLUNT INJURY—MINOR SOFT TISSUE INJURY
   1. DESCRIPTION
      a. Generally results from a fall
      b. Etiologies include hemorrhage into subcutaneous, adipose, or muscle tissue.
      c. Usually self-limiting through absorption of the excess fluid
   2. ASSESSMENT
      a. The area is swollen and painful, with limited movement.
      b. The skin usually remains intact.
   3. DIAGNOSTIC TESTS
      a. X-ray to rule out fracture
      b. Arthrocentesis, which would indicate sanguineous or bloody fluid if the test is positive
   4. NURSING INTERVENTIONS
      a. See the nursing interventions for sprain (page 216).
   5. SURGICAL MANAGEMENT
      a. Generally none

E. DISLOCATION
   1. DESCRIPTION
      a. Severe injury, generally a trauma to ligaments surrounding a joint resulting in complete displacement of articular surfaces of the joint
      b. Usually joints—thumb, elbow, shoulder, hip, patella
      c. Etiology can also be congenital deformity or pathologic manifestation.
      d. Complications—open joint injuries, intra-articular fractures, avascular necrosis (bone cell death), damage to neurovascular tissues, repeat dislocations to affected joint

2. ASSESSMENT
   a. Asymmetry such as shorter on the affected side
   b. Pain
   c. Tenderness
   d. Functional loss
   e. Edema
3. DIAGNOSTIC TESTS
   a. X-ray to determine amount the joint shifted
   b. Aspiration to assess for the presence of hemarthrosis or fat cells, which may indicate intra-articular fracture
4. NURSING INTERVENTIONS
   a. Instruct the client that realignment is performed by closed or open reduction.
   b. Facilitate immobilization and protection of the affected part.
   c. Administer prescribed analgesia to relieve pain.
   d. Perform gentle range-of-motion exercises to avoid contractures if the joint is stable and supported.
   e. Perform a complete neurological assessment, which is crucial in this injury to assess for avascular necrosis.
      1) Assess circulation, movement, and sensation (CMS) every 15 to 30 minutes for several hours, then every 3 to 4 hours.
      2) Assess the 5 Ps.
         a) Pain
         b) Pallor
         c) Paresthesia
         d) Puffiness
         e) Pulselessness
5. SURGICAL MANAGEMENT
   a. Immediate realignment by closed or open reduction

F. SUBLUXATION
   1. DESCRIPTION
      a. Injury to the joint surfaces resulting in an incomplete dislocation of a joint, most generally the thumb, elbow, shoulder, hip, patella
      b. Etiology can also be congenital deformity or pathologic manifestation.
      c. Complications
         1) Open joint injuries
         2) Intra-articular fractures
         3) Avascular necrosis or bone cell death
         4) Damage to neurovascular tissues
         5) Repeat dislocations to the affected joint
   2. ASSESSMENT
      a. Similar to dislocation but less severe
      b. Asymmetry on the affected side
      c. Pain
      d. Tenderness

e. Functional loss

f. Swelling

3. DIAGNOSTIC TESTS

a. X-ray to determine amount the joint shifted

b. Aspiration to assess for presence of hemarthrosis or fat cells, which would indicate intra-articular fracture

4. NURSING INTERVENTIONS

a. Assist with realignment by closed or open reduction.

b. Maintain immobilization and protection of the affected part.

c. Administer prescribed analgesia to relieve pain.

d. Perform gentle range-of-motion exercises to avoid contractures if the joint is stable and supported.

5. SURGICAL MANAGEMENT

a. Immediate realignment by closed or open reduction

G. FRACTURES

1. DESCRIPTION

a. Disruption or break in the bone structure, generally caused by a trauma

b. Highest incidence in young males 15 to 24 years; incidence in older adults is often associated with osteoporosis.

2. TYPES OF FRACTURES

a. Comminuted—shattered portion of the bone with two or more bone fragments

b. Displaced—sometimes referred to as an overriding fracture, in which a portion of bone is overriding another portion of bone

c. Greenstick—an incomplete fracture resulting in one side being splintered and the other side bent

d. Impacted—two or more bone fragments are forced into another portion of bone

e. Interarticular—fracture that extends to the articular surface

f. Longitudinal—fracture running along the longitudinal axis of the bone

g. Oblique—fracture extending in an oblique direction

h. Pathological—spontaneous fracture generally occurring at a site of bone disease

i. Spiral—fracture extending in a spiral direction along the shaft of the bone

j. Stress—occurs in either normal or abnormal bone in which there is stress on the bone

k. Transverse—fracture extending over the bone shaft at a right angle to the longitudinal axis

3. FRACTURE HEALING

a. Bone goes through remarkable reparative process of self-healing occurring in stages known as union.

b. Many factors influence the time required for fracture healing to be complete, such as age, initial displacement of the fracture, site of the fracture, and blood supply to the area.

c. Stages of healing:

1) Fracture hematoma—occurs in first 72 hours

2) Granulation tissue is formed from the hematoma.

3) Callus formation (an unorganized network of bone) occurs when important minerals such as calcium, phosphorus, and magnesium are present, indicating healing is occurring.

4) Ossification of the callus occurs in 3 to 6 weeks.

5) Consolidation occurs when the bone fragments meet.

6) Remodeling occurs when excess bone tissue is reabsorbed in the final stage of bone healing.

4. FRACTURES DESCRIBED AND CLASSIFIED ACCORDING TO:

a. Type, communication or noncommunication with the external environment

b. Location

c. Stability

1) Stable fracture—transverse, spiral, or greenstick

2) Unstable—comminuted or oblique

5. FRACTURES DESCRIBED ACCORDING TO LOCATION AND SPECIFIC CONSIDERATIONS:

a. Colles' fracture—fracture of the distal radius (ulna may be involved)

1) One of the most common fractures in adults

2) Frequently occurs in women over age 50 with osteoporosis

3) Assess for vascular insufficiency.

4) Usually managed by closed manipulation and immobilization

5) Sugar-tong splint or a long arm cast used for immobilization

6) Encourage active movement of the thumb, fingers, shoulder.

b. Humerus fracture:

1) Common injury among young and middle-aged adults

2) Major complications include radial nerve injury and vascular injury to the brachial artery as a result of laceration, transaction, or spasm.

3) Treatment is a hanging arm cast, shoulder immobilizer, sling, and swathe.

c. Pelvis fracture:
   1) The usual etiology is trauma.
   2) In older adults, etiology is osteoporosis or fall.
   3) High mortality rate
   4) Treatment depends on the severity of injury.
   5) Client is only turned in bed when specifically ordered by the health care provider.

d. Hip fracture:
   1) Common trauma in older adults
   2) More frequent in women than men older than 65 years because of osteoporosis
   3) Medical complications associated with fracture and immobility
   4) Clinical manifestations include external rotation, muscle spasm, shortening of the affected extremity, severe pain, and tenderness.
   5) Surgical repair is preferred and may include hardware insertion.
   6) May be treated with traction initially
   7) Postoperative management includes an abduction pillow.

e. Femoral shaft fracture:
   1) Common injury occurring particularly in young adults
   2) Severe direct force is required to produce this injury.
   3) Frequently causes damage to the adjacent soft tissue
   4) Frequently results in open fracture
   5) Surgical intervention may include hardware insertion.

f. Tibia fracture:
   1) Strong force required to produce this fracture
   2) Soft tissue damage and other complications occur due to the strong force.

g. Vertebral fracture—stable or unstable:
   1) Usual etiology is trauma or athletic injuries.
   2) Compression type of fracture is common.
   3) Log roll precautions
   4) Back brace is usual treatment.
   5) Surgical intervention may be required if unstable.

h. Maxillofacial fractures:
   1) Ensure patent airway and adequate ventilation.
   2) Artificial airway (tracheostomy) may be required.
   3) May also have a cervical spine injury (cervical collar)

6. FRACTURE COMPLICATIONS (SEE TABLE 9-3)
  a. Direct
    1) Alteration in union: delayed union, malunion, nonunion, and etiologies include:
      a) Inadequate immobilization
      b) Inadequate reduction
      c) Excess movement
      d) Infection
      e) Poor nutrition
      f) Age—healing time for fractures increases with age.
    2) Avascular necrosis—death of cells from no blood supply
    3) Osteomyelitis—bone infection
  b. Indirect
    1) Associated with blood vessel and nerve damage; etiologies include:
      a) Compartment syndrome—distal humerus and proximal tibia are the most frequent sites for this syndrome.
      b) Venous thrombosis
      c) Fat embolism
      d) Hypovolemic shock

7. ASSESSMENT
  a. Immediate localized pain
  b. Decreased function
  c. Inability to use the affected part
  d. Visible deformity, although a fracture may not be accompanied by obvious bone deformity.
  e. Ecchymosis
  f. Limited sensation distal to the site
  g. Crepitus or clicking sounds on movement

8. DIAGNOSTIC TESTS
  a. X-ray to confirm fracture
  b. Blood studies specific to the fracture
  c. Client-specific history

9. NURSING INTERVENTIONS
  a. Maintain anatomic realignment of bone fragments, known as reduction.
  b. Maintain immobilization to maintain realignment.
  c. Restore function of the injured part.
  d. Administer prescribed muscle relaxants or analgesics for pain and muscle spasms.
  e. Encourage a diet that is high protein, high calorie, high fiber (protein = 1 g/kg of body weight: calories = 1500 or more per day depending on individual needs).
  f. Encourage vitamins B, C, and D.
  g. Ensure an adequate intake of calcium (immobility and callus formation increases calcium needs).
  h. Increase fluid intake to 2000–3000 ml per day to promote bowel and bladder

function and prevent constipation or renal calculi.

   i. Administer prescribed stool softeners such as docusate sodium (Colace) to prevent constipation.

   j. Apply a trapeze bar to the bed frame.

   k. Apply direct pressure if active bleeding occurs.

   l. Obtain a complete client history to rule out abuse.

  10. SURGICAL MANAGEMENT

   a. Immediate realignment of bones if possible

   b. An open reduction internal fixation (ORIF) of a fracture may be necessary when no other realignment method can be completed.

H. OSTEOMYELITIS

  1. DESCRIPTION

   a. Infection of bone by direct or indirect invasion of an organism

    1) Direct etiologies—open fracture or surgery

    2) Indirect etiologies—blood-borne infection from a distant site such as teeth, infected tonsils, diabetic ulcers, and furuncles

    3) Organisms responsible:

     a) Most common is *Staphylococcus aureus*

     b) *Streptococcus pyogenes*

     c) Pneumococcus species

     d) *Pseudomonas aeruginosa*

     e) *Escherichia coli*

     f) *Proteus vulgaris*

     g) *Pasturella multicida* (from cat and dog saliva)

   b. Children are most often affected.

    1) Occurs more often in boys

    2) Sites most seen include the femur, proximal tibia, humerus, and radius.

  2. ASSESSMENT

   a. Systemic and local signs of infection

   b. Sudden pain and tenderness in the affected bone

   c. Edema around the affected bone

   d. Restricted movement around the affected bone

  3. DIAGNOSTIC TESTS

   a. Blood studies such as white blood count (WBC) and erythrocyte sedimentation rate (ESR)

   b. Wound cultures to identify type of infection and determine proper treatment choice

   c. Bone or tissue biopsy to identify type of infection and determine proper treatment choice

   d. Bone scans to assist with diagnosis

   e. Magnetic resonance imaging (MRI) or computerized tomography (CT) scan to identify the extent of the infection, including any soft tissue involvement

  4. NURSING INTERVENTIONS

   a. Promote rest and support of the affected bone using sandbags, splints, and a cast.

   b. Administer antibiotics, possibly on a long-term basis. Provide immediate treatment with broad-spectrum antibiotics until the organism is identified.

   c. Administer prescribed analgesics.

   d. Hyperbaric oxygen therapy as appropriate (wound healing center)

   e. Irrigate wound with antiseptics and antibiotics.

  5. SURGICAL MANAGEMENT

   a. May include flaps, skin and bone grafting, removal of infected hardware; amputation only as a last resort

I. OSTEOPOROSIS

  1. DESCRIPTION

   a. Metabolic bone disorder where low bone mass and structural deterioration of bone tissue results in increased bone fragility

   b. More common in postmenopausal women

   c. Major etiology of fractures in postmenopausal women and older adults in general

   d. Estrogen levels help the body maintain strong bones, and these levels decrease after menopause.

   e. When bone density is decreased, as with osteoporosis, the fracture risk increases.

   f. One in two women and one in eight men over age 50 will have an osteoporotic-produced fracture in their lifetime.

   g. Complications include deformity, loss of height, fractures, or death.

  2. THREE FRACTURE LOCATIONS GENERALLY REFERRED TO AS OSTEOPOROSIS FRACTURES ARE THE HIP, SPINE, WRIST.

   a. Hip fractures:

    1) Most often related to a fall

    2) Generally occurs in the upper narrow part of the thigh closer to the pelvic bone

    3) Mobility issues may lead to serious complications in older adults.

   b. Spine compression fractures:

    1) Occur as the vertebrae collapse on each other

    2) Cause tremendous pain

3) Curving of the spine as the person loses height

c. Wrist fractures:

1) Generally occurs when a person is trying to break a fall

2) May be an early sign of decreased bone density

3. RISK FACTORS FOR WOMEN INCLUDE:

a. Consuming less calcium over the lifetime

b. Having less bone mass

c. Bone resorption increased at an earlier age in women and is accelerated after menopause

d. Pregnancy and breastfeeding decrease calcium reserves.

e. Living longer (osteoporosis risk increases with age)

4. RISK FACTORS FOR BOTH MEN AND WOMEN INCLUDE:

a. Being thin or "small boned"

b. Aging

c. Smoking

d. Alcohol use

e. Long-term use of corticosteroids, heparin, and anticonvulsants

f. Lack of exercise

g. Low intake of dietary calcium

h. Family history

i. Medical abnormalities such as thyroid disease, rheumatoid arthritis, problems that block intestinal absorption of calcium

j. Malnutrition

5. ASSESSMENT

a. Common sign is the outward-curved thoracic spine.

b. May have no clinical manifestations until fracture occurs or vertebrae collapse

c. If fracture occurs, there is:

1) Immediate localized pain

2) Decreased function

3) Inability to use the affected part

4) Deformity is a cardinal sign of fracture but fracture may not be accompanied by obvious bone deformity.

6. DIAGNOSTIC TESTS

a. Dual-energy x-ray absorptiometry (DEXA) scan

1) A special type of x-ray that measures bone density

2) Score is determined by the density of bone based on a 21-year-old's density score known as bone mineral density, or BMD.

b. Blood studies

1) Serum calcium, phosphorus, and parathyroid hormone should be normal (if decreased, suspect osteomalacia or thyroid disease).

2) Alkaline phosphate may be elevated if fracture is present (if decreased, suspect osteomalacia).

3) 25 Hydroxyvitamin D should be normal; if not, rule out osteomalacia.

7. NURSING INTERVENTIONS

a. Encourage proper nutrition.

b. Discourage alcohol and tobacco use.

c. Encourage calcium supplements (1000–1500 mg/day) and vitamin D (400–800 international units per day).

d. Encourage moderate exercise using weight bearing and strength training.

e. Administer drugs that may help to increase bone density, including:

1) Estrogen (hormone) replacement therapy (HRT)

2) Bisphosphonates—alendronate, raloxifene, etidronate, and calcitonin (see Chapter 6, musculoskeletal medications section, for details).

3) There are new indications that parathyroid hormone may help to increase bone density.

f. Apply supportive devices to assist in proper alignment and to protect hips.

8. SURGICAL MANAGEMENT

a. Hip arthroplasty

b. Fracture repair

c. Possible fusion of vertebrae

J. AMPUTATION

1. DESCRIPTION

a. Surgical removal of infected or partially amputated part

b. Etiologies of amputation include:

1) Osteomyelitis

2) Peripheral vascular disease

3) Atherosclerosis

4) Vascular changes related to diabetes mellitus

5) Traumatic injury

6) Hazardous occupations (seen more in men)

7) Bone cancer (osteogenic sarcoma)

8) Burn trauma (heat, extreme cold, electrical)

9) Congenital disorders

c. Complications:

1) Limb sensation and pain (phantom pain occurs in 80% of clients with an amputation)

2) Severe infection leading to another amputation with greater extremity loss

3) Wound dehiscence or the separation of previously joined

wound edges. Three contributing factors in dehiscence are:

a) Infection
b) Granulation tissue is not strong enough to withstand the force placed on the wound.
c) Obesity, which interferes with healing

4) Hip contractures—the most common contracture in a client with an amputation is a hip flexion contracture and can be avoided in three ways:

a) Restrict sitting in a chair to 30 minutes at a time.
b) Avoid elevating the residual limb on pillows.
c) Have the client lie on his abdomen with the hips extended at least 3 times a day for 30 minutes at a time.

5) Death from gangrene or systemic infection

2. ASSESSMENT
   a. Severely and unrepairably damaged limb
3. DIAGNOSTIC TESTS
   a. Blood studies—WBC increased with infection, RBC decreased with anemia; electrolytes—fluid and electrolyte balances
   b. Vascular studies to determine circulatory status such as arteriography and transcutaneous ultrasound
4. NURSING INTERVENTIONS
   a. Management of underlying etiology
   b. Implement appropriate preoperative and postoperative management.
   c. Administer prescribed analgesic and muscle relaxants.
   d. Assist with immediate or delayed prosthetic fitting.
   e. Assist with physical therapy for muscle strengthening and gait training.
   f. Assist with psychosocial issues related to body image disturbances and lifestyle changes.
5. SURGICAL MANAGEMENT
   a. Reserve extremity length and function.
   b. Remove all infected, pathologic, or ischemic tissue.

K. OSTEOMALACIA
   1. DESCRIPTION
      a. Metabolic bone disease
      b. A rare condition related to vitamin D deficiency, with adult bones resulting in soft bones from decalcification
      c. Known as rickets in children, in which the epiphyseal growth plates are still open
      d. Vitamin D is required for calcium to be absorbed in the intestines.
      e. Etiologies include:
         1) Lack of sunlight (exposure to ultraviolet rays)
         2) Malabsorption
         3) Extensive burns
         4) Chronic diarrhea
         5) Pregnancy
         6) Renal disease
         7) Certain medications
      f. Mineralization of bone increased, generally taking 10 days to 2–3 months
      g. Complications:
         1) If left untreated, fractures of vertebrae, ribs, long bones
         2) May be misdiagnosed as cancer or osteoporosis
   2. ASSESSMENT
      a. Skeletal pain, especially during walking
      b. Progressive muscle weakness
      c. Weight loss
      d. Progressive deformities of the spine and extremities
   3. DIAGNOSTIC TESTS
      a. Blood studies
         1) Serum calcium and phosphorus—decreased in the disease
         2) Serum alkaline phosphatase—increased in the disease
         3) 25 Hydroxyvitamin D—decreased in the disease
      b. X-rays to indicate extent of bone demineralization; however, extensive disease may be present without changes on x-ray noted.
   4. NURSING INTERVENTIONS
      a. Administer vitamin D to correct vitamin D deficiency.
      b. Administer calcium salts and phosphorus supplements.
      c. Encourage the client to include eggs, milk, fish, and vegetables in his diet.
      d. Encourage weight-bearing exercise such as walking.
      e. Encourage exposure to sunlight.

L. PAGET'S DISEASE (OSTEITIS DEFORMANS)
   1. DESCRIPTION
      a. Progressive metabolic bone disorder resulting in deformity related to increased bone resorption accompanied by abnormal regeneration
      b. Etiology is unknown but may be due to virus acquired 20 to 40 years prior to its onset.
      c. May have familial risk associated, such as 30% found in clients with family history

    d. Older adults are more susceptible (1 to 3 million in the United States have disease).

    e. Cultural considerations—seen more in European descent (not frequently seen in Asian and Scandinavian countries)

    f. Complications:

      1) Gout

      2) Hyperparathyroidism

      3) Renal stones

      4) Heart failure

      5) Osteogenic sarcoma

      6) If untreated, deafness or blindness

2. ASSESSMENT

    a. Asymptomatic in 80% of clients.

    b. Pain is usually in the lower back and extremities and nerves.

    c. Posture changes

    d. Bowing of long bones

    e. Enlarged skull

    f. Pathologic fractures

    g. Flushed warm skin

    h. Fatigue

3. DIAGNOSTIC TESTS

    a. Blood studies

      1) Serum alkaline phosphatase is elevated in disease.

      2) Serum calcium is normal or elevated in disease.

      3) Uric acid is elevated and may be misdiagnosed as primary gout.

    b. Urine studies

      1) Hydroxyproline—the greater the value, the greater the severity of the disease.

      2) Calcium is normal or elevated.

    c. X-ray—identifies increased bone resorption. Bone mass is increased and deformities, fractures, and arthritic changes may be present.

    d. MRI/CT scan—to detect sarcomas, changes in skull and spinal cord, and nerve compression

    e. Bone biopsy—if no other method detects disease

4. NURSING INTERVENTIONS

    a. Administer analgesics such as nonsteroidal anti-inflammatory drugs (generally the first choice) for pain relief.

    b. Administer suppressive drugs to reduce bone resorption such as Calcitonin, etidronate (Didronel), mithramycin (Mithracin), and biphosphonates.

    c. Administer heat.

    d. Implement massage therapy.

    e. Encourage exercise.

    f. Encourage orthotic device to support or immobilize.

    g. Provide information for Paget's Disease Foundation and Arthritis Foundation for support.

5. SURGICAL MANAGEMENT

    a. Partial or total arthroplasty may be necessary.

M. RHEUMATOID ARTHRITIS

1. DESCRIPTION

    a. Systemic chronic disease characterized by inflammation of the synovial joints leading to joint destruction

    b. Etiology unknown but some theories support the possibility of infection, autoimmunity, or genetic factors

    c. Affects women three times more than men

    d. Usually diagnosed between the ages of 20 to 55 years

    e. Onset may be slow and insidious.

    f. Complications include infections, osteoporosis, amyloidosis, carpal tunnel syndrome, and vasculitis.

2. FOUR STAGES OF THE DISEASE

    a. First stage—synovitis (joint inflammation and swelling)

    b. Second stage—pannus (inflammatory granulation tissue)

    c. Third stage—tough fibrous connective tissue

    d. Fourth stage—calcification of bone

3. CLASSIFICATION OF RHEUMATOID ARTHRITIS ACCORDING TO SEVERITY OF SEVEN CRITERIA

    a. Morning stiffness

    b. Three or more joints with observable tissue swelling

    c. At least one of the three or more joints involves the wrist.

    d. Symmetrical joints involved

    e. Subcutaneous nodules

    f. Abnormal rheumatoid factor blood study findings

    g. Typical rheumatoid arthritis radiologic findings

4. ASSESSMENT

    a. Tender and swollen joints

    b. Morning stiffness

    c. Fatigue

    d. Anorexia

    e. Weight loss

    f. Limited range of motion

    g. Signs of inflammation

    h. Subluxation

    i. Ulnar drift

    j. Swan-neck deformities

    k. Muscle wasting

l. Extra articular manifestations such as anemia, osteoporosis, or rheumatoid nodules

m. Clinical manifestations generally symmetrical See Table 9-4.

5. DIAGNOSTIC TESTS

    a. Blood studies (helpful but not diagnostic)

      1) ESR elevation

      2) Serum rheumatoid factor titer greater than 1:160

      3) Antinuclear antibody (ANA) and lupus cell test may be positive.

      4) Hemoglobin and hematocrit decreased in anemia

      5) WBC normal or slightly elevated

      6) Platelets elevated in active disease

      7) C-reactive protein usually elevated

      8) Immunoglobulins (IgG, IgA, IgB) usually elevated

    b. Arthrocentesis of synovial fluid

    c. White blood cell count and increased volume with decreased viscosity will be present in active disease.

    d. X-rays, in early stages, show joint swelling and osteoporosis. Later stages show joint space narrowing, bony erosions at articular margins, and eventual malalignment.

6. NURSING INTERVENTIONS

    a. Inform the client that the goal of treatment is to reduce inflammation and pain, maintain function and muscle strength, and prevent deformity.

    b. Administer prescribed drugs such as:

      1) Nonsteroidal anti-inflammatory drugs (NSAIDs; initial drug given)

      2) Disease-modifying antirheumatic drugs (DMARDs)

      3) Immunosuppressive agents

      4) Systemic corticosteroids

      5) Biologic agents

      6) Analgesics

      7) Antidepressants

      8) Intra-articular steroid injections

    c. Protect joints.

    d. Implement heat and cold therapy.

    e. Encourage a balance between exercise and rest.

    f. Promote physical comfort.

    g. Instruct the client on self-management.

    h. Promote a good body image with the client.

    i. Instruct the client on the use of assistive devices.

    j. Encourage a well-balanced diet and nutrition.

    k. Question the client about complementary and alternative therapies such as:

      1) Transcutaneous electrical nerve stimulation (TENS)

      2) Hypnosis

      3) Acupuncture

      4) Magnet therapy

      5) Imagery

      6) Music therapy

    l. Inform the client on the Arthritis Foundation as a support and information source (http://www.arthritis.org).

    m. Perform a psychosocial assessment on these clients—within 10 years, 50% of clients will lose their independence.

7. SURGICAL MANAGEMENT

    a. Used as a last resort when other therapies are ineffective

    b. Osteomy—bone is cut and realigned to reduce pain or correct deformity.

    c. Synovectomy—removal of the synovial membrane from the joint (can only be done if no cartilage or bone destruction has occurred)

    d. Arthrocentesis

    e. Arthroscopy—partial or total joint replacement

N. OSTEOARTHRITIS OR DEGENERATIVE JOINT DISEASE (DJD)

1. DESCRIPTION

    a. Most common type of arthritis that is a noninflammatory disease

    b. Prevalence increases with age but changes from osteoarthritis are different than those associated with the aging process.

    c. Begins with degeneration in the cartilage and progresses to:

      1) Loss of cartilage

      2) Joint malalignments

      3) Abnormal wear and tear

      4) Abnormal use of the tendons and ligaments

      5) Damage to the bone

    d. Etiologies include age, genetics, trauma, excessive repetitive stress, mechanical, and metabolic processes.

    e. Older adult considerations—almost everyone over 60 years old has some radiologic changes suggestive of DJD.

    f. Ethnic considerations:

      1) Native Americans, African Americans, and South African blacks are affected more than Caucasians.

      2) Hip DJD occurs less in Asian descent.

      3) Knee DJD is highest in African Americans.

    g. Women considerations:

1) After age 50, women have higher prevalence than men.

2) Usually have hand involvement and have more joints involved than men

2. ASSESSMENT

   a. Pain provoked by activity and stiffness by rest

   b. Degeneration of cartilage

   c. Osteophyte or spur formation

   d. Heberden's nodes can form on the distal interphalangeal joints.

   e. Bouchard's nodes form on the proximal joints.

   f. Asymmetrical joint involvement

   g. Inflammation is not a major part of DJD.

   h. There are no associated systemic features. See Table 9-4.

3. DIAGNOSTIC TESTS

   a. Blood studies—ESR is elevated if synovial inflammation is present.

   b. X-ray—can have joint space narrowing, bony sclerosis, osteophytes, and, in some cases subluxation.

     1) In the early stages, degenerative changes in cartilage and reactive new bone present

     2) In the late stages, loss of cartilage and bone hypertrophy present

   c. MRI—to detect bone changes in the spine

   d. Bone scan—can show early signs of DJD years before an x-ray

4. NURSING INTERVENTIONS

   a. Instruct the client to lose weight if overweight.

   b. Administer analgesics and muscle relaxants to relieve pain or muscle spasms.

     1) Initially, try topical agents and acetaminophen.

     2) If not controlled, second line of drug therapy consists of NSAIDs.

     3) Steroid injections may be used in a single joint.

     4) Opioid analgesics are not appropriate therapy due to the chronic nature of pain in DJD.

   c. Instruct the client on exercise to strengthen muscle, muscle tone, and joint range of motion.

   d. Instruct the client on assistive devices such as a cane, a walker, or crutches.

   e. Encourage the client to get adequate rest.

   f. Maintain proper positioning of the affected joint.

   g. Implement heat and cold therapy as appropriate.

     1) Heat is used unless the joint is severely inflamed.

     2) Hot showers, compresses, and moist heating pads

   h. Question the client on complementary and alternative therapies such as:

     1) Transcutaneous electrical nerve stimulation (TENS)

     2) Hypnosis

     3) Acupuncture

     4) Magnet therapy

     5) Imagery

     6) Music therapy

     7) Tai chi

     8) Therapeutic touch

     9) Dietary supplements such as cayenne pepper, gamma linolenic acid, glucosamine, chondroitin

   i. Inform the client on the Arthritis Foundation as a support and information source (http://www.arthritis.org).

5. SURGICAL MANAGEMENT

   a. Partial or total arthroplasty if conservative treatments are ineffective.

Table 9-4 Comparison of Rheumatoid Arthritis and Osteoarthritis

Variable	Rheumatoid Arthritis	Osteoarthritis
Age	Middle aged	> 40 years
Gender	Female > male	Same
Weight	Weight loss	Overweight
Illness	Systemic	Local
Joints	Symmetric	Asymmetric
Effusions	Common	Uncommon
Nodules	Rheumatoid	Heberden and Bouchard
Synovial	Inflammatory	Noninflammatory
X-rays	Osteoporosis, narrow space, erosions	Narrow space, osteophytes, subchondral cysts
Anemia	Common	Uncommon
Rheumatoid factor	Positive	Negative
Erythrocyte sedimentation rate (ESR)	Elevated	Normal

O. LUPUS ERYTHEMATOSUS (SLE)
   1. DESCRIPTION
      a. Clinical manifestations result from immune complex invasion of body systems.
      b. Etiology is unknown but there is some theory on the possibility of genetics, sex hormones, race, environmental factors, virus, infections, immunologic abnormalities, and stress.
      c. Pathogenesis—autoimmune reactions, lupus vasculitis, fibrinoid degeneration, and thrombus generation
      d. Women considerations—diagnosed in women between 15 and 40 years old (occurs up to 10 times more often in women)
      e. Cultural considerations—1 in 250 African-American women affected compared to 1 in 700 women of other ethnicities
      f. Complications—Multisystem involvement that includes the possibility of death
         1) Protein in the urine indicates renal failure.
         2) Lupus nephritis is the number one cause of death in SLE.
   2. ASSESSMENT
      a. Butterfly rash called erythematous rash
      b. Fever
      c. Unexplained weight loss
      d. Abdominal pain
      e. Arthralgias (aching muscles and joints)
      f. Excessive fatigue
      g. Cutaneous and muscle tissue involvement
      h. Organ involvement includes the lining of the lungs, heart, nervous tissue, and the kidneys.
      i. Alternating periods of remission and exacerbations
   3. DIAGNOSTIC TESTS
      a. Blood studies—ANA, anti-DNA, ESR, anti-Sm antibody, rheumatoid factor, serum complement (C3 and C4), immunoglobulin, antiphospholipid antibodies
         1) To assess multisystem involvement—CBC, electrolytes, renal function, cardiac and liver enzymes, and clotting factor
      b. Skin biopsy—skin is gently scraped and the cells viewed under a microscope.
         1) Presence of characteristic lupus cells and inflammatory cells confirm the diagnosis.
   4. NURSING INTERVENTIONS
      a. Administer prescribed drugs such as:
         1) Topical cortisone
         2) Plaquenil
         3) Corticosteroids
         4) Immunosuppressive agents (azathioprine, Imuran)
         5) Cytoxan
         6) Cyclophosphamide
         7) Plasmapheresis
      b. Instruct the client to minimize sun exposure, eliminate activities that produce exacerbations, and maintain a positive self-image.
   5. SURGICAL MANAGEMENT
      a. Renal transplant may be required with renal involvement.

P. GOUT
   1. DESCRIPTION
      a. Systemic disease where urate crystal deposits in the joints and tissues, causing inflammation
      b. Primary pathogenesis—hereditary error of purine metabolism, occurs in 90% of middle-aged men
      c. Secondary pathogenesis—hyperuricemia (excessive uric acid in the blood) caused by another acquired disorder such as alcoholism, diabetes mellitus, obesity, cytotoxic drugs, hypertension
      d. Etiology—increased serum uric acid precipitated by trauma, surgery, alcohol ingestion, and infection
      e. Complications include slowly progressive disability, joint deformity, predisposition to osteoarthritis, infection, or renal calculi.
   2. ASSESSMENT
      a. One or more joints, generally less than four, appear dusky or cyanotic and are extremely tender.
         1) Great toe is the most common site.
         2) Onset—usually rapid swelling and pain peaking in several hours, and subsides, treated or not, in 7 to 10 days
         3) Tophi (sodium urate crystal deposited under the skin)
   3. FOUR PHASES OF PRIMARY GOUT
      a. Asymptomatic hyperuricemic—uric acid elevated with no apparent symptoms
      b. Acute—the first symptoms of pain occur in this phase. In 75%, the great toe is the initial location (called podogra).
      c. Intercritical—client is asymptomatic after the acute attack is over. This phase may last for years.
      d. Chronic or tophaceous gout—after years of acute attacks, urate crystal deposits under the skin and in major organs (particularly the kidneys).

4. DIAGNOSTIC TESTS
   a. Blood studies
      1) Serum uric acid levels (because uric acid levels are altered with foods, this test is usually done in a series, and a consistent level above 8 mg/100 ml is abnormal)
      2) Blood urea nitrogen and creatinine to assess renal involvement
   b. Urine study
      1) 24-hour urine to examine for over- or undersecretion of uric acid (600 mg/24 hr is overproduction)
      2) This test is measured after a 5-day restriction of purine intake.
   c. Arthrocentesis—for definitive diagnosis of gout, do joint aspiration, which will show crystals in the synovial fluid of the inflamed joint.

5. NURSING INTERVENTIONS
   a. Drugs used for acute gout are different from those used in chronic gout.
      1) Colchicines and nonsteroidal anti-inflammatory drugs are used for acute gout to relieve the pain.
      2) The goal in chronic gout is to increase secretion of uric acid with probenecid (Benemid) or prevent production of uric acid with allopurinol (Zyloprim).
      3) Corticosteriods may be used only when other drugs are not effective.
      4) Avoid aspirin and diuretics because they precipitate attacks or may inactivate the other drugs.
   b. Immobilize the affected part with a sling or splint.
      1) Use a footboard or bed cradle to protect the painful toe.
   c. Apply heat or cold to relieve the pain.
   d. Inform the client that the dietary restriction of protein is controversial.
      1) Some advocate restricting all protein.
      2) Some restrict only red and organ meats.
      3) Some do not advocate a restriction at all.
      4) All believe alcohol use and fad diets must be restricted.
   e. Increase fluid to 3000 ml per day to prevent formation of renal calculi.

Q. REACTIVE ARTHRITIS
   1. DESCRIPTION
      a. Three types of reactive arthritis include:
         1) Ankylosing spondylitis (AS), affecting the sacroiliac joints, apophyseal and costovertebral joints of the spine, and adjacent soft tissue

         a) Caucasian, adolescent, or young adults are 90% of clients.
         b) More common in men, with possible genetic etiology
         c) Treatment includes methotrexate or sulfasalazine (Azulfidine).
      2) Psoriatic, which affects the skin, producing a psoriatic rash usually present around the back of the ear and polyarticular clinical manifestations
         a) Treatment includes methotrexate and steroids.
      3) Reiter's syndrome is a self-limiting disease characterized by urethritis, arthralgias, conjunctivitis, and mucocutaneous lesions that may be caused by *Shigella* or *Chlamydia* that generally affects males.
         a) There may be a genetic predisposition.
         b) ESR may be elevated.
         c) Symptomatic treatment
         d) Tetracycline (Doxycycline) is administered.

   2. ASSESSMENT
      a. Spine pain in ankylosing spondylitis
      b. Arthritis of the small joints of the hands and feet in psoriatic arthritis
      c. Urethritis, low-grade fever, conjunctivitis, and arthritis in Reiter's syndrome

   3. DIAGNOSTIC TESTS
      a. Spine x-ray
      b. ESR
      c. Complete blood count
      d. Blood uric acid

   4. NURSING INTERVENTIONS
      a. Goal is to manage clinical manifestations.

R. ARTHROPLASTY (TOTAL KNEE ARTHROPLASTY [TKA] AND TOTAL HIP ARTHROPLASTY [THA])
   1. DESCRIPTION
      a. Replacement of a joint, either partially or totally
      b. Goal for surgical intervention is the relief of pain, improve or maintain range of motion, and correct deformity.
      c. Types of prosthesis include metal or plastic ball-and-socket joints.
      d. Most common joints replaced include the knee, hip, shoulder, elbow, finger, wrist, ankle, and toes.

   2. NURSING INTERVENTIONS FOR THA
      a. Instruct the client on the immediate post-op care, which includes maintenance of proper alignment, drugs for pain and nausea and vomiting, and adequate nutrition.

b. Maintain compression dressing.

c. Instruct the client to avoid tub baths and driving for 4–6 weeks.

d. Instruct the client to avoid bending over and to use a "reacher" to pick things up.

e. Instruct the client to avoid crossing the legs.

f. Inform the client that physical therapy will begin assistance with ambulation on the first day postoperative.

g. Instruct the client on range-of-motion exercises.

h. Administer enoxaparin (Lovenox) as prescribed to prevent deep vein thrombosis.

3. NURSING INTERVENTIONS FOR TKA

a. Instruct the client on isometric exercises.

b. Progress to straight leg raises and range-of-motion exercises.

c. Use the CPM machine.

d. Inform the client that physical therapy will begin with ambulation before discharge.

e. Inform the client that a stationary bicycle may be used at home.

PRACTICE QUESTIONS

1. The nurse is caring for a client who just returned from surgery with a long leg cast. Which of the following interventions is the priority in the first 24 hours?
   1. Position the client supine to facilitate drying of the cast
   2. Dangle the client on the side of the bed in the evening
   3. Elevate the leg on a pillow above heart level
   4. Assess the cast for rough edges and smoothness

2. Immediately after application of a plaster of paris cast, the client asks the nurse when weight bearing may begin. The most appropriate response by the nurse is which of the following?
   1. "I do not know. I will ask your physician."
   2. "It is all individualized based on how you feel."
   3. "Within 8 hours, you will be standing next to the bed."
   4. "Generally after 24 to 48 hours."

3. The client asks the nurse after a total hip replacement with a cemented prosthesis when ambulation and weight bearing may begin. The nurse bases the answer on the knowledge that weight bearing and ambulation
   1. are permitted after 4 weeks.
   2. are individualized and difficult to predict.
   3. may begin with a walker the first postoperative day.
   4. occur within 3 to 5 months.

4. The nurse is caring for a client who has a compression dressing in place after an amputation. The nurse appropriately removes the dressing
   1. for bathing and physical therapy.
   2. when getting the client into a chair.

   3. for 2 hours once a shift.
   4. when the pain has stopped.

5. The nurse is discharging a client with rheumatoid arthritis who complains of morning stiffness. Which of the following measures should the nurse include in the discharge instructions?
   1. Encourage the client to sleep with pillows under the knees
   2. Instruct the client to apply ice packs to the joints before getting out of bed
   3. Instruct the client to take a warm shower in the morning when getting up
   4. Teach the client to perform all of the household chores at one time

6. Before a client has skin traction applied, which of the following should the nurse include in the instructions given to the client?
   1. Skin traction may be used for long periods of time
   2. Skin traction is applied until surgery can be performed
   3. A pin will be put in the bone
   4. Weights up to 45 pounds will be applied

7. In planning the post-op care for a client with a hip spica cast, the nurse should know that the best method of positioning this client would be to
   1. maintain the client in a prone position.
   2. use the support bar between the thighs to turn the client.
   3. turn the client side to side and support with pillows.
   4. allow the client to turn into any position that offers comfort.

8. Which of the following dietary guidelines should the nurse provide to a client with a fracture?
   1. Three large, high-calorie meals

2. High-fiber foods and 2000 to 3000 ml of fluids daily
3. Low-protein and low-fat foods
4. Limit milk and milk products to two servings daily

9. Which of the following changes in a client's neurovascular assessment should be reported as a critical sign of arterial insufficiency?
   1. Pale extremity that is cool to touch
   2. Hypersensation below the injury
   3. Pain unrelieved by analgesic
   4. Reduced motion in affected extremity

10. In planning the postoperative care for a client with a cast, the nurse would select which of the following as an appropriate nursing diagnosis?
    1. Risk for deficient fluid volume related to excess fluid loss
    2. Total urinary incontinence: related to aging process
    3. Constipation related to decreased mobility
    4. Imbalanced nutrition: less than body requirements related to lack of knowledge of appropriate food choices

11. The nurse assesses a client over what age to commonly have osteoarthritis? _____

12. Which of the following interventions would be appropriate for the nurse to include in the treatment plan of a client with a stump?
    1. Expose the stump to air for 20 minutes
    2. Generously apply lotion to the stump
    3. Administer skin care by rubbing with alcohol
    4. Scrub the stump daily to prevent infection

13. The nurse is assisting a client to walk with a crutch for the first time after an amputation. Which of the following indicates the nurse correctly understands the principles of crutch walking after an amputation?
    1. Instruct the client to remove the compression dressing before crutch walking
    2. Encourage the client to place the weight of the body on the axilla
    3. Administer an analgesic 30 minutes prior to crutch walking
    4. Assist the client to crutch walk for no more than 5 minutes

14. Because a client has bursitis, plans for nursing interventions should include
    1. aggressive antibiotic therapy.
    2. rest.
    3. range-of-motion activities.
    4. a high-protein diet.

15. The nurse is admitting a client with rheumatoid arthritis. Which of the following laboratory test results would the nurse evaluate as being elevated and used to monitor disease activity?
    1. Serum uric acid
    2. Erythrocyte sedimentation rate

3. Bence Jones protein
4. White blood cell count

16. The nurse is caring for a client with gout. Which of the following dietary selections should the nurse include in the dietary instructions?

    Select all that apply:
    [ ] 1. Salmon
    [ ] 2. Macaroni
    [ ] 3. Sardines
    [ ] 4. Cheese
    [ ] 5. Spinach
    [ ] 6. Venison

17. The nurse assesses which of the following clinical manifestations in a client with osteomyelitis?

    Select all that apply:
    [ ] 1. Night sweats
    [ ] 2. Cool extremities
    [ ] 3. Petechiae
    [ ] 4. Fever
    [ ] 5. Nausea
    [ ] 6. Restlessness

18. The nurse assists a client with osteoporosis to make which of the following menu selections?
    1. Scrambled eggs and a banana
    2. Bagel with cream cheese and half a grapefruit
    3. 3 oz grilled chicken and a baked potato
    4. Sardines and cooked broccoli

19. The nurse expects to find which of the characteristic clinical manifestations in a client with osteoarthritis?
    1. Loss of function from Bouchard's and Heberden's nodes
    2. Joint pain that is relieved by rest
    3. Joint stiffness that is worse with activity
    4. Pain and stiffness that improve with humidity and low barometric pressure

20. The nurse is admitting a client for possible systemic lupus erythematosus (SLE). When assessing this client, the nurse understands that the most significant clinical manifestation present in SLE is
    1. petechiae on the abdomen.
    2. low-grade afternoon fever.
    3. discoid rash over the face and upper chest.
    4. multiple ecchymoses over the body.

21. The nurse evaluates a serum potassium of 4.0 mEq/L to be in the normal range of _____.

22. The nurse is caring for a client with an open fracture. Which of the following would be the priority to include in this client's treatment plan?
    1. A high-protein diet
    2. Insertion of a Foley catheter

3. Tetanus toxoid
4. Passive range-of-motion exercises

23. The nurse should instruct a client that which of the following concepts are necessary to achieve good body mechanics and prevent pain and injury in a client at risk for falls and back pain?

Select all that apply
[ ] 1. Stamina
[ ] 2. Body alignment
[ ] 3. Nutrition
[ ] 4. Balance
[ ] 5. Coordinated movement
[ ] 6. Hydration

24. A client is scheduled for an open reduction internal fixation (ORIF) of a fracture. The nurse is explaining to the client why this procedure is necessary. Which of the following is the primary reason for the nurse to give a client that best describes the purpose of the ORIF?
1. "It is used when the client is in too much pain to do a closed reduction."
2. "It is completed whenever a client cannot maintain long-term immobility."
3. "It is necessary when no other realignment method can be completed."
4. "It is necessary when a cast would be too large to provide adequate mobility."

25. Which of the following neurovascular complications should the nurse assess for after a fracture?

Select all that apply:
[ ] 1. Petechiae over all extremities
[ ] 2. Pallor
[ ] 3. Exaggerated extremity movement
[ ] 4. Decreased sensation distal to the fracture site
[ ] 5. Purulent drainage at the site of an open fracture
[ ] 6. Pulselessness

26. A client with a fractured pelvis has a nursing diagnosis of impaired mobility related to bed rest, weakness, and traction. The nurse should inform the client that the rationale for maintaining good body alignment in the bed is to
1. decrease protein catabolism.
2. minimize the workload on the heart.
3. increase body strength and muscle mass.
4. reduce musculoskeletal strain and enhance lung expansion.

27. A nurse is developing a care plan for a client with an open fracture of the femur. Which of the following nursing diagnoses would the nurse choose as the priority nursing diagnosis?
1. Risk for constipation related to immobilization

2. Activity intolerance related to prolonged immobility
3. Risk for impaired skin integrity related to immobility
4. Impaired neurovascular status related to compression of nerves

28. The nurse has given discharge instructions to a client with an above-the-knee amputation who will be fitted with a prosthesis when healing is complete. Which of the following statements by the client would indicate that the client has understood the instructions?
1. "I should lie on my abdomen for 30 minutes three or four times a day."
2. "I should change the limb sock when it becomes soiled or stretched out."
3. "I should use lotion on the stump to prevent drying and cracking of the skin."
4. "I should elevate the residual limb on a pillow several times a day to decrease edema."

29. The nurse assesses that a client has lower-extremity weakness on the left. What should the nurse observe the client doing to evaluate the client's ability to use a walker?
1. Moving both the walker and the left leg forward 6 inches, then moving the right leg while the body weight is supported by the arms and the left leg
2. Moving both the walker and the right leg forward 6 inches, then moving the left leg while the body weight is supported by the arms and the right leg
3. Moving the walker forward 12 inches, bearing the body weight on the arms and extremities, then walking up to the walker
4. Moving both the walker and the left leg forward 12 inches, then moving the right leg while the body weight is supported by the arms and the left leg

30. A client has been admitted to the hospital with a diagnosis of osteoporosis resulting in a compression fracture of the spine. The physician has ordered complete bed rest and has ordered a dietician consultation. Which of the following is the priority for the dietician to include in the nutritional counseling?
1. Protein intake should be increased to 50% of the calorie intake daily
2. Vitamin D should be taken in the diet as food, not as an oral medication
3. Calcium intake should be 1500 mg daily
4. Calorie and fat intake should not exceed 1500 calories daily

31. A student nurse asks the nurse what the normal serum sodium level is. The most appropriate response by the nurse is _____.

32. Which of the following is a priority for the nurse to include in the preoperative teaching plan for a client scheduled for a total hip arthroplasty?
    1. Signs of prosthetic dislocation
    2. Methods to prevent dehydration
    3. Exercises to promote hip flexion
    4. Measures to prevent malnutrition

33. Which of the following would be the priority nursing action after being unable to palpate the client's pedal pulse after an open reduction of a tibia fracture?
    1. Notify the physician of the inability to detect the pedal pulse
    2. Check the lower extremity for pallor
    3. Use a Doppler to check for the pedal pulse
    4. Measure both extremities for comparison

34. A client has received teaching on the use of a cane to assist with ambulation. Which of the following statements by the client would indicate to the nurse that further teaching is needed?
    1. "My elbows should be slightly bent when I use the cane."
    2. "I should hold the cane on my unaffected side."
    3. "A walker would be more difficult to use than a cane."
    4. "While walking, I should have shoes and socks on at all times."

35. During an exercise session, the nurse assists the client to dorsiflex and plantarflex the foot. The client asks what kind of exercise this is. Which of the following is the appropriate response by the nurse?
    1. Active range of motion
    2. Passive range of motion
    3. Isometric
    4. Isotonic

36. A client with systemic lupus erythematosus (SLE) is admitted to a nursing unit. Which of the following would indicate to the nurse that the client's condition is deteriorating?
    1. A serum sodium of 145 mEq/L
    2. A serum potassium of 5.5 mEq/L
    3. Large amounts of glucose in the urine
    4. Large amounts of protein in the urine

37. The registered nurse delegates which of the following nursing tasks to unlicensed assistive personnel?
    1. Perform active range-of-motion activities on a client who had a hip arthroplasty
    2. Reinforce the instruction given on how to perform a two-point crutch walk
    3. Instruct a client on how to use a walker
    4. Walk a client who has an ankle sprain to the bathroom

38. Which of the following crutch gaits should the nurse instruct the client to use who has bilateral paralysis of the hips and legs?
    1. Swing-to gait
    2. Four-point gait
    3. Three-point gait
    4. Two-point gait

39. Which of the following should the nurse include when instructing a client with crutches on the two-point gait?
    1. Move the right crutch followed by the left foot, then move the left crutch forward followed by the right foot
    2. Move both crutches forward together and bring the legs through beyond the crutches
    3. Move the left crutch and right foot forward together, followed by moving the right crutch and the left foot forward together
    4. Move both crutches and the weaker leg forward, followed by moving the stronger leg forward

40. The nurse should include which of the following in the teaching plan for a client who has a cane prescribed?
    1. Move the cane forward 2 feet to ensure that the body weight is supported on both legs
    2. Hold the cane with the hand on the weaker side of the body
    3. Position the arm holding the cane so the elbow is completely straight to ensure maximum support
    4. Position the cane 6 inches to the side and 6 inches to the front of the foot of the strongest leg

ANSWERS AND RATIONALES

1. 3. The priority nursing intervention for a client with a long leg cast in the first 24 hours is to elevate the extremity above the level of the heart by placing the leg on several pillows to prevent edema. The edges of the cast may be checked for smoothness or roughness.

2. 4. Generally for 24 to 48 hours after direct cast application, direct weight bearing is contraindicated. After the 24- to 48-hour time frame, a walking heel will be applied to the cast.

3. 3. Weight bearing and ambulation following a total hip replacement with a cemented

prosthesis may begin with a walker the first postoperative day.

4. 1. The compression dressing that is applied immediately following surgery is only removed for bathing and physical therapy. The purpose of the compression dressing is to support the soft tissues while reducing edema and promoting limb shrinkage to ensure a good prosthetic fit at a later date.

5. 3. Morning stiffness is a common complaint of clients with rheumatoid arthritis because of the limited joint movements. A warm shower upon arising is recommended to increase mobility and decrease discomfort associated with the limited mobility. Cold packs may be used during exacerbations of the disease, but heat is most effective to relieve stiffness. The work of cleaning the house should be spread out throughout the week and not done at one time.

6. 2. The purpose of skin traction such as Buck's, Bryant's, Russell, a pelvic belt, or a sling is simply to stabilize the affected part and maintain alignment until surgery or skeletal traction can be performed. Skin traction is only a short-term treatment and generally for no longer than 48 to 72 hours. Generally the weight for skin traction does not exceed 7 to 10 pounds.

7. 3. A client with a hip spica cast should be turned from side to side and supported with pillows. The prone position and turning the client by using the support bar are contraindicated because they can cause the cast to break.

8. 2. Although three well-balanced meals are encouraged following a fracture, an excessive calorie intake is to be avoided because of the limited mobility that predisposes the client to weight gain. A high-fiber diet and increased fluid intake are necessary to prevent constipation. Adequate protein and calcium intake must be maintained to ensure adequate healing.

9. 1. A pale and cool extremity following a musculoskeletal injury is the classic indication of arterial insufficiency and must be immediately reported. Hypersensation below the injury as well as other abnormal sensations may be experienced, but they are not the priority finding. An evaluation of a potential problem including a comparison of the affected and unaffected extremity will prove beneficial. Pain unrelieved by analgesics is indicative of compartment syndrome. Reduced movement in the affected extremity should be investigated as potential damage to the motor component of the affected nerves.

10. 3. Constipation related to decreased mobility is an appropriate nursing diagnosis for a client with a cast.

11. 65. Almost everyone over the age of 65 years has osteoarthritis.

12. 1. Following an amputation, the stump is exposed to air for 20 minutes daily after washing to promote adequate drying. Lotion and alcohol are contraindicated unless specifically prescribed by the physician. Scrubbing a stump is strictly contraindicated. The stump should be gently cleansed.

13. 4. Initially following an amputation, crutch walking is limited to 5 minutes to avoid dependent edema. A client should never place weight on the axilla. This can compromise the nerve passing through the axilla. A compression dressing would not be removed prior to ambulation. Administration of an analgesic 30 minutes prior to ambulation could cause sedation and predispose a client to a fall.

14. 2. Bursitis is inflammation of the bursa (small sacs of the connective tissues lined with synovial fluid). Bursitis is generally the result of some kind of mechanical injury and is most successfully treated by rest.

15. 2. Although no single laboratory test is used for rheumatoid arthritis, the erythrocyte sedimentation rate (ERS) is elevated in over 80% of clients and is used to monitor disease activity and the response to treatment.

16. 2. 4. Foods high in purine are limited for a client with gout. Gout is repeat arthritic episodes associated with high levels of serum uric acid. Uric acid is the end product of purine catabolism. Liver, salmon, sardines, venison, and sweetbreads are high in purine content. Macaroni and cheese are lower-purine food choices.

17. 1. 4. 5. 6. Osteomyelitis is an infection of the bone characterized by both local and systemic manifestations. Systemic manifestations include fever, chills, night sweats, nausea, malaise, and restlessness.

18. 4. Osteoporosis is characterized by a deterioration of bone and increased bone fragility. An adequate intake of calcium is essential in both the prevention and treatment of osteoporosis. Foods high in calcium include milk and milk products, sardines, salmon, and certain green leafy vegetables such as broccoli. Eggs, fruits, poultry, and potatoes are poor calcium food choices.

19. 2. Joint pain that is relieved by rest is characteristic of osteoarthritis. Pain and stiffness are made worse with increased humidity and a low barometric pressure. Heberden's nodes are bony overgrowths at the distal interphalangeal joints. Bouchard's nodes involve the proximal interphalangeal joints. Although these nodes are generally red, swollen, and tender, they do not cause a significant loss of function.

20. 3. A discoid (coinlike) rash is the classic dermatologic manifestation of systemic lupus erythematosus. It characteristically takes on a butterfly appearance.

21. 3.5–5.4 mEq/L A normal serum potassium level is 3.5–5.4 mEq/L.

22. 3. The priority nursing intervention for an open fracture in which the skin integrity is broken is to administer a tetanus toxoid. A high-protein diet would be important but not the priority.

23. 2. 4. 5 Body alignment, balance, and coordinated movement—sensors in muscles and joints tell the cerebellum and other parts of the brain where and how the arm or leg is moving and what position it is in (feedback results in balance with smooth, coordinated motion).

24. 3. When no other method, such as long-term immobility, can accomplish realignment for a fracture, open reduction internal fixation (ORIF) will be completed. Pain is evident in a fracture; however, with the medications available today, pain can usually be controlled enough to complete a closed reduction either under IV conscious sedation or with general anesthesia.

25. 2. 4. 6. Neurovascular complications are assessed by a neurovascular check. Clinical manifestations of a possible neurovascular problem include pain with passive motion, pallor, pulselessness, paresthesia, pressure, and paralysis. Loss of sensation is an indication of paresthesia.

26. 4. Fractures cause damage to the affected bone, placing additional strain on the surrounding tissues, ligaments, and joints. Traction places the affected bone in proper alignment to reduce the strain on the surrounding parts. A client who has bed rest ordered may have a rapid deconditioning resulting in decreased lung capacity and orthostatic hypotension. Proper body alignment reduces the strain and increases lung expansion.

27. 4. Compression of the nerves is the most serious complication from an open fracture and is caused by edema or bone displacement. Compression of nerves can cause cell death. Risk for constipation, activity intolerance, and risk for impaired skin integrity are all important nursing diagnoses, but they are not the priority.

28. 1. Lying on the abdomen will help to make a well-rounded stump and prevent hip contractures. The limb sock should always be changed daily. Lotion is never used on a stump. Elevation is not a treatment of amputation. Pressure on the stump and hip contractures are to be avoided.

29. 1. A walker is a mechanical aid used for walking assistance by clients who need more support than a cane. Instructions for use of a walker are to move the walker and affected leg ahead 6 inches, then move the stronger leg ahead, and repeat. Arms bear the weight in the second step after the affected leg is moved forward 6 inches.

30. 3. Calorie, protein, and fat intake if adequate for sustaining health are not a concern in osteoporosis. It is true that getting vitamins in the food is best; however, if additional vitamin D is required, a supplement is good if the client gets at least 15 minutes of sunlight per day. Calcium intake for women before menopause should be at least 1000 mg/day and after menopause should increase to at least 1500 mg/day. In a client with osteoporosis at any age, adequate calcium intake is at least 1500 mg/day.

31. 135–147 mEq/L. A normal serum range is between 135 and 147 mEq/L.

32. 1. When a hip is replaced, dislocation is a real problem; it is very important to teach the signs of dislocation to the client both preoperatively and postoperatively. Dehydration and malnutrition are not usual manifestations of hip arthroplasty, and hip flexion is not a desired outcome. Hip flexion can cause dislocation of the arthroplasty.

33. 3. To ensure that the circulation is intact when the pulse is not palpable, the nurse should use a Doppler. It is inappropriate to notify the physician without collecting all the appropriate data. Although checking the lower extremity pallor and measuring circumference will provide data of circulation, it does not ensure that a pedal pulse is present.

34. 3. The client should use the cane on the unaffected side. The elbow is held slightly flexed. There are different reasons to use a walker versus a cane; however, neither one is "better." Shoes must be worn. Never use socks alone. Socks may be optional to wear with the shoes.

35. 2. Passive range-of-motion is exercise conducted with the assistance of another individual. Active range of motion is done by the client alone. Isometric exercise involves resistance, and isotonic exercise does not use resistance.

36. 4. Protein in the urine indicates renal failure, and lupus nephritis is the number one cause of death in SLE. Serum sodium and potassium and glucose in the urine are not indicative of complications resulting from SLE. A serum sodium level of 145 mEq/L and a serum potassium level of 5.5 mEq/L are normal.

37. 4. Unlicensed assistive personnel cannot reinforce instruction or provide instruction. Performing active range-of-motion exercises on a client who had a hip arthroplasty is not an appropriate job assignment for unlicensed assistive personnel, and active range of motion is likely to dislocate the hip (particularly adduction). Unlicensed

assistive personnel may walk a client who has an ankle sprain to the bathroom.

38. 1. A swing-to gait is a crutch gait that is used by clients who have paralysis of the hips and legs or wear bilateral braces on the legs. A four-point gait may be used by arthritic clients. A three-point gait may be used by a client with a broken leg or sprained ankle. A two-point gait requires more weight bearing on each foot. It is a faster crutch gait than a four-point gait.

39. 3. When using the two-point gait, the left crutch and right foot are moved forward together, followed by moving the right crutch and left foot forward together. The crutch walk requires some weight bearing on each foot. During the four-point gait, the right crutch is moved forward followed by the left foot, then the left crutch is moved forward followed by the right foot. This is the most stable of all crutch walks. It provides the most support while requiring

weight bearing on both legs. This gait may be used for some types of paralysis, such as in children with cerebral palsy. In the three-point gait, both crutches are moved forward with the weaker leg, followed by moving the stronger leg forward. In this gait, the client is required to bear all weight on the unaffected leg. In the swing-to gait, both crutches are moved forward together followed by bringing the legs through beyond the crutches. This gait is used by clients who have a paralysis of their lower extremities.

40. 4. To provide a wide base of support, the cane should be positioned both 6 inches to the side and 6 inches to the front of the foot of the strongest leg. The cane should be held on the stronger side of the body. The elbow is bent to correctly use a cane. A cane is not an appropriate assistive device for someone with bilateral leg weakness.

REFERENCES

Daniels, R. (2010). *Delmar's manual of laboratory and diagnostic tests* (2nd ed.). Clifton Park, NY: Delmar Cengage Learning.

Daniels, R., & Nicoll, L. (2012). *Contemporary medical-surgical nursing.* Clifton Park, NY: Delmar Cengage Learning.

DeLaune, S. C., & Ladner, P. K. (2011). *Fundamentals of nursing:* Standard and practice (4th ed.). Clifton Park, NY: Delmar Cengage Learning.

Estes, M. (2010). *Health assessment and physical examination* (4th ed.). Clifton Park, NY: Delmar Cengage Learning.

Spratto, G. R., & Woods, A. L. (2012). *PDR nurse's drug handbook 2012.* Clifton Park, NY: Delmar Cengage Learning.

CHAPTER 10

GENITOURINARY DISORDERS

I. **ANATOMY AND PHYSIOLOGY**
   A. FUNCTIONS OF THE URINARY SYSTEM
      1. URINE FORMATION
      2. URINE STORAGE
      3. URINE DRAINAGE
      4. ACID-BASE BALANCE
      5. ACTIVATION OF VITAMIN D
      6. PRODUCTION OF ERYTHROPOIETIN AND RENIN
      7. CONTROL OF BLOOD PRESSURE
      8. REGULATION OF FLUID AND ELECTROLYTES
   B. MAIN STRUCTURES (SEE FIGURE 10-1)
      1. TWO KIDNEYS
      2. TWO URETERS
      3. BLADDER
      4. URETHRA
   C. KIDNEYS
      1. LOCATED BEHIND THE PERITONEUM ON THE RIGHT AND LEFT OF THE VERTEBRAL COLUMN
      2. POSITIONED AT THORACIC 12 TO LUMBAR 3 VERTEBRAE LEVEL
      3. COMPOSED OF THREE REGIONS: RENAL CORTEX (OUTER), RENAL MEDULLA (MIDDLE), AND RENAL PELVIS (INNER)
         a. Renal cortex has the mechanism that filters blood.
         b. Renal medulla has 8 to 12 renal pyramids that empty into the renal calyx.
         c. Renal pyramid directs urine to the renal pelvis.
      4. PROTECTED BY A LAYER OF FAT AND CONNECTIVE TISSUE CALLED CAPSULE
      5. FLOW OF BLOOD: RENAL ARTERY, RENAL CORTEX, RENAL MEDULLA, RENAL PYRAMID, RENAL CALYX, RENAL PELVIS, AND RENAL VEIN
      6. ADRENAL GLANDS ARE LOCATED ON TOP OF THE KIDNEYS.
      7. ALDOSTERONE IS SECRETED BY THE ADRENAL GLANDS.
      8. FUNCTIONS OF THE KIDNEYS
         a. Water elimination
         b. Blood filtration
         c. Fluid-electrolyte regulation
         d. Acid-base balance maintenance
         e. Erythropoietin and renin production
         f. Vitamin D activation
   D. NEPHRONS
      1. FUNCTIONAL UNITS OF THE KIDNEYS
      2. CONSIST OF THE GLOMERULUS, BOWMAN'S CAPSULE, AND TUBULAR SYSTEM
      3. TUBULAR SYSTEM CONSISTS OF PROXIMAL CONVOLUTED TUBULE, LOOP OF HENLE, AND DISTAL CONVOLUTED TUBE.
      4. URETERS
      5. CONNECT THE KIDNEYS TO THE BLADDER
      6. FIBROMUSCULAR TUBES
      7. CARRY URINE FROM THE KIDNEY TO THE BLADDER
   E. BLADDER
      1. LOCATED BEHIND THE SYMPHYSIS PUBIS
      2. MUSCULAR, DISTENSIBLE ORGAN
      3. STORES AND ASSISTS IN THE ELIMINATION OF URINE
      4. TOTAL BLADDER CAPACITY IS BETWEEN 600 ML AND 1000 ML.
      5. APPROXIMATELY 1500 ML PER DAY IS AVERAGE ADULT URINE OUTPUT.
      6. HAVING 200–250 ML OF URINE IN THE BLADDER RESULTS IN MODERATE DISTENSION AND THE URGE TO VOID (MICTURATE).
   F. URETHRA
      1. CONNECTS THE NECK OF THE BLADDER TO THE EXTERNAL MEATUS
      2. PASSAGEWAY FOR URINE TO LEAVE THE BODY
      3. THE FEMALE URETHRA IS 1–2 INCHES LONG, WITH THE EXTERNAL MEATUS POSITIONED ANTERIOR TO THE VAGINA.

Figure 10-1 The urinary system with inset of a nephron.

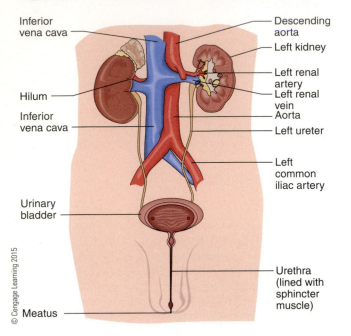

Inferior vena cava
Descending aorta
Left kidney
Left renal artery
Left renal vein
Aorta
Hilum
Inferior vena cava
Left ureter
Left common iliac artery
Urinary bladder
Urethra (lined with sphincter muscle)
Meatus

© Cengage Learning 2015

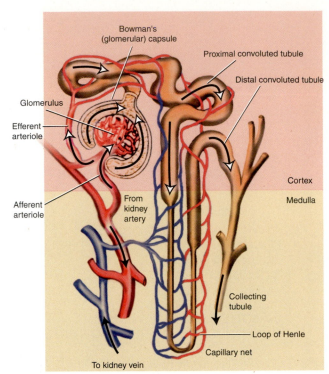

Bowman's (glomerular) capsule
Proximal convoluted tubule
Distal convoluted tubule
Glomerulus
Efferent arteriole
Afferent arteriole
From kidney artery
Cortex
Medulla
Collecting tubule
Loop of Henle
Capillary net
To kidney vein

4. THE MALE URETHRA IS 8–10 INCHES LONG, AND PASSES THROUGH THE PROSTATE GLAND, UROGENITAL DIAPHRAGM, AND PENIS.
5. FUNCTIONS AS THE PASSAGEWAY FOR URINE AND SEMEN IN MEN

G. URINE FORMATION
1. URINE IS FORMED THROUGH THREE PROCESSES: GLOMERULAR FILTRATION, TUBULAR REABSORPTION, AND TUBULAR SECRETION.
   a. Glomerular filtration: blood flows into the glomerulus and is filtered.
   b. Tubular reabsorption: proximal tubule and loop of Henle reabsorb water and electrolytes back into the capillaries through active and passive transport.
   c. Tubular secretion: in the distal tubule, potassium, hydrogen, and ammonia are secreted from the capillaries by active transport.

H. BLOOD PRESSURE REGULATION
1. DECREASE IN EXTRACELLULAR FLUID VOLUME, LOWERED BLOOD PRESSURE, AND DECREASED AMOUNT OF SALT STIMULATE THE KIDNEYS.
2. KIDNEYS SECRETE RENIN INTO THE BLOOD.
3. RENIN IS CARRIED TO THE LUNGS.
4. RENIN FORMS ANGIOTENSIN I IN THE LUNGS.

5. ANGIOTENSIN I IS CONVERTED TO ANGIOTENSIN II BY ANGIOTENSIN-CONVERTING ENZYME.
6. ANGIOTENSIN II INCREASES PERIPHERAL VASOCONSTRICTION.
7. VASOCONSTRICTION INCREASES BLOOD PRESSURE.
8. ANGIOTENSIN II STIMULATES SECRETION OF ALDOSTERONE FROM THE ADRENAL GLAND.
9. ALDOSTERONE CONTROLS POTASSIUM SECRETION IN THE TUBULES.
10. ADRENAL GLAND SECRETES MORE ALDOSTERONE AS A RESULT OF HIGHER POTASSIUM LEVELS.
11. ALDOSTERONE HELPS WITH SODIUM RETENTION THROUGH CONTROL OF TUBULAR REABSORPTION.
12. SODIUM RETENTION INCREASES EXTRACELLULAR FLUID VOLUME AND INCREASES BLOOD PRESSURE.

I. RED BLOOD CELL (RBC) PRODUCTION
1. LOWER RED BLOOD CELLS IN THE BLOOD REDUCE THE OXYGEN CARRIED TO THE KIDNEYS.
2. REDUCED OXYGEN TRIGGERS THE KIDNEYS TO PRODUCE ERYTHROPOIETIN.
3. THE HORMONE ERYTHROPOIETIN TRAVELS TO THE BONE MARROW.

4. BONE MARROW IS STIMULATED TO PRODUCE ERYTHROPOIETIN.
5. RED BLOOD CELLS CARRY OXYGEN TO THE KIDNEYS.

J. ANTIDIURETIC HORMONE
1. DECREASED BLOOD VOLUME INCREASES SERUM OSMOLARITY.
2. HYPOTHALAMUS IS TRIGGERED.
3. HYPOTHALAMUS SENDS SIGNALS TO THE PITUITARY GLAND.
4. PITUITARY GLAND SECRETES ANTIDIURETIC HORMONE (ADH).
5. ADH CIRCULATES IN THE BLOOD TO THE KIDNEYS.
6. DISTAL CONVOLUTED TUBULES AND COLLECTING DUCTS BECOME PERMEABLE TO WATER.
7. WATER IS REABSORBED INTO THE PERITUBULAR CAPILLARIES.
8. INCREASED VOLUME OF WATER IN THE CIRCULATION INCREASES BLOOD VOLUME AND DECREASES SERUM OSMOLARITY.

K. ACID-BASE BALANCE
1. ACID IS PRODUCED AS A RESULT OF METABOLIC PROCESSES.
2. THREE MECHANISMS TO NEUTRALIZE ACID ARE: BUFFER SYSTEM (IMMEDIATE ACTING), RESPIRATORY SYSTEM (FAST ACTING), AND RENAL SYSTEM (SLOW ACTING).
3. RENAL MECHANISM TAKES 2 TO 3 DAYS TO RESPOND.
4. KIDNEYS REABSORB THE FILTERED BICARBONATE.
5. KIDNEYS PRODUCE MORE BICARBONATE WHEN NEEDED.
6. HYDROGEN IONS ARE EXCRETED IN THE URINE.
7. HYDROGEN IONS ARE COMBINED WITH AMMONIA (NH_4) IN THE KIDNEYS TO PRODUCE AMMONIUM (NH_{41}).
8. OTHER WEAK ACIDS ARE EXCRETED BY THE KIDNEYS.
9. URINE PH VARIES BETWEEN 4 AND 8, INDICATING HOW MUCH ACID IS ELIMINATED.

II. **ASSESSMENT**
A. HEALTH HISTORY
1. PAST MEDICAL HISTORY
2. HISTORY OF SMOKING
3. MEDICATION (NEPHROTOXIC DRUGS)
4. SURGERIES
5. SEXUAL AND REPRODUCTIVE HISTORY
B. PHYSICAL EXAMINATION
1. INSPECTION
a. Inspect the skin around the kidneys, bladder, and perineum (meatus) for texture, turgor, bruises, edema.
b. Edema and weight gain
c. Urine for frequency, color, amount, odor, and clarity
d. Distention of the bladder
e. Incontinence
2. PALPATION
a. Palpate the kidneys in supine position for location.
b. Palpate the bladder when distended.
c. Kidneys are palpable when enlarged.
3. PERCUSSION
a. To detect tenderness
b. Dull sound if the bladder contains more than 150 ml of urine
4. AUSCULTATION
a. Abdominal aorta and renal arteries for bruit

III. **DIAGNOSTIC STUDIES**
A. URINE TESTS AND URINALYSIS
1. DESCRIPTION: EXAMINATION OF THE URINE FOR COLOR, ODOR, PH, SPECIFIC GRAVITY, OSMOLARITY, GLUCOSE, PROTEIN, NITRATE, BLOOD, WHITE BLOOD CELLS, RED BLOOD CELLS, AND MICROORGANISMS
2. PROCEDURE
a. Provide the client a urine collection container.
b. Instruct the client to wash the perineal area with warm, soapy water.
c. Instruct the client to collect first-voiding morning urine.
d. Instruct the client on the correct technique of obtaining a midstream sample if a clean catch sample is required.
3. POSTPROCEDURE
a. Instruct the client to wash hands.
b. Label the container and send to the lab.
B. URINE CULTURE AND SENSITIVITY (MIDSTREAM)
1. DESCRIPTION
a. Specimen is obtained to confirm presence of microorganisms.
b. Result of less than 10,000 organisms per milliliter is negative for infection; 10,000–100,000 organisms per milliliter generally is not significant.
c. Organisms greater than 100,000 per milliliter significant for infection
2. PREPROCEDURE
a. Instruct the female client to separate the labia and cleanse the meatus from front to back with 3–4 antiseptic wipes.
b. Instruct the male client to cleanse the tip of the penis (retracting the foreskin, if present) with 3–4 antiseptic wipes.
c. Instruct the client to begin the urinary stream in the toilet to flush out the urethra, followed by urinating in the sterile collection container.

3. PROCEDURE

   a. If the client is unable to urinate, insert a urinary catheter to obtain the sample.

   b. If the client has an indwelling urinary catheter, remove a sample with a syringe and needle.

   c. For infants and young children, collect the sample using a U bag.

   d. For clients with urinary diversion, insert a urinary catheter into the stoma to obtain a sample.

4. POSTPROCEDURE

   a. Instruct the client to wash hands.

   b. Indicate any medications the client is taking that may affect the test results on the slip sent to the lab.

C. CREATININE CLEARANCE

  1. DESCRIPTION

   a. Creatinine used in skeletal muscle contraction is the end product of creatinine phosphate.

   b. Measures glomerular filtration rate (GFR) in the diagnosis of renal disease

   c. Normal measurement is 87–107 ml/min (female), 107–139 ml/min (male).

  2. PREPROCEDURE

   a. Provide the client with a large urine container to collect all urine for 24 hours.

   b. Instruct the client to keep all collected urine on ice or in the refrigerator during the 24-hour period.

   c. Instruct the client not to put any toilet paper in the urine.

   d. Instruct the client to void prior to defecation so urine is not contaminated with feces.

   e. Advise the client that vigorous activity or exercise increases creatinine clearance levels.

  3. PROCEDURE

   a. Instruct the client to save all urine for 24 hours after discarding the first voided specimen.

   b. Label the container, including the start and end time of urine collection.

   c. Place a 24-hour urine collection sign in the bathroom to avoid accidental discarding.

   d. Encourage the client to drink 2 to 3 liters of fluid unless contraindicated.

   e. Ensure serum creatinine is done during the 24-hour period.

  4. POSTPROCEDURE

   a. Instruct the client to wash hands after each voiding.

   b. Send the urine container to the lab for analysis.

D. BLOOD CHEMISTRIES

  1. BLOOD UREA NITROGEN (BUN)

   a. Reflects urea nitrogen in the blood; urea is the product of protein metabolism.

   b. Renal diseases decrease the excretion of urea, thus increasing the BUN level.

   c. Formed in the liver and excreted by the kidneys

   d. Used to diagnose impaired renal function

   e. Normal level is 10–20 mg/dl.

   f. Strenuous activity, gastrointestinal (GI) bleed, fever, and steroids may increase levels.

  2. CREATININE

   a. Measures creatinine, a by-product of protein metabolism in the blood

   b. Results are more reliable and diagnostic of renal function than BUN.

   c. Normal level is 0.5–1.2 mg/dl.

  3. URIC ACID

   a. Product of purine metabolism used to primarily detect disorders of purine metabolism such as gout

   b. Excreted by the kidneys and intestines

   c. May also be used in the detection of kidney disease

   d. Ask the client about intake of foods high in purines.

   e. Normal male level is 4–8.5 mg/dl (0.24–0.51 mmol/L).

   f. Normal female level is 2.7–7.3 mg/dl (0.16–0.43 mmol/L).

  4. SODIUM

   a. Major cation in the extracellular space

   b. Level remains constant until end-stage renal disease.

   c. Ask about intake of foods high in sodium content.

   d. Normal level is 135–145 mEq/L (134–145 mmol/L).

  5. POTASSIUM

   a. Major cation in the intracellular space

   b. Excreted primarily by the kidneys

   c. Altered level is the first indication of renal disease.

   d. Abnormalities also indicative of cardiac disease

   e. Normal level is 3.5–5 mEq/L (3.5–5.5 mmol/L).

  6. CALCIUM

   a. Major mineral in bone

   b. Responsible for the contraction of muscle, neurotransmission, and clotting factors

   c. Evaluate parathyroid function and calcium metabolism

   d. Used in monitoring renal failure

   e. Absorption is decreased in renal disease.

f. Normal level is 9–10.5 mg/dl (2.25–2.75 mmol/L).

7. PHOSPHORUS
   a. Inverse relationship between phosphorus and calcium balance
   b. Primarily excreted by the kidneys
   c. Levels increase with renal failure.
   d. Normal level is 3–4.5 mg/dl (0.97–1.45 mmol/L).

8. BICARBONATE
   a. Kidneys reabsorb filtered bicarbonate.
   b. Kidneys produce more bicarbonate when needed.
   c. Metabolic acidosis and low bicarbonate levels result from renal failure.
   d. Normal level is 20–30 mg/dl (20–30 mmol/L).

IV. **RADIOLOGIC STUDIES**
   A. KIDNEY, URETERS, BLADDER (KUB) X-RAY
      1. DESCRIPTION
         a. X-ray study of the pelvis and abdomen
         b. Used in diagnosing renal stones, malformations of kidneys and bladder, and other intra-abdominal diseases
      2. PREPROCEDURE
         a. Instruct the client that fasting is not required.
         b. Instruct the client that the procedure has no associated discomfort.
         c. Shield the testicles of a male client with a lead shield to protect them from radiation.
         d. Unable to shield the female client's ovaries from radiation because of their location near the kidneys, ureter, and bladder
      3. PROCEDURE
         a. Place the client in supine position on the examination table with the arms extended.
      4. POSTPROCEDURE
         a. No special care is necessary.
   B. INTRAVENOUS PYELOGRAPHY (IVP) OR EXCRETORY UROGRAM
      1. DESCRIPTION
         a. X-ray study of the pelvis and abdomen
         b. Contrast dye is injected intravenously.
      2. PREPROCEDURE
         a. Obtain written consent.
         b. Assess for allergies to iodine and shellfish.
         c. Administer laxative the evening before the procedure.
         d. May be NPO for 8 hours
         e. Ensure adequate or IV hydration to prevent dye-induced renal failure.
         f. Assess serum levels of BUN and creatinine to prevent a deterioration of an already abnormal renal function.
         g. Clients receiving high volumes of IV solutions may have IV rate

decreased to increase concentration of the dye within the urinary system.
      3. PROCEDURE
         a. Place the client in supine position.
         b. Take an x-ray film of the pelvis and abdomen to ensure there is no stool obstructing the visualization or the renal system. Also assesses for renal calculi.
         c. Insert peripheral IV line.
         d. Administer contrast dye via the IV line.
         e. Inform the client that a warm, flushed sensation may be experienced when contrast is injected.
         f. Obtain x-ray films at 1-, 5-, 10-, 20-, and 30-minute intervals to monitor the path of the dye from the kidneys to the bladder.
         g. Instruct the client to void after all interval films are obtained.
         h. Obtain final x-ray film after voiding to assess the empty bladder.
      4. POSTPROCEDURE
         a. Monitor the client's urine output.
         b. Ensure adequate IV fluids or oral fluids to facilitate excretion of the contrast dye.
   C. NEPHROTOMOGRAM
      1. DESCRIPTION
         a. X-ray examination of kidneys
         b. Uses tomographic technique
         c. Contrast dye is injected.
         d. A single layer of the organ is examined.
      2. PROCEDURE
         a. Same as IVP (see pages 239 & 240)
   D. RETROGRADE PYELOGRAM
      1. DESCRIPTION
         a. X-ray of the urinary tract
         b. Contrast dye is administered through urethral catheters.
         c. Cystoscopy is done.
      2. PREPROCEDURE
         a. Explain the procedure.
         b. Obtain informed consent.
         c. Administer enemas as ordered.
         d. Keep NPO after midnight.
         e. Administer medications as ordered.
         f. Inform the client that contrast dye injected into the ureters is not absorbed.
      3. PROCEDURE
         a. Insert ureteral catheter by cystoscopy.
         b. Inject contrast dye.
         c. Obtain an x-ray.
         d. Withdraw the catheters while injecting the dye and obtaining x-ray films.
         e. Obtain x-ray 5 minutes after the last injection to assess emptying of the ureter.
         f. Place a stent in the ureter if an obstruction is found.

4. POSTPROCEDURE

    a. Assess the client and monitor vital signs for evidence of bleeding (hypotension, tachycardia).

    b. Assess the client for an indication of sepsis (elevated temperature, flushing, chills).

    c. Administer prescribed analgesics.

    d. Monitor the client's urine output.

    e. Increase fluid intake to promote the excretion of the dye.

    f. Monitor for bladder spasms, ability to void, and urinary retention.

E. CYSTOGRAPHY

  1. DESCRIPTION

    a. X-ray of the bladder

    b. Bladder is filled with contrast dye.

  2. PREPROCEDURE

    a. Explain the procedure.

    b. Obtain informed consent.

    c. Clear liquids for breakfast

    d. Insert a Foley catheter.

  3. PROCEDURE

    a. Place the client supine or in lithotomy position.

    b. Administer contrast dye into the bladder.

    c. Clamp the catheter.

    d. Obtain x-ray films.

    e. Remove the catheter if the client is able to void.

    f. Obtain an x-ray as the client is emptying the bladder.

    g. Protect the male client's gonads with a lead shield.

    h. Unable to protect female client's ovaries with a lead shield without obstructing visualization of bladder

  4. POSTPROCEDURE

    a. Assess the client for urinary tract infection.

    b. Administer IV fluids or encourage increased fluid intake to excrete the dye.

F. RENAL ANGIOGRAM

  1. DESCRIPTION

    a. X-ray examination of the renal blood vessels

    b. Contrast dye is injected into the renal artery by a catheter inserted into the femoral artery.

  2. PREPROCEDURE

    a. Explain the procedure.

    b. Obtain informed consent.

    c. Assess the client for allergies to iodine dye and shellfish.

    d. Assess the client's medication for anticoagulation therapy.

    e. NPO after midnight

    f. Mark the peripheral pulses.

    g. Encourage the client to void before the procedure.

    h. Remove valuables, dentures, and contact lenses.

    i. Shave the groin on both sides.

    j. Administer prescribed preprocedure medications.

    k. Inform the client that some discomfort such as bladder distension and a warm, flushed sensation associated with the injected contrast dye may be experienced.

  3. PROCEDURE

    a. Place the client supine.

    b. Administer sedatives as ordered.

    c. Prepare and drape the groin using sterile technique.

    d. Make an incision in the groin and place the catheter into the femoral artery.

    e. Inject the contrast dye into the catheter and obtain x-ray films.

    f. Monitor the client and vital signs for malignant hypertension.

  4. POSTPROCEDURE

    a. Apply a pressure dressing to the incision site.

    b. Monitor the client's vital signs and dressing for indications of hemorrhage.

    c. Monitor the peripheral pulses in the leg used for vascular access to rule out occluded blood flow.

    d. Encourage fluid intake to promote excretion of the dye.

    e. Maintain bed rest for 4–6 hours.

    f. Assess the client for any adverse reaction to the contrast dye.

    g. Monitor the client's lower extremities for circulation, motion, and sensation.

    h. Administer prescribed analgesics.

G. ULTRASOUND

  1. DESCRIPTION

    a. Noninvasive procedure facilitating visualization of the kidneys, ureters, and bladder through the use of sound waves

    b. May be safely performed on clients in renal failure

  2. PREPROCEDURE

    a. Explain the procedure.

    b. Inform the client that fasting is not required.

  3. PROCEDURE

    a. Place the client supine.

    b. Apply a conductive gel to the skin to enhance sensitivity of the sound waves by the transducer.

  4. POSTPROCEDURE

    a. Cleanse the conductive gel off the client's skin.

H. COMPUTERIZED TOMOGRAPHY (CT) SCAN

  1. DESCRIPTION

    a. Noninvasive cross-sectional x-ray

    b. Contrast dye is used.

    c. Organs are viewed from many angles.

2. PREPROCEDURE
   a. Explain the procedure.
   b. Obtain informed consent.
   c. Assess the client for allergies to iodine and shellfish.
   d. NPO 4 hours prior to the procedure
   e. Insert an IV.
   f. Inform the client that a warm, flushed sensation may be experienced with the injected contrast dye.
   g. Inform the client to remain motionless throughout the procedure.

3. PROCEDURE
   a. Place the client supine on the CT scan table.
   b. Inject IV contrast dye.
   c. Obtain CT scan images on x-ray film.

4. POSTPROCEDURE
   a. Assess the client for allergic reaction to contrast dye.
   b. Encourage fluid intake to promote excretion of the dye.

I. MAGNETIC RESONANCE IMAGING (MRI)
1. DESCRIPTION
   a. Noninvasive scan
   b. The client is placed in a magnetic field.
   c. Films are obtained.

2. PREPROCEDURE
   a. Explain the procedure.
   b. Obtain informed consent.
   c. Inform the client that fasting is not required.
   d. Inform the client there is no exposure to radiation.
   e. Ask the client to remove any metal objects due to damage to items, production of artifacts on the images, and danger to the client.
   f. Instruct the client to remain motionless during the procedure.
   g. Instruct the client to void before the procedure.
   h. Administer sedative medications as ordered if the client is claustrophobic.

3. PROCEDURE
   a. Place the client supine on the MRI table.
   b. Inform the client that a thumping sound will be heard during the procedure and that earplugs are available.
   c. Inform the client that the ability to speak to procedure personnel is maintained.

4. POSTPROCEDURE
   a. No special care is necessary.

J. RENAL SCAN
1. DESCRIPTION
   a. Nuclear scan with IV injection of a radioscope
   b. Scintillator camera monitors gamma rays produced by a radionuclide.
   c. Used to view the kidneys
   d. Detects normal structure, function, and blood perfusion in the kidneys
   e. Can detect any abnormalities in the kidneys, such as cysts, tumors, or abscesses
   f. Several kinds of renal scanning are done, such as: perfusion scan, structure scan, function scan, renal hypertension scan, and obstruction scan.

2. PREPROCEDURE
   a. Explain the procedure.
   b. Inform the client that fasting is not required.
   c. Encourage the client to drink fluid (2–3 glasses) before the procedure for hydration.
   d. Inform the client that no pain or discomfort is associated with this procedure.
   e. Ask the client to void before the procedure.
   f. Insert an IV access.
   g. Instruct the client to lie still during the procedure.

3. PROCEDURE
   a. Place the client in a sitting (prone) position.
   b. Administer the IV radionuclide.
   c. Pass the scintography camera over the kidneys.
   d. Record the radioactive uptake.

4. POSTPROCEDURE
   a. Encourage fluid intake to promote excretion of the radioactive substance.

K. CYSTOSCOPY
1. DESCRIPTION
   a. Urethra and bladder are visualized.
   b. Cystoscope is inserted into the bladder through the urethra.
   c. Used diagnostically and therapeutically
   d. May be done under general or local anesthesia

2. PREPROCEDURE
   a. Explain the procedure.
   b. Obtain informed consent.
   c. Administer cleansing enemas if ordered.
   d. NPO after midnight for general anesthesia
   e. Provide clear liquid breakfast for local anesthesia
   f. Administer IV fluids or encourage oral fluid intake several hours before the procedure.
   g. Administer prescribed medications.
   h. Instruct the client to lie still during the procedure.

3. PROCEDURE
   a. Place the client in lithotomy position.
   b. Instill local anesthesia into the urethra or administer general anesthesia.

    c. Insert the cystoscope into the bladder.

    d. Perform the diagnostic or therapeutic studies.

    e. Inform the client that the urge to void may be felt.

  4. POSTPROCEDURE

    a. Assess the client for back pain and bladder spasms.

    b. Offer warm sitz baths.

    c. Administer prescribed analgesics.

    d. Administer prescribed antibiotics generally 1 day preprocedure and 3 days postprocedure.

    e. Maintain bed rest immediately postprocedure (orthostatic hypotension may be experienced).

    f. Assess urinary output for 24 hours because urinary retention may occur.

    g. Inform the client that urine will initially be pink-tinged.

L. CYSTOMETROGRAM (CMG)

  1. DESCRIPTION

    a. Measures pressure in the bladder

    b. Sensory and motor functions of the bladder are tested when incontinence is present and neurogenic bladder is suspected.

  2. PREPROCEDURE

    a. Explain the procedure.

    b. Inform the client that fasting is not required.

    c. Instruct the client to avoid straining while voiding because test results can be altered.

  3. PROCEDURE

    a. Instruct the client to void and measure the amount, time, and any straining, hesitancy, and dribbling experienced.

    b. Place the client supine or in the lithotomy position.

    c. Insert a catheter into the bladder.

    d. Measure residual volume.

    e. Instill 30 ml of saline into the bladder followed by 30 ml of warm water.

    f. Withdraw the fluid.

    g. Connect the catheter to a cystometer.

    h. Instill normal saline, sterile water, or carbon dioxide gas into the bladder.

    i. Inform the client to indicate when the urge to void is experienced.

    j. Measurements are recorded on a graph.

    k. Administer prescribed drugs into the bladder (anticholinergics are given to relax a hyperactive bladder and cholinergics to increase tone when flaccid bladder is present).

    l. The bladder is emptied of any residual urine.

  4. POSTPROCEDURE

    a. Monitor the client for increased temperature and chills, indicating presence of infection.

    b. Assess the client's urine for hematuria.

    c. Offer the client sitz baths to relieve discomfort.

M. RENAL BIOPSY

  1. DESCRIPTION

    a. Examination of renal tissue

    b. Sample is obtained percutaneously.

  2. PREPROCEDURE

    a. Explain the procedure.

    b. Obtain informed consent.

    c. NPO after midnight

    d. Assess the client's hemoglobin, hematocrit, and coagulation studies.

    e. Type and cross-match the client.

  3. PROCEDURE

    a. Place the client prone with a pillow under the abdomen.

    b. Cleanse the skin over the area.

    c. Administer local anesthesia.

    d. Instruct the client to hold the breath during the insertion of the biopsy needle.

    e. Apply pressure to the area for 20 minutes after withdrawing the needle.

    f. Apply pressure dressing to the site.

  4. POSTPROCEDURE

    a. Maintain flat bed rest for 24 hours.

    b. Monitor the client for signs of hemorrhage such as hypotension, tachycardia, pallor, dizziness, and shoulder, flank, and back pain.

    c. Assess the client for signs of damage to the liver or bowel such as abdominal pain, guarding, and decreased bowel sounds.

    d. Inform the client to avoid strenuous activities and those that increase abdominal pressure, such as coughing and straining at stool.

    e. Encourage fluids to reduce the risk of blood clots and urine retention.

    f. Monitor the client's hemoglobin and hematocrit.

    g. Monitor the client's urine for hematuria, which should cease after the first 24 hours.

    h. Administer prescribed analgesics.

V. **URINARY AND RENAL TUBES**

  A. DESCRIPTION: PLASTIC OR RUBBER TUBE INSERTED FOR THE PURPOSE OF DRAINING URINE.

  B. URETHRAL CATHETERIZATION

    1. DESCRIPTION: CATHETER INSERTED INTO THE BLADDER THROUGH THE URINARY MEATUS INTO THE URETHRA FOR THE PURPOSE OF DRAINING URINE

2. TYPES
   a. Indwelling (Foley)
   b. Intermittent
3. INSERTION
   a. Assist the female client to a supine position with the knees flexed (dorsal recumbent position).
   b. A side-lying position with the upper leg flexed at the knee and hip (Sims' position) may be used for the female client who has severe arthritic joints or has had a total hip replacement and can assume a supine position or abduct the leg.
   c. Assist the male client to a supine position with the legs slightly abducted.
   d. Drape the client and ensure adequate lighting of the perineum.
   e. Don disposable gloves and cleanse the perineal area with warm, soapy water. Remove the gloves and wash hands.
   f. Using aseptic technique, open the catheterization tray, maintaining sterility of the inside wrapper.
   g. Don sterile gloves, open the sterile packages and lubricant, and pour antiseptic solution over sterile cotton balls.
   h. Attach a prefilled syringe to the balloon port to ensure patency of the balloon.
   i. Generously lubricate the end of the catheter (approximately 2 inches for female and 7 inches for male).
   j. For the female client: (1) cuff both corners of the drape over the hands and place the cuffed edges under the client's buttocks, with the remainder of the drape between the legs; (2) place a fenestrated drape over the perineum.
   k. For the male client: place a drape over the thighs and fenestrated drape over the penis.
   l. For the female client, spread and firmly hold the labia apart with the nondominant hand. With the dominant hand, pick up a new povidone-iodine-soaked cotton ball with forceps to cleanse from top to bottom first the far labia followed by the near labia and ending with the urethral meatus.
   m. For the male client, with the nondominant hand, retract the foreskin, if present, and firmly grasp the penis. With the dominant hand, pick up a new povidone-iodine-soaked cotton ball with forceps and cleanse the glans penis in a circular motion until all cotton balls are used.
   n. With the dominant hand, pick up a lubricated catheter 3–4 inches from the tip and insert until urine begins to flow, or 2–3 inches in the female client and 7–9 inches in the male client.
   o. If ordered, collect a urine specimen or drain the bladder of urine.
   p. If an indwelling catheter is ordered, inflate the retention balloon with the prefilled syringe according to manufacturer guidelines, being careful to avoid overinflating or underinflating the balloon (generally a 5-ml balloon).
   q. Securely tape the catheter to the inner thigh or lower abdomen.

C. URETERAL CATHETERS
   1. DESCRIPTION: CATHETER IS INSERTED INTO THE RENAL PELVIS THROUGH THE URETERS EITHER THROUGH A SURGICAL INCISION OR CYSTOSCOPY FOR THE PURPOSE OF DRAINING URINE.
   2. PURPOSE: TO SPLINT THE URETERS FOLLOWING SURGERY TO DECREASE THE INCIDENCE OF OBSTRUCTION FROM EDEMA
   3. USES: FOLLOWING SURGERY, FOR THE REMOVAL OF A TUMOR OBSTRUCTING THE URETER
   4. NURSING INTERVENTIONS
      a. Maintain the client on bed rest until ambulation is permitted.
      b. Record output separate from other urinary catheters.
      c. Monitor drainage every hour.
      d. Avoid damaging the catheter.
      e. Report output greater than 3 to 5 ml.
      f. Irrigate with normal saline if prescribed.
      g. Avoid kinking and tension on the tubing.

D. SUPRAPUBIC CATHETER
   1. DESCRIPTION: CATHETER INSERTED PERCUTANEOUSLY AND DIRECTLY INTO THE BLADDER FROM THE ABDOMEN FOR THE PURPOSE OF DRAINING URINE
   2. USES
      a. Short-term placement following bladder, urethral, or prostate surgery
      b. Long-term placement in paralyzed clients such as a quadriplegic to decrease the incidence of penoscrotal fistulas
      c. May be used in young males if unable to insert a urethral catheter
   3. NURSING INTERVENTIONS
      a. Meticulous care is required because suprapubic catheter is prone to poor drainage.

b. Avoid kinking of tube to facilitate gravity drainage.

c. Encourage the client to turn from side to side, promoting tube drainage.

d. Milk or irrigate the tubing if previous measures fail.

e. Administer prescribed antispasmodics if bladder spasms occur.

f. Frequently monitor and record drainage.

g. Apply protective skin barrier such as stomahesive to prevent skin breakdown.

E. NEPHROSTOMY TUBES

1. DESCRIPTION: TUBE INSERTED DIRECTLY INTO THE KIDNEY FOR THE PURPOSE OF DRAINING URINE

2. PURPOSE

a. To preserve renal function

3. USES

a. Short-term placement following a ureteral obstruction

4. NURSING INTERVENTIONS

a. Maintain strict aseptic technique when caring for the tube.

b. Avoid clamping or kinks in the tube.

c. Assess the tube for patency when the client complains of pain in the area of the tube or excessive drainage is noted around the tube.

d. If prescribed, irrigate the tube with no more than 5 ml to prevent renal damage from overdistending the kidney parenchyma.

e. Monitor and record the drainage.

f. Report indications of infection or stone formation.

VI. NURSING DIAGNOSES

A. IMPAIRED URINARY ELIMINATION

B. ACUTE PAIN

C. RISK FOR INFECTION

D. INEFFECTIVE THERAPEUTIC REGIMEN MANAGEMENT

E. IMPAIRED SKIN INTEGRITY

F. EXCESS FLUID VOLUME (RENAL FAILURE)

Nursing Diagnoses: Definitions and Classification 2012–2014. Copyright © 2012, 1994–2012 by NANDA International. Used by arrangement with John Wiley & Sons Limited.

VII. URINARY DISORDERS

A. URINARY TRACT INFECTIONS

1. INFECTION OCCURRING AT DIFFERENT LOCATIONS THROUGHOUT THE URINARY TRACT

2. NOSOCOMIAL URINARY INFECTIONS OR HOSPITAL-ACQUIRED URINARY INFECTIONS MOST COMMONLY CAUSED BY URINARY CATHETERIZATION

3. GRAM-NEGATIVE ENTERIC BACTERIA *(ESCHERICHIA COLI)* MOST COMMON CAUSATIVE ORGANISM

4. FUNGAL, PARASITIC, AND VIRAL INFECTIONS MAY BE RESPONSIBLE FOR URINARY TRACT INFECTIONS (UTIs) IN CLIENTS WHO HAVE TAKEN ANTIBIOTICS LONG TERM, HAVE DIABETES MELLITUS, OR ARE IMMUNOCOMPROMISED.

B. CYSTITIS

1. DESCRIPTION

a. Infection of the lower urinary tract involving the bladder

b. More common in women, children, and older men

2. ASSESSMENT

a. Increased urgency and frequency of urination

b. Dysuria

c. Foul-smelling urine

d. Pyuria

3. DIAGNOSTIC TESTS

a. Urinalysis

b. Urine culture and sensitivity

c. Urine Gram stain

4. NURSING INTERVENTIONS

a. Administer prescribed antibiotics such as sulfamethaxazole, trimethoprim (Bactrim, Septra), cephalexin (Keflex), and nitrofurantoin (Macrodantin), and fluoroquinolones such as ciprofloxacin (Cipro) and ofloxacin (Floxin).

b. Administer prescribed urinary analgesic such as phenazopyridine (Pyridium).

c. Increase fluid intake to 2500–3000 ml per day unless contraindicated.

d. Avoid caffeinated beverages, citrus juices, chocolate, alcohol, and spices, which may irritate the bladder.

e. Instruct female clients to wipe from front to back after elimination.

f. Instruct the client on the importance of taking the prescribed antibiotics for the prescribed period of time.

g. Instruct the client to avoid taking bubble baths and using perineal products.

h. Encourage the client to urinate when the urge is present and to fully empty the bladder with each voiding.

C. ACUTE PYELONEPHRITIS

1. DESCRIPTION

a. Infection of the upper urinary tract involving the kidney

b. Generally ascends from the lower urinary tract

c. Preexisting conditions such as vesicoureteral reflux in children and

structural abnormalities such as prostatic hyperplasia, tumor, urinary stones, or pregnancy are frequently present.
   d. Complications include bacteremia leading to septic shock.
   e. Chronic pyelonephritis may result from repeated episodes of acute pyelonephritis.

2. ASSESSMENT
   a. Fever
   b. Chills
   c. Fatigue
   d. Dysuria
   e. Increased urgency and frequency of urination
   f. Costovertebral tenderness and flank pain

3. DIAGNOSTIC TESTS
   a. Urinalysis
   b. Urine culture and sensitivity
   c. Urine Gram stain
   d. White blood cell count
   e. IVP
   f. Blood culture

4. NURSING INTERVENTIONS
   a. IV antibiotics may be prescribed initially followed by 2- to 3-week course of oral antibiotics.
   b. Same as nursing interventions listed for cystitis (see page 244)

D. URETHRITIS

1. DESCRIPTION
   a. Inflammation of the urethra
   b. Causes include *Trichomonas, Chlamydia*, gonorrhea, and monilial infections.
   c. May be present with cystitis

2. ASSESSMENT
   a. Urethral discharge
   b. Dysuria
   c. Increased urgency and frequency of urination
   d. Foul-smelling urine
   e. Pyuria

3. DIAGNOSTIC TESTS
   a. Split urine collections taken at the beginning of the flow of urine and again in the middle of the flow of urine.
   b. Urethral or cervical tissue culture to detect the presence of *Chlamydia*

4. NURSING INTERVENTIONS
   a. Administer prescribed antibiotics for bacterial infections, nystatin (Mycostatin) or fluconazole (Diflucan) for monilial infections, or metronidazole (Flagyl) and clotrimazole (Mycelex) for *Trichomonas*.
   b. Instruct female clients to avoid perineal deodorant sprays.

   c. Offer hot sitz baths.
   d. Instruct the client on proper cleansing of the perineal area after elimination.
   e. Encourage the client to avoid sexual intercourse until symptoms subside.

E. GLOMERULONEPHRITIS

1. DESCRIPTION
   a. Immunologic disorder of the kidney that may be caused by systemic lupus erythematosus, scleroderma, or streptococcal infection
   b. Primary inflammation of glomeruli with accompanying tubular, interstitial, and vascular changes
   c. May be focal or diffuse depending on the extent of the involvement
   d. Changes that occur may be minimal or widespread.
   e. Complications include renal tissue damage or severe renal insufficiency from chronic glomerulonephritis.

2. DIAGNOSTIC TESTS
   a. Renal biopsy to detect the presence of antiglomerular basement membrane antibodies (anti-GBM antibody)
   b. Urinalysis
   c. BUN and creatinine
   d. KUB x-ray

3. ASSESSMENT
   a. Mild to gross hematuria
   b. Presence of red blood cells (RBCs) and white blood cells (WBCs) in the urine

4. NURSING INTERVENTIONS
   a. Assess the client's exposure to drugs, immunizations, and viral and bacterial infections.
   b. Evaluate and monitor the client's preexisting autoimmune disorder.

F. RENAL CALCULI

1. DESCRIPTION
   a. Stones in the urinary tract that produce clinical manifestations when the flow of urine becomes obstructed
   b. Majority of stones are composed of calcium.
   c. Most commonly affects Caucasians between the ages of 20 and 55 years with a familial history
   d. Contributing factors include a sedentary lifestyle, high-protein dietary intake, decreased fluid intake, decreased urinary output and increased perspiration during warm weather months, or metabolic abnormalities resulting in increased levels of calcium, uric acid, and citric or oxaluric acid.

2. TYPES
   a. Calcium oxalate stones
     1) Account for over 30% of the urinary calculi

    2) Characteristically small stones that may become trapped in a ureter
    3) More common in men
  b. Struvite (magnesium-ammonium phosphate stones)
    1) Account for approximately 10% of the urinary calculi
    2) More common in women who experience frequent urinary tract infections
    3) Generally take on a staghorn appearance
    4) Contributing factors include *Proteus* urinary tract infection.
  c. Calcium phosphate stones
    1) Account for only 8% of the urinary calculi
    2) Most commonly are a combination struvite or oxalate mixed stone
  d. Uric acid stones
    1) Account for less than 5% of all urinary calculi
    2) More common in Jewish men who have a family history or an incidence of gout
  e. Cystine stones
    1) Account for less than 2% of all urinary calculi
3. ASSESSMENT
  a. Flank or abdominal pain that is generally severe
  b. Nausea
  c. Vomiting
  d. Pain that becomes colicky in nature when the stone passes into the ureter
  e. Cool, moist skin
  f. Chills
4. DIAGNOSTIC TESTS
  a. Excretory urography
  b. Urinalysis
  c. Urine culture
  d. KUB x-ray
  e. Serum calcium, phosphorus, and protein
  f. 24-hour urine collection
  g. Ultrasound
  h. IVP or retrograde pyelogram
  i. Cystoscopy
  j. CT scan
  k. BUN and creatinine
  l. Urine pH
5. NURSING INTERVENTIONS
  a. Administer prescribed analgesics.
  b. Reassure the client that most stones smaller than 4 mm pass spontaneously.
  c. Provide education to prevent future stones.
  d. Encourage increased daily fluid intake.
  e. Instruct the client to avoid foods that contribute to the diagnosed type of urinary stone (see Table 10-1).

Table 10-1 Therapeutic/Dietary Management for Specific Urinary Calculi

Type of Urinary Stone	Therapeutic Management	Dietary Management
Calcium oxalate	Goal of therapy is to increase hydration and reduce dietary oxalate. Urinary pH is not a factor in the development of calcium oxalate calculi. Administer prescribed thiazide diuretic such as cholorothiazide (Diuril) or hydrochlorothiazide (HydroDIURIL) to promote calcium reabsorption in the urine. Administer sodium cellulose phosphate to reduce intestinal absorption of calcium.	Encourage acid-ash diet, including meats, whole grains, eggs, cheese, plums, prunes, and cranberries. Instruct the client to avoid foods high in oxalate, such as spinach, tomatoes, celery, parsley, beets, asparagus, rhubarb, cabbage, okra, chocolate, cocoa, tea, instant coffee, and peanuts.
Calcium phosphate	Goal of therapy is to reduce dietary calcium.	Instruct the client to avoid foods high in calcium, such as milk and other dairy products.
Struvite (magnesium-ammonium phosphate)	Goal of therapy is to control infection. Administer prescribed antibiotics. May require surgical removal of stones.	Instruct the client to avoid high-phosphate foods, such as red meats, organ meats, dairy products, and whole grains, to help prevent the formation of these stones.
Uric acid	Goal of therapy is to reduce the urinary concentration of uric acid and make urine more alkaline. Administer prescribed allopurinol (Zyloprim) to decrease uric acid levels frequently seen in clients with gout.	Encourage alkaline-ash foods such as tea, milk, vegetables, and fruits except plums, prunes, and cranberries. Instruct the client to avoid foods containing purine, such as organ meats, boned fish, whole-grain breads, red wine, and pastries. Encourage the client to increase fluid intake to 2500–3000 ml daily.
Cystine	Goal of therapy is to increase hydration to 3000–4000 ml daily to dilute the urine and prevent cystine crystals from developing.	Encourage alkaline-ash foods, such as vegetables and most fruits except plums, prunes, and cranberries. Instruct the client to avoid foods that result in acidic urine to prevent the formation of future stones.

6. SURGICAL MANAGEMENT
   a. Surgery may become the treatment of choice if the stone fails to spontaneously pass or impaired renal function, severe infection, or bacteriuria is present, and the client has continual pain or is unable to be treated medically.
   b. The type of surgical procedure depends on the location of the stone (see Figure 10-2).
7. TYPES OF NONSURGICAL MANAGEMENT
   a. Cystoscopy
      1) Endoscopic procedure to remove small stones lodged in the bladder or lower ureter
      2) After inserting a ureteral catheter, the stone is dislodged, with the goal of removing the stone.
      3) The ureteral catheter is left in place to dilate the ureter, facilitate complete passage of stone, and ensure drainage of urine.
   b. Lithotripsy
      1) Types of lithotripsy that break up calculi include extracorporeal shock-wave lithotripsy, laser lithotripsy, electrohydraulic lithotripsy, and percutaneous lithotripsy.

Figure 10-2 Common locations of urinary calculi formation.

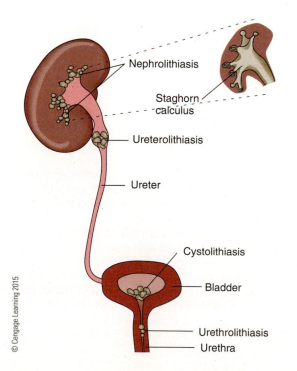

Nephrolithiasis

Staghorn calculus

Ureterolithiasis

Ureter

Cystolithiasis

Bladder

Urethrolithiasis
Urethra

© Cengage Learning 2015

      2) Extracorporeal shock-wave lithotripsy
         a) Noninvasive procedure utilizing ultrasound delivered with the client submersed in a warm bath or shock waves delivered by electrohydraulic, electromagnetic, or piezoelectric to fragment the calculus.
         b) The client receives anesthesia, whether it is conscious sedation, a spinal, or general, to facilitate lying very still during the procedure.
         c) High-energy shock waves are delivered by a lithotripter to the affected kidney through the use of a fluoroscopy or ultrasound to disintegrate the calculus.
         d) The urine is strained following the procedure to monitor the elimination of the calculus, which generally occurs within a few days of the procedure.
         e) A stent may be placed in the ureter to promote the passage of the calculus fragments.
         f) The urine is monitored for hematuria, which may occur postprocedure.
      3) Laser lithotripsy
         a) Common noninvasive procedure in which the interaction between a wavelength and the dye used results in fragmentation of large bladder and lower ureteral calculus
      4) Electrohydraulic lithotripsy
         a) Utilizes a probe that is placed over the location of the calculi to fragment the calculi to facilitate the removal of the fragments by either a continuous saline irrigation suction or through the use of forceps
         b) The client may experience colicky pain postprocedure.
         c) The urine may be bright red initially followed by a dark-red or smoky-colored urine.
         d) Antibiotics may be prescribed postprocedure to prevent infection.
      5) Percutaneous lithotripsy
         a) Invasive procedure that positions an ultrasonic probe directly into the renal pelvis to fragment large calculi into minute particles that may be easily removed

     b) Reserved for calculi that have been unsuccessfully removed by other lithotripsy procedures

     c) Types of surgical procedures

        1. A ureterolithotomy (incision into the ureter), pyelolithotomy (incision into the renal pelvis), cystotomy (incision into the bladder), or nephrolithotomy (incision into the kidney) is reserved for clients who have abnormalities in the calyces and at the ureteropelvic junction or are extremely obese.

G. RENAL TRAUMA

  1. DESCRIPTION

    a. Variety of traumatic injuries that occur as a result of violent crime, increased speed in transportation, or sports

    b. More common in men under the age of 30 years

  2. ASSESSMENT

    a. Reported injury to the abdomen, flank, or back area

    b. Hematuria

  3. DIAGNOSTIC TESTS

    a. Urinalysis

    b. Hemoglobin, hematocrit, and WBC count

    c. Intravenous urography

    d. Renal arteriography

    e. Computed tomography

  4. NURSING INTERVENTIONS

    a. Restore fluid volume.

    b. IV fluid and electrolyte replacement

    c. Plasma volume expanders such as albumin or dextran

    d. Frequent monitoring of vital signs

    e. Hourly urine output

    f. Instruct the client on safety measures to prevent future renal trauma, such as wearing seat belts, avoiding excessive vehicle speeds, wearing protective clothing for contact sports, and avoiding contact sports when only one kidney is present.

H. URINARY INCONTINENCE

  1. DESCRIPTION

    a. Involuntary loss of urine

    b. Embarrassment associated with incontinence results in the failure to seek medical care and costly physical and psychosocial consequences.

    c. Not a normal physiological response to aging

    d. Causes include abnormalities in bladder contraction, urethral contraction, or conditions outside of the urinary system.

  2. TYPES (SEE TABLE 10-2)

    a. Urge incontinence

    b. Overflow incontinence

    c. Stress incontinence

    d. Reflex incontinence

    e. Trauma- or surgically-induced incontinence

  3. DIAGNOSTIC TESTS

    a. Urinalysis

    b. IVP

    c. Cystoscopy

    d. Cystometrogram

    e. Ultrasound

I. URINARY RETENTION

  1. DESCRIPTION

    a. Inability to void, even the presence of an urge to void

    b. Causes include

      1) A response to stress

      2) Obstruction of the urethra by cancer, tumors, benign prostatic hyperplasia, fecal impaction

      3) Side effects of medications such as sedatives, anticholinergics, antihistamines, antiparkinsonians, antispasmodics, certain antihypertensives

      4) Reaction to anesthesia

      5) Postoperatively due to a decreased fluid intake, decreased activity, and medications given before and after surgery

  2. ASSESSMENT

    a. Abdominal discomfort from an overdistended bladder

    b. Frequent voiding but in small amounts

    c. Palpable bladder above the symphysis pubis

  3. DIAGNOSTIC TESTS

    a. Complete history, including drug history, changes in activity, diet, surgery, and stressful events

    b. Urinalysis

  4. NURSING INTERVENTIONS

    a. Insert a urinary catheter to empty the bladder.

    b. Perform intermittent catheterization after the client voids to measure residual urine (should be less than 50 ml).

    c. Encourage the client to increase ambulation and oral fluid intake unless contraindicated.

J. RENAL FAILURE

  1. DESCRIPTION: KIDNEY DISEASE IN WHICH THE FUNCTION OF THE KIDNEYS IS SEVERELY COMPROMISED OR THE KIDNEYS CEASE TO FUNCTION.

Table 10-2 Types of Urinary Incontinence

Type	Description	Causes	Assessment	Nursing Intervention
Urge incontinence	Inability to suppress a strong desire to urinate	Abnormal detrusor muscle contractions

Associated with:

Neurological conditions such as cerebrovascular disorder, Parkinson's disease, spinal cord lesions, and Alzheimer's disease

Bladder conditions such as cancer of the bladder, interstitial cystitis, and bladder outlet obstruction | Involuntary and uncontrollable loss of urine

Nocturnal incontinence | Encourage a timed voiding schedule.

Instruct the client to wear incontinence pads or undergarments.

Administer prescribed anticholinergics such as propantheline (Pro-Banthine).

Administer prescribed tricyclic antidepressants such as imipramine (Tofranil) at bedtime.

Instruct the client to avoid fluids that contain caffeine and alcohol that have a diuretic effect.

Instruct the client to perform Kegel exercises to strengthen the pelvic floor muscles. |
| Overflow incontinence | Involuntary loss of urine in the presence of an overdistended bladder | Inability of detrusor muscle to contract and expel urine in the presence of an overdistended bladder

Associated with

Bladder conditions such as bladder outlet obstruction, enlarged prostate, and urethral stricture

Neurological conditions such as diabetic neuropathy, herniated discs, and neurogenic bladder

Surgery or radiation to lower abdomen

Anesthesia | Distended bladder

Frequent dribbling of urine | Perform intermittent catheterization as ordered.

Administer prescribed bethanechol (Urecholine).

Instruct the client on bladder compression techniques to empty the bladder, such as the Crede method, Valsalva maneuver, double voiding, or splinting. |
| Stress incontinence | Involuntary expulsion of urine during activities such as coughing, laughing, jogging, dancing, sneezing, or lifting

Most common type of incontinence; more likely to affect women | Relaxed pelvic wall musculature occurring in conditions such as cystocele and rectocele, multiple pregnancies, or gynecological and obstetrical surgical procedures

Conditions occurring as a result of decreased estrogen production and vaginal atrophy

Conditions affecting the prostate in men | Involuntary loss of urine during periods of increased intra-abdominal pressure | Instruct the client to perform Kegel exercises.

Encourage weight reduction if necessary.

Administer prescribed estrogen.

Instruct the client on bladder training.

Instruct the client to avoid fluids containing caffeine and alcohol.

Instruct the client on procedures such as vaginal cones, urethral inserts, patches, pessaries, or devices that fit into the bladder neck for support.

Care for the client following surgery if indicated to correct the problem. |

(continues)

Table 10-2 Types of Urinary Incontinence *(continued)*

Reflex incontinence	Involuntary passage of urine with no advanced warning	Detrusor muscle hyperreflexia preventing normal detrusor muscle contraction and relaxation Associated with neurological conditions resulting in spinal cord lesions	Involuntary urination at any time during the day or night	Administer prescribed prazosin, baclofen (Lioresal), or diazepam (Valium) to relax urinary sphincters. Perform intermittent catheterization as ordered. Administer postoperative care if sphincterotomy was performed.
Trauma-induced or surgically-induced incontinence	Involuntary expression of urine after genitourinary surgical procedures	Gynecological cancers, surgical procedures, and radiation resulting in vesicovaginal or urethrovaginal	Uncontrollable loss of urine at unpredictable times	Administer appropriate postoperative care for surgery correcting the fistula or creating a urinary diversion. Perform intermittent catheterization.

© Cengage Learning 2015

2. TYPES
   a. Acute
      1) Rapid onset generally occurring over hours to day that has the potential to be reversible with supportive care
      2) Causes include hypovolemia or hypotension over an extended period of time, contact with nephrotoxic agent, glomerulonephritis, pyelonephritis, benign prostatic hyperplasia, prostatic cancer, tumors, and cancer.
      3) Clinical manifestations initially include a decreased urinary output that may be less than 400 ml in a 24-hour period associated with proteinuria, fluid retention, decreased serum bicarbonate and increased serum potassium, sodium, creatinine, and BUN (see Table 10-3).
      4) Complications depend on the client's overall state of health, before renal failure, with hyperkalemia being the most severe.
   b. Chronic
      1) Multisystem disease with a gradual onset over months to years resulting in an irreversible destruction of as much as 95% of the nephrons in end-stage renal disease (ESRD)
      2) Causes include unsuccessful treatment of acute renal failure, diabetic nephropathy, hypertension, glomerulonephritis, and cystic kidney disease.

      3) Complications include progressive azotemia and uremia (increased nitrogenous wastes in the blood), leading to ESRD.
3. DIAGNOSTIC TESTS
   a. Serum electrolytes
   b. Serum creatinine and BUN
   c. Urinalysis
   d. 24-hour urine for creatinine
   e. Renal ultrasound
   f. CT scan
4. NURSING INTERVENTIONS
   a. Administer prescribed IV insulin, promoting the movement of potassium into the cells.
   b. Administer prescribed IV glucose concurrently with insulin to prevent hypoglycemia.
   c. Instruct the client to avoid foods high in potassium, such as bananas, oranges, melon, prunes, potatoes, deep-yellow and deep-green vegetables, legumes, and salt substitutes.
   d. Administer prescribed oral or rectal sodium polystyrene sulfonate (Kayexalate), a cation-exchange agent generally mixed with sorbitol (a bulk laxative) to ensure excretion of potassium in the stool.
   e. Administer prescribed antihypertensives, generally calcium-channel blockers, to control the hypertension but also to improve the GFR and renal blood flow.
   f. Monitor the blood pressure frequently in supine, sitting, and standing positions.
   g. Assess the client's weight at the same time each day.

Table 10-3 Clinical Manifestations of Chronic Renal Failure

Neurological	Lethargy
	Decreased concentration
	Muscular irritability
	Seizures
	Confusion
	Coma
Cardiovascular	Hypertension
	Cardiomyopathy
	Congestive heart failure
	Pericarditis
	Pleural effusion
	Arrhythmias (fatal arrhythmia may occur with potassium greater than 7 to 8 mEq/L)
Respiratory	Uremic fetor or halitosis (urine-like breath odor)
	Tachypnea
	Hyperpnea
	Suppressed cough reflex
	Pulmonary edema
	Uremic lung or pneumonitis
Metabolic	Increased BUN
	Increased serum creatinine
	Hyperglycemia
	Hyperinsulinemia
	Hyperkalemia
	Hypernatremia
	Metabolic acidosis
Hematologic	Anemia
	Bleeding
Integumentary	Yellow discoloration of skin
	Dry skin
	Pruritus
	Ecchymosis
	Purpura
	Uremic frost (urea crystals occurring on the face, axilla, and groin from evaporated perspiration)
Musculoskeletal	Renal osteodystrophy (skeletal changes including osteomalacia [lack of bone mineralization]), osteitis fibrosa [bone resorption], and calcification of the soft tissues of the body)
Gastrointestinal	Stomatitis
	Nausea vomiting
	Metallic taste in the mouth
	Diarrhea or constipation
	Uremic gastritis
Urinary	Polyuria and nocturia (early)
	Oliguria leading to anuria (late)
	Proteinuria
	Hematuria
	Dilute pale-yellow urine
Reproductive	Decreased libido
	Infertility
	Amenorrhea

h. Instruct the client to avoid foods high in protein and sodium.

i. Instruct the client to avoid foods high in phosphorus, such as beef, pork, chicken, tuna, dairy products, bran, whole grains, and legumes.

j. Administer prescribed vitamins to supplement a low-protein diet deficient in vitamins.

k. Instruct the client to avoid over-the-counter nonsteroidal anti-inflammatory drugs (NSAIDs), which may result in renal hypoperfusion.

l. Instruct the client to avoid over-the-counter antacid and laxative products containing magnesium due to an impaired renal excretion of magnesium.

m. Restrict fluid intake to equal urinary output plus 500–600 ml for insensible loss.

n. Instruct the client on methods to reduce thirst, such as sucking on hard candy and ice chips.

o. Provide skin care using warm water and bath oils to prevent dry skin and relieve pruritus.

p. Trim the client's nails to prevent skin breakdown from scratching.

5. DIALYSIS

a. Movement of fluid and waste products in the blood across a semipermeable membrane into a dialysis solution, dialysate that is designed to restore chemical and electrolyte balance

b. A general criterion for dialysis is when the client's GFR is less than 5–10 ml per minute.

c. Involves the principles of diffusion (solutes that move from an area of greater concentration to an area of lesser concentration) and osmosis (fluid that moves from an area of lesser concentration to an area of greater concentration)

d. Peritoneal dialysis

  1) Catheter inserted into the anterior abdominal wall, which serves as an excellent semipermeable membrane because of its large surface area

  2) Three phases of the dialysis cycle

    a) Fill: 1–2 liters of dialysate is infused in approximately 10 minutes into the peritoneal cavity.

    b) Dwell: the fluid remains in the peritoneal cavity from 30 minutes to 8 hours after clamping the catheter.

    c) Drain: the fluid drains from the peritoneal cavity generally within 15–30 minutes.

  3) Types of peritoneal dialysis

    a) Automated peritoneal dialysis

      1. Utilizes a machine called a cycler

      2. The 2-hour exchanges occur four to eight times a night, allowing the client to sleep during the exchanges.

      3. The client is free of dialysis during the day, allowing the client to carry on with normal activities.

    b) Continuous ambulatory peritoneal dialysis

      1. Does not require a machine

      2. Four 2-liter exchanges are performed daily with 4- to 8-hour dwell times.

      3. During the dwell time, the client may roll up the empty dialysate bag and tubing under the clothing or remove the catheter tubing and place a protective cap over the peritoneal catheter junction, permitting normal activities.

      4. After the dwell time, the dialysate solution is drained from the peritoneal cavity followed by the instillation of more dialysate solution and application of an empty bag.

  4) Nursing interventions during peritoneal dialysis

    a) Obtain baseline vital signs and laboratory tests, especially glucose and electrolyte tests, prior to initiating dialysis.

    b) Weigh the client before the dialysis treatment and every 24 hours.

    c) Continually monitor the vital signs throughout the treatment.

    d) Monitor the client for respiratory distress and abdominal pain.

    e) Assess the abdominal dressing for wetness or bleeding.

    f) Maintain a strict intake and output—dialysate inflow should equal dialysate outflow (if dialysate outflow is less than inflow, the difference is equal to the amount that was absorbed or retained by the client and should be recorded as intake).

g) Maintain precise dwell time and routine blood glucose assessments to prevent predisposition to hyperglycemia because glucose is absorbed by some clients.

h) Monitor the color and clarity of the outflow.

5) Complications of peritoneal dialysis

a) Peritonitis

1. Major complication of peritoneal dialysis is caused by a contaminated connection site during the exchange manifested by a cloudy or opaque dialysate outflow, fever, malaise, nausea, vomiting, abdominal tenderness, and pain.

2. Maintaining meticulous sterile technique during connection and clamping of dialysate bags is the priority nursing intervention to prevent peritonitis.

3. Obtain Gram stain and cell count to identify the organism prior to initiating antibiotics.

b) Abdominal pain

1. May be common during initial exchanges as a result of peritoneal irritation, generally resolving within 2 weeks

2. Warm dialysate solution with a specific dialysate warming pad or in the warming chamber of the automated cycling machine, not in a microwave oven, to prevent this complication.

c) Dialysate leakage

1. May occur 1–2 weeks after initial peritoneal dialysis is started

2. More commonly occurs in clients who are diabetic, obese, or receiving steroid medications

3. Administer small volumes of dialysate initially to facilitate tolerating the full 2-liter exchange without leakage and the development of infection.

d) Insufficient flow of the dialysate

1. Results from constipation, twisted or kinked connection tubing, migration of the peritoneal catheter, and prolonged sitting or standing position

2. Ensure bowel evacuation prior to initiating catheter placement and establishment of bowel program, including a high-fiber diet and stool softeners.

3. Maintain tubing that is free from kinks or twisting.

4. Obtain x-ray to confirm catheter placement.

5. Turn the client side to side to maintain inflow and outflow of drainage.

6. Encourage low-Fowler's position and avoiding coughing to prevent increased intra-abdominal pressure.

e) Colored outflow

1. Initially, outflow is bloody followed by a normal clear outflow.

2. Report outflow that is brown as a possible bowel perforation, yellow as a possible bladder perforation, and cloudy or opaque as a possible infection.

f) Bronchitis, pneumonia, or atelectasis

1. May occur from a long dwell time, resulting in a decreased ability of the lungs to expand and a repeated upward displacement of the diaphragm

2. Elevating the head of the bed, frequent position changes, and deep breathing exercises will help prevent respiratory complications.

g) Increased protein loss

1. Occurs as a result of proteins and amino acids crossing the peritoneal membrane and being lost in the dialysate fluid

2. Optimal protein intake for peritoneal dialysis is 1.3 g/kg body weight/day.

6. HEMODIALYSIS

a. Requires the use of a machine with an artificial semipermeable membrane that may be referred to as an artificial kidney and a surgically created graft or fistula allowing access to the client's circulatory system

b. With each treatment, a catheter must be inserted into the graft or fistula, facilitating the circulation of the blood through a semipermeable membrane, promoting the removal of excess fluids by osmosis and the by-products of protein metabolism and electrolytes by diffusion or filtration, and allowing fluids, electrolytes, and blood to be returned to the client.

c. Types of vascular access (see Figure 10-3)

  1) Arteriovenous (AV) shunt

   a) Two cannulas are subcutaneously inserted, one into the artery and one into the vein, that are connected by a silicone rubber tubing exiting the skin, creating an external shunt.

   b) A U-shaped shunt device connects the two ends at the midpoint, creating vascular access. It may be used immediately after insertion.

   c) Most common site is the forearm.

   d) Not commonly used since the development of special catheters allowing temporary vascular access

---

Figure 10-3 Hemodialysis access sites.

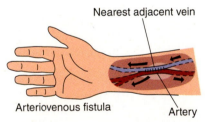

Nearest adjacent vein

Arteriovenous fistula   Artery

Edges of incision in artery and vein are
sutured together to form a common opening

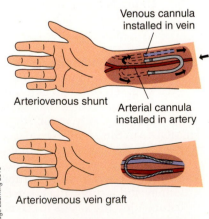

Venous cannula
installed in vein

Arteriovenous shunt   Arterial cannula
installed in artery

Arteriovenous vein graft

Ends of natural or synthetic graft sutured
into an artery and a vein

2) Arteriovenous fistula

   a) An artery and a vein are anastomosed, allowing arterial blood to flow through the vein, facilitating an increased pressure in the arterial blood flow, which creates thick and tough veins appropriate for circulation of rapid and large volumes.

   b) Requires weeks to months for maturation of fistula

   c) The most common site is the forearm.

   d) Most frequently vascular access is used, promoting patency with a lower incidence of complications such as infection and clotting.

   e) Requires two large-gauge needles to create access (one withdraws the client's blood and one returns the dialyzed blood)

3) AV grafts

   a) Grafts made of synthetic materials, generally polytetrafluoroethylene (PTEE) and Gore-Tex, form a bridge between the arterial and venous systems.

   b) Requires 1–2 weeks to 1 month for maturation of graft

   c) May be inserted into the forearm, upper arm, and inner thigh

   d) Most frequently reserved for older adult clients

   e) Requires the use of two large-gauge needles to create access

   f) The access site is capable of closing over the puncture site when the needle is removed.

   g) High incidence of infection because of artificial materials used to make grafts

d. Complications of vascular access routes

  1) Thrombosis

   a) Most common complication seen with grafts

   b) Anticoagulants may be needed with clotting-prone clients.

   c) May require surgical declotting or excision of stenotic area after formation of clot

   d) Avoid intravenous starts, venipunctures, and blood pressures in the extremity with the vascular access route.

   e) Assess for thrill and bruit over the vascular access site.

   f) Avoid constrictive devices over the vascular access route.

2) Infection
   a) Most common complication in AV grafts and shunts
   b) Frequently, *Staphylococcus aureus* is introduced during needle puncture for access.
   c) Strict aseptic technique is essential for cannulation, site care, and dressing changes.
   d) Avoid intravenous starts, venipunctures, and blood pressures in the extremity with the vascular access route.
   e) Extent of infection may necessitate removal of the graft.
3) Bleeding
   a) More common in AV shunts
   b) May occur at needle puncture sites
   c) Have clamps available for dressing changes with the AV shunt.
4) Aneurysms
   a) Result from repeated needle sticks in the same location in the AV fistula, rendering it nonfunctional
   b) May require surgical repair
5) Ischemia
   a) More common in AV fistulas
   b) Results from a decreased arterial blood flow distal to the AV fistula
6) Arterial steal syndrome
   a) Occurs from persistent ischemia in the AV fistula
   b) Clinical manifestations include pale, cold, and numb fingers, which may progress to gangrene.
   c) To preserve the extremity, the AV fistula may require ligation if collateral circulation does not develop.
e. Complications of hemodialysis
   1) Dialysis disequilibrium syndrome
      a) The precise cause is unknown but is thought to be due to the rapid decrease in the BUN levels that occur during hemodialysis.
      b) Cerebral edema and increased intracranial pressure may occur from changes in urea.
      c) Monitor the client closely for nausea, vomiting, headache, restlessness, altered level of consciousness, and seizures.
      d) Early recognition may prevent coma and death.
      e) Start hemodialysis treatments initially for short periods of time with low blood flows to

prevent rapid plasma composition changes.
      f) Administer prescribed mannitol and anticonvulsants.
      g) Slow or stop the hemodialysis treatment.
   2) Hepatitis
      a) Significantly reduced as a result of testing clients for hepatitis B surface antigen (Hbs-Ag), appropriate disposal of contaminated needles and equipment, administration of hepatitis B vaccine to all dialysis clients and staff, and utilizing isolation precautions as necessary.
      b) Maintain strict adherence to all hepatitis preventive measures.
   3) Muscle cramps
      a) May occur from a rapid change in the sodium and water levels
      b) Administer hypertonic IV solution or a bolus of normal saline.
   4) Bleeding
      a) Most commonly results from the presence of residual blood left in the dialysis machine, or if the client is receiving too much heparin.
      b) Thoroughly rinse the dialyzer after each treatment.
      c) Closely monitor heparinization and signs of bleeding.
      d) Apply pressure on the access site when the needle is removed.
   5) Renal transplantation
      a) May be used in ESRD
      b) Although not considered "a cure," it may reverse pathophysiological changes in the diseased kidney, eliminate the need for dialysis, and restore a more normal lifestyle.
      c) Stringent conditions must be met by the donor and recipient.
      d) Recipient
         1. Generally between the ages of 4 and 70 years of age
         2. Must be in relatively good health, free of conditions that would increase the risk of complications
         3. Renal transplantation contraindicated in advanced cardiac disease
         4. Risk versus benefits must be evaluated in metabolic diseases such as diabetes

mellitus, certain cancers, obesity, and gastrointestinal disorders.

e) Donor
1. May be living donor or cadaver donor
2. Most living donors are related to the recipient and in good health, with no diagnosed kidney disease.
3. Most cadaver donors were young and in good health prior to being the victim of a trauma that left the potential donor brain dead.

f) Pretransplanation
1. ABO blood group, histocompatibility, human leukocyte antigens, and cross-matching are performed.
2. Removal of the donor kidney may take 3–4 hours.
3. Transplantation of the kidney into the recipient may take 4–5 hours.
4. Recipient must receive dialysis treatment within 2 hours of transplantation.

g) Post-transplantation
1. Maintain strict adherence to immunosuppressive drug therapy to prevent tissue rejection.
2. Monitor the client for signs of infection that may occur from impaired wound healing from immunosuppressive therapy.
3. Maintain strict intake and output.
4. Perform meticulous catheter care.
5. Monitor the urinary drainage hourly—initially it will be pink and bloody but should return to normal within several days to weeks.
6. Perform continuous bladder irrigations as prescribed to remove blood clots.
7. Monitor daily urine laboratory test such as BUN, creatinine, glucose, and cultures.
8. Remove the Foley catheter as soon as possible to prevent infection.
9. Administer prescribed antibiotics, corticosteroids, and immunosuppressant agents.
10. Monitor daily weights and blood pressure readings.
11. Monitor oral and intravenous fluid intake closely to prevent fluid overload.
12. Assess the client frequently for indications of complications.

h) Rejection
1. Hyperacute rejection occurs within 48 hours of transplantation and results in the removal of the transplanted kidney.
2. Acute rejection is the most common, occurring 6 weeks to 2 years after transplantation, and may be successfully treated with immunosuppressant drug therapy.
3. Chronic rejection may occur months to years after transplantation and may be irreversible, placing the client in chronic renal failure again.

i) Renal artery stenosis
1. Bruit develops over the renal artery anastomosis site, resulting in decreased renal function and hypertension.
2. Stenotic artery must be resected and new anastomosis created.
3. Instruct the client to adhere to immunosuppressant therapy, avoid individuals with infections, and avoid contact sports.

K. HYDRONEPHRITIS
1. DESCRIPTION
   a. Renal pelvis and renal calyces dilate.
   b. Urine flow is obstructed.
   c. May involve one or both kidneys
2. ASSESSMENT
   a. Pain
   b. Nausea
   c. Vomiting
   d. Pain with voiding
   e. Blood in urine
   f. Difficulty urinating
3. DIAGNOSTIC TESTS
   a. Ultrasound
   b. Excretory urography
   c. Renal function tests
4. NURSING INTERVENTIONS
   a. Surgery to remove obstruction
   b. Low protein diet
   c. Antibiotics

5. SURGICAL MANAGEMENT
   a. Nephrostomy tube placement
L. RENOVASCULAR HYPERTENSION
   1. DESCRIPTION: SCLEROSIS AND RISE IN ARTERIAL RENAL BLOOD PRESSURE
   2. ASSESSMENT
      a. Hypertension
      b. Renal failure
      c. Headache
      d. Tachycardia
      e. Anxiety
   3. DIAGNOSTIC TESTS
      a. Venous renin assay
      b. Duplex Doppler ultrasound
      c. MRI
      d. Angiography
   4. NURSING INTERVENTIONS
      a. Antihypertensives
      b. Low-sodium diet
      c. Diuretics
   5. SURGICAL MANAGEMENT
      a. Surgery: renal artery bypass or nephrectomy
      b. Renal artery dilation via balloon catheter
M. ACUTE TUBULAR NECROSIS/ACUTE TUBULOINTERSTITIAL NEPHRITIS
   1. DESCRIPTION
      a. Injury or ischemia from surgery, trauma, dehydration, septic shock, anesthesia, or ingestion of nephrotoxic agents
      b. Causes acute renal failure, uremia, necrosis, lesions, or obstruction in tubules
   2. ASSESSMENT
      a. Low urine output
      b. Increased serum potassium
      c. Pulmonary edema
      d. HEART failure
      e. Anemia
      f. Nausea, vomiting
      g. Confusion, mental status changes
      h. Fever

3. DIAGNOSTIC TESTS
   a. Arterial blood gases
   b. Urine analysis
   c. Complete blood count
   d. Serum electrolytes, bun, and creatinine
4. NURSING INTERVENTIONS
   a. Intravenous fluids
   b. Diuretics
   c. Packed RBCs
   d. Decreased serum potassium with medication
   e. Dialysis
   f. Antibiotics for infection
N. RENAL CANCER (SEE CHAPTER 11)
O. POLYCYSTIC KIDNEY DISEASE
   1. DESCRIPTION
      a. Formations of cysts in the cortex and medulla
      b. The cysts contain fluid.
      c. The kidneys become enlarged, are compressed, and become nonfunctioning.
      d. May be accompanied by hepatic fibrosis
   2. ASSESSMENT
      a. Hypertension
      b. Hematuria
      c. Urinary tract infection
      d. Pain in the lumbar region
      e. Enlarged kidneys
      f. Increased abdominal girth and swelling
   3. DIAGNOSTIC TESTS
      a. Urinalysis
      b. Ultrasound
      c. CT scan
      d. MRI
   4. NURSING INTERVENTIONS
      a. Fluid restriction
      b. Dialysis if renal failure develops
      c. Antibiotics
      d. Antihypertensives
      e. Analgesics
   5. SURGICAL MANAGEMENT
      a. Nephrectomy
      b. Surgery to drain the cysts

PRACTICE QUESTIONS

1. The nurse is teaching a class on urinary infections. Which of the following should the nurse include?
   1. The urinary tract below the urethra is sterile
   2. Pyelonephritis is a common infection of the lower urinary tract
   3. *E. coli* is the most common cause of urinary infections

4. Males are more prone to urinary tract infections than females

2. The nurse tells a student nurse that the normal constituents of urine are the following. Select all that apply:
   [ ] 1. Protein
   [ ] 2. Sodium chloride
   [ ] 3. Ketones

[ ] 4. Urea
[ ] 5. Epithelial cells
[ ] 6. Water

3. The nurse assesses a client's hourly output of urine to be 70 ml. Which of the following is the most appropriate action by the nurse?
   1. Notify the physician immediately
   2. Encourage the client to drink more fluids
   3. Instruct the client on the importance of ambulation
   4. Recognize this as a normal hourly output

4. The nurse instructs a client with pyelonephritis to drink 3000 ml of fluids per day. The nurse understands that the rationale for this intervention is to
   1. prevent reflux of urine.
   2. prevent stasis of urine.
   3. decrease urine output.
   4. decrease residual urine.

5. A nurse is discharging a client who was hospitalized with calcium oxalate calculi. The nurse instructs the client that which of the following food selections contribute to the development of calcium oxalate calculi? Select all that apply:
   [ ] 1. Celery
   [ ] 2. Salmon
   [ ] 3. Beets
   [ ] 4. Bacon
   [ ] 5. Whole-wheat bread
   [ ] 6. Asparagus

6. The nurse is teaching a class on renal disease. Which of the following should the nurse include?
   1. Involvement of 90% of the nephrons is found in acute renal failure
   2. There is a direct correlation between the amount of urine produced and the severity of renal failure
   3. Acute renal failure follows prolonged hypotension
   4. The most diagnostic lab test for renal failure is the blood urea nitrogen

7. The nurse administers which of the following prescribed medications to a client with recurrent urinary tract infections caused by *Escherichia coli*?
   1. Hyoscyamine sulfate (Levsin)
   2. Bethanechol chloride (Urecholine)
   3. Sulfamethoxazole and trimethoprim (Bactrim DS)
   4. Phenazopyridine hydrochloride (Pyridium)

8. The nurse is caring for a client experiencing renal colic associated with nephrolithiasis. Which of the following nursing measures should receive priority in the client's plan of care?

1. Strain urine
2. Administer morphine sulfate
3. Monitor intake and output
4. Encourage ambulation

9. The nurse is caring for a client suspected of sustaining renal trauma following an automobile accident. It is a priority that the nurse monitor and report which of the following findings?
   1. Lethargy
   2. Hypertension
   3. Hematuria
   4. Bradycardia

10. The nurse is caring for a client in acute renal failure. Which of the following clinical manifestations is a priority for the nurse to monitor in this client?
    1. Infection
    2. Pain
    3. Oliguria
    4. Anemia

11. The nurse is caring for a client in acute renal failure. Which of the following would indicate to the nurse that the client is uremic?
    1. BUN of 32 mg/dl
    2. Serum calcium of 10.5 mg/dl
    3. Serum potassium of 2.8 mg/dl
    4. Urine specific gravity of 1.030

12. The nurse is preparing a client for an intravenous pyelogram (IVP). Which of the following would be essential for the nurse to include?
    1. Instruct the client that no fasting is required
    2. Inform the client that a ureteral catheter will be inserted during the procedure
    3. Administer a laxative the night before the procedure
    4. Monitor for bladder spasms after the procedure

13. The nurse identifies which of the following hospitalized clients to be at greatest risk for the development of a nosocomial urinary tract infection?
    1. A 48-year-old male suspected of Parkinson's disease who had been jogging prior to admission
    2. A 75-year-old male who has pancreatic cancer
    3. A 34-year-old male who drinks 2500 ml of fluids daily, following a fracture of the fibula
    4. A 60-year-old obese female with cholecystitis

14. The nurse correctly collects urine by which of the following methods to establish the diagnosis of urethritis?

1. Obtain a specimen in the beginning and in the middle of the urine flow
2. Obtain the first voided specimen in the morning
3. Collect all urine for 24 hours
4. Collect any voided specimen during the day

15. The nurse identifies which of the following diagnostic laboratory tests as the one the nurse should assess first to establish a diagnosis for renal disease?
    1. Blood urea nitrogen (BUN)
    2. Serum creatinine
    3. Serum uric acid
    4. Serum potassium

16. The nurse is collecting a nursing history from a client admitted with acute pyelonephritis. Which of the following questions should the nurse ask?
    1. "Have you noticed any blood in your urine?"
    2. "Have you experienced a decrease in your urinary output?"
    3. "Do you have pain when urinating?"
    4. "Do you find you are experiencing dribbling at the end of urinating?"

17. The nurse identifies which of the following clients to be at greatest risk for the development of struvite calculi?
    1. A Jewish male with a history of gout
    2. A male with idiopathic hypercalcuria
    3. A female with an autosomal recessive defect
    4. A female with a urinary tract infection

18. The nurse monitors a client who has chronic renal failure and a potassium level of 5.8 mEq/L for which of the following clinical manifestations?
    Select all that apply:
    [ ] 1. Dry skin
    [ ] 2. Lethargy
    [ ] 3. Weakness
    [ ] 4. Muscle irritability
    [ ] 5. Loss of deep tendon reflexes
    [ ] 6. Diarrhea

19. When preparing a client for a renal biopsy, it would be essential for the nurse to explain which of the following aspects of the procedure?
    1. Inform the client that the procedure involves insertion of a catheter and installation of saline solution into the bladder
    2. Explain to the client that burning on urination following the procedure is expected
    3. Inform the client that prior to the procedure, typing and cross-matching blood will be done

    4. Explain to the client that before the procedure, a cathartic or enema will be administered

20. The nurse monitors an increased incidence of stress incontinence in a client during which of the following activities?
    1. Eating
    2. Sleeping
    3. Walking
    4. Laughing

21. After inserting an indwelling Foley catheter, the nurse begins to inflate the balloon and the client complains of pain. Which of the following would be the priority action for the nurse to implement?
    1. Aspirate back solution from the balloon and remove the catheter
    2. Insert the remainder of the solution in the balloon and pull back gently until resistance is felt
    3. Aspirate back solution from the balloon and advance the catheter further
    4. Withdraw the catheter slightly and insert an additional 1 ml into the balloon

22. Which of the following principles of catheter care should the nurse consider before catheterizing a client?
    1. Place a urinary catheter in a client who is geriatric to prevent urinary incontinence
    2. Use catheterization as a last resort
    3. Keep the catheter bag on the bed and at the level of the bladder
    4. Sprinkle powder in the perineal area and around the catheter insertion site

23. The nurse should include which of the following in the procedure for female urinary catheterization?
    1. Expose the urinary meatus with the dominant hand
    2. Lubricate 2 inches of the catheter
    3. Insert the catheter 8 inches with the sterile gloved hand
    4. Allow the labia to relax after the meatus is cleansed

24. Before calculating the urinary output of a client suspected of decreased renal perfusion and possible renal failure, the nurse understands that the minimum hourly urinary output must not fall below how many milliliters per hour? _____

25. When preparing a client for an intravenous pyelography (IVP), the nurse should explain which of the following aspects of the procedure?

Select all that apply:

[ ] 1. Fasting is not required

[ ] 2. A laxative will be given the evening before the procedure

[ ] 3. A contrast dye will be given intravenously

[ ] 4. A ureteral catheter will be inserted during the procedure

[ ] 5. A sedative will be given

[ ] 6. Mild discomfort may be experienced during the procedure

26. The registered nurse may delegate which of the following nursing tasks to unlicensed assistive personnel (UAP)?

Select all that apply:

[ ] 1. Perform a glucose test on a urine specimen for a client who has diabetes mellitus

[ ] 2. Monitor a client's intravenous line for patency

[ ] 3. Provide teaching to a client on how to prevent urinary tract infections

[ ] 4. Assist a client who has calcium oxalate calculi in making appropriate menu selections

[ ] 5. Take the vital signs of a client in renal failure

[ ] 6. Record the intake and output of a client experiencing urinary incontinence

27. The nurse evaluates a client with a diagnosis of dehydration to have which of the following specific gravity readings?

1. 1.000
2. 1.017
3. 1.023
4. 1.035

28. The nurse is reviewing the normal limits for a urinalysis. Which of the following findings would indicate to the nurse the need for additional investigation?

1. Dark, amber-colored urine
2. Faint, aromatic odor
3. Specific gravity of 1.015
4. pH of 6.0

29. Which of the following should the nurse include to correctly collect a timed urine specimen?

1. Instruct the client to save the first voided specimen when the urine collection time starts

2. Instruct the client on the importance of continuing to save all urine even if one specimen is missed

3. Place the collection container in a location that is room temperature and away from accidental spillage

4. Encourage the client to empty the bladder and save this specimen at the end of the collection time

ANSWERS AND RATIONALES

1. 3. *E. coli* is the most common organism causing urinary infections. The urinary tract above the urethra is sterile. Pyelonephritis is an infection of the kidneys or upper urinary tract. The incidence of urinary tract infections is greater in the female because the urethra is shorter than that of the male and also is closer to the vagina and rectum.

2. 2. 4. 6. Urine is normally made up of sodium chloride, urea, and water. Protein is an abnormal constituent of urine indicating renal disease. Ketones may be found in a client who is in diabetic ketoacidosis. The presence of epithelial cells is found in a urinary tract infection.

3. 4. The average 24-hour daily output for an adult is approximately 1500 ml or 62.5 ml per hour, so 70 ml is considered normal and no further action is necessary.

4. 2. Increasing the fluid intake promotes the flushing out of the urinary tract and prevents stasis of urine. Preventing reflux of urine and

decreasing urinary output or residual urine do not provide rationales for increasing fluid intake in pyelonephritis.

5. 1. 3. 6. The goal of dietary management in calcium oxalate calculi is to encourage an acid-ash diet and reduce dietary oxalate. Celery, beets, and asparagus are all high in dietary oxalate. Salmon, bacon, and whole-wheat bread are all meats or whole grains that are permitted on an acid-ash diet.

6. 3. Acute renal failure does occur after prolonged hypovolemia or hypotension. Involvement of 95% of the nephrons is found in end-stage renal disease. There is no direct correlation between the amount of urine produced and the severity of renal failure. Even though acute renal failure is often associated with a urinary output of less than 400 ml per day, it is possible to have a normal or even an increased urinary output. Creatinine is the most diagnostic test for renal failure.

7. 3. Sulfamethoxazole and trimethoprim (Bactrim DS) is an antibiotic and a drug of choice in the treatment of urinary tract infections. Hyoscyamine sulfate (Levsin) is an anticholinergic used in specific spastic disorders. Bethanechol chloride (Urecholine) is a cholinergic agonist used in urinary retention. Phenazopyridine hydrochloride (Pyridium) is a urinary analgesic given to produce an analgesic effect on the urinary mucosa.

8. 2. Straining the urine, monitoring intake and output, and encouraging ambulation are all appropriate interventions in the management of renal calculi, but administering an analgesic is the priority intervention for a client experiencing renal colic. Renal colic is an excruciating pain that occurs when a stone passes into the ureter.

9. 3. When monitoring a client for hematuria who has sustained a renal trauma, it is important to detect hemorrhage, which can be a life-threatening complication.

10. 1. The nurse should closely monitor a client in acute renal failure for the presence of an infection, which constitutes the greatest risk for mortality. The incidence may be as high as 70% in clients who developed acute renal failure resulting from an infection following trauma or surgery. Pain is generally not a clinical manifestation in acute renal failure. Although a client may die from oliguria, it is generally reversible and the mortality rate is approximately 50%. Anemia occurs in chronic, not acute, renal failure.

11. 1. An elevated BUN, or increased nitrogenous wastes in the blood, is classic uremia in a client in acute renal failure. A normal BUN is 10 to 20 mg/dl. A serum calcium of 10.5 mg/dl and a urine specific gravity of 1.030 are at the upper range for normal calcium (9 to 10.5 mg/dl) and specific gravity (1.010 to 1.030). A serum potassium of 2.8 mg/dl is low (3.5 to 5.5 mEq/L) and is not indicative of acute renal failure.

12. 3. Administering a laxative the evening before an IVP is correct. Fasting for 8 hours is required. There is no fasting before a KUB (kidneys, ureters, bladder) x-ray. Inserting a ureteral catheter occurs during a retrograde pyelogram, not an IVP. Bladder spasms occur after a retrograde pyelogram, not an IVP.

13. 2. Although nosocomial urinary infections may occur in any hospitalized client, the incidence is significantly impacted by the client's overall state of health. A client who is male, older, and has a terminal cancer and is receiving chemotherapy is immunosuppressed and at the greatest risk.

14. 1. Obtaining a urine specimen in the beginning and again in the middle of the urine flow (split urine collections) for the purpose of performing a culture is the correct procedure for diagnosing urethritis.

15. 2. Although serum potassium, uric acid, and blood urea nitrogen are all useful diagnostic tests in the diagnosis of renal disease, the serum creatinine is the most diagnostic.

16. 3. Dysuria, or painful urination, does occur in acute pyelonephritis. Blood in the urine and dribbling at the end of urinating are not clinical manifestations. An increased urinary output, and not a decreased output, occurs in pyelonephritis.

17. 4. Women who experience frequent urinary tract infections are more likely to develop struvite calculi that take on a staghorn appearance from repeated *Proteus* urinary tract infections. A Jewish male with a history of gout is at risk for uric acid calculi. A male with idiopathic hypercalcuria is at risk for calcium oxalate. A female with an autosomal recessive defect is at risk for cystine calculi.

18. 3. 4. 6. Weakness, muscle irritability, and diarrhea are all indications of hyperkalemia. Confusion, lethargy, and depression occur in hyponatremia. Hypotension, drowsiness, and loss of deep tendon reflexes occur in hypermagnesemia. Dry skin, nausea, and vomiting occur in hypernatremia.

19. 3. A client scheduled for a renal biopsy will routinely be typed and cross-matched for blood because of the risk of bleeding. The insertion of a catheter and installation of saline solution into the bladder occur with a cystometrogram. Burning on urination is an anticipated outcome following a cystoscopy. Administering an enema or cathartic before the procedure may occur with several procedures, such as intravenous pyelography, retrograde pyelogram, or a cystoscopy.

20. 4. Stress incontinence occurs during periods of increased abdominal pressure such as that which occurs with laughing. Eating, sleeping, and walking do not alter the abdominal pressure.

21. 3. When a client complains of pain during inflation of the balloon after inserting an indwelling catheter, the nurse should aspirate back the inserted solution and advance the catheter further to ensure the catheter is in the bladder and not lodged in the urethra.

22. 2. Catheterization may be used as a last resort after all noninvasive measures to promote urination, such as encouraging ambulation and fluids, have failed. Catheterization should never be used for clients who are geriatric to prevent urinary incontinence. The catheter bag

should always be kept below the level of the bladder. Powder should never be applied to the perineal area and around the catheter insertion site, because this practice promotes infection.

23. 2. For the female client, the urinary catheter should be lubricated 2 inches to facilitate easy insertion. The urinary meatus is exposed with the gloved nondominant hand. The catheter is inserted until urine begins to flow, which is generally 2 to 3 inches. Allowing the labia to relax after the meatus is cleansed results in contamination and increases the risk of infection.

24. 30. An hourly urinary output less than 30 ml per hour is indicative of decreased blood flow to the kidneys and should be reported.

25. 2. 3. A laxative is given the evening before an IVP and a contrast dye is administered intravenously. The client should be NPO for 8 hours. No fasting is required for a renal scan, a nephrotomogram, an MRI, an ultrasound, and a KUB (kidney, ureters, bladder) x-ray. A ureteral catheter is inserted by cystoscopy during a retrograde pyelogram. Sedation medication may be administered before an MRI if a client is claustrophobic. Discomfort may be associated with a retrograde pyelogram, renal angiogram, renal biopsy, and cystoscopy.

26. 1. 5. 6. It is the responsibility of the registered nurse to know or reasonably believe that unlicensed assistive personnel have the appropriate training, orientation, and documented competencies. The UAP cannot do assessments or evaluate responses.

27. 4. Normal specific gravity is 1.003 to 1.030. An elevated specific gravity occurs with albuminuria, glycosuria, and dehydration. A decreased specific gravity occurs with diabetes insipidus.

28. 1. Normal urine specific gravity is 1.003 to 1.030. Normal urine pH is 4.0 to 8.0. Urine is normally yellow in color and faint in odor. Dark, amber-colored urine may indicate dehydration, infection, or blood in the urine.

29. 4. The first voided specimen for a timed urinary test should be discarded. The collection container should be kept in the refrigerator or on ice in the bathroom. If a urine specimen is missed, the whole timed test must start again. It is helpful to have a sign on the bathroom door and above the toilet to save all urine. At the conclusion of the test, the client should be encouraged to empty the bladder and save this specimen.

REFERENCES

Daniels, R. (2010). *Delmar's manual of laboratory and diagnostic tests* (2nd ed.). Clifton Park, NY: Delmar Cengage Learning.

Daniels, R., & Nicoll, L. (2012). *Contemporary medical-surgical nursing.* Clifton Park, NY: Delmar Cengage Learning.

DeLaune, S. C., & Ladner, P. K. (2011). *Fundamentals of nursing: Standard and practice* (4th ed.). Clifton Park, NY: Delmar Cengage Learning.

Estes, M. (2010). *Health assessment and physical examination* (4th ed.). Clifton Park, NY: Delmar Cengage Learning.

Spratto, G. R., & Woods, A. L. (2012). *PDR nurse's drug handbook 2012.* Clifton Park, NY: Delmar Cengage Learning.

CHAPTER 1

ONCOLOGY DISORDERS

I. OVERVIEW

A. DEFINITION
   1. CANCER IS THE UNREGULATED GROWTH OF CELLS.
   2. IT OCCURS IN PERSONS OF BOTH GENDERS, ALL RACES, AND ALL AGES.

B. EPIDEMIOLOGY
   1. INCIDENCE (SEE TABLE 11-1)
      a. Annually, over 1 million Americans are diagnosed with cancer.
      b. Men more likely than women
      c. African American more likely than Caucasian
      d. Most diagnosed after age 55 years
      e. Approximately 5 million Americans are cancer-free for 5 or more years.
      f. Overall, skin cancer is the most frequently diagnosed.
   2. SURVIVAL
      a. Second most common cause of adult death in the United States (first is heart disease)
      b. The number of cancer deaths is decreasing or remaining stable (except for lung cancer in women).
      c. Annually, over 500,000 Americans die from cancer.
      d. The death rate from cancer is higher in African Americans.

II. CANCER BIOLOGY

A. CARCINOGENESIS
   1. CAN OCCUR IN ANY CELL OF THE BODY
   2. DEVELOPMENT AND GROWTH ARE THOUGHT TO BE MULTIFACTORIAL: CHEMICAL, VIRAL/BACTERIAL, PHYSICAL, AND FAMILIAL, ALL TERMED "CARCINOGENS" AND CAPABLE OF CAUSING CELLULAR CHANGES.
   3. DIVIDED INTO THREE STAGES:
      a. Initiation—often irreversible alteration in cells' genetic structure
      b. Promotion—reversible growth of initiated cells
      c. Progression—increased growth of cells, invasion, and metastasis
   4. MULTIPLE CARCINOGENS, INITIATING AND PROMOTING, ARE NEEDED FOR CANCER DEVELOPMENT (SEE TABLE 11-2).

Table 11-2 Carcinogens

Type	Examples
Chemical	Coal tar, tobacco, benzene, chemotherapy agents, estrogen, diethylstilbestrol (DES)
Viral/bacterial	Epstein-Barr virus (EBV), hepatitis B virus (HBV), human papilloma virus (HPV), human immunodeficiency virus (HIV), *Helicobacter pylori*
Physical	Ultraviolet and ionizing radiation, asbestos, secondhand smoke
Familial	• Few cancers actually "inherited"
	• Mutations in tumor suppressor genes (e.g., *BRCA1* and *BRCA2* in breast cancer)
	• Familial syndromes (e.g., familial polyposis and *APC* gene)
Diet	• Plays role in cancer development
	• Research ongoing

© Cengage Learning 2015

Table 11-1 Cancer Incidence in the United States by Gender

Most Common in Women	Most Common in Men
Breast	Prostate
Lung	Lung
Colon and rectum	Colon and rectum
Uterine	Urinary bladder
Non-Hodgkin's lymphoma	Non-Hodgkin's lymphoma

© Cengage Learning 2015

5. A COMPLETE CARCINOGEN BOTH INITIATES AND PROMOTES.
6. THERE MAY BE A GAP OF MANY YEARS BETWEEN THESE STAGES.

B. CELL CYCLE
1. CANCER IS THE CONTINUOUS OPERATION OF THE CELL CYCLE (SEE FIGURE 11-1).

C. CANCER CELLS VS. NORMAL CELLS
1. NORMAL CELLS KNOW WHEN AND WHAT TISSUE TO GROW INTO AND WHEN TO DIE.
2. CANCER CELLS USUALLY GROW AT THE SAME RATE AS TISSUE BUT WITHOUT THE USUAL CONTROLS.
3. CANCER CELLS HAVE SPECIFIC CHARACTERISTICS:
   a. Do not die at planned time
   b. Do not stop growing when cells touch (lose contact inhibition)
   c. Do not stick together (lose adhesion)
   d. Do not stop growing (continue in cell cycle)
   e. Need fewer nutrients
   f. Do not need a surface on which to grow
   g. Less differentiated (less specific), similar to embryonic state

Figure 11-1 Cell cycle.

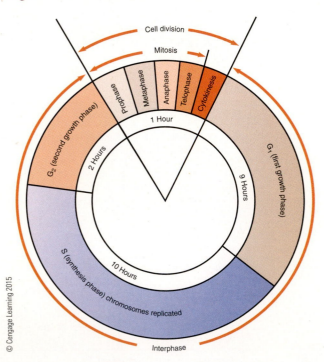

D. METASTASIS
1. TUMOR METASTASIS (CANCER SPREAD) IS A SEVERAL-STEP PROCESS:
   a. Growth and development of blood vessels (angiogenesis)
   b. Invasion through the membrane of the tissue of origin
   c. Cells travel through lymph or blood vessels (many are destroyed here).
   d. Evasion of the immune system (most do not survive this)
   e. Invasion into the blood vessels of a distant organ
   f. Cells break through vessels in the organ.
   g. Growth of cancer cells within the organ
2. MOST COMMON SITES OF METASTASIS:
   a. Lungs
   b. Brain
   c. Bones
   d. Liver
3. MULTIPLE ORGANS MAY BE INVOLVED.

E. CLASSIFICATION OF CANCER
1. BENIGN
   a. Well differentiated, nonspreading
   b. Term ends in "oma" (e.g., papilloma)
2. METASTATIC
   a. Term ending based on anatomic origin (e.g., osteosarcoma)
3. ANATOMIC
   a. Carcinoma—from skin, glands, or mucous membrane linings
   b. Sarcoma—from connective tissue, muscle, bone, or fat
   c. Lymphoma/leukemia—from the hematopoietic system
4. HISTOLOGIC (SEVERAL GRADING SYSTEMS EXIST AND DIFFER SOMEWHAT ACCORDING TO THE CANCER)
   a. Grade I—well differentiated, similar to normal cells
   b. Grade II—moderately differentiated, more abnormal
   c. Grade III—poorly differentiated, very abnormal
   d. Grade IV—very immature, anaplastic; hard to determine the tissue of origin
5. STAGING (EXTENT OF DISEASE RATHER THAN APPEARANCE; VARIOUS STAGING SYSTEMS EXIST)
   a. Stage 0—carcinoma in situ; all characteristics of cancer except metastatic capability
   b. Stage I—localized; limited to tissue of origin

c. Stage II—limited local spread (e.g., possibly to lymph nodes)

d. Stage III—extensive local and regional spread (e.g., large tumor with lymph node involvement)

e. Stage IV—metastasis to other tissue

6. TNM STAGING SYSTEM

a. T1, T2, T3, T4—tumor of increasing size

b. N0, N1, N2, N3—increasing lymph node involvement

c. M0, M1—negative or positive metastasis

III. SCREENING

A. EARLY DETECTION AND TREATMENT ARE THE CORNERSTONES OF CANCER SURVIVAL.

B. EDUCATING THE PUBLIC ABOUT A HEALTHY LIFESTYLE AND EARLY DETECTION

1. REDUCE AND AVOID EXPOSURES TO KNOWN CARCINOGENS SUCH AS CIGARETTES AND THE SUN.

2. EAT A BALANCED DIET OF VEGETABLES, FRUITS, AND WHOLE GRAINS, REDUCING INTAKE OF FAT AND RED, SMOKED, AND CURED MEAT.

3. LIMIT ALCOHOLIC BEVERAGES IF USED.

4. EXERCISE REGULARLY.

5. REDUCE STRESS AND ENCOURAGE ADEQUATE REST AND RELAXATION.

6. FOLLOW SCREENING RECOMMENDATIONS OF THE AMERICAN CANCER SOCIETY AS WELL AS PRACTICING SELF-EXAMINATION SUCH AS BREAST AND TESTICULAR SELF-EXAM.

7. KNOW THE SEVEN WARNING SIGNS OF CANCER.

8. SEEK MEDICAL ATTENTION IF ANY OF THE SEVEN WARNING SIGNS ARE PRESENT.

C. BREAST SELF-EXAMINATION

1. DESCRIPTION: MONTHLY EXAMINATION OF BREAST TISSUE (INCLUDING THE NIPPLE) PERFORMED BY THE CLIENT, AGE 20 YEARS AND OVER, FOR DETECTION OF LUMPS OR COLOR OR TEXTURE CHANGES

2. INSPECTION

a. Stand in front of the mirror with the arms relaxed at the sides, arms pulled back, hands on the hips and the chest thrust out, and arms overhead.

b. Observe the breasts for unilateral dimpling, prominent vein pattern, flat nipple, puckered skin, or scaly nipple in all of these positions.

3. PALPATION

a. Perform in the shower or lying down, or both.

b. Raise the arm near the breast to be examined overhead.

c. Use the pads of the first three fingers of the opposite hand.

d. Use light, medium, and deep pressure while making small circles with the fingers.

e. Palpate the entire breast from the clavicle to the inframammary crease and sternum to the axilla.

f. Circular pattern beginning at the nipple or a vertical pattern may be used.

D. TESTICULAR SELF-EXAMINATION

1. DESCRIPTION: MALES AGE 40 YEARS OF AGE OR MORE SHOULD PERFORM MONTHLY EXAMINATION OF THE TESTES FOR NODULES.

2. PALPATION

a. Perform in the shower with soapy hands.

b. Hold the scrotum in the palm of the hand; compare the weight of each testicle.

c. Use gentle pressure to roll each testicle individually between the first two fingers and thumb.

d. Identify the spermatic cord, epididymis, and testis.

E. SKIN SELF-EXAMINATION

1. DESCRIPTION: PERIODIC VISUAL ASSESSMENT OF THE ENTIRE INTEGUMENT BY CLIENTS OVER 30 YEARS OF AGE WITH RISK FACTORS FOR SKIN CANCER

2. INSPECTION

a. Well-lighted room with full-length mirror and hand mirror

b. Systematic visualization of the entire skin surface, including the scalp, palms of hands, soles of feet

c. Monitor for changes in the size, shape, color, and borders of moles, or new moles.

IV. DIAGNOSTIC TESTS

A. BIOPSY

1. DESCRIPTION

a. Removal of tissue for histologic examination by a pathologist

b. Essential for choosing appropriate treatment

c. Types
   1) Needle aspiration: cells obtained
   2) Incisional: removal of less than whole tumor
   3) Excisional: removal of tumor but may not obtain cancer-free margin
   4) Punch
   5) Bone marrow aspiration
d. May be guided by computerized tomography (CT), magnetic resonance imaging (MRI), or ultrasound

2. PREPROCEDURE
   a. Depends on location and type of biopsy
   b. May need to be NPO if sedation or contrast agent is used
   c. Inform the client about the procedure.

3. POSTPROCEDURE
   a. Control bleeding.
   b. Monitor for infection.
   c. Manage pain.
   d. Inform the client how to obtain results.

B. IMAGING
   1. DESCRIPTION
      a. X-ray, nuclear medicine, ultrasonographic, or magnetic resonance methods of obtaining information about the presence, location, and extent of a tumor
      b. Method chosen based on:
         1) Ability to visualize tumor
         2) Risk
         3) Client comfort
         4) Cost
   2. PREPROCEDURE
      a. Assess for allergy to contrast if to be used.
      b. NPO depending on the area being imaged, use of sedation or contrast
      c. Prepare the client for length of imaging (30–120 minutes), possible noise of machinery, need to remain still.
      d. Most imaging studies are painless.
      e. Monitor the client for flushing, itching, or nausea, indicating allergy to contrast.
   3. POSTPROCEDURE
      a. Inform the client that transportation home is necessary if sedation was used.
      b. Provide the client the means of obtaining test results.

C. LABORATORY TESTING
   1. DESCRIPTION
      a. Testing of blood, urine, or other body fluids for enzymes, hormones, antigens, and proteins altered or produced by the presence of cancer (tumor markers)
      b. No single test can specifically diagnose a cancer.
      c. Used to substantiate diagnosis, monitor response to treatment, identify recurrence

V. **NURSING DIAGNOSES**
   A. INEFFECTIVE COPING
   B. GRIEVING
   C. DISTURBED BODY IMAGE
   D. FATIGUE
   E. IMPAIRED URINARY ELIMINATION
   F. DYSFUNCTIONAL GASTROINTESTINAL MOTILITY
   G. HOPELESSNESS
   H. IMPAIRED ORAL MUCOUS MEMBRANES
   I. NAUSEA
   J. IMBALANCED NUTRITION: LESS THAN BODY REQUIREMENTS
   K. ACUTE PAIN
   L. IMPAIRED SKIN INTEGRITY
   Nursing Diagnoses: Definitions and Classification 2012–2014. Copyright © 2012, 1994–2012 by NANDA International. Used by arrangement with John Wiley & Sons Limited.

VI. **TREATMENT MODALITIES**
   A. SURGERY
      1. DESCRIPTION
         a. Removal of tissue for diagnosis, staging, palliation, or treatment of cancer
         b. Most frequently used cancer therapy
         c. Most successful single therapy if cancer has not spread
         d. Very often performed on an outpatient or brief-stay basis
      2. TYPES
         a. Curative—tumor removed with cancer-free margin; adjuvant treatment as needed
         b. Control—less than entire tumor removed; augments effectiveness of adjuvant therapy
         c. Supportive—insertion of devices to assist in providing adjuvant therapy
         d. Palliative—procedure with goal of maintaining quality of life
         e. Rehabilitative/reconstructive—goal is to maintain quality of life by improving body image after cancer surgery
   B. RADIATION THERAPY
      1. DESCRIPTION
         a. Energy sufficient to break DNA bonds, interrupting mitosis
         b. Localized ionizing radiation used for cure, control, or palliation for over 50% of clients
         c. Cancer cells and proliferative normal cells more susceptible due to frequent division

d. Cells most sensitive during M and G2 phases

e. Radiosensitivity

  1) Highly sensitive—ovaries, testes, bone marrow/blood, intestines

  2) Low sensitivity—muscle, brain, and spinal cord

f. Normal tissue has a maximum tolerable radiation dose.

2. TYPES

  a. Teletherapy (external) beam

  1) Used more commonly

  2) Simulation—x-ray or CT planning session to identify the field that delivers maximum radiation to the tumor and minimal to normal tissue prior to treatment; involves skin markings or immobilization devices

  3) Client is not radioactive during treatment.

  4) Administered in fractions of the full dose, 5 days a week for 4 to 6 weeks

  b. Brachytherapy (internal)

  1) Used primarily in head and neck, gynecologic, and prostate cancers

  2) High dose to the tumor from a sealed internal container with minimal exposure to normal tissue

  3) Client is radioactive only when implant is in place.

  4) Plan care efficiently to minimize nurses' exposure to implant, use shielding, wear a film badge, and maintain safe distance.

  5) Pregnant nurses should not care for clients with implanted radiation.

  6) Pick up dislodged implants with long forceps; place in a special room container.

  7) Body fluids of clients treated with systemic radioactive iodine are radioactive; fluids of clients with implants are not.

3. ADVERSE REACTIONS

  a. Seen only in the organs in the radiation field, except for systemic effects of nausea, anorexia, and fatigue (common) related to the toxins resulting from tumor death and their metabolism (rare)

  b. Skin reactions are common and expected with external beam; however, "burns" or severe skin reactions are uncommon and should not occur with today's technology.

  c. Acute: during and up to 6 months posttreatment (depending on the area radiated)—skin, gastrointestinal (GI), esophageal, mucous membranes, lung, and bone marrow suppression; fatigue; alopecia

  d. Late: post 6 months (depending on the area radiated)—bone and central or peripheral nervous tissue necrosis, sterility, second malignancy, pulmonary fibrosis, pericarditis, skin fibrosis or poor healing

C. CHEMOTHERAPY

  1. DESCRIPTION

  a. Systemic treatment with chemicals that destroy rapidly proliferating cells

  b. Used for cure in testicular cancer, Hodgkin's disease, acute lymphocystic leukemia (ALL), neuroblastoma, and Wilms' and Burkitt's lymphoma

  c. Used to control breast, non-Hodgkin's lymphoma, small cell lung, and ovarian cancer

  d. May also be used palliatively for relief of pain, obstruction, and to improve comfort

  2. TYPES

  a. Cell cycle specific—effective during certain phases of the cell cycle

  b. Cell cycle nonspecific—effective during all phases of the cell cycle

D. BIOLOGIC THERAPY

  1. DESCRIPTION

  a. Agents that change the body's response to the tumor

  b. Based on the principle that a functioning immune system will recognize cancer cells as foreign and destroy them

  c. The mechanism of action is not thoroughly understood; it may be used for cure, control, or maintenance alone, or in combination with surgery, chemotherapy, or radiation therapy.

  2. TYPES

  a. Change the client's immune response

  b. Kill tumors directly

  c. Affect the tumor cell's growth and spread

E. BONE MARROW AND STEM CELL TRANSPLANT

  1. DESCRIPTION

  a. Used for malignant such as acute myelogenous leukemia (AML), chronic myelogenous (granulocytic) leukemia (CML), ALL, Hodgkin's disease, non-Hodgkin's lymphoma, multiple myeloma, ovarian and testicular cancer, and nonmalignant diseases such as sickle cell, thalassemia, aplastic anemia, and immunodeficiency diseases

   b. Permits the use of high-dose chemotherapy with marrow or stem cell rescue (solid tumors), or replacement of diseased marrow (hematologic cancers)

   c. Primarily used for curative intentions

   d. Bone marrow biopsy is performed to confirm remission in hematologic cancers (most likely timing for successful transplant).

   e. Stem cells collected by leukapheresis after the client's cells are stimulated with growth factor (GCSF)

2. TYPES

   a. Allogeneic—stem cells or marrow from family or unrelated donor who is a human leukocyte antigen (HLA) match

     1) If an identical twin is the donor, syngeneic transplant

     2) Umbilical cord blood may be used as stem cell source, although it may not have enough cells for an adult client.

     3) Used to treat leukemias, lymphomas, hematologic and genetic disorders, and immune deficiencies

     4) Client receives high-dose chemotherapy with or without radiation; donor's marrow is harvested from the iliac crest, filtered, and transfused to the client via a central venous catheter.

   b. Autologous—use of the client's own marrow or stem cells

     1) Marrow or stem cells are harvested from the client and processed (including purging of tumor cells), the client receives high-dose chemotherapy with or without radiation, the marrow or cells are transfused back to the client through a central venous catheter.

     2) Used to treat leukemias, lymphomas, and a variety of solid tumors

3. COMPLICATIONS

   a. Failure to engraft

   b. Life-threatening bacteria, viral, and fungal infection, especially for the first 100 days posttransplant

   c. Graft vs. host disease (GVHD): T lymphocytes in the transplanted donor marrow recognize the new host (client) as foreign and attack, particularly the skin, liver, and intestines (acute), or almost any organ (chronic).

     1) Occurs in 25% to 70% of clients

     2) Risk increased when not a perfect six-of-six HLA match

     3) Acute (first 100 days posttransplant) and chronic (> 100 days posttransplant)

     4) Potentially life threatening (10% of bone marrow transplant [BMT] deaths)

   d. GI toxicity

     1) Oral, esophageal, gastric, and intestinal mucositis

     2) Nausea, vomiting, diarrhea

   e. Veno-occlusive disease of the liver: 10% to 60% of clients during the first 30 days

   f. Pulmonary complications: 40% to 60% of clients

     1) Interstitial pneumonia: 8% to 25% develop in the first 100 days; 50% due to cytomeglovirus (CMV)

   g. Neurologic: 60% to 70% of clients; neuropathies, somnolence, confusion, leukoencephalopathy

   h. Gonadal dysfunction

     1) Total body irradiation (TBI), often used in conjunction with BMT, results in sterility.

     2) Men who do not have TBI may retain the ability to father children; women < 26 years old may be fertile.

     3) Counseling and sperm or ova storage should be offered.

   i. Multiple psychosocial issues for the client and family

   j. Second malignancy: rate is four times greater than in the general population

F. GENE THERAPY

   1. DESCRIPTION

     a. Newer therapy, although concept of genes being related to some cancers has been known for about 30 years.

     b. The goal is to treat cancer by inserting new gene into the client's nonreproductive cells to replace a malfunctioning gene or perform a counterfunction.

     c. Currently performed primarily in clinical trials

     d. Raises many ethical issues

     e. Roles of nurses involve educating clients, observing for adverse reactions, and participating in conduct of clinical trials.

2. TYPES
   a. Gene marking or labeling for future identification of source of cancer recurrence in autologous BMT
   b. Gene therapy—deliver chemotherapy directly to the tumor, vaccine, nucleic binding

VII. MANAGING EFFECTS OF CANCER AND TREATMENT
A. PAIN
1. DESCRIPTION
   a. Whatever the client says it is, whenever the client says it exists
   b. May be caused by treatment, cancer destruction of tissue or pressure on nearby structures, and cancer progression
   c. Acute or chronic
   d. Deep tissue pain characterized by aching or gnawing; may or may not be localized
   e. Nerve pain characterized by burning, tingling, shooting, or numbness
   f. Bone metastases are a very common cause of cancer pain.
2. ASSESSMENT
   a. Location
   b. Duration
   c. Severity
      1) What has pain prevented the client from doing?
   d. Quality
      1) Client's description of the pain sensation
   e. Intensity
      1) Use the method appropriate for the age and culture of the client.
      2) Common assessment tools include the 0–10 scale, color scale, faces scale, and observation of the client.
   f. Exacerbating factors
   g. Relieving factors
   h. Client and family beliefs about pain and pain management
3. NURSING INTERVENTIONS
   a. Assess all clients for pain even if they do not appear to be experiencing it.
   b. Educate clients and families about narcotic use.
      1) Correct use of narcotics results in addiction in < 1% of clients.
      2) Narcotic dose may be increased with increasing pain and therefore does not have be reserved for last-resort use.
   c. Instruct clients on nonpharmacologic methods of pain management such as imagery, distraction, healing touch, heat or cold therapy, and massage.
   d. Administer pain medication as ordered, utilizing a combination of nonnarcotic and narcotic analgesics according to the World Health Organization (WHO) analgesic ladder.
   e. Oral route is preferred if possible.

B. FATIGUE
1. DESCRIPTION
   a. Most common adverse reaction of cancer and its treatment
   b. Profound lack of energy often unrelieved by rest
2. ASSESSMENT
   a. Assess all clients.
   b. Use tools as appropriate, such as the Piper Fatigue Questionnaire.
   c. Duration
   d. Severity
      1) What is the client prevented from doing?
   e. Exacerbating factors
   f. Relieving factors
   g. Mental health; stress
   h. Client and family beliefs and fatigue's effect on self-image, work, and relationships
   i. Nutrition
   j. Assess sleep patterns and reasons for disturbances.
   k. Ability to exercise and activities performed
   l. Laboratory values (e.g., low hemoglobin)
   m. Respiratory and cardiovascular status
   n. Pain
3. NURSING INTERVENTIONS
   a. Instruct the client and family that fatigue is an expected adverse reaction that may be worse approximately 10–14 days postchemotherapy administration.
   b. For prevention and treatment, encourage moderate exercise, proper nutrition, keeping a fatigue diary, pacing activities to correspond with higher-energy times, prioritizing activities, and obtaining adequate sleep each night.
   c. Administer medications as ordered, such as erythropoietin to stimulate red blood cells (RBCs), blood products, and oxygen.

C. MYELOSUPPRESSION
   1. DESCRIPTION
      a. Reduced numbers of white blood cells (WBCs), RBCs, and platelets associated with cancer or treatment
      b. Neutropenia—absolute neutrophil count $< 1000/mm^3$
      c. Thrombocytopenia— $< 100,000$ platelets/mm^3
      d. More profound at certain points during treatment (e.g., nadir 5–14 days postchemotherapy or while waiting for engraftment during bone marrow or stem cell transplant)
      e. May result in infection and bleeding
      f. The oral cavity is a primary site of infection in clients undergoing cancer treatment.
   2. ASSESSMENT
      a. Monitor for clinical manifestations of infection:
         1) Erythema, warmth, swelling at an incision or other site
         2) Fever (may be as little as 1° elevation for 24 hours)—most reliable indicator of infection
         3) Shaking chills
         4) Pain
         5) Foul-smelling drainage or urine
         6) Subtle change in mentation
         7) White oral plaque
         8) Monitor laboratory values.
      b. Monitor for clinical manifestations of bleeding:
         1) Bruising and petechiae
         2) Blood in the urine, stool, vomitus, and sputum
         3) Changes in mentation
         4) Pain
         5) Weak, rapid pulse; low blood pressure; pale, cool skin
   3. NURSING INTERVENTIONS
      a. Instruct the client and family to practice careful handwashing technique (hand washing is the most important precaution).
      b. Perform oral and perineum care.
      c. Implement meticulous hand washing between clients and aseptic technique.
      d. Place clients in protective isolation as necessary.
      e. Administer antibiotics and acetaminophen as ordered for fever and infection.
      f. Avoid aspirin and nonsteroidal anti-inflammatories (NSAIDs) in clients who are or may become thrombocytopenic.
      g. Administer meperidine (Demerol) as ordered to relieve shaking chills.
      h. Clients should avoid contact with infected persons, crowds, hospitals, and day care facilities when neutropenic.
      i. Clients should avoid becoming injured, especially in situations where microorganisms may be high, such as gardening, animal bites, and excrement, by wearing protective clothing or taking precautions.
      j. Instruct the client and family to monitor for signs of infection and bleeding.
      k. Avoid any unnecessary invasive procedures such as enemas, suppositories, catheterization, and so forth to prevent bleeding and infection.
      l. Avoid shaving with straightedge razor if thrombocytopenic.
      m. Avoid activities that require straining or impact when thrombocytopenic.
      n. Administer ice lavage through a nasogastric tube, as ordered, for gastric bleeding.

D. ALTERATIONS IN NUTRITION
   1. DESCRIPTION
      a. May be caused by cancer, cancer progression, or treatment
      b. Includes nausea, vomiting, mucositis, alteration in taste, and cachexia
      c. Young women, and those with histories of motion or morning sickness, are at increased risk for chemotherapy-related nausea.
      d. Anticipatory nausea may occur due to anxiety, especially if previous treatments caused nausea and vomiting.
      e. Vomiting may occur within hours to days (delayed) of chemotherapy.
      f. Mucositis may occur throughout the digestive tract because cells are unable to replace those worn away by normal use because of the effects of chemotherapy or radiation therapy (most often occurs during WBC nadir at 1–2 weeks postchemotherapy).
      g. Taste alterations can result from head- and neck-radiation-induced saliva reduction and destruction of taste buds, metallic taste of some chemotherapy, and oral infection.
      h. Cachexia is significant, progressive wasting due to anorexia from a variety of disease- and treatment-related causes that may result in death.

2. ASSESSMENT
   a. History of previous experience with chemotherapy or propensity for nausea and vomiting
   b. Current diet and food preferences (special attention to cultural difference)
   c. Regular measurement of height and weight
   d. Socioeconomic, mental, and physical status related to ability to shop for, purchase, and prepare healthy meals
   e. Coping and mental status related to appetite, meaning of food and weight loss or gain to the client
   f. Pattern of posttreatment nausea and vomiting
   g. Precipitating factors of nausea and vomiting
   h. Laboratory studies to assess for electrolyte imbalances
   i. Vital signs and examination to assess for dehydration such as dry skin, poor skin turgor, low blood pressure, weakness, thirst, weak and rapid pulse
   j. Frequent examination of oral mucosa for signs of infection and tissue breakdown

3. NURSING INTERVENTIONS
   a. Administer prescribed antiemetic drugs.
   b. Encourage the client to take oral antiemetics on an around-the-clock schedule for several days following chemotherapy.
   c. Instruct the client on relaxation, distraction, music therapy, and other complementary therapies to reduce nausea and vomiting.
   d. Encourage client to avoid smells that stimulate nausea, such as by eating in a cool, relaxed atmosphere.
   e. Instruct the client to sit up for 30 minutes following a meal.
   f. Encourage small, frequent meals, especially avoiding sweet, greasy, and spicy foods for at least several days postchemotherapy.
   g. Encourage fluids throughout the day unless the client has restriction (sports drinks, popsicles, and fruit bars may be alternatives to water if the taste is unpleasant).
   h. Encourage frequent rinsing of the mouth with saline solution for reduction of stomatitis during head and neck radiation and chemotherapy cycle.
   i. Recommend rinsing the mouth or sucking on mints prior to meals to improve taste and stimulate taste buds and salivation.
   j. Encourage food choices that do not irritate the oral mucosa (e.g., discourage nuts, popcorn, and spicy, hot food).
   k. Encourage careful and thorough oral care with a soft toothbrush or sponge swabs.
   l. Avoid mouthwashes containing alcohol and use of alcohol and tobacco, which are drying to the oral mucosa.
   m. Encourage use of lip balm to reduce tissue breakdown.
   n. Administer viscous xylocaine (or other analgesics) as ordered for pain relief associated with stomatitis.
   o. Encourage small-quantity and high-calorie nutritional supplements for clients with cachexia.
   p. Encourage moderate exercise, as abilities permit, to stimulate appetite.
   q. Administer appetite-stimulant medications (e.g., dexamethasone, megestrol acetate) as ordered for cachexia.

E. ALTERATIONS IN ELIMINATION
   1. DESCRIPTION
      a. Primarily includes diarrhea and constipation
      b. May be caused by cancer, cancer progression, or treatment
      c. Diarrhea may be stress or food related as well.
      d. Diarrhea may also occur in the presence of fecal impaction.
      e. Electrolyte imbalances, dehydration, and impaired tissue integrity of the perineum can be serious consequences of diarrhea.
      f. Dehydration, narcotic analgesics, and spinal cord compression may also be causes of constipation.
      g. Constipation may potentially lead to serious sequelae, including paralytic ileus and bowel obstruction.
   2. ASSESSMENT
      a. Obtain a history of the client's usual bowel pattern.
      b. If excessive diarrhea is present, obtain order to culture stool for *C. difficile*.
      c. Monitor the client's weight.
      d. Assess the color, odor, consistency, amount, and frequency of stools.
      e. Assess the client's diet.
      f. Obtain a history of recent treatment.
      g. Assess laboratory values for electrolytes.

3. NURSING INTERVENTIONS
   a. Assist the client in modifying the diet appropriately.
      1) Diarrhea—avoid excessive fiber and residue-producing foods, including dairy products, coffee, alcohol, and fried foods.
      2) Constipation—increase dietary fiber, fruits, vegetables, and whole grains.
   b. Encourage fluids to replace losses associated with diarrhea, or maintain softer stool related to constipation.
   c. Administer antibiotics as ordered for positive stool culture.
   d. Administer antidiarrheal medications as ordered (e.g., bismuth subsalicylate or loperamide).
   e. Instruct the client that narcotic analgesic use and surgery will promote constipation, and obtain an order for a stool softener.
   f. Administer laxatives or enemas for constipation as ordered.
   g. Design and encourage a bowel training program to prevent constipation.
      1) Keep a bowel diary.
      2) Void at the same time of day.
      3) Manually stimulate the bowel with a finger or suppository.
      4) Maintain privacy.
      5) Administer the prescribed stool softener.
      6) Encourage physical activity.

F. INEFFECTIVE COPING
   1. DESCRIPTION: DEPRESSION, ANXIETY, GRIEF, LOSS OF CONTROL, ALTERED BODY IMAGE, AND RELATIONSHIP CHANGES ARE COMMONLY ASSOCIATED WITH A CANCER DIAGNOSIS AND TREATMENT FOR BOTH CLIENT AND FAMILY.
   2. ASSESSMENT
      a. Assess how the client usually manages major life changes.
      b. Life stage of the client
      c. Client's usual coping mechanisms and support systems
      d. History of psychiatric disorders, suicide attempts, substance abuse
      e. Other life stressors concurrent with cancer diagnosis
      f. Monitor the client for agitation, difficulty concentrating, hopelessness, weight loss or gain, insomnia or hypersomnia, and lack of pleasure in activities.
      g. Assess for suicide plan and means.
      h. Identify clients who may have body image changes, such as women undergoing breast cancer surgery.
      i. Identify clients who may have sexual functioning issues, such as those with prostate, breast, gynecologic, urinary tract, and testicular cancers.
   3. NURSING INTERVENTIONS
      a. Promote active listening, build honesty, and develop a trusting relationship.
      b. Use touch, as appropriate, to demonstrate caring.
      c. Encourage the client to communicate concerns to staff and family.
      d. Provide access to counseling, support groups, and/or a chaplain.
      e. Validate feelings and provide realistic reassurance without false hope.
      f. Assist in maintaining hope and setting realistic goals.
      g. Administer antidepressant or anxiolytic drugs as ordered.
      h. Instruct clients that antidepressants will take several weeks to reach their full effectiveness and that once on them they should not be stopped abruptly.
      i. Instruct clients that anxiolytic and antidepressants may cause dry mouth, constipation, and drowsiness (or insomnia).
      j. Treat the client and family with respect, communicate care plan, provide information, and offer choices and participation in decision making to the extent desired, whenever possible, to assist in restoring control.
      k. Prepare the client in advance for alterations in body image and sexual functioning, such as suggesting modifications to maintain sexual relationships despite adverse reactions to treatment.
      l. Counsel the client to use a birth control method during treatment and provide resources related to sperm banking as appropriate.
      m. Provide resources related to purchasing head coverings such as wigs and hats due to treatment-related alopecia prior to hair loss.
      n. Reassure the client that hair does grow back after treatment is discontinued and may be a different texture and color.

o. Instruct on relaxation techniques and assess for complementary therapy providers.

VIII. SELECTED ONCOLOGY EMERGENCIES

A. HYPERCALCEMIA

1. DESCRIPTION

a. Greater than 11 mg/dl of serum calcium

b. Occurs in up to 40% of clients with cancer

c. Most common oncologic emergency but may become less common due to use of biphosphonates

d. Occurs in clients with bone metastasis, multiple melanoma, kidney failure, or when the tumor releases factors that encourage bone resorption

e. Most commonly seen in clients with breast, head and neck, lung, and renal cancers

f. Immobility also contributes to calcium loss from the bone.

2. ASSESSMENT

a. Muscle weakness

b. Fatigue; confusion

c. Nausea, vomiting, constipation

d. Cardiac bradycardia and other dysrhythmias (increased sensitivity to digoxin)

e. Potentially lethal late effects include coma, cardiac arrest, ileus, and renal failure.

3. NURSING INTERVENTIONS

a. Monitor serum calcium, blood urea nitrogen (BUN), creatinine level, and electrocardiogram (ECG) and notify the provider as indicated.

b. Administer IV fluids (normal saline 3–4 liters in 24 hours) as ordered.

c. Administer a diuretic (if indicated) as ordered following rehydration.

d. Administer biphosphonates or other medications that inhibit bone resorption, as ordered.

e. Assist the client to maintain his or her level of physical functioning through exercise or referral to physical therapy (encourage weight-bearing exercise as able).

B. SUPERIOR VENA CAVA SYNDROME

1. DESCRIPTION

a. Compression of the superior vena cava by a tumor, enlarged lymph nodes, or a clot interfering with the return of blood from the head, neck, and upper body back to the heart

b. Client needs emergency care.

c. Uncommon overall

d. Most at risk are clients with lymphoma of the mediastinal lymph nodes and lung cancer.

e. Clients who have had radiation to the chest or have central venous catheters or pacemakers are also at risk.

2. ASSESSMENT

a. Most common clinical manifestation is shortness of breath.

b. Swelling of the head, orbits, neck, arms

c. Late clinical manifestations include respiratory distress, change in level of consciousness, severe headache.

3. NURSING INTERVENTIONS

a. Monitor for signs of upper body swelling unrelated to other factors.

b. Assess respiratory status.

c. Assess tissue perfusion.

d. Elevate the head of the bed.

e. Pace activities to conserve energy.

f. Instruct the client to avoid activities that involve straining, such as the Valsalva maneuver.

g. Administer prescribed oxygen, steroids, diuretics, and chemotherapy.

h. Avoid venipuncture and taking of blood pressure in the upper extremities.

i. Assist the client with activities of daily living and ambulation.

j. Reassure the client and provide resources to decrease anxiety.

k. Instruct the client about the use of radiation and chemotherapy to shrink the tumor and decrease superior vena cava pressure.

C. SYNDROME OF INAPPROPRIATE ANTIDIURETIC HORMONE (SIADH)

1. DESCRIPTION

a. Abnormally elevated serum levels of antidiuretic hormone resulting in fluid retention by the kidneys

b. Rare

c. Clients most at risk are those with primarily small-cell lung cancer as well as those with cancer of the pancreas, duodenum, prostate, brain, ovary, and head and neck.

d. Clients with central nervous system or pulmonary infections, and those being treated with chemotherapy, are also at risk.

2. ASSESSMENT

a. Decreased urinary output

b. Weight gain greater than 5 pounds/day

c. Nausea and vomiting

d. Confusion and fatigue

e. Dilutional hyponatremia (serum sodium less 130 mEq/L)

3. NURSING INTERVENTIONS
    a. Follow orders for fluid restriction.
    b. Obtain daily weights.
    c. Test urine specific gravity.
    d. Monitor blood for electrolyte imbalances.
    e. Offer sugarless candy and mouth rinses for oral comfort during fluid restriction.
    f. Orient the client to person, place, time, and environment; perform neurologic assessments.
    g. Maintain a safe environment for the client such as placing the bed in a low position, giving the client the call light, and so on.
    h. Implement seizure precautions.
    i. Administer demeclocycline as ordered for moderate hyponatremia.
    j. Administer vasopressin receptor agonists as ordered (new experimental therapy).
    k. Administer 3% to 5% saline solution IV, if ordered, for severe SIADH.
    l. Administer cancer therapy as ordered (only way to cure SIADH).

D. TUMOR LYSIS SYNDROME
  1. DESCRIPTION
    a. Rapid entry of potassium, phosphorus, and uric acid into the blood from dead tumor cells
    b. Results in hyperkalemia, hyperphosphatemia, hyperuricemia, and hypocalcemia
    c. May result in acute renal failure, arrhythmias, and acute respiratory distress syndrome (ARDS)
    d. Most often occurs in clients with leukemia, lymphoma, or small-cell lung cancer
    e. Occurs within 24 to 48 hours of chemotherapy administration
  2. ASSESSMENT
    a. Clinical manifestations of electrolyte imbalances occur, including:
        1) Muscle weakness, twitching, seizure
        2) Lethargy, confusion
        3) Cardiac arrhythmias, arrest
        4) Nausea and vomiting
    b. Clinical manifestations of renal failure
        1) Flank pain
        2) Oliguria
        3) Edema and weight gain
  3. NURSING INTERVENTIONS
    a. Assess for clinical manifestations of electrolyte imbalances.
    b. Monitor intake and output (I & O).
    c. Obtain daily weights.
    d. Maintain client safety.
    e. Administer fluids and maintain hydration as ordered (primary treatment).
    f. Administer allopurinol as ordered.
    g. Monitor urine pH and notify the physician if < 7.0.

IX. ONCOLOGY DISORDERS
  A. BLADDER CANCER
    1. DESCRIPTION
      a. Transitional cell carcinoma most common (90–95%)
      b. In situ (noninvasive)—has not invaded basement membrane; distant spread unlikely (5-year survival = 94%)
      c. Incidence in the United States approximately 54,300 new cases; 12,400 deaths
      d. Risk factors include:
          1) Smoking
          2) Occupational exposures including dyes, rubber, leather industry
          3) Caucasian males over age 50
      e. Metastatic sites include:
          1) Pelvic lymph nodes and adjacent organs, including the uterus, vagina, colon, rectum, sigmoid colon, prostate
          2) Distant spread—bones, liver, lungs
      f. No screening for early detection
    2. ASSESSMENT
      a. Gross, painless hematuria
      b. Dysuria
      c. Urinary frequency
      d. Urgency
      e. Urinary hesitancy
      f. Suprapubic, rectum, back pain
    3. DIAGNOSTIC STUDIES
      a. Urinary cytology—late morning or early afternoon urine
      b. Bladder washings—more reliable
      c. Flow cytometry—examine DNA content of urine cells
      d. Excretory urogram—evaluate hematuria
      e. Intravenous pyelography—evaluate upper urinary tracts (perform before cystoscopy)
      f. Cystoscopy—tumor visualization and biopsy
      g. CT, transurethral ultrasound, MRI
      h. Tumor marker—p53 and epidermal growth factor (EGF) in late stage
    4. SURGICAL MANAGEMENT
      a. Transurethral resection (TUR) and fulguration (destruction of surrounding tissue with electricity) are most common for in situ and low-grade cancers.

    b. Radical cystectomy (bladder, prostate, seminal vesicles, urethra, uterus, ovaries, fallopian tubes, anterior vaginal wall removed) is most common for high-stage and high-grade tumors.

  5. ADJUVANT THERAPY

    a. Radiation therapy—external beam or brachytherapy may be used for invasive cancer.

    b. Chemotherapy—cisplatin or methotrexate, vincristine, doxorubicin, cisplatin (MVAC) for invasive cancer; BCG may be given intravesically over 6 weeks for superficial disease.

  6. NURSING INTERVENTIONS

    a. Instruct the client on pre-op low-residue and clear liquid diet, antibiotics, and cathartics.

    b. Assess the urinary stoma and teach maintenance of the ileal conduit and appliance.

    c. Assess urinary output (device should produce urine immediately) for urinary tract infection, electrolytes, and signs of peritonitis.

    d. Instruct a client with continent ileal reservoir on care of Kock pouch.

    e. Monitor nasogastric suction (2–3 days post-op).

    f. Assess the client and family for emotional well-being and willingness to learn stoma care.

    g. Discuss possible sexual dysfunction and its treatment.

B. KIDNEY (RENAL) CANCER

  1. DESCRIPTION

    a. Kidney cancer is uncommon in the United States.

    b. Renal cell—most common—85% of kidney cancers

    c. Poor prognostic indicators—lymph node involvement, invasion of renal capsule, and metastasis

    d. Risk factors include:

      1) Male gender

      2) Hispanic

      3) Over 55 years old

      4) Cigarette smoking

      5) Occupational exposures—asbestos, lead cadmium

      6) Heavy use of aspirin

    e. Metastatic sites

      1) Spread through venous and lymphatic route to the lungs, bones, liver

      2) Direct extension to the renal vein or vena cava

      3) 5-year survival less than 10% for Stage IV disease

      4) At diagnosis, 30% to 50% of kidney cancers have metastasized.

    f. No screening for early detection

  2. ASSESSMENT

    a. Gross hematuria

    b. Dull, aching pain

    c. Abdominal mass

  3. DIAGNOSTIC STUDIES

    a. CT

    b. MRI

    c. DNA flow cytometry

    d. Excretory urogram

    e. Intravenous pyelogram

    f. Renal ultrasound and arteriography

  4. SURGICAL MANAGEMENT

    a. Radical nephrectomy and renal hilar lymph node dissection

  5. ADJUVANT THERAPY

    a. Radiation therapy

    b. Chemotherapy including cisplatin (Platinol), vinblastine (Velban), doxorubicin (Adriamycin), and methotrexate

    c. Intravesical therapy

  6. NURSING INTERVENTIONS

    a. Atelectasis and pneumonia prevention (nephrectomy close to the diaphragm)

    b. Assess for signs of hemorrhage.

    c. Monitor urine output and renal function of the remaining kidney.

    d. Pain management

    e. Assessment for and prevention of paralytic ileus

    f. Support the client and family in appropriate follow-up tests for metastasis, hypertension, and kidney function.

C. BREAST CANCER

  1. DESCRIPTION

    a. Most common cancer in women, approximately 200,000/year in the United States; 1% occur in men.

    b. Majority of breast cancers originate in the upper outer quadrant.

    c. Stages I and II are between 70% and 90% curable.

    d. Noninvasive (in situ, DCIS, or precancer)—confined to the duct or lobule; not capable of metastasis; over 90% curable

    e. Invasive or infiltrating—capable of metastasis; no longer contained in the duct or lobule

      1) Ductal—70% of all breast cancers

      2) Lobular—10% of all breast cancers, higher incidence of contralateral breast cancer

      3) Inflammatory (rare)—presents with erythema, pain, edema due to invasion of cancer cells into the skin; poor prognosis

f. Risk factors
   1) Female gender
   2) Over age 50
   3) Previous breast cancer history
   4) Family history—first-degree relatives (especially premenopausal at diagnosis)
   5) *BRCA1* or *BRCA2* gene mutation (5% of breast cancers)
   6) Never having children; having them after age 30
   7) Menarche before age 12; menopause after age 50
   8) Use of estrogens
   9) Atypical hyperplasia on biopsy
   10) History of endometrial, ovarian, or colon cancer
   11) Majority of women have no identifiable risk factors.

g. Metastatic sites
   1) Bone
   2) Lung
   3) Liver
   4) Brain

h. Screen the client.

2. ASSESSMENT
   a. Past history of previous biopsies, family and personal history of breast and other cancers, screening history, current symptoms
   b. Early breast cancer presents with no symptoms and may only be detectable by mammography.
   c. Dimpling, nipple retraction, asymmetry, peau d'orange (edema with orange peel appearance), nipple discharge, ulceration
   d. Inspect with the arms down, over the head, and at the waist with the chest thrust out.
   e. Examine all breast tissue with the pads of the first three fingers. Make dime-size circles, pressing with light, medium, and deep pressure, using a circular or vertical pattern.
   f. Majority present with painless lump or thickening; however, 75% of lumps are benign.

3. DIAGNOSTIC STUDIES
   a. Mammography, ultrasound, MRI, scintimammography, positron emission tomography (PET)
   b. Only diagnosed definitively via biopsy
      1) Needle core, stereotactic—mammographic/computer guided

   2) Ultrasound guided
   3) Fine-needle aspiration—attempt to differentiate benign cyst from solid lesion; may not provide sufficient cells for diagnosis
   4) Open biopsy—wire localized excisional or incisional

c. Tumor marker CA2729

4. SURGICAL MANAGEMENT
   a. Primary treatment for breast cancer
   b. Breast conservation (lumpectomy, segmental resection)
      1) Removal of cancer with margin of healthy tissue
      2) If followed by radiation therapy, has equivalent 5-year survival to mastectomy
   c. Mastectomy
      1) Simple—removal of all breast tissue, nipple, and skin
      2) Modified radical—axillary lymph nodes also removed
      3) Radical mastectomy—pectoral muscles also removed (very seldom performed)
      4) Plastic surgery breast reconstruction may usually be performed at the time of mastectomy.
   d. Lymph node biopsy
      1) Diagnostic evaluation for metastasis
      2) Sentinel lymph node biopsy—injection of radiopharmaceutical or dye, or both, to isolate first draining axillary lymph node for removal and pathology evaluation
      3) Axillary dissection—removal of several levels of lymph nodes in the axilla for cancer evaluation
         a) Risk of lymphedema—chronic fluid collection, pain, and swelling of the arm on the surgical side, which may occur years after surgery

5. ADJUVANT THERAPY
   a. External beam radiation therapy approximately 3 weeks postlumpectomy or after mastectomy when the tumor is large with lymph node involvement; most frequently used
   b. Brachytherapy may also be used.
   c. Chemotherapy—doxorubicin (Adriamycin), cyclophosphamide (Cytoxan), and paclitaxel (Taxol) or docetaxel (Taxotere)

d. Monoclonal antibody therapy (herceptin) may also be used in clients who have tumors that overexpress the protooncogene *HER2*

e. Hormonal therapy (for estrogen receptor positive tumors)—tamoxifen (Nolvadex), progestins, aromatase inhibitors, and ovarian oblation

f. From a sea sponge for metastatic breast cancer—eribulin mesylate (Halaven)

6. NURSING INTERVENTIONS

a. Assist the client and family with adjustment to the cancer diagnosis and decision making.

b. Instruct the client on surgical drain care (e.g., Jackson Pratt) and range-of-motion arm exercises postoperatively.

c. Instruct the client on postoperative sensations in the breast (mastectomy site) and axilla, prevention and reporting of early lymphedema.

d. Support the client and family with body image change and sexuality issues, and provide resources related to breast prostheses.

e. Instruct the client on breast cancer risk reduction and screening.

f. Monitor for adverse reactions of chemotherapy and radiation.

D. CENTRAL NERVOUS SYSTEM CANCERS

1. DESCRIPTION

a. Approximately 17,000 malignant primary brain tumors are diagnosed in the United States annually.

b. Metastatic tumors from primary cancers originating elsewhere are more common (> 100,000 annually).

c. Prognosis for malignant tumors varies greatly by type of tumor and location, although generally very poor; even histologically benign tumors can cause death due to location and damage to structures.

d. Risk factors—very little known

e. Metastatic sites

1) Distant metastasis from the brain are rare; possibly lung or bone if metastasis occurs.

2) Spinal tumors usually do not metastasize distantly but may invade the dura and nearby structures

f. No screening programs exist.

2. ASSESSMENT

a. Clinical manifestations vary greatly depending on location of the tumor; may be related to displacement of the brain, impairment of function, increased intracranial pressure, or spinal cord compression.

b. Change in level of consciousness

c. Change in cognition, memory, personality, ability to communicate

d. Headache

e. Pupil changes or papilledema, or both; changes in vision

f. Motor or sensory deficits

g. Weakness (spinal cord tumors)

h. Vomiting

i. Seizures

j. Vital sign changes

k. Pain—most common clinical manifestations of spinal cord tumors

l. Bowel or bladder dysfunction (spinal cord tumors), or both

3. DIAGNOSTIC STUDIES

a. CT, MRI (preferred method)

b. PET and single-photon emission computed tomography (SPECT); both used as complements to CT and MRI

c. Cerebral angiography

d. Lumbar puncture

4. SURGICAL MANAGEMENT

a. Initial treatment for most brain and spinal cord tumors

b. The goal is to remove all or as much as possible of the tumor.

c. Biopsy may be used for diagnosis or primary surgical treatment.

1) CT or MRI guided needle biopsy through burr hole

2) Open biopsy via craniotomy

3) Stereotactic biopsy—tumor located with three-dimensional coordinates then biopsied or removed; most widely used method

5. ADJUVANT THERAPY

a. Radiation therapy

1) Standard treatment for metastatic brain tumors

2) Used when primary tumors cannot be completely resected or recur despite aggressive surgical intervention and spinal cord tumors

3) Some tumors may be resistant to radiation (e.g., malignant gliomas).

4) Brachytherapy and stereotactic radiosurgery may also be used.

b. Chemotherapy

1) Use is limited by the blood–brain barrier.

2) Not curative, but may contribute to survival time

        3) Plays little role in spinal cord tumors

        4) Ommaya reservoir may be used to deliver chemotherapy directly into the cerebrospinal fluid (CSF); preferred method

  6. NURSING INTERVENTIONS

    a. Will depend on location of the tumor and symptoms exhibited

    b. Ongoing neurologic assessment for changes in mental and functional status, seizure, infection, hemorrhage at the operative site or within the brain, cerebral edema, or increasing intracranial pressure (ICP)

    c. Prevent ICP.

    d. Administer drugs as ordered to treat cerebral edema (e.g., corticosteroids), prevent seizures (anticonvulsants).

    e. If mobility is impaired, maintain a safe environment.

        1) Obtain appropriate assistive devices and equipment such as a cane, walker, wheelchair, commode, bathroom guardrail, shower stool, or safe footwear.

        2) Assess the home for safety, such as the stairs and rugs.

        3) Obtain an occupational therapist's input.

    f. If cognition is impaired:

        1) Reorient the client.

        2) Encourage use of functional ability.

        3) Provide visual cues or reminders (e.g., calendars, clocks, photos).

        4) Encourage social activity.

    g. Pain management

        1) Administer analgesics as ordered and monitor side effects.

        2) Encourage and teach relaxation and distraction methods.

    h. Prevent tissue breakdown.

        1) Assess the skin of pressure points (and peri area if incontinent) frequently.

        2) Assist with position changes.

        3) Utilize pressure relief and comfort methods such as sheepskin, lotion, massage.

    i. Provide education, support, and referral to resources to the client and family.

    j. Management of side effects related to chemotherapy and radiation

E.   CERVICAL CANCER

  1. DESCRIPTION

    a. Approximately 13,000 cancers and 4000 deaths in the United States annually

    b. Mortality from cervical cancer has decreased greatly over the last several decades in the United States.

    c. Very treatable and curable if detected early

    d. Squamous cell carcinomas are 80% to 90% of cases.

    e. Risk factors

        1) Sexual intercourse before age 17, multiple partners

        2) Sexual partner who has multiple partners

        3) Cigarette smoking

        4) Human papilloma virus

        5) Lower socioeconomic status

    f. Metastatic sites

        1) Abdomen and pelvis

        2) Lung

        3) Liver

        4) Bone

    g. Screening

        1) Papanicolaou (Pap) smear beginning at age 18 or on becoming sexually active

        2) Screen the client as appropriate.

  2. ASSESSMENT

    a. Asymptomatic in early stages

    b. Watery vaginal discharge

    c. Late clinical manifestations include postcoital, heavy, or intermenstrual bleeding.

  3. DIAGNOSTIC STUDIES

    a. Colposcopy—application of acetic acid followed by magnified examination of the cervix

    b. Biopsy

    c. Endocervical curettage

    d. Cone biopsy

  4. SURGICAL MANAGEMENT

    a. Total abdominal hysterectomy and lymphadenectomy

    b. Depends on the stage of the disease, physician preferences, and desire for childbearing

  5. ADJUVANT THERAPY

    a. External beam and brachytherapy radiation may be used alone or in combination with surgery.

    b. Chemotherapy for advanced disease only (wide variety of possible regimens)

  6. NURSING INTERVENTIONS

    a. Assess for changes in bowel and bladder pattern related to both surgery and radiation therapy.

    b. Bladder training by clamping suprapubic catheter, if used, at several-hour intervals and measuring postvoid residuals as ordered by the physician

  c. If laser surgery for early disease is used, instruct the client to avoid douching, tampons, and sexual intercourse for 2–4 weeks.

  d. Assess for sexual dysfunction concerns related to surgical shortening of the vagina, vaginal dryness associated with radiation, and posttreatment anxiety.

  e. During radiation, instruct the client on the use of vaginal dilators or lubricant, especially if not sexually active.

  f. Encourage open communication between the client and her partner.

F. COLON CANCER

 1. DESCRIPTION

  a. Approximately 107,000 cases and 48,000 deaths annually in the United States

  b. Adenocarcinoma is the predominant histological type.

  c. Ascending and sigmoid colon are the most common locations.

  d. Ascending colon cancers usually have a better prognosis.

  e. Survival 92% for localized, 63% for regional spread, 7% for distant metastasis

  f. Risk factors

   1) Men or women over age 50 years

   2) Family history

   3) History of Crohn's disease or ulcerative colitis

   4) Physical inactivity

   5) Obesity

   6) Diet high in red meat and low in vegetables

   7) Smoking

   8) More than one alcohol-containing drink per day

  g. Metastatic sites

   1) Liver (most common site)

   2) Peritoneal surfaces

   3) Spread via lymphatics to the lung, bones, brain

  h. Screening

   1) Early detection via screening is key to favorable prognosis.

 2. ASSESSMENT

  a. Early colorectal cancer is symptom-free.

  b. Bleeding from the rectum

  c. Blood in stool

  d. Change in the caliber of stool

  e. Cramping, lower abdominal pain

  f. Urge for bowel movement, feeling of inability to empty the rectum

  g. Constipation alternating with diarrhea

 3. DIAGNOSTIC STUDIES

  a. Stool sample for occult blood

  b. Sigmoidoscopy and colonoscopy

  c. Double-contrast barium enema

  d. CT

  e. Endoscopic ultrasound and biopsy

 4. SURGICAL MANAGEMENT

  a. Primary therapy for colorectal cancer

  b. Preoperative colon cleansing with isotonic lavage (e.g., Goytely); client drinks 4 liters the evening before surgery plus oral antibiotics the day before; IV antibiotic on surgical day

  c. Right hemicolectomy—primary surgery for cancers of the ascending colon

   1) Removal of the terminal ileum, cecum, and right transverse colon

  d. Left hemicolectomy—primary surgery for cancers of the descending and sigmoid colon

   1) Removal of the distal transverse, descending, and sigmoid colon

  e. Ends of the colon remaining may be able to be anastomosed, or the bowel is brought to the surface and colostomy is formed.

   1) Single-barrel colostomy—proximal colon is brought to the surface, forming one stoma.

   2) Double barrel, two stomas—proximal excretes stool; distal secretes mucus.

   3) Stool formation depends on the area of the colon forming the colostomy.

    a) Ascending—loose, liquid stool

    b) Transverse—semisolid stool

    c) Descending—soft, formed stool

  f. Sexual dysfunction affects 15% to 100% depending on client age, surgical technique, and preexisting conditions.

 5. ADJUVANT THERAPY

  a. Postoperative external beam radiation therapy is used primarily in rectal cancer.

  b. Radiation may also be used pre- and intraoperatively.

  c. 5-fluorouracil (5-FU) is the most common chemotherapy used, usually in combination with leucovorin (folic acid derivative)

 6. NURSING INTERVENTIONS

  a. Preoperative education and surgical preparation (colon cleansing)

  b. Postoperative monitoring for:

   1) Anastomotic leak—intra-abdominal pain

   2) Infection—fever

   3) Bowel obstruction—constipation, abdominal pain

c. Instruct the client to access available resources related to sexual dysfunction.

d. Monitor the stoma and skin surrounding for complications such as stomal retraction, narrowing, redness, edema, bleeding.

e. Participate with the enterostomal therapist in the care of and education related to the stoma and appliance.

G. ENDOMETRIAL CANCER

1. DESCRIPTION
   a. Approximately 39,000 cancers and 7000 deaths in the United States annually
   b. Highest incidence among Caucasian women
   c. Death is twice as likely among African-American women than Caucasians.
   d. Of cases, 90% are adenocarcinomas.
   e. The 5-year survival is 96% for earliest stages, 26% for late stage.
   f. Risk factors
      1) Female over age 50
      2) High cumulative exposure to endogenous or exogenous estrogen
      3) Nulliparity
      4) Family or personal history of breast or ovarian cancer
      5) Infertility
      6) Diabetes
      7) Hypertension
      8) Obesity
   g. Metastatic sites
      1) Cervix and vagina
      2) Lymph nodes
   h. Screen the client as appropriate.

2. ASSESSMENT
   a. Abnormal vaginal bleeding
   b. Pain in later stages

3. DIAGNOSTIC STUDIES
   a. Pelvic examination
   b. Pap smear (primarily for diagnosis of cervical cancer, however)
   c. Endometrial biopsy is 90% effective.
   d. Dilatation and curettage (D & C)

4. SURGICAL MANAGEMENT
   a. Used for staging
   b. Total abdominal hysterectomy, bilateral salpingo-oophorectomy, possible omentectomy, and peritoneal washings

5. ADJUVANT THERAPY
   a. Not required in the earliest stage—surgery is curative.
   b. Intravaginal radiation for early-stage, low-grade tumors
   c. Pelvic external beam radiation for high-grade tumors
   d. Hormonal therapy (progestins) and chemotherapy reserved for advanced disease and lack efficacy

6. NURSING INTERVENTIONS
   a. Encourage and instruct the client regarding the importance of regular pelvic examination in women with early-stage disease cured by surgery alone.
   b. Instruct the client on healthy lifestyle modifications such as weight management and exercise.
   c. Support the client with concerns over loss of femininity and childbearing ability (if applicable).
   d. Postsurgical and radiation assessment of bowel, bladder, and sexual function (instruct the client regarding use of vaginal lubricant during intercourse)
   e. Postsurgical pain management
   f. Management of concurrent medical problems (e.g., hypertension, diabetes)
   g. Prevention of postsurgical venous stasis
      1) Encourage turning and ambulation.
      2) Antiembolic stockings
   h. Instruct the client on the clinical manifestations of recurrence such as:
      1) Vaginal bleeding
      2) Pelvic pain
      3) Constipation

H. GASTRIC CANCER

1. DESCRIPTION
   a. Approximately 22,000 cancers and 13,000 deaths in the United States annually
   b. African Americans, Japanese, Chinese, and native Hawaiian persons in the United States have a higher incidence than do Caucasian persons.
   c. Of cases, 95% are adenocarcinomas.
   d. Prognosis is poor; 5-year survival is 5% to 15%.
   e. Risk factors
      1) Male, greater than 40 years of age
      2) Low-socioeconomic status
      3) Poor nutritional habits and vitamin A deficiency
      4) Family history
      5) Previous gastric resection for benign disease
      6) Pernicious anemia
      7) Helicobacter pylori infection
      8) Gastric atrophy and chronic gastritis
      9) Rubber workers and coal miners

f. Metastatic sites
   1) Direct extension to the pancreas, liver, or esophagus
   2) Intraperitoneal dissemination to the ovary
   3) Nodal spread to the neck
   4) Bloodstream metastasis to the lung, adrenal glands, liver, bone, peritoneal cavity
g. Screening
   1) Among high-risk persons only
   2) Barium x-ray or endoscopy

2. ASSESSMENT
   a. Early clinical manifestations are nonspecific.
   b. Upper epigastrium, retrosternal pain
   c. Uneasy sense of fullness after meals
   d. As disease progresses:
      1) Loss of appetite
      2) Nausea and vomiting
      3) Weakness
      4) Fatigue
      5) Anemia

3. DIAGNOSTIC STUDIES
   a. Upper endoscopic gastroduodenoscopy (EGD)
   b. Biopsy can be performed during EGD.
   c. Endoscopic ultrasound
   d. Double-contrast upper gastrointestinal series
   e. CT scanning (most common)

4. SURGICAL MANAGEMENT
   a. Only treatment that is potentially curative
   b. Total gastrectomy
   c. Radical subtotal gastrectomy
      1) Billroth I
      2) Billroth II
   d. Proximal subtotal gastrectomy
   e. Palliation of symptoms

5. ADJUVANT THERAPY
   a. External beam radiation adds control of unresectable tumor, palliation, and increased survival; intraoperative radiation is used in some centers, although its usefulness is not known.
   b. Chemotherapy has little impact—5-FU, doxorubicin, mitomycin C, Platinol, etoposide, and cisplatin are used most commonly in various combinations.

6. NURSING INTERVENTIONS
   a. Goal is control of clinical manifestations and supporting optimal functioning.
   b. Assess the nutritional status and administer a diet as ordered.
      1) Small, frequent feedings of low-carbohydrate, high-fat, high-protein foods and restricting fluids 30 minutes before and after a meal are useful in preventing dumping syndrome.
   c. Postoperatively assess for:
      1) Respiratory status; reflux aspiration
      2) Infection
      3) Pain—potential anastomotic leak obstruction
      4) Bezoar (food clumping) formation, causing gastric outlet obstruction
      5) Bleeding
      6) Dumping syndrome
      7) Weight loss
      8) Anemia
   d. Provide emotional support for the client and family.

I. HEAD AND NECK CANCERS
   1. DESCRIPTION
      a. Approximately 71,000 cancers and 19,000 deaths in the United States annually
      b. Of cases, 40% are found in the oral cavity but may be found in the larynx, oro-/hypopharynx, sinuses, nasopharynx, nasal cavity, and salivary glands.
      c. More prevalent in other nations (e.g., China)
      d. Of cases, 95% are squamous cell carcinomas.
      e. The 5-year survival for earliest stage is 95%; late stage, less than 50%.
      f. Most clients will present with advanced disease due to substance abuse, denial of clinical manifestations, and a delay in seeking medical intervention.
      g. Risk factors
         1) Male over age 50
         2) Tobacco use of all forms (primary risk factor)
         3) Heavy alcohol consumption (combined with tobacco use, accounts for 95% of these cancers)
         4) Poor oral hygiene
      h. Metastatic sites
         1) Neck lymph nodes (common)
         2) Local and regional spread within the head and neck
         3) Distant metastasis is rarer but may be found in the lung, liver, and bone.
      i. Screening
         1) No screening guidelines exist.
         2) High-risk clients should have thorough head and neck

examinations and referral to smoking and alcohol cessation programs.

2. ASSESSMENT
  a. Clinical manifestations vary depending on location of the cancer.
  b. Throat pain
  c. Persistent hoarseness
  d. A painless mass
  e. Pain
  f. White or red spots in the oral cavity
  g. Nasal stuffiness

3. DIAGNOSTIC STUDIES
  a. Thorough physical examination of the neck and oral cavity
  b. Fiberoptic nasopharyngoscopy
  c. Direct laryngoscopy
  d. X-rays, barium swallow and x-ray, CT, MRI, PET
  e. Biopsy of suspicious areas

4. SURGICAL MANAGEMENT
  a. Surgery and radiation, alone or in combination, is the primary treatment.
  b. Reconstructive (plastic) surgery may be needed to restore form and function.
  c. Radiation therapy and chemotherapy may be used to debulk unresectable tumors.

5. ADJUVANT THERAPY
  a. External beam radiation 4–6 weeks postoperatively
  b. Radiation is the primary treatment for nasopharynx tumors.
  c. Brachytherapy may be used for various areas of the oral cavity.
  d. Chemotherapy is used for:
    1) Recurrent and metastatic tumors
    2) Making the tumor more sensitive to radiation
  e. Single agents such as cisplatin (Platinol), bleomycin (Blenoxane), 5-FU (Adrucil), paclitaxel (Taxol), and methotrexate may be used.
  f. Biologic response modifiers such as interleukin-2 may also be used, although studies are ongoing in this area.

6. NURSING INTERVENTIONS
  a. Primary role is assisting clients in coping with issues of dysfunction, losses, and body image changes associated with difficult and disfiguring treatments.
  b. Monitor during hospitalization for delirium tremens in clients with history of alcohol abuse.
  c. Prepare the client and family preoperatively with information about tracheostomy tubes, drains, suction, and alternative methods of communication (e.g., picture board, paper and pencil, etc.) as appropriate to surgery.
  d. Airway management
    1) Tracheostomy care
    2) Humidity
    3) Suctioning
    4) Stoma care
  e. Provide oral care with saline or peroxide solution with toothettes (avoid mouthwashes that are drying to the mucosa).
  f. Assess for and obtain orders for adequate nutrition intake.
  g. Assess the ability to swallow and ensure safety when eating.
  h. Encourage gradual interaction with others and support group participation, as well as smoking cessation and Alcoholics Anonymous, as appropriate.
  i. Involve therapists and social workers in rehabilitation (e.g., swallowing, speaking, work, financial issues).

J. HEMATOLOGIC MALIGNANCIES
  1. DESCRIPTION
    a. Leukemias, lymphoma, and multiple myeloma
    b. Approximately 31,000 leukemia cases and 22,000 deaths in the United States annually
    c. Leukemias are divided into acute and chronic categories.
      1) AML—acute myelogenous
      2) ALL—acute lymphocytic (80% of childhood leukemias)
      3) CML—chronic myelogenous (Philadelphia chromosome)
      4) CLL—chronic lymphocytic
    d. Excessive numbers of these WBCs cause tissue damage and decrease the number of functioning WBCs, RBCs, and platelets.
    e. Median survival for all treated leukemias is 1–6 years.
    f. Survival of children treated for ALL approaches 90%.
    g. Approximately 61,000 lymphoma cases and 26,000 deaths in the United States annually
    h. Lymphomas are divided in categories:
      1) Hodgkin's disease
        a) Presence of Reed-Sternberg cell
      2) Non-Hodgkin's lymphoma (NHL)
        a) Uncontrolled proliferation of the T and B lymphocytes (majority are B cell)
        b) More common and more fatal than Hodgkin's disease

       c) Can involve any organ or tissue
       d) May be indolent to rapidly growing and quickly fatal
  i. The 5-year survival is 83% for Hodgkin's and 53% for NHL.
  j. Multiple myeloma is a malignancy of the plasma cell (derived from the B lymphocyte).
    1) Cells produce M protein, which does not function in immunity.
    2) Osteoclast factor that causes lytic bone lesions
  k. Approximately 15,000 cases of myeloma and 11,000 deaths in the United States annually; myeloma is a fatal disease.
  l. Risk factors
    1) Leukemias
      a) Men, women, and children of all ages
      b) Down syndrome
      c) Ionizing radiation
      d) Benzene exposure
      e) Previous cancer treatment
      f) Viruses
    2) Lymphomas
      a) Young adults and persons over 70 years
      b) Non-Hodgkin's lymphoma—white males
      c) Reduced immune function
      d) Organ transplantation
      e) HIV and HTLV-I
      f) Epstein-Barr virus
    3) Multiple myeloma
      a) Twice as common in African Americans than Caucasians
      b) Male, 60 years of age
  m. Metastatic sites
    1) NHL and multiple myeloma are widely disseminated at presentation.
    2) Gastrointestinal, bone marrow, and the liver are common areas of spread for NHL.
    3) Multiple myeloma can affect the hematologic, skeletal, renal, and nervous systems.
  n. Screening
    1) No screening programs exist.

2. ASSESSMENT
  a. Leukemias
    1) Varies somewhat based on the type
    2) Splenomegaly
    3) Infection
    4) Low hemoglobin and platelets
    5) WBC count variable to very high
    6) Fatigue
    7) Weight loss
    8) Anorexia
    9) Recurrent infections
    10) Unexplained bleeding
    11) Bone pain
  b. Hodgkin's lymphoma
    1) Enlarged cervical, supraclavicular, or mediastinal lymph nodes
    2) Weight loss, fever, night sweats, pruritus, malaise
  c. Non-Hodgkin's lymphoma
    1) Wide variety of symptoms based on location of the tumor
    2) Lymphadenopathy
    3) Night sweats, weight loss, fatigue
    4) Abdominal, pelvic mass

3. DIAGNOSTIC STUDIES
  a. Leukemias
    1) Complete blood count
    2) Bone marrow aspiration and biopsy
    3) Cerebrospinal fluid analysis
  b. Lymphomas
    1) Excisional lymph node biopsy
  c. Multiple myeloma
    1) Bone marrow biopsy
    2) Serum protein electrophoresis
    3) Urine immunoelectrophoresis

4. SURGICAL MANAGEMENT
  a. Not used in the treatment of hematologic malignancies

5. ADJUVANT THERAPY
  a. Chemotherapy followed by bone marrow transplant is the primary treatment for most leukemias and multiple myeloma.
  b. Treatment is delayed in CLL until the client is symptomatic—steroids and radiation may be the first line of treatment, followed by chemotherapy in late disease.
  c. Radiation to reduce adenopathy is the primary treatment for early Hodgkin's lymphoma and early-stage NHL.
  d. Chemotherapy is used in advanced Hodgkin's disease or in combination with radiation in early NHL and Hodgkin's disease.
  e. Bone marrow or stem cell transplant is used in recurrent NHL.
  f. Rituximab (Rituxan) (monoclonal antibody) is available for certain B-cell NHL.

6. NURSING INTERVENTIONS
  a. Based on the hematologic malignancy being treated
  b. Administer chemotherapy as ordered.

c. Institute precautions for myelosuppressed and thrombocytopenic clients.

d. Monitor for signs of bleeding if the client has thrombocytopenia.

e. Perform neurologic assessment every 2–4 hours when the WBC count is over 50,000.

f. Instruct the client and family on the function of various blood cells and disease processes.

g. Assess for signs of tumor lysis syndrome (common in lymphoma treatment).

h. Assess for signs of hypercalcemia in clients with multiple myeloma.

i. Assess for signs of superior vena cava syndrome in clients with mediastinal lymphadenopathy.

K. LUNG CANCER

1. DESCRIPTION

a. Approximately 170,000 cancers and 155,000 deaths in the United States annually

b. Incidence and deaths among men have declined, while both have increased among women.

c. Repeated exposure of the bronchial epithelium to carcinogens results in increased cell growth, change in cell type, and loss of function.

d. Two primary categories

   1) Small cell (25% of lung cancers)
      a) Oat cell (90%)
      b) Intermediate
      c) Combined
      d) Usually form along a main bronchus
      e) All subtypes are very aggressive and usually metastasized at diagnosis

   2) Non-small cell
      a) Squamous cell (30%)
      b) Adenocarcinoma
         1. Most common overall (even in nonsmokers)
         2. 40% of all lung cancers
         3. Slowest growing, although metastasizes early
      c) Large cell
         1. Rarest type
         2. Divided further into clear cell and giant cell categories
         3. Giant cell has the worst prognosis.

e. The 5-year survival is 48% if detected early and localized, which is very rare.

f. Overall 5-year survival is 15%.

g. Risk factors

   1) Cigarette smoking (primary)
   2) Exposure to arsenic, radon, asbestos (risk increased among smokers)
   3) Radiation
   4) Secondhand smoke in nonsmokers

h. Metastatic sites
   1) Brain
   2) Liver
   3) Bone
   4) Lymph nodes

i. Screening
   1) No screening program currently exists.

2. ASSESSMENT

a. Clients are very rarely symptomatic at the time of diagnosis.

b. Persistent cough and dyspnea

c. Recurrent bronchitis or pneumonia

d. Blood-streaked sputum

e. Chest pain

3. DIAGNOSTIC STUDIES

a. Chest x-ray

b. Sputum cytology

c. CT scan

d. Bronchoscopy with biopsy

e. Transthoracic needle biopsy

f. Video-assisted thoracoscopic surgery

4. SURGICAL MANAGEMENT

a. Dependent on whether the tumor is resectable

b. May be cure for non-small cell if no metastasis has occurred to the other lung or elsewhere in body and lung function is sufficient on removal of all or part of the lung (only about 50% of clients)

c. Lobectomy—removal of the lobe of the lung (most common if confined to one lobe)

d. Pneumonectomy—removal of the lung (only if a lobectomy cannot be done)

e. Segmentectomy—partial removal of the lung lobe

f. May be used in selected clients after chemotherapy

5. ADJUVANT THERAPY

a. Chemotherapy may be used prior to surgery in some clients.

b. Chemotherapy is the primary treatment for small cell.

c. Radiation is standard post-op for advanced non-small cell; may be only treatment for clients with early non-small cell.

d. Chemotherapy and radiation, used alone or in combination, frequently are used to treat small cell.

6. NURSING INTERVENTIONS

a. Assess for signs of superior vena cava syndrome.

b. Postlobectomy—manage chest tubes (chest tube is not used in pneumonectomy).

c. Assess respiration and for presence of pneumothorax or atelectasis.

d. Position properly postoperatively.
   1) Lobectomy—avoid prolonged lying on the operative side.
   2) Pneumonectomy—position on the back or operative side only.

e. Instruct the client on postoperative deep breathing, coughing, and ambulation.

f. Pain management to promote deep breathing

g. Refer the client to smoking cessation programs.

h. Provide support and education to the family and client, especially important for this often fatal disease.

i. Monitor and provide care for adverse reactions related to chemotherapy and radiation depending on the drugs used.

L. OVARIAN CANCER
   1. DESCRIPTION
      a. Approximately 23,000 cancers and 14,000 deaths in the United States annually
      b. Second most common gynecologic cancer after uterine
      c. Most common cause of gynecologic cancer death
      d. Most develop from the epithelial surface of the ovary
      e. Industrial countries (except Japan) have higher incidence.
      f. The 5-year survival is 30% to 35%.
      g. Of cases, 60% to 70% are diagnosed at Stage III or IV.
      h. Risk factors
         1) No clearly defined high-risk population
         2) Women in their mid-50s to 70 years of age (peak 55–59 years)
         3) Higher education and socioeconomic status
         4) No pregnancies, nonuse of oral contraceptives, and infertility
         5) Family history of ovarian cancer
         6) Breast or endometrial cancer in self or family members
         7) Mutation in *BRCA 1* or *BRCA 2*
         8) Hereditary nonpolyposis colon cancer
         9) Use of talc on the peritoneum
      i. Metastatic sites
         1) Direct extension to the fallopian tubes, uterus, bladder, and peritoneum
         2) Peritoneal seeding to the diaphragmatic surface, liver, bladder, bowel
         3) Distant to the liver, lungs, and pleura
      j. Screening
         1) No specific screening program exists.
         2) Pelvic examination
         3) Transvaginal ultrasound and tumor marker CA 125 for high-risk women or with symptoms (not routine screening)
   2. ASSESSMENT
      a. Usually no early clinical manifestations
      b. Abdominal discomfort or enlargement
      c. Indigestion and flatulence that persists without explanation
   3. DIAGNOSTIC STUDIES
      a. Pelvic examination
      b. Ultrasound and CT scan
      c. Blood test for tumor marker CA 125 (although not specific to ovarian cancer only)
      d. Barium enema, sigmoidoscopy, cystoscopy, and IVP may all be used to make diagnosis and stage the cancer.
   4. SURGICAL MANAGEMENT
      a. Peritoneal washings to find cancer cells in fluid
      b. Primary treatment is tumor removal with TAH-BSO, omentectomy, lymph node sampling, and removal of any other visible tumor.
      c. Creation of a colostomy may be necessary.
      d. Surgery may be the only treatment for Stage I.
      e. "Second look" exploration after apparent complete response to adjuvant therapy to evaluate response (does not improve survival and is not standard of care outside of a clinical trial)
   5. ADJUVANT THERAPY
      a. Combination chemotherapy with intravenous paclitaxel (Taxol) and cisplatin (Platinol), and carboplatin (Paraplatin)
      b. Various chemotherapy may be administered intraperitoneally.
      c. Hormone therapy (tamoxifen [Nolvadex] or megestrol [Megace]) may be used after chemotherapy.
      d. External beam radiation to the pelvis and abdomen may be used.
      e. Radioactive isotopes may be placed intraperitoneally.

6. NURSING INTERVENTIONS
   a. Major role involves assisting the client and family in maintaining hope and coping with this often fatal disease.
   b. Post-op TAH-BSO care
   c. Assess for constipation, nausea, and vomiting related to the disease or treatment and treat as ordered.
   d. Assess for increasing abdominal ascites by daily weights, abdominal girth measurements, and palpation for fluid wave.
   e. Assess respiratory function and possible pleural effusion; elevate the head of the bed, pace activities, administer oxygen and analgesics as ordered.
   f. Assess and treat fluid and electrolyte imbalances by monitoring blood tests, daily weights, I & O, and vital signs; administer diuretics, low-sodium diet; maintain mobility as ordered.
   g. Maintain patency of the peritoneovenous shunt.
   h. Assist the client and family with body image and sexuality issues related to persistent (possibly lifelong) ascites and issues related to TAH-BSO.
   i. Pain management
   j. Home care or hospice referral

M. PROSTATE CANCER
   1. DESCRIPTION
      a. Approximately 190,000 cancers and 30,000 deaths in the United States annually
      b. Incidence significantly higher in African-American men (highest in the world)
      c. Second leading cause of cancer death in men
      d. Mortality for African-American men is greater than twice that of Caucasian men.
      e. Of cases, 95% are adenocarcinoma.
      f. Over 80% are diagnosed in early stages, allowing an almost 100% 5-year survival; survival overall for all stages is 96%.
      g. Risk factors
         1) Male over age 65 years
         2) Black men have highest incidence worldwide.
         3) North American or Northwest European
         4) Strong family history
         5) High-fat diet may play a role.
         6) Having had a vasectomy may play a role.

      h. Metastatic sites
         1) Typically slow-growing cancer
         2) Lymphatic spread
         3) Bones, lungs, bladder, liver via the bloodstream
      i. Screening
         1) Screen the client as appropriate.
   2. ASSESSMENT
      a. Early stages may be asymptomatic.
      b. Weak or hesitant urine stream
      c. Inability to start or stop flow of urine
      d. Frequent nocturia
      e. Hematuria
      f. Pain on urination
      g. Pain in the lower back, pelvis, upper thighs in advanced disease
   3. DIAGNOSTIC STUDIES
      a. Digital rectal examination
      b. Transrectal or perineal fine-needle biopsy
      c. Open biopsy in some cases
      d. Prostate specific antigen (PSA) blood test
      e. Abdominal and pelvic CT/MRI
   4. SURGICAL MANAGEMENT
      a. Radical prostatectomy (removal of the prostate gland, capsule ejaculatory ducts, seminal vesicles, plus possible lymph node sampling); surgery of choice in early stage
      b. Nerve-sparing technique can be used in early stages to reduce impotence.
      c. Later stage—transurethral resection of the prostate (TURP) followed by external beam radiation
      d. "Watchful waiting" without intervention may be appropriate treatment in men over 70 years of age with small, early-stage cancers.
   5. ADJUVANT THERAPY
      a. External beam radiation following surgery for early stages
      b. Radiation may be used instead of surgery in some cases.
      c. Brachytherapy—radioactive seeds placed in the prostate gland
      d. Hormonal manipulation (leuprolide, goserelin, estrogen, surgical orchiectomy) alone used in advanced disease
      e. Chemotherapy usually reserved for hormone-refractory prostate cancers
   6. NURSING INTERVENTIONS
      a. Postoperative care
         1) Maintain urinary catheter with aseptic technique and teach the client to manage on discharge (in place several weeks).

2) Maintain continuous bladder irrigation as prescribed; keep normal saline at all times for the first 24 hours post-op or as ordered.

3) Encourage fluids.

4) Ambulation; cough and deep breathing

5) Administer pain medications and antispasmodics as ordered.

6) Administer stool softeners as ordered to reduce constipation and straining with stool.

7) Administer cabazitaxel (Jevtana), which is used to treat hormone refractory prostate cancer.

8) Report inability to void and signs of infection to the physician if brachytherapy was used.

   a) Client is hospitalized until radioactivity decays sufficiently.

   b) Follow radioactivity precautions.

   c) Client should avoid close contact with children and pregnant women following discharge but is not a radioactive source posing risk to others.

   d) Strain urine for dislodged seeds.

   e) Wear a condom for 2 months during intercourse to catch any remaining seeds.

b. Instruct the client on urinary incontinence management techniques.

1) Undergarment liners to absorb urine

2) Variety of catheters

3) Kegel exercises

c. Instruct the client on methods of restarting sexual activity following complete healing, and support coping with body image changes.

1) Open communication with partner

2) Sexual expression alternatives to penile penetration

3) Inform the client that erection may not return in some men.

4) Inform the client about external and internal erection devices.

N. SKIN CANCER

  1. DESCRIPTION

a. Over 1 million basal and squamous cell carcinomas in the United States annually

b. Approximately 54,000 melanomas resulting in 7500 deaths in the United States annually

c. Basal and squamous cell carcinomas are highly curable when treated early.

d. Basal cell carcinoma is the most common skin cancer of Caucasians.

e. Kaposi's sarcoma is a type of skin cancer found among clients with AIDS and cutaneous T-cell lymphoma.

f. Melanoma is 10 times more prevalent in Caucasians than in African Americans.

g. Melanoma has increased among women more than any other cancer except lung cancer.

h. Most melanomas arise from the melanocytes in the skin (cutaneous).

i. Most skin cancers can be prevented by limiting or avoiding midday sun exposure and wearing a hat, sunglasses, and protective clothing and using sunscreen with a solar protective factor (SPF) of 15 or greater.

j. Overall 5-year survival for melanoma is 89%, 96% for localized disease.

k. Risk factors

1) Excessive UVA and UVB radiation exposure (sun or tanning beds)

2) Severe sunburn in childhood

3) Fair complexion

4) Family history

5) Multiple or atypical nevi (moles)

6) Occupational exposure to various chemicals

7) X-ray therapy

8) HIV

l. Metastatic sites (melanoma)

1) Skin

2) Subcutaneous tissue

3) Lymph nodes

4) Lung, liver, brain, and bone

m. Screening

1) Screen the client as appropriate.

  2. ASSESSMENT

a. Basal and squamous cell carcinomas can present as a variety of flat or raised fleshy, pearly white to dark, shiny, scaly, or ulcerated plaques or papules.

b. Melanomas are characterized by:

1) Asymmetry

2) Border irregularity

3) Nonuniform color (may be tan, brown, black, blue, red)

4) Diameter of more than 6 mm

c. Assess for:

1) Change in size or color of a mole

2) New darkly pigmented growth with irregular borders

3) Oozing or bleeding or change in sensation of a mole or nodule

4) Blue-black- or red-colored mole

3. DIAGNOSTIC STUDIES
   a. Careful physical examination of the skin
   b. Biopsy—punch, shave, incisional or excisional with wide margin
   c. Measurement of depth of invasion is essential for staging of melanoma.
4. SURGICAL MANAGEMENT
   a. Excision with a wide margin is the primary treatment if anatomically possible.
   b. Electrodesiccation (heat), cryosurgery (freezing), or laser surgery may be used for nonmelanoma skin cancers.
   c. Lymph node dissection may also be performed for melanoma to determine extent of spread.
5. ADJUVANT THERAPY
   a. External beam radiation is used postoperatively for melanoma.
   b. Radiation is also recommended for nonmelanoma lesions that are inoperable and between 1 cm and 10 cm.
   c. Radiation is used for palliation of inoperable metastases.
   d. Metastatic melanoma is resistant to many chemotherapies, although single agents may be used.
6. NURSING INTERVENTIONS
   a. Provide education related to prevention and early warning signs to the public and client's posttreatment.
   b. Encourage self-exams and health professional screening examinations.
   c. Provide postoperative care of the surgical wound.
   d. Assess for signs of infection, bleeding, and loss (sloughing) of skin graft or flap if used.
   e. Assess the area from which the graft or flap was taken for signs of infection and bleeding.

O. SOFT TISSUE AND BONE CANCER
   1. DESCRIPTION
      a. Osteosarcoma (bone tissue), chondrosarcoma (cartilage), fibrosarcoma (fibrous tissue), Ewing's sarcoma (reticuloendothelial tissue), plus sarcomas of fat, muscle, and vasculature make up this category.
      b. Very rare cancers; approximately 11,000 of all types annually in the United States resulting in 5000 deaths (this does not include cancer that metastasizes to the bone from distant sites)
      c. Osteosarcoma is the most common bone tumor; 5-year survival is approximately 50% with addition of chemotherapy.
      d. The 5-year survival for soft tissue sarcomas ranges from 30% to 90% based on the subtype and grade; prognosis is poor if metastasis has occurred.
      e. Risk factors (osteosarcoma)
         1) Male between 10 and 25 years of age
         2) Older adults with history of Paget's disease
         3) Previous radiation
         4) Ewing's sarcoma is most diagnosed in males ages 5–15 years.
         5) Chondrosarcomas are more common in men ages 30–60 years.
         6) Due to the variety and uncommon nature of these cancers, few risk factors have been identified.
      f. Metastatic sites
         1) Osteosarcoma—lungs (early)
         2) Ewing's sarcoma—lungs, lymph nodes, and bones
      g. Screening
         1) No screening program exists.
   2. ASSESSMENT
      a. Pain and swelling of the affected area (bone cancers)
      b. Painless, swollen mass in the affected area that may go on to cause additional symptoms as its growth presses on nearby nerves and vessels (soft tissue cancers)
   3. DIAGNOSTIC STUDIES
      a. Physical examination
      b. X-rays
      c. Bone scan
      d. CT, MRI
      e. Open or needle biopsy is essential.
   4. SURGICAL MANAGEMENT
      a. Highly individualized based on histology
      b. Amputation including the joint above the tumor
      c. Reconstruction with bone grafts, metal, or synthetic materials, or fitting of prosthesis
      d. Limb salvage resections in eligible clients
   5. ADJUVANT THERAPY
      a. Radiation is most often used for palliation or in conjunction with surgery and chemotherapy because bone cancers are somewhat resistant.
      b. External radiation and brachytherapy are used for Ewing's and soft tissue sarcomas.
      c. Chemotherapy may be given both pre- and postoperatively for both bone and soft tissue cancers.
   6. NURSING INTERVENTIONS
      a. Prepare the client and family for changes in body image and function associated with amputation.

b. Preoperative preparation of the client for phantom limb pain associated with amputation

c. Collaboration with physical and occupational therapy pre- and postoperatively to teach the client transfer techniques and begin strengthening and mobility exercises and use of assistive devices

d. Pain management

e. Monitor for clinical manifestations of infection and wound necrosis following reconstruction procedures.

f. Assess for anemia through vital signs and blood test.

g. Assist the client and family in coping and maintaining hope in the face of an often grim prognosis.

h. Assist the client with strategies for reentry to work, school, and other activities of daily living (e.g., assist in procurement of handicapped parking privileges).

P. TESTICULAR CANCER
1. DESCRIPTION
   a. Approximately 7500 cases resulting in 400 deaths annually in the United States
   b. Most common cancer of men between 15 and 35 years of age
   c. Aggressive and spreads quickly although highly curable when found in early stage
   d. Rare cancer, although incidence is increasing in Caucasians
   e. Scandinavian countries have the highest incidence.
   f. Of cases, 93% are of the classic seminomatous histological type, which are slower spreading than nonseminomas.
   g. Over 90% cure rate for early stage or limited advanced disease
   h. Risk factors
      1) Male between ages 20 and 30 years
      2) Family or personal history of testicular cancer
      3) History of undescended testicle
      4) Infertility (may aid discovery of diagnosis)
   i. Metastatic sites
      1) Direct extension to nearby structures
      2) Lymphatic or hematologic spread to the lung (most common), brain, bone, or liver
   j. Screening
      1) Screen the client as appropriate.

2. ASSESSMENT
   a. Small, hard scrotal mass (most common sign)
   b. Scrotal pain, swelling, pulling sensation
   c. Low back pain (lymph node spread)
   d. Cough, hemoptysis (pulmonary spread)
   e. Gynecomastia (due to elevated serum beta HCG)

3. DIAGNOSTIC STUDIES
   a. Bimanual scrotal palpation
   b. Ultrasound (used commonly)
   c. Inguinal orchiectomy for pathologic diagnosis
   d. Chest x-ray or CT scan, or both, for staging
   e. Blood tests for alpha-fetoprotein (AFP) and beta human chorionic gonadotropin (BHCG) (either or both elevated in 85%)

4. SURGICAL MANAGEMENT
   a. Primary treatment involves transinguinal orchiectomy and retroperitoneal lymph node dissection for early-stage nonseminomas.
   b. Nerve-sparing techniques may be used to preserve fertility.

5. ADJUVANT THERAPY
   a. Cisplatin (Platinol)-based chemotherapy prior to surgery is the primary treatment for men with advanced disease.
   b. Cisplatin-based regimen also is used in men with metastasis to lymph nodes or elsewhere.
   c. Recurrent testicular cancer may also be potentially cured with chemotherapy.
   d. Early-stage seminomas are very sensitive to external beam radiation therapy; combine with chemotherapy for later stage.

6. NURSING INTERVENTIONS
   a. Instruct the public and clients to perform testicular self-exam.
   b. Offer sperm banking prior to treatment if chemotherapy, radiation, and lymph node dissection are planned.
   c. Postoperatively (inguinal orchiectomy)
      1) Typically outpatient procedure
      2) Instruct the client on incisional wound care.
      3) Pain management ice to the scrotal area as ordered
      4) Instruct the client to wear an athletic supporter when ambulating, avoid heavy lifting for 4–6 weeks, and avoid standing for long periods.
      5) Provide support to the client related to altered body image.

6) Instruct the client that fertility and sexual function are not altered by this procedure; fertility may be lost (although the ability to have orgasm remains) if lymph node dissection was performed.

d. Assess respiratory status postoperatively, especially in clients who have received neoadjuvant bleomycin chemotherapy.

e. Assess for ileus; auscultate for bowel sounds; assess patency and placement of the nasogastric tube.

PRACTICE QUESTIONS

1. A client asks the nurse, "Does everyone who gets cancer die of it?" The nurse's best response is based on which of the following?
   1. About 5 million people in the United States survive cancer for 5 or more years
   2. All 1 million people diagnosed in the United States annually will eventually die of their disease
   3. Cancer is the leading cause of adult death in the United States
   4. It destroys hope to discuss dying with a client with cancer

2. The client states, "I heard that all men get prostate cancer sometime in their lives." In teaching the client about cancer incidence, the best response is based on which of the following?
   1. Lung cancer is the most frequently diagnosed cancer in men
   2. Prostate cancer is the most frequently diagnosed cancer in men
   3. Prostate cancer is the most prevalent in Caucasian men
   4. There is no way to screen for prostate cancer, so it is the most common cause of cancer death in men

3. When planning the discharge of a client with cancer, which of the following should the nurse include as a priority?
   1. Encouragement to drink no alcoholic beverages
   2. Information on all local hospices
   3. Plans for a visiting nurse
   4. Information on stress reduction techniques

4. While assessing a client's skin, the nurse should report which of the following findings as a possible skin cancer?
   1. Red, swollen plaques
   2. A bull's-eye rash
   3. A blue-black appearing mole
   4. Spider angiomas

5. The nurse is collecting a health history on a client admitted for colon cancer. Which of the following questions would be a priority to ask this client?
   1. "Have you noticed any blood in the stool?"
   2. "Have you been experiencing nausea?"
   3. "Do you have any back pain?"
   4. "Have you noticed your abdomen has swollen?"

6. A nurse is educating a group of clients on cancer screening practices. Which of the following instructions should the nurse include as a recommended screening pattern?
   1. Annual Pap and pelvic examination should begin at age 40
   2. Annual cancer check-ups for all persons over age 40
   3. Annual mammography should begin at age 30
   4. Annual fecal occult blood test and colonoscopy at age 40

7. The client with cancer states, "My pain is a 10!" on a 0-to-10 scale (10 being worst possible pain). Which of the following is the appropriate nursing intervention?
   1. Instruct the client that no more narcotic analgesia can be given at this time in order to prevent addiction
   2. Ask the client if the pain is really that bad, as narcotic analgesia will be given as a last resort for severe pain
   3. Assure that a strong opioid, nonopioid, and adjuvant are ordered and administer per order
   4. Administer another dose of meperidine (Demerol) as prescribed

8. In planning the care of a client experiencing fatigue related to chemotherapy, which of the following is the most appropriate nursing intervention?
   1. Prioritize and administer nursing care throughout the day
   2. Accomplish all the nursing cares early in the day so the client can rest the remainder of the day

3. Perform all nursing cares during the evening shift when the client is the most rested
4. Limit the number of visitors, promoting a maximum opportunity for sleep

9. The nurse is caring for a client who underwent a bone marrow transplant 10 days ago. The nurse should monitor the client for which of the following clinical manifestations that indicates a potentially life-threatening situation?
   1. Mucositis
   2. Confusion
   3. Depression
   4. Mild temperature elevation

10. Six days after receiving chemotherapy, the client reports that, "My mouth feels like it's on fire!" Which of the following is the priority nursing action?
    1. Encourage rinsing the mouth several times per day with an over-the-counter mouthwash
    2. Administer analgesics as ordered
    3. Assess the oral mucosa for signs of infection and tissue breakdown
    4. Instruct the client to eat small, frequent meals of soft food such as applesauce

11. The nurse finds the client vomiting on the second day after chemotherapy. Antiemetics and IV fluids have been administered as ordered. The nurse should include which of the following as an appropriate intervention for this client?
    1. Offer music therapy to decrease nausea
    2. Encourage the client to remain in an upright position for 2 hours after eating
    3. Obtain an order for a tube feeding to assure adequate nutrition
    4. Discuss decreasing the next dose of chemotherapy with the physician

12. In preparing a client on oral narcotic analgesics for discharge after a mastectomy, the nurse should include which of the following in postoperative teaching?
    1. Use oral narcotics sparingly to avoid constipation
    2. Bowel-training program
    3. High-protein, low-carbohydrate diet plan
    4. Upper extremity weight-training program

13. While caring for the client with superior vena cava syndrome, the nurse should include which of the following interventions?
    1. Restrict visitors, as the client will be anxious
    2. Withhold chemotherapy until the syndrome resolves
    3. Instruct the client in Valsalva's maneuver
    4. Elevate the head of the bed

14. The nurse is caring for a client with small-cell lung cancer. Which of the following observations would be a priority that the nurse should report immediately?
    1. Weight loss
    2. Serum sodium less than 130 mEq/L
    3. Headache
    4. Urinary output greater than 60 ml/hour

15. The nurse is caring for a client who received chemotherapy for leukemia 24 hours ago and is now complaining of flank pain. The client's urinary output has decreased to less than 30 ml/hour. The nurse evaluates which of the following conditions as the most likely cause of the client's clinical manifestations?
    1. Syndrome of inappropriate antidiuretic hormone (SIADH)
    2. Tumor lysis syndrome
    3. Superior vena cava syndrome
    4. Hypercalcemia

16. The nurse should instruct a client that which of the following is the most effective prevention against bladder cancer?
    1. Drink 8 to 10 glasses of fluid per day
    2. Void at least five times per day
    3. Stop smoking
    4. Take herbal supplements

17. Which of the following should the nurse include in the preoperative care plan of a client with head and neck cancer?
    1. Instruct the client and family in communicating with a picture board
    2. Assess the client's favorite foods to assure these are provided postoperatively
    3. Plan for a volunteer to take the client outside for cigarette breaks
    4. Provide frequent oral care, including rinsing with mouthwash

18. A client who has been treated for lung cancer returns to the clinic and during the nursing assessment reports recent problems with balance and memory. Based on the nurse's understanding of lung cancer, the appropriate action would be which of the following?
    1. Reassure the client that these are just common signs of aging
    2. Recommend that the client obtain gingko from the health food store
    3. Perform a more thorough assessment
    4. Call for an ambulance, as this is an oncology emergency

19. The nurse is caring for a client following lobectomy lung cancer. Which of the following should the nurse include in the plan of care for this client?
    1. Position the client on the operative side only

2. Avoid administering narcotic pain medication
3. Maintain strict bed rest
4. Instruct the client on the importance of coughing and deep breathing

20. The spouse of a client with early-stage prostate cancer asks the nurse, "Why isn't the physician treating my husband's cancer?" The nurse's best response should be based on which of the following?
   1. Watchful waiting is often appropriate for men over age 70
   2. The client must really have Stage IV cancer, which is not curable
   3. All prostate cancer should be treated, and this client should get another opinion
   4. The client is being treated with hormonal manipulation, which isn't perceived as treatment by clients

21. While performing a nursing assessment, a female client informs the nurse of vague abdominal discomfort, bloating, and unexplained indigestion and flatulence for the last few months. What should the nurse ask in order to elicit the most important information for completing the assessment?
   1. "Do you often eat spicy food?"
   2. "Tell me about your family's medical history."
   3. "Have you had weight loss recently?"
   4. "Are you experiencing unusual menstrual bleeding?"

22. A client asks the nurse what percent of noninvasive breast cancer is curable. The most appropriate response by the nurse is _____

23. A nurse is teaching a class on breast self-examination. Which of the following should the nurse include in the class?
   1. Use only deep pressure when palpating the breast
   2. Include both inspection and palpation of the breast in the exam
   3. Use the fingertips while palpating the breast
   4. Perform the breast palpation exam in front of a mirror

24. A client states, "I'm worried about being burned by radiation therapy." The most appropriate response is based on the nurse's understanding that
   1. applying hand lotion to the area being radiated will reduce the chance of burns.
   2. darker-skinned persons burn more easily during radiation therapy.
   3. burns are very rare with today's technology.

4. washing the radiated area with strong soap will reduce the chance of burns.

25. When planning care for a client being treated for cervical cancer, it would be a priority for the nurse to include which of the following in the plan of care?
   1. Instruction on birth control methods
   2. Vigorous fluid hydration
   3. Assessment of sexual function
   4. Daily weights

26. The registered nurse is making out the nursing tasks for the day. Which of the following nursing tasks may be delegated to a licensed practical nurse?
   1. Administer 3% saline solution IV to a client with severe syndrome of inappropriate antidiuretic hormone (SIADH)
   2. Assess for an electrolyte imbalance in a client with tumor lysis syndrome
   3. Administer prescribed anticonvulsant to prevent seizure in a client who has a central nervous system tumor
   4. Monitor the serum calcium level in a client who has hypercalcemia

27. The nurse is teaching a class on breast cancer. Which of the following should the nurse include as risk factors?
   1. Menopause at an early age and excessive caffeine use
   2. Slender build and first birth before the age of 20 years
   3. Menarche at an early age and nulliparous
   4. Asian descent and lower-socioeconomic status

28. Which of the following findings on a female breast exam should the nurse report as suspicious of breast cancer?
   1. Multiple, bilateral, round, lumpy tissue that is tender
   2. A soft, mobile, single lobular nodule that is nontender
   3. A poorly defined, firm lump that is nontender and fixed to the skin
   4. A single soft lump that is well defined and tender

29. The nurse is admitting a client with vaginal cancer. Which of the following questions should the nurse ask to elicit the most likely causative factor?
   1. "Did you experience your first menses before the age of 11 years?"
   2. "Did your mother take diethylstilbestrol (DES) during pregnancy?"
   3. "Have you ever taken tamoxifen?"
   4. "Do you have a history of a sexually transmitted disease?"

30. The nurse should instruct a female client that the best time to perform a breast self-examination is which of the following?
    1. At the onset of menstruation
    2. The last day of the menstrual period
    3. Every month during ovulation
    4. Weekly at the same time of day

31. Which of the following instructions should the nurse give a male client on how to perform a testicular self-examination (TSE)?
    1. Examine the testicle while lying down
    2. Gently feel the testicle with one finger to feel for a growth
    3. The best time to examine the testicle is after a shower
    4. A testicular exam should be done once every 6 months

ANSWERS AND RATIONALES

1. 1. Over 1 million Americans are diagnosed with cancer each year. However, only 500,000 die annually and approximately 5 million are cancer-free for 5 or more years. Heart disease, not cancer, is the leading cause of adult death in the United States.

2. 2. Prostate cancer is the most common cancer in U.S. men, with lung cancer being second. The incidence of prostate cancer is significantly higher in black men worldwide. Screening is available for prostate cancer.

3. 4. Reducing stress in a person's life is one of the recommended methods of cancer risk reduction. Clients with cancer are at a higher risk of a new cancer or recurrence, and therefore should be instructed in risk-reduction methods. Limiting alcoholic beverages is encouraged to reduce cancer risk, but it is not required that the client abstain completely unless there are other medical reasons to do so. Not all clients will require home or hospice care after discharge, as many clients with cancer lead long, productive lives.

4. 3. A blue-black appearing mole is one of the cardinal signs of melanoma skin cancer. Red, swollen plaques, bull's-eye rash, and spider angiomas are not indicative of skin cancer, but other dermatologic abnormalities.

5. 1. Although early colon cancer is asymptomatic, occult or frank blood in the stool is often an assessment finding in a client diagnosed with colon cancer. If pain is present, it is usually lower abdominal cramping. Constipation and diarrhea are more frequent findings than nausea, and ascites is more likely to be present in very advanced disease stages of ovarian and liver cancers.

6. 2. Nationally recognized cancer screening guidelines recommend everyone over age 40 visit the doctor annually for cancer assessment. Pap and pelvic examinations and screening for cervical and uterine cancer should begin at age 18. Mammographic screening for breast cancer is not recommended on an annual basis until at least age 40, and colorectal screening is recommended beginning at age 50, with colonoscopy only every 5 to 10 years.

7. 3. Fewer than 1% of clients become addicted to narcotic analgesics when used appropriately for pain management; therefore, in this case, addiction should not be a concern. Narcotic doses can be increased as pain increases, and therefore do not need to be reserved for fear of using them too early. Meperidine (Demerol) is seldom used to treat cancer pain because of metabolites that accumulate with continued use. If this is ordered, the nurse should consult with the physician regarding a change. According to the World Health Organization analgesic ladder for pain management, severe pain should be treated with a strong opioid (e.g., morphine), with a nonopioid analgesic (e.g., acetaminophen), and an adjuvant (e.g., nonsteroidal anti-inflammatory).

8. 1. Clients should be taught to pace their activities throughout the day in order to conserve energy; therefore, nursing care should be paced as well. Fatigue is the most common side effect of cancer and its treatment; therefore, it needs to be appropriately managed. Although adequate sleep is important, maximal sleep will not completely resolve clinical manifestations. Completely restricting visitors does not promote healthy coping and may result in isolation.

9. 4. During the first 100 days posttransplant, clients are at high risk for life-threatening infections. This is especially true prior to marrow engraftment, which occurs at approximately 2 to 3 weeks posttransplant. The earliest sign of infection in an immunocompromised client may be a mild fever. Mucositis, confusion, and depression are possible clinical manifestations but represent less life-threatening complications.

10. 3. Adverse reactions of chemotherapy include stomatitis and mucositis in some clients. The nurse should always first assess the client's oral mucosa for signs of breakdown and infection. Pain medication may be necessary to administer, but this is not the first action the nurse should take. Rinsing the oral mucosa is encouraged, but with salt or soda solution, not over-the-counter mouthwashes, which can be drying. Clients should eat small, frequent meals of soothing foods after chemotherapy, but usually this is not required after the first week, and, again, the nurse should perform an assessment before implementing a plan of care.

11. 1. The addition of complementary therapies, such as music therapy, relaxation techniques, distraction, and imagery, has been shown to provide additional relief from nausea and vomiting. The client should remain in an upright position after eating, but 30 minutes is usually sufficient. A tube feeding would be inappropriate because nausea and vomiting after chemotherapy are usually short-term problems, after which the client will be able to return to normal eating patterns. Unless extremely severe and unmanageable, it would not be appropriate to decrease the dose of chemotherapy at the next administration.

12. 2. Surgery, narcotic analgesics, and client immobility promote constipation postoperatively. Therefore, clients should be instructed in a bowel-training program that includes use of suppositories or oral stool softener as needed, physical activity such as walking, and intake of fruits, fiber, and fluid. Oral narcotics should be used as needed for pain while managing the adverse reaction of constipation. The diet should be high in fiber, not necessarily protein. A weight-training program would not be appropriate until surgical drains are removed, although use of the affected side with gentle arm motion is advocated.

13. 4. Superior vena cava syndrome is compression of the superior vena cava by enlarged lymph nodes, clot, or tumor, thus restricting the flow of blood out of the head, neck, and upper extremities. This results in swelling of these areas and shortness of breath. Elevating the head of the bed decreases the pressure in the head and upper body by allowing gravity to assist in blood flow. The client should not perform Valsalva's maneuver, as this increases that pressure. The client will be anxious about this, so providing resources to decrease anxiety, including supportive friends and family, would be advocated. Chemotherapy or radiation to decrease the size of a tumor or lymph node is one of the treatments for superior vena cava

syndrome, so chemotherapy should be administered as ordered, and not withheld.

14. 2. Clients most at risk for syndrome of inappropriate antidiuretic hormone (SIADH) are those with small-cell lung cancer, as well as several other cancers. Therefore, the nurse should be alert for clinical manifestations of this, such as weight gain, decreased urinary output, and dilutional hyponatremia. Headache may occur, but this is not a common clinical manifestation of SIADH.

15. 2. Tumor lysis is most common in clients who have received chemotherapy for leukemia, lymphoma, or small cell lung cancer, within 24 to 48 hours of administration. Flank pain is a clinical manifestation of renal failure associated with tumor lysis syndrome. Flank pain is not a typical clinical manifestation of syndrome of inappropriate antidiuretic hormone (SIADH), superior vena cava syndrome, or hypercalcemia.

16. 3. Persons at greatest risk for bladder cancer are Caucasian men over 50 years of age who have had occupational exposures to dyes, rubber, and leather industries, and who smoke. Because age, race, and occupation are not alterable, the best alternative is to stop smoking. Clients should be provided with smoking cessation information and support to reduce their risk of several cancers and other health problems.

17. 1. Surgery is the primary treatment for head and neck cancer and may involve removal of part of the tongue, larynx, and other structures. This surgery is often disfiguring and often makes eating and communicating with staff and family very difficult. Losses can lead to difficulties in coping, so nursing interventions to lessen losses and promote coping (such as communicating with a picture board) have a major role for the nurse in this setting. Mouthwash should not be used because it is drying to the oral mucosa. Smoking should be highly discouraged; it is one of the leading risk factors for this cancer and it dries the oral mucosa. The diet for this client should be developed in collaboration with the physician and therapists and often includes tube feeding followed by soft mechanical diet, due to swallowing difficulties. Unfortunately, the client will not be able to have favorite foods for a while.

18. 3. Lung cancer often metastasizes to the brain, causing neurologic symptoms as the client is describing. Providing reassurance is minimizing the client's concerns, and making recommendations for herbal supplements without a thorough assessment is not an appropriate nursing intervention. The client is not in immediate danger, so calling an ambulance is not appropriate either.

19. 4. Postoperatively, deep breathing is important to promote oxygenation and clear secretions, so strict bed rest is discouraged and ambulation is encouraged. Additionally, administration of pain medication to lessen pain and promote deep breathing is essential and should not be avoided. After a lobectomy, prolonged lying on the operative side is to be avoided.

20. 1. Prostate cancer is very slow growing in older men, and therefore no intervention is recommended. "Watchful waiting" is appropriate for men over age 70 with small, early-stage cancers. Transurethral resection of the prostate and external beam radiation are used to treat advanced disease. The client may be receiving hormonal therapy, but it is primarily used for advanced disease.

21. 2. Vague abdominal discomfort, bloating, and unexplained indigestion and flatulence are unfortunately the only clinical manifestations of ovarian cancer, and the reason it is often overlooked. Therefore, to more thoroughly complete the assessment, the nurse should take a complete family cancer history to aid in determining the client's risk of ovarian cancer. Women with a family history of ovarian cancer are at higher risk. If anything, the client would probably be gaining weight, not losing, from abdominal ascites. Unusual menstrual bleeding is an important clinical manifestation related to uterine, rather than ovarian, cancer.

22. 90% Noninvasive breast cancers, such as in situ, are 90% curable because they are not capable of metastasis.

23. 2. Breast self-exam should include inspection of the breasts in front of a mirror. According to national authorities, it should also include palpation using light, medium, and deep pressure with the pads of the first three fingers (not the fingertips) while in the shower and while lying down. It is not necessary to perform the palpation exam in front of a mirror.

24. 3. The equipment and techniques used to deliver radiation therapy today very rarely result in skin burns. Local skin reaction such as redness, dryness, desquamation, and irritation may occur. These reactions occur most often in fair-skinned persons, and are potentially worse if there are oils on the skin from hand lotion, soap, or deodorant; therefore, application of these is discouraged. Washing the area receiving radiation with plain water and patting dry is preferred to strong soap.

25. 3. Surgery and radiation therapy for cervical cancer often result in shortening of the vagina, vaginal dryness, and loss of libido due to emotional issues related to sexuality and femininity. Therefore, the client's feelings about sexuality and the partner's feelings should be assessed. If a client is not sexually active, instructions should be given in the use of a vaginal dilator and lubricant to prevent adhesion of the vaginal walls. Although instruction about birth control methods may be needed for some clients, treatment for cervical cancer may include total abdominal hysterectomy, so this would not be appropriate for all clients. Encouraging fluids and daily weights are not priorities in cervical cancer care.

26. 3. Syndrome of inappropriate antidiuretic hormone (SIADH), tumor lysis syndrome, and hypercalcemia are all oncology medical emergencies, requiring the attention of a registered nurse. Administering an IV solution, assessing for an electrolyte imbalance, and monitoring the serum calcium are all nursing tasks reserved for the registered nurse. Hypercalcemia is also an oncology medical emergency, so monitoring the serum calcium is a nursing task reserved for the registered nurse. A licensed practical nurse may administer an anticonvulsant to a client who has a central nervous system tumor.

27. 3. Risk factors for breast cancer include being white over being nonwhite. The incidence of breast cancer is higher in obese females. Additional risk factors include menarche at an early age and being nulliparous.

28. 3. A poorly defined, firm lump that is nontender and fixed to the skin is characteristic of breast cancer.

29. 2. A client whose mother had taken diethylstilbestrol (DES) during pregnancy is more likely to develop vaginal cancer. There is no correlation with the age of the first menses, having taken tamoxifen, or having had a history of a sexually transmitted disease.

30. 2. The best time to perform a breast self-examination is the last day of the menstrual period.

31. 3. The best time to perform a testicular self-examination is after a shower. The warmth of the shower causes the testes to position themselves lower in the scrotum. The testes should be examined by both hands by rolling each testis between the thumb and first three fingers until the surface has been covered. The examination should be performed each month at a consistent time such as the first of the month.

REFERENCES

American Cancer Society. (2011). *Cancer facts and figures 2011* [Brochure]. Atlanta, GA: Author.

Daniels, R. (2010). *Delmar's manual of laboratory and diagnostic tests* (2nd ed.). Clifton Park, NY: Delmar Cengage Learning.

Daniels, R., & Nicoll, L. (2012). *Contemporary medical-surgical nursing*, Clifton Park, NY: Delmar Cengage Learning.

Estes, M. (2010). *Health assessment and physical examination* (4th ed.). Clifton Park, NY: Delmar Cengage Learning.

Spratto, G. R., & Woods, A. L. (2012). *PDR nurse's drug handbook 2012*. Clifton Park, NY: Delmar Cengage Learning.

Yarbro, C. H., Frogge, M. H., Goodman, M., & Groenwald, S. L. (2011). *Cancer nursing: Principles and practice* (7th ed.). Sudbury, MA: Jones and Bartlett.

CHAPTER 12

HEMATOLOGICAL DISORDERS

I. ANATOMY AND PHYSIOLOGY

A. FUNCTIONS OF THE HEMATOLOGIC SYSTEM (SEE TABLE 12-1)
   1. TRANSPORTATION OF OXYGEN AND CARBON DIOXIDE TO AND FROM CELLS
   2. TRANSPORTATION OF HORMONES, ELECTROLYTES, AND NUTRIENTS TO CELLS
   3. TRANSPORTATION OF WASTE PRODUCTS TO THE LIVER AND KIDNEYS
   4. COAGULATION AND CLOTTING OF THE BLOOD
   5. IMMUNE RESPONSE

B. BONE MARROW (SEE FIGURE 12-1)
   1. SOFT MATERIAL THAT FILLS THE CENTRAL CORE OF BONES AND IS THE BLOOD-FORMING TISSUE THAT PRODUCES THREE TYPES OF BLOOD CELLS (ERYTHROCYTES, LEUKOCYTES, AND PLATELETS) FROM ONE STEM CELL

C. BLOOD CELLS
   1. ERYTHROCYTES
      a. Enucleated concave discs
      b. Carry hemoglobin that transports oxygen to the tissues of the body

Figure 12-1 Stem cell maturation

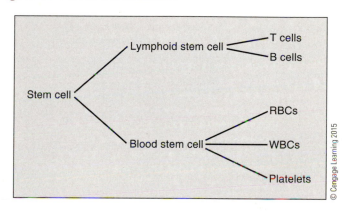

c. Circulates approximately 120 days and is eliminated in the liver and spleen
      d. Whole blood contains 14–15 grams of hemoglobin per 100 ml blood.
   2. LEUKOCYTES (SEE TABLE 12-2)
      a. Function by phagocytosis to rid the body of foreign particles, mutations in cell division, or bacteria in the immune response
   3. PLATELETS
      a. Primary function is to aid the body in clot formation

Table 12-1 Components of Blood

Plasma	Cellular Components
55% of blood volume	Derived from stem cells
Water 92%	Erythrocytes (red blood cells)
Protein 7%	Leukocytes (white blood cells and lymphocytes)
Hormones Albumin Fibrinogen Globulins Inorganic salts 1%	Platelets

© Cengage Learning 2015

Table 12-2 Types of Leukocytes

Granulocytes (70% of leukocytes)	Neutrophil—ingest and destroy microorganisms (phagocytosis)
	Basophils—activate allergic response
	Eosinophils—activate allergic response
Mononuclear cells	Monocytes—active in phagocytosis Lymphocytes— B cells: humoral immunity; produce antibodies (immunoglobulins) T cells: cellular immunity includes helper(T_4) and suppressor cells (T_8)

© Cengage Learning 2015

   b. Thrombocytes are derived from megakaryocytes in the bone marrow.
   c. Normal platelet count range is 150,000/mm^3–450,000/mm^3.
   d. Life span is 8–12 days.
   e. Stored in the spleen and destroyed there by phagocytosis

D. SPLEEN
   1. VASCULAR, BEAN-SHAPED ORGAN LOCATED IN THE LEFT UPPER QUADRANT OF THE ABDOMEN BEHIND THE STOMACH
   2. HEMATOPOIETIC FUNCTION—PRODUCES RED BLOOD CELLS (RBCS) DURING FETAL DEVELOPMENT
   3. FILTER FUNCTION—REMOVES OLD DEFECTIVE CELLS FROM CIRCULATION AND BREAKS DOWN RBCS AND RECYCLES THE IRON TO THE BONE MARROW
   4. IMMUNE FUNCTION—CONTAINS A SUPPLY OF LYMPHOCYTES AND MONOCYTES
   5. STORES PLATELETS

E. LYMPHATICS
   1. CARRIES LYMPH FLUID VIA DUCTS AND LYMPH NODES FROM THE INTERSTITIAL SPACES TO THE BLOOD
   2. LYMPH FLUID MOVES THROUGH DUCTS PUMPED BY THE ACTION OF THE MUSCLES THAT SURROUND THEM.
   3. LYMPHATIC CAPILLARIES
      a. Join to form lymphatic ducts that carry the lymph to either the right lymphatic duct or the thoracic duct
      b. Drain into the subclavian vein in the chest
   4. LYMPH NODES
      a. Small rounded or bean-shaped structures that filter bacteria and foreign particles from the lymph
      b. Distributed all over the body, both superficially and deep

F. LIVER
   1. LARGE ORGAN LOCATED IN THE RIGHT UPPER QUADRANT AND EPIGASTRIC REGION OF THE ABDOMEN
   2. RECEIVES BLOOD FROM THE SPLEEN THROUGH PORTAL CIRCULATION
   3. FUNCTIONS:
      a. Production of procoagulants necessary for hemostasis and blood coagulation
      b. Storage of iron and vitamin B$_{12}$
      c. Detoxification of drugs
      d. Kupffer cells carry out phagocytosis.
      e. Bile production from erythrocyte destruction

G. CLOTTING MECHANISMS
   1. CLOTTING MECHANISMS DECREASE BLOOD LOSS WHEN THE BODY SUSTAINS INJURY.

   a. Vascular response
      1) Immediate vasoconstriction
      2) Vascular spasm lasting 30 minutes, allowing time for platelet response
   b. Platelet response
      1) Activated by exposure to interstitial collagen
      2) Aggregation or clumping of platelets occurs.
   c. Plasma clotting factors
      1) Plasma protein that circulates in inactive forms to initiate clotting
      2) Thrombin essential enzyme in coagulation process converting fibrinogen to fibrin, which is essential in the formation of a blood clot

H. ANTICOAGULATION
   1. COUNTERMECHANISM TO BLOOD CLOTTING
   2. MAINTAINS BLOOD IN ITS LIQUID STATE
   3. ANTITHROMBINS AND FIBRINOLYSIS MECHANISMS RESPONSIBLE FOR ANTICOAGULATION
      a. Antithrombin antagonizes thrombin, maintaining blood in a liquid state
      b. Fibrinolysis occurs when plasminogen is activated to plasmin, often initiated by thrombin.

II. **ASSESSMENT**
A. HEALTH HISTORY
   1. PAST MEDICAL HISTORY
      a. Age, gender, race, and ethnic background
      b. Family history of hematologic health problems (e.g., bleeding or clotting tendency, jaundice, genetic disorders)
      c. History of, or beliefs about, blood transfusions or other potential treatments; some cultures and religious beliefs prohibit transfusion of blood products.
      d. Nutritional status
         1) Note intake of iron, vitamins, and fluids.
         2) Dietary beliefs of the client
         3) Ingestion of quinine-containing beverages
      e. Drug or alcohol abuse, cigarette smoking, exposure to pesticides or radiation
      f. Elimination pattern—any blood in stool, urine, or emesis
      g. For women—reproduction history, menstrual flow, amenorrhea
      h. Respiratory clinical manifestations—shortness of breath at rest or with exertion, cough
      i. Neurologic clinical manifestations—lightheadedness, tingling, numbness, headache, confusion, fatigue, syncope

2. MEDICATIONS
   a. Allergies and reactions
   b. Past, present, and any over-the-counter medications, vitamins, herbs, or other supplements
   c. Prescription medications (when and for how long)—antibiotics, aspirin, nonsteroidal anti-inflammatory pain medication use, cardiac and blood pressure medications, antineoplastics, corticosteroids, and hormones
3. SURGERIES, INJURIES, AND EXPOSURES
   a. Any complications such as blood clots or excessive bleeding after a surgical procedure, including dental surgeries
   b. Reactions to blood transfusions
   c. Injuries to the spleen, splenectomy, cardiac valve replacement, serious infection (HIV), radiation or chemical exposure

B. PHYSICAL EXAMINATION
   1. INSPECTION
      a. Mouth—color, dentition, symmetry, ulcers, shiny smooth tongue, ulcers on mucous membranes, cracking at the corners of the mouth (cheilosis)
      b. Skin—color, rashes, bruising, texture, petechiae
      c. Nail beds—pallor, spooning of nails (koilonychia)
      d. Eyes—sclera color, jaundice, condition and color of conjunctiva
      e. Chest and abdomen symmetry, size
      f. Lymph nodes note size, location of enlarged nodes
   2. AUSCULTATION
      a. Neck—carotid bruits
      b. Lungs—tachypnea, abnormal or absent breath sounds
      c. Heart—murmurs, tachycardia, widened pulse pressure
      d. Abdomen—listen over the spleen, bowel sounds.
   3. PERCUSSION
      a. Lungs—note areas of tenderness, dullness.
      b. Abdomen—note areas of tenderness, splenomegaly, hepatomegaly.
   4. PALPATION
      a. Skin—note temperature, degree of dryness or moisture, turgor.
      b. Lymph nodes—especially the neck, axillary, and groin; note texture, size, and degree of fixation and tenderness.
      c. Abdomen—spleen and liver size and tenderness

III. DIAGNOSTIC STUDIES (SEE TABLE 12-3)
   A. BONE MARROW BIOPSY AND ASPIRATION
      1. DESCRIPTION: ASPIRATION OR BIOPSY, OR BOTH, OF THE BONE MARROW WITH A NEEDLE AND SYRINGE (IN ADULTS THE POSTERIOR ILIAC CREST IS THE BEST BONE SITE FOR THIS TEST.)

Table 12-3 Commonly Used Blood Tests in Hematology

Test	Significance
Hemoglobin (Hb)	Measurement of gas-carrying capacity of RBCs Normal range is higher in men than in women Low levels in anemias High levels in smokers, polycythemia vera
Hematocrit (Hct)	RBC volume as a percentage of the total blood volume Normally about three times the hemoglobin Ratio 4
Total RBC count	Number of circulating RBCs
Mean corpuscular volume (MCV)	Relative size of RBCs Low in anemia Low MCV = microcytosis (iron deficiency, thalassemia) High MCV = macrocytosis (folate and vitamin B_{12} deficiency)
Mean corpuscular hemoglobin (MCH)	Average weight of Hb/RBC Low MCH = microcytosis High MCH = macrocytosis
Mean corpuscular hemoglobin concentration (MCHC)	RBC saturation with Hb Low in very severe anemia

(continues)

Table 12-3 Commonly Used Blood Tests in Hematology *(continued)*

Test	Significance
White blood cell (WBC) count	Absolute number of leukocytes Decreased–leukopenia, neutropenia Increased–leukocytosis
Differential count:	Percentage of total WBC of each kind of WBC An absolute count can be determined by multiplying total WBC 3 × Cell% 100
Neutrophils	50–70%
Lymphocytes	20–40%
Monocytes	4–8%
Eosinophils	2–8%
Basophils	0–2%
Platelet count	Number of platelets Low–thrombocytopenia High–thrombocytosis Not a measurement of the quality of function in clotting blood
Reticulocyte count	Measure of immature RBCs in the circulating blood High in hemolytic anemia and sickle cell disease
Erythrocyte sedimentation rate (ESR)	Settling of RBCs Faster rate occurs in inflammatory processes

Iron studies:
  Serum iron
  total iron-binding capacity (TIBC)
  Ferritin
	Low in iron deficiency anemia; may be influenced by other coexisting conditions
	Measurement of the amount of extra iron that can be carried
	Measurement of iron stores
	Low in iron deficiency anemia
	High in hemochromatosis

Coombs' test
  Direct
  Indirect
	
	Detection of antibodies on RBCs
	Detection of antibodies in serum

Bilirubin	Measures the degree of hemolysis Elevated in sickle cell anemia, hemolytic anemias
Folic acid	Water-soluble vitamin not produced in the body Low levels in alcoholism, poor diet, anemia
Vitamin B$_{12}$ (serum)	Water-soluble vitamin not produced by the body Decreased level in anemia, intestinal malabsorption, diet lacking in meat, milk, eggs, shellfish Diagnostic of pernicious anemia

2. PREPROCEDURE
   a. Inform the client about the procedure.
   b. Inform the client that a written consent will be obtained.
   c. Administer prescribed systemic analgesic.
   d. Position the client comfortably on the abdomen with the arms toward the head.
   e. Inform the client that a local anesthetic will be given by the physician.
3. POSTPROCEDURE
   a. Apply pressure dressing to the site.
   b. Instruct the client to lie on the back for 20–30 minutes.
   c. Monitor a heavily anesthetized client frequently.
   d. Assess for bleeding at the site and dizziness before ambulating the client.
B. LYMPH NODE BIOPSY
   1. DESCRIPTION
      a. Obtain lymph node tissue for histologic examination performed to determine the reason for enlarged lymph node.
      b. Open biopsy—removal of the entire node
      c. Closed (needle) biopsy performed at the bedside or with the assistance of computerized tomography (CT). A portion of the lymph node is removed

and may not be enough tissue to be diagnostic.

2. PREPROCEDURE
   a. Inform the client about the procedure.
   b. Inform the client that an informed consent will be obtained.
   c. Inform the client that a local anesthesia is generally administered.

3. POSTPROCEDURE
   a. Monitor for bleeding.
   b. Change the sterile dressing as ordered by the surgeon.
   c. Inspect the wound for infection.

C. RADIOLOGIC IMAGING
   1. PLAIN X-RAYS
      a. Evaluate bone abnormalities or fractures.
      b. No prep
   2. COMPUTERIZED TOMOGRAPHY (CT)
      a. Description: noninvasive, using computer-assisted x-ray to evaluate internal organs such as the liver, spleen, or lymph nodes for masses or hemorrhage
      b. Preprocedure
         1) Ask the client about past reactions to intravenous CT contrast.
         2) Nothing by mouth for 8 or more hours for abdominal test.
         3) Administer contrast solution 1 and 2 hours before the procedure.
         4) Encourage fluids.
      c. Postprocedure
         1) Maintain oral hydration.
         2) Administer the prescribed laxative.
   3. MAGNETIC RESONANCE IMAGING (MRI)
      a. Description: noninvasive test that produces sensitive images of soft tissue without using contrast dyes
      b. Preprocedure
         1) Clients must be "MRI safe." Ask about any recent surgeries and surgically implanted metals in the eyes or brain or claustrophobia. If claustrophobic, the client may want to consider sedation.
      c. Postprocedure
         1) Inform a sedated client that a designated driver must drive home.
   4. LYMPHANGIOGRAM
      a. Description
         1) Used to evaluate deep lymph nodes
         2) Radiopaque oil-based dye is infused slowly into lymph vessels via small needles in the dorsum of each foot.
         3) Radiographs are taken immediately and on the next day.
         4) Less commonly used because of improvements such as CT

b. Preprocedure
   1) Inform the client that an informed consent will be obtained.
   2) Assess for iodine sensitivity.
   3) NPO
   4) Inform the client that he or she may need to take laxatives to clear the bowel of its contents for better imaging.
   5) Sedate the client as ordered.
c. Postprocedure
   1) Inform the client that the urine and the skin on the feet will be blue from the dye.
   2) Monitor for fever, general malaise, and muscle aches for 12–24 hours.
   3) Monitor for signs of oil embolus to the lungs, hacking cough, dyspnea, pleuritic pain, and hemoptysis.

D. RADIOISOTOPE SCANS
   1. DESCRIPTION: RADIOACTIVE ISOTOPE IS INJECTED INTRAVENOUSLY TO ASSESS THE STRUCTURE OF THE LIVER, SPLEEN, BONES, OR LYMPH NODES.
   2. PREPROCEDURE
      a. Inform the client that after the isotope is injected, there will be a delay of about 3 hours to allow the tracer to circulate before the scan can be done.
   3. POSTPROCEDURE
      a. None

IV. NURSING DIAGNOSES
   A. INEFFECTIVE THERAPEUTIC REGIMEN MANAGEMENT
   B. ACTIVITY INTOLERANCE
   C. IMBALANCED NUTRITION: LESS THAN BODY REQUIREMENTS
   D. RISK FOR INFECTION
   E. FATIGUE

Nursing Diagnoses: Definitions and Classification 2012–2014. Copyright © 2012, 1994–2012 by NANDA International. Used by arrangement with John Wiley & Sons Limited.

V. HEMATOLOGIC DISEASES
   A. ANEMIA
      1. DESCRIPTION
         a. A reduction below normal in the number of erythrocytes, the quantity of hemoglobin, and the volume of erythrocytes (hematocrit)
         b. Results from decreased erythrocyte production, increased erythrocyte destruction, or acute or chronic blood loss
      2. IRON DEFICIENCY ANEMIA
         a. Description
            1) Most common type of anemia; 10% to 30% of all adults in the United States have iron deficiency anemia.

2) Causes include insufficient intake, chronic blood loss, excessive menstrual bleeding, iron malabsorption, or increased needs for iron such as that which occurs in pregnancy

b. Assessment
  1) May be asymptomatic
  2) Pallor, cracking at the corners of the mouth (cheilosis)
  3) Spoon-shaped nails (koilonychias)
  4) Glossitis (inflammation of the tongue); smooth, shiny tongue
  5) Lethargy, headaches, fatigue, shortness of breath
  6) Compulsive ingestion of laundry starch, clay, or ice (pica) may precede development of anemia.
  7) Tachycardia, palpitations, chest pain
  8) Paresthesias, tinnitus
  9) Menorrhagia
  10) History of blood loss—surgery, gastrointestinal (GI) bleeding, or uterine bleeding
  11) Regular blood donation or frequent venipunctures for laboratory tests, especially in the critically ill hospitalized client

c. Diagnostic tests
  1) Complete blood count (CBC)
  2) Iron studies and ferritin
  3) Reticulocyte count
  4) Sedimentation rate

d. Nursing interventions
  1) Identify at-risk groups, such as infants, women who are pregnant, older adults, persons from a low-socioeconomic background, and individuals experiencing blood loss.
  2) Instruct the client and family about coping with and reducing fatigue and strategies to optimize energy level, such as rest periods between activities.
  3) Increase iron intake.
    a) Provide nutritional education about foods high in iron content such as liver and green leafy vegetables (spinach).
    b) Administer supplemental oral iron as ordered, especially for women who are pregnant.
    c) Administer iron with orange juice before meals because the body can only absorb small quantities of iron at a time. An acidic environment is best for absorption.
    d) Monitor a client receiving iron for adverse reactions such as pyrosis (heartburn), constipation, diarrhea, and dark stools.
    e) Inform the client that parenteral iron therapy may stain the skin.
    f) Administer parenteral iron Z-track method and avoid massaging the site of injection.
    g) Inform the client that IV iron is iron dextran and a test dose will be administered first. Then continue the infusion slowly, monitoring the client closely for an adverse reaction.
    h) Administer packed red blood cell transfusion if the client is symptomatic.

3. THALASSEMIA
  a. Description
    1) Decreased production of hemoglobin due to abnormal hemoglobin synthesis
    2) Autosomal recessive genetic disorder commonly found in persons whose origins are near the Mediterranean Sea
    3) May be thalassemia minor or thalassemia major
      a) Thalassemia minor or trait has one thalassemic and one normal gene with mild clinical manifestations and requires no treatment.
      b) Thalassemia major has two thalassemic genes causing a severe condition.
  b. Assessment
    1) Skin: pale or jaundiced
    2) Splenomegaly and hepatomegaly
    3) Thickened cranium and maxillary sinus space from bone marrow hyperplasia
  c. Diagnostic tests
    1) CBC
      a) Anemia; mean cell volume (MCV) will be lower in thalassemia than in iron-deficiency states
    2) Hemoglobin electrophoresis
  d. Nursing interventions
    1) Administration of blood transfusions and chelations therapy to reduce iron overload
    2) Monitor the client receiving a transfusion for manifestations of transfusion reactions or diseases acquired through transfusions.

3) Instruct the client about treatments, medications, and physical energy conservation techniques.

4) Strengthen the client support and family systems, which may include family members who may also have thalassemia or the trait.

4. MEGALOBLASTIC ANEMIA

a. Description

1) Defective erythrocyte (megaloblast) structure caused by impaired DNA synthesis caused by cobalamin (vitamin B_{12}) or folate deficiency

2) The erythrocytes are large with fragile membranes that rupture easily.

b. Pernicious anemia

1) Description

a) The gastric mucosal lining atrophies after years of gastritis.

b) Intrinsic factor (IF), which is secreted by the parietal cells of the gastric mucosa and is essential for cobalamin absorption, becomes defective or stops functioning.

c) Cobalamin deficiency may also occur after small bowel resection and in Crohn's disease.

d) Populations most affected are Northern European ancestry over age 40 and young African Americans.

2) Assessment

a) Mouth—sore tongue

b) Nausea and vomiting, anorexia, diarrhea

c) Muscle weakness

d) Neurologic changes such as paresthesias, ataxia, mental confusion

3) Diagnostic tests

a) CBC and blood smear— erythrocytes are large (macrocytic) and abnormally shaped.

b) Low serum cobalamine, normal or increased folate levels

c) Antibody to IF in serum

d) Direct gastric analysis for IF or achlorhydria (the absence of hydrochloric acid [HCl]), gastroscopy, and biopsy of the gastric mucosa

e) Schilling test: Radioactive vitamin B_{12} malabsorption is measured by the small amount secreted in the urine. When vitamin B_{12} is administered with gastric IF parenterally, its absence in urine will diagnose pernicious anemia.

4) Nursing interventions

a) Protect the client's extremities from injury and burns.

b) Promote compliance with monthly vitamin B_{12} injections or weekly self-administered intranasal gel form.

c) Monitor the client for neuromuscular complications that may be permanent, requiring modifications in the home environment.

d) Assess the client for an increased risk of gastric and thyroid cancers.

c. Folic acid deficiency

1) Description: folic acid is required for DNA synthesis in erythrocyte formation.

2) Assessment

a) Poor nutrition

b) Alcohol abuse

c) Anorexia

d) Impaired absorption in the small intestine

e) Clients undergoing hemodialysis (folic acid is dialyzable)

f) Certain drugs such as oral contraceptives, antiseizure drugs, and antibiotics, which can block the absorption of folic acid

g) Certain conditions such as pregnancy, chronic hemolytic anemia, and sickle cell disease, which may increase the need for folic acid

3) Diagnostic tests

a) CBC: RBCs, hemoglobin, and hematocrit are decreased and the MCV is increased.

b) Serum folate levels are low.

c) Serum cobalamin level is normal.

4) Nursing interventions

a) Promote compliance with replacement therapy (1–5 mg oral folate per day).

b) Administer prenatal vitamins in pregnancy.

c) Instruct the client on foods high in folic acid, such as leafy greens, liver, citrus fruits, nuts, and grains.

5. ANEMIA OF CHRONIC DISEASE

a. Description: a decrease in erythrocyte precursor production that occurs in some chronic conditions such as end-stage renal failure, chronic liver disease, alcohol abuse, or hypothyroidism

  b. Assessment

    1) All assessments for anemia apply. Look for an underlying, coexisting chronic condition in an older adult client.

  c. Diagnostic tests

    1) Ferritin: Iron stores may be high in contrast to iron deficiency anemia.

    2) CBC

  d. Nursing interventions

    1) Facilitate diagnosis and treatment of underlying, contributory condition.

    2) Inform the client that this type of anemia does not respond to folic acid, iron, or Vitamin B_{12}.

    3) Erythropoietin therapy is administered to a client with anemia related to renal failure.

6. APLASTIC ANEMIA

  a. Description

    1) A life-threatening stem cell disorder with many possible etiological mechanisms characterized by a hypoplastic, fatty bone marrow and pancytopenia

    2) Cause is most often immune mediated but can be congenital (Fanconi's anemia) or acquired from radiation, chemical exposures such as from solvents like benzene, viral or bacterial infections, pregnancy, or, usually, idiopathic.

  b. Assessment

    1) Insidious development of clinical manifestations, including fatigue, dyspnea, pallor, fever, infections from neutropenia, easy bleeding from thrombocytopenia (petechiae, epistaxis)

  c. Diagnostic tests

    1) All blood counts are decreased.

    2) Reticulocyte count is low.

    3) Iron studies: serum iron and TIBC may be elevated initially.

    4) Bone marrow aspirate and biopsy-hypo-cellular bone marrow aspiration may be difficult because of lack of bone marrow cellularity ("dry tap").

  d. Nursing interventions

    1) Pancytopenia plan of care to prevent complications such as infection and bleeding, including private room, strict hand washing, and minimizing invasive procedures

    2) Provide the client and family with a lot of support for the lengthy hospitalization and treatment.

  e. Medical management

    1) Antithymocyte globulin and cyclosporine therapy with steroids requires specialized nursing care to observe for serum sickness and complications from steroid use and cyclosporine.

    2) Bone marrow transplant with a donor matched for human leukocyte antigen (HLA) also requires specialized nursing care. Complications include graft vs. host disease (the donor bone marrow rejects the host, resulting in severe rash, diarrhea, and may result in death), transfusion and drug reactions, infection, and bleeding.

  f. Anemia from blood loss

    1) Description (may be acute or chronic)

      a) Sudden and rapid loss of blood

      b) Causes include trauma, complications from surgery, pregnancy, and diseases that disrupt vascular integrity.

      c) May result in hypovolemic shock or if blood loss is relatively slow, plasma volume may be preserved but erythrocyte levels are decreased.

    2) Assessment

      a) Clinical findings may vary depending on the rate and quantity of blood loss.

      b) 10% of blood volume loss: no findings

      c) 20% of blood volume lost: no findings at rest; tachycardia with exertion and slight hypotension

      d) 30% of blood volume lost: normal supine blood pressure and pulse at rest; postural hypotension and tachycardia with exercise

      e) 40% of blood volume lost: rapid, thready pulse, cold and clammy skin; blood pressure below normal at rest

      f) 50% of blood volume lost: shock and potential death

      g) Assessment should include pain clinical manifestations such as signs or history of trauma, dizziness, syncope, swelling, or abdominal distension.

3) Diagnostic studies
   a) Hemoglobin and hematocrit may be normal initially. After hours to days, the erythrocyte volume is replaced by endogenous or exogenous intravenous solutions means the red cell mass is diluted and the hemoglobin level drops.
4) Nursing interventions
   a) Identify the source of bleeding; check dressings and drainage tubes in postoperative clients.
   b) Administer prescribed intravenous fluids.
   c) Monitor for signs of hypovolemic shock and loss of consciousness.
   d) Perform frequent vital signs.
   e) Administer prescribed blood products and iron supplementation.

g. Anemia caused by increased erythrocyte destruction (see Table 12-4)
   1) Description
      a) Two sites of hemolysis:
         1. Intravascular destruction occurs within the circulation.
         2. Extravascular destruction occurs in the spleen, liver, or bone marrow.
      b) Intrinsic hemolytic anemias: usually hereditary; defects in the erythrocytes themselves
         1. Abnormal hemoglobins such as with sickle cell disease
         2. Enzyme deficiencies such as with glucose-6 phosphate dehydrogenase deficiency, or G6PD
         3. Cell membrane abnormalities

      c) Extrinsic hemolytic anemias: normal erythrocytes are damaged by external factors such as antibodies, toxins, mechanical injury (prosthetic heart valves), dialysis, transfusion reaction (ABO blood typing mismatch), and trapping of cells within the liver and spleen.
   2) Assessment of hemolytic anemias
      a) Jaundice due to increased bilirubin levels from destruction of the erythrocytes, pallor, chills, fever, irritability
      b) Enlarged liver and spleen due to sequestration of defective erythrocytes in these organs; abdominal pain, vomiting, melena, diarrhea, hematuria
   3) Diagnostic tests
      a) CBC
      b) Reticulocyte count elevated in the absence of bleeding
      c) Haptoglobin (plasma protein that binds hemoglobin in plasma) is low. It can be abnormal for other reasons besides hemolysis.
      d) Bilirubin: indirect bili is elevated and so is total bili.
      e) Indirect Coombs' test will be elevated in the case of immune hemolysis.
      f) LDH elevated
      g) Renal function and urinalysis; urine hemosiderin is positive if iron is lost in urine. This could also lead to iron deficiency.
   4) Medical management
      a) Identify and treat the underlying cause.
      b) Drug treatments include corticosteroid to combat immune response, folic acid, and iron supplements.
      c) Blood transfusions if anemia is severe
      d) Splenectomy
   5) Nursing interventions
      a) Encourage compliance with medical treatments and medications.
      b) Instruct a client with jaundice to avoid soaps while bathing, use tepid or cool water to minimize pruritus, and administer good skin care; provide regular turning of the client in bed.

Table 12-4 Classification of Hemolytic Anemias

Intrinsic	Examples: • G6PD deficiency • Hemoglobinopathies: Sickle cell anemia
Extrinsic	Examples: • Autoimmune, drug toxicity • Thrombotic thrombocytopenic purpura (TTP) • Disseminated intravascular coagulation (DIC) • Infection: malaria, *Clostridium* • Hypersplenism • Burns

c) Assist the client to adapt to fatigue from the anemia; provide adequate rest periods.

d) Instruct the client and family about the nature of the disease and the rationale for treatments given.

e) Offer pre-op teaching and pneumoccal vaccine before splenectomy.

h. Sickle cell disease

1) Description

a) A group of inherited disorders caused by the genetic mutation and structural change in globin (hemoglobin A) genes, resulting in defective or nonfunctioning hemoglobin molecules such as hemoglobin S or C

b) In sickle cell anemia, the amino acid valine is changed to glutamine.

c) Oxygen-bonding capacity of the cell is reduced. The lack of oxygen in the cell causes the erythrocyte to become rigid, sticky, and form an elongated crescent (sickle) shape that breaks apart easily. Life expectancy of a sickle red blood cell is 7–45 days. (Normal RBCs live about 120 days.)

d) Affects more than 50,000 Americans, mostly African Americans, occurring in 1 out of 375 live births. There is no cure, except for bone marrow transplant in childhood. Adults can survive past middle age with proper treatment.

e) Hemoglobin S gene is prevalent in Africa. Protective against falciparum, the organism that causes malaria.

f) Vaso-occlusive aspect of the disease

1. Sickled cells flow poorly through small capillaries, causing hemostasis, occlusion, hypoxia, deoxygenation of more red blood cells, and more sickling.

2. Severe pain results, causing chronic, progressive organ damage, especially to the kidneys, liver, and spleen.

g) Sickle cell trait is heterozygous and has few ill effects. If both parents have this trait there is a 25% chance with each

pregnancy of producing a child with sickle cell disease.

h) Complications vary between individuals and may be mild or severe and life threatening, precipitated by heat from weather or exertion, dehydration, pregnancy, stress, and infection.

2) Assessment (see Table 12-5)

a) Painful episodes, sudden onset of severe pain in the chest, back, abdomen, and extremities, precipitated by heat from weather or exertion, dehydration, pregnancy, stress, and infection

b) Chronic anemia

c) Organ damage to the kidney, liver, spleen (autosplenectomy); cardiomegaly and congestive heart failure

d) Chronic leg ulcers

e) Priapism: a prolonged painful penile erection

f) Chest syndrome

g) Retinopathy

h) Skin: pallor of the mucous membranes, ulcers on the legs

i) Short stature, fingers may have swellings (dactylitis)

j) Shortness of breath, fatigue, frequent pneumonias

3) Diagnostic tests

a) CBC: hemoglobin levels can vary within a range of 5–11 g/dl, and peripheral blood smear (sickled cells not present

Table 12-5 Clinical Manifestations of Sickle Cell Disease

Organ	Clinical Manifestations
Brain	Thrombosis or hemorrhage may cause sensory or mobility deficits and/or death.
Eye	Retinopathy, retinal detachment, hemorrhage, blindness
Lung	Acute chest syndrome, pulmonary hypertension, pneumonia
Heart	Cardiomegaly leading to congestive heart failure
Kidney	Inability to concentrate urine (specific gravity of 1.000), hematuria, renal failure
Spleen	Autosplenectomy or splenomegaly (Hgb SC)
Bones and joints	Dactylitis (hand-foot syndrome), osteonecrosis
Penis	Priapism—a painful prolonged erection
Liver-gallbladder	Hepatomegaly, gallstones (may require cholecystectomy)
Skin	Ulcers on lower extremities (difficult to heal)

© Cengage Learning 2015

in the trait) may show evidence of hemolysis, with an increase in reticulocytes.

b) Sickledex: normally used only in newborn screening; positive in both trait and diseased individuals

c) Hemoglobin electrophoresis: the blood specimen is subjected to electrical field. The different kinds of hemoglobin separate into predictable patterns; may be used to determine effect of an exchange transfusion of RBCs on the percent of sickle hemoglobin in the client.

d) Skeletal x-rays will show bone and joint abnormalities. A chest x-ray is used to determine lung abnormalities such as pneumonia and sickle chest syndrome.

e) MRI may be used to diagnose brain injury following a cerebrovascular accident.

4) Nursing interventions

a) Provide rest.

b) Monitor vital signs.

c) Instruct the client to report a fever immediately.

d) Administer pain medications as ordered, monitor for effect on pain and oversedation. Facilitate nonmedicinal forms of pain relief such as distraction (television or radio, heating pads, tub soaks, or massage).

e) Encourage fluids; client cannot concentrate urine in the kidney and requires extra fluids when exercising or in warm weather.

f) Create a care plan with the client for use during repeated hospitalizations or outpatient treatment of painful episodes.

g) Administer prescribed drugs.

1. Penicillin: prevents infection with encapsulated organisms of splenectomized persons

2. Folic acid: vitamin supplement needed to replenish bone marrow stores

3. Hydroxyurea: an oral cancer drug that can increase the percent of fetal hemoglobin in adults and protects against sickle cell crises

4. Desferrioxamine (Desferal): subcutaneous injection or infusion of iron chelator that helps decrease the iron overload

h) Administer vaccinations: influenza, pneumococcal, and hepatitis B.

i) Administer oxygen to hospitalized clients to help decrease sickling from hypoxia.

j) Administer blood transfusions when ordered. Note that sickling can be enhanced by increased viscosity of the blood following packed cell transfusion. Exchange transfusions maintain viscosity and blood volume, increases the ratio of normal to sickle blood, and do not contribute to iron overload.

k) Provide the client and family education and counseling regarding the disease, prevention of complications, depression from coping with a chronic illness, and self-care for painful episodes.

l) Encourage genetic counseling and testing of carriers and diseased clients and partners.

i. Glucose-6-phosphate dehydrogenase (G6PD) deficiency

1) Description

a) A group of X-linked familial hemolytic mutations of the gene for G6PD

b) Deficiency leads to erythrocyte destruction when older erythrocytes are exposed to oxidative drugs or foods or infection, which increase metabolism and stress the cells.

c) More common in males of Mediterranean or African descent

2) Assessment

a) Jaundice

b) Headache, dizziness, easy fatigability

3) Diagnostic tests

a) Quantification of G6PD levels during nonhemolytic phase

b) Indirect tests for hemolysis following administration of an oxidative substance

4) Nursing interventions

a) Provide periods of rest.

b) Provide adequate hydration.

c) Administer antibiotics and other treatments as ordered to minimize complications.

B. HEMOCHROMATOSIS
1. DESCRIPTION
   a. Autosomal recessive, increased iron absorption, and increased iron storage in tissue
   b. Incidence is 1 in 300 and is the most common genetic disease in Caucasians.
2. ASSESSMENT
   a. Onset of clinical manifestations is at 50 years of age and in those with periodic blood loss, such as premenopausal or multigravida women and frequent blood donors.
   b. Skin pigmentation changes ("bronzing")
   c. Cardiomyopathy
   d. Diabetes mellitus
   e. Enlarged liver and spleen
3. DIAGNOSTIC TESTS
   a. Elevations of serum iron, TIBC, transferrin saturation, and ferritin (may not be elevated in younger adults)
   b. Liver biopsy shows increased iron in hepatocytes
   c. HLA testing—linked to HLA-A3, HLA-B7, and HLA-B14
4. NURSING INTERVENTIONS
   a. Goal is to remove iron from the body. Periodic phlebotomy of 500 ml of blood, weekly then maintenance schedule of every 3–6 months; check hematocrit before each phlebotomy.
   b. Detection and management of organ involvement as appropriate
   c. Limit dietary and iron supplements.
C. POLYCYTHEMIA
1. DESCRIPTION
   a. Increased production of erythrocytes resulting in an increase in circulating RBCs
   b. Primary erythrocytosis: polycythemia vera (PV), a neoplastic disorder arising from a single pluripotent stem cell; increase in all three types of blood cells: granulocytes, platelets, as well as erythrocytes.
   c. Secondary erythrocytosis: caused by presence of hypoxia; this stimulates erythropoietin production and results in an increase in erythrocytes.
2. ASSESSMENT
   a. Headache, dizziness, tinnitus, and visual disturbances
   b. Vascular: angina, congestive heart failure, intermittent claudication and thrombophlebitis, stroke
   c. Skin: plethoric and pruritic (secondary to histamine release)
   d. Hemorrhage from vessel distention or alteration in platelet function

   e. Gastrointestinal clinical manifestations such as pain and fullness
   f. Splenomegaly in primary polycythemia only
3. DIAGNOSTIC TESTS
   a. CBC
   b. Elevated uric acid, leukocyte alkaline phosphatase
   c. Bone marrow biopsy in PV shows hypercellularity.
4. NURSING INTERVENTIONS
   a. Assist with a phlebotomy to decrease blood volume.
   b. Maintain adequate hydration to decrease viscosity.
   c. In polycythemia vera, administer myelosuppressive agents such as hydroxyurea (Hydrea), melphalan (Alkeran), allopurinol (Zyloprim) to reduce gout.
   d. Maintain adequate oxygenation and encourage smoking cessation.
   e. Assess nutritional intake.
   f. Prevent clot formation by encouraging range of motion activity, and assess for signs of clot or cerebrovascular disease.
D. THROMBOCYTOSIS OR ESSENTIAL THROMBOCYTHEMIA
1. DESCRIPTION: INCREASED PLATELET FORMATION
2. ASSESSMENT
   a. Many may have no clinical findings.
   b. Gastrointestinal bleeding such as splenomegaly and hepatomegaly
   c. Vascular manifestations such as clots and headaches
   d. Paresthesias and burning feet sensation
3. DIAGNOSTIC TESTS
   a. CBC—platelet count over $600,000/mm^3$
   b. Bone marrow is hypercellular with increased megakaryocytes
4. NURSING INTERVENTIONS
   a. Symptomatic treatment
   b. Assess for life-threatening bleeding or thrombosis.
   c. Encourage smoking cessation measures.
   d. Inform the client that platelet apheresis may be ordered to reduce platelet count emergently.
   e. Ensure medication compliance. Medications may include, hydroxyurea (Hydrea), anagrelide (Agrylin), interferon alpha, or 32P (phosphate) IV every 6 months to 2 years.
E. DISORDERS OF HEMOSTASIS
1. THROMBOCYTOPENIA
   a. Description
      1) Platelet count is lower than normal.
      2) Most are acquired, not inherited.

Table 12-6 Coagulation Studies

Study	Significance
International normalized ratio (INR)	Standardized system of PT reporting; useful in monitoring and dosing warfarin
Prothrombin time (PT)	Extrinsic coagulation factor assessment: Factors I, II, V, VII, X
Activated partial thromboplastin time (APTT)	Intrinsic coagulation factor assessment: Factors I, II, V, VIII, IX, X, XI, XII
Bleeding time	Time to clot when a small slit is made in the skin; Prolonged in Von Willebrand's disease; normal in hemophilia
Thrombin time	Adequacy of thrombin
Fibrinogen	Level of fibrinogen: Increased = hypercoagulability Decreased = predisposed to bleed
Fibrin split products (FSP) or fibrin degradation products (FDP)	Degree of fibrinolysis; increased in disseminated intravascular coagulation (DIC)

3) Types have similar manifestations but have different causes and treatments.
   b. Assessment
     1) See individual types.
   c. Diagnostic tests (see Table 12-6)
   d. Nursing interventions
     1) See individual types.
   e. Immune thrombocytopenic purpura (ITP)
     1) Description: below-normal platelet count caused by destruction of mature platelets in the peripheral blood or spleen by immune processes
     2) Assessment: history and physical exam for signs of bleeding, specifically in mucous membranes
     3) Diagnostic tests: complete blood count and peripheral smear morphology
     4) Nursing interventions: assess for bleeding; administer intravenous immunoglobulin and glucocorticoids safely; and administer pre- and postsurgical care for a client undergoing a splenectomy.
   f. Thrombotic thrombocytopenic purpura (TTP)
     1) Description

     a) An uncommon syndrome with five clinical components: microangiopathic hemolytic anemia, thrombocytopenia, mental status changes, fever, and kidney failure. Platelet agglutination causes microthrombi in tiny vessels.
     b) Causes bleeding and clotting at the same time; medical emergency
    2) Assessment
     a) Bleeding is more prolonged than in thrombocytopenia.
     b) Skin manifestations include bruising, petechiae, and purple patches (purpura).
     c) Heavy menstruation
     d) Nosebleeds
     e) Blood in stool and vomit
     f) Mental status changes, confusion
     g) Renal failure, decreased urine output, blood in urine
    3) Diagnostic tests
     a) CBC—low platelet count
     b) Coagulation tests
     c) Urinalysis
     d) Bone marrow biopsy to look for platelet precursors
    4) Medical management
     a) Corticosteroids
     b) Plasma exchange
     c) Aspirin
     d) Dialysis in severe renal failure
    5) Nursing interventions
     a) Instruct the client and family about the condition and rationale for interventions.
     b) Maintain good venous access for plasma exchange, dialysis.
     c) Frequently monitor for signs of bleeding.
     d) Implement safety precautions for the confused client to ensure that the client is not injured.
   g. Heparin-induced thrombocytopenia and thrombosis syndrome (HITTS)
    1) Description
     a) An immune mechanism that results in destruction of platelets and vessel wall lining injury, causing bleeding
     b) Peripheral arterial clotting can lead to ischemia in the extremities and gangrene.
     c) Incidence varies from 5% to 25%, less common in porcine heparin.

2) Assessment
   a) Skin: petechiae, purpura, and ecchymoses; prolonged bleeding from venipuncture sites
   b) Extremities: pulses, skin color and temperature changes, pain in joints
   c) Cardiac: tachycardia, hypotension
   d) GI: abdominal pain or distension, tarry stools
   e) Neurological: dizziness, loss of consciousness
3) Diagnostic tests
   a) CBC and platelet count—thrombocytopenia and anemia
   b) Clotting studies, bleeding time
   c) Assay for antiheparin antibodies
4) Nursing interventions
   a) Assess the medication history, especially any recent use of heparin, including small amounts used to keep IV access catheters open.
   b) Discontinue heparin; document as an allergy on the client identification arm band, medication, and medical records.
   c) Use alternative solutions to keep IV catheters open (saline or citrate flushes).
   d) Monitor for bleeding and thrombosis.
   e) Instruct the client and family regarding bleeding precautions such as shaving with an electric razor.
   f) Maintain IV access in a client receiving plasmapheresis treatment to remove IGG.
   g) Inform the client on the uses of other treatments such as steroids and thrombin inhibitors and that platelet transfusions are not therapeutic and may increase the thrombosis.

2. HEMOPHILIA
   a. Description
      1) Hereditary bleeding disorder caused by a lack of coagulation factors
      2) Two major forms of hemophilia:
         a) Hemophilia A, or classic hemophilia: deficiency of factor VIII, most common type, incidence is 1 in 10,000 males
         b) Hemophilia B or Christmas disease: deficiency of factor IX, incidence is 1 in 100,000 males
      3) Early in the twentieth century, survival was normally to 11 years. By the 1970s it rose to 68 years median survival. Infection with HIV from factor gathered from pools of donors decreased the life expectancy to 49 years in the 1980s. Life expectancy is improving because of tests now available for HIV and hepatitis, better screening of donors, and heat treatment of some products.
   b. Assessment
      1) Skin bruising or ecchymoses
      2) Neurological manifestations such as pain, lack of sensation in a limb, paralysis
      3) Musculoskeletal manifestations such as joint swelling from bleeding internally (hemarthrosis); may have deformities of joints, causing mobility problems
   c. Diagnostic tests
      1) Blood tests for intrinsic factors VIII, IX, XI, or XII deficiency
      2) Coagulation tests: partial thromboplastin time may be prolonged. Others may be normal because the extrinsic system is not involved.
   d. Medical management
      1) Before 1986, HIV infection from factor transfusion gathered from many donors was common. Factor safety has been increased with heat and chemical treatment of factor concentrates, and recombinant DNA technologies for making factor that does not use donors.
      2) The body can produce inhibitors to factors VIII and IX, making these treatments less effective. One strategy is to suppress the immune system to slow this response.
   e. Nursing interventions
      1) Assess the client's history and physical, family, or personal history for excessive or delayed bleeding from minor skin trauma, dental extraction, or hematuria.
      2) Acute intervention focus is to stop bleeding.
      3) Administer coagulation factor; concentrate on time and for long enough time.
      4) Encourage bed rest for joint or major muscle bleed.
      5) Administer prescribed drugs for pain.
      6) Prevent airway compromise.
      7) Assess for intracranial bleeding.

8) Provide referral to genetic counseling, psychosocial counseling, and support.

9) Instruct the client and family regarding prevention and early signs of bleeding, home administration of factors, pain management, and rehabilitation considerations.

10) Instruct the client to wear a Medic Alert bracelet, participate in noncontact sports, and avoid injury from tools in the home.

3. VON WILLEBRAND'S DISEASE
   a. Description
      1) Hereditary bleeding disorder caused by the deficiency of the von Willebrand coagulation protein (vWF) and platelet dysfunction; most common type of bleeding disorder (1 in 100); can range from mild to severe
      2) Autosomal dominant; occurs in both sexes
   b. Assessment
      1) Same as hemophilia (see page 310)
   c. Diagnostic tests
      1) Bleeding time: prolonged due to dysfunctional platelets
      2) Reduction in factor VIII
   d. Medical management
      1) Desmopressin acetate (DDAVP) given intravenously or as a nasal spray increases factor VIII and vWf concentration; decreases bleeding time but the effect is short-lived; useful to control bleeding from a dental procedure or surgery
   e. Nursing interventions
      1) Same as hemophilia (see page 310)

4. DISSEMINATED INTRAVASCULAR COAGULATION (DIC)
   a. Description
      1) A serious bleeding disorder that results in both thrombosis and bleeding
      2) Triggered by another abnormal process or illness in the body
      3) Initially thrombin production is increased. Fibrinogen is converted to fibrin and platelet aggregation is enhanced. Clotting ensues and becomes excessive; clotting factors and platelets are consumed.
      4) The fibrinolytic system is stimulated to break up clots and produce fibrin-split products.
      5) The effect on the client is an inability to form clots at any injury site (including venipuncture sites).
      6) Chronic DIC can occur in some malignancies or autoimmune disorders, causing a range of abnormal laboratory findings, bleeding, and hypercoagulability.
   b. Assessment
      1) Skin manifestations such as pallor, petechiae, bleeding from venipuncture sites and mucous membranes, and ecchymosis
      2) Lung manifestations such as shortness of breath and hemoptysis
      3) Gastrointestinal manifestations such as blood in stools, abdominal distention
      4) Urinary manifestations such as hematuria and oliguria
      5) Neurological manifestations such as mental status changes, headache, visual changes, and dizziness
      6) Musculoskeletal manifestations such as bone or joint pain
   c. Diagnostic tests (see Table 12-7)
      1) Clotting time is generally prolonged, and materials such as platelets to make clots are decreased in number.
   d. Medical management
      1) Treat the underlying cause (malignancy, infection, trauma, etc.).
      2) Heparin and antithrombin III (AT III) to prevent and treat thrombosis
      3) Epsion-aminocaproic acid (Amicar) to inhibit fibrinolysis

Table 12-7 Diagnostic Laboratory Tests and Findings for Acute Disseminated Intravascular Coagulation

Test	Laboratory Value
Prothrombin time	Increased (75%) Normal or shortened (25%)
Partial thromboplastin time	Increased
Thrombin time	Increased
Fibrinogen	Decreased
Platelets	Decreased
Fibrin-split products (FSPs) or fibrin-degradation products (FDPs)	Increased
Coagulation factors	Factors V, VII, VIII, X, XIII decreased
D-dimers (cross-linked fibrin fragments)	Increased (more reliable than FSP)
Antithrombin III	Decreased
Bleeding time	Increased

© Cengage Learning 2015

4) Clotting factor and platelet replacement, blood transfusion
5) Supportive care (e.g., hemodialysis)
   e. Nursing interventions
      1) Acute DIC is a medical emergency and the nurse should do everything possible to facilitate procedures for appropriate testing.
      2) Ongoing assessment for external and internal bleeding
      3) Minimize damage to tissues to prevent new sites of bleeding.
      4) Administer blood products, cryoprecipitate, and fresh frozen plasma promptly and safely.
      5) Instruct the client about the entity of DIC and the rationale for seemingly paradoxical therapies.
5. HYPERCOAGULABILITY LEADING TO VENOUS CLOT FORMATION
   a. Description
      1) A disorder or condition that renders the client more likely to form clots
      2) Occurs in some cancers, Trousseau's syndrome, inherited disorders such as factor V Leiden, protein C or S deficiencies, antithrombin III deficiency, elevated homocysteine, thrombocytosis, polycythemia vera, estrogen therapy
   b. Assessment
      1) Skin manifestations such as swelling in the lower extremities; erythema; tenderness; warmth over the area; or cyanosis, which is a late sign
      2) Palpation of firm cord along the vein
      3) Prominent superficial veins in the same limb
   c. Diagnostic tests: ultrasound of the area assessing patency of the vein
   d. Medical management
      1) Heparin therapy given IV bolus then as a continuous infusion; PTT should be 1.5–2 times normal.
      2) Low-molecular-weight heparin may be administered s.q. by the nurse or client. Complication rate is less than with heparin.
      3) Warfarin sodium (Coumadin) given orally initiated after heparin infusion and overlapping with heparin until the INR is 2–3. Vitamin K interferes with warfarin and can be used to counteract its effects if bleeding occurs.
      4) Inferior vena cava filter may be surgically placed to prevent pulmonary embolism and recurrent thromboembolism.
      5) Thrombolytic agents dissolve the clot. This treatment can result in bleeding and is not used as a first course of action for venous clots.
   e. Nursing interventions
      1) Assess personal or family history and a history of recent immobilization or surgery.
      2) Elevate the affected limb and apply antithrombosis stockings.
      3) Measure and document the circumference of the limb.
      4) Assess for signs of additional clot extension, pulmonary embolism.
      5) Assess for bleeding as a complication of medical treatments.
      6) Instruct the client about reducing risk of clotting and signs of bleeding.
      7) Instruct the client about interactions between drugs and diet, such as leafy green vegetables, which contain vitamin K and can interfere with warfarin activity.

F. NEUTROPENIA
   1. DESCRIPTION
      a. Syndrome of leukopenia (decreased WBC) or granulocytopenia that occurs in a variety of conditions or as a reaction to medications and other chemicals
      b. Neutropenia is a neutrophil count of < 1000 to 1500/ml.
      c. A complication of neutropenia is infection. The risk of infection depends on the rate of decline in the WBC, the degree of neutropenia, and the duration.
      d. Causes (see Table 12-8) are numerous but usually iatrogenic as a result of chemicals, medicines, or disease.
   2. ASSESSMENT
      a. Fever
         1) Without neutrophils, the body cannot produce normal inflammatory responses to infection such as pus, erythema, and swelling.
      b. Malaise and chills
      c. Pain may be present at the site of infection, such as sore throat, rectal pain, chest pain, pain or burning with urination.
      d. Lung manifestations such as dry cough or shortness of breath
      e. Assess for signs of septic shock, including decrease in urinary output,

Table 12-8 Causes of Neutropenia

Autoimmune disorders, such as
Rheumatoid arthritis
Systemic lupus erythematosus
Drugs that cause neutropenia, such as
Antitumor drugs (doxorubicin, cychlophosphamide)
Antimetabolites (methotrexate, 6-mercaptopurine)
Anti-inflammatory drugs (phenylbutazone)
Antibiotics (Chloramphenicol, triethoprimsulfamethoxazole, penicillins)
Antiseizure drugs (phenytoin)
Hypoglycemics (tolbutamide)
Phenothiazines (chlorpromazine)
Psychotropic and antidepressants (imipramine)
Anti-HIV (Zidovudine)
Hematologic disorders, such as
Aplastic anemia
Leukemia
Cyclic neutropenia
Infections, such as
Viral (hepatitis, influenza, HIV)
Fulminant bacterial infection (typhoid fever, milliary tuberculosis)
Miscellaneous
Overwhelming sepsis
Involvement of the bone marrow by disease or infectious agent (carcinoma, lymphoma, tuberculosis)
Hypersplenism
Nutritional deficiencies (cobalamin, folic acid)
Exposure to high doses of radioactivity

© Cengage Learning 2015

drop in blood pressure, mental confusion, and loss of consciousness.

3. DIAGNOSTIC TESTS
  a. CBC with differential
  b. Bone marrow biopsy and aspiration
  c. If infection is suspected, obtain a chest x-ray, urinary analysis and culture, stool cultures, and blood cultures from two different sites.

4. NURSING INTERVENTIONS
  a. Instruct the client on the importance of strict hand washing, private room, protective isolation, and no visitors who have illness manifestations. Some facilities have high-efficiency particulate air (HEPA) filtration or laminar airflow (LAF) rooms for protection of severely immunocompromised clients.
  b. Monitor for clinical manifestations of infection and septic shock, reporting abnormal vital signs immediately.
  c. Promptly obtain cultures and administer antibiotics as ordered. Combination broad-spectrum antibiotics are usually given IV to clients who are febrile and neutropenic. Delay in this therapy can lead to shock and death in a matter of hours. Prophylactic oral antibiotic therapy can be effective in prevention of more serious infections.
  d. Monitor for adverse reactions of the antibiotics.
  e. Administer prescribed granulocytic growth factors.
  f. Administer prescribed antipyretics.
  g. Avoid invasive procedures as much as possible (rectal temperatures, suppositories, enemas, urinary catheters). Minimize venipunctures.
  h. Instruct the client and family about good hygienic practices and infection prevention measures. Support the client, who may be anxious and afraid of getting an infection.

G. DISORDERS OF THE SPLEEN
  1. DESCRIPTION
    a. Hypersplenism is an enlarged spleen that occurs in a variety of diseases and is accompanied by changes in the peripheral blood counts of platelets, RBCs, and WBCs.
    b. Examples of diseases with hypersplenism: sickle cell disease (hemoglobin SC), thalassemia major, ITP, hemolytic anemia, polycythemia vera, leukemia, liver disease, infections such as infectious mononucleosis, AIDS

  2. ASSESSMENT
    a. Abdominal distension, asymptomatic enlargement of the spleen detected on the physical exam
    b. Early satiety due to pressure on the stomach from massive splenomegaly
    c. Abdominal pain

  3. DIAGNOSTIC TESTS
    a. CBC, platelet count and differential
    b. Liver-spleen scan
    c. CT scan of the abdomen
    d. Ultrasound of the spleen
    e. Laparotomy and splenectomy to assess the spleen

  4. NURSING INTERVENTIONS
    a. Administer analgesics for splenomegaly.
    b. Position the client for lung expansion and comfort and that will not injure the spleen.
    c. Encourage several small meals a day.
    d. In splenectomized client:
      1) Presplenectomy: giving pneumococcal vaccine several days to weeks before surgery is best.

2) Postsplenectomy: administer analgesic; observe for hemorrhage, infection (especially encapsulated organisms such as *Pneumococcus*), and abdominal distension.

3) Monitor CBC: splenectomy can result in sudden rebound in blood counts.

4) Instruct the client about dressing changes, activity, and manifestations of infection before discharge from the hospital.

VI. BLOOD COMPONENT THERAPY

A. SEE MEDICATION THERAPY (CHAPTER 15)

PRACTICE QUESTIONS

1. The nurse is admitting a client suspected of having sickle cell anemia. The client has a fever of 38.9°C or 102°F, faint yellow-tinged sclera, and is complaining of abdominal pain. Which of the following clinical manifestations further support this diagnosis?

   Select all that apply:
   [ ] 1. Rapid but regular breathing
   [ ] 2. Pale, dilute urine
   [ ] 3. Skin ulcers on the lower extremities
   [ ] 4. Swollen fingers
   [ ] 5. Pallor
   [ ] 6. Fatigue

2. The nurse making a care plan for a client with severe thrombocytopenia should include which of the following?
   1. Careful examination of spinal fluid obtained by lumbar puncture
   2. A private room with reverse isolation precautions
   3. Avoid intramuscular administration of medications
   4. Careful monitoring of urinary output while titrating the dosage of furosemide (Lasix)

3. A client with lung cancer is admitted with a new diagnosis of acute disseminated intravascular coagulation (DIC). Which of the following actions is a priority?
   1. Obtain a diet history from the client for the last 3 days
   2. Assess the client for any indications of internal or external bleeding
   3. Take the family to the family lounge and discuss home care for a client with DIC
   4. Call the dialysis unit to determine when the client may be transferred

4. The nurse has instructed a client with a hematological disorder about the functions of the hematologic system. The client indicates a need for further teaching by describing the function of the hematologic system as
   1. "the coagulation and clotting of blood."
   2. "the exchange of oxygen and carbon dioxide at the alveoli."
   3. "the transportation of oxygen and carbon dioxide to cells of the body."
   4. "to fight infection."

5. The nurse is admitting a client with severe shortness of breath. The nurse assesses which of the following clinical manifestations to be present in the client with pernicious anemia?

   Select all that apply:
   [ ] 1. Oral temperature greater than 38°C or 100.5°F
   [ ] 2. Dark-brown urine
   [ ] 3. Paresthesia
   [ ] 4. White and yellow patches on the tongue
   [ ] 5. Mental confusion
   [ ] 6. Muscle weakness

6. The nurse is discharging a client with aplastic anemia. Which of the following statements made by the client would demonstrate the need for additional teaching by the nurse?
   1. "I'm a little nervous about the side effects of my medicines and will call if I have questions."
   2. "I have a lot of sisters and brothers. I hope one of them will match for my bone marrow transplant."
   3. "I'm going back to my job in the toddler room at a day care center tomorrow."
   4. "Diabetes runs in my family, so we will be checking my glucose levels while I am on the prednisone."

7. A client with a chronic bleeding duodenal ulcer is admitted to the hospital. What clinical manifestations should the nurse assess for in a client with a 30% blood volume loss?

   Select all that apply:
   [ ] 1. Postural hypotension
   [ ] 2. Dizziness
   [ ] 3. Tachycardia with activity
   [ ] 4. Swelling
   [ ] 5. Blood pressure below normal at rest
   [ ] 6. Pain

8. Which of the following should the nurse include in the instructions provided to a client with sickle cell anemia?

   Select all that apply:
   [ ] 1. Administer pain medications
   [ ] 2. Encourage fluids
   [ ] 3. Treat the presence of infection
   [ ] 4. Avoid informing others of the condition
   [ ] 5. Vigorous exercise is permitted
   [ ] 6. Inform the client that the disorder is not hereditary

9. The nurse is evaluating a client with an enlarged spleen. Which of the following diagnostic tests would confirm the diagnosis?
   1. Urinalysis
   2. CAT scan of the chest
   3. Blood cultures
   4. CAT scan of the abdomen

10. The nurse has started a transfusion of packed red blood cells. The nurse should immediately stop the transfusion when which of the following occurs?
    1. Fever and back pain
    2. Dry mouth
    3. Hypothermia and pallor
    4. Heart rate of 74 beats per minute

11. The nurse is caring for a client with neutropenia. Which of the following blood tests would indicate to the nurse the desired response to treatment?
    1. Increased granulocytes
    2. Decrease in platelet count
    3. Normal hemoglobin
    4. Liver functions above normal

12. The nurse is preparing to administer a red blood cell transfusion to a client. The client tells the nurse of being terrified of contracting HIV from the transfusion. Which of the following statements is the most appropriate by the nurse?
    1. "Don't worry. I've given a lot of transfusions and I've never had a client get HIV, yet."
    2. "I understand your concerns. The blood supply is not 100% safe. Why don't you get someone in your family to donate blood for you?"
    3. "This blood was given by screened donors and tested for HIV. The chances of getting HIV from a blood transfusion are very small."
    4. "You are much more likely to die if you don't get this transfusion than if you do."

13. Which of the following is essential for the nurse to assess in the health history of a client with a hematologic disorder?
    1. The client's occupation
    2. The client's recreational activities
    3. The client's menstrual history
    4. The client's recent trip to Canada

14. A student nurse is reviewing the chart of a client with a long-standing anemia. The student asks the nurse what the term *koilonychias* means. The nurse should inform the student that *koilonychias* means the
    1. fingernails are spoon-shaped.
    2. skin is flushed.
    3. mucous membranes are pink and moist.
    4. WBC count is elevated.

15. A client returns to the clinic after a procedure complaining of pain in the left lower back. The nurse suspects the client most likely is experiencing
    1. a hematoma from a bone marrow biopsy and aspiration performed 2 days ago.
    2. splenomegaly following a Schilling test.
    3. viral hepatitis B infection from a blood transfusion.
    4. folic acid deficiency.

16. A client with an enlarged lymph node in the neck is scheduled to have an open biopsy of the node. Which of the following client statements would alert the nurse to an inadequate understanding of the procedure?
    1. "I have to go to the hospital really early in the morning and I can't drink or eat anything after midnight."
    2. "My husband will have to drive me home after the biopsy."
    3. "They are going to find cancer and I have to stay in the hospital overnight."
    4. "I will know the results of my biopsy within a couple of days."

17. The nurse should instruct a client to lay on the back after a bone marrow biopsy for how long? _____

18. The admitting nurse is making room assignments for a client admitted with aplastic anemia. The nurse appropriately selects which of the following room assignments for this client?
    1. Semiprivate room with strict hand washing
    2. Private room, protective isolation, and HEPA filtration
    3. Semiprivate room with no special precautions
    4. Private room with ECG monitoring on a cardiac care unit

19. During an IV antibiotic administration, the nurse inspects a 2-day-old IV site on a client who is neutropenic and observes redness without swelling. The client complains of tenderness. Which of the following

interventions is the priority for the nurse to implement?

1. Check the client's vital signs before going to care for another client
2. Inform the client that the IV will need to be changed to a new site
3. Administer prescribed pain medications
4. Inform the client that medication is causing a rash

20. A client with iron deficiency anemia is very pale, has shortness of breath, and records a hemoglobin level of 7.5 grams. Which of the following is a priority for the nurse to implement?

1. Administer an iron supplement
2. Instruct the client on a diet high in iron
3. Administer packed red blood cells
4. Instruct the client to conserve energy

21. During a therapeutic phlebotomy of a client with hemochromatosis, the nurse explains the rationale for the procedure by telling the client which of the following?

1. "You may need several phlebotomies during your lifetime to keep the iron from damaging your pancreas and heart."
2. "The blood is being removed so your blood is available for future transfusions."
3. "If you hadn't been a vegetarian you wouldn't have gotten this disease."
4. "You have too much blood, and some of it has to be removed to make you less prone to infections."

22. Which of the following should the nurse include in the plan of care for a client scheduled for a bone marrow biopsy?

1. Assist the client on the abdomen with arms toward the head preprocedure
2. Place the client NPO preprocedure
3. Position the client on the abdomen for 1 hour postprocedure
4. Place a light gauze dressing on the insertion site

23. A nurse caring for a client with acute disseminated intravascular coagulation (DIC) should monitor the client for which of the following clinical manifestations?

Select all that apply:
[ ] 1. Bleeding from the nose and mouth
[ ] 2. Hypertension
[ ] 3. Jaundiced sclera
[ ] 4. Elevated platelet count
[ ] 5. Oliguria
[ ] 6. Dizziness

24. The nurse should monitor a client with blood type A who received a transfusion from a type O donor for which of the following?

1. A febrile reaction because of the blood type mismatch
2. An expected rise in hemoglobin and hematocrit
3. A conversion from Rh negative to Rh positive because of the mismatched blood type
4. Fluid overload symptoms

25. A client is experiencing blood loss from anemia and is exhibiting rapid and thready pulse, cold and clammy skin, and a blood pressure below normal at rest. The nurse anticipates what percent of blood loss?_____

ANSWERS AND RATIONALES

1. 3. 4. 5. 6. The client with sickle cell anemia develops skin ulcers on the lower extremities from the vaso-occlusive aspects of the disease. The client would have shortness of breath and be fatigued and pale. The client may have swollen fingers. The hemolysis of red blood cells results in bilirubinuria. The client's urine is dark colored.

2. 3. Severe thrombocytopenia is a platelet count of < 10,000 to 20,000/mm³. The client with this low number of platelets is at great risk of bleeding from any invasive procedure. Intramuscular injections can cause a hematoma in the muscle and should be avoided if possible. A lumbar puncture would put the client at an unnecessary risk of bleeding.

A private room is not indicated unless there are other reasons for isolation (infection, neutropenia). Furosemide is a diuretic and not used as therapy for thrombocytopenia.

3. 2. Acute disseminated intravascular coagulation (DIC) is a serious disorder resulting in bleeding and clotting. It is a priority that the client must be assessed frequently by the nurse for bleeding. After ensuring that there is no active bleeding, the nurse may obtain a detailed diet history or implement family teaching. A delay to do family teaching away from the client or to dwell on diet history would not be appropriate. Some clients with chronic DIC may eventually require dialysis.

4. 2. Oxygen and carbon dioxide are transported in the blood. Air exchange occurs in the lungs, which are a part of the respiratory system. The blood also contains substances that help to form clots and mount immune responses to infectious agents.

5. 3. 5. 6. Pernicious anemia results from a deficiency of the vitamin cobalamin. The client may be short of breath and have muscle weakness. Neurology changes, such as paresthesia and mental confusion, can also occur in severe cases. Elevated temperature and dark-colored urine may be present in sickle cell anemia. A client with pernicious anemia may have a sore tongue but not white patches, which is characteristic of candidiasis.

6. 3. A client newly treated for aplastic anemia may be immunocompromised for weeks, at risk of bleeding, and fatigued. Returning to work in a day care center may be unrealistic and risky to the client. The nurse should be sure the client and family understand the risks before discharge.

7. 1. 3. An acute blood loss of 30% may appear more severe than a slower rate of blood loss. The client would not be showing signs of shock (clammy skin) and the vital signs would not be completely normal. It is important for the nurse to assess the client in various positions and states of activity in order to elicit the signs of significant blood loss. Pain, dizziness, and swelling occur with a 50% blood loss.

8. 1. 2. 3. Recognition of the signs of a vaso-occlusive crisis and knowledge of the measures to prevent it are very important in keeping the health of a client with sickle cell anemia in control. It is essential to administer pain medications, encourage fluids, and treat infections. Individuals may fear the disease, but educating friends of the client is a healthy approach to the disease. Dehydration from excessive exercise or heat can precipitate a cycle of pain. Sickle cell anemia is a genetic disorder, and counseling of couples before they have offspring is recommended.

9. 4. Complications from an enlarged spleen can be reflected in the complete blood count. Cell morphology may be abnormal in certain conditions that are associated with splenomegaly. The spleen is located in the abdomen, and visualization of the spleen and surrounding structures with a CAT scanner may be helpful in finding an etiology.

10. 1. Fever and back pain can occur in hemolytic blood transfusion reaction caused by the mismatch of blood types. If the transfusion is not stopped immediately, the client could go into shock and die. Dry mouth could be caused by an antihistamine given as a premedication or from dehydration, but it is not a reason to stop the transfusion. Blood products expire in a few hours and interruptions should be minimized. A heart beat of 74 beats per minute is not too high or too low. The client may also spike a temperature and have flushed skin.

11. 1. Neutropenia is an abnormally low white blood cell or granulocyte count. The goal of treatment would be an increase in the granulocyte count. Platelets, hemoglobin level, and liver function test changes may indicate response to some treatments, but are not measures of neutrophil count.

12. 3. Informing the client of the blood donation process is an objective way to reduce the fear of transfusion. Blood from related donors is not safer because of a family member's motivation to hide a possible health history.

13. 3. A woman's reproductive history can help explain if the client is anemic from an abnormal menstrual flow. Transfusion reactions (alloimmunization from multiple pregnancies) may also occur. Occupation, recreational activities, and travel to Canada would have little relevance to the hematologic health history.

14. 1. Spoon-shaped fingernails, or koilonychias, is a sign of long-standing chronic anemia.

15. 1. The most common site for biopsy and aspiration of the bone marrow is the posterior iliac crest bone. A hematoma from inadequate pressure applied to the site postprocedure could cause pain. Splenomegaly does not cause pain in this area and does not result from a Schilling test for pernicious anemia. Hepatitis from a blood transfusion would typically take weeks to cause symptoms, and pain in this specific site is unlikely. Folic acid deficiency is not painful and usually is the result of poor dietary intake and not of a procedure.

16. 3. Open biopsies of lymph nodes may be done in the operating room under local anesthesia. The client may be told to be NPO as a precaution. The client should be able to go home that same day if someone else drives. The biopsy is being done to determine why the lymph node is swollen. Cancer could be found on a lymph node biopsy, but there may be other causes of an enlarged node. Usually the pathological results are available within 2 days.

17. 20 to 30 minutes

It is recommended that a client lie on the back for 20–30 minutes after a bone marrow biopsy.

18. 2. The aplastic anemia client has neutropenia and needs protection from other clients and staff. A private room with protective isolation and special air filtration is ideal.

19. 2. A client who is neutropenic is susceptible to infection. In the absence of white blood cells, the inflammatory response to infection and the ability to produce pus is suppressed. Redness and pain may be the only clinical manifestations. Changing the 2-day-old IV site is appropriate. Vital signs may further indicate infection if abnormal, but not always. Administering pain medications will ease the pain but not the infection, which could become rapidly severe. Notifying the physician is not a priority.

20. 3. A client with a hemoglobin of 7.5 grams classifies as severe anemia. The client is symptomatic and the administration of packed red blood cells is the priority. Administering an iron supplement, instructing the client on a diet high in iron, and conserving energy are all important interventions but not the priority.

21. 1. Hemochromatosis is a genetic disorder that may require periodic series of phlebotomies to remove iron from the body. The purpose is not to save the blood for later transfusion back to the client. Diet cannot cause the disease. Having too much blood does not cause infections.

22. 1. The bone marrow biopsy is an aspiration of bone marrow performed with a needle and syringe. The posterior iliac crest is the best bone site for this test. The client does not have to be NPO. The client should lie on the back for 20 to 30 minutes postprocedure. A pressure dressing should be applied to the area.

23. 1. 5. 6. Disseminated intravascular coagulation (DIC) is a serious bleeding disorder that results in both thrombosis and bleeding. Bleeding occurs due to a very low platelet count. The client would be most likely to have hypotension rather than hypertension. Jaundiced sclera indicates hemolysis or liver disease.

24. 2. The type O blood would not cause a febrile transfusion reaction because it contains neither A nor B antigens to which the recipient's antibodies react. Type O is a universal donor for this reason. Nothing in the case was mentioned about the Rh status of the donor or recipient, thus no conclusion about this can be made. A fluid overload reaction is caused by volume and rate of transfusion, not by the blood type.

25.   40%

A rapid and thready pulse, cold and clammy skin, and a blood pressure below normal at rest are the result of anemia from a 40% blood loss.

REFERENCES

Daniels, R. (2010). *Delmar's manual of laboratory and diagnostic tests* (2nd ed.). Clifton Park, NY: Delmar Cengage Learning.

Daniels, R., & Nicoll, L. (2012). *Contemporary medical-surgical nursing*. Clifton Park, NY: Delmar Cengage Learning.

Estes, M. (2010). *Health assessment and physical examination* (4th ed.). Clifton Park, NY: Delmar Cengage Learning.

Spratto, G. R., & Woods, A. L. (2012). *PDR nurse's drug handbook 2012*. Clifton Park, NY: Delmar Cengage Learning.

CHAPTER 13

FLUID, ELECTROLYTE, AND ACID-BASE DISORDERS

I. **PRINCIPLES OF FLUIDS AND ELECTROLYTES**
   A. BODY FLUID
      1. WATER CONTENT OF THE BODY
         a. The body is composed of a variety of fluid spaces.
         b. The volume and composition of the various spaces remain constant in a healthy person.
         c. The maintenance of a constant environment despite continuous changes is called homeostasis.
         d. Water accounts for approximately 60% of the adult's body weight.
         e. Older adults' bodies contain approximately 45% to 55% water, which puts them at risk for fluid and electrolyte imbalances.
         f. The infant's body contains 70% to 80% water.
      2. BODY FLUID COMPARTMENTS
         a. Fluid found inside the cell is called intracellular fluid (ICF).
         b. Fluid found outside of the cell is called extracellular fluid (ECF).
         c. Extracellular fluid consists of interstitial fluid (ISF) and intravascular fluid (IVF) or plasma.
         d. Plasma accounts for 5% of adult body weight, ISF accounts for approximately 15%, and ICF accounts for the remaining 40%.
         e. Transcellular fluid is the fluid contained within the cerebrospinal, pericardial, pleural, and synovial spaces, as well as the intraocular and digestive secretions. It is usually approximately 1 liter in volume.
      3. MECHANISMS AFFECTING THE MOVEMENT OF WATER AND SOLUTES
         a. Membranes
            1) A selectively permeable membrane separates fluid compartments.
            2) Water and small molecules can move between compartments through the membrane.
            3) The membrane restricts certain large molecules such as plasma proteins from leaving the IVF.
         b. Transport processes
            1) Diffusion is the movement of molecules from an area of high concentration to an area of low concentration.
            2) Facilitated diffusion is the movement of molecules from an area of high concentration to an area of low concentration by means of a carrier substance.
            3) Active transport is the mechanism by which molecules move across a selectively permeable membrane against a concentration gradient. It requires external energy.
            4) Osmosis is the movement of water across a selectively permeable membrane from an area of lower solute concentration to an area of high solute concentration.
            5) Hydrostatic pressure is the force of the fluid against the walls of the compartment.
            6) Filtration is the movement of water and solutes from an area of high hydrostatic pressure to an area of low hydrostatic pressure.
         c. Concentration of body fluids
            1) Changes in the concentration of body fluids affect the movement of water between the two compartments.
            2) Osmolality is the measure of a solution's ability to create osmotic pressure or pull water into a compartment across a selectively permeable membrane.

3) Osmolality is reported in milliosmoles/kilogram (mOsm/kg).

4) Normal serum value is 275–295 mOsm/kg.

5) Water will continue to move across the semipermeable membrane until the osmolality of both compartments is equal.

6) Plasma proteins such as albumin maintain plasma volume by holding fluid in the IVF.

4. REGULATION OF FLUID BALANCE

a. Renin-angiotensin system

1) Renin is produced in and released from the kidneys.

2) Renin leads to the production of angiotensin II.

3) Angiotensin II is a powerful vasoconstrictor.

4) Angiotensin II also stimulates the production of aldosterone.

b. Aldosterone

1) Mineralocorticoid released by the adrenal cortex

2) Acts on the distal portion of the renal tubule to increase reabsorption of sodium and increase excretion of potassium and hydrogen ion

3) Water follows the reabsorbed sodium to increase the IVF volume.

4) Aldosterone is released in response to increased renin levels, increased plasma potassium levels, and decreased plasma sodium levels.

5) Stress and trauma stimulate the release of adrenocorticotropic hormone (ACTH), which in turn causes an increase in aldosterone levels.

c. Antidiuretic hormone (ADH)

1) Produced by the hypothalamus and excreted into circulation by the posterior pituitary

2) Acts on the distal tubule and collecting duct in the kidneys to cause water reabsorption

3) Water retention increases intravascular volume and decreases serum osmolality.

4) Stimulates vasoconstriction in the presence of rapidly declining blood pressure

5) Release is stimulated by increased serum osmolality and decreased circulating volume as sensed by baroreceptors.

6) Also known as vasopressin

d. Atrial natriuretic hormone

1) Cardiac hormone stored in the atria

2) Dilates the arteries and veins and increases the glomerular filtration rate, resulting in a decreased blood pressure

3) Released in response to increased venous return and increased atrial pressure

e. Thirst

1) Thirst receptors are located in the hypothalamus.

2) The thirst mechanism is stimulated by low blood pressure and increased serum osmolality.

3) The sensitivity of the thirst mechanism is decreased in older adults, leaving them prone to dehydration.

f. Kidneys

1) Play a vital role in regulating fluid and electrolyte balance

2) Nephrons filter blood at 180 liters/day or 125 milliliters/minute.

3) The average adult kidneys reabsorb approximately 99% of this filtrate and produce 1.5 liters of urine/day.

4) Normal urine output is 30 ml/hr.

5) As filtrate moves through the renal tubule, water and electrolytes are either secreted into the urine or reabsorbed into the bloodstream.

6) ADH and aldosterone act on the renal tubules to affect fluid and electrolyte balance.

7) Renal function is often decreased in the older adult.

g. Gastrointestinal

1) Fluid is gained by consumption of liquids and from solid foods.

2) In homeostasis, only 100–200 ml of fluid is lost through the gastrointestinal tract per day.

3) The gut secretes and reabsorbs 3–6 liters of isotonic fluid per day.

4) Fluids above the pylorus are isotonic and contain chiefly sodium, potassium, chloride, and hydrogen.

5) Fluids below the pylorus are isotonic and contain sodium, potassium, and bicarbonate.

6) Diarrhea losses from the large intestine are hypotonic.

5. INTRAVENOUS THERAPY (SEE TABLE 13-1)

a. Crystalloids

1) Solutions containing only electrolytes and glucose

2) Able to cross capillary membranes

3) May be isotonic, hypotonic, or hypertonic

Table 13-1 Summary of Intravenous Fluids

Solution	Composition (per liter)	Indications	Considerations
Isotonic Solutions			
0.9 normal saline (NS) 0.9 NaCl	154 mEq Na$^+$ 154 mEq Cl$^-$	Intravascular volume expander Blood transfusions Hypercalcemia Fluid replacement in diabetic ketoacidosis Hyponatremia Dehydration	Administer cautiously, because it may cause intravascular volume overload and pulmonary edema in clients with heart failure and renal failure.
D5W	50 g dextrose	Replacement of water losses in dehydration Hypernatremia Diluent for medication administration	Initially isotonic, but becomes hypotonic as glucose is metabolized
Lactated Ringer's solution	130 mEq Na$^+$ 4 mEq K$^+$ 3 mEq Ca^{++} 109 mEq Cl$^-$ 28 mEq lactate	Burns Gastrointestinal fluid losses, especially below the pylorus Dehydration Blood loss Hypovolemia secondary to third spacing	Similar to serum except it does not contain magnesium Contraindicated in renal failure and liver disease Do not administer if pH is > 7.5.
Hypotonic Solutions			
0.45 NaCl	77 mEq Na$^+$ 77 mEa Cl$^-$	Hypertonic dehydration Replacement of gastric fluid loss due to nasogastric (NG) suctioning or vomiting Diabetic ketoacidosis after NS infusion if blood glucose (BG) is still > 250 mg/dl	May cause increase in intracranial pressure if administered too quickly
Hypertonic Solutions			
D$_5$0.45% NaCl	77 mEq Na$^+$ 77 mEq Cl$^-$ 50 g dextrose	Diabetic ketoacidosis once glucose falls below 250 mg/dl Provides both free water and replaces sodium and chloride losses	Becomes hypotonic once glucose is metabolized
D$_5$0.9% NaCl	154 mEq Na$^+$ 154 mEq Cl$^-$ 50 g dextrose	Hypotonic dehydration SIADH Addisonian crisis	Administer cautiously in clients with heart failure or renal failure.
Dextrose 10%	100 g dextrose	Free water replacement Calories	Monitor for hyperglycemia. May dilute plasma electrolytes and lead to imbalances Monitor for water excess. May stimulate overproduction of insulin

© Cengage Learning 2015

b. Colloids
   1) Contain cells, proteins, or large molecules that expand plasma volume by pulling fluid into the bloodstream
   2) Always hypertonic
c. Tonicity
   1) Isotonic fluids have the same tonicity as body fluids and tend to stay in the intravascular space.
   2) Hypotonic fluids have tonicity less than that of body fluids and are drawn from the intravascular space into intracellular and interstitial spaces.
   3) Hypertonic fluids have a tonicity greater than that of body fluids and draw fluid into the intravascular space.
B. ELECTROLYTES
   1. DESCRIPTION
      a. Compounds that, when placed in solution, separate into electrically charged particles called ions
      b. Ions have either a positive or negative charge.

    c. Positively charged ions are called cations.

    d. Negatively charged ions are called anions.

2. MEASUREMENT OF ELECTROLYTES

    a. The weight of ions or chemical particles in a solution is measured in milligrams per 100 milliliters, or mg/dl.

    b. The number of electrically charged ions is measured in milliequivilents per liter, or mEq/L.

    c. The total cations measured in mEq/L must equal the total anions in mEq/L in homeostasis.

    d. Electrolytes exist in all body fluid compartments, but only the levels of electrolytes outside the cell can be measured.

3. ELECTROLYTE COMPOSITION OF BODY FLUIDS

    a. Extracellular electrolytes

      1) Sodium is the major cation in the ECF.

      2) Chloride is the major anion in the ECF.

    b. Intracellular electrolytes

      1) Potassium is the major cation in the ICF.

      2) Phosphate is the major anion in the ICF.

4. FUNCTIONS OF MAJOR ELECTROLYTES

    a. Potassium

      1) Conduction of nerve impulses

      2) Contraction of the myocardium, smooth muscle, and skeletal muscle

      3) Provides enzyme action for cellular energy production

      4) Regulates osmolality of ICF

    b. Sodium

      1) Governs ECF osmolality and volume

      2) Regulates acid-base balance by combining with Cl^- or HCO_{3-} (bicarbonate)

      3) Influences conduction and transmission of nerve impulses

    c. Calcium

      1) Transmission of nerve impulses

      2) Contraction of myocardium

      3) Regulation of blood pressure

      4) Building blocks of bones and teeth

      5) Blood clotting

    d. Phosphorus or phosphate

      1) 85% combined with calcium in bones and teeth

      2) Found in adenosine triphosphate (ATP), which is necessary for transport of substances in and out of cells

      3) Regulates acid-base balance as the primary urinary buffer

      4) Acidifies urine to prevent stone formation and urinary tract infections

      5) Nerve and muscle function

      6) Backbone of nucleic acids

      7) Necessary for metabolism of carbohydrates, proteins, and fats

    e. Magnesium

      1) Coenzyme in metabolism of carbohydrates and protein

      2) Transmission of nerve impulses in the central nervous system (CNS)

      3) Contraction of myocardium

      4) Transmission of sodium and potassium across all membranes

      5) Vasodilation

      6) Formation of healthy bones

      7) Activates B-complex vitamins

      8) Cofactor in blood clotting cascade

C. ACIDS AND BASES

    1. PH

      a. pH refers to the concentration of hydrogen ions in a solution.

      b. A pH higher than 7 indicates the solution is basic and contains a smaller concentration of hydrogen ions.

      c. A pH less than 7 indicates the solution is an acid and contains a higher concentration of hydrogen ions.

      d. Arterial blood is slightly basic or alkaline with a pH of 7.35–7.45.

      e. Arterial blood pH falls below 7.35 when acids accumulate or bases such as bicarbonate are lost. This condition is called acidosis.

      f. Arterial blood pH rises above 7.45 if bicarbonate levels increase or hydrogen ions are lost. This condition is called alkalosis.

    2. REGULATION OF ACIDS AND BASES

      a. Chemical buffers

        1) Fastest-acting system and major regulator of acid-base balance

        2) Act to combine with excess acids or bases to prevent large changes in pH

        3) Found in IVF, ISF, and ICF

        4) Main systems are the carbonic acid-bicarbonate system, the monohydrogen-dihydrogen phosphate system, the plasma protein buffers, and hemoglobin buffers.

      b. Respiratory system

        1) Regulates pH within minutes of pH change

        2) Lungs regulate levels of carbon dioxide (CO_2) in the blood.

3) Excess levels of CO_2 lead to higher hydrogen ion concentration and lower pH.

4) Chemoreceptors in the brain detect pH changes and signal the respiratory center to change the rate and depth of respirations.

5) If increased levels of CO_2 or hydrogen ions are present (acidosis), the respiratory center increases the rate and depth of breaths, resulting in a loss of CO_2 and a lower hydrogen ion concentration.

6) If decreased levels of CO_2 are present, the respiratory center decreases rate and depth of breaths to retain CO_2 and increase hydrogen ion concentration.

7) The lungs lose their ability to compensate for acid-base imbalance in cases of respiratory failure.

c. Renal system

1) Kidneys respond to changes in pH within hours or days.

2) They respond to decreases in pH by reabsorbing bicarbonate and excreting hydrogen ion (H^+) in the renal tubule.

3) They respond to increases in pH by conserving H^+ and excreting sodium bicarbonate ($NaHCO_3$).

4) The pH of urine in homeostasis is around 6 due to excretion of acidic by-products of cellular metabolism.

5) Kidneys lose their ability to compensate for acid-base imbalances in cases of renal failure.

3. INTERPRETING ARTERIAL BLOOD GASSES (SEE TABLE 13-2)

a. Check pH.

1) Determine if it is normal, high, or low.

2) If it is above 7.4 and below 7.45, consider the possibility of a compensated alkalosis.

3) If it is below 7.4 and above 7.35, consider the possibility of a compensated acidosis.

4) Mixed acid-base disorders may also result in a normal pH.

b. Check $PaCO_2$.

1) Provides information about the respiratory component of acid-base balance

2) Determine if it is low, normal, or high.

3) Determine if alteration is due to a primary respiratory disturbance or a compensatory response to a metabolic disturbance. Ask, "Does the $PaCO_2$ fit the pH?"

4) If imbalance is due to respiratory disturbance, a high $PaCO_2$ will correspond with a low or low-normal pH, and a low $PaCO_2$ will correspond with a high or high-normal pH.

5) If alteration is due to a compensatory response to a metabolic disturbance, HCO_3_- (bicarbonate) and $PaCO_2$ will move in the same direction (either both elevated or both below normal).

6) Expect pH to be normal to high-normal for a compensated alkalosis or normal to low-normal for a compensated acidosis. The body will not overcompensate.

c. Check HCO_3_- (bicarbonate).

1) Metabolic component of acid-base balance

2) Determine if level is normal, low, or high.

3) If abnormal, determine if alteration is due to a primary metabolic disturbance or a compensatory response to a respiratory disturbance. Ask, "Does the HCO_3_- match the pH?"

4) If the primary problem is metabolic, the pH and the bicarbonate level will move in the same direction (both elevated or both decreased).

5) If alteration is compensation for respiratory disturbance, HCO_3_- will move in the direction of CO_2 level.

6) Expect pH to be normal to high-normal for a compensated alkalosis and normal to low-normal for a compensated acidosis. The body will not overcompensate.

d. Check PaO_2 and SaO_2.

1) Provides information about the body's ability to pick up oxygen from the lungs

2) Consider making adjustments to oxygen delivery rate or concentration if levels are low or high.

Table 13-2 Normal Arterial Blood Gas Values

pH	7.35–7.45
$PaCO_2$	35–45 mm Hg
HCO_3_-	22–26 mEq/L
PaO_2	80–95 mm Hg
O_2 saturation	95–99%

e. Base excess
   1) Indicates the amount of hemoglobin and plasma bicarbonate present as buffers in blood
   2) High levels indicate alkalosis.
   3) Low levels indicate acidosis.

II. FLUID VOLUME DISORDERS

A. HYPOVOLEMIA
   1. DESCRIPTION
      a. Loss of isotonic fluids from the extracellular space
      b. May be caused by an extracellular fluid loss or by a third-space fluid shift (movement of fluid out of the intravascular space into a space other than the intracellular space)
      c. Common etiologies (see Table 13-3)
   2. ASSESSMENT
      a. Mild hypovolemia (2–5% weight loss)—fatigue, anorexia, weakness
      b. Moderate hypovolemia (5–10% weight loss)—confusion, thirst, orthostatic hypotension, tachycardia, urine output < 30 ml/hr, delayed capillary refill (.2 seconds)
      c. Severe hypovolemia (10–15% weight loss)—decreased cardiac output; rapid, thready pulse; hypotension; weak peripheral pulses; cool, mottled skin; decreased level of consciousness; urine output < 10 ml/hr, coma; arrhythmias; myocardial ischemia

Table 13-3 Causes of Fluid Volume Disorders

Hypovolemia	Hypervolemia
Extracellular losses	Chronic renal failure
Diuresis (diuretic therapy or in diabetes mellitus)	Acute renal failure
Sweating	Fluid and sodium retention
Fever	Hyperaldosteronism
Blood loss	Heart failure
NG drainage	Nephrotic syndrome
Vomiting	Cirrhoses of the liver
Diarrhea	Glucocorticosteroid therapy
Fistulas	Excessive intake of fluid and sodium
Renal failure	Administration of normal saline or lactated Ringer's solution
Third-space fluid shift	Excessive dietary sodium intake
Peritonitis	Administration of blood products
Burns	Fluid shifts
Ascites	Administration of hypertonic solutions (3% saline or mannitol)
Fractured hip (bleeding into joint)	Administration of albumin
Bowel obstruction	Burns (remobilization of fluids after treatment)
Pleural effusion	
Crush injuries	
Hypoalbuminemia	

© Cengage Learning 2015

3. DIAGNOSTIC TESTS
   a. Serum sodium—may be high or low (see sodium imbalances)
   b. Hematocrit—may be high with dehydration or low with hemorrhage
   c. Blood urea nitrogen (BUN)—may be high due to dehydration or decreased renal function
   d. Urine specific gravity—may be high as kidneys attempt to conserve water
4. NURSING INTERVENTIONS
   a. Administer isotonic fluids or blood products as ordered.
   b. Place a large-bore IV catheter to deliver fluid bolus or blood products quickly.
   c. Lower the client's head or place the client in supine position with the legs elevated at 45 degrees. Avoid the Trendelenburg position, because it places pressure on the diaphragm and inhibits respirations.
   d. If bleeding is present, apply pressure or elevate the area.
   e. Monitor neurological status, vital signs, and skin temperature for signs of impending shock. Notify the physician immediately if status deteriorates.
   f. Insert a Foley catheter if ordered.
   g. Monitor input, output, and daily weight.
   h. Monitor for fluid overload in a client receiving fluids and blood products.
   i. Place the bed in low position and keep the side rails up.
   j. Prevent falls by instructing the client to rise slowly and to call for assistance when getting up.

B. HYPERVOLEMIA
   1. DESCRIPTION
      a. Accumulation of excess isotonic fluid in the extracellular compartment
      b. Causes include fluid and sodium retention, excessive intake of fluid and sodium, acute or chronic renal failure, or fluid shifts from the interstitial space to plasma.
      c. Common etiologies (see Table 13-3)
   2. ASSESSMENT
      a. Cardiovascular—increased blood pressure; edema; weight gain; rapid, bounding pulse; distended neck veins; S3 gallop; decreased blood pressure (with heart failure)
      b. Pulmonary—dyspnea, rales, rhonchi, wheezes, tachypnea, frothy sputum
      c. Integumentary—dependent edema, anasarca, cool skin temperature

3. DIAGNOSTIC TESTS
   a. Serum sodium—may be decreased (see sodium imbalances)
   b. Serum osmolality—may be decreased
   c. Hematocrit—decreased as a result of hemodilution
   d. BUN—increased in renal failure
   e. Arterial blood gases (ABGs)—hypoxemia or respiratory alkalosis
   f. Chest x-ray—may reveal pulmonary congestion
4. NURSING INTERVENTIONS
   a. Administer diuretics as ordered by the physician.
   b. Restrict sodium and fluids as ordered by the physician.
   c. Monitor lung sounds and respiratory patterns for signs of pulmonary edema.
   d. Administer prescribed oxygen, morphine, or nitroglycerin if the client has pulmonary edema.
   e. Monitor vital signs. Be alert for signs of hypovolemia due to overcorrection. Report changes to the physician.
   f. Monitor and record accurate intake, output, and daily weights.
   g. Assess edema and document using the 1–4 scale.
   h. Monitor ABGs for hypoxemia or respiratory alkalosis.
   i. Insert a Foley catheter as ordered to facilitate accurate monitoring of output and for client comfort during diuresis.
   j. Place the client in a semi-Fowler's position if the blood pressure remains stable.
   k. Administer oxygen as needed.
   l. Monitor for signs and symptoms of hypokalemia if loop or thiazide diuretics are administered. Monitor for hyperkalemia if potassium-sparing diuretics are administered.
   m. Instruct the client to avoid foods high in sodium (see Table 13-8).
   n. Instruct the client on fluid restriction. Offer ice chips or hard candy to relieve thirst. Instruct the client how to measure and record intake.
   o. Provide skin care to clients with edema to prevent breakdown.
   p. Turn and reposition every 2 hours and assess bony prominences for breakdown.
   q. Instruct the client to check daily weight at home and which changes warrant physician notification.

III. ELECTROLYTE DISORDERS
A. HYPOKALEMIA
   1. DESCRIPTION
      a. Serum potassium level less than 3.5 mEq/L

   b. Can result from shifting of potassium from ECF to ICF or abnormal losses through the kidneys and GI tract
   c. Common etiologies (see Table 13-4)
2. ASSESSMENT
   a. Major concerns include ventricular arrhythmias, paralytic ileus, digitalis toxicity, and respiratory muscle weakness.
   b. Clinical manifestations
      1) Neuromuscular—skeletal muscle weakness, leg cramps, decreased reflexes, paresthesias
      2) Cardiovascular—weak, irregular pulse; orthostatic hypotension; ventricular arrhythmias;

Table 13-4 Causes of Potassium Imbalances

Hypokalemia	Hyperkalemia
Decreased intake	Increased intake
• Starvation	• Excessive or rapid IV administration
• Alcoholism	• Potassium salt substitutes
• Malnutrition	• Transfusion of blood that is 1–3 weeks old
Increased losses	Decreased excretion
• GI: vomiting, diarrhea, gastric or intestinal suctioning, fistulas, bulimia, laxative abuse	• Acute and chronic renal failure
• Renal: diuretic phase of acute renal failure, hyperaldosteronism, magnesium depletion	• Addison's disease (adrenal insufficiency)
• Integumentary: diaphoresis in fever or increased environmental temperature	Shift of potassium from ICF to ECF
• Hemodialysis or peritoneal dialysis	• Injury
Shift of potassium from ECF to ICF	• Sepsis
• Increased insulin (resulting from administration of total parenteral nutrition [TPN] or fluids containing dextrose)	• Burns
• Alkalosis	• Acidosis
• Treatment of metabolic acidosis	Medications
• Increased beta adrenergic agonist activity (from stress, myocardial ischemia, or exogenous administration)	• Potassium-sparing diuretics (e.g., spironolactone)
• Tissue repair	• Beta blockers
Medications	• ACE inhibitors
• Diuretics (thiazide and loop diuretics)	• Potassium-containing drugs (e.g., potassium-penicillin)
• Antibiotics (e.g., gentamicin, amphotericin B)	• NSAIDs
• Corticosteroids	
• Insulin	
• Beta-adrenergic agents (e.g., dobutamine, albuterol, epinephrine)	

© Cengage Learning 2015

electrocardiogram (ECG) changes, digoxin toxicity

    3) Gastrointestinal—nausea, constipation, abdominal distention, decreased bowel sounds, paralytic ileus

3. DIAGNOSTIC TESTS
- **a.** Serum potassium less than 3.5 mEq/L
- **b.** ABGs may reveal metabolic alkalosis (elevated pH and bicarbonate levels).
- **c.** ECG—flattened T wave, depressed ST segment, U wave

4. NURSING INTERVENTIONS
- **a.** Instruct the client to increase intake of foods high in potassium (see Table 13-8).
- **b.** Inform the client of the clinical manifestations of hypokalemia and which ones should be reported to the physician.
- **c.** Assess renal function, including intake and output and serum creatinine. Notify the physician of a decrease in function if the client is receiving potassium supplementation.
- **d.** Administer oral supplements with meals or with 4 oz liquid to avoid gastric irritation.
- **e.** Administer IV replacement no faster than 10 mEq/hr peripherally or 20 mEq/hr through a central line.
- **f.** Never give IV potassium as a bolus.
- **g.** Assess IV site for phlebitis and infiltration.
- **h.** Provide a safe environment for the client who is weak or experiencing orthostatic hypotension from hypokalemia.
- **i.** Assess for risk factors for hypokalemia, especially medications (see Table 13-4).
- **j.** Monitor and document urine output. Approximately 40 mEq of potassium is lost in each liter of urine.
- **k.** Monitor for constipation and decreased bowel sounds.
- **l.** Monitor respiratory rate and depth. Notify the physician if breaths become shallow and rapid.
- **m.** Monitor ECG for characteristic changes.

B. HYPERKALEMIA
1. DESCRIPTION
- **a.** Serum potassium level greater than 5 mEq/L
- **b.** Can result from impaired renal excretion, massive intake of potassium, or shift of potassium from ICF to ECF
- **c.** Common etiologies (see Table 13-4)

2. ASSESSMENT
- **a.** Major concerns include heart block, ventricular arrhythmias, and cardiac arrest

- **b.** Clinical manifestations
  - 1) Neuromuscular—irritability, weakness of lower extremities, paresthesias
  - 2) Cardiovascular—irregular pulse, decreased heart rate, hypotension
  - 3) Gastrointestinal—nausea, vomiting, diarrhea, abdominal cramping
  - 4) Other—oliguria or anuria

3. DIAGNOSTIC TESTS
- **a.** Serum potassium—greater than 5 mEq/L
- **b.** ABGs—decreased arterial pH and decreased bicarbonate in cases of metabolic acidosis
- **c.** ECG—tall, peaked T waves, prolonged PR interval, ST depression, flattened or absent P wave, and widened QRS

4. NURSING INTERVENTIONS
- **a.** Instruct the client to restrict foods high in potassium (see Table 13-8).
- **b.** Administer cation exchange resins such as polystyrene sulfonate (Kayexelate) orally, nasogastrically, or rectally as ordered.
- **c.** Monitor bowel movements when administering Kayexalate, as potassium is lost through the stools (often sorbitol is given to promote diarrhea and increase potassium loss).
- **d.** Encourage a client receiving rectal polystyrene sulfonate (Kayexalate) to retain enema for 30–60 minutes to ensure adequate potassium exchange.
- **e.** Monitor serum sodium, magnesium, and calcium levels. Understand that cation exchange resins also bind with magnesium and calcium. Serum sodium levels may rise. Watch for signs of fluid overload.
- **f.** Administer 10% calcium gluconate (usually 10 ml) over 3 minutes to counteract neuromuscular and cardiac effects of hyperkalemia. Effects are temporary.
- **g.** Anticipate the administration of intravenous glucose and insulin in acute cases of hyperkalemia. Administer in the order prescribed.
- **h.** If sodium bicarbonate or insulin and glucose are prescribed to temporarily shift potassium into cells, anticipate further therapy, such as dialysis or cation exchange resins, which will permanently remove potassium from the body.
- **i.** Monitor ECG for characteristic changes and notify the physician of any changes immediately.
- **j.** Monitor urine output and report output less than 0.5 ml/kg/hr.

k. Monitor vital signs.

l. Monitor serum potassium levels and watch for hypokalemia in clients receiving Kayexelate for 2 or more days.

m. Instruct the client on the clinical manifestations of hyperkalemia and importance of reporting them to the physician.

C. HYPONATREMIA

1. DESCRIPTION

a. Serum sodium less than 135 mEq/L

b. Can result from inadequate sodium intake, increase in sodium excretion, or dilution of serum sodium in cases of fluid excess

c. Common etiologies (see Table 13-5)

2. ASSESSMENT

a. Major concerns are neurological symptoms that do not occur until sodium level has dropped to around 120–125 mEq/L

b. Clinical manifestations

1) Hyponatremia with decreased ECF volume (sodium loss hyponatremia)—nausea; vomiting; diarrhea; dry mucous membranes; weight loss; postural hypotension; thready pulse; tachycardia; flattened neck veins; cold, clammy skin; tremors; seizures; irritability; apprehension, or coma

2) Hyponatremia with normal or increased ECF volume—weight gain, nausea, vomiting, increased blood pressure, edema, distended neck veins, muscle spasms, headache, lassitude, weakness, confusion seizures, coma

3. DIAGNOSTIC TESTS

a. Serum sodium—less than 135 mEq/L

b. Serum osmolality—decreased (< 275 mOm/kg) except in cases of hyponatremia associated with hyperglycemia, hyperlipidemia, and hyperproteinemia

c. Urine osmolality—generally decreased due to the body's attempt to excrete excess fluid. Urine osmolality is increased in syndrome of inappropriate antidiuretic hormone (SIADH).

d. Urine sodium—usually decreased (< 20 mEq/L) but increased in syndrome of inappropriate antidiuretic hormone (SIADH) and adrenal insufficiency

4. NURSING INTERVENTIONS

a. Measure and record intake and output.

b. Monitor daily weight.

c. Monitor lab values, especially serum sodium, serum chloride, serum glucose, and serum osmolality. Also monitor urine osmolality and urine sodium.

d. Restrict fluid for mild hyponatremia, especially that caused by water excess.

e. Inform the client that commercially available hydrating fluids may be used in the home setting.

f. Administer sodium-containing IV fluids in hyponatremia associated with fluid loss.

g. If the client receives hypertonic saline solutions (3% NS) for dangerously low sodium, monitor serum sodium levels closely and use an infusion pump, and assess carefully for signs of IVF overload (crackles in the lungs, shortness of breath, tachypnea, tachycardia, or increased blood pressure).

h. Administer hypertonic saline solutions slowly and with an infusion pump in order to prevent crenation (shriveling) of red blood cells and permanent neurological damage secondary to the destruction of myelin.

i. Administer loop diuretics as ordered to correct hyponatremia with increased ECF.

j. Instruct the client and family about fluid restrictions and help develop a

Table 13-5 Causes of Sodium Imbalances

Hyponatremia	Hypernatremia
Sodium loss with decreased ECF	Water loss with decreased ECF
GI—vomiting, diarrhea, NG suctioning, bulimia, wound drainage, fistulas	Insensible water loss (heat stroke, fever, perspiration, pulmonary infections)
Renal—adrenal insufficiency, salt-wasting kidney disease	Severe watery diarrhea
Skin—burns, excessive sweating, wound drainage	Osmotic diuresis (from HHNK, iodinated contrast, or high-protein tube feedings)
Water gain with increased ECF	Diabetes insipidus
CHF	Sodium gain with increased ECF
Cirrhosis	Hypertonic saline solutions
Nephrotic syndrome	Primary hyperaldosteronism
Excessive hypotonic fluid administration, SIADH	Cushing's syndrome
Primary polydipsia (excessive ingestion of water)	Saltwater near-drowning
Medications	Medications
Loop diuretics	Sodium bicarbonate (IV or oral antacids)
Thiazide diuretics	Sodium polystyrene sulfonate (Kayexelate)
Barbiturates	Salt tablets
Morphine	Cortisone injections
Carbamazepine	Sodium-containing antibiotics (e.g., Timentin)
Some antineoplastics	
Some antipsychotics	

© Cengage Learning 2015

plan to distribute fluid intake throughout the day.

k. Assess the client for risk factors for hyponatremia, including medications.

D. HYPERNATREMIA

1. DESCRIPTION

a. Serum sodium greater than 145 mEq/L
b. Caused by either an increase in sodium intake or excessive water losses
c. Common etiologies (see Table 13-5)

2. ASSESSMENT

a. Neurological symptoms result when fluid moves by osmosis from inside the cell to outside of the cell in order to balance the concentrations of sodium in the two compartments.

b. Clinical manifestations

   1) Hypernatremia with decreased ECF (due to water loss)—intense thirst; restlessness; agitation; twitching; seizures; weakness; coma; dry, swollen tongue; postural hypotension; weight loss

   2) Hypernatremia with increased ECF (due to sodium gain)—intense thirst, flushed skin, restlessness, agitation, twitching, seizures, weakness, coma, weight gain, peripheral or pulmonary edema, increased blood pressure

c. Infants, older adults, and comatose individuals are at highest risk for hypernatremia due to an impaired thirst mechanism.

3. DIAGNOSTIC TESTS

a. Serum sodium—greater than 145 mEq/L
b. Serum osmolality—increased (.295 mOsm/kg) due to elevated serum sodium
c. Urine osmolality—usually increased due to the kidney's attempt to conserve water, but it is decreased in diabetes insipidus

4. NURSING INTERVENTIONS

a. Assess for clinical manifestations of hypernatremia in clients who are at high risk for diabetes insipidus (such as those with tumors or surgery near the pituitary gland).
b. Monitor lab values, especially serum sodium, serum chloride, and urine osmolality.
c. Monitor vital signs, especially blood pressure and pulse.
d. Measure and record intake, output, and daily weights.
e. Monitor for signs of cerebral edema if the client is receiving D5% or hypotonic saline solutions.

f. Notify the physician of significant neurological changes.
g. Administer fluids slowly and closely watch serum sodium levels to prevent rapid shift of fluid from ECF to ICF, causing cerebral edema or pulmonary edema.
h. Instruct the client with hypernatremia to avoid foods rich in sodium (see Table 13-8).
i. Review the client's medications and identify those that may cause increased sodium levels.
j. Keep the bed in low position and the side rails up.
k. Assess for hypokalemia in a client being treated with diuretics or IV fluids.

E. HYPOCALCEMIA

1. DESCRIPTION

a. Serum calcium less than 9 mg/dl or less than 2.25 mmol/L
b. The principal cause of hypocalcemia is renal failure.
c. Common etiologies (see Table 13-6)

2. ASSESSMENT

a. Calcium deficit affects peripheral nerves, skeletal and smooth muscle, and cardiac muscle, resulting in neuromuscular excitability.

Table 13-6 Causes of Calcium Imbalances

Hypocalcemia	Hypercalcemia
Gastrointestinal	**Dietary**
• Inadequate vitamin D intake	• Excessive use of calcium supplements
• Low protein diet	• Increased intestinal absorption (from excessive vitamin D or vitamin A intake)
• Laxative abuse	
• Malabsorption syndrome	
• Chronic diarrhea	**Increased release of calcium from bone**
• Chronic pancreatitis (results in secondary hypoparathyroidism)	• Multiple myeloma
• Chronic alcoholism	• Lymphoma
Renal	• Bone metastasis
• Phosphorus retention and subsequent calcium loss through urine resulting from chronic renal failure	• Tumors producing parathyroid-related proteins (e.g., ovarian, lung, and kidney)
	• Prolonged immobilization
Decreased release of calcium from bone	• Paget's disease
• Decreased parathyroid hormone	• Hyperparathyroidism
• Increased calcitonin	**Acid-base balance**
Electrolyte and acid-base balance	• Acidosis
• Increased phosphorus	
• Decreased magnesium	
• Alkalosis	

© Cengage Learning 2015

b. Clinical manifestations
   1) Neuromuscular—anxiety, irritability, tetany, twitching and numbness around the mouth, numbness and tingling in the extremities, hyperreflexia, positive Trousseau's sign, positive Chvostek's sign, laryngeal spasm, insomnia
   2) Cardiovascular—ventricular tachycardia, ECG changes, prolonged clotting times secondary to reduction of prothrombin
   3) Gastrointestinal—increased peristalsis, diarrhea
   4) Skeletal—fractures with prolonged hypocalcemia
3. DIAGNOSTIC TESTS
   a. Total serum calcium level—less than 9 mg/dl
   b. Serum albumin should always be evaluated with serum calcium, because a drop in serum albumin will result in a drop in total calcium levels. Clients with hypoalbuminemia should be treated according to ionized calcium levels.
   c. Ionized serum calcium—less than 4.5 mg/dl
   d. Serum magnesium—may be decreased (< 1.5 mEq/L)
   e. Serum phosphorus—may be increased (> 2.6 mEq/L)
   f. ECG—prolonged ST segment, prolonged QT interval
4. NURSING INTERVENTIONS
   a. Administer oral calcium to an asymptomatic client.
   b. Instruct the client that calcium supplements with vitamin D should be taken 30 minutes before meals to increase absorption.
   c. Instruct the client to increase intake of high-calcium foods (see Table 13-8).
   d. Acute hypocalcemia in the presence of tetany, seizures, arrhythmias, or laryngospasm is treated initially with 10–20 ml of 10% calcium gluconate IV given 0.5–1 ml/min to avoid hypotension and bradycardia.
   e. Administer a continuous infusion of 100 ml 10% calcium gluconate diluted in 1000 ml D_5W over 4 hours.
   f. Clarify the type of calcium solution ordered (one ampule of calcium gluconate contains around 4.5 mEq of calcium and one ampule of calcium chloride contains 13.6 mEq of calcium).
   g. Assess the IV site frequently. Calcium gluconate and calcium chloride may cause tissue necrosis. Administer through the central line if possible.
   h. Monitor a client taking digoxin (Lanoxin) who is receiving calcium supplementation. Elevated calcium levels enhance the action of digoxin, causing digoxin toxicity.
   i. Monitor for signs of hypercalcemia when administering IV calcium such as lethargy, confusion, or nausea.
   j. Never administer calcium IM.
   k. Keep the tracheostomy tray at the bedside for clients with thyroid surgery in case of sudden hypocalcemia and subsequent laryngospasm.
   l. Place a client who is symptomatic on seizure precautions and reduce environmental stimuli.
   m. Monitor serum total calcium and serum ionized calcium levels.
F. HYPERCALCEMIA
   1. DESCRIPTION
      a. Serum calcium level greater than 11 mg/dl or greater than 2.75 mmol/L
      b. Hypercalcemia is frequently caused by calcium loss from bones.
      c. Common etiologies (see Table 13-6)
   2. ASSESSMENT
      a. Hypercalcemia decreases the activity of cardiac muscle, skeletal muscle, and smooth muscle.
      b. Clinical manifestations
         1) Neuromuscular—flabby muscles, weakness, depressed reflexes, decreased memory, confusion, psychosis, depression, apathy
         2) Cardiovascular—bradycardia, heart block, increased digitalis effect, ventricular arrhythmias, cardiac arrest
         3) Gastrointestinal—anorexia, nausea, vomiting, paralytic ileus, constipation
         4) Skeletal—pathologic fractures, bone pain
         5) Renal—flank pain (from urinary calculi)
   3. DIAGNOSTIC TESTS
      a. Total serum calcium level—greater than 11 mg/dl or 2.75 mmol/L
      b. Ionized calcium—greater than 5.5 mg/dl
      c. ECG—shortened ST segment and QT interval, prolonged PR
      d. X-ray—osteoporosis, pathologic fractures, or urinary calculi
   4. NURSING INTERVENTIONS
      a. Instruct the client to drink 3–4 liters of fluid per day in cases of mild hypercalcemia to prevent formation of renal calculi.

b. Review the client's medication history for those causing hypercalcemia.

c. Encourage an intake of foods that are high in acid content, such as cranberry juice, meat, fish, poultry, eggs, peanuts, and cereals, to prevent renal calculi.

d. Administer normal saline with a loop diuretic to increase urinary calcium excretion.

e. Anticipate that serum calcium levels will decrease over several days when IV biphosphonates such as pamidronate and etidronate are ordered to obstruct calcium release from bone.

f. If IV calcitonin is given, assess the IV site for erythema and pain.

g. Assess for and treat bone pain.

h. Promote client safety in the presence of clinical manifestations that may cause injury.

i. Monitor for digoxin toxicity in clients receiving digoxin (Lanoxin).

j. Monitor ECG and report changes to the physician.

k. Assess the client's level of consciousness and report changes to the physician.

l. Record accurate intake and output. Be alert to polyuria caused by increased calcium excretion through the urine.

m. Encourage increased activity to promote bone resorption of calcium.

n. Promote active and passive range of motion exercises for a client who is bedridden.

G. HYPOPHOSPHATEMIA
  1. DESCRIPTION
    a. Serum phosphorus less than 2.5 mg/dl or less than 1.8 mEq/L
    b. Causes are related to inadequate intake, malabsorption, increased urinary losses, increased cellular use, or shift from ECF to ICF.
    c. Common etiologies (see Table 13-7)
  2. ASSESSMENT
    a. Clinical manifestations differ, depending in whether the client is experiencing an acute loss of phosphorus or has developed hypophosphatemia over time.
    b. Most clinical manifestations are the result of decreases in adenosine triphosphate (ATP) and 2,3 biphosphoglycerate (BPG), an energy-storing substance in red blood cells (RBCs) that helps transfer oxygen from RBCs to tissues.

Table 13-7 Causes of Phosphorus Imbalances

Hypophosphatemia	Hyperphosphatemia
Malnutrition	Acute or chronic renal failure
Malabsorption	Hypoparathyroidism
Alcoholism	Large ingestion of milk
Recovery from malnutrition	Extracellular shifts
Diabetic ketoacidosis (with treatment)	Diabetic ketoacidosis (before treatment)
Intracellular shifts	Respiratory acidosis
Intravenous glucose administration or TPN	Cellular destruction
Recovery from burns	Myelogenous leukemia or lymphoma treated with chemotherapeutic agents
Respiratory alkalosis	Rhabdomyolysis
Recovery from hypothermia	Trauma
Increased urinary losses	Infection
Hyperparathyroidism	Heatstroke
Osmotic diuresis during diabetic ketoacidosis	Medications
Medications	Excess intake of vitamin D supplements
Acetazolamide	Fleets enema
Thiazide diuretics	Laxatives containing phosphate
Loop diuretics	Oral phosphorus supplements
Insulin	IV phosphorus supplements
Laxatives	
Phosphorus-binding antacids (aluminum carbonate, aluminum hydroxide, calcium carbonate, or magnesium oxide)	

© Cengage Learning 2015

c. Clinical manifestations of acute hypophosphatemia
  1) Neuromuscular—confusion, coma, seizures, numbness and tingling of the fingers and around the mouth, muscle pain, muscle weakness
  2) Cardiovascular—chest pain (from inadequate oxygenation of the myocardium), decreased blood pressure, decreased stroke volume, cyanosis
  3) Pulmonary—respiratory muscle weakness resulting in increased respiratory rate
  4) Hematological—increased susceptibility to infection

d. Clinical manifestations of chronic hypophosphatemia
  1) Neuromuscular—lethargy, weakness, stiffness of joints, memory loss
  2) Skeletal—bone pain, osteomalacia
  3) Hematological—decreased platelet function (resulting in bruising, bleeding, or GI bleed)

3. DIAGNOSTIC TESTS
  a. Serum phosphorus—less than 2.5 mg/dl or less than 1.8 mEq/L

    b. ABGs—metabolic or respiratory alkalosis

    c. Parathyroid hormone (PTH)—elevated

    d. X-ray—skeletal changes

4. NURSING INTERVENTIONS

    a. Monitor phosphorus levels in an at-risk client such as one receiving TPN or suffering burns.

    b. Instruct a client with mild-to-moderate hypophosphatemia (1–2.5 mg/dl) to increase intake of high-phosphorus foods (see Table 13-8).

    c. Instruct a client taking an oral supplement to ensure the powder is completely dissolved before drinking.

    d. Administer IV potassium phosphate or sodium phosphate slowly and with an infusion pump. Potassium phosphate should not be given faster than 10 mEq/hr.

    e. Monitor the IV site for infiltration, because potassium phosphate may result in sloughing of tissue and necrosis.

    f. Monitor for complications of IV replacement therapy, including hypocalcemia, hyperphosphatemia, and tetany.

    g. Never administer phosphorus IM.

    h. Monitor the rate and depth of respirations. Try to prevent hyperventilation. Report signs of hypoxemia to the physician (confusion, restlessness, or cyanosis).

    i. Monitor neurological status, including level of consciousness, orientation, muscle strength, and restlessness. Document carefully for comparison on future shifts. Notify the physician of changes.

    j. Monitor for signs of heart failure such as crackles in the lungs, decreased blood pressure (BP), increased heart rate (HR), or shortness of breath.

    k. Maintain client safety by keeping the bedrails up and placing the bed in the lowest position.

    l. Implement seizure precautions in cases of acute hypophosphatemia.

    m. Ensure the client has adequate pain relief.

    n. Monitor temperature and use aseptic technique when changing dressings or working with intravenous access.

    o. Inform the client's family that the client's confusion will subside as phosphorus levels return to normal.

    p. Orient the client and keep clocks, calendars, and familiar objects at the bedside.

Table 13-8 Food Sources of Major Electrolytes

Electrolyte	Food Source
Potassium	Dried beans and peas
	Meat
	Bananas
	Oranges
	Melon
	Nuts
	Salt substitute
	Tomatoes
	Potatoes
Sodium	Smoked or canned meat
	Canned fish
	Frozen dinners
	Lunch meats
	Processed cheese
	Canned soups or broth, bouillon cubes
	Canned vegetables
	Chips, pretzels, crackers
	Soy sauce
	Seasoning salt
Calcium	Dairy products
	Leafy green vegetables (e.g., greens, spinach)
	Broccoli
	Legumes
	Nuts
	Whole grains
	Molasses
	Canned salmon
	Tofu
Phosphorus	Dairy products
	Whole grains
	Dried beans and peas
	Seeds (e.g., sesame, sunflower)
	Fish
	Poultry
	Eggs
	Organ meats
Magnesium	Whole grains
	Meat
	Fish
	Nuts
	Dried beans and peas
	Leafy, green vegetables
	Bananas
	Oranges
	Chocolate

H. HYPERPHOSPHATEMIA

    1. DESCRIPTION

      a. Serum phosphorus > 4.5 mg/dl

      b. Most commonly caused by acute or chronic renal failure

c. Also may be caused by malignancies, movement of phosphorus from ICF to ECF, excessive ingestion of phosphate, or large intake of vitamin D
d. Common etiologies (see Table 13-7)

2. ASSESSMENT
a. Most manifestations are the result of concomitant hypocalcemia or calcium phosphate precipitates in soft tissue, joints, arteries, or skin.
b. Clinical manifestations
　1) Neuromuscular—tetany, hyperreflexia, muscular weakness or paralysis, irritability
　2) Cardiovascular—tachycardia; calcium phosphate deposits in the arteries; calcium phosphate deposits in the heart, resulting in conduction disturbances or arrhythmias
　3) Gastrointestinal—nausea, vomiting, diarrhea, cramping
　4) Skeletal—renal osteodystrophy (pathological changes in bone)
　5) Soft tissue calcifications resulting in corneal haziness, conjunctivitis, or papular eruptions

3. DIAGNOSTIC TESTS
a. Serum phosphorus greater than 4.5 mg/dl or greater than 2.6 mEq/L
b. Serum calcium—may be decreased
c. X-ray—skeletal changes
d. Parathyroid hormone—may be decreased

4. NURSING INTERVENTIONS
a. Instruct the client to limit foods high in phosphorus (see Table 13-8).
b. Administer phosphate-binding agents as ordered such as aluminum, magnesium, or calcium gels or antacids.
c. Instruct the client to take phosphate binders with or after meals and 1–2 hours apart from other oral medications.
d. Assess and treat constipation to facilitate excretion of phosphorus through the gastrointestinal tract.
e. Advise the client that the feces may be white from the drugs.
f. Monitor serum phosphorus and calcium levels and report abnormalities to the physician.
g. Monitor for hypocalcemia and report clinical manifestations to the physician.
h. Monitor renal function, including BUN, creatinine, and urine output.
i. Instruct the client to avoid phosphate-containing laxatives and enemas.
j. Instruct the client taking phosphate-binding antacids to notify the physician

if he experiences signs of hypocalcemia such as numbness and tingling in the fingers or around the mouth, muscle cramps, or weakness.
k. Be aware that administration of glucose-containing IV fluids causes false-low phosphorus levels.

I. HYPOMAGNESEMIA
1. DESCRIPTION
a. Serum magnesium less than 1.5 mEq/L
b. Chronic alcoholism and uncontrolled diabetes mellitus are leading causes of hypomagnesemia.
c. Can be associated with hypokalemia that does not resolve with potassium replacement
d. Common etiologies (see Table 13-9)

2. ASSESSMENT
a. Signs and symptoms are primarily the result of neuromuscular and central nervous system irritability.
b. Clinical manifestations
　1) Neuromuscular—hyperirritability, confusion, hyperactive deep tendon reflexes, tremors, seizures, leg cramps
　2) Cardiovascular—hypertension, premature ventricular contractions, ventricular tachycardia, Torsades de pointes, atrial fibrillation
　3) Gastrointestinal—nausea, vomiting, difficulty swallowing

3. DIAGNOSTIC TESTS
a. Serum magnesium less than 1.5 mEq/L
b. Serum albumin may result in a low total serum magnesium level because one-third of magnesium is protein-bound. Clients with a low albumin should have serum ionized magnesium evaluated.
c. Serum potassium—may be low, because magnesium is required for the sodium-potassium pump to move potassium into cells.
d. Serum calcium—may be low because magnesium is necessary for parathyroid hormone release.
e. ECG—flat or inverted T wave, depressed ST segment, prolonged PR, prolonged QT, heart block, dysrhythmias

4. NURSING INTERVENTIONS
a. Monitor serum magnesium levels in a high-risk client, such as one with alcoholism, receiving magnesium-free IV fluids, or with an NG suctioning, vomiting or diarrhea.
b. Administer oral replacement as prescribed in cases of mild or chronic hypomagnesemia.

Table 13-9 Causes of Magnesium Imbalances

Hypomagnesemia	Hypermagnesemia
Decreased intake • Malnutrition • Malabsorption (e.g., irritable bowel syndrome, pancreatitis, cancer, or bowel resection) • Alcoholism (poor diet or decreased absorption) **Increased losses** • Fistulas, vomiting, NG suction, diarrhea • Acute renal failure (diuretic phase) • Diabetic ketoacidosis or uncontrolled diabetes mellitus (from osmotic diuresis) • CHF (during diuresis) • Hyperaldosteronism • Alcoholism (vomiting and increased urinary losses) • Prolonged TPN administration **Medications** • Loop or thiazide diuretics • Cortisone • Digitalis • Aminoglycosides (e.g., gentamicin, tobramycin) • Insulin • Amphotericin B • Laxatives • Cyclosporine **Medications** • Prolonged NS administration • Citrated blood transfusions • Phenytoin • Phenobarbital • Calcitonin • Loop diuretics • Phosphates (oral or IV) • Gentamicin (lowers magnesium level)	**Increased intake** • Use of magnesium-containing antacids in clients with renal failure • Magnesium-sulfate infusions for preterm labor, pregnancy-induced hypertension, or seizures **Decreased excretion** • Renal failure • Adrenocortical insufficiency • Addison's disease **Medications** • Antacids (e.g., Maalox, Mylanta, Gaviscon, Riopan, Tempo, Gelusil) • Vitamin and mineral supplements with magnesium • Laxatives (e.g., milk of magnesia, magnesium citrate, magnesium sulfate) **Medications** • Calcium-containing antacids • Thiazide diuretics • Lithium • Vitamin D • Vitamin A

c. Instruct the client that diarrhea is a common adverse reaction of magnesium supplementation and to notify the physician if it occurs.

d. Instruct the client to increase intake of foods high in magnesium (see Table 13-8).

e. Never administer IV magnesium as a bolus, because it may cause cardiac or respiratory arrest.

f. Monitor for digitalis toxicity. Hypomagnesemia enhances the effects of digitalis.

g. Initiate seizure precautions and decrease environmental stimuli for a client who is symptomatic.

h. Monitor reflexes in a client receiving IV replacement. Notify the physician of decreased patellar reflex caused by dangerously high magnesium levels.

i. Monitor vital signs in a client receiving IV magnesium and notify the physician of decreasing blood pressure or labored respirations.

j. Monitor heart rate and ECG for characteristic changes.

k. Test the client's swallowing ability before administering food or liquids.

l. Monitor serum calcium and potassium levels. Consult with the physician to correct low levels once magnesium is replaced.

J. HYPERMAGNESEMIA
1. DESCRIPTION
   a. Serum magnesium greater than 2.5 mEq/L
   b. Frequently occurs in clients with renal failure who have received excessive amounts of magnesium
   c. Common etiologies (see Table 13-9)
2. ASSESSMENT
   a. Primary clinical manifestations are the result of depressed peripheral and central nervous system transmission.
   b. Client does not usually exhibit clinical manifestations until serum levels are greater than 4 mEq/L.
   c. Clinical manifestations
      1) Neuromuscular—CNS depression, lethargy, drowsiness, loss of deep tendon reflexes, muscular weakness
      2) Integumentary—flushing, increased perspiration
      3) Gastrointestinal—nausea, vomiting
      4) Cardiovascular—hypotension, bradycardia
3. DIAGNOSTIC TESTS
   a. Serum magnesium .2.5 mEq/L
   b. ECG—may show prolonged QT or A-V block if serum levels are severely elevated
4. NURSING INTERVENTIONS
   a. Monitor serum magnesium levels in a high-risk client, such as one who is receiving IV magnesium sulfate for preterm labor or a client with renal failure.
   b. Avoid use of magnesium-containing drugs in a client with decreased renal function.

c. Administer 0.45% NS and diuretics in a client with adequate renal function in order to promote renal excretion of magnesium.

d. Treat potentially lethal magnesium level with 10 ml of 10% calcium gluconate IV in order to block the neuromuscular effects. Effects are temporary.

e. Monitor for respiratory depression and hypotension.

f. Perform and document neurological assessment, including mental status, reflexes, and muscle strength (absent reflexes indicate a serum level > 7 mEq/L).

g. Provide a safe environment by keeping the side rails up and the bed down.

h. Anticipate dialysis for clients with renal failure.

i. Provide the client with a list of common magnesium-containing over-the-counter products, and instruct him to avoid these products.

j. Instruct the client to avoid vitamin supplements with minerals, because these may contain magnesium.

IV. ACID-BASE IMBALANCES (SEE TABLE 13-10)

A. RESPIRATORY ACIDOSIS
  1. DESCRIPTION
    a. Caused by alveolar hypoventilation resulting in increased PCO_2
    b. Carbon dioxide (CO_2) combines with water to form carbonic acid (H_2CO_3).
    c. Carbonic acid disassociates into hydrogen ion (H^+) and bicarbonate (HCO_{3-}), thus increasing the hydrogen ion concentration in the blood and lowering pH.
    d. The kidneys compensate for increased PCO_2 by conserving bicarbonate.
    e. The kidneys usually respond to acute respiratory acidosis within 24 hours.
    f. Common etiologies (see Table 13-10)
  2. ASSESSMENT
    a. Neurological—drowsiness, restlessness, disorientation, apprehension, headache, decreased deep tendon reflexes, seizures, coma
    b. Cardiovascular—decreased blood pressure, peripheral vasodilatation, ventricular fibrillation
    c. Respiratory—rapid shallow breathing or bradypnea
    d. Other—diaphoresis; warm, flushed skin; nausea; vomiting
  3. DIAGNOSTIC TESTS
    a. Arterial blood gases
      1) Uncompensated respiratory acidosis—decreased pH, normal bicarbonate, increased PCO_2
      2) Compensated respiratory acidosis—pH normal, increased bicarbonate, increased PCO_2, urine pH < 6
    b. Chest x-ray—may indicate underlying respiratory disease or trauma (e.g., pneumonia, pulmonary edema, chronic obstructive pulmonary disease [COPD], pneumothorax)
    c. Drug screen—indicated in suspected overdose

Table 13-10 Causes of Acid-Base Imbalances

Respiratory Acidosis	Metabolic Acidosis
Pneumonia	Renal failure
Pneumothorax	Hypoaldosteronism
Acute respiratory distress syndrome (ARDS)	Salicylate, methanol toluene, or ethylene glycol poisoning
Pulmonary embolus	Excess ketone production
Bronchospasm	• Diabetic ketoacidosis
Acute asthma attack	• Alcohol-induced ketoacidosis
Pulmonary edema	• Starvation
Cardiac arrest	Lactic acidosis
Central nervous system trauma	• Shock
Guillain-Barré syndrome	• Heart failure
Hypophosphatemia	• Pulmonary disease
Hypokalemia	• Hepatic disorders
Overdose	Loss of HCO_{3-}
Medications	• Diarrhea
• Narcotics	• Ileostomy
• Curare	• Biliary or pancreatic drainage
• Anesthetics	Medications
• Sedatives	• Carbonic anhydrase inhibitors
• Aminoglycosides	• Potassium-sparing diuretics
Respiratory Alkalosis	**Metabolic Alkalosis**
Hyperventilation	Hypercalcemia
• Anxiety	Hypokalemia
• Pain	Hypochloremia (from gastric losses)
• Mechanical ventilation	Vomiting
Stimulation of respiratory control center in the medulla resulting in	NG suctioning
• Stroke	Cushing's disease
• Trauma	Respiratory acidosis
• Ischemia	Blood transfusions
• Fever	Medications
• Sepsis	• Thiazides
Acute hypoxia from	• Furosemide
• High altitude	• Ethacrynic acid
• Pulmonary disease	• Sodium bicarbonate administration
• Anemia	• Steroids
• Congestive heart failure	• Bicarbonate-containing antacids
Medications	
• Catecholamines	
• Salicylates	
• Nicotine	
• Xanthines	

© Cengage Learning 2015

4. NURSING INTERVENTIONS
   a. Collaborative intervention to treat underlying cause of alveolar hypoventilation
   b. Monitor cardiac function for tachycardia, hypotension, and arrhythmias. Respiratory acidosis may lead to shock or cardiac arrest.
   c. Report changes in respiratory rate, rhythm, and use of accessory muscles. Keep equipment for intubation close at hand.
   d. Monitor serum electrolytes and all ABG results. Report significant changes to the physician.
   e. Monitor neurological status such as level of consciousness and orientation. Report changes to the physician.
   f. Position the client for optimal gas exchange and comfort. In many cases, semi-Fowler's position helps increase expansion of the chest wall.
   g. An intubated client with unilateral lung disease may benefit from a side-lying position with the unaffected lung down.
   h. Assist a client with secretion removal by encouraging coughing, deep breathing, or suctioning as needed.
   i. Ensure client safety by keeping the bed rails up and the bed in low position.
   j. Provide reassurance to the client's family that confusion will subside with treatment.
   k. Administer oxygen as ordered, keeping in mind that high concentrations of oxygen suppress hypoxic drive in some clients with COPD and depress respiratory efforts.
   l. Monitor intake and output. Provide adequate hydration through oral or parenteral fluids.
   m. Use sedatives or narcotics cautiously, because they suppress the respiratory effort.

B. RESPIRATORY ALKALOSIS
   1. DESCRIPTION
      a. PCO_2 decreased as a result of alveolar hyperventilation.
      b. Decreased PCO_2 results in decreased carbonic acid concentration in the blood and increased pH.
      c. Compensation is rare unless the cause is chronic such as in long-term ventilation or central nervous system pathology.
      d. Common etiologies (see Table 13-10)
   2. ASSESSMENT
      a. Neuromuscular—lethargy, lightheadedness, confusion, restlessness, tetany, numbness, tingling, hyperreflexia, seizures
      b. Cardiovascular—tachycardia, arrhythmias
      c. Gastrointestinal—nausea, vomiting, epigastric pain
      d. Respiratory—tachypnea, increased depth of respirations
   3. DIAGNOSTIC TESTS
      a. ABGs
         1) Uncompensated respiratory alkalosis—increased pH, decreased PCO_2, normal bicarbonate
         2) Compensated respiratory alkalosis—normal pH, decreased PCO_2, decreased bicarbonate, urine pH > 6
      b. ECG—prolonged PR interval, flattened T wave, depressed ST segment
      c. Serum ionized calcium—may be decreased in severe alkalosis as calcium ionization is inhibited
      d. Serum potassium—may be decreased as a result of the hydrogen ion moving out of the cell and the potassium shifting into the cell
   4. NURSING INTERVENTIONS
      a. Collaborative interventions to treat an underlying disorder
      b. Administer oxygen as needed if hypoxemia is the cause.
      c. Administer sedatives as ordered and help reassure the client if anxiety is the underlying cause.
      d. Instruct the client on controlled breathing techniques or assist the client to breathe into a paper bag (this forces the client to rebreathe exhaled carbon dioxide).
      e. Monitor ABGs for metabolic acidosis as PCO_2 returns to normal range.
      f. Allow the client to rest undisturbed, because the client may be fatigued from hyperventilation.
      g. Monitor cardiac rhythm and report dysrhythmias.
      h. Monitor serum ionized calcium levels. Assess for signs of hypocalcemia due to increased binding of calcium.
      i. Monitor ABGs frequently if the client is on mechanical ventilation. Check ABGs after making changes to settings.

C. METABOLIC ACIDOSIS
   1. DESCRIPTION
      a. Gain of fixed acid other than carbonic acid
      b. Inability to excrete acid by the kidneys
      c. Loss of base bicarbonate in body fluids
      d. Respiratory system compensates by increasing CO_2 excretion by the lungs.

e. Renal system attempts to compensate by excreting additional acid through urine.

f. Common etiologies (see Table 13-10)

2. ASSESSMENT

   a. Neurological—drowsiness, confusion, headache, coma

   b. Cardiovascular—decreased blood pressure, arrhythmias, peripheral vasodilatation

   c. Gastrointestinal—nausea, vomiting, diarrhea, abdominal pain

   d. Respiratory—deep, rapid (Kussmaul's) respirations

   e. Other—cold, clammy skin, fruity odor on the breath (if the cause is ketoacidosis)

3. DIAGNOSTIC TESTS

   a. ABGs

     1) Uncompensated metabolic acidosis—decreased pH, PCO_2 normal, decreased bicarbonate, increased anion gap (> 14 mEq/L) in cases of lactic or ketoacidosis, normal anion gap with loss of bicarbonate

     2) Compensated metabolic acidosis—normal pH, PCO_2 decreased, decreased bicarbonate, urine pH < 6

   b. Serum potassium—increased as the hydrogen ion moves into the cell and potassium moves out of the cell in exchange

   c. Plasma lactate—increased in lactic acidosis

   d. Serum ketone bodies—elevated in ketoacidosis

   e. ECG—tall T waves, prolonged PR interval, and wide QRS interval due to hyperkalemia

4. NURSING INTERVENTIONS

   a. Administer sodium bicarbonate as ordered. Sodium bicarbonate is sometimes indicated if pH is < 7.2.

   b. Monitor serum sodium levels and for signs of fluid overload if sodium bicarbonate is ordered.

   c. Monitor ABGs throughout bicarbonate replacement. Be alert for metabolic alkalosis.

   d. Flush the IV line thoroughly with normal saline before and after administering sodium bicarbonate, because it forms precipitates with many medications.

   e. Monitor serum potassium levels. Anticipate a fall in potassium as acidosis is corrected and potassium moves back into the intracellular spaces.

f. Replace potassium as ordered.

g. Monitor cardiac rhythm and report changes.

h. Monitor vital signs. Be alert for decreases in blood pressure as a result of hypovolemia.

i. Monitor respiratory rate and effort. Be aware that hyperventilation is a compensatory mechanism to blow off carbon dioxide.

j. Monitor intake and output carefully.

k. Anticipate hemodialysis for a client with renal failure or drug overdose.

l. Monitor neurological status and report changes.

m. Provide a safe environment for a confused client and reorient.

n. Instruct a client admitted with ketoacidosis the importance of blood glucose testing and management of diabetes on sick days. Ensure that the client is aware of the clinical manifestations of hyperglycemia.

D. METABOLIC ALKALOSIS

1. DESCRIPTION

   a. Loss of strong acid or gain of base (HCO_{3-}), resulting in decreased H^{++} concentration, increased pH, and increased serum bicarbonate levels

   b. Carbon dioxide is retained by the respiratory system in order to compensate.

   c. Renal system may also compensate by excreting excess bicarbonate.

   d. Common etiologies (see Table 13-10)

2. ASSESSMENT

   a. Neurological—dizziness, irritability, nervousness, confusion, tremors, hypertonic muscles, muscle cramps, tetany, tingling of the feet and toes, seizures

   b. Cardiovascular—tachycardia, arrhythmias, postural hypotension

   c. Gastrointestinal—anorexia, nausea, vomiting

   d. Respiratory—slow, shallow respirations

   e. Other—poor skin turgor, polyuria, dry mucous membranes

3. DIAGNOSTIC TESTS

   a. Arterial blood gases

     1) Uncompensated metabolic alkalosis—increased pH, PCO_2 normal, increased bicarbonate

     2) Compensated metabolic alkalosis—normal pH, PCO_2 increased, increased bicarbonate, urine pH > 6

   b. Serum potassium—decreased

   c. Serum chloride—less than 95 mEq/L

   d. Total CO_2—greater than 28 mEq/L

e. ECG—flattened T wave and dysrhythmias resulting from cardiac irritability

4. NURSING INTERVENTIONS

a. Monitor a client who is at risk for developing metabolic alkalosis, such as one with gastric suctioning or who is receiving IV bicarbonate.

b. For losses caused by gastric suctioning, administer saline infusions as ordered to correct hypovolemia and replace chloride losses.

c. Administer acetazolamide (Diamox) as ordered in order to promote excretion of renal bicarbonate (HCO_3-). Monitor serum potassium levels and replace as necessary, since acetazolamide also increases potassium loss.

d. Administer histamine-blocking agents such as famotidine (Pepcid) as ordered

in order to decrease production of gastric acid and subsequent losses from gastric suctioning or vomiting.

e. Monitor vital signs, cardiac rhythm, and respiratory rate and rhythm. Notify the physician of changes.

f. Monitor ABGs throughout treatment.

g. Monitor serum potassium, chloride, and total CO_2. Notify the physician of significant changes.

h. Administer potassium chloride supplements as ordered to correct low potassium and chloride levels.

i. Monitor intake and output.

j. Use normal saline to irrigate gastric tubes to prevent loss of electrolytes.

k. Monitor neurological status and report changes.

PRACTICE QUESTIONS

1. The nurse evaluates which of the following arterial blood gases for normal values?

   Select all that apply:
   [ ] 1. pH of 7.30
   [ ] 2. $PaCO_2$ of 36 mm Hg
   [ ] 3. HCO_3- of 20 mEq/L
   [ ] 4. PaO_2 of 84 mm Hg
   [ ] 5. $PaCO_2$ of 30 mm Hg
   [ ] 6. pH of 7.43

2. The nurse evaluates which of the following clients to be at risk for developing hypernatremia?
   1. 50-year-old with pneumonia, diaphoresis, and high fevers
   2. 62-year-old with congestive heart failure taking loop diuretics
   3. 39-year-old with diarrhea and vomiting
   4. 60-year-old with lung cancer and syndrome of inappropriate antidiuretic hormone (SIADH)

3. A client is admitted with diabetic ketoacidosis who, with treatment, has a normal blood glucose, pH, and serum osmolality. During assessment, the client complains of weakness in the legs. Which of the following is a priority nursing intervention?
   1. Request a physical therapy consult from the physician
   2. Ensure the client is safe from falls and check the most recent potassium level
   3. Allow uninterrupted rest periods throughout the day

4. Encourage the client to increase intake of dairy products and green, leafy vegetables

4. A client with a potassium level of 5.5 mEq/L is to receive sodium polystyrene sulfonate (Kayexalate) orally. After administering the drug, the priority nursing action is to monitor
   1. urine output.
   2. blood pressure.
   3. bowel movements.
   4. ECG for tall, peaked T waves.

5. The nurse is caring for a client who has been in good health up to the present and is admitted with cellulitis of the hand. The client's serum potassium level was 4.5 mEq/L yesterday. Today the level is 7 mEq/L. Which of the following is the next appropriate nursing action?
   1. Call the physician and report results
   2. Question the results and redraw the specimen
   3. Encourage the client to increase the intake of bananas
   4. Initiate seizure precautions

6. A client is receiving an intravenous magnesium infusion to correct a serum level of 1.4 mEq/L. Which of the following assessments would alert the nurse to immediately stop the infusion?
   1. Absent patellar reflex
   2. Diarrhea
   3. Premature ventricular contractions
   4. Increase in blood pressure

7. A client with chronic renal failure reports a 10-pound weight loss over 3 months and has had difficulty taking calcium supplements. The total calcium is 6.9 mg/dl. Which of the following would be the first nursing action?
   1. Assess for depressed deep tendon reflexes
   2. Call the physician to report calcium level
   3. Place an intravenous catheter in anticipation of administering calcium gluconate
   4. Check to see if a serum albumin level is available

8. A client with heart failure is complaining of nausea. The client has received IV furosemide (Lasix), and the urine output has been 2500 ml over the past 12 hours. The client's home drugs include metoprolol (Lopressor), digoxin (Lanoxin), furosemide, and multivitamins. Which of the following are the appropriate nursing actions before administering the digoxin?

   Select all that apply:
   [ ] 1. Administer an antiemetic prior to giving the digoxin
   [ ] 2. Encourage the client to increase fluid intake
   [ ] 3. Call the physician
   [ ] 4. Report the urine output
   [ ] 5. Report indications of nausea
   [ ] 6. Monitor continuous ECG for peaked T waves and widened QRS

9. The nurse is caring for a bedridden client admitted with multiple myeloma and a serum calcium level of 13 mg/dl. Which of the following is the most appropriate nursing action?
   1. Provide passive range-of-motion exercises and encourage fluid intake
   2. Teach the client to increase intake of whole grains and nuts
   3. Place a tracheostomy tray at the bedside
   4. Administer calcium gluconate IM as ordered

10. An older adult client admitted with heart failure and a sodium level of 113 mEq/L is behaving aggressively toward staff and does not recognize family members. When the family expresses concern about the client's behavior, the nurse would respond most appropriately by stating which of the following?
    1. "The client may be suffering from dementia, and the hospitalization has worsened the confusion."
    2. "Most older adults get confused in the hospital."
    3. "The sodium level is low, and the confusion will resolve as the levels normalize."
    4. "The sodium level is high, and the behavior is a result of dehydration."

11. A client with a serum sodium of 115 mEq/L has been receiving 3% NS at 50 ml/hr for 16 hours. This morning the client feels tired and short of breath. Which of the following interventions is a priority?
    1. Turn down the infusion
    2. Check the latest sodium level
    3. Assess for signs of fluid overload
    4. Place a call to the physician

12. A client with chronic renal failure receiving dialysis complains of frequent constipation. When performing discharge teaching, which over-the-counter products should the nurse instruct the client to avoid at home?
    1. Bisacodyl (Dulcolax) suppository
    2. Fiber supplements
    3. Docusate sodium
    4. Milk of magnesia

13. A client is receiving intravenous potassium supplementation in addition to maintenance fluids. The urine output has been 120 ml every 8 hours for the past 16 hours and the next dose is due. Before administering the next potassium dose, which of the following is the priority nursing action?
    1. Encourage the client to increase fluid intake
    2. Administer the dose as ordered
    3. Draw a potassium level and administer the dose if the level is low or normal
    4. Notify the physician of the urine output and hold the dose

14. The nurse should monitor for clinical manifestations of hypophosphatemia in which of the following clients?
    1. A client with osteoporosis taking vitamin D and calcium supplements
    2. A client who is alcoholic receiving total parenteral nutrition
    3. A client with chronic renal failure awaiting the first dialysis run
    4. A client with hypoparathyroidism secondary to thyroid surgery

15. A client admitted with squamous cell carcinoma of the lung has a serum calcium level of 14 mg/dl. The nurse should instruct the client to avoid which of the following foods upon discharge?

    Select all that apply:
    [ ] 1. Fish
    [ ] 2. Eggs
    [ ] 3. Broccoli
    [ ] 4. Organ meats
    [ ] 5. Nuts
    [ ] 6. Canned salmon

16. A client with pancreatitis has been receiving potassium supplementation for 4 days since being admitted with a serum potassium of 3.0 mEq/L. Today the potassium level is 3.1 mEq/L. Which of the following laboratory values should the nurse check before notifying the physician of the client's failure to respond to treatment?
   1. Sodium
   2. Phosphorus
   3. Calcium
   4. Magnesium

17. The nurse should include which of the following instructions to assist in controlling phosphorus levels for a client in renal failure?
   1. Increase intake of dairy products and nuts
   2. Take aluminum-based antacids such as aluminum hydroxide (Amphojel) with or after meals
   3. Reduce intake of chocolate, meats, and whole grains
   4. Avoid calcium supplements

18. A client with pneumonia presents with the following arterial blood gases: pH of 7.28, $PaCO_2$ of 74, HCO_3 of 28 mEq/L, and PO_2 of 45. Which of the following is the most appropriate nursing intervention?
   1. Administer a sedative
   2. Place client in left lateral position
   3. Place client in high-Fowler's position
   4. Assist the client to breathe into a paper bag

19. A client with COPD feels short of breath after walking to the bathroom on 2 liters of oxygen nasal cannula. The morning's ABGs were pH of 7.36, $PaCO_2$ of 62, HCO_3 of 35 mEq/L, O_2 at 88% on 2 liters. Which of the following should be the nurse's first intervention?
   1. Call the physician and report the change in client's condition
   2. Turn the client's O_2 up to 4 liters nasal cannula
   3. Encourage the client to sit down and to take deep breaths
   4. Encourage the client to rest and to use pursed-lip breathing technique

20. A client who had a recent surgery has been vomiting and becomes dizzy while standing up to go to the bathroom. After assisting the client back to bed, the nurse notes that the blood pressure is 55/30 and the pulse is 140. The nurse hangs which of the following IV fluids to correct this condition?
   1. D5.45 NS at 50 ml/hr
   2. 0.9 NS at an open rate
   3. D_5W at 125 ml/hr
   4. 0.45 NS at open rate

21. A client with renal failure enters the emergency room after skipping three dialysis treatments to visit family out of town. Which set of ABGs would indicate to the nurse that the client is in a state of metabolic acidosis?
   1. pH of 7.43, PCO_2 of 36, HCO_3 of 26
   2. pH of 7.41, PCO_2 of 49, HCO_3 of 30
   3. pH of 7.33, PCO_2 of 35, HCO_3 of 17
   4. pH of 7.25, PCO_2 of 56, HCO_3 of 28

22. A client with a small bowel obstruction has had an NG tube connected to low intermittent suction for 2 days. The nurse should monitor for clinical manifestations of which acid-base disorder?
   1. Respiratory alkalosis
   2. Respiratory acidosis
   3. Metabolic alkalosis
   4. Metabolic acidosis

23. A client who suffers from an anxiety disorder is very upset, has a respiratory rate of 32, and is complaining of lightheadedness and tingling in the fingers. ABG values are pH of 7.48, $PaCO_2$ of 29, and HCO_3 of 24, and O_2 is at 93% on room air. The nurse performs which of the following as a priority nursing intervention?
   1. Monitor intake and output
   2. Encourage client to increase activity
   3. Institute deep breathing exercises every hour
   4. Provide reassurance to the client and administer sedatives

24. Which of the following assessment findings would indicate to the nurse that a client's diabetic ketoacidosis is deteriorating?
   1. Deep tendon reflexes decreasing from 12 to 11
   2. Bicarbonate rising from 20 mEq/L to 22 mEq/L
   3. Urine pH less than 6
   4. Serum potassium decreasing from 6.0 mEq/L to 4.5 mEq/L

25. A client who is admitted with malnutrition and anorexia secondary to chemotherapy is also exhibiting generalized edema. The client asks the nurse for an explanation for the edema. Which of the following is the most appropriate response by the nurse?
   1. "The fluid is an adverse reaction to the chemotherapy."
   2. "A decrease in activity has allowed extra fluid to accumulate in the tissues."
   3. "Poor nutrition has caused decreased blood protein levels, and fluid has moved from the blood vessels into the tissues."
   4. "Chemotherapy has increased your blood pressure, and fluid was forced out into the tissues."

26. A client with a recent thyroidectomy complains of numbness and tingling around the mouth. Which of the following findings indicates the serum calcium is low?
    1. Bone pain
    2. Depressed deep tendon reflexes
    3. Positive Chvostek's sign
    4. Nausea

27. A client recently diagnosed with syndrome of inappropriate antidiuretic hormone (SIADH) complains of headache, weight gain, and nausea. Which of the following is an appropriate nursing diagnosis for this client?
    1. Deficient fluid volume related to decreased fluid intake
    2. Excess fluid volume related to increased water retention
    3. Deficient fluid volume related to excessive fluid loss
    4. Risk for injury related to fluid volume loss

28. The registered nurse is delegating nursing tasks for the day. Which of the following tasks may the nurse delegate to a licensed practical nurse?
    1. Assess a client for metabolic acidosis
    2. Evaluate the blood gases of a client with respiratory alkalosis
    3. Obtain a glucose level on a client admitted with diabetes mellitus
    4. Perform a neurological assessment on a client suspected of having hypocalcemia

29. A client who is post-gallbladder surgery has a nasogastric tube, decreased reflexes, pulse of 110 weak and irregular, and blood pressure of 80/50 and is weak, mildly confused, and has a serum of potassium of 3.0 mEq/L. Based on the assessment data, which of the following is the priority intervention?
    1. Withhold furosemide (Lasix)
    2. Notify the physician
    3. Administer the prescribed potassium supplement
    4. Instruct the client on foods high in potassium

30. The nurse is admitting a client with a potassium level of 6.0 mEq/L. The nurse reports this finding as a result of
    1. acute renal failure.
    2. malabsorption syndrome.
    3. nasogastric drainage.
    4. laxative abuse.

31. Which of the following should the nurse include in the diet teaching for a client with a sodium level of 158 mEq/L?

    Select all that apply:
    [ ] 1. Peanut butter sandwich
    [ ] 2. Pretzels
    [ ] 3. Baked chicken
    [ ] 4. Chicken bouillon
    [ ] 5. Baked potato
    [ ] 6. Baked ham

32. The nurse assesses a client to be experiencing muscle cramps, numbness, and tingling of the extremities, and twitching of the facial muscle and eyelid when the facial nerve is tapped. The nurse reports this assessment as consistent with which of the following?
    1. Hypokalemia
    2. Hypernatremia
    3. Hypermagnesemia
    4. Hypocalcemia

33. Which of the following should the nurse include when preparing to teach a class on the regulation and functions of electrolytes?
    1. Sodium is essential to maintain intracellular fluid water balance
    2. Magnesium is essential to the function of muscle, red blood cells, and nervous system
    3. Less calcium is excreted with aging
    4. Chloride is lost in hydrochloride acid

34. The nurse assists a client with a serum potassium of 3.2 mEq/L to make which of the following menu selections?

    Select all that apply:
    [ ] 1. Baked cod
    [ ] 2. Ham and cheese omelet
    [ ] 3. Fried eggs
    [ ] 4. Baked potato
    [ ] 5. Whole-grain muffin
    [ ] 6. Spinach

35. The nurse evaluates which of the following clients to have hypermagnesemia?
    1. A client who has chronic alcoholism and a magnesium level of 1.3 mEq/L
    2. A client who has hyperthyroidism and a magnesium level of 1.6 mEq/L
    3. A client who has renal failure, takes antacids, and has a magnesium level of 2.9 mEq/L
    4. A client who has congestive heart disease, takes a diuretic, and has a magnesium level of 2.3 mEq/L

36. The nurse is evaluating the serum laboratory results on the following four clients. Which of the following laboratory results is a priority for the nurse to report first?
    1. A client with osteoporosis and a calcium level of 10.6 mg/dl
    2. A client with renal failure and a magnesium level of 2.5 mEq/L
    3. A client with bulimia and a potassium level of 3.6 mEq/L
    4. A client with dehydration and a sodium level of 149 mEq/L

37. The registered nurse is delegating client assignments to unlicensed assistive personnel. Which of the following clients does not require additional monitoring and assessment and may be delegated to unlicensed assistive personnel?
1. A client who has been experiencing diarrhea and has a serum chloride level of 100 mEq/L
2. A client with renal failure who has a serum magnesium level of 3.0 mEq/L
3. A client who has experienced a fracture of the femur and has a serum phosphate of 5.0 mg/dl
4. A client with dehydration who has a serum sodium level of 128 mEq/L

ANSWERS AND RATIONALES

1. 2. 4. 6. Normal pH is 7.35. Normal $PaCO_2$ is 35–45 mm Hg. Normal HCO_3 is 22–26 mEq/l. Normal $PaCO_2$ is 80–95 mm Hg. Normal O_2 saturation is 95–99%. Arterial blood is slightly basic or alkaline with a pH of 7.35–7.45. Arterial blood pH rises above 7.45 if bicarbonate levels increase or hydrogen ions are lost. This condition is called alkalosis. Increased CO_2 levels are present in acidosis. When decreased levels of CO_2 are present, the respiratory center decreases the rate and depth of breaths to retain CO_2 and increase hydrogen ion concentration.

2. 1. Diaphoresis and a high fever can lead to free water loss through the skin, resulting in hypernatremia. Loop diuretics are more likely to result in a hypovolemic hyponatremia. Diarrhea and vomiting cause both sodium and water losses. Clients with syndrome of inappropriate antidiuretic hormone (SIADH) have hyponatremia, due to increased water reabsorption in the renal tubules.

3. 2. In the treatment of diabetic ketoacidosis, the blood sugar is lowered, the pH is corrected, and potassium moves back into the cells, resulting in low serum potassium. Client safety and the correction of low potassium levels are a priority. The weakness in the legs is a clinical manifestation of the hypokalemia. Dairy products and green, leafy vegetables are a source of calcium.

4. 3. Kayexalate causes potassium to be exchanged for sodium in the intestines and excreted through bowel movements. If client does not have stools, the drug cannot work properly. Blood pressure and urine output are not of primary importance. The nurse would already expect changes in T waves with hyperkalemia. Normal serum potassium is 3.5 to 5.5 mEq/L.

5. 2. When the serum potassium goes from 4.5 mEq/L to 7.0 mEq/L with no risk factors for hyperkalemia, false high results should be suspected because of hemolysis of the specimen. The physician would likely question results as well. Bananas are a food high in potassium. Seizures are not a clinical manifestation of hyperkalemia.

6. 1. An intravenous magnesium infusion may be used to treat a low serum magnesium level. Normal serum magnesium is 1.5 to 2.5 mEq/L. Clinical manifestations of hypermagnesemia are the result of depressed neuromuscular transmission. Absent reflexes indicate a magnesium level around 7 mEq/L. Diarrhea and PVCs are not clinical manifestations of high magnesium levels. Hypermagnesemia causes hypotension.

7. 4. A client with chronic renal failure who reports a 10-pound weight loss over 3 months and has difficulty taking calcium supplements is poorly nourished and likely to have hypoalbuminemia. A drop in serum albumin will result in a false low total calcium level. Placing an IV is not a priority action. Depressed reflexes are a sign of hypercalcemia. Normal serum calcium is 9 to 11 mg/dl.

8. 3. 4. 5. Potassium is lost during diuresis with a loop diuretic such as furosemide (Lasix). Hypokalemia can cause digitalis toxicity, which often results in nausea. The physician should be notified, and digoxin should be held until potassium levels and digoxin levels are checked. Peaked T waves and widened QRS are manifestations of hyperkalemia.

9. 1. A client who has a serum calcium of 13 mg/dl has hypercalcemia. Normal serum calcium is 9 to 11 mg/dl. Fluid intake promotes renal excretion of excess calcium. ROM exercises promote reabsorption of calcium into bone. Placing a tracheostomy at the bedside is a nursing intervention for hypocalcemia. Although calcium gluconate may be administered in hypocalcemia, it is never administered IM.

10. 3. Normal serum level is 135 to 145 mEq/L. Neurological symptoms occur when sodium levels fall below 120 mEq/L. The confusion is an acute condition that will go away as the sodium levels normalize. Dementia is an irreversible condition.

11. 3. A complication of hypertonic sodium solution administration is fluid overload. Although turning down the infusion, checking the latest sodium level, and notifying the physician may all be reasonable, the priority intervention is to assess for manifestations of fluid overload. Assessment is always the priority to determine what action to take next.

12. 4. Milk of magnesia contains magnesium, an electrolyte that is excreted by kidneys. Clients with renal failure are at risk for hypermagnesemia, as their bodies cannot excrete the excess magnesium. The client should avoid magnesium-containing laxatives.

13. 4. Urine output is an indication of renal function. Normal urine output is at least 30 ml/hour. Clients with impaired renal function are at risk for hyperkalemia. Initiating a lab draw requires a physician order.

14. 2. A client with osteoporosis taking vitamin and calcium supplements, a client with chronic renal failure awaiting dialysis, and a client with hypoparathyroidism secondary to thyroid surgery are at risk for hyperphosphatemia. Alcoholics and clients receiving total parenteral nutrition (TPN) are at risk for low phosphorus levels, due to poor intestinal absorption and shifting of phosphorus into cells along with insulin and glucose.

15. 3. 5. 6. Fish, eggs, and organ meats are high in phosphorus. Broccoli, nuts, and canned salmon are high in calcium. Clients with lung or breast cancer often have elevated calcium levels due to tumor-induced hyperparathyroidism.

16. 4. Low serum magnesium levels can inhibit potassium ions from crossing cell membranes, resulting in potassium loss through the urine. Generally, low magnesium levels must be corrected before potassium replacement is effective.

17. 2. Aluminum-based antacids are often prescribed in the treatment of renal failure to bind with phosphate and increase elimination through the GI tract. Dairy products and nuts are foods high in phosphorus. Chocolate, meats, and whole grains are foods high in magnesium. Clients with renal failure often require calcium supplements as a result of poor vitamin D metabolism and in order to prevent hyperphosphatemia.

18. 3. The client with a pH of 7.28, $PaCO_2$ of 74, HCO_3 of 28 mEq/L, and PO_2 of 45 is in a state of respiratory acidosis. Placing the client in high-Fowler's position will facilitate the expansion of the lungs and help the client blow off the excess CO_2. Sedatives would impede respirations. The question does not indicate which is the affected lung, so left lateral

position would not be a first choice. Breathing into a paper bag will cause the PCO_2 to rise higher.

19. 4. Clients with COPD, especially those who are in a chronic compensated respiratory acidosis, are very sensitive to changes in O_2 flow, because hypoxemia rather than high CO_2 levels stimulates respirations. Deep breaths are not helpful, because clients with COPD have difficulty with air trapping in alveoli. There is no need to call the physician, since this client is presently most likely at baseline.

20. 2. A client who recently had surgery is vomiting, becomes dizzy when standing up, has a blood pressure of 55/30, and has a pulse of 140 is hypovolemic and requires plasma volume expansion. Isotonic fluids such as 0.9 NS will expand volume. Hypotonic fluids such as 0.45 NS will leave the intravascular space. D_5W will metabolize into free water and leave the intravascular space. D5.45 NS is a good maintenance fluid but a rate of 50 ml per hour is not sufficient to expand the vascular volume quickly.

21. 3. A pH of 7.33, PCO_2 of 35, and HCO_3 of 17 and a pH of 7.25, PCO_2 of 56, and HCO_3 of 28 both indicate acidosis. The pH of 7.25 is a respiratory acidosis. A pH of 7.41, PCO_2 of 49, and HCO_3 of 30 is a compensated metabolic alkalosis. A pH of 7.43, PCO_2 of 36, and HCO_3 of 26 is normal.

22. 3. Clients with gastric suctioning can lose hydrogen ions, resulting in a metabolic alkalosis.

23. 4. A client who is anxious and upset, gets lightheaded, and has tingling in the fingers is in respiratory alkalosis. The arterial blood gases include a pH of 7.48, $PaCO_2$ of 29, and HCO_3 of 24. Administering sedatives will assist the client to slow breathe and retain more CO_2, thus bringing the pH back into normal range. Deep breathing exercises may worsen the client's condition. Encouraging the client to increase activity is contraindicated because clients are often exhausted and require rest after expending so much energy in breathing. Monitoring intake and output is not a priority.

24. 1. A decrease in deep tendon reflexes is a sign that pH is dropping and that metabolic acidosis is worsening in diabetic ketoacidosis. An increase in bicarbonate would indicate that the acidosis is being corrected. A urine pH less than 6 indicates the kidneys are excreting acid. Serum potassium levels are expected to fall because acidosis is corrected and potassium moves back into the intracellular space.

25. 3. Generalized edema, or anasarca, is often seen in clients with low albumin levels secondary to poor nutrition. Decreased oncotic pressure within the blood vessels allows fluid to move from the intravascular space to the interstitial space.

26. 3. Numbness and tingling around the mouth indicate hypocalcemia, which results in neuromuscular irritability. A positive Chvostek's sign is the contraction of facial muscles when the facial nerve in front of the ear is tapped. Bone pain, nausea, and depressed deep tendon reflexes are signs of hypercalcemia.

27. 2. The client exhibits signs of excess fluid volume. Syndrome of inappropriate antidiuretic hormone (SIADH) is the release of excess ADH by the pituitary gland, which results in hypervolemic hyponatremia and clinical manifestations of headache, weight gain, and nausea.

28. 3. A licensed practical nurse may obtain a finger-stick glucose on a client with diabetes mellitus. A licensed practical nurse may not assess a client for metabolic acidosis, evaluate blood gases on a client with respiratory alkalosis, or perform a neurological assessment on a client suspected of hypocalcemia.

29. 2. The priority intervention for a client who had gallbladder surgery and has a nasogastric tube, decreased reflexes, pulse of 110 weak and irregular, and blood pressure of 80/50 and is weak, mildly confused, and has a serum potassium of 3.0 mEq/L would be to notify the physician that the potassium level is low. After notifying the physician, the furosemide (Lasix) may be withheld and potassium supplement should be administered as prescribed and may even be increased after talking with the physician. The client may also be instructed on foods high in potassium. These are all appropriate interventions but not the priority.

30. 2. A serum potassium level of 6.0 mEq/L is indicative of acute renal failure. Malabsorption syndrome, nasogastric drainage, and laxative abuse may result in a low serum potassium level, because output may be greater than input. Diarrhea results in malabsorption syndrome and can come from laxative abuse. Fluids and electrolytes may be lost in the nasogastric drainage. Normal serum potassium is 3.5 to 5.5 mEq/L.

31. 3. 5. Normal serum sodium is between 135 and 145 mEq/L. A sodium level of 158 mEq/L is elevated and a low-sodium diet should be prescribed. A peanut butter sandwich, pretzels, chicken bouillon, and baked ham are all foods high in sodium content. Baked chicken and baked potato are low-sodium food choices.

32. 4. Normal serum calcium is 9 to 11 mg/dl. A client who has hypocalcemia would experience muscle cramps, numbness, and twitching of the facial muscles and eyelid when the facial nerve is tapped. Hypocalcemia may result from renal failure, hypoparathyroidism, acute pancreatitis, liver disease, malabsorption syndrome, and vitamin D deficiency. Normal serum potassium level is 3.5 to 5.5 mEq/L. Normal serum sodium is 135 to 145 mEq/L. Normal serum magnesium is 1.5 to 2.5 mEq/L.

33. 4. Sodium is essential to maintain extracellular fluid water balance. Phosphate is the major anion in intracellular fluid water balance that is essential in the function of muscle, red blood cells, and nervous system. A person tends to excrete more calcium with age. Chloride is lost through hydrochloride acid.

34. 1. 4. 6. Normal serum potassium is 3.5 to 5.5 mEq/L. A client who has a potassium of 3.2 mEq/L would benefit from a diet high in potassium. Baked cod, baked potato, and spinach are all food selections high in potassium. A ham and cheese omelet is high in sodium. Fried eggs are high in cholesterol. A whole-grain muffin is high in grains.

35. 3. Normal serum magnesium is 1.5 to 2.5 mEq/L. Clients who have chronic alcoholism and hyperthyroidism are prone to hypomagnesemia. A client who has congestive heart failure, takes a diuretic, and has a magnesium level of 2.3 mEq/L falls within the normal magnesium range.

36. 4. Although a client with acute osteoporosis may have a high serum calcium, a level of 10.6 mg/dl is normal. Normal serum calcium is 9 to 11 mg/dl. Normal serum magnesium is 1.5 to 2.5 mEq/L. A client who has renal failure is prone to hypermagnesemia, but a level of 2.5 mEq/L is at the upper limit of normal. A client who has bulimia generally vomits enough to result in a low potassium level, but a potassium level of 3.6 mEq/L is low-normal. Normal serum potassium is 3.5 to 5.5 mEq/L. Normal serum sodium is 135 to 145 mEq/L. The sodium level generally goes up with dehydration. A sodium level of 149 mEq/L is elevated.

37. 1. Normal serum chloride is 95 to 105 mEq/L. A client with diarrhea may experience a low chloride level, but 100 mEq/L is within the normal range and may be delegated to unlicensed assistive personnel. Normal serum magnesium is 1.5 to 2.5 mEq/L. A magnesium level of 3.0 mEq/L is elevated and may occur in renal failure. Phosphate levels may be elevated with healing fractures. A phosphate level of 5.0 mg/dl is elevated. Normal serum phosphate is 2.8 to 4.5 mg/dl. A sodium level of 128 mEq/L is decreased and may be found with dehydration. Normal serum sodium is 135 to 145 mEq/L.

REFERENCES

Daniels, R. (2010). *Delmar's manual of laboratory and diagnostic tests*. Clifton Park, NY: Delmar Cengage Learning.

Daniels, R., & Nicoll, L. (2012). *Contemporary medical-surgical nursing*. Clifton Park, NY: Delmar Cengage Learning.

DeLaune, S.C., & Ladner, P.K. (2011). *Fundamentals of nursing: Standard and practice* (4th ed.). Clifton Park, NY: Delmar Cengage Learning.

Kee, J. L., Paulanka, B. J., & Purnell, L. (2010a). *Fluids and electrolytes with clinical applications: A programmed approach* (8th ed.). Clifton Park, NY: Cengage Delmar Learning.

Kee, J. L., Paulanka, B. J., & Purnell, L. L. (2010b). *Handbook of fluids, electrolytes and acid-base imbalances* (3rd ed.). Clifton Park, NY: Delmar Cengage Learning.

Spratto, G. R., & Woods, A. L. (2012). *PDR nurse's drug handbook 2012*. Clifton Park, NY: Delmar Cengage Learning.

CHAPTER 14

PERIOPERATIVE NURSING

I. PERIOPERATIVE NURSING
  A. DEFINITION
  1. DELIVERY OF NURSING CARE IN THE PREOPERATIVE, INTRAOPERATIVE, OR POSTOPERATIVE PERIODS OF A CLIENT'S SURGICAL EXPERIENCE
  2. CARE MAY OCCUR IN A VARIETY OF SETTINGS, RANGING FROM OPERATING ROOM SUITES TO THE CLIENTS' HOMES, PHYSICIANS' OFFICES, TO FREESTANDING AMBULATORY CARE SETTINGS.
  3. PERIOPERATIVE NURSING CARE IS UNDERSCORED BY THE NURSING PROCESS.

II. IDENTIFICATION OF PREOPERATIVE, INTRAOPERATIVE, AND POSTOPERATIVE CARE
  A. PREOPERATIVE NURSING CARE: BEGINS AT THE TIME SURGERY IS SCHEDULED AND ENDS AT THE TIME THAT THE CLIENT IS TRANSFERRED TO THE OPERATING ROOM SUITE
  B. INTRAOPERATIVE NURSING CARE: BEGINS AT THE TIME THAT THE CLIENT ENTERS THE OPERATING ROOM AND ENDS AT THE TIME THE CLIENT IS TRANSFERRED TO THE POSTANESTHESIA CARE UNIT
  C. POSTOPERATIVE NURSING CARE: BEGINS WHEN THE CLIENT'S SURGICAL PROCEDURE IS COMPLETED AND THE CLIENT IS TRANSFERRED TO EITHER THE POSTANESTHESIA CARE UNIT OR THE INTENSIVE CARE UNIT

III. PREOPERATIVE ASSESSMENT
  A. REVIEW THE CLIENT'S MEDICAL CHART TO IDENTIFY:
  1. PROPOSED SURGICAL PROCEDURE
  2. PERTINENT CLIENT HISTORY, INCLUDING:
    a. Previous hospitalizations or surgeries, or both, and any complications
    b. Any implanted devices, including metal hardware and pacemakers
    c. Smoking, alcohol, or drug use
    d. Possibility of pregnancy
    e. Client allergies, including latex allergy
  3. SIGNED SURGICAL CONSENT AND BLOOD ADMINISTRATION CONSENT IF INDICATED
  4. ANESTHESIA NOTE/PERMIT (EVIDENCE THAT CLIENT HAS BEEN EVALUATED BY ANESTHESIA)
  5. HISTORY AND PHYSICAL
  6. HEIGHT, WEIGHT, AND VITAL SIGNS CHARTED
  7. PREOPERATIVE MEDICATIONS, INCLUDING ASSESSMENT OF RECENT ADMINISTRATION OF ASPIRIN OR BLOOD THINNERS
  B. VERIFY WITH THE CLIENT THAT:
  1. IDENTIFICATION BAND IS IN PLACE
  2. DENTURES, PARTIAL PLATES, AND RETAINERS ARE REMOVED
  3. JEWELRY IS REMOVED OR SECURED
  4. NOTHING BY MOUTH (NPO) STATUS IS MAINTAINED (USED TO REDUCE ASPIRATION RISK)

IV. PREOPERATIVE NURSING DIAGNOSES
  A. SELF-CARE DEFICIT
  1. ASSESSMENT OF LIVING CONDITIONS
  2. HOME CARE OF EQUIPMENT NEEDS
  3. SOCIAL SUPPORT
  4. ANY EDUCATION NEEDS
  B. DEFICIENT KNOWLEDGE RELATED TO UPCOMING PROCEDURE
  1. NPO STATUS
  2. ADMINISTRATION OF PREOPERATIVE MEDICATIONS
  3. REMOVAL OF MAKEUP, JEWELRY, CONTACT LENS, AND NAIL POLISH
  4. APPROPRIATE PREOPERATIVE PREPS, TESTS, AND TREATMENTS

Table 14-1 Preoperative Nursing Responsibilities

Nursing Responsibilities	Nursing Interventions
Potential risk factors for surgical experience	Identify clients who may be at risk due to their age (clients at the extremes of the age spectrum are at increased risk).
	Identify clients who are at risk due to nutritional status (clients who are obese or undernourished are at increased risk).
	Identify clients who are at risk due to past medical history (clients with chronic cardiac or respiratory conditions may be at increased risk).
	Identify clients who have diabetes (these clients may need modification of their medication regime on the day of the procedure).
	Identify clients who are extremely anxious (these clients may need extra support or medications prior to their surgical experience).
	Assess clients' medication history and document all medications, paying attention to those medications that may increase operative risks, including anticoagulants (including nonsteroidal analgesics and aspirin), steroids, and antibiotics.
	Assess for history of allergies to any medications, skin preparation products (betadine, iodine), and to latex or tape.
Preoperative physical assessment	Assess skin integrity—identify lesions or areas of concern and document.
	Assess baseline neurological status.
	Assess cardiac status, noting baseline pulse and blood pressure. Assess for peripheral edema for a history of chest pain.
	Assess respiratory status, noting baseline lung sounds and respiratory rate. Check for adequate oxygenation status by examining skin color.
	Assess for baseline fluid volume status. Assess for adequate hydration by examining skin turgor.
	Assess patency of IV site—initiate IV placement as ordered.
Preoperative client teaching	Instruct the client about the expected postoperative course—initial stay in postanesthesia care unit, expected tubes and drains, and parameters for dismissal if outpatient surgery.
	Instruct the client about the following:
	• Deep breathing and coughing exercises
	• Postoperative exercise of lower extremities
	• Pain control techniques, including both pharmacological and alternative treatments (relaxation, imagery, etc.)
	• Incentive spirometry usage
	• Splinting of incision
Preoperative preparation	Review preoperative orders and verify special preparations (gastrointestinal prep, skin preparation, preoperative medications).
	Verify NPO status orders.
	Verify signed surgical consent.
	Complete preoperative checklist—the following is usually included:
	• Preoperative vital signs
	• Verification of identification
	• Verification of signed surgical permit
	• Verification of procedure, including correct extremity if appropriate
	• Verification of removal of dentures, contact lenses, jewelry, and nail polish
	• Documentation of implanted metal, pacemaker, implanted defibrillator
	• Have client void on call to surgical suite.
	• Administer preoperative sedatives as ordered.

© Cengage Learning 2015

V. PREOPERATIVE NURSING RESPONSIBILITIES (SEE TABLE 14-1)

VI. INTRAOPERATIVE CARE
  A. SELECTION OF TYPES OF ANESTHESIA
    1. SELECTION OF APPROPRIATE CHOICE OF ANESTHESIA MADE BY THE CLIENT IN CONJUNCTION WITH THE ANESTHESIA PROVIDER AND SURGEON

  B. GENERAL ANESTHESIA
    1. COMPLICATIONS:
      a. Latex allergy
      b. Hypoxia or other respiratory dysfunction
      c. Aspiration
      d. Cardiovascular dysfunction—including problems with hypertension

e. Renal dysfunction

f. Fluid or electrolyte imbalances

g. Dental damage

h. Malignant hyperthermia—a rare life-threatening reaction to a "triggering" agent used in general anesthesia (typically succinylcholine or inhalation anesthetics)

j. Dark blood in the surgical field (due to desaturated blood)

k. Hypertension or lability in blood pressure

l. Late manifestation in rising body temperature (1–2 Celsius degrees every 5 minutes)

C. REGIONAL ANESTHESIA
   1. REVERSIBLE LOSS OF SENSATION IN A SPECIFIC REGION OF THE BODY BY INJECTING A LOCAL ANESTHETIC ALONG THE PATHWAY OF A NERVE—COMMON ANESTHETIC TECHNIQUES INCLUDE CAUDAL, EPIDURAL, SPINAL, AND MAJOR PERIPHERAL NERVE BLOCKS

D. MONITORED ANESTHESIA CARE (MAC)
   1. COMBINATION OF INFILTRATION OF SURGICAL SITE WITH LOCAL ANESTHETIC IN COMBINATION WITH IV SEDATION

E. CONSCIOUS SEDATION
   1. A TYPE OF ANESTHESIA THAT ALLOWS CLIENTS TO TOLERATE UNPLEASANT PROCEDURES WHILE MAINTAINING ADEQUATE CARDIORESPIRATORY FUNCTION

F. LOCAL ANESTHESIA
   1. ADMINISTRATION OF ANESTHETIC AGENT TO THE SURGICAL SITE BY LOCAL INFILTRATION OF ANESTHESIA OR TOPICAL APPLICATION OF AN ANESTHETIC

VII. **NURSING ASSESSMENT OF ANESTHETIC COMPLICATIONS**
   A. BRONCHOSPASM
   B. HYPOTENSION
   C. HYPERTENSION
   D. DYSRHYTHMIAS
   E. HYPOTHERMIA
   F. ALTERED THOUGHT PROCESSES
   G. NAUSEA AND VOMITING
   H. ASPIRATION
   I. PAIN
   J. URINARY RETENTION

VIII. **INTRAOPERATIVE NURSING DIAGNOSES**
   A. RISK FOR INJURY RELATED TO SENSORY OR MOTOR DEFICITS SECONDARY TO SEDATION AND ANESTHESIA
      1. POSITION FOR SURGERY
      2. SAFETY PRECAUTIONS FOR ELECTROCAUTERY DEVICES

USED TO CAUTERIZE BLOOD VESSELS AND TO CUT TISSUE AND LASER
   3. USE OF TOURNIQUET
   4. ABILITY TO MOVE THE EXTREMITIES
   5. DERMATOME LEVEL—DOCUMENTATION OF FULL SENSATION
   6. PULSE
   7. CIRCULATION
   8. CAPILLARY REFILL
   9. SENSATION
   10. ELEVATION OF LIMB
   11. WOUND/DRESSING

B. RISK FOR IMPAIRED GAS EXCHANGE RELATED TO INEFFECTIVE AIRWAY CLEARANCE
   1. BREATH SOUNDS
   2. RESPIRATIONS
   3. CARDIAC RHYTHM

C. RISK FOR INFECTION RELATED TO A BREAK IN SKIN INTEGRITY
   1. DRESSING
   2. SKIN PREP

D. FLUID VOLUME, EXCESS OR DEFICIENT, RELATED TO PHYSIOLOGICAL RESPONSE TO STRESS SECONDARY TO SURGICAL PROCEDURE
   1. IRRIGATION OFTEN ACCOUNTED FOR
   2. DURING CONSCIOUS SEDATION—VITAL SIGNS, O_2 SATURATION LEVEL, LEVEL OF CONSCIOUSNESS MONITORED

E. PAIN RELATED TO PHYSIOLOGICAL RESPONSE TO SURGERY
   1. PAIN SCALES MONITORED, ESPECIALLY DURING CONSCIOUS SEDATION

F. INEFFECTIVE THERMOREGULATION RELATED TO ENVIRONMENTAL TEMPERATURES AND EFFECTS OF SEDATION
   1. SKIN STATUS MONITORED
   2. SKIN COLOR MONITORED

G. ANXIETY RELATED TO POST-OP STATUS, UNFAMILIARITY WITH ENVIRONMENT, AND SEPARATION FROM FAMILY/SIGNIFICANT OTHER
   1. MONITOR EMOTIONAL RESPONSE

H. RISK FOR IMPAIRED MOBILITY RELATED TO PROCEDURE OR PAIN, OR BOTH
   1. ACTIVITY
   2. TOLERANCE

Nursing Diagnoses: Definitions and Classification 2012–2014.
Copyright © 2012, 1994–2012 by NANDA International.
Used by arrangement with John Wiley & Sons Limited.

IX. **PERIOPERATIVE NURSING RESPONSIBILITIES (SEE TABLE 14-2)**

Table 14-2 Perioperative Nursing Responsibilities

Nursing Responsibilities	Nursing Interventions
Preoperative assessment	Review preoperative orders and verify their completion. Verify the client's identity. Verify the client's allergy status, including allergies to medications, prep solutions, and latex. Verify NPO status. Verify signed surgical consent and appropriate procedure, including correct extremity if appropriate. Verify completed preoperative checklist. Verify anesthesia assessment.
Client safety	Assist in the client's transfer from cart to operating room table at the beginning and completion of the operative procedure. Assist anesthesia during the induction process as needed. Always stand by the client until induction of anesthesia is completed. Assist the surgical team in proper positioning of the client; pad bony prominences as necessary. Assess for appropriate location of electrocautery grounding pad and apply to the appropriate location. Perform instrument, sponge, and needle counts prior to the surgical procedure and at its completion. Monitor the client for hypothermia and assist in maintenance of normothermia as appropriate (use of Baer hugger, heated IV solutions, and warm blankets).
Collaborative responsibilities	Assist the surgical team as needed by gathering and opening sterile supplies on the surgical field. Monitor the client's condition and provide updates to the family as necessary. Assist anesthesia as needed. Provide report to the postanesthesia care unit, emphasizing the procedure performed, estimated blood loss and blood transfusions, the client's condition, and any complications.

© Cengage Learning 2015

X. POSTOPERATIVE NURSING DIAGNOSES

A. RISK FOR IMPAIRED GAS EXCHANGE RELATED TO INEFFECTIVE AIRWAY CLEARANCE

1. THE FIRST PRIORITY IS TO ESTABLISH A PATENT AIRWAY.

   a. Check for snoring, decreased air movement, retraction of intercostal muscles, asynchronous movements of the chest and abdomen, and decreased oxygen saturation level.

   1) Client may need stimulation to breathe.
   2) Repositioning the client—often to lateral position
   3) Open the airway with a chin lift or jaw thrust.
   4) Artificial airway may need to be inserted.
   5) In certain situations, intubation and ventilation may be required.

2. LARYNGOSPASM: SERIOUS COMPLICATION IN WHICH MUSCLES OF THE LARYNX CONTRACT AND CAUSE PARTIAL OR COMPLETE OBSTRUCTION OF THE AIRWAY

   a. Usually the result of an irritable airway
   b. Nursing interventions include:

   1) Removing irritating stimulus to the airway
   2) Suctioning secretions that may be causing airway irritation
   3) Opening airway
   4) May require administration of inhaled aerosol with racemic epinephrine
   5) With prolonged clinical manifestations (longer than 1 minute), may require administration of muscle relaxant (succinylcholine) to relax the muscles of the larynx
   6) Reintubation is used only as a last resort.

3. BRONCHOSPASM

   a. Lower airway obstruction caused by spasms of the muscles surrounding the bronchi

B. RISK FOR IMPAIRED MOBILITY RELATED TO SURGICAL PROCEDURE

C. DECREASED CARDIAC OUTPUT

1. HYPOTENSION

   a. Blood pressure of less than 20% of baseline blood pressure
   b. Often indicates hypovolemia
   c. In addition to decreased blood pressure, watch for tachycardia; disorientation; restlessness; decreased urine output; or cold, pale skin.

d. Assess for cardiac dysfunction (myocardial infarction, congestive heart failure, ischemia, dysrhythmias, or reaction to drugs).

2. HYPOVOLEMIA
   a. Reduces cardiac output
   b. May be caused by dehydration, blood loss, or increased positive end-expiratory pressure (PEEP)
   c. Treat with fluid resuscitation or blood replacement.
   d. Assess for decreased vascular resistance related to anaphylaxis, response to drugs, or anesthesia.

3. HYPERTENSION
   a. Causes an increase in cardiac output
   b. Increase in blood pressure from the client's baseline
   c. Very common postoperative complication
   d. May be caused by volume overload
   e. Common causes are pain, anxiety, or other conditions that may increase vascular resistance.

4. DYSRHYTHMIAS
   a. Sinus tachycardia
      1) Common dysrhythmia often caused by anxiety, pain, hypovolemia, or hypoxia
      2) Treatment involves treating the underlying cause
      3) Beta blockers may be given.
   b. Sinus bradycardia
      1) Common dysrhythmia; can be caused by vagal stimulation, hypoxemia, hypothermia, high spinal anesthesia, and certain anesthetic drugs
      2) Atropine is usually the medication of choice.

D. RISK FOR IMBALANCED BODY TEMPERATURE
   1. WIDESPREAD PROBLEM IN THE POSTANESTHESIA CARE UNIT (PACU) AFFECTING AS MANY AS 60% OF CLIENTS
   2. CAUSES PHYSIOLOGIC STRESS
   3. CAN PROLONG RECOVERY TIME AND CONTRIBUTES TO POSTOPERATIVE MORBIDITY
   4. REWARM CLIENTS BY REMOVING WET GOWNS AND BLANKETS, APPLYING WARM BLANKETS, AND USING FORCED-WARM-AIR DEVICES THAT BLOW WARM AIR INTO SPECIAL PLASTIC OR PAPER BLANKETS THAT COVER THE CLIENT.

E. DISTURBED THOUGHT PROCESSES
   1. WIDE RANGES OF CAUSES, INCLUDING EFFECTS OF ANESTHESIA, PAIN, OR ANXIETY
   2. MUST ALWAYS RULE OUT HYPOXEMIA FIRST
   3. CLIENTS WITH PROBLEMS OF CHEMICAL OR SUBSTANCE ABUSE MAY EMERGE FROM ANESTHESIA AGITATED.

F. NAUSEA
   1. AFFECTS LARGE NUMBERS OF PATIENTS IN THE PACU
   2. ANTIEMETIC THERAPY IS OFTEN GIVEN INTRAOPERATIVELY AS A PREVENTIVE MEASURE.
   3. COMMONLY USED MEDICATIONS INCLUDE ONDANSETRON (ZOFRAN), PROCHLORPERAZINE (COMPAZINE), AND PROMETHAZINE (PHENERGAN).

G. RISK FOR ASPIRATION
   1. OCCURS WHEN GASTRIC CONTENTS ENTER THE LUNGS
   2. RISK FACTORS INCLUDE TRACHEAL INTUBATION, OBESITY, PREGNANCY, RECENT ORAL INTAKE, AND DEPRESSED LEVEL OF CONSCIOUSNESS.
   3. CLINICAL MANIFESTATIONS INCLUDE:
      a. Coughing
      b. Wheezing
      c. Dyspnea
      d. Apnea
      e. Bradycardia
      f. Hypotension

H. PAIN
   1. UP TO 75% OF POSTOPERATIVE CLIENTS MAY BE UNDERTREATED FOR PAIN.
   2. ALL CLIENTS MUST BE ASSESSED FOR POSTOPERATIVE PAIN.
   3. MULTIPLE PHARMACOLOGICAL OPTIONS INCLUDE PATIENT-CONTROLLED ANALGESIA (PCA), USE OF SPINAL OR EPIDURAL ANESTHESIA, OR INFILTRATION OF SURGICAL SITE WITH LOCAL ANESTHETIC.
   4. NONPHARMACOLOGICAL INTERVENTIONS INCLUDE APPLICATIONS OF HEAT OR COLD, POSITIONING, VERBAL REASSURANCE, TRANSCUTANEOUS ELECTRICAL NERVE STIMULATION (TENS), RELAXATION, BIOFEEDBACK, AND MUSIC.

Nursing Diagnoses: Definitions and Classification 2012–2014. Copyright © 2012, 1994–2012 by NANDA International. Used by arrangement with John Wiley & Sons Limited.

XI. **POSTOPERATIVE NURSING RESPONSIBILITIES (SEE TABLE 14-3)**

Table 14-3 Postoperative Nursing Responsibilities

Nursing Responsibilities	Nursing Interventions
Client safety	Monitor the client's vital signs for signs of hypovolemia, hypertension, hypotension, and hypothermia.
	Monitor the client's incision for drainage, bleeding, and wound dehiscence.
	Monitor the client's skin for break in the integrity, paying special attention to the pressure areas (coccyx, occiput) and to the area where electrocautery pad was applied.
	Monitor for any signs of neurological damage related to positioning.
	Monitor the client's urinary output for a minimum of 30 ml/hr and palpate the bladder to detect urinary retention.
	Monitor the client's bowel sounds to rule out postoperative ileus.
Pain assessment	Monitor the client for the presence of pain, including assessment of nonverbal cues.
	Monitor the client for adverse reaction to pain medications, including decreased respirations, decreased pulse oximeter readings, and nausea or vomiting.
	Administer prescribed analgesics and antiemetics as ordered.
	Ask the client to rate pain and evaluate pain management strategies frequently.
	Provide emotional support to the client.
	Reposition the client for comfort.
Promote adequate oxygenation	Monitor the client's airway at all times.
	Ascertain oxygenation status by monitoring respirations, skin color, and pulse oximetry.
	Auscultate lung sounds.
	Encourage coughing, deep breathing, and the use of incentive spirometry.
	Reposition the client frequently; encourage ambulation as tolerated and prescribed.
	Provide adequate pain relief to promote lung expansion.
	Have the client splint the incision as needed.
Prevention of deep vein thrombosis	Administer prescribed anticoagulants as ordered.
	Apply and monitor sequential compression devices, TED stockings, or plexipulses as ordered.
	Encourage leg exercises if not contraindicated.
	Monitor for clinical manifestations of deep vein thrombosis—calf tenderness, swelling, and redness.

© Cengage Learning 2015

PRACTICE QUESTIONS

1. The nurse evaluates which of the following drugs to place the surgical client at risk for perioperative complications?
   Select all that apply:
   [ ] 1. Acetaminophen (Tylenol)
   [ ] 2. Acetylsalicylic acid (aspirin)
   [ ] 3. Omeprazole (Prilosec)
   [ ] 4. Diphenhydramine (Sominex)
   [ ] 5. Ibuprofen (Motrin)
   [ ] 6. Sertraline (Zoloft)

2. Which of the following should the nurse include when teaching a client about an upcoming outpatient surgery?
   1. Postoperative nursing interventions
   2. Risk for postoperative complications
   3. Risks and benefits of proposed surgical procedure
   4. Risks and benefits of anesthetic choices

3. In reviewing the chart of a client about to undergo general anesthesia, which of the following is the greatest risk factor? The client who
   1. expresses anxiety about the upcoming procedure.
   2. ate a snack within the last three hours.
   3. smokes and states his last cigarette was 24 hours ago.
   4. has a history of hypertension controlled by diet and exercise.

4. Which of the following is a priority in the nursing assessment of a client preoperatively?
   1. Question the client about any known allergies
   2. Verification of client identification
   3. Determination of client's nutritional status
   4. Verification of client's neurological status

5. The nurse is obtaining a nursing history from a client suspected to be at risk for malignant hyperthermia. Which of the following should the nurse assess first to elicit the most accurate risk assessment?

1. Previous history of complications associated with surgery
2. Drug allergies
3. Over-the-counter medication usage
4. History of unexplained fevers

6. The nurse is concerned about a client's risk for impaired gas exchange related to ineffective airway clearance. Which of the following would be a priority assessment?
   1. Number of respirations per minute
   2. Number of liters of oxygen per minute inspired
   3. Decreased air movement
   4. Capillary refill

7. The nurse is caring for a postoperative client who has received a general anesthetic. Which of the following observations is the priority to be immediately reported?
   1. Complaints of nausea
   2. Mild hypertension
   3. Decreased urine output
   4. Rising body temperature

8. The nurse is caring for a client who is perioperative. Which of the following is a priority nursing intervention utilized to prevent infection in this client?
   1. Preparation of the skin overlying the surgical site
   2. Maintenance of hemodynamic status
   3. Maintenance of client's temperature
   4. Determination of estimated blood loss

9. When caring for a client receiving conscious sedation, which of the following should the perioperative nurse routinely monitor?
   1. Temperature
   2. Level of consciousness
   3. Dermatome level
   4. Urine output

10. Which of the following should the perioperative nurse monitor when evaluating the presence of ineffective thermoregulation in a client?
    1. Cardiac rhythm
    2. Blood pressure
    3. Oxygen saturation level
    4. Temperature

11. Which of the following is the priority nursing intervention that the nurse should perform for a client in the postoperative period after surgery?
    1. Establish a patent airway
    2. Maintain adequate blood pressure
    3. Establish level of consciousness
    4. Assess level of pain

12. The nurse is caring for a client postoperatively. Which of the following would indicate that the client has a compromised airway? The client
    1. complains of anxiety.
    2. complains of pain.

3. has a pulse oximetry reading of 90%.
4. is slightly cool and clammy.

13. The nurse is caring for a client who developed a compromised airway. Which of the following interventions is the priority to perform first?
    1. Reposition the client in a supine position
    2. Open the airway with a chin lift or jaw thrust
    3. Prepare for reintubation of the client
    4. Notify the surgeon

14. Which of the following nursing measures should the nurse include in the plan of care to help reduce the clinical manifestations of laryngospasm?
    1. Administer atropine
    2. Reposition the client in a supine position
    3. Administer high-flow oxygen via face mask
    4. Administer succinylcholine (Anectine)

15. The nurse is caring for a client in the immediate postoperative period. Which of the following would indicate that the client is becoming hypovolemic?
    1. A diastolic blood pressure of 100 mm Hg
    2. The client complains of excruciating pain
    3. The client complains of anxiety
    4. Blood loss of 500 ml

16. The nurse is caring for a client postoperatively who develops sinus tachycardia. Which of the following interventions should the nurse perform?
    1. Apply warmed blankets
    2. Administer atropine sulfate
    3. Position the client in a left lateral position
    4. Manage the client's anxiety

17. The nurse is caring for a client postoperatively who has become hypothermic. The nurse's best action would be to
    1. position the client in a left lateral position.
    2. administer an analgesic.
    3. remove clothing saturated with blood.
    4. monitor the intake and output.

18. A client is experiencing confusion in the immediate postoperative period. Which of the following assessments is essential to determine the reason for the confusion?
    1. Airway status
    2. Cardiac rhythm
    3. Level of consciousness
    4. Level of anxiety

19. The nurse admits a client scheduled for surgery. Which of the following findings should the nurse report as a risk factor for aspiration?
    1. Obesity
    2. Cigarette smoking
    3. An elevated serum sodium level
    4. A history of sleep apnea

20. Which of the following is a priority in the plan of care for a client who has had abdominal surgery and complains of pain in the immediate postoperative period?
    1. Monitor the client's blood pressure
    2. Teach the client to splint the abdomen
    3. Reposition the client for comfort
    4. Ask the client to describe the pain

21. A 16-year-old client has a medical history of anorexia nervosa. The nurse is preparing the client for abdominal surgery. The nurse is most concerned about the client's risk for
    1. aspiration.
    2. infection.
    3. hypovolemia.
    4. tissue perfusion.

22. A client is scheduled for an operative procedure to rule out cancer. When the nurse assesses the client, the nurse observes tears in the client's eyes. Which of the following would be the most therapeutic nursing intervention?
    1. Contact the surgeon to alleviate the client's concerns
    2. Ask the client to describe his or her feelings
    3. Medicate the client with a preoperative analgesic
    4. Reassure the client that there is nothing to be concerned about

23. A client is admitted for emergency surgery for a bowel obstruction. The perioperative nurse understands that the client is at greatest risk during the perioperative period for
    1. infection.
    2. electrolyte imbalances.
    3. aspiration.
    4. airway obstruction.

24. A client admitted to the postanesthesia care unit (PACU) after abdominal surgery complains of "feeling a pop" and a gush of warm fluid at the incision site. The nurse concludes that the client has experienced a wound dehiscence. The priority nursing interventions would be to Select all that apply:
    [ ] 1. Position the client in a supine position
    [ ] 2. Obtain a complete set of vital signs
    [ ] 3. Cover the incision with a sterile dressing
    [ ] 4. Apply oxygen via nasal cannula at 8 L per minute
    [ ] 5. Contact the surgical team
    [ ] 6. Increase the IV fluid rate

25. A client has a PCA (patient-controlled analgesia) machine ordered to manage postoperative pain. The PACU (postanesthesia care unit) nurse determines that the best time to initiate the PCA machine is
    1. when the client complains of pain.
    2. when the client arrives at the PACU.
    3. just prior to transfer of the client to the floor.
    4. when the client shows evidence of nonverbal signs of pain.

26. The registered nurse is preparing the clinical assignments for the day. Which of the following may the nurse delegate to a licensed practical nurse?
    1. Inform a client scheduled for surgery on the surgical procedure
    2. Instruct a client scheduled for surgery on the preoperative preparation
    3. Obtain an informed consent from a client
    4. Administer the preoperative intramuscular medication

ANSWERS AND RATIONALES

1. 2. 4. 5. 6. Drugs that place clients at risk during the perioperative period include aspirin, antidepressants, anticholinergics, steroids, nonsteroidal anti-inflammatory, antihypertensives, tranquilizers, diuretics, and drugs containing bromide. Acetylsalicylic acid (aspirin) may increase bleeding during surgery. Diphenhydramine (Sominex) contains bromide, which can accumulate in the body and produce manifestations of dementia. Nonsteroidal anti-inflammatory drugs such as ibuprofen (Motrin) may increase the risk of stress ulcers and displace other drugs from blood proteins. Antidepressants such as sertraline (Zoloft) may lower blood pressure during anesthesia.

Acetaminophen (Tylenol) and omeprazole (Prilosec) have no effect on the surgical process.

2. 1. Preoperative teaching involves educating the client about anticipated postoperative nursing interventions, including turning, coughing, deep breathing, and leg exercises. Risks of complications, proposed surgical procedures, and anesthetic choices are primarily discussed with the client by the surgical and anesthetic team.

3. 2. Aspiration poses a risk during general anesthesia. Clients are instructed not to eat or drink anything prior to general anesthesia in order to reduce the risk of aspiration. Although cigarette smoking and controlled hypertension may increase risks of complications

postoperatively, aspiration poses a more significant risk in this situation. Anxiety does not pose a risk factor for general anesthesia.

4. 2. Prior to completing any assessment of a client preoperatively, it is imperative to correctly verify the client's identity. After verification of client identity, the nursing assessment can continue; this would include assessing the client's allergies, nutritional status, and neurological status.

5. 1. An integral part of the preoperative nursing assessment is the determination of previous complications associated with surgery. Drug allergies, over-the-counter medication usage, and a history of unexplained fevers are not associated with malignant hyperthermia. Malignant hyperthermia is a potentially life-threatening syndrome characterized by a hypermetabolic state caused by certain anesthetic agents, such as succinylcholine.

6. 3. Decreased air movement may indicate a significant respiratory compromise. Assessing the client's ability to move air is a priority nursing assessment. The number of respirations per minute, number of liters of oxygen inspired, and capillary refill are important assessment data, but are not priority assessments.

7. 4. A rising body temperature can indicate malignant hyperthermia, a rare but life-threatening complication of general anesthesia. Complaints of nausea, mild hypertension, and decreased urine output would need to be conveyed to the anesthesia or surgical team, but are not emergent complaints.

8. 1. Preparation of the skin is a priority nursing intervention utilized to prevent infection. Maintenance of hemodynamic status, temperature, and estimated blood loss do not impact on a client's risk for infection.

9. 2. Level of consciousness is routinely monitored in the provision of conscious sedation. Temperature and urine output are monitored in the postoperative phase. Dermatome level is monitored postoperatively after the provision of regional anesthesia.

10. 4. Body temperature is the primary method of assessment utilized by nurses to determine the client's thermoregulation. Cardiac rhythm, blood pressure, and oxygen saturation levels are all monitored, but give little indication of the client's risk for altered body temperature.

11. 1. The first priority in caring for a client in the postoperative period is the establishment of a patent airway. Maintenance of hemodynamic stability, determination of level of consciousness, and assessment of pain are all important aspects in postoperative care, but are not the priorities.

12. 1. Hypoxemia is often associated with complaints of anxiety. A complaint of pain is a common postoperative complaint but is not associated with airway compromise. Normal pulse oximetry levels are above 90%. The assessment finding of coolness and clamminess is a nonspecific assessment finding that may indicate a wide variety of problems.

13. 2. The initial priority nursing intervention for a client experiencing a compromised airway is the reestablishment of the airway. The client may need to be repositioned but often to a Fowler's or lateral position. The client may need to be reintubated and the surgeon should be notified, but these are not the priority interventions.

14. 4. With severe laryngospasm, a client may require the administration of a muscle relaxant such as succinylcholine (Anectine) to relax the muscles of the larynx. Clients experiencing laryngospasm are often repositioned into a semi-Fowler's position. The administration of high-flow oxygen is based upon client's oxygen saturation levels and may be used to treat hypoxia, but will not directly reduce the clinical manifestations of laryngospasm.

15. 4. Blood loss and resulting low fluid volume may result in hypovolemia in the postoperative period. Anxiety and pain may cause hypertension in the perioperative client, but would not cause hypovolemia. An elevated diastolic blood pressure is not indicative of hypovolemia.

16. 4. Treatment of sinus tachycardia involves treating the underlying cause. Sinus tachycardia is a common dysrhythmia often caused by anxiety. Atropine is a drug commonly used to treat sinus bradycardia. Applying warmed blankets and positioning a client in the left lateral position would not be performed for sinus tachycardia.

17. 3. The nurse removes clothing saturated with blood and reapplies clean and dry clothing in order to maintain a client's body temperature. Repositioning a client, medicating a client for pain, or monitoring intake and output do not treat a client's low body temperature.

18. 1. The nurse must first rule out hypoxemia as being the cause of a client's confusion. A client with an impaired airway may be experiencing confusion due to hypoxemia. Cardiac rhythm, level of consciousness, and anxiety are all important assessments in the postoperative period, but are not the initial assessment in a client presenting with confusion.

19. 1. Obesity increases a client's risk for aspiration due to increased pressure of abdominal contents on the lower esophageal sphincter. Cigarette smoking, an elevated serum sodium level, or a history of sleep apnea do not increase the risk of aspiration.

20. 4. A priority assessment for a client's pain includes a description of the severity and nature of the pain as experienced by the client. Monitoring blood pressure, repositioning of the client, and teaching the client to splint the abdomen are all important postoperative nursing interventions, but are not priority interventions in the management of the client's postoperative pain.

21. 2. Clients who have experienced anorexia nervosa are at risk for malnutrition and lowered immune function, and may experience an increased risk of infection and tissue healing. A history of anorexia nervosa does not pose a greater-than-average risk for aspiration, hypovolemia, or altered tissue perfusion.

22. 2. Assessing what the client is actually experiencing will assist the nurse in selecting the most appropriate nursing intervention. Supporting and advocating for the client are nursing responsibilities. The surgeon may be contacted if the client has specific concerns, but would not be contacted prior to an initial assessment. Medicating the client with a preoperative analgesic would be inappropriate without first addressing the client's concerns or questions.

23. 3. Clients who have bowel obstructions are at increased risk of aspiration because the intestinal contents can be vomited and aspirated during induction of anesthesia. Clients who have bowel obstructions are

not at an increased risk during the perioperative period for infection or airway obstruction. Fluid shifts may occur in the client with a bowel obstruction, but aspiration presents a greater risk for the client.

24. 1. 3. 5. The priority nursing interventions include repositioning the client in a supine position to prevent evisceration of abdominal contents, covering the wound with a sterile dressing, and notifying the surgical team immediately. Administering oxygen may be applied if the client's oxygen saturation is low. The IV rate may be increased if there is an indication to do so, but is not a priority intervention.

25. 2. PCA (patient-controlled analgesia) is an effective mechanism for the management of client pain. It is initiated upon arrival to the postanesthesia care unit (PACU) and client education is reinforced during the client's stay in the PACU. A delay in initiation of the PCA device may cause an increase in client pain.

26. 4. A licensed practical nurse may administer a preoperative intramuscular medication to a client scheduled for surgery. Informing a client scheduled for surgery on the surgical procedure and instructing a client scheduled for surgery on the preoperative preparation are job tasks reserved for the registered nurse. A licensed practical nurse may not obtain an informed consent because the surgeon must inform the client about the surgical procedure and obtain the informed consent.

REFERENCES

Daniels, R., & Nicoll, L. (2012). *Contemporary medical-surgical nursing.* Clifton Park, NY: Delmar Cengage Learning.

DeLaune, S. C., & Ladner, P. K. (2011). *Fundamentals of nursing: Standard and practice* (4th ed.). Clifton Park, NY: Delmar Cengage Learning.

Spratto, G. R., & Woods, A. L. (2012). *PDR nurse's drug handbook 2012.* Clifton Park, NY: Delmar Cengage Learning.

UNIT III

PHARMACOLOGY

CHAPTER 15

MEDICATION THERAPY

I. SAFE DRUG ADMINISTRATION
  A. PHARMACOLOGY
   1. THE STUDY OF DRUGS, THEIR USES (PHARMACOLOGY), HOW THE BODY RESPONDS TO DRUGS (PHARMACODYNAMICS), AND THE ABSORPTION, DISTRIBUTION, METABOLISM, AND EXCRETION OF DRUGS (PHARMACOKINETICS) IS ESSENTIAL FOR THE SAFE ADMINISTRATION OF DRUGS.
  B. DRUG USES
   1. RELIEF OF THE DISEASE MANIFESTATIONS IS THE MOST COMMON USE OF DRUGS, SUCH AS ANTIHISTAMINES USED IN THE TREATMENT OF ALLERGIES.
   2. CURATIVE DRUGS SUCH AS ANTIBIOTICS ARE USED TO CURE DISEASES.
   3. DIAGNOSTIC DRUGS SUCH AS RADIOPAQUE DYES ARE CONSIDERED DRUGS BECAUSE THEY ALLOW THE DETECTION OF DISEASE.
   4. HEALTH MAINTENANCE DRUGS SUCH AS INSULIN, VITAMINS, AND MINERALS ARE USED TO KEEP THE BODY HEALTHY.
   5. PREVENTIVE DRUGS SUCH AS THE HEPATITIS VACCINE ARE USED TO PREVENT DISEASE.
   6. CONTRACEPTIVE DRUGS SUCH AS ORAL CONTRACEPTIVES ARE USED TO PREVENT PREGNANCY.
  C. DRUG NAMES
   1. CHEMICAL NAMES SUCH AS ACETYLSALICYLIC ACID DESCRIBE THE CHEMICAL COMPOSITION AND MOLECULAR STRUCTURE OF THE DRUG.
   2. GENERIC OR NONPROPRIETARY DRUGS SUCH AS ASPIRIN HAVE A SIMPLER NAME THAN A CHEMICAL NAME AND ARE MUCH LESS EXPENSIVE THAN A BRAND-NAME DRUG.
   3. TRADE, BRAND, OR PROPRIETARY NAMES SUCH AS NITRO-BID, NITRONG, AND NITROSTAT ARE KNOWN BY SEVERAL NAMES AND SOLD BY DRUG MANUFACTURERS.
  D. DRUG LAWS
   1. FOOD AND DRUG ACT OF 1906
      a. Required that all drugs in the United States meet minimal standards of strength, purity, and quality
      b. Established the U.S. Pharmacopoeia (USP) and the National Formulary (NF) as the legal standards for drugs in the United States
   2. FOOD, DRUG, AND COSMETIC ACT (FDCA) OF 1938
      a. Regulates sale and content of drugs and cosmetics
      b. Requires specific labeling and cautions against unsafe use
      c. Mandates governmental review of safety studies before selling new drugs
   3. DURHAM-HUMPHREY AMENDMENT OF 1952
      a. Requires that certain drugs be dispensed and refilled only by a prescription
      b. Recognizes that certain drugs may be sold without a prescription (over the counter [OTC])
      c. Mandates that certain drugs be classified as legend drugs
   4. KEFAUVER-HARRIS AMENDMENT OF 1962
      a. Requires that both prescription and nonprescription drugs be effective and

safely distributed with information on the uses, action, adverse reactions, and contraindications

5. COMPREHENSIVE DRUG ABUSE PREVENTION AND CONTROL ACT OF 1970 (CONTROLLED SUBSTANCE ACT) (SEE TABLE 15-1)
   a. Classifies drugs according to their potential for abuse
   b. Regulates the manufacture and distribution of drugs that have the potential to cause dependency

E. DRUG ORDER
   1. NAME OF THE CLIENT
   2. DATE AND TIME OF WRITTEN ORDER
   3. NAME OF DRUG TO BE GIVEN
   4. DOSE OF DRUG
   5. ROUTE OF ADMINISTRATION
   6. TIME OF ADMINISTRATION
   7. SIGNATURE OF THE PERSON WRITING THE ORDER

F. RIGHTS OF MEDICATION ADMINISTRATION
   1. RIGHT DRUG
   2. RIGHT DOSE
   3. RIGHT CLIENT
   4. RIGHT TIME
   5. RIGHT ROUTE
   6. RIGHT DOCUMENTATION
   7. RIGHT TECHNIQUE

II. DRUG ASSESSMENT
   A. ASSESSMENT
      1. OBTAIN A COMPLETE MEDICAL HISTORY, INCLUDING CHRONIC DISEASES AND SURGERIES.
      2. QUESTION THE CLIENT REGARDING CURRENT PRESCRIPTION DRUGS, OVER-THE-COUNTER DRUGS, HERBAL SUPPLEMENTATION, AND ILLICIT DRUGS.
      3. QUESTION THE CLIENT REGARDING DRUG AND FOOD ALLERGIES (IODINE CONTRAINDICATED IN CLIENTS ALLERGIC TO SHELLFISH AND SOME VACCINES CONTRAINDICATED IN CLIENTS ALLERGIC TO EGGS).
      4. ASSESS ANY ADVERSE REACTIONS THE CLIENT MAY EXPERIENCE WITH DRUGS TAKEN.
      5. OBTAIN THE CLIENT'S BIOGRAPHICAL DATA TO ASCERTAIN AGE, EDUCATION, OCCUPATION, AND DRUG

Table 15-1 Controlled Substances Schedules

Schedule	Characteristics	Examples
Schedule I	High potential for abuse; No accepted medical use; Research purposes only; Unsafe	Heroin, lysergic acid diethylamide (LSD), marijuana, methaqualone (Quaalude)
Schedule II	High potential for abuse; Does have medical use; Prescription only; No phone refills	Meperidine (Demerol), morphine, methylphenidate (Ritalin), hydromorphone (Dilaudid), cocaine, oxycodone (OxyContin), amphetamines
Schedule III	Moderate potential for abuse; Does have medical use; Prescription only; May be filled five times in 6 months; High psychological dependence; Low physical dependence	Glutethimide (Doriden), secobarbital (Seconal), Tylenol with codeine, hydrocodone with acetaminophen (Vicodin), butabarbital (Butisol), barbiturates
Schedule IV	Lower potential for abuse over Schedule III; Does have medical use; Limited dependence; May be filled five times in 6 months	Chlordiazepoxide (Librium), diazepam (Valium), flurazepam (Dalmane), oxazepam (Serax), phenobarbital, lorazepam (Ativan), pentazocine (Talwin), alprazolam (Xanax)
Schedule V	Low potential for abuse; Does have medical use; Over-the-counter narcotic drugs that must be sold by a registered pharmacist	Cough syrup with codeine, guaifenesin (Naldecon DX), diphenoxylate HCl with atropine sulfate (Lomotil), Novahistine Expectorant
Schedule VI	Some states such as North Carolina have adopted a Schedule VI	Marijuana is the only drug in this schedule; it has limited medicinal use by prescription in certain situations

INSURANCE COVERAGE THAT MAY INFLUENCE DRUG COMPLIANCE.

6. ASSESS THE CLIENT'S LIFESTYLE BEHAVIORS (DIET, SMOKING, ALCOHOL, ILLEGAL DRUGS) AND CULTURAL BELIEFS THAT MAY INFLUENCE COMPLIANCE WITH DRUG REGIMEN.

7. ASSESS THE CLIENT'S SENSORY AND COGNITIVE STATUS, INCLUDING HEARING, VISION, WEAKNESS, PARALYSIS, AND MEMORY IMPAIRMENT, WHICH MAY INTERFERE WITH CORRECT DRUG ADMINISTRATION.

8. PERFORM A COMPLETE PHYSICAL HISTORY, INCLUDING AN EVALUATION OF BODY SYSTEMS, HEIGHT, WEIGHT, AND VITAL SIGNS.

9. MONITOR DIAGNOSTIC AND LABORATORY DATA THAT MAY EITHER EVALUATE THE BODY'S RESPONSE TO MEDICATIONS OR MAY BE AFFECTED WITH DRUG ADMINISTRATION.

B. PLANNING
1. DEVELOP A TEACHING PLAN ON THE ACTION, USES, ADVERSE REACTIONS, AND INTERVENTIONS FOR PRESCRIBED DRUGS.

2. EVALUATE LABORATORY DATA ON WHICH SAFE DRUG ADMINISTRATION IS DEPENDENT (SERUM GLUCOSE FOR INSULIN, DIGOXIN LEVEL FOR DIGOXIN [LANOXIN]).

3. DETERMINE APPROPRIATE NURSING DIAGNOSES FOR SAFE DRUG ADMINISTRATION.

C. IMPLEMENTATION
1. REVIEW THE AGENCY'S POLICIES FOR DRUG ADMINISTRATION PROCEDURE.

2. INITIATE DISCHARGE TEACHING ON SAFE DRUG ADMINISTRATION.

3. IMPLEMENT A TEACHING PLAN ON THE DRUG'S ACTION, USE, ADVERSE REACTIONS, AND INTERVENTIONS.

4. INCLUDE A FAMILY MEMBER IN THE DRUG TEACHING WHEN APPROPRIATE.

5. INSTRUCT THE CLIENT ON THE APPROPRIATE METHOD OF DRUG SELF-ADMINISTRATION.

6. USE ONLY ACCEPTABLE ABBREVIATIONS IN DRUG ORDERS AND DOCUMENTATION (SEE TABLE 15-2).

7. ADMINISTER THE DRUG BY THE APPROPRIATE ROUTE AND METHOD.

D. EVALUATION
1. EVALUATE CLIENT OUTCOME FROM DRUG ADMINISTRATION.

III. **REVIEW PRINCIPLES OF DRUG ADMINISTRATION**
A. ORAL
1. REVIEW THE PROCEDURE FOR ORAL DRUG ADMINISTRATION.

2. ENSURE THAT THE CLIENT HAS THE ABILITY TO SAFELY SWALLOW THE DRUG.

3. MAINTAIN THE CLIENT IN AN UPRIGHT POSITION AFTER ADMINISTERING THE DRUG TO PREVENT ASPIRATION.

4. SAVE THE EMESIS AND NEVER READMINISTER A DRUG WITHOUT AN ORDER IF THE CLIENT VOMITED AFTER TAKING A DOSE.

5. AVOID TOUCHING THE DRUG WHEN SETTING IT UP.

6. NEVER CRUSH OR DISRUPT ENTERIC-COATED, SUSTAINED-ACTION, SUBLINGUAL, AND BUCCAL DRUGS.

7. PLACE A SUBLINGUAL DRUG UNDER THE TONGUE AND INSTRUCT THE CLIENT TO AVOID CHEWING THE DRUG OR SMOKING UNTIL THE DRUG IS DISSOLVED.

8. AVOID ADMINISTERING TABLETS AND CAPSULES TO CHILDREN UNDER THE AGE OF 5 YEARS (LIQUID DRUGS ARE THE PREFERRED ROUTE).

9. UNLESS CONTRAINDICATED, MIX A SMALL AMOUNT OF FLAVORING WITH DRUGS TO ENSURE PALATABILITY.

10. OFFER FINELY CRUSHED ICE WITH A CARBONATED BEVERAGE POURED OVER IT FOLLOWING ADMINISTRATION OF A DRUG TO DECREASE NAUSEA.

11. MEASURE LIQUID DRUGS IN AN ORAL SYRINGE, PLASTIC CUP, OR TEASPOON TO ENSURE AN ACCURATE DOSE.

12. MONITOR OLDER ADULT CLIENTS FOR FLUID OVERLOAD.

13. ADMINISTER ONE DRUG AT A TIME TO OLDER ADULT CLIENTS.

14. CONSIDER DECREASED GASTRIC ACIDITY, DECREASED PERISTALSIS, AND DELAYED GASTRIC MOTILITY, WHICH MAY DECREASE ABSORPTION AND EXCRETION.

15. INSTRUCT THE CLIENT TO USE A DAY AND TIME PILL BOX FOR ORGANIZATION OF DRUGS AT HOME.

16. CRUSH DIFFICULT-TO-SWALLOW DRUGS UNLESS CONTRAINDICATED, OR MIX WITH APPLESAUCE TO FACILITATE SWALLOWING.

B. NASOGASTRIC
1. ENSURE CORRECT PLACEMENT OF THE NASOGASTRIC (NG) TUBE BEFORE

Table 15-2 Abbreviations Commonly Found in Drug Orders

Abbreviation	English Meaning	Abbreviation	English Meaning
āā.	of each	NGT	nasogastric tube
ad lib	freely, as desired	p̄	after
a.c.	before meals	p.c.	after meals
b.i.d., B.I.D.	twice a day	p.o., PO	by mouth
c̄	with	p.r.n., PRN	as the occasion arises, when needed or requested
Caps.	capsule(s)	Q	every
Cc	cubic centimeter	q.h.	every hour
dl, dL	deciliter	Q2h	every 2 hours
elix.	elixir	Q4h	every 4 hours
ext.	extract	Q6h	every 6 hours
g, gm, G, Gm	gram	Q8h	every 8 hours
Gr	grain	Q12h	every 12 hours
Gtt	drop(s)	s̄	without
h, hr	hour	Subcut	subcutaneously
ID	intradermal	S.L.	sublingually
IM	intramuscularly	Sol.	solution
inj.	by injection	s̄s̄	one-half
I.U.	International Units	Stat	immediately
IV or I.V.	intravenously	susp.	suspension
IVPB	intravenous piggyback	tab.	tablet
Kg	kilogram	t.i.d., T.I.D.	three times a day
Kvo	keep vein open	TPN	total parenteral nutrition
L	liter	tr.	tincture
Mcq	micrograms	tsp.	teaspoon
mEq	milliequivalents	U	unit
Mg	milligram		
ml, mL	milliliter		
n, noc	night		

DRUG ADMINISTRATION THROUGH THE TUBE.
2. AVOID ADDING DRUGS TO THE FEEDING TUBE UNLESS THERE IS AN ORDER.
3. UNLESS CONTRAINDICATED, ADMINISTER ONE DRUG AT A TIME WITH APPROXIMATELY 30 ML OF WATER. FLUSH BETWEEN DRUGS WITH 5 TO 30 ML WATER AND FOLLOW WITH 30 TO 50 ML (FOR ADULTS) OR 20 TO 25 ML (FOR CHILDREN) AT THE END AND CLAMP FOR APPROXIMATELY 30 MINUTES.
4. MAINTAIN THE CLIENT IN AN UPRIGHT POSITION FOR AT LEAST 30 MINUTES FOLLOWING DRUG INSTILLATION.
C. TOPICAL (EYE, EAR, NOSE, THROAT, VAGINA, RECTUM, AND SKIN)
   1. REVIEW THE PROCEDURE FOR EYE, EAR, NOSE, THROAT, RECTAL, AND SKIN DRUG ADMINISTRATION.

2. INSTRUCT THE CLIENT THAT TOPICAL DRUGS PRODUCE A LOCALIZED OR SYSTEMIC EFFECT, PROVIDE A CONTINUOUS ABSORPTION, AND PROTECT THE SKIN.

3. ASSESS THE AREA THAT THE TOPICAL DRUG IS TO BE ADMINISTERED FOR ERYTHEMA OR ANY BREAKS IN THE SKIN.

4. WEAR GLOVES WHEN ADMINISTERING TOPICAL DRUGS.

5. USE AN APPLICATOR TO REMOVE A PASTE, CREAM, OR OINTMENT TO PREVENT CROSS CONTAMINATION BETWEEN CLIENTS FOLLOWED BY APPLYING THE DRUG WITH LONG SMOOTH STROKES IN THE DIRECTION OF THE HAIR FOLLICLES.

6. INSTRUCT THE CLIENT TO AVOID SHARING OF EYEDROP OR EARDROP BOTTLES.

7. AVOID TOUCHING THE EYE DROPPER TO ANY PART OF THE CLIENT'S EYE AND DISCARD THE DROPPER IF IT BECOMES CONTAMINATED.

8. CLEARLY LABEL EYE AND EAR DROPPER BOTTLES WITH LARGE PRINT FOR CLIENTS WITH GLAUCOMA OR CATARACTS TO PREVENT INSTILLING THE DRUG IN THE WRONG EYE OR EAR.

9. INSTRUCT THE OLDER ADULT CLIENT ON WAYS TO ADMINISTER EYEDROPS BY BRACING THE UNUSED FINGERS ON THE FACE OR ON THE SIDE OF THE HEAD.

10. ENCOURAGE THE PARENTS OF A CHILD WITH AN EYE INFECTION TO DISCOURAGE THE CHILD FROM RUBBING THE EYES TO PREVENT CROSS CONTAMINATION AND TO WASH HANDS FREQUENTLY.

11. INSTRUCT THE CLIENT WITH CONTACT LENS TO CLEARLY LABEL EYEDROP BOTTLES TO PREVENT CONFUSION WITH SIMILAR SIZE BOTTLES SUCH AS LIQUID GLUE OR NAIL POLISH.

12. INSTRUCT THE PARENTS AND CLIENTS TO ENSURE GOOD LIGHTING IN THE HOME AT ALL TIMES TO AVOID MISTAKES IN BOTTLE IDENTIFICATION.

13. INSTRUCT THE CLIENT USING A NASAL SPRAY TO INHALE WHEN ADMINISTERING THE NASAL SPRAY.

14. INSERT THE NASAL DROPPER 3/8 INCH INTO THE NOSTRIL WITHOUT TOUCHING THE SIDES OF THE NOSTRIL AND REMAIN IN AN APPROPRIATE POSITION FOR 5 MINUTES AFTER ADMINISTRATION.

15. INSTRUCT THE CLIENT WITH NASAL CONGESTION THAT SALINE NASAL SPRAYS MAY BE USED IN CONJUNCTION WITH DECONGESTANTS FOR THE CONGESTION.

16. PLACE THE OLDER ADULT CLIENT IN AN ALTERNATIVE POSITION IF THE SIMS' OR RECUMBENT POSITION IS DIFFICULT FOR VAGINAL DRUGS.

17. INSTRUCT THE CLIENT WHO RECEIVED A VAGINAL DRUG TO LIE DOWN FOR 20 MINUTES AFTER ADMINISTRATION OF THE DRUG TO PREVENT LEAKAGE OF THE DRUG.

18. ADJUST THE DOSE OF TOPICAL (SKIN) DRUGS FOR OLDER ADULT CLIENTS AS PRESCRIBED BECAUSE OF THIN SKIN.

D. PARENTERAL INJECTIONS

1. REVIEW THE PROCEDURE FOR PARENTERAL DRUG ADMINISTRATION.

2. WEAR GLOVES FOR ALL PARENTERAL DRUG INJECTIONS.

3. NEVER RECAP A NEEDLE AFTER GIVING AN INJECTION.

4. SELECT THE APPROPRIATE-SIZE SYRINGE FOR PARENTERAL DRUG ADMINISTRATION (SEE TABLE 15-3).

5. SELECT THE APPROPRIATE-SIZE NEEDLE FOR PARENTERAL DRUG ADMINISTRATION (SEE TABLE 15-4).

6. ADMINISTER AN INTRADERMAL INJECTION TO THE FOREARM OR UPPER BACK.

7. INSERT THE INTRADERMAL NEEDLE AT A 5- TO 15-DEGREE ANGLE; AVOID ASPIRATION. INJECT THE DRUG TO FORM A SMALL BLEB AND AVOID MASSAGING THE SITE.

8. ADMINISTER SUBCUTANEOUS INJECTION TO THE VASCULAR AREAS AROUND THE POSTERIOR ASPECT OF THE UPPER ARMS, ABDOMEN, OR ANTERIOR THIGH.

9. INSERT THE NEEDLE FOR A SUBCUTANEOUS INJECTION AT A 45-DEGREE ANGLE (DRUGS OTHER THAN INSULIN AND HEPARIN) TO A 90-DEGREE ANGLE (INSULIN, HEPARIN). INJECT THE DRUG AND MASSAGE THE SITE IF APPROPRIATE.

10. ADMINISTER INTRAMUSCULAR INJECTION TO THE VASTUS LATERALIS, VENTROGLUTEAL, DORSOGLUTEAL, AND DELTOID MUSCLES.

11. INSERT THE NEEDLE FOR AN INTRAMUSCULAR INJECTION AT A 90-DEGREE ANGLE, ASPIRATE, AND MASSAGE THE SITE AFTER ADMINISTRATION OF THE DRUG.

Table 15-3 Types of Syringes

Syringe	Size	Scale	General Uses	
Tuberculin (TB)	1 ml	0.01 ml	Intradermal injections Allergy injections Injectable medications for infants and young children Heparin injections Other situations requiring precise measurement of a small volume of medication (less than 1 ml)	
Insulin	0.3 ml 0.5 ml 1 ml	units	Administration of insulin of a specified strength	
General purpose	2–50 ml	ml	For use in administering 0.5–50 mL of medication; for example, the administration of antibiotics and pain medication	

© Cengage Learning 2015

Table 15-4 Selection of Needles for Injection

Type of Injection	Suggested Needle Gauge (G)	Suggested Needle Length	Nursing Implications
Intradermal	26 or 27 G	¼" or ⅜"	Used for diagnostic purposes and to determine sensitivity to injectable medications Most frequent site of injection is the inner aspect of the forearm
Subcutaneous	25 to 28 G	½" or ⅝" ⅞" in obese people	Used most frequently for administration of insulin and heparin Can be used for administration of fluids by clysis, when 22-G, 1½ ≤ needles are preferred
Intramuscular	21–23 G	1" to ½"	Longer needles are preferred for irritating medications. Larger-gauge needles (20 G) are preferred for viscous injectable products (e.g., those in an oil vehicle).
Intravenous	18–24 G 16 G	Various lengths depending on the type of equipment preferred (½"–1½")	Used for blood tests and administration of most fluids and electrolyte solutions Used for blood transfusions
Intracardiac	26 G	4"	For emergency use only by physician

© Cengage Learning 2015

12. SELECT THE DELTOID MUSCLE FOR AN INTRAMUSCULAR INJECTION OF 1 ML OR LESS OF A CLEAR, NONIRRITATING SOLUTION.
13. AVOID SELECTING THE DORSOGLUTEAL OR VENTROGLUTEAL SITES FOR INTRAMUSCULAR INJECTIONS IN INFANTS AND CHILDREN WHO HAVE NOT BEEN WALKING FOR 1 YEAR.
14. SELECT THE VASTUS LATERALIS AS THE PREFERRED SITE OF INTRAMUSCULAR DRUG ADMINISTRATION IN CHILDREN UNDER 3 YEARS OF AGE.
15. APPLY EMLA (LIDOCAINE 2.5% AND PRILOCAINE 2.5%) TO THE INTRAMUSCULAR INJECTION SITE 1–2 HOURS BEFORE ADMINISTERING AN INJECTION TO A CHILD.
16. AVOID ADMINISTERING MORE THAN 2 ML OF AN INTRAMUSCULAR DRUG TO ONE SITE FOR AN OLDER ADULT CLIENT, 1 ML FOR A CHILD, OR 0.5 ML FOR AN INFANT.
17. SELECT A TUBERCULIN SYRINGE (½ TO 1 INCH, 25- TO 27-GAUGE NEEDLE) FOR A SMALL DOSE OF AN INTRAMUSCULAR (IM) DRUG TO BE GIVEN TO A SMALL INFANT.
18. SELECT THE Z-TRACK INTRAMUSCULAR INJECTION METHOD FOR IRRITATING DRUGS SUCH AS IRON DEXTRAN AND HYDRALAZINE HYDROCHLORIDE (APRESOLINE).
19. DRAW UP THE DRUG TO BE GIVEN Z-TRACK WITH A LARGE-BORE NEEDLE, REPLACE IT WITH THE APPROPRIATE SIZE AND NEEDLE LENGTH FOR THE CLIENT, AND ADD 0.1 TO 0.2 ML OF AIR TO THE SYRINGE TO ENSURE ALL OF THE DRUG IS PUSHED OUT OF THE SYRINGE.
20. DISPLACE THE UPPER LAYER OF SKIN BEFORE INJECTING THE NEEDLE. INJECT THE DRUG SLOWLY AT A 90-DEGREE ANGLE, LEAVE THE NEEDLE IN PLACE FOR 10 SECONDS, AND AVOID RUBBING THE SITE AFTER ADMINISTRATION.
21. AFTER DISTRACTING THE CHILD, TAP THE INJECTION SITE LIGHTLY SO THE CHILD WILL FOCUS ON THE TAP AND NOT THE INJECTION.

IV. INTRAVENOUS THERAPY

A. PURPOSES AND USES
　1. MAINTAINS THE FLUID VOLUME WHEN THE CLIENT CANNOT TOLERATE ORAL OR TUBE FEEDINGS
　2. USED WHEN FLUID LOSSES ARE SEVERE
　3. REPLACEMENT OF FLUIDS, ELECTROLYTES, AND NUTRIENTS BY THE VENOUS ROUTE
　4. FACILITATES A VASCULAR ROUTE FOR DRUGS, BLOOD, OR BLOOD COMPONENTS

B. TYPES OF INTRAVENOUS SOLUTIONS (SEE TABLE 13-1)

C. LOCATION OF SITES
　1. PERIPHERAL (SEE FIGURE 15-1)
　2. VASCULAR ACCESS DEVICES

D. EQUIPMENT
　1. ALL EQUIPMENT IS PREPACKED, STERILE, AND DISPOSABLE.
　2. BUTTERFLY (SCALP VEIN OR WING-TIPPED)
　3. BEVELED SHORT NEEDLES WITH PLASTIC FLAPS ATTACHED TO THE SHAFT
　4. USED FOR SHORT-TERM (COUPLE HOURS WITH ENDOSCOPY) OR INTERMITTENT IV ACCESS IN INFANTS AND CHILDREN

E. ANGIOCATHETER (OVER-THE-NEEDLE)
　1. INTRACATH (PLASTIC TUBE INSERTED INTO A VEIN) INSERTED INTO THE SKIN AFTER PIERCING THE SKIN WITH A METAL STYLET INSIDE THE INTRACATH, FOLLOWED BY WITHDRAWAL OF THE STYLET WHEN CORRECT VEIN PLACEMENT IS SECURED
　2. GENERALLY USED FOR SHORT-TERM IV THERAPY
　3. SITE SHOULD BE CHANGED EVERY 72 HOURS.

F. SALINE LOCK
　1. THE HUB OF A PERIPHERAL CATHETER INSERTED INTO A VEIN IS CAPPED WITH A LOCK CALLED A LUER LOCK INJECTION SITE AND MUST BE CHANGED EVERY 72 HOURS.

G. NEEDLE-FREE SYSTEM
　1. NEEDLELESS SYSTEMS THAT PREVENT ACCIDENTAL NEEDLE STICKS (SEE FIGURE 15-2)

H. VASCULAR ACCESS DEVICES (CENTRAL VENOUS CATHETERS) (SEE TABLE 15-5)
　1. INCLUDES A VARIETY OF CATHETERS, CANNULAS, AND INFUSION PORTS
　2. USED FOR LONG-TERM IV THERAPY OR THE NECESSITY OF REPEATED ACCESS TO THE CENTRAL VENOUS SYSTEM
　3. ALL CENTRAL CATHETERS MUST BE RADIOPAQUE TO ALLOW CORRECT PLACEMENT BY RADIOGRAPHY BEFORE INITIATING ANY SOLUTION.

Figure 15-1 Peripheral veins used in intravenous therapy: A. Arm and forearm; B. Dorsum of the hand; C. Dorsal plexus of the foot

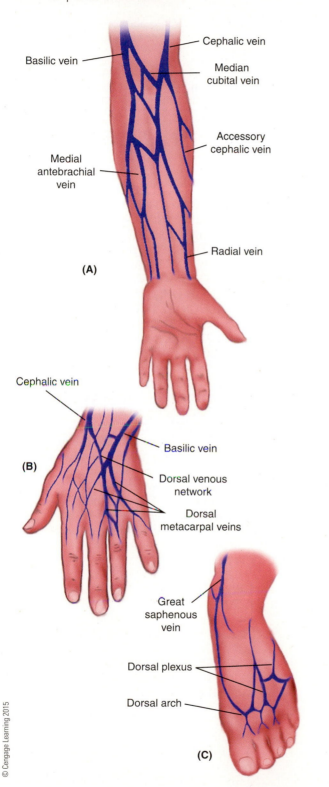

Figure 15-2 Needle-free system

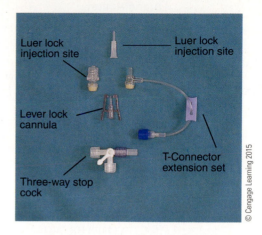

4. GENERALLY INSERTED INTO THE INTERNAL JUGULAR OR SUBCLAVIAN VEIN, WITH THE DISTAL TIP LOCATED IN THE SUPERIOR VENA CAVA TO MINIMIZE IRRITATION TO THE VESSEL AND SCLEROSIS (OCCASIONALLY, THE FEMORAL VEIN IS USED WHEN THROMBOSIS OF INTERNAL JUGULAR OR SUBCLAVIAN VEIN IS PRESENT)

5. SURGICALLY IMPLANTED CATHETERS MAY BE IMPLANTED (ENTIRELY UNDER THE SKIN) OR TUNNELED (CATHETER PARTIALLY EXITS THE SKIN).

6. TUNNELED CATHETERS SUCH AS THE HICKMAN CATHETER ARE INSERTED THROUGH SUBCUTANEOUS TISSUE, GENERALLY BETWEEN THE NIPPLE AND CLAVICLE, WITH THE CATHETER TIP INSERTED THROUGH THE CEPHALIC OR EXTERNAL JUGULAR VEIN AND THREADED TO THE RIGHT ATRIUM.

7. AN IMPLANTABLE PORT SUCH AS THE PORTACATH IS A RADIOPAQUE SILICONE CATHETER ATTACHED TO A PLASTIC OR STAINLESS STEEL INJECTION PORT WITH A SILICONE-RUBBER SELF-SEALING SEPTUM THAT ONLY SPECIALLY TRAINED NURSES MAY ACCESS BECAUSE OF THE RISK OF INFECTION IF THE NEEDLE IS INCORRECTLY PLACED.

8. NONCORING NEEDLES SUCH AS THE HUBER NEEDLE ARE USED TO ACCESS THE IMPLANTABLE PORT AND SHOULD BE CHANGED EVERY 7 DAYS.

9. PERIPHERALLY INSERTED CENTRAL CATHETER (PICC) IS A GENERIC NAME FOR SEVERAL DIFFERENT DEVICES THAT ARE INSERTED INTO ONE OF THE MAJOR VEINS OF THE ANTECUBITAL FOSSA.

© Cengage Learning 2015

Table 15-5 Vascular Access Devices

Type	Brand Name	Use
Nontunneled central venous catheter	Hohn, Deseret	Short-term fluid or blood administration, obtaining blood specimens, and (triple-lumen) administering medications
Tunneled central venous catheter (single or double lumen)	Hickman, Broviac, Groshong	Long-term (months to years) fluid replacement therapy, medication administration, nutritional supplement, and blood specimen withdrawal
Implanted infusion port	Chemo-Port, Infuse-a-Port, Mediport, Port-a-Cath	Long-term (months to years) fluid replacement therapy, medication administration (especially chemotherapy), blood or blood product administration, and blood specimen withdrawal
Peripherally inserted central catheter (PICC)	C-PICC, Groshong PICC, Solo PICC	Long-term fluid replacement therapy, medication administration (chemotherapy, antibiotics, controlled narcotics), blood or blood product administration, and blood specimen withdrawal

© Cengage Learning 2015

10. GENERALLY, THE PICC IS A 52-CM-LONG CATHETER WHOSE TIP IS PLACED IN THE LOWER THIRD OF THE SUPERIOR VENA CAVA.

11. MONITOR A CLIENT RECEIVING A CENTRAL VENOUS CATHETER FOR MANIFESTATIONS OF PNEUMOTHORAX, INCLUDING A SUDDEN SHORTNESS OF BREATH, SHARP CHEST PAIN, ANXIOUSNESS, A WEAK RAPID PULSE, HYPOTENSION, PALLOR, OR CYANOSIS, WHICH INDICATES PUNCTURE OF THE PLEURAL MEMBRANE.

V. ADMINISTRATION OF INTRAVENOUS THERAPY

A. SELECTION OF PERIPHERAL VEIN

1. ASSESS THE CLIENT'S AGE, BODY SIZE, AND CLINICAL CONDITION.
2. SELECT THE MOST DISTAL VEIN IN THE HAND, FOREARM, OR ANTECUBITAL FOSSA.
3. AVOID LOWER EXTREMITY VEINS BECAUSE THE BLOOD TENDS TO POOL, CLOT, AND RESULT IN AN EMBOLISM.
4. SELECT SCALP VEINS FOR AN INFANT.
5. SELECT THE MOST DISTAL END OF THE VEIN, MAINTAINING VEIN INTEGRITY AND AVOIDING INTERFERENCE WITH THE UPWARD VENOUS BLOOD FLOW TOWARD THE HEART.
6. IF AN INFILTRATION OCCURS, SELECT A PUNCTURE SITE ABOVE THE PREVIOUS PUNCTURE SITE ONLY.
7. CLEANSE THE SELECTED PUNCTURE SITE WITH BETADINE ONLY; AVOID USING ALCOHOL IN COMBINATION WITH BETADINE BECAUSE A TOXIC REACTION OCCURS THAT MAY BE ABSORBED INTO THE SKIN.
8. IDEALLY SELECT THE NONDOMINANT ARM OR HAND FOR VEIN SELECTION.

9. AVOID TAKING BLOOD PRESSURE IN THE ARM WITH THE IV.
10. AVOID SELECTING AN IV SITE IN AN AREA OF INFECTION, INFILTRATION, THROMBOSIS, ON THE SAME SIDE AS A MASTECTOMY, PARALYZED ARM, ARM WITH A SHUNT, OR WITH ANY INDICATION OF A CIRCULATORY OR NEUROLOGICAL IMPAIRMENT.
11. PLACE AN ARMBOARD UNDER THE IV SITE IN AN AREA OF FLEXION.
12. AVOID COVERING THE IV SITE WITH A RESTRAINT.
13. USE A VENOSCOPE (VEIN FINDER) TO FIND DIFFICULT VEINS SUCH AS THOSE THAT MAY OCCUR IN AN OBESE CLIENT.
    a. Fiberoptic arm used to detect an appropriate vein (dark, shadowy line)
    b. A vein may be assessed for sclerosis by applying downward pressure over the fiberoptic arm. Observe the vein when applying and releasing pressure.
    c. A nonsclerotic vein disappears with pressure and reappears when pressure is released.

B. PREPARING INTRAVENOUS THERAPY

1. REVIEW THE AGENCY'S POLICY ON PREPARING AN INTRAVENOUS SOLUTION.
2. CHECK THE EXPIRATION DATE OF THE BAG AND TUBING.
3. COMPARE THE SELECTED INTRAVENOUS SOLUTION AGAINST THE PHYSICIAN'S ORDER.
4. DATE AND TIME THE BAG AND TUBING WITH APPROPRIATE LABELS.
5. NEVER USE A FELT-TIPPED PEN TO MARK THE IV BAG OR MAKE A TIME STRIP WITH ADHESIVE TAPE BECAUSE INK AND ADHESIVE MAY LEACH THROUGH THE PLASTIC AND CONTAMINATE THE SOLUTION.

C. ADMINISTERING INTRAVENOUS THERAPY
1. REVIEW THE AGENCY'S POLICY ON ADMINISTERING AN INTRAVENOUS SOLUTION.
2. AVOID LETTING THE IV BAG HANG FOR MORE THAN 24 HOURS.
3. CHANGE THE IV TUBING EVERY 48 TO 72 HOURS.
4. ADMINISTER FLUIDS CONTINUOUSLY OR INTERMITTENTLY.
5. ASSESS BACKFLOW OF BLOOD INTO THE CATHETER HUB TO ENSURE PATENCY BY LOWERING THE IV BAG BELOW THE INFUSION SITE.
6. CALCULATE AND REGULATE THE RATE OF INTRAVENOUS INFUSION MANUALLY, BY A DIAL-A-FLO, PUMP REGULATOR, INFUSION CONTROLLER, OR VOLUME CONTROLLER.
7. AS A SAFETY FEATURE, SET THE END TIME WHEN AN INFUSION CONTROLLER IS USED TO INITIATE THE ALARM AT APPROXIMATELY 50 ML SHORT OF THE REQUIRED VOLUME TO ALLOW WARMING OF IV FLUIDS THAT NEED WARMING OR ALLOW SUFFICIENT TIME TO PREPARE THE NEXT SOLUTION.
8. USE A MACRODRIP CHAMBER FOR MOST ADULT CLIENTS (DROP FACTOR GENERALLY BETWEEN 10 TO 20 DROPS PER MILLILITER).
9. SELECT A MICRODRIP CHAMBER FOR MEDICATIONS THAT NEED TO BE TITRATED OR FOR OLDER ADULT OR PEDIATRIC CLIENTS (DROP FACTOR IS 60 DROPS PER MILLILITER).

D. ADMINISTERING INTRAVENOUS DRUGS
1. MAY BE ADMINISTERED BY VOLUME-CONTROL ADMINISTRATION SET, INTERMITTENT INFUSION SET, OR IV PUSH
2. REVIEW THE AGENCY'S POLICY FOR ADMINISTRATION OF INTRAVENOUS DRUGS BY VOLUME-CONTROL ADMINISTRATION SET, INTERMITTENT INFUSION SET, AND IV PUSH.
3. BEFORE ADDING DRUGS TO AN IV BAG, CHECK COMPATIBILITY WITH THE IV SOLUTION SUCH AS AVOIDING ADDING DIAZEPAM (VALIUM) OR CHLORDIAZEPOXIDE HYDROCHLORIDE (LIBRIUM) TO SALINE SOLUTIONS AND ADDING INSULIN TO INFUSION BAGS BECAUSE THE INSULIN ADHERES TO THE INSIDE OF THE BAG.
4. VOLUME-CONTROL ADMINISTRATION SET (SOLUSET, METRISET, VOLUTROL, OR BURETROL) DELIVERS A SMALL AMOUNT OF IV FLUID IN A PEDIATRIC CLIENT OR IN A CRITICAL CARE SITUATION.
5. INTERMITTENT INFUSION ALLOWS PERIODIC DRUG ADMINISTRATION BY A SECONDARY TUBING PIGGYBACKED INTO THE PRIMARY LINE.
6. FLUSH PRIMARY TUBING WITH NORMAL SALINE IF INTERMITTENT DRUG IS INCOMPATIBLE WITH THE PRIMARY SOLUTION.
7. INTERMITTENT INFUSION DEVICES SUCH AS SALINE LOCKS ALLOW THE DELIVERY OF AN INTERMITTENT INFUSION OR AN IV PUSH DRUG WITHOUT THE NEED FOR ADDITIONAL FLUIDS AND MUST BE FLUSHED EVERY 8 HOURS TO MAINTAIN PATENCY.
8. IV PUSH DRUG ALLOWS PERIODIC ADMINISTRATION OR EMERGENCY ADMINISTRATION OF A DRUG BY A CONTINUOUS INFUSION LINE OR SALINE LOCK.
9. PRIMARY LINE FLUIDS MUST BE STOPPED BY PINCHING OFF THE TUBING ABOVE THE INJECTION PORT WHEN ADMINISTERING IV PUSH DRUG TO PREVENT THE BACKUP OF THE DRUG.

E. COMPLICATIONS OF INTRAVENOUS THERAPY
1. HYPERVOLEMIA (CIRCULATORY OVERLOAD)
    a. Description
        1) Increased circulating fluid volume generally occurring from too rapid an infusion of fluids
        2) May lead to pulmonary edema and cardiac failure
        3) Clients at high risk include those with cardiac decompensation.
    b. Clinical manifestations
        1) Dyspnea
        2) Tachycardia
        3) Hypertension
        4) Coughing
        5) Pulmonary edema
        6) Cyanosis
        7) Rales
        8) Increased venous pressure
    c. Nursing interventions
        1) Slow the rate of the IV fluid to keep vein open (KVO).
        2) Immediately notify the physician.
        3) Raise the head of the bed to aid breathing.
        4) Frequently monitor the vital signs and central venous pressure.
        5) Document.

2. INFILTRATION
   a. Description: Seepage of intravenous fluid into surrounding interstitial tissue by inserting the wrong gauge of needle, high-pressure drug or solution administered by a pump, or dislodgment of the device from the vein
   b. Clinical manifestations
      1) Pain at the IV site
      2) Edema at the IV site
      3) Coolness and paleness at the IV site
   c. Nursing interventions
      1) Discontinue the infusion and apply a dressing.
      2) Monitor the infusion site for bleeding.
      3) Elevate the affected extremity and apply a cold compress.
      4) Avoid rubbing the infiltrated site because a hematoma may result.
      5) Monitor for vesicant (medication that causes blistering and tissue injury after it escapes into the surrounding tissues).
      6) Assess for infiltration by lowering the IV fluid bag below the IV site and observe for lack of blood backflow into the tubing.
      7) Document.
3. PHLEBITIS
   a. Description
      1) May be the result of mechanical or chemical trauma
      2) Mechanical trauma includes inserting too large a gauge of needle, using a vein that is too small or fragile, or leaving the catheter in too long.
      3) Chemical trauma includes infusing solutions that are hypertonic, acidic, or contain electrolytes such as potassium and magnesium, or infusing solutions too rapidly.
   b. Clinical manifestations
      1) Tenderness at the IV site
      2) Redness at the IV site
      3) Pink or red stripe along the vein
      4) Warmth at the IV site
      5) Swelling at the IV site
   c. Nursing interventions
      1) Discontinue the IV.
      2) Check the agency's policy to determine if the tip of the catheter needs to be cultured and send to the lab.
      3) Apply warm, moist compresses to the area.
      4) Change the IV site appropriately, every 48 to 72 hours, depending on the agency's policy.
      5) Document.

4. PYROGENIC REACTION
   a. Description: microorganisms enter the body through a contaminated tube, solution, or needle.
   b. Clinical manifestations
      1) Sudden increased temperature
      2) Severe chills generally within 30 minutes of initiating an infusion
      3) Backache
      4) Headache
      5) General malaise
      6) Nausea and vomiting
      7) Vascular collapse with hypertension and cyanosis if the reaction is severe
   c. Nursing interventions
      1) Discontinue the IV.
      2) Assess vital signs.
      3) Notify the physician.
      4) Send the entire administration set to the pharmacy.
      5) Obtain a culture and sensitivity as prescribed.
      6) Document.
5. THROMBOPHLEBITIS
   a. Description: Formation of a blood clot and inflammation of the vein
   b. Clinical manifestations
      1) Pain at the IV site
      2) Warmth at the IV site
      3) Redness at the IV site
      4) Swelling at the IV site
      5) Loss of motion of the body part
   c. Nursing interventions
      1) Discontinue the IV.
      2) Apply warm compresses to the area.
      3) Notify the physician.
      4) Restart the IV in another vein.
      5) Document.
6. AIR EMBOLISM
   a. Description
      1) Entrance of air into the vein as a result of a loose connection, during a tubing change, or an inadequately primed IV tubing
      2) As little as 10 ml of air may be fatal.
   b. Clinical manifestations
      1) Cyanosis
      2) Dyspnea
      3) Hypotension
      4) Weak rapid pulse
      5) Decreased level of consciousness
      6) Tachycardia
   c. Nursing interventions
      1) Immediately stop the entrance of air into the vein.
      2) Notify the physician.

3) Place the client on the left side with the head lowered (Trendelenburg) to raise the air into the right atrium and allow blood to empty into the left side of the heart.

4) Administer oxygen.

5) Prevention is the key—adequately prime the IV tubing, secure all connections, and hang another IV bag before the existing bag goes dry.

F. DISCONTINUATION OF INTRAVENOUS THERAPY

1. PERIPHERAL IV CATHETER SHOULD BE DISCONTINUED WHEN CONTAMINATION IS SUSPECTED, COMPLICATIONS ARE PRESENT, OR TO CHANGE THE SITE EVERY 48–72 HOURS DEPENDING ON THE AGENCY'S POLICY.

2. APPLY A PRESSURE STERILE DRESSING TO THE SITE.

3. PICCS ARE REMOVED ONLY BY A SPECIALLY TRAINED NURSE.

4. AS A RESULT OF PICC BEING COMPLETELY INVISIBLE AND INSERTED INTO THE VASCULAR SYSTEM, RESISTANCE MUST BE ASSESSED DURING REMOVAL (IF RESISTANCE IS FELT, ASSESS FOR COMPLICATIONS SUCH AS VENOUS SPASM, VAGAL REACTION, PHLEBITIS, THROMBOSIS, OR KNOTTING OF THE CATHETER).

VI. BLOOD THERAPY

A. PURPOSES AND USES

1. REPLACE BLOOD LOSS WITH BLOOD OR BLOOD PRODUCTS.

B. TYPES

1. RED BLOOD CELLS (RBCS)

a. Used to replace erythrocytes in conditions such as anemia and blood loss

b. Generally delivered in 1-unit 250-ml bags through a Y tubing and primed with normal saline

c. One unit increases the hemoglobin by 1g/dl and hematocrit by 2% to 3% over a period of 4 to 6 hours.

d. May be stored for 5 to 6 weeks or several years if frozen

2. WHOLE BLOOD

a. Used in cases when the client needs all components of blood, such as in cases of hemorrhage or to restore the ability to carry oxygen

b. Generally delivered in 1-unit 500-ml bags

c. Not used as much as packed RBCs

d. Has a refrigerator shelf-life of 35 days

3. FRESH OR FROZEN PLASMA

a. Used to replace clotting factors and increase the intravascular compartment

b. Generally infused within 6 hours after thawing with a straight-line administration set

c. Delivered in 1-unit 250- or 500-ml bags

d. Does not contain platelets

e. Rh and ABO compatibility must be performed prior to infusion.

f. Hepatitis is a risk.

g. Monitor prothrombin (PT) and partial thromboplastin (PTT) for evaluation of therapy.

4. PLATELETS

a. Used to replace platelets and correct bleeding disorders such as thrombocytopenia

b. Delivered in a variety of unit sizes, such as 50-, 70-, 200-, and 400-ml bags

c. Infuse immediately upon receipt from the blood bank at a rate of 10 minutes per unit with a platelet administration set.

d. Monitor the platelet level for evaluation of therapy.

e. Must be used within 3 days of being extracted from whole blood

5. ALBUMIN

a. Used to restore intravascular volume; treat shock and hypoproteinemia

b. Delivered in 5% and 25% solutions

c. Slowly infused with tubing that comes with albumin

6. GRANULOCYTES (WHITE BLOOD CELLS [WBCS])

a. Used to restore WBCs, usually after chemotherapy

b. Slowly infuse over 2 to 4 hours with Y-type blood filter after being primed with normal saline.

7. CRYOPRECIPITATE

a. Used to replace factors VIII and fibrinogen in the treatment of hemophilia A

b. Administer with a straight-line administration set.

c. Monitor for febrile reactions.

C. PRINCIPLES OF BLOOD THERAPY

1. ABO TYPE AND RH TYPE ARE DONE ON ALL CLIENT AND DONOR BLOOD.

2. ANTIBODY SCREEN IS DONE TO EVALUATE IF ANTIBODIES OTHER THAN ANTI-A AND ANTI-B ARE PRESENT (BLOOD TYPE A HAS ANTI-A ANTIBODIES, BLOOD TYPE AB HAS NEITHER ANTI-A NOR ANTI-B ANTIBODIES, AND BLOOD TYPE O HAS BOTH ANTI-A AND ANTI-B ANTIBODIES AND MUST RECEIVE ONLY TYPE O BLOOD).

3. CROSS-MATCHING IS DONE ON ALL BLOOD IN WHICH DONOR RBCS ARE COMBINED WITH THE SERUM OF THE CLIENT AND COOMBS' SERUM

(COMPATIBILITY IS DETERMINED IF NO AGGLUTINATION OF RBCS OCCURS).

4. SIX TYPES OF RH ANTIGEN ARE POSSIBLE BUT TYPE D IS THE MOST COMMON AND INDICATES IMMUNE RESPONSE (PRESENCE OF TYPE D DETERMINES RH TYPE—WHEN D ANTIGEN IS PRESENT, THE CLIENT IS RH POSITIVE; WHEN D ANTIGEN IS ABSENT, IT INDICATES RH NEGATIVE).

5. RH-NEGATIVE CLIENTS MUST BE EXPOSED TO RH-POSITIVE BLOOD BEFORE RH ANTIBODIES ARE FORMED (RH-POSITIVE BLOOD MAY BE GIVEN TO A CLIENT WITH RH-NEGATIVE BLOOD IF NO EXPOSURE TO RH-POSITIVE BLOOD HAS OCCURRED AND THE POSTTRANSFUSION RISK IS PRESENT AND EXPOSURE OCCURRED).

6. RH-NEGATIVE MOTHER EXPOSED TO RH ANTIGEN MAY TRANSFER RH ANTIBODIES ACROSS THE PLACENTA TO RH-POSITIVE FETUS AND CAUSE FETAL HEMOLYSIS (ANEMIA AND JAUNDICE).

7. O-NEGATIVE RBCS AND AB PLASMA MAY BE ADMINISTERED TO MOST CLIENTS WITHOUT TESTING IN AN EMERGENCY.

8. CAUTION IS TO BE USED WHEN USING AN INFUSION PUMP OR CONTROL BECAUSE NEGATIVE MACHINE PRESSURE MAY CAUSE HEMOLYSIS OF RBCS (ABO BLOOD TYPING DETERMINES THE PRESENCE OF ANTIGENS ON THE SURFACE OF RBCS—BLOOD TYPE A HAS TYPE A ANTIGEN PRESENT, BLOOD TYPE B HAS TYPE B ANTIGEN PRESENT, AND BLOOD TYPE O HAS NEITHER A NOR B ANTIGEN PRESENT).

9. WARM BLOOD TO PREVENT HYPOTHERMIA (NEVER WARM BLOOD IN THE MICROWAVE OR HOT WATER).

D. TYPES OF BLOOD DONATIONS
　1. AUTOLOGOUS
　　a. Donation of the client's own blood, generally for a surgery within 5 weeks of the transfusion date but not closer than 72 hours of the transfusion
　　b. Multiple units may be donated at intervals of generally 3 days if hemoglobin is above 11 g/dl.
　2. ALLOGENIC
　　a. Donation of blood, generally for a blood bank, with an unknown recipient
　3. DIRECT ALLOGENIC
　　a. Donation of blood designated for an identified blood type and compatible recipient

　　b. Disadvantage may be pressure on the donor to donate blood
　　c. No safer than the general population of allogenic donations because compatible friends and family may also engage in practices that place the recipient at risk for hepatitis and HIV and because of uncomfortableness in disclosing practices

E. PREPARING TO ADMINISTER BLOOD THERAPY
　1. HAVE THE CLIENT SIGN A CONSENT FORM.
　2. INSERT AN 18- OR 19-GAUGE NEEDLE IN A VEIN OF AN ADULT CLIENT (14- OR 15-GAUGE NEEDLE IF THE BLOOD IS TO BE INFUSED QUICKLY) OR A 23-GAUGE NEEDLE IN A PEDIATRIC OR OLDER ADULT CLIENT WITH SMALL, FRAGILE VEINS.
　3. USE Y TUBING PRIMED WITH NORMAL SALINE.
　4. PERFORM A TYPE AND CROSS-MATCH.
　5. OBTAIN A BASELINE SET OF VITAL SIGNS.
　6. ASSESS A PEDIATRIC, OLDER ADULT CLIENT, OR MALNOURISHED CLIENT FOR CIRCULATORY OVERLOAD (MAY NEED TO DIVIDE VOLUME OF BLOOD ADMINISTERED OR ADMINISTER PACKED RBCS INSTEAD OF WHOLE BLOOD).
　7. INFUSE ALL IV DRUGS BEFORE BLOOD ADMINISTRATION TO PREVENT A DRUG REACTION WHILE THE BLOOD IS INFUSING (IT WOULD BE DIFFICULT TO DETERMINE IF THE REACTION WAS DRUG OR BLOOD INDUCED).

F. ADMINISTERING BLOOD THERAPY
　1. REVIEW THE PROCEDURE FOR BLOOD ADMINISTRATION.
　2. LICENSED PERSONNEL MUST SIGN A RELEASE OF BLOOD FORM TO RELEASE BLOOD FROM THE BLOOD BANK.
　3. UNIT OF BLOOD MUST BE CHECKED AND SIGNED FOR BY TWO LICENSED PERSONNEL PRIOR TO HANGING BLOOD.
　4. CHECK THE ACCURACY OF THE BLOOD LABEL AGAINST THE UNIT OF BLOOD (INCLUDE THE CLIENT'S NAME, IDENTIFICATION NUMBER, ABO NUMBER, RH FACTOR, DONOR NUMBER, TYPE OF BLOOD ORDERED BY THE PHYSICIAN, AND THE EXPIRATION DATE OF THE BLOOD).
　5. DRAW THE CLIENT'S BLOOD SAMPLE AND LABEL IT AT THE BEDSIDE.

6. ASSESS THE BAG FOR CLEARNESS, COLOR, CONSISTENCY, OR BUBBLES.
7. HANG A BAG OF NORMAL SALINE WITH A Y-SET TUBING WITH IN-LINE FILTER TO FLUSH THE EXISTING CATHETER.
8. HANG A SECOND BAG OR NORMAL SALINE TO PREVENT HEMOLYSIS OF BLOOD.
9. HANG BLOOD WITHIN 30 MINUTES OF RECEIVING IT FROM THE BLOOD BANK TO PREVENT LYSIS OF RBCS AND INFECTION (WHOLE BLOOD SHOULD NEVER BE UNREFRIGERATED FOR MORE THAN 4 HOURS—RELEASES POTASSIUM AND CAUSES HYPERKALEMIA).
10. TAKE A BASELINE SET OF VITAL SIGNS.
11. ADMINISTER BLOOD AT A RATE OF 20 GTTS/MIN FOR THE FIRST 15 MINUTES.
12. ASSESS VITAL SIGNS EVERY 15 MINUTES FOR THE FIRST HOUR.
13. AVOID LETTING BLOOD HANG FOR 4 HOURS OR MORE (IDEALLY INFUSE IN 2 HOURS BECAUSE DETERIORATION OF BLOOD OCCURS AFTER BLOOD IS AT ROOM TEMPERATURE FOR 2 HOURS).
14. MONITOR THE IV SITE FOR HEMATOMA AND DISCONTINUE IF IT OCCURS.
15. DOCUMENT PROCESS OF ADMINISTERING BLOOD.
  G. COMPLICATIONS OF BLOOD THERAPY
   1. ACUTE HEMOLYTIC REACTION
      a. Description
         1) Rare
         2) Caused by mismatched client and donor blood
         3) Results in hemolysis of RBCs
         4) Occurs within 15 minutes after starting the transfusion
      b. Clinical manifestations
         1) Headache
         2) Dyspnea
         3) Cyanosis
         4) Tachycardia
         5) Chest pain
         6) Back pain
         7) Hypotension
      c. Nursing interventions
         1) Discontinue the IV.
         2) Maintain the IV patency with normal saline.
         3) Send the blood tubing and bag back to the blood bank.
         4) Obtain urine and blood samples and send to the laboratory labeled "blood transfusion reaction."
         5) Monitor vital signs.
         6) Monitor intake and output.
         7) Document.
   2. DELAYED HEMOLYTIC REACTION
      a. Description
         1) Caused by mismatched anti-A and anti-B agglutinins of the donor and client's blood or improper storage of the unit of blood
         2) Results in cell clumping and small blood vessel plugs
         3) Occurs within 2 to 14 days after receiving the transfusion
      b. Clinical manifestations
         1) Jaundice
         2) Anemia
         3) Fever
         4) Oliguria
         5) Flank pain
         6) Bleeding
      c. Nursing interventions
         1) May receive no specific treatment but recognition is essential to prevent an acute hemolytic reaction.
         2) Monitor the client for anemia.
         3) Notify the physician.
         4) Notify the blood bank.
         5) Prevention includes careful cross-matching.
         6) Document.
   3. MILD ALLERGIC REACTION
      a. Description
         1) Caused by sensitivity to plasma proteins
         2) Occurs immediately or up to 1 hour after the transfusion
      b. Clinical manifestations
         1) Rash
         2) Itching
         3) Urticaria
         4) Wheezing
      c. Nursing interventions
         1) Discontinue the IV.
         2) Monitor the client for anaphylactic shock.
         3) Administer prescribed antihistamine.
         4) Monitor the vital signs.
         5) Document.
   4. SEVERE ALLERGIC REACTION
      a. Description
         1) Caused by antibody-antigen response
         2) Results in agglutination of red blood cells and multisystem manifestations

  b. Clinical manifestations
  1) Shortness of breath
  2) Chest pain
  3) Hypotension
  4) Nausea
  5) Vomiting
  6) Decreased level of consciousness
  7) Cardiac arrest
  c. Nursing interventions
  1) Discontinue the IV.
  2) Maintain the patency of the IV.
  3) Notify the physician.
  4) Notify the blood bank.
  5) Monitor the vital signs.
  6) Administer prescribed antihistamines, corticosteroids, epinephrine, and antipyretics.
  7) Monitor for cardiovascular collapse and cardiac arrest.
  8) Begin cardiopulmonary resuscitation (CPR) if cardiac arrest occurs.
  9) Document.
5. FEBRILE REACTION
  a. Description
  1) Caused by a sensitivity to the WBCs, platelets, and plasma proteins
  2) Occurs within 30 minutes after initiating the blood transfusion or 6 hours after the transfusion is completed
  b. Clinical manifestations
  1) Warm, flushed skin
  2) Headache
  3) Muscle pain
  4) Anxiety
  c. Nursing interventions
  1) Discontinue the IV.
  2) Administer prescribed antipyretics.
  3) Monitor the temperature.
  4) Document.
6. SEPSIS
  a. Description
  1) Serious reaction

  2) Caused by the administration of contaminated blood
  3) Occurs during the transfusion or up to 2 hours after the transfusion
  b. Clinical manifestations
  1) Chills
  2) Fever
  3) Abdominal cramping
  4) Vomiting
  5) Diarrhea
  6) Shock
  7) Renal failure
  c. Nursing interventions
  1) Discontinue the IV.
  2) Maintain the IV patency with new tubing and a bag of normal saline.
  3) Notify the physician.
  4) Monitor the vital signs.
  5) Obtain blood cultures.
  6) Administer prescribed antibiotics.
  7) Monitor the intake and output.
7. HYPERVOLEMIA
  a. Description
  1) Caused by too rapid transfusion rate or too great a blood volume
  2) Occurs during the transfusion or up to 2 hours after the transfusion
  b. Clinical manifestations
  1) Dyspnea
  2) Cough
  3) Rales
  4) Distended neck veins
  5) Hypertension
  6) Tachycardia
  c. Nursing interventions
  1) Slow or discontinue the transfusion.
  2) Elevate the head of the bed.
  3) Notify the physician.
  4) Administer prescribed diuretics.
  5) Administer prescribed oxygen.
  6) Document.

PRACTICE QUESTIONS

1. The nurse is preparing to administer insulin to a client with diabetes mellitus for which of the following purposes?
1. Relief of disease manifestations
2. Preventive
3. Health maintenance
4. Curative

2. The nurse is collecting a medication history. Which of the following questions would elicit the most accurate information?
Select all that apply:
[ ] 1. "Do you take any herbal supplements?"
[ ] 2. "What time of day do you go to bed?"
[ ] 3. "What is the highest level of education you completed?"

[ ] 4. "Do you have a vision or hearing impairment?"

[ ] 5. "Where do you eat most of your meals?"

[ ] 6. "Do you have drug insurance coverage?"

3. Which of the following should the nurse include in the oral drug administration procedure?

1. Administer a drug to a 3-year-old child as a capsule
2. Administer two drugs at a time to an older adult client
3. Administer a carbonated beverage over ice following a drug
4. Administer a sustained action buccal drug under the tongue

4. The nurse evaluates a client who is experiencing an acute hemolytic reaction when which of the following are present? Select all that apply:

[ ] 1. Occurs within 2 to 14 days after receiving the transfusion

[ ] 2. Headache, dyspnea, cyanosis

[ ] 3. Jaundice, oliguria, bleeding

[ ] 4. Fever, anemia, flank pain

[ ] 5. Tachycardia, chest pain, back pain

[ ] 6. Occurs within 15 minutes after starting the transfusion

5. Which of the following should the nurse include when administering drugs by a nasogastric tube?

1. Crush the drug before administering through a feeding tube
2. Flush between drugs with 10 ml of sterile water
3. Administer one drug with 30 ml of water
4. Maintain the client in an upright position for 15 minutes following drug administration

6. Which of the following principles of parenteral drug administration is a priority for the nurse to consider before administering a parenteral injection to a 2-year-old child?

1. Apply EMLA (lidocaine 2.5% and prilocaine 2.5%) to the injection site 1 hour before administering the injection
2. Lightly tap the injection site before administering the injection
3. Administer up to 1 ml of the prescribed drug to the injection site
4. Select the vastus lateralis for the administration of the drug

7. The nurse selects which of the following isotonic intravenous solutions for the primary purpose of promoting rehydration and elimination, while providing a good vehicle for potassium replacement?

1. Sodium chloride 0.45%

2. Dextrose 5% in water
3. Dextrose 5% in 0.45% saline
4. Ringer's lactate

8. The nurse selects which of the following IV site locations when starting an IV in the medial antebrachial vein? (Label the medial antebrachial vein on the accompanying figure.)

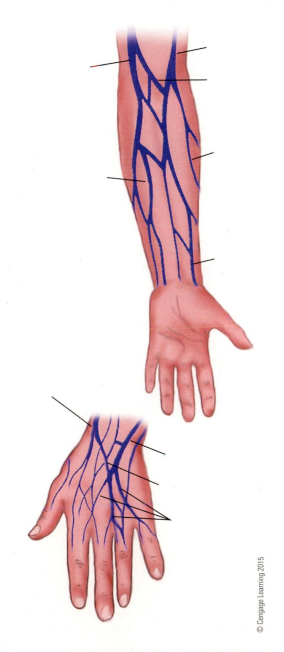

© Cengage Learning 2015

9. The nurse is preparing the client assignments for the day. Which of the following assignments would be appropriate for the registered nurse (RN) to assign to a licensed practical nurse (LPN)?

1. Administer a drug to a client who has an implantable intravenous infusion port

2. Insert an angiocath into the medial antebrachial vein of a client going to surgery

3. Instruct a client on the advantages of an autologous blood transfusion

4. Discontinue a client's peripheral IV site

10. The nurse prepares to hang which of the following for a client with thrombocytopenia?
    1. Whole blood
    2. Packed red blood cells
    3. Platelets
    4. Albumin

11. The nurse is caring for a client with a peripheral IV. Which of the following would indicate the client is experiencing hypervolemia?
    Select all that apply:
    [ ] 1. Nausea and vomiting
    [ ] 2. Headache
    [ ] 3. Dyspnea
    [ ] 4. Hypertension
    [ ] 5. Fever
    [ ] 6. Tachycardia

12. The nurse is caring for a client with an IV who is experiencing dyspnea, hypotension, a weak and rapid pulse, and a decreased level of consciousness, and who is becoming cyanotic. The priority nursing intervention is to
    1. notify the physician.
    2. place the client in a Trendelenburg position.
    3. administer oxygen.
    4. discontinue the IV.

13. Because a client is receiving fresh plasma, the nurse should evaluate which of the following laboratory results for the effectiveness of therapy?
    1. Hemoglobin and hematocrit
    2. Platelets
    3. Prothrombin (PT) and partial thromboplastin (PTT)
    4. White blood cells

14. The nurse is teaching a class on controlled substances. Which of the following should the nurse include in the class?
    1. There is no accepted medical use for Schedule I controlled substances
    2. Examples of Schedule II drugs include glutethimide (Doriden), secobarbital (Seconal), and hydrocodone with acetaminophen (Vicodin)
    3. Schedule III controlled substances have a high potential for abuse
    4. Schedule IV controlled substances are over-the-counter narcotics that must be sold by a registered pharmacist

15. The nurse prepares to administer a heparin injection with a tuberculin syringe with what volume? _____

16. The nurse prepares to administer meperidine (Demerol) intramuscularly to an adult client by selecting which of the following needles?
    1. 16 gauge
    2. 18 gauge
    3. 23 gauge
    4. 26 gauge

17. The client is receiving a unit of packed red blood cells. Which of the following observations indicate to the nurse that the client is having an acute hemolytic reaction?
    Select all that apply:
    [ ] 1. Tachycardia
    [ ] 2. Headache
    [ ] 3. Fever
    [ ] 4. Hypertension
    [ ] 5. Dyspnea
    [ ] 6. Back pain

18. The nurse should select what gauge of needle to administer blood? _____

19. The nurse should instruct a client receiving a blood transfusion to notify the nurse if itching, urticaria, wheezing, or a rash appears for how many hours after completion of the transfusion? _____

20. When administering intravenous therapy to a client, it would be essential for the nurse to include which of the following aspects of the procedure?
    1. Make a time strip on the bag with a felt-tip marker
    2. Change the tubing every 24 hours
    3. Replace the intravenous solution with the same solution when the current solution runs out
    4. Avoid letting the intravenous solution hang more than 24 hours

21. The nurse should include which of the following in the administration of an intravenous solution?
    1. Select a microdrip chamber for medications administered to a pediatric client
    2. Set the end time of an infusion on a controller to initiate the alarm 20 minutes before the scheduled end time
    3. Select a macrodrip chamber for medications administered to a geriatric client
    4. Choose a volume-control administration set to deliver a large amount of an intravenous solution

22. After initiating intravenous therapy, a client experiences chills, headaches, backache, and a temperature of 38.3°C, or 101°F. The nurse should report this as which of the following types of intravenous reactions?
    1. Phlebitis
    2. Pyrogenic reaction
    3. Thrombophlebitis
    4. Air embolism

23. Which of the following is a priority for the nurse to perform on a client who has a thrombophlebitis?
    1. Apply warm, moist compresses to the area
    2. Document the appearance of the IV site
    3. Discontinue the IV
    4. Notify the physician

24. The nurse is observing another nurse start an intravenous infusion. Which of the following would indicate the nurse starting the IV does not understand the procedure?
    1. Select a butterfly needle for an endoscopy procedure
    2. Select the scalp vein for an infant
    3. Cleanse the selected IV site with Betadine followed by alcohol
    4. Use a venoscope to find a difficult vein

25. The nurse should monitor a client with a central venous catheter for which of the following manifestations of a pneumothorax? Select all that apply:
    [ ] 1. Hypertension
    [ ] 2. Shortness of breath
    [ ] 3. Flushing
    [ ] 4. Lethargy
    [ ] 5. Chest pain
    [ ] 6. Weak, rapid pulse

26. A client receiving a blood transfusion complains of chills, headache, backache, and sudden spikes in temperature. The priority nursing action is to
    1. flush the tubing with normal saline.
    2. slow the transfusion.
    3. discontinue the transfusion.
    4. continue to monitor the client.

27. The nurse identifies which of the following orders as an intermittent intravenous infusion?
    1. Diazepam (Valium) 5-mg IV push
    2. 500 ml intralipids IV in 6 hours
    3. Potassium chloride 20 mEq in 1000 ml every 8 hours
    4. Ranitidine (Zantac) 0.5 mg in 50 ml 0.9% NaCl over 20 minutes every 6 hours

28. Which of the following principles of intravenous push does the nurse consider before administering a drug by this route?
    1. There is less of a risk of adverse reactions with the IV push route
    2. The rate of IV push administration must be verified in a drug book
    3. All IV push drugs must be diluted in 50 ml of NaCl before administration
    4. All IV push drugs should be administered within 1 minute or less

29. The nurse knows that gauifensin belongs to what schedule of drugs having the lowest potential of abuse? _____

30. The nurse is observing another nurse administer blood. Which of the following indicates to the observing nurse that the administering nurse does not understand blood administration?
    1. Run the blood slowly for the first 15 minutes at 20 drops per minute
    2. Establish the required flow rate after 15 minutes if no signs of a reaction
    3. Infuse the transfusion slowly over 6 hours
    4. Assess the vital signs every 30 minutes until 1 hour posttransfusion

31. The nurse assesses which of the following clients to be most appropriate for the selection of the central venous catheter?
    1. A client who is dehydrated with hypokalemia, requiring fluid and electrolyte replacement
    2. A client who has cancer of the esophagus and is receiving chemotherapy
    3. A client who has an infection and needs short-term antibiotics
    4. A client who had gallbladder surgery and is experiencing post-op nausea

32. Which of the following should the nurse include when caring for a client with a peripherally inserted central venous catheter (PICC)?
    1. Weigh the client daily
    2. Avoid taking the blood pressure in the arm on the side of the PICC
    3. Take the temperature every 4 hours
    4. Monitor the client's response to fluid and electrolyte therapy

33. The nurse is caring for a client with a central venous access device. Which of the following clinical manifestations does the nurse interpret as indicative of a dislodged catheter? Select all that apply:
    [ ] 1. Pain in the neck
    [ ] 2. Bleeding from the site
    [ ] 3. Gurgling sounds
    [ ] 4. Skin that is pale and cool to touch
    [ ] 5. Palpitations
    [ ] 6. Chills

34. The nurse is caring for a client with a central venous catheter who is experiencing chest pain, dyspnea, coughing, and apprehension. The nurse reports this as indicative of a(n)
    1. infection.
    2. thrombus.
    3. phlebitis.
    4. air embolism.

35. A student nurse asks the nurse where a peripherally inserted central catheter is inserted. Which of the following is the appropriate response by the nurse?
    1. Subclavian vein
    2. Jugular vein
    3. Antecubital area of the basilic vein
    4. Directly into the superior vena cava

36. The nurse selects which of the following intravenous fluids to administer to a client who is very dehydrated with a serum potassium of 2.2 mEq/L, sodium of 129 mEq/L, and calcium of 7.5 mg/dl?
    1. Sodium chloride 0.45%
    2. Ringer's lactate
    3. Dextrose 5% in water
    4. Dextrose 10% in water

37. Which of the following evaluations does the nurse make when the venipuncture site has an observable swelling and is tender and cool to touch?
    1. An infection has developed
    2. Bleeding into the surrounding tissue has occurred
    3. The IV site has infiltrated
    4. A phlebitis is developing

38. A client receiving continuous intravenous therapy is complaining of dyspnea, cough, and tachycardia. The nurse auscultates crackles bilaterally. In determining what action to take next, which of the following factors should the nurse consider?
    1. The client is apprehensive about receiving continuous IV fluids
    2. The client has developed a respiratory infection or pneumonia
    3. The client is exhibiting signs of hypervolemia
    4. The client is experiencing internal bleeding

39. Which of the following solutions should the nurse administer to correct an excessive fluid loss and provide sodium chloride to a client?
    1. Dextrose 5% in water
    2. Sodium chloride 0.45%
    3. Ringer's lactate
    4. Dextrose 5% in 0.45% normal saline

40. The nurse should perform which of the following Centers for Disease Control and Prevention (CDC) guidelines to decrease intravascular infection resulting from intravenous therapy in adult clients?
    1. Routinely apply topical antimicrobial ointment to the insertion site of peripheral venous catheter
    2. Replace the IV tubing, including secondary tubing, and stopcocks every 24 hours
    3. Cleanse the skin site before the venipuncture with warm, soapy water
    4. Replace short peripheral venous catheter and rotate sites every 48 to 72 hours

41. Which of the following should the nurse consider when selecting a site for venipuncture?
    1. Shave the insertion site and surrounding area
    2. Select a vein distal to a previously used venipuncture site
    3. Use the same finger to palpate a vein by pressing downward
    4. Apply the tourniquet 2 inches above the selected venipuncture site

42. Which of the following gerontological considerations should the nurse include when selecting a venipuncture site and initiating intravenous therapy for an older adult client?
    1. Use a 22- to 24-gauge needle for the venipuncture
    2. Apply the tourniquet tightly and vigorously massage the selected vein
    3. Select a vein on the back of the dominant hand
    4. Secure the needle after the venipuncture with an adhesive tape and avoid covering the site

ANSWERS AND RATIONALES

1. 3. Health maintenance drugs, such as insulin, vitamins, and minerals, are used to keep the body healthy. Relief of disease manifestations, such as with antihistamines, is the most common use of drugs used in treatment. Preventive drugs, such as a hepatitis vaccine, are used to prevent disease. Curative drugs, such as antibiotics, are used to cure disease.

2. 1. 3. 4. 6. When obtaining a medication history, it is important to assess if herbal supplements are taken because of drug–herb interactions.

Assessing an impairment of vision or hearing would evaluate the client's inability to correctly administer the drugs. Drug insurance coverage assures that the client is more likely to obtain the drug and comply with the treatment plan. It is important to assess the client's level of education to facilitate appropriate teaching.

3. 3.   Pouring a carbonated beverage over ice and administering it after a drug will decrease nausea. Drugs should be administered in liquid form to children under the age of 5 years. Administering one drug at a time is recommended for an older adult client because of a possibility of impaired swallowing. A buccal drug is a drug to be placed inside the mouth or cheek.

4. 2. 5. 6.   Headache, dyspnea, cyanosis, tachycardia, chest pain, and back pain are adverse reactions of an acute hemolytic reaction. An acute hemolytic reaction also occurs within 15 minutes after starting the transfusion. Adverse reactions of a delayed hemolytic reaction include jaundice, oliguria, and bleeding. It occurs within 2 to 14 days after receiving the transfusion.

5. 3.   One drug should be administered at a time through a nasogastric tube, but it is better to avoid administering drugs through a feeding tube because the lumen is much smaller than a nasogastric tube. Administer each drug with 5 to 30 ml of water and flush with 5 to 30 ml of water between drugs. The client should be placed in an upright position for at least 30 minutes following drug administration.

6. 4.   The priority of any intramuscular injection is the selection of the appropriate site. The vastus lateralis is the preferred site of drug administration in children under the age of 3. EMLA (lidocaine 2.5% and prilocaine 2.5%) may be applied to an intramuscular injection site one to two hours before administering an injection to a child, but the priority is site selection. Tapping the injection site before administering an injection to a child is helpful because it distracts the child (who then focuses on the tap and not the injection). No more than 1 ml should be administered to a child.

7. 2.   Dextrose 5% in water is an isotonic intravenous solution with the primary purpose of promoting rehydration and elimination, while providing a good vehicle for potassium replacement. Sodium chloride 0.45% is a hypotonic solution that moves fluids into the cells. It is used to provide daily maintenance of body fluid and establishment of renal function. The client should be monitored for water intoxication. Dextrose 5% in 0.45% saline is a hypertonic solution that draws fluids from the cells. The client should be monitored for dehydration. Ringer's lactate is an isotonic solution that resembles the normal composition of blood serum and plasma. It contains sodium, potassium, calcium, chloride, and lactate, but no dextrose.

8.   The nurse selects which of the following IV site locations when starting an IV in the medial antebrachial vein? (Label the medial antebrachial vein on the accompanying figure.)

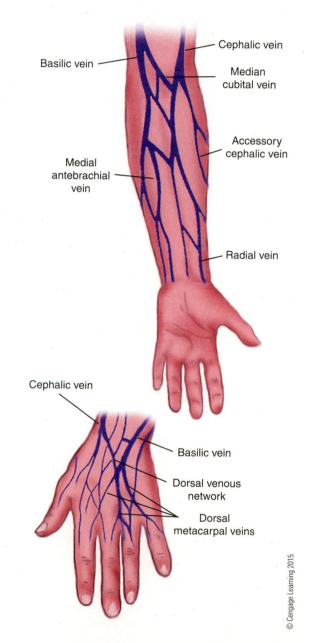

© Cengage Learning 2015

9. 4.   A licensed practical nurse may discontinue an uncomplicated peripheral IV site. An LPN or any RN who has not been specially trained may not access an implantable intravenous infusion port, because of the risk of infection. Only an RN may insert an IV line such as an angiocath.

An LPN may not instruct a client on the various types of blood transfusions. That is a task for an RN.

10. 3. Platelets are administered in the treatment of bleeding disorders, such as thrombocytopenia. Whole blood is not used as much as packed red blood cells but may be used in cases of hemorrhage. Red blood cells are used to replace erythrocytes in conditions such as anemia or blood loss. Albumin is used to restore intravascular volume in the treatment of shock and hypoproteinemia.

11. 3. 4. 6. Clinical manifestations of hypervolemia with intravenous therapy include dyspnea, hypertension, tachycardia, coughing, pulmonary edema, cyanosis, rales, and increased venous pressure. Nausea, vomiting, and fever are clinical manifestations of a pyrogenic reaction.

12. 4. A client who is dyspneic; has hypotension; has a weak, rapid pulse; has a decreased level of consciousness; and is cyanotic is experiencing an air embolism. Administering oxygen, notifying the physician, and placing the client in a Trendelenburg position are all appropriate interventions, but the priority intervention is to immediately stop the entrance of air into the vein. As little as 10 ml of air may be fatal. An air embolism may result from a loose connection, tubing change, or inappropriately primed tubing. To assure that the entrance of air is stopped from entering the vein, it is safest and quickest to discontinue the IV instead of risking further air entering the vein.

13. 3. The prothrombin (PT) and partial thromboplastin (PTT) laboratory tests should be evaluated to determine the effectiveness of receiving fresh plasma. The hematocrit and hemoglobin are evaluated to indicate successful red blood cell therapy. The platelets should be monitored to evaluate successful platelet therapy. The white blood cell count would be evaluated to determine effective granulocyte therapy.

14. 1. Schedule I controlled substances have no acceptable medical use and are used for research purposes only. Glutethimide (Doriden), secobarbital (Seconal), and hydrocodone with acetaminophen (Vicodin) are examples of Schedule III drugs. Schedule II controlled substances have a high potential for abuse, and Schedule III drugs have a moderate potential for abuse. Schedule V controlled substances are over-the-counter narcotics that must be sold by a registered pharmacist.

15. 1 ml. A tuberculin syringe has a volume of 1 ml with a scale of 0.01 ml and is used for heparin injections.

16. 3. The appropriate gauge needle to administer an intramuscular injection to an adult client is 21 to 23 gauge.

17. 1. 2. 5. 6. Clinical manifestations of an acute hemolytic reaction include tachycardia, headache, hypotension, dyspnea, back pain, chest pain, and cyanosis.

18. 6. Blood is administered with a 16-gauge needle.

19. One. Itching, urticaria, wheezing, or a rash are all clinical manifestations of a mild allergic reaction to a blood transfusion and may occur immediately or up to 1 hour after the transfusion.

20. 4. An intravenous solution should not hang more than 24 to 72 hours. Intravenous tubing should be changed every 48 to 72 hours. The IV solution to be hung should always be checked against the current doctor's order. It is unsafe practice to just hang the solution running out, because the order may have been changed. A time strip should never be made with a felt-tip marker because the ink from the marker may leech through the plastic bag and contaminate the solution.

21. 1. A microdrip chamber should be selected when administering medications to both pediatric and geriatric clients. As a safety feature, the infusion controller alarm should be set to go off 50 ml before the volume is infused. A volume-control administration set delivers a small amount of IV fluid to a pediatric client or in a critical care situation.

22. 2. Clinical manifestations of a pyrogenic reaction include a sudden increased temperature, chills, backache, headache, general malaise, and nausea and vomiting.

23. 3. Discontinuing the IV is the priority nursing intervention when a thrombophlebitis is present. After discontinuing an intravenous solution, warm, moist compresses are applied to the area, the physician is notified, the incident is documented, and the IV is restarted at another site.

24. 3. Cleansing the selected IV with Betadine followed by alcohol may form a toxic material that may be absorbed through the skin. It is appropriate to select a butterfly needle for an endoscopy procedure, use the scalp vein for an infant, or find a difficult vein with a venoscope.

25. 2. 5. 6. Clinical manifestations of a pneumothorax include sudden shortness of breath, sharp chest pain, hypotension, pallor, cyanosis, and a weak and rapid pulse, which may indicate the pleural membrane has been punctured.

26. 3. Blood administration reactions generally occur within the first 15 minutes. Chills, headache, backache, and a sudden spike in temperature indicate a reaction. The priority nursing action is to discontinue the transfusion and notify the physician immediately.

27. 4.   An intermittent intravenous infusion is the administration of an IV drug without the infusion of solution. These infusions are administered at regularly scheduled times. An example of an intermittent intravenous infusion is ranitidine (Zantac) 0.5 mg in 50 ml 0.9% NaCl over 20 minutes every 6 hours.

28. 2.   Administering a drug by the IV push rate is a way to administer a small amount of a drug in a short period of time. The rate of any IV drug must be verified in a drug book before administration. Because this is a rapid way of administering drugs to a client, there is a high risk of adverse reactions. If the drug is given too quickly, such as in 1 minute or less, there is no opportunity to discontinue the drug should a reaction occur.

29.   5.   Schedule V controlled substances have the lowest potential of abuse. Guaifenesin is an example.

30. 3.   Blood should not hang for more than 4 hours. If it hangs for more than 4 hours, there is a risk of bacterial growth. Blood should be run slowly for the first 15 minutes at 20 drops per minute. If no reaction occurs after 15 minutes, the flow rate may be established. The vital signs should be assessed every 30 minutes until 1 hour after transfusion to make sure that no reaction is occurring.

31. 2.   A central venous catheter is generally inserted into the internal jugular and subclavian veins with the distal tip located in the superior vena cava to minimize vessel irritation and sclerosis. It is used for long-term therapy, such as for a client who has cancer of the esophagus and is receiving chemotherapy.

32. 2.   The taking of blood pressure should be avoided in the arm on the side of a peripherally inserted central catheter (PICC).

33. 1. 3. 5.   Clinical manifestations of a dislodged catheter in a client with a central venous access device include pain in the neck, gurgling sounds, and palpitations.

34. 4.   Clinical manifestations of an air embolism in a client with a central venous catheter include chest pain, dyspnea, coughing, and apprehension.

35. 3.   A peripherally inserted central catheter is inserted into the antecubital area of the basilic vein.

36. 2.   A client who has a serum potassium of 2.2 mEq/L, sodium of 129 mEq/L, and a calcium of 7.5 mg/dl would benefit from an intravenous solution that resembles the normal composition of the blood serum and plasma with a potassium level below the daily requirement. Ringer's lactate is an isotonic solution that provides sodium, potassium, calcium, chloride, and lactate.

Sodium chloride 0.45% is an isotonic solution that may be used for daily maintenance of body fluid and establishment of renal function. Dextrose 5% in water is an isotonic solution that promotes rehydration and elimination. Administering D_5W may cause a sodium loss but does provide a good medium for administration of potassium. Dextrose 10% in water also contains a higher percentage of dextrose.

37. 3.   An intravenous solution that has infiltrated develops a noticeable swelling and is tender and cool to touch. Infiltration may be caused by using a catheter of the wrong gauge, using the wrong type of device, or by dislodgement of the device from the vein. A phlebitis results from a mechanical or chemical trauma. Tenderness is the first indication. Other clinical manifestations include a reddened area or pink or red stripe along the vein, warmth, and swelling. If the IV site develops an infection, the area becomes red and warm to the touch, and may have an observable drainage. Bleeding into the surrounding tissue around an IV site may cause the area to become swollen and red.

38. 3.   A client receiving a continuous intravenous solution who is complaining of dyspnea, cough, and tachycardia and who has crackles auscultated bilaterally is exhibiting clinical manifestations of hypervolemia, or an increased circulating volume. This may cause cardiac overload that can lead to pulmonary edema and cardiac failure. Hypervolemia may be caused by an intravenous solution running at too rapid a rate. Upon detection, the IV should be slowed to a keep-open rate and the physician should be notified.

39. 4.   Dextrose 5% in 0.45% normal saline promotes renal function and urinary output while providing calories and sodium to a client. It also corrects an excessive fluid loss. Although sodium chloride 0.45% establishes renal function while providing daily maintenance of body fluids, it does not provide a source of calories. Ringer's lactate resembles the normal composition of blood and serum while replacing potassium in a client who is hypokalemic. Ringer's lactate contains sodium, potassium, calcium, chloride, and lactate. Dextrose 5% in water promotes rehydration and elimination, and serves as a good medium for the administration of potassium. It may also cause a loss of urinary sodium. D_5W is a source of calories, but does not provide a source of sodium.

40. 4.   In an adult client, short peripheral venous catheters should be replaced and the site rotated every 48 to 72 hours. Topical antimicrobial ointment should not be applied to the insertion site of a peripheral or central venous catheter. Prior to insertion, the insertion

site should be cleansed with 70% alcohol or 10% povidone-iodine. IV tubing, including secondary tubing, and stopcocks should not be changed more frequently than every 72 hours.

41. 3. The nurse should use the same finger to palpate the vein by pressing downward to determine resilience of the vein. The insertion site should not be shaved, because shaving may cause abrasions that predispose the site to infection. The tourniquet should be applied 4 to 5 inches above the proposed insertion site. An insertion site should not be selected if it is distal to a previous insertion site. This may cause the new IV to infiltrate.

42. 1. When initiating an intravenous solution in an older adult client, a 22- to 24-gauge needle is the best. A 22- to 24-gauge needle is used for the delivery of fluid and drugs. The dorsal metacarpal veins are the best veins. Because the veins of an older adult client are fragile, a loosely applied tourniquet or no tourniquet should be used. Adhesive tape should be avoided because the older adult client has fragile skin that can be easily torn. Paper tape is recommended.

REFERENCES

Broyles, B., Reiss, B., & Evans, M. (2013). *Pharmacological aspects of nursing care* (8th ed.). Clifton Park, NY: Delmar Cengage Learning.

Daniels, R., & Nicoll, L. (2012). *Contemporary medical-surgical Nursing.* Clifton Park, NY: Delmar Cengage Learning.

DeLaune, S. C., & Ladner, P. K. (2011). *Fundamentals of nursing: Standard and practice* (4th ed.). Clifton Park, NY: Delmar Cengage Learning.

Josephson, D. L. (2004). *Intravenous infusion therapy for nurses* (2nd ed.). Clifton Park, NY: Delmar Cengage Learning.

Spratto, G. R., & Woods, A. L. (2012). *PDR nurse's drug handbook 2012.* Clifton Park, NY: Thomson Delmar Learning.

CHAPTER 16

MEASUREMENT AND DRUG CALCULATIONS

I. SYSTEMS OF MEASUREMENT

A. METRIC SYSTEM
  1. THE METRIC SYSTEM IS THE INTERNATIONAL SYSTEM OF UNITS. IT USES DECIMALS MULTIPLIED OR DIVIDED BY MULTIPLES OF 10.
  2. COMMON MEASUREMENTS USED IN HEALTH CARE FIELDS:
     a. Weight:
        1 mg (milligram) = 1000 mcg (micrograms) also µg
        1 g (gram)   = 1000 mg (milligrams)
        1 kg (kilogram) = 1000 g (grams) also GM
     b. Volume:
        1 L (liter) = 1000 ml (milliliters) or cc (cubic centimeters)
  3. SOME METRIC CONVERSION EXAMPLES:
     a. To convert from a larger unit to a smaller one, move x decimal places to the right.
     b. To convert from a smaller unit to a larger one, move x decimal places to the left.
     c. Conversion examples:
        200 mg = 0.2 g
        5.8 L   = 5800 ml
        0.78 g = 780 mg
        750 ml = 0.75 L
        6 mcg   = 0.006 mg
        72 mg   = 7200 mcg

B. APOTHECARIES SYSTEM
  1. THE APOTHECARIES SYSTEM USES BOTH ARABIC AND ROMAN NUMERALS AND FRACTIONS RATHER THAN DECIMALS.
  2. THE SYMBOL OR ABBREVIATION IS WRITTEN FIRST, FOLLOWED BY THE QUANTITY.
  3. CONVERSIONS ARE NOT EQUAL AS MEASUREMENTS IN THIS SYSTEM BUT ARE APPROXIMATIONS. THEREFORE, DISCREPANCIES WILL EXIST.
  4. COMMON USEFUL MEASUREMENTS:
     a. Weight measurements are in grains (gr), drams (dr) or (ʒ), ounces (oz) or (ξ), and pounds (lb).
     b. When Roman numerals are used to write doses, symbols such as ss = ½ and iiiss = 3½ are used.
     c. Volume measurements are in minims (m) or (min), drams (dr) or (ʒ), ounces (oz) or (ξ), pints (pt), and quarts (qt).
  5. WEIGHT CONVERSION FOR MEDICATION ADMINISTRATION ONLY UTILIZES THE GRAIN MEASUREMENT: 60 GRAINS (GR 60) = 1 DRAM.
  6. COMMON VOLUME CONVERSIONS:
     60 minims = 1 fluid dram
     4 drams   = ½ ounce
     8 drams   = 1 ounce
     16 ounces = 1 pint
     32 ounces = 1 quart
     2 pints   = 1 quart
     4 quarts = 1 gallon

C. HOUSEHOLD SYSTEM
  1. THE HOUSEHOLD SYSTEM IS THE LEAST ACCURATE OF THE SYSTEMS AND IS WHAT IS USED BY MOST PEOPLE AT HOME. IT IS THE STANDARD COOKBOOK MEASUREMENT SYSTEM.
  2. THE HOUSEHOLD SYSTEM USES ARABIC NUMBERS AND FRACTIONS.
  3. THE NURSE SHOULD UTILIZE ANOTHER SYSTEM OF MEASURE WHENEVER POSSIBLE BUT SHOULD BE PREPARED TO MAKE CONVERSIONS FOR HOME USE WHEN NECESSARY.

4. COMMON USEFUL MEASUREMENTS:

60 drops (gtts)	= 1 teaspoon (tsp)
3 teaspoons (tsp)	= 1 tablespoon (tbsp or T)
3 tsp or 1 T	= ½ ounce (oz)
2 tablespoons	= 1 ounce (oz)
8 ounces (oz)	= 1 cup (c)
16 ounces (oz)	= 2 cups or 1 pint (pt)
32 ounces (oz)	= 4 cups or 1 quart (qt)
2 pints (pt)	= 1 quart (qt)

5. EQUIVALENTS FROM HOUSEHOLD TO APOTHECARIES TO METRIC (SEE TABLE 16-1)

II. MEASUREMENT CONVERSIONS

A. USING THE RATIO-PROPORTION METHOD
   1. CARRY DECIMALS OUT TO TWO DECIMAL PLACES FOR ACCURACY.
   2. RATIOS MAY BE STATED AS FRACTIONS AND CROSS MULTIPLIED TO SOLVE FOR X. OR USE RATIO-PROPORTIONS TO SOLVE BY MULTIPLYING THE MEANS AND THE EXTREMES. THE PRODUCT OF THE MEANS EQUALS THE PRODUCT OF THE EXTREMES.
   3. WHEN USING RATIO-PROPORTIONS, IT IS PREFERABLE TO PLACE THE KNOWN EQUIVALENT IN THE FIRST RATIO AND THE UNKNOWN EQUIVALENT IN THE SECOND RATIO.

Table 16-1 Household to Apothecaries, and Metric Equivalencies

Household	Apothecaries	Metric
1 gtt	minim 1 (m i)	
minim 15 (m xv)	1 ml	
1 tsp	60 gtts	5 ml
1 tsp	dram i (3 i)	5 ml
3 tsp	½ ounce (ξ ss)	
1 tbsp	½ ounce (ξ ss)	15 ml
1 tbsp	dram iv (3 iv)	15 ml
2 tbsp	dr viii (3 viii)	30 ml
2 tbsp	1 ounce (ξ i)	30 ml
1 cup	8 ounces (ξ viii)	240 ml
1 pint	16 ounces (ξ xvi)	500 ml
1 quart	32 ounces (ξ xxxii)	1000 ml
	grains 15 (gr xv)	1 gram (1000 mg)
	grains 1 (gr i)	60 mg
	2.2 lb	1 kg (1000 g)

© Cengage Learning 2015

B. EXAMPLES OF CONVERSIONS BETWEEN SYSTEMS USING RATIO-PROPORTION METHOD
   1. YOU MUST KNOW AT LEAST ONE CONVERSION FACTOR BETWEEN THE TWO SYSTEMS.
   2. FOR EXAMPLE, WHEN CONVERTING POUNDS TO KILOGRAMS, YOU KNOW THAT 1 KG IS EQUAL TO 2.2 POUNDS.
   3. EXAMPLE PROBLEM 1 : 50 LB = x KG
      a. The known equivalent ratio 2.2 lb : 1 kg is placed first.
      b. The unknown equivalent ratio 50 lb : x is placed second.
      c. In ratio format, the problem looks like this:
         2.2 lb : 1 kg :: 50 lb : x kg
         The product of the means is 50.
         The product of the extremes is 2.2x.
      d. Then solve for x by dividing 50 by 2.2.
         1) x = 50 ÷ 2.2
         2) x = 22.7 kg
      e. Or in fraction format, the problem looks like this:
         1) 2.2 lb/1 kg = 50 lb/x kg
         2) Cross multiplied 1 × 50 = 50 and 2.2 × x = 2.2x
         3) 50 ÷ 2.2 = 22.7 kg
   4. EXAMPLE PROBLEM 2 : 5 = ML = X MINIMS
      a. Conversion factor for converting milliliters to minims is 1 ml = 15 m.
      b. The known equivalent ratio 1 ml : 15 m is placed first.
      c. The unknown equivalent ratio : = ml : x is placed second.
      d. In ratio format, the problem looks like this:
         1) 1 ml : 15 m :: 5 = ml : x m
         2) Multiply the means: 15 × 5 = 75
         3) Multiply the extremes: 1 × x = 1x
      e. Solve for x by dividing 75 by 1. The answer is 75 minims.
      f. In fraction format, the problem looks like this:
         1) 1 ml/15 m = 5 ml/x m
         2) Cross multiply 15 × 5 = 75
         3) Cross multiply 1 × x = 1x
         4) Solve for x: 75 ÷ 1 = 75.
      g. The answer is 75 minims.

III. DRUG CALCULATION METHODS

A. ANY OF THE FOLLOWING METHODS ARE APPROPRIATE TO USE IN CALCULATING DRUG DOSAGES; HOWEVER, IT IS RECOMMENDED THAT YOU USE WHAT YOU ARE MOST FAMILIAR WITH.

B. DRUG CALCULATIONS USING THE RATIO-PROPORTION METHOD

1. EXAMPLE 1
   a. One form of digoxin (Lanoxin) comes in 0.125-mg tablets.
   b. The medication order reads digoxin (Lanoxin) 0.0625 mg p.o. every day.
   c. How many tablets do you administer?
   d. Calculation:
      1) First, set up the problem using the ratio or the fraction format.
      2) 1 tab/0.125 = X/0.0625 and solve for x
      3) 0.125x = 0.0625 × 1
      4) 0.125x = 0.0625
      5) x = 0.0625/0.125
      6) x = ½ tab
      7) Or: 1 : 0.125 :: x : 0.0625
      8) 0.125x = 1 × 0.0625
      9) x = 0.0625/0.125
      10) x = ½ tab
2. EXAMPLE 2
   a. One form of phenytoin (Dilantin) comes in 100-mg capsules.
   b. The medication order reads phenytoin (Dilantin) 0.3 g p.o. every day.
   c. How many capsules will you administer?
   d. Calculation
      1) First convert grams to mg, then you are able to set up the problem properly.
         a) 0.3 g = x mg
         b) 1 g : 1000 mg :: 0.3 g : x mg
         c) 1x = 0.3 × 1000
         d) x = 300 mg
      2) Then set up the problem knowing that 0.3 g = 300 mg. How many capsules will you administer?
         a) 100 mg : 1 capsule :: 300 mg : x capsules
         b) 300 mg ÷ 100 mg x
         c) x = 3 capsules
      3) You will administer three 100-mg capsules of phenytoin (Dilantin).
C. DRUG CALCULATIONS USING THE FORMULA METHOD
   1. FORMULAS MAY BE USED WHEN THE DOSES CALCULATED ARE OF THE SAME MEASUREMENT SYSTEM.
   2. THEREFORE, BOTH THE DESIRED DOSE AND THE DOSE ON HAND MUST BE CONVERTED TO THE SAME SYSTEM BEFORE A FORMULA CAN BE APPLIED.
   3. FORMULA 1:
      a. $\dfrac{D}{H} \times Q = X$
      b. D = the desired dose
      c. H = the strength available
      d. Q = the quantity of measure (unit of measure)
      e. x = the unknown

4. FORMULA 2:
   a. DW/SW = DV/SV
   b. This formula is a proportion set up as a fraction and is functionally the same as the ratio-proportion method.
   c. DW is the dose weight (desired dose).
   d. SW is the stock weight (what is on hand).
   e. DV is the dose volume (the unknown).
   f. SV is the stock volume (the quantity or volume that contains the available dose).

IV. ORAL MEDICATION CALCULATION EXAMPLES
   A. RATIO-PROPORTION METHOD
      1. ORDERED: WARFARIN SODIUM (COUMADIN) 7.5 MG P.O. EVERY DAY
      2. AVAILABLE: WARFARIN SODIUM (COUMADIN) 2.5 MG TABS
      3. CALCULATION:
         a. 2.5 mg/1 tab = 7.5 mg/x tabs
         b. Cross multiply: 7.5 × 1 = 7.5 and 2.5 × x
         c. 7.5 mg/2.5x
         d. x = 3 tabs
      4. YOU WILL ADMINISTER THREE 2.5-MG TABLETS OF WARFARIN SODIUM (COUMADIN).
   B. FORMULA 1 METHOD
      1. ORDERED: AMPICILLIN (OMNIPEN) 1 G P.O. EVERY 6 HOURS
      2. AVAILABLE: AMPICILLIN (OMNIPEN) 250-MG CAPSULES
      3. CALCULATION:
         a. First convert grams to milligrams: 1 g = 1000 mg
         b. $\dfrac{D}{H} \times Q = X$
         c. $\dfrac{1000 \text{ mg}}{250 \text{ mg}} \times 1 = X$
         d. 4 = X
      4. YOU WILL ADMINISTER FOUR 250-MG CAPSULES OF AMPICILLIN (OMNIPEN).
   C. FORMULA 2 METHOD
      1. ORDERED: PHENOBARBITAL (SOLFOTON) GR ISS P.O. QAM
      2. AVAILABLE: PHENOBARBITAL (SOLFOTON) 15 MG TABLETS
      3. CALCULATION
         a. First convert grains to milligrams.
         b. gr i = 60 mg
         c. gr iss = 90 mg
         d. Then use the formula: DW/SW = DV/SV.
         e. 90 mg = DV (x tabs)
         f. 15 mg 1 tab
         g. 15x = 90 mg
         h. x = 90/15
         i. x = 6 tablets
      4. YOU WILL ADMINISTER SIX TABLETS OF PHENOBARBITAL (SOLFOTON).

V. PARENTERAL MEDICATION CALCULATION
A. EXAMPLE 1
   1. ORDER: MORPHINE SULFATE (DURAMORPH) GR ¼ IM EVERY 4 HOURS P.R.N.
   2. AVAILABLE: MORPHINE SULFATE (DURAMORPH) 10 MG/ML
   3. HOW MANY MILLIGRAMS AND HOW MANY MILLILITERS WILL YOU ADMINISTER?
   4. CALCULATION:
      a. First convert gr ¼ to milligrams: gr i/60 mg = gr ¼ / x, x = 15 mg.
      b. If the desired dose is 15 mg, then what is the volume to be administered IM?
      c. 10 mg/1 ml = 15 mg/x ml
      d. 10x = 15
      e. x = 15/10
      f. x = 1.5 ml
   5. YOU WILL ADMINISTER 1.5 ML OF THE MORPHINE SULFATE (DURAMORPH) SOLUTION IM.
B. EXAMPLE 2
   1. ORDER: MEPERIDINE (DEMEROL HCL) 50 MG IM EVERY 4 HOURS P.R.N.
   2. AVAILABLE: MEPERIDINE (DEMEROL HCL) 75 MG/ML
   3. WHAT VOLUME OF THE MEPERIDINE (DEMEROL HCL) SOLUTION WILL YOU ADMINISTER?
   4. CALCULATION:
      a. 75 mg/1 ml = 50 mg/x ml
      b. 75x = 50
      c. x = 50/75
      d. x = 2/3 or 0.66 ml or 0.67 ml of the meperidine (Demerol HCl) solution.
   5. YOU WILL ADMINISTER 0.67 ML OF MEPERIDINE (DEMEROL HCL) SOLUTION.

VI. POWDERED DRUG CALCULATION EXAMPLES
A. RECONSTITUTED ORAL MEDICATIONS
   1. THE POWDERED AMOXICILLIN (AMOXIL) BOTTLE READS: ADD 85 ML WATER TO MAKE 100 ML OF AMOXICILLIN SUSPENSION.
   2. WHEN RECONSTITUTED, THE AVAILABLE SUSPENSION WILL HAVE A CONCENTRATION OF 125 MG/5 ML.
   3. THE ORDER READS: AMOXICILLIN SUSPENSION (AMOXIL) 200 MG P.O. EVERY 6 HOURS.
   4. HOW MANY MILLILITERS PER DOSE WILL YOU ADMINISTER? HOW MANY DOSES ARE THERE IN THE BOTTLE?
   5. CALCULATION
      a. 125 mg/5 ml = 200 mg/x ml
      b. 125x = 1000
      c. 1000/125 = 8

6. YOU WILL ADMINISTER 8 ML PER DOSE. TO DETERMINE THE NUMBER OF DOSES PER BOTTLE, DIVIDE 100 ML BY THE 8-ML DOSE = 12.5 DOSES.
B. RECONSTITUTED PARENTERAL MEDICATIONS
   1. THREE (3) MILLION UNITS PENICILLIN G POTASSIUM (PFIZERPEN) COMES IN DRY CRYSTAL FORM IN A BOTTLE FOR RECONSTITUTION.
   2. THE BOTTLE READS: DILUTE WITH 4.2 ML NORMAL SALINE TO MAKE = ML.
   3. THE ORDER READS: PENICILLIN G POTASSIUM (PFIZERPEN) 300,000 UNITS IM NOW.
   4. AVAILABLE: PENICILLIN G POTASSIUM (PFIZERPEN) × MILLION UNITS IN = ML
   5. HOW MANY MILLILITERS WILL YOU ADMINISTER TO EQUAL 300,000 UNITS?
   6. CALCULATION:
      a. First, write out millions: × million = 3,000,000
      b. Set up the ratio: 3,000,000/5 ml = 300,000/x ml
      c. 3,000,000 × x = 5 × 300,000
      d. 3,000,000x = 1,500,000
      e. x = 3,000,000/1,500,000
      f. x = 1/2 or 0.5 ml
   7. YOU WILL ADMINISTER 0.5 ML OF SOLUTION.

VII. INTRAVENOUS DRUG CALCULATION EXAMPLES
A. MANUAL REGULATION: FORMULAS FOR DROPS PER MINUTE
   1. FORMULA: $V_1/T_1 \times V_2/V_2 = $ GTT/MIN
      a. $V_1 = $ Volume to infuse
      b. $V_2 = $ drop factor of the tubing (10, 15, or 20)
      c. $T_1 = $ Time in hours to infuse
      d. $T_2 = $ time in minutes (usually 60)
      e. Example:
         1) Run 750 ml D_5 0.9 NS over 4 hours, with a tubing drop factor of 10 gtts/ml.
         2) $V_1 = 750$, $V_2 = 10$, $T_1 = 4$ hours, and $T_2 = 60$
         3) 750/4 × 10/60 5
         4) 7500/240 5
         5) 31.25 gtts/min or 31 gtts/min
   2. FORMULA: $V/T \times C = R$
      a. This formula requires that you already know the hourly rate.
         1) V = volume ordered to be infused in 1 hour.
         2) C = drop factor (gtts ml).
         3) T = time ordered by the physician converted to minutes.

b. Example:
  1) The physician has ordered D_5 0.45 at 75 ml per hour.
  2) The tubing drop factor is 10 gtts/ml.
  3) Use the following steps to calculate the IV flow rate in drops per minute.
     a) 75 ml/60 min × 10 gtts/1 ml 5
     b) Cancel the zeros out, leaving 75/6 × 1/1.
     c) Cancel the 1s, leaving 75/6.
     d) The answer is 12.5 gtts/min or 13 gtts/min.

B. THREE-STEP METHOD FOR IV DRIP CALCULATIONS
  1. TO DETERMINE ML/HR, DIVIDE TOTAL FLUIDS BY HOURS TO RUN.
  2. TO DETERMINE ML/MIN, DIVIDE ML/HR BY 60 MINUTES.
  3. TO DETERMINE DROPS/MINUTE, MULTIPLY ML/MIN AND GTTS/ML.
  4. EXAMPLE:
     a. The order states: run 100 ml D_5W over 30 minutes.
     b. The tubing drop factor is 10 gtts/ml.
     c. Figure ml/hr: 100 ml/½ hr = 100 × 2 divided by 1 = 200 ml/hr
     d. Figure ml/min: 200 ml/hr divided by 60 minutes = 3.3 ml/min
     e. Figure drops/minute: 3.3 ml/min × 10 gtt/ml = 33 gtts/min

C. ELECTRONIC FLOW REGULATORS
  1. ELECTRONIC FLOW REGULATORS OR PUMPS MUST BE SET AT AN HOURLY RATE IN MILLILITER PER HOUR.
  2. THEREFORE, ALL VOLUME ORDERS MUST BE CONVERTED TO ML/HR BEFORE SETTING THE REGULATOR.
  3. EXAMPLE USING THE RATIO-PROPORTION METHOD
     a. The order states: administer nafcillin sodium (Nafcil) IVPB, 1 Gm diluted in 50 ml. Run over 15 minutes.
     b. The tubing drop factor is 15 gtts/ml.
     c. For what rate will you set the electronic regulator?
     d. Using the ratio-proportion method, set up the equation:
        1) 50 ml/15 min = x ml/60 min
                        (1 hr)
        2) 15x = 3000
        3) x = 3000/15
        4) x = 200 ml/hr
     e. You will set the electronic regulator for 200 ml/hr.
  4. EXAMPLE USING THE THREE-STEP METHOD
     a. The order reads: Administer 250 ml of D_5 0.45 over 6 hours per microdrip.
     b. Microdrip tubing drop factor is 60 gtts/ml.

c. Figure ml/hr: 250 ml/6 hr = 41.5 or 42 ml/hr set on the electronic regulator
d. Figure ml/min: 42 ml/hr divided by 60 minutes = 0.7 ml/min
e. Figure gtts/min: 0.7 ml/min × 60 gtts/ml = 42 gtts/min via microdrip tubing

VIII. **HEPARIN CALCULATION EXAMPLES**
  A. SUBCUTANEOUS HEPARIN DOSAGES
    1. THE ORDER READS: HEPARIN SODIUM (HEPARIN) 2500 UNITS S.Q. STAT.
    2. THE AVAILABLE CONCENTRATION IS HEPARIN SODIUM (HEPARIN) 5000 UNITS/ML.
    3. SET UP THE RATIO:
       a. 5000 units/1 ml = 2500 units/x ml
       b. 5000x = 2500
       c. x = 2500/5000
       d. x = ½
    4. YOU WILL ADMINISTER 0.5 ML OF THE AVAILABLE CONCENTRATION OF HEPARIN SODIUM (HEPARIN).
  B. INTRAVENOUS INFUSION HEPARIN
    1. THE ORDER READS: INFUSE 1000 UNITS/HOUR OF HEPARIN SODIUM (HEPARIN) IV.
    2. AVAILABLE IS 1 L NS WITH 40,000 UNITS OF HEPARIN SODIUM (HEPARIN) ADDED.
    3. THE DROP FACTOR FOR THE ADMINISTRATION IV SET IS 15 GTTS/ML.
    4. CONVERT TO UNITS/ML: 40,000 UNITS/1000 ML = 40 UNITS/1 ML
    5. SET UP THE EQUATION:
       a. 40 units/1 ml = 1000 units/x ml
       b. 40x = 1000
       c. x = 1000/40
       d. x = 25 ml/hour
    6. YOU WILL SET THE ELECTRONIC REGULATOR TO 25 ML/HOUR.

IX. **PEDIATRIC DOSAGE CALCULATION METHODS AND EXAMPLES**
  A. CALCULATION OF PEDIATRIC DOSAGES BASED ON THE CHILD'S WEIGHT
    1. ALWAYS CONVERT POUNDS TO KILOGRAMS FIRST. REMEMBER THAT 2.2 LB = 1 KG.
    2. MULTIPLY THE WEIGHT IN KILOGRAMS BY THE RECOMMENDED DOSE PER KILOGRAMS.
       a. An appropriate dose for a drug is 10 mg/kg/24 hrs.
       b. The child weighs 20 kg.
       c. Therefore, 10 mg × 20 kg = 200 mg/24 hr.
    3. DIVIDE THE 24-HOUR DOSE BY THE NUMBER OF RECOMMENDED DOSES PER DAY.
       a. 200 mg/day divided by 4 doses = 50 mg per dose.

4. FINALLY, CALCULATE THE VOLUME OR AMOUNT TO BE ADMINISTERED FROM WHAT IS IN STOCK.

B. CALCULATION OF PEDIATRIC DOSES BASED ON A RECOMMENDED SAFE DOSE RANGE
1. EXAMPLE:
   a. The order states: cephalexin (Keflex) oral suspension 150 mg p.o. every 6 hours.
   b. The child weighs 20 kg.
   c. The medication package states that the recommended dose is 25–50 mg/kg/day in 4 divided doses.
   d. Is the ordered dose within safe limits?
   e. Calculation
      1) First figure out what the safe range is for this child.
         a) 25 mg × 20 kg = 500 mg/day
         b) 50 mg × 20 kg = 1000 mg/day
      2) The safe range for this child is 500 mg to 1000 mg per 24-hour period.
      3) The actual dose ordered is 150 mg every 6 hours
      4) To determine if it falls within the range, either multiply the actual dose by 4 (every 6 hours is 4 doses per day) or divide the range dosages by 4 to determine the range for the individual dosages.
         a) 150 mg × 4 doses = 600 mg/day, which is within the range of 500 mg to 1000 mg per day.
         b) Thus, the dose is determined to be safe.
      5) Also, dividing the recommended daily dosages gives a dose range of:
         a) 500 mg ÷ 4 doses = 125 mg/dose, and
         b) 1000 mg ÷ 4 doses = 250 mg/dose
      6) The dose of 150 mg falls within the recommended range of 125 mg to 250 mg per dose for this child.

C. PEDIATRIC DOSAGE CALCULATIONS BASED ON BODY SURFACE AREA
1. THREE WAYS TO DETERMINE DOSAGES BASED ON BODY SURFACE AREA (BSA).
   a. One is based on the height and the weight of the child using a formula.
   b. The second method calculates BSA based on only the child's weight.
   c. The third method is based on the use of a tool called a West Nomogram chart. The nomogram is used only for children of normal height and weight and is also a method that requires some skill. It is not addressed in this review.

2. BSA CALCULATIONS USING HEIGHT AND WEIGHT
Either of the following formulas, one using metric measurements and one using English measurements, may be used.
   a. $\sqrt{\dfrac{kg \cdot cm/3600}{3600}} = BSA\,(m^2)$
   b. Example:
      1) A child weighs 20 kg and is 70 cm tall
      2) $\sqrt{20\ kg \times 70\ cm/3600} = \sqrt{1400/3600}$
         $= \sqrt{0.388}$
         $= 0.62\,m^2\ BSA$
      3) $\sqrt{lb \times in/3131} = BSA\,(m^2)$
   c. Using the same measurements converted to pounds and inches:
      1) The child weighs 44 lb and is 28 in. tall.
      2) $\sqrt{44\ lb \times 28\ in/3131} = BSA$
      3) $\sqrt{1231/3131} = BSA$
      4) $\sqrt{0.39} = BSA$
      5) $0.63 = BSA\,(m^2)$

3. BODY SURFACE AREA CALCULATION USING WEIGHT ONLY
   a. Formula:
   $$\dfrac{(4 \times child's\ weight\ in\ kg) + 7}{(child's\ wt\ in\ kg) + 90} = m^2 BSA$$
   b. Example: A child weighs 45 pounds.
      1) Convert pounds to kg: 45 ÷ 2.2 = 20.4 kg
         a) $\dfrac{(4 + 20.4) + 7}{20.4 + 90} = \dfrac{81.8 + 7}{110.4} =$
         $\dfrac{88.8}{110.4} = 0.80\ m^2$

4. CALCULATION OF PEDIATRIC DOSAGES USING BSA
   a. The formula for calculation of dosages using BSA is:
   (BSA in m^2/1.7 m^2) × 50 = the estimated pediatric dose
   b. Example:
      1) A child is 34 inches tall and weighs 28 pounds.
      2) The adult dose for a medication is 50 mg.
      3) First figure the BSA for the child:
         a) $\sqrt{34 \times 28/3131}$
         b) $\sqrt{0.30}$
         c) $0.55\ m^2$

4) Then use the formula to determine the estimated pediatric dose.

    a) $(0.55 \text{ m}^2/1.7 \text{ m}^2) \times 50 = 16.21$

5) The estimated pediatric dose for this child is 16 mg per dose.

  c. Example:

    1) A child weighs 35 kg and is 120 cm tall.

    2) The adult dose for the ordered medication is 500 mg.

3) First determine the child's BSA:

    a) $\sqrt{120 \times 35/3600} =$

    b) $\sqrt{1.16}$

    c) 1.08 m^2

4) Then utilize the dosage formula.

    a) $(1.08 \text{ m}^2/1.7 \text{ m}^2) \times 500 = 318$

5) The estimated dose for this child is 320 mg per dose.

PRACTICE QUESTIONS

1. A physician has ordered acetylsalicylic acid (aspirin) 10 gr every 4 hours p.r.n. The available dose for aspirin is 325 mg per tablet. What will the nurse administer?
   1. 2 tabs
   2. 1 tab
   3. 6.6 tabs
   4. 1.5 tabs

2. The physician has ordered guaifenesin (Robitussin) expectorant syrup 1½ ounces p.o. every 4 hours. One 90-ml bottle of guaifenesin (Robitussin) syrup is available. What will the nurse administer?
   1. 30 ml
   2. 45 ml
   3. 15 ml
   4. 10 ml

3. The physician's order reads phenytoin sodium (Dilantin) 0.1 g p.o. now. On hand are phenytoin sodium (Dilantin) capsules, 100 mg per capsule. The nurse will give
   1. 1 capsule.
   2. 3 capsules.
   3. 2 capsules.
   4. 1½ capsules.

4. The order reads levodopa (Dopar) 1.5 g p.o. b.i.d. On hand are levodopa (Dopar) tablets in a 500-mg strength. The nurse will give
   1. 1.5 tablets.
   2. 3 tablets.
   3. ½ tablet.
   4. 2 tablets.

5. The doctor's order states glipizide (Glucotrol) 5000 mcg daily. On hand the nurse has glipizide (Glucotrol) 2.5 mg tablets. How many tablets will the nurse administer?
   1. 1 tablet
   2. 2.5 tablets
   3. 0.2 tablets
   4. 2 tablets

6. The nurse reads a physician's order, which states atropine sulfate 0.5 mg IM stat. The nurse has atropine sulfate 0.3 mg/0.5 ml for injection available. What volume of the atropine solution should the nurse administer IM?
   1. 0.1 ml
   2. 0.5 ml
   3. 0.8 ml
   4. 1.0 ml

7. The order reads hydromorphone HCl (Dilaudid) 1.5 mg s.q. every 4 to 6 hours p.r.n. The nurse has injectable hydromorphone HCl (Dilaudid) ampules gr 1/30 per ml. What volume will the nurse administer?
   1. 0.9 ml
   2. 7.5 ml
   3. 0.5 ml
   4. 0.75 ml

8. The doctor's order reads vitamin B_{12} injection 1000 mcg once a month. The nurse has injectable vitamin B_{12} available in a concentration of 0.5 mg/ml. What volume should the nurse administer?
   1. 2.5 ml
   2. 2 ml
   3. 0.5 ml
   4. 1 ml

9. The doctor has ordered furosemide (Lasix) 40-mg IV push. The nurse has injectable furosemide (Lasix) 20 mg in 2 ml available. What should the nurse administer?
   1. 4 ml
   2. 0.4 ml
   3. 2 ml
   4. 3 ml

10. The doctor has ordered diazepam (Valium) 2.5-mg IV push stat. Available is injectable diazepam (Valium) = mg/ml. How much will the nurse administer?
    1. 0.75 ml
    2. 1 ml
    3. 0.5 ml
    4. 5 ml

11. The order reads ceftriaxone (Rocephin) 1.4 g IM b.i.d. Available is a ceftriaxone (Rocephin) 1-vial; when reconstituted with 2.1 ml, it results in a concentration of 350 mg per ml. What volume will the nurse administer?
    1. 3 ml/1 vial
    2. 4 ml/2 vials
    3. add more diluent to yield 4 ml in 1 vial
    4. 5 ml total/2 vials

12. Amoxicillin with clavulanic acid (Augmentin) powder reconstituted with 69 ml water results in a 75-ml suspension with a 200-mg/5-ml concentration. The doctor's order reads Augmentin 600-mg oral suspension p.o. every 12 hours. What volume of the suspension will the nurse administer?
    1. 30 ml
    2. 10 ml
    3. 15 ml
    4. 20 ml

13. Administer 800 ml IV D_5W at 75 ml/hour. The drop factor is 10 gtt/ml. What is the drops-per-minute rate?
    1. 13
    2. 10
    3. 17
    4. 21

14. Infuse heparin 40,000 units in 1000 ml of normal saline IV over 24 hours. The administration set has a drop factor of 10 gtt/ml. The nurse will set the gtt per minute at what rate?
    1. 14 gtt
    2. 42 gtt
    3. 17 gtt
    4. 7 gtt

15. The order reads heparin 2000 units s.q. The nurse has on hand heparin 2500 units/ml. How much will the nurse administer?
    1. 0.8 ml
    2. 0.5 ml
    3. 0.6 ml
    4. 0.9 ml

16. Heparin 30,000 units in 1000 ml of normal saline is to be administered IV over 24 hours via microdrip. How many units of heparin is the client receiving per hour?
    1. 635
    2. 1000
    3. 1250
    4. 125

17. Infuse 2000 ml of lactated Ringer's over 12 hours. The drop factor is 15 gtt/ml. The nurse will regulate the IV to how many gtt per minute?
    1. 28
    2. 42
    3. 56
    4. 14

18. Use an electronic regulator to administer 1500 ml of D_5W in 6 hours. The nurse will set the machine for
    1. 150 ml/hour.
    2. 200 ml/hour.
    3. 250 ml/hour.
    4. 275 ml/hour.

19. The physician has ordered morphine sulfate (Duramorph) 10 mg s.q. every 4 hours p.r.n. The child weighs 80 lb. The recommended maximum dose of morphine sulfate (Duramorph) is 0.1 mg to 0.2 mg/kg/dose. To determine the safety of this dose, what is the safe dose range for this child?
    1. 3.6 mg to 7.3 mg/dose
    2. 5 mg to 10 mg/dose
    3. 36 mg to 73 mg/dose
    4. 2.8 mg to 6 mg/dose

20. The nurse determines a 23-kg child to weigh how many pounds?

21. The recommended dosage for cefaclor (Ceclor) suspension is 20 to 40 mg/kg/day divided into 2 or 3 doses. The child receiving the cefaclor (Ceclor) weighs 22 kg. What is the recommended range for the individual dose ordered as twice daily for this child?
    1. 330 to 660 mg
    2. 440 to 880 mg
    3. 220 to 440 mg
    4. 200 to 400 mg

22. The recommended dosage for furosemide (Lasix) oral solution is a single dose of 2 mg/kg, and subsequent doses of 1 to 2 mg/kg every 6 hours until suitable response, up to a maximum of 6 mg/kg/day. What is the minimum to maximum 24-hour dose range for a child weighing 26 kg?
    1. 52 mg to 156 mg/24 hours
    2. 52 mg to 104 mg/24 hours

3. 26 mg to 52 mg/24 hours
4. 46 mg to 100 mg/24 hours

23. Using the child's weight, determine what the pediatric dose for digoxin (Lanoxin) would be if the usual adult dose is 0.15 mg p.o. every day. The child weighs 13 kg. The nurse will administer
1. 0.15 mg.
2. 0.05 mg.
3. 0.1 mg.
4. 0.07 mg.

24. An adult dose of doxycycline (Vibramycin) is 100 mg b.i.d. The child who is to take doxycycline (Vibramycin) is 32 inches tall and

weighs 48 pounds. Determine the child's dose based on BSA.
1. 30 mg/dose
2. 25 mg/dose
3. 50 mg/dose
4. 40 mg/dose

25. The recommended adult dose of acyclovir is 200 mg every 4 hours. What would an appropriate dose be for a child weighing 8 kg and standing 57 cm tall?
1. 40 mg
2. 60 mg
3. 30 mg
4. 50 mg

ANSWERS AND RATIONALES

1. 1. Find the number of tablets to be administered:

1 gr = 60 mg and 1 tablet = 325 mg
First convert grains to milligrams:

1 gr = 60 mg, 10 gr = 600 mg
660 mg is the desired dose.
Set up the ratio:

$$\frac{325 \text{ mg}}{1 \text{ tab}} = \frac{660 \text{ mg}}{x}$$

$$x = \frac{660}{325}$$

$$x = 2.03$$

Because conversions between apothecary and metric systems are not exact, two 325-mg tablets may be administered for the 600-mg grains. The nurse will administer 2 tablets.

2. 2. Find the amount of expectorant that should be administered.

1 ounce = 30 ml
Convert ounces to milliliters:

1 ounce = 30 ml, 1½ ounces = 45 ml, x = 45 ml
The nurse will administer 45 ml.

3. 1. Find the number of capsules to be administered. The order is for 0.1 g and each capsule = 100 mg.
Convert grams to milligrams:

1 gram = 1000 mg, 0.1 g = 100 mg, x = 1 capsule
The nurse will administer 1 capsule.

4. 2. Find the number of tablets to be administered. The order is for 1.5 g, and the tablets on hand are 500 mg.
First convert 1.5 g to milligrams:

1 gram = 1000 mg, 1.5 g = 1500 mg
Determine the number of tablets to be administered:

$$\frac{500 \text{ mg}}{1 \text{ tablet}} = \frac{1500 \text{ mg}}{x}$$

$$x = \frac{1500 \text{ mg}}{500 \text{ mg}} \text{ tablets}$$

$$x = 3 \text{ tablets}$$

The nurse will administer 3 tablets of levodopa (Dopar).

5. 4. Find the number of tablets to be administered. The order is for 5000 mcg, and the tablets on hand are 2.5 mg.
Convert 5000 mcg to milligrams:

1000 mcg = 1 mg, then 5000 mcg = 5 mg
Set up the ratio to determine the number of tablets to deliver:

$$\frac{2.5 \text{ mg}}{1 \text{ tab}} = \frac{5 \text{ mg}}{x}$$

$$x = \frac{5 \text{ mg}}{2.5 \text{ mg}} \text{ tablets}$$

$$x = 2 \text{ tablets}$$

The nurse will administer 2 tablets of glipizide (Glucotrol).

6. 3. Find the volume for this injection.
Set up a ratio:

$$\frac{0.3 \text{ mg}}{5 \text{ ml}} = \frac{5.0 \text{ mg}}{x}$$

$$x = 5 \text{ ml} \times \frac{0.5 \text{ mg}}{3.0 \text{ mg}}$$

$$x = \frac{2.5}{0.3} \text{ ml,}$$

$$x = 0.8 \text{ ml}$$

The nurse will administer 0.8 ml of the injectable solution intramuscularly.

7. 4.   Find the volume to inject.
Conversion: 1 gr = 60 mg, and the drug has 1/30 grain per ml.
Convert 1/30 grain and 1.5 mg to the same units.
Note: It is generally easier to convert grains to milligrams.

$$1 \text{ gr} = 60 \text{ mg}, \ 1/30 \text{ gr} = \frac{60}{30} \text{ mg}$$

The medicine has a strength of 2 mg/ml.
Then set up the ratio:

$$2 \text{ mg/ml} = \frac{1.5 \text{ mg}}{x}$$

$$x = \frac{1.2 \text{ mg}}{2 \text{ mg}} \text{ ml} = .75 \text{ ml}$$

The nurse will administer 0.75 ml of the injectable solution.

8. 2.   Find the volume for this injection.
The concentration available is 0.5 mg/ml.
Convert mcg to mg:

1 mg = 1000 mcg
Then set up the ratio:

$$\frac{0.5 \text{ mg}}{1 \text{ ml}} = \frac{1 \text{ mg}}{x}$$

$$x = \frac{1 \text{ mg}}{0.5 \text{ mg}} \text{ ml}$$

$$x = 2 \text{ ml}$$

The nurse will administer 2 ml injectable vitamin B_{12}.

9. 1.   Find the volume to inject.
The order is for 40 mg; available is 20 mg/2 ml.
Set up the ratio:

$$\frac{20 \text{ mg}}{2 \text{ ml}} = \frac{40 \text{ mg}}{x}$$

$$x = \frac{40 \times 2}{20 \text{ ml}}$$

$$x = 4 \text{ ml}$$

The nurse will administer 4 ml of injectable furosemide (Lasix) IV push.

10. 3.   Find the volume to be injected.
The order is for 2.5 mg; the available solution is = mg/ml.
Set up a ratio:

$$\frac{5 \text{ mg}}{1 \text{ ml}} = \frac{2.5 \text{ mg}}{x}$$

$$x = \frac{2.5 \text{ mg}}{5 \text{ mg}} \text{ ml}$$

$$x = 0.5 \text{ ml}$$

The nurse will administer 0.5 ml of the injectable furosemide (Valium) solution.

11. 2.   Find the volume to be administered.
The order is for 1.4 g; the available solution is 350 mg/ml.

Convert the grams to mg:

1 g = 1000 mg, 1.4 g = 1400 mg
Convert 1.4 g to milligrams (move the decimal point three places) to equal 1400 mg.
Set up a ratio:

$$350 \text{ mg/ml} = \frac{1400 \text{ mg}}{x},$$

$$x = \frac{1400 \text{ mg}}{350 \text{ mg}} \text{ ml},$$

$$x = 4 \text{ ml}$$

The nurse will need to administer 4 ml of the ceftriaxone (Rocephin). There is not enough medication in 1 vial to administer 4 ml. Therefore the nurse will need to reconstitute 2 vials for the prescribed dose.

12. 3.   Determine the volume to be administered.
The order is for 600 mg; available is 200 mg/5 ml.
Set up a ratio:

$$\frac{200 \text{ mg}}{5 \text{ ml}} = \frac{600 \text{ mg}}{x}$$

$$x = \frac{5 \times 600 \text{ mg}}{200 \text{ mg}} \text{ ml}$$

$$x = 15 \text{ ml}$$

The nurse will administer 15 ml of the reconstituted Augmentin suspension.

13. 1.   Determine the drip rate per minute in gtt.
The order is for a rate of 75 ml/hr; the drop factor is 10 gtt/ml.
Convert the order to ml/minute:

1 hour = 60 minutes, 1/60 × 75 ml/hr = 1.25 ml/minute
Determine the drip rate:

x = order × drop factor

x = 1.25 ml/min × 10 gtt/ml

x = 12.5 gtt/min, rounded to 13
The nurse will administer 13 gtt/minute.

14. 4.   Determine the gtt/minute rate.
The order is for a rate of 1000 ml/day; the drop factor is 10 gtt/ml.
Convert the order to ml/minute:

1 day = 24 hours/day × 60 minutes/hour

$$1000 \text{ ml / day} = \frac{1000}{24 \times 60} = 0.69 \text{ ml / minute}$$
minutes/day

Determine the drip rate:

x = order × drop factor

x = 0.69 ml/minute × 10 gtt/ml

x = 6.9 gtt/minute, rounded to 7
The nurse will administer 7 gtt/minute.

15. 1.   What volume will the nurse administer?
The order is for 2000 units and available is a 2500-units/ml solution.

Set up a ratio:

$$\frac{2500 \text{ units}}{1 \text{ ml}} = \frac{2000 \text{ units}}{x}$$

$$x = \frac{2000}{2500}$$

$$x = 4/5 \text{ or } 0.8 \text{ ml}$$

The nurse will administer 0.8 ml.

16. 1. Determine the units to be administered per hour.
The rate is 30,000 units over 24 hours.
Note: The mention of "microdrip" does not enter into this calculation at all; you only need to convert units per day to units per hour. The microdrip calculation is only a factor when determining the setting for delivery of the order.

The order is for $\dfrac{30,000 \text{ units}}{24 \text{ hours}} = \dfrac{x}{1 \text{ hour}}$

$$x = \frac{30,000 \text{ units}}{24 \text{ hours}}$$

$$x = 1249.9 \text{ units per hour, or } 1250 \text{ units per hour}$$

The nurse will administer 1250 units per hour.

17. 2. Determine the drip rate in gtt/minute.
The order is for 2000 ml/12 hours; the drop factor is 15 gtt/minute.
Convert the prescription to a rate per minute:

$$\frac{2000 \text{ ml}}{12 \text{ hours}} = 167 \text{ml/hours}$$

$$\frac{167 \text{ ml}}{60 \text{ minutes}} = 2.78 \text{ ml/hours}$$

Now calculate the drip rate:

$$2.78 \text{ ml/minute} \times 15 \text{ gtt/ml} = 41.7 \text{ gtt/minute}$$
$$\text{or } 42 \text{ gtt/minute}$$

The nurse will administer 42 gtt/minute.

18. 3. Determine the setting in ml/hour for an electronic regulator.
The order is for 1500 ml/6 hours.

$$x = \frac{1500 \text{ ml}}{6 \text{ hours}} = 250 \text{ ml/hour}$$

The nurse will set the machine to administer 250 ml/hour.

19. 1. Determine the safety of this order.
The recommended dose is from 0.1 mg/kg to 0.2 mg/kg; the child's weight is 80 pounds.
Convert the child's weight to kilograms:

$$1 \text{ pound} = \frac{1}{2.2} \text{ kilograms,}$$

$$80 \text{ lb} = \frac{80}{2.2} \text{ kg} = 36.4 \text{kg}$$

Calculate the recommended upper and lower thresholds for this child.

Lower threshold: 0.1 mg/kg × 36.4 kg = 3.6 mg

Upper threshold: 0.2 mg/kg × 36.4 kg = 7.3 mg

10 mg per dose is not within the safe dose range for this child.

20. 51. A 23-kg child weighs 50.6 pounds or 51. Multiply the 23 kg by 2.2 to convert from kg to lbs.

21. 3. Determine the recommended safety range of this drug.
The recommended dosage is from 20 mg/kg/day to 40 mg/kg/day.
The child's weight is 22 kg; the drug will be administered 2 times per day.
Calculate the recommended upper and lower thresholds for this child.

Lower threshold: 20 mg/kg/day × 22 kg = 440 mg/day

2 doses per day, lower threshold per dose = 1/2 × 440 mg = 220 mg

Upper threshold: 40 mg/kg/day × 22 kg = 880 mg/day

2 doses per day, upper threshold per dose = 1/2 × 880 mg = 440 mg
The range for this child is 220 mg to 440 mg.

22. 1. Determine the range of daily safe dosages for a 26-kg child.
The safe dosage range has a minimum of 2 mg/kg as a single application, and a maximum of 6 mg/kg/day
Determine the lower threshold for this child: If the first 2 mg/kg shows results, there would be no further application.

For a child of 26 kg, the lower threshold is 26 kg × 2 mg/kg = 52 mg.
Determine the upper threshold:
The daily upper limit is given as 6 mg/kg/day.

For a child of 26 kg, the upper threshold is 26 kg × 6 mg/kg = 156 mg.
The range for this child is 52 mg to 156 mg.

23. 2. Find the amount of digoxin the nurse should administer based on BSA.
The usual adult dose is for 0.15 mg, and the child weighs 13 kg.

S = log W × 0.425 + log H × 0.725 + 1.8564, where
S is in cm²; W is in kg; and H is in cm.
Determine the child's BSA using weight:

$$\frac{(4 \times 13) + 7}{13 + 90} = \frac{52 + 7}{103} = \frac{59}{103} = 0.57 \text{ m}^2 \text{ BSA}$$

Determine the child's dose based on BSA:

$$\frac{0.57 \text{ m}^2}{1.7} \times 0.15 \text{ mg} = 0.34 \times 0.15 = 0.05 \text{ mg}$$

The nurse will administer a 0.05-mg dose.

24. 4. Determine a child's dose of Vibramycin using BSA.

An adult dose is 100 mg; the child is 32 inches tall and weighs 48 pounds.

$S = \log W \times 0.425 + \log H \times 0.725 + 1.8564$, S is in cm^2; W is in kg; and H is in cm.
Determine the child's BSA:

$$\sqrt{\frac{48 \times 32}{3131}} = \sqrt{\frac{1536}{3131}} = \sqrt{0.49} = 0.70 \text{ m}^2$$

Determine the child's dose based on the BSA:

$$\frac{0.70 \text{ m}^2}{1.7} \times 100 \text{ mg} = 41 \text{ mg/dose}$$

The nurse will administer 40 mg per dose.

25. 1. Determine a child's dose of acyclovir using BSA. The adult dose is 200 mg; the child is 57 cm tall and weighs 8 kg.
Determine the child's BSA:

$$\sqrt{\frac{8 \text{ kg} \times 57 \text{ cm}}{3600}} = \sqrt{\frac{456}{3600}} = \sqrt{0.12} = 0.35 \text{ m}^2$$

Determine the child's dose:

$$\frac{0.35 \text{ m}^2}{1.7} \times 200 \text{ mg} = \text{child's dose}$$

$$0.21 \times 200 = 42 \text{ mg}$$

The nurse will administer 40 mg every 4 hours.

REFERENCES

Broyles, B. E. (2009). *Dosage calculation practice for nurses* (2nd ed.). Clifton Park, NY: Delmar Cengage Learning.

Curren, A. M. (2009). *Math for meds: Dosages and solutions* (10th ed.). Clifton Park, NY: Delmar Cengage Learning.

Gray Morris, D. C. (2009). *Calculate with confidence* (5th ed.). St. Louis, MO: Mosby.

Pickar, G. D. (2012). *Dosage calculations* (10th ed.). Clifton Park, NY: Delmar Cengage Learning.

Saxton, D. F., Ercolano-O'Neill, N., & Glavinspiehs, C. (2005). *Math and meds for nurses* (2nd ed.). Clifton Park, NY: Delmar Cengage Learning.

CHAPTER 17

DRUGS FOR THE EYES, EARS, NOSE, AND THROAT

I. **OPHTHALMIC MEDICATIONS**
   A. PRINCIPLES FOR ADMINISTRATION OF EYE MEDICATIONS
      1. EYE MEDICATIONS ARE USUALLY AVAILABLE IN DROP FORM OR OINTMENTS.
      2. TO PREVENT THE OVERFLOW OF MEDICATION INTO THE NASAL PASSAGES, INSTRUCT THE CLIENT TO OCCLUDE THE NASOLACRIMAL DUCT WITH ONE FINGER FOR 1–2 MINUTES AFTER INSTILLING THE MEDICATION.
      3. WHEN SEVERAL EYE MEDICATIONS ARE TO BE ADMINISTERED, WAIT AT LEAST 3 MINUTES BETWEEN MEDICATIONS.
      4. PERFORM GOOD HAND WASHING BEFORE ADMINISTRATION OF EYE MEDICATIONS TO AVOID CONTAMINATING THE EYE OR APPLICATOR.
      5. GOOD HAND WASHING AFTER THE ADMINISTRATION WILL RINSE OFF ANY RESIDUE ON THE HANDS.
      6. USE A SEPARATE BOTTLE OR TUBE OF MEDICATION FOR EACH CLIENT TO AVOID ACCIDENTAL CROSS CONTAMINATION.
      7. INSTILL THE DOSE OF EYE MEDICATION IN THE LOWER CONJUNCTIVAL SAC, NEVER DIRECTLY ONTO THE CORNEA.
      8. AVOID TOUCHING ANY PART OF THE EYE WITH THE DROPPER OR APPLICATOR.
      9. ADMINISTER EYEDROPS OR LIQUIDS BEFORE ANY ORDERED OINTMENTS.
      10. IN A CLIENT RECEIVING A BETA BLOCKER, WITHHOLD THE NEXT DOSE IF THE PULSE IS BELOW 50 TO 60 BEATS PER MINUTE AND REPORT TO THE PHYSICIAN.
      11. INSTRUCT THE CLIENT ON CORRECT INSTILLATION OF THE MEDICATION AND SUPERVISE THE INSTILLATION TO ASSESS IF THE CLIENT IS ABLE TO COMPLY SAFELY.
      12. INSTRUCT THE CLIENT TO CAREFULLY READ LABELS TO ENSURE ADMINISTRATION OF THE CORRECT STRENGTH AND MEDICATION.
      13. INSTRUCT THE CLIENT IF HIS VISION IS BLURRED TO AVOID DRIVING OR OPERATING HAZARDOUS EQUIPMENT.
      14. INSTRUCT THE CLIENT THAT HE OR SHE MAY BE UNABLE TO DRIVE HOME FOLLOWING AN EYE EXAMINATION WHEN MEDICATIONS TO DILATE THE PUPIL OR PARALYZE THE CILIARY BODY ARE ADMINISTERED.
      15. INSTRUCT THE CLIENT TO WEAR SUNGLASSES AND AVOID BRIGHT LIGHTS IF PHOTOPHOBIA OCCURS.
      16. INSTRUCT THAT A MISSED DOSE SHOULD BE ADMINISTERED AS SOON AS RECALLED, UNLESS THE NEXT DOSE IS DUE IN 1–2 HOURS.
      17. INSTRUCT THE CLIENT WITH GLAUCOMA THAT THE DISORDER CAN ONLY BE CONTROLLED WITH A REGULAR SCHEDULED DOSAGE.
      18. INFORM THE CLIENT THAT THE TREATMENT FOR GLAUCOMA MAY INITIALLY CAUSE PAIN AND BLURRED VISION.
      19. INFORM THE CLIENT TO REPORT ANY EYE IRRITATION THAT MAY DEVELOP.
      20. INSTRUCT THE CLIENT TO STORE THE EYE MEDICATIONS AS DIRECTED.
      21. INFORM THE CLIENT WITH SOFT CONTACT LENSES THAT CERTAIN

MEDICATIONS MAY DISCOLOR THE LENSES.

22. ADVISE THE CLIENT WITH CONTACT LENSES TO ASK ABOUT ANY SPECIAL PRECAUTIONS WITH MEDICATION.

23. ADVISE THE CLIENT TO KEEP THESE AND ALL MEDICATIONS OUT OF THE REACH OF CHILDREN.

B. PROCEDURE FOR THE ADMINISTRATION OF EYE MEDICATIONS

1. WASH THE HANDS THOROUGHLY AND APPLY CLEAN GLOVES.

2. VERIFY THE NAME, STRENGTH, DOSE, AND EXPIRATION DATE ON THE MEDICATION.

3. VERIFY THE CLIENT BY CHECKING THE IDENTIFICATION BAND AND ASKING TO STATE AND SPELL NAME.

4. VERIFY ANY ALLERGIES WITH THE CLIENT AND ALLERGY BAND.

5. POSITION THE CLIENT IN A SUPINE OR SITTING POSITION WITH THE HEAD TILTED BACK AND INSTRUCT TO OPEN EYES AND LOOK UP.

6. RETRACT THE LOWER LID DOWNWARD TOWARD THE CHEEKBONE.

7. GRASP THE BOTTLE LIKE A PENCIL WITH THE TIP DOWNWARD.

8. GENTLY REST YOUR HAND ON THE CLIENT'S FOREHEAD WHILE HOLDING THE BOTTLE ABOVE THE EYE.

9. GENTLY SQUEEZE THE BOTTLE TO ADMINISTER THE DROP INTO THE CONJUNCTIVAL SAC.

10. INSTRUCT THE CLIENT TO GENTLY CLOSE HIS EYES AND AVOID SQUEEZING SHUT.

11. INSTRUCT THE CLIENT TO ROTATE THE CLOSED EYE IN A CIRCLE TO DISTRIBUTE MEDICATION.

12. ALLOW 3–5 MINUTES BEFORE THE INSTILLATION OF ANOTHER DROP TO PROMOTE ABSORPTION.

13. WITH A GLOVED HAND, OCCLUDE THE NASOLACRIMAL DUCT TO AVOID SYSTEMIC ABSORPTION.

14. AVOID CONTACT BETWEEN THE MEDICATION BOTTLE AND THE EYEBALL.

15. ADMINISTER THE OINTMENT BY HOLDING THE TUBE NEAR, BUT NOT TOUCHING, THE EYE.

16. AFTER RETRACTING THE EYELID DOWNWARD, SQUEEZE A THIN RIBBON OF OINTMENT ALONG THE SAC FROM THE INNER TO OUTER CANTHUS.

17. INSTRUCT THE CLIENT TO GENTLY CLOSE HIS EYE AND ROTATE THE EYES FOR APPLICATION.

18. INSTRUCT THE CLIENT THAT AN OINTMENT MAY CAUSE BLURRED VISION.

II. **TOPICAL ANTI-INFECTIVE MEDICATIONS**

A. DESCRIPTION: THESE ARE USED TO KILL OR INHIBIT THE GROWTH OF BACTERIA, FUNGI, OR VIRUSES.

B. USES

1. ANTIBACTERIAL, ANTIFUNGAL, AND ANTIVIRAL INFECTIONS OF THE EYE

C. ADVERSE REACTIONS

1. BURNING, STINGING; ITCHING
2. PHOTOPHOBIA, TEARING, SENSITIVITY
3. HEADACHE, RASH
4. BLURRED VISION, PRURITUS
5. EDEMA, CORNEAL CLOUDING
6. SUPERINFECTIONS
7. INCREASED TOXICITY MAY OCCUR WITH TOPICAL CORTICOSTEROIDS.

D. CONTRAINDICATIONS/PRECAUTIONS

1. HYPERSENSITIVITY SUCH AS AN ALLERGY TO QUINOLONES (CIPRO)

E. NURSING INTERVENTIONS

1. METICULOUS EYELID HYGIENE WITH BABY SHAMPOO OR PLAIN WATER SOFTENS AND REMOVES CRUSTING.
2. GOOD HANDWASHING PRACTICES DECREASE THE SPREAD OF THE INFECTION OR VIRUS.
3. WARM COMPRESSES SEVERAL TIMES A DAY
4. INSTRUCT THE CLIENT NOT TO SHARE TOWELS OR OTHER PERSONAL ITEMS.
5. TREATMENT VARIES FROM 3 TO 21 DAYS FOR EFFECTIVENESS.
6. MAY NEED TO BE STORED IN THE REFRIGERATOR

F. TYPES (SEE TABLE 17-1)

III. **ANTI-INFLAMMATORY EYE MEDICATIONS**

A. DESCRIPTION

1. CONTROL ALLERGIC CONJUNCTIVITIS CAUSED BY ALLERGENS
2. CONTROL SWELLING AND EDEMA OF THE CONJUNCTIVA BEYOND THE EYELIDS
3. CONTROL INFLAMMATION, REDUCING VISION LOSS AND SCARRING

B. USES

1. SWELLING OF THE EYELIDS DUE TO ALLERGY

Table 17-1 Topical Anti-Infective Medications

Type	Medication	Uses
Antibacterial	Bacitracin Chloramphenicol (Chloromycetin) Ciprofloxacin (Cipro) Erythromycin Gentamicin Floxacin (Besivance)	*Staphylococcus aureus* *Streptococcus pneumoniae* *Haemophilus influenzae* Bacterial conjunctivitis
Antiviral	Vidarabine (Vira-A) Trifluridine (Viroptic) Acyclovir (Zovirax)	Herpes simplex virus 1 Herpes simplex virus 2
Antifungal	Natamycin (Natacyn) Trifluridine (Viroptic)	Herpes simplex virus Herpes simplex virus 1 and 2

© Cengage Learning 2015

2. ITCHING, BURNING, REDNESS, AND TEARING WITH ALLERGY RESPONSE
C. ADVERSE REACTIONS
   1. STINGING, BURNING, TEARING, ITCHY EYES
   2. BLURRED VISION, FOREIGN BODY SENSATION
D. NURSING INTERVENTIONS
   1. SHAKE THE MEDICATION WELL BEFORE USE.
   2. INSTRUCT THE CLIENT TO AVOID USE OF CONTACT LENSES DURING TREATMENT.
   3. INSTRUCT THE CLIENT TO AVOID ALLERGEN IF KNOWN.
   4. INSTRUCT THE CLIENT TO STOP THE USE OF CORTICOSTEROIDS IF THE INFECTION PROCESS IS PRESENT.
E. TYPES (SEE TABLE 17-2)
   1. CROMOLYN (INTAL): FOR CONJUNCTIVITIS
   2. LEVOCABASTINE (LIVOSTIN): FOR ALLERGIC CONJUNCTIVITIS
   3. LODOXAMIDE (ALOMIDE): FOR KERATOCONJUNCTIVITIS

Table 17-2 Anti-Inflammatory Eye Medications

Type	Medication	Uses
Topical antihistamines	Cromolyn Levocabastine (Livostin) Lodoxamide (Alomide)	Conjunctivitis Allergic conjunctivitis Kerato conjunctivitis
Topical corticosteroids	Prednisolone acetate Prednisolone sodium phosphate Dexamethasone (Decadron)	Postoperative care Conjunctivitis

© Cengage Learning 2015

IV. **MYDRIATICS**
A. DESCRIPTION
   1. CAUSE DILATION OF THE PUPIL FOR VISUALIZATION OF INNER EYE STRUCTURES
   2. PREVENT CONTRACTION OF THE PUPIL WHEN IN BRIGHT LIGHT FOR EXAMINATION
B. USES
   1. DILATION OF THE PUPIL FOR DIAGNOSTIC EYE EXAMINATION
   2. DIFFERENTIATE BETWEEN VARIOUS TYPES OF HORNER'S SYNDROME
C. ADVERSE REACTIONS
   1. TACHYCARDIA
   2. ELEVATED BLOOD PRESSURE
D. CONTRAINDICATIONS/PRECAUTIONS
   1. CARDIAC ARRHYTHMIA
   2. CEREBRAL ATHEROSCLEROSIS
   3. OLDER ADULT CLIENT
   4. PROSTATIC HYPERTROPHY
   5. DIABETES MELLITUS
   6. PARKINSON'S DISEASE
   7. GLAUCOMA (MAY INCREASE THE RISK OF INCREASED INTRAOCULAR PRESSURE)
E. NURSING INTERVENTIONS
   1. INSTRUCT THE CLIENT TO WEAR DARK GLASSES FOR COMFORT IN DAYLIGHT.
   2. INSTRUCT THE CLIENT THAT MEDICATION EFFECTS MAY LAST 4–6 HOURS.
F. TYPES
   1. ATROPINE SULFATE
   2. CYCLOPENTOLATE (CYCLOGYL)
   3. HOMATROPINE (ISOPTO HOMATROPINE)
   4. SCOPOLAMINE (ISOPTO HYOSCINE)
   5. TROPICAMIDE (MYDRIACYL)

V. **CYCLOPLEGICS**
A. DESCRIPTION
   1. RELAX THE CILIARY MUSCLE, CAUSING BLURRED VISION
   2. BLOCK THE RESPONSES OF THE SPHINCTER MUSCLE IN THE CILIARY BODY
B. USES
   1. IN THE PREPARATION OF A CLIENT FOR AN OPHTHALMIC EXAMINATION
   2. PREOPERATIVELY TO RELAX THE CILIARY MUSCLES
C. ADVERSE REACTIONS
   1. IRRITATION
   2. BLURRED VISION
   3. PHOTOPHOBIA
D. CONTRAINDICATIONS/PRECAUTIONS
   1. GLAUCOMA

E. NURSING INTERVENTIONS
   1. INSTRUCT THE CLIENT THAT THE EFFECTS MAY LAST UP TO 7–12 HOURS.
   2. INSTRUCT THE CLIENT TO WEAR DARK GLASSES FOR COMFORT IN DAYLIGHT.
F. TYPES
   1. TROPICAMIDE (MYDRIACYL)
   2. CYCLOPENTOLATE (CYCLOGYL)
   3. SCOPOLOMINE (ISOPTO HYOSCINE)
   4. HOMATROPINE

VI. NONSTEROIDAL ANTI-INFLAMMATORY EYE MEDICATIONS
A. DESCRIPTION
   1. REDUCE OR PREVENT OCULAR INFLAMMATION AND INCREASE COMFORT
   2. AVOID THE EFFECTS OF CORTISONE-TYPE PREPARATIONS
B. USES
   1. FOR POSTOPERATIVE INFLAMMATION
   2. TO INHIBIT INTRAOPERATIVE MIOSIS
C. ADVERSE REACTIONS
   1. BURNING, STINGING OF THE EYES
   2. OCULAR ALLERGY RESPONSE
   3. BLURRED VISION
D. CONTRAINDICATIONS/PRECAUTIONS
   1. AN ABRASION OR WOUND OF THE EYE
E. NURSING INTERVENTIONS
   1. INSTRUCT THE CLIENT TO INSTILL AS PRESCRIBED.
   2. INSTRUCT THE CLIENT TO USE CAUTION WITH AN ABRASION OR WOUND OF THE EYE.
F. TYPES
   1. DICLOFENAC (VOLTAREN): FOR POSTOPERATIVE INFLAMMATION
   2. KETOROLAC: FOR POSTOPERATIVE INFLAMMATION
   3. FLURBIPROFEN (OCUFEN): INHIBIT INTRAOPERATIVE MIOSIS
   4. SUPROFEN (PROFENAL): INHIBIT INTRAOPERATIVE MIOSIS

VII. CORTICOSTEROIDS EYE MEDICATIONS
A. DESCRIPTION
   1. CONTROL CHRONIC ALLERGY RESPONSE IN THE EYE
   2. CONTROL INFLAMMATION IN THE EYE
B. USES
   1. ACUTE AND CHRONIC ALLERGIC EYE CONDITIONS
   2. INFLAMMATORY CONDITIONS OF THE EYE, INCLUDING CONJUNCTIVITIS AND KERATITIS
   3. OPTIC NEURITIS, SYMPATHETIC OPTHALMIA, AND ALLERGIC CORNEAL ULCERS

C. ADVERSE REACTIONS
   1. ELEVATED INTRAOCULAR PRESSURE (IOP)
   2. CATARACT FORMATION
   3. SECONDARY OCULAR INFECTION
D. CONTRAINDICATIONS/PRECAUTIONS
   1. USE FOR SHORT PERIODS OF TIME (PROLONGED USE MAY RESULT IN GLAUCOMA OR DAMAGE TO THE STRUCTURE OF THE EYE).
E. NURSING INTERVENTIONS
   1. ASSESS THE CLIENT FOR SIGNS OF INFLAMMATION OR INFECTION.
   2. SHAKE THE SUSPENSION BEFORE INSTILLATION OF THE MEDICATION.
   3. MAY INSTRUCT THE CLIENT TO TAPER DOSAGE OVER SEVERAL DAYS
F. TYPES
   1. DEXAMETHASONE (DECADRON): ACUTE AND CHRONIC INFLAMMATIONS
   2. PREDNISOLONE (PREDNISOL): FOR POSTOPERATIVE INTRAOCULAR EDEMA AND PRESSURE

VIII. BETA-ADRENERGIC BLOCKING MEDICATIONS
A. DESCRIPTION
   1. DECREASE AQUEOUS HUMOR PRODUCTION WITHOUT AFFECTING PUPIL SIZE
   2. DECREASE INTRAOCULAR PRESSURE (IOP)
B. USES
   1. CHRONIC OPEN-ANGLE GLAUCOMA
C. ADVERSE REACTIONS
   1. TRANSIENT DISCOMFORT
   2. RARE SYSTEMIC REACTIONS (BRADYCARDIA, HEART BLOCK, HEADACHE, DEPRESSION)
   3. PHOTOPHOBIA
D. CONTRAINDICATIONS/PRECAUTIONS
   1. ASTHMA
   2. CAUTION WITH USE IN CLIENTS RECEIVING BETA BLOCKERS
   3. BRADYCARDIA
   4. HEART FAILURE
E. NURSING INTERVENTIONS
   1. MONITOR THE PULSE AND BLOOD PRESSURE.
   2. ENCOURAGE THE CLIENT TO WEAR DARK SUNGLASSES.
F. TYPES
   1. BETAXOLOL HCL (BETOPTIC): TO DECREASE INTRAOCULAR PRESSURE
   2. LEVOBUNOLOL HCL (BETAGON LIQUIFILM); TO DECREASE INTRAOCULAR PRESSURE
   2. TIMOLOL MALEATE (TIMOPTIC): TO TREAT GLAUCOMA

IX.   **CARBONIC ANHYDRASE INHIBITORS**
A.   DESCRIPTION
1.   DECREASE AQUEOUS HUMOR PRODUCTION
2.   ENHANCE FLUID OUTFLOW AND DECREASES PRESSURE
B.   USES
1.   LONG-TERM TREATMENT OF OPEN-ANGLE GLAUCOMA
C.   ADVERSE REACTIONS
1.   ANOREXIA AND GASTROINTESTINAL DISTURBANCES
2.   PHOTOSENSITIVITY
3.   POLYURIA
4.   RENAL CALCULI
5.   HYPOKALEMIA
6.   PARESTHESIAS (TINGLING IN THE EXTREMITIES)
D.   CONTRAINDICATIONS/PRECAUTIONS
1.   HYPERSENSITIVITY TO SULFONAMIDES
E.   NURSING INTERVENTIONS
1.   INSTRUCT THE CLIENT TO AVOID PROLONGED SUNLIGHT EXPOSURE.
2.   INSTRUCT THE CLIENT THAT THE MEDICATION CAN ALTER ELECTROLYTE LEVELS.
3.   MONITOR SERUM ELECTROLYTES.
F.   TYPES
1.   BRINZOLAMIDE (AZOPT)
2.   ACETAZOLAMIDE (DIAMOX)
3.   DICHLORPHENAMIDE (DARANIDE)

X.   **OSMOTIC EYE MEDICATIONS**
A.   DESCRIPTION
1.   INHIBIT CARBONIC ANHYDRATE ACTIVITY
2.   REDUCE INTRAOCULAR PRESSURE IN THE EYE
B.   USES
1.   REDUCE INTRAOCULAR PRESSURE IN THE EYE
2.   EMERGENCY TREATMENT OF ACUTE CLOSED-ANGLE GLAUCOMA
3.   PREOPERATIVELY AND POSTOPERATIVELY TO DECREASE VITREOUS HUMOR VOLUME
C.   ADVERSE REACTIONS
1.   HEADACHE
2.   NAUSEA, VOMITING, AND DIARRHEA
3.   DISORIENTATION
4.   ELECTROLYTE IMBALANCE
D.   NURSING INTERVENTIONS
1.   MONITOR FOR CHANGES IN ELECTROLYTE IMBALANCE.
2.   MONITOR FOR CHANGES IN LEVEL OF ORIENTATION.
3.   MONITOR VISUAL ACUITY.
4.   ASSESS RISK FOR INJURY DUE TO ELECTROLYTE CHANGES.

E.   TYPES
1.   MANNITOL (OSMITROL)
2.   ISOSORBIDE (ISMOTIC)
3.   GLYCERIN (OPHTHALGAN)

XI.   **OTIC MEDICATIONS**
A.   PRINCIPLES FOR ADMINISTRATION OF EAR MEDICATIONS
1.   EAR MEDICATIONS ARE USUALLY IN THE FORM OF DROPS.
2.   TREATMENT SHOULD BE INITIATED AT THE TIME OF DIAGNOSIS.
3.   MEDICATIONS ARE CONTINUED FOR 1 WEEK, OR IF RECURRENT, 2 WEEKS.
4.   IF THE EAR CANAL IS VERY EDEMATOUS, A WICK MAY BE INSERTED ON WHICH THE SOLUTION IS DROPPED AND THE MEDICATION IS MORE EFFECTIVELY DISTRIBUTED IN THE CANAL.
5.   IN AN ADULT, PULL THE AURICLE UP AND BACK TO STRAIGHTEN THE EAR CANAL TO INSTILL EARDROPS.
6.   PULL THE AURICLE DOWN AND BACK FOR INFANTS AND CHILDREN UNDER 3 YEARS OF AGE.
7.   THE EAR MUST BE INSPECTED FOR PERFORATION PRIOR TO EAR IRRIGATION.
8.   WITH EAR IRRIGATION, PREPARE THE SOLUTION TO 100°F (37.7°C) BECAUSE COOLER SOLUTIONS MAY CAUSE EAR INJURY, NAUSEA, OR VERTIGO.
9.   IF EARDROPS ARE STORED IN THE REFRIGERATOR, ALLOW TO WARM TO ROOM TEMPERATURE.
10.   MAINTAIN STERILITY OF THE DROPPER APPLICATOR.
11.   CAREFUL HANDLING AND DISPOSAL OF MATERIAL SATURATED WITH DRAINAGE IS IMPORTANT.
12.   ANIMATE OBJECTS MUST BE IMMOBILIZED BEFORE REMOVAL.
13.   MINERAL OIL OR ALCOHOL MAY BE USED TO DROWN AN INSECT.
14.   INANIMATE OBJECT REMOVAL SHOULD BE DONE BY AN OTOLARYNGOLOGIST.
B.   PROCEDURES FOR ADMINISTRATION OF EAR MEDICATIONS
1.   ASSESS THE EAR CANAL AND TYMPANIC MEMBRANE FOR POSSIBLE PERFORATION.
2.   A TYMPANIC MEMBRANE THAT MOVES, EVEN SLIGHTLY, CANNOT BE PERFORATED.

3. POSITION THE CLIENT WITH THE HEAD TO THE SIDE SO THAT THE AFFECTED EAR IS UPWARD.
4. PULL THE AURICLE GENTLY UP FOR ADULTS AND DOWN FOR A CHILD LESS THAN 3 YEARS OF AGE.
5. AFTER ADMINISTRATION, ENCOURAGE THE CLIENT TO REMAIN WITH THE HEAD UPWARD AND GENTLY MASSAGE THE FRONT OF THE EAR TO FACILITATE ENTRY OF THE EARDROPS INTO THE CANAL.
6. A COTTON BALL MAY BE PLACED IN THE EAR CANAL TO PREVENT ESCAPE OF THE DROPS.

XII.   **ANTI-INFECTIVE EAR MEDICATIONS**
    A. DESCRIPTION
      1. KILL OR INHIBIT THE GROWTH OF *PSEUDOMONAS AERUGINOSA, PROTEUS VULGARIS, ESCHERICHIA COLI,* AND *STAPHYLOCOCCUS AUREUS*
      2. REDUCTION OF DISCOMFORT AND INFLAMMATION IN THE EAR CANAL
    B. USES
      1. SUPERFICIAL INFECTION IN THE EAR CANAL DUE TO BACTERIA
      2. SYSTEMIC TREATMENT OF OTITIS MEDIA OR TOPICAL TREATMENT OF OTITIS EXTERNA
    C. ADVERSE REACTIONS
      1. TOPICAL: BURNING, ITCHING, URTICARIA; VESICLE DERMATITIS WITH SENSITIVITY
      2. SYSTEMIC: INCREASED RISK OF SUPERINFECTION WITH PROLONGED USE, HYPERSENSITIVITY, URTICARIA, NAUSEA, AND DIARRHEA
    D. CONTRAINDICATIONS/PRECAUTIONS
      1. IN CONJUNCTION WITH TETRACYCLINE
    E. NURSING INTERVENTIONS
      1. ASSESS FOR RUPTURED TYMPANIC MEMBRANE.
      2. ASSESS FOR HISTORY OF ALLERGY OR HYPERSENSITIVITY REACTIONS.
      3. INSTRUCT THE CLIENT THAT SYSTEMIC MEDICATION MAY DECREASE THE EFFECT OF ORAL CONTRACEPTION.
      4. INSTRUCT THE CLIENT THAT THE ACTION OF TETRACYCLINES MAY INTERFERE WITH DRUG EFFECTS.
      5. INSTRUCT THE CLIENT NOT TO "SAVE" OR "SHARE" MEDICATIONS WITH OTHERS.
      6. INSTRUCT THE CLIENT TO TAKE THE MEDICATION AS DIRECTED THROUGHOUT THE DAY, NOT AS A SINGLE DOSE.
    F. TYPES (SEE TABLE 17-3)

Table 17-3 Anti-Infective Ear Medications

Type	Medication	Uses
Topical anti-infectives	Polymixin B Colistin (Polymyxin E) Neomycin Chloramphenicol (Chloromycetin)	Otitis externa bacterial infection *Pseudomonas aeruginosa* *Proteus vulgaris* *Escherichia coli* *Staphylococcus aureus*
Systemic anti-infectives	Amoxicillin Polycillin Cefaclor (Ceclor) Clindamycin (Cleocin) Erythromycin Clarithromycin (Biaxin)	Otitis media bacterial infection Following recent upper respiratory infections Bottle feeding

© Cengage Learning 2015

XIII.   **TOPICAL ANTIFUNGAL EAR MEDICATIONS**
    A. DESCRIPTION: INHIBIT GROWTH OF FUNGAL INFECTION
    B. USES
      1. FUNGAL INFECTIONS OF THE EXTERNAL EAR
    C. ADVERSE REACTIONS
      1. REDNESS, ITCHING
    D. CONTRAINDICATIONS/PRECAUTIONS
      1. HYPERSENSITIVITY
    E. NURSING INTERVENTIONS
      1. ASSESS FOR AN ALLERGY OR PREVIOUS HISTORY OF HYPERSENSITIVITY.
      2. PROTECT THE MEDICATION FROM HEAT, LIGHT, MOISTURE, AND AIR.
    F. TYPES
      1. NYSTATIN

XIV.   **CERUMINOLYTIC EAR MEDICATIONS**
    A. DESCRIPTION
      1. EMULSIFY AND DISPERSE EARWAX IN THE EAR CANAL
    B. USES
      1. IMPACTED EARWAX IN THE EAR CANAL
    C. ADVERSE REACTIONS
      1. IRRITATION
      2. REDNESS OR SWELLING OF THE EAR CANAL
    D. NURSING INTERVENTIONS
      1. INSTRUCT THE CLIENT NOT TO USE DROPS MORE OFTEN THAN PRESCRIBED.
      2. INSTRUCT THE CLIENT TO FOLLOW PHYSICIAN DIRECTIONS REGARDING CERUMEN REMOVAL.
      3. INSTRUCT THE CLIENT TO NOTIFY THE PHYSICIAN IF REDNESS, PAIN, OR SWELLING PERSISTS.
    E. TYPES
      1. DEBROX
      2. BORIC ACID
      3. CERUMENEX

XV. ANTIHISTAMINE AND DECONGESTANT EAR MEDICATIONS
- A. DESCRIPTION
  1. PRODUCE VASOCONSTRICTION
  2. REDUCE RESPIRATORY TISSUE EDEMA TO OPEN OBSTRUCTED EUSTACHIAN TUBES
  3. DRY FLUID COLLECTION IN THE TISSUES OF THE MIDDLE EAR
  4. FLUID REDUCTION IMPROVES HEARING.
- B. USES
  1. ACUTE AND SEROUS OTITIS MEDIA
- C. ADVERSE REACTIONS
  1. DROWSINESS
  2. BLURRED VISION
  3. DRY MUCOUS MEMBRANES
- D. NURSING INTERVENTIONS
  1. INSTRUCT THE CLIENT TO AVOID HAZARDOUS ACTIVITIES IF DROWSINESS OCCURS.
  2. INFORM THE CLIENT THAT DROWSINESS, BLURRED VISION, AND A DRY MOUTH MAY OCCUR.
  3. INSTRUCT THE CLIENT TO INCREASE FLUID INTAKE UNLESS CONTRAINDICATED.
  4. INSTRUCT THE CLIENT THAT SUCKING ON HARD CANDY MAY ALLEVIATE DRY MOUTH.
- E. TYPES
  1. TRIPROLIDINE AND PSEUDOEPHEDRINE (ACTIFED)
  2. NAPHAZOLINE HCL (ALLEREST)
  3. CHLORPHENIRAMINE (CHLOR-TRIMETON)
  4. BROMPHENIRAMINE (DIMETANE)

XVI. ANTIEMETIC EAR MEDICATIONS
- A. DESCRIPTION
  1. SUPPRESSION OF NOXIOUS STIMULI THAT PROMOTE NAUSEA
  2. SUPPRESSION OF LABYRINTH EDEMA
- B. USES
  1. MIDDLE EAR DISORDERS THAT CREATE NAUSEA AND VOMITING
  2. DECREASE PRESSURE AND TINNITUS IN THE EAR TISSUES
- C. ADVERSE REACTIONS
  1. DROWSINESS
  2. GASTROINTESTINAL UPSET; CONSTIPATION
  3. DRY MOUTH
  4. THICKENING OF BRONCHIAL SECRETIONS
  5. URINARY RETENTION
- D. CONTRAINDICATIONS/PRECAUTIONS
  1. ALCOHOL
  2. CENTRAL NERVOUS SYSTEM DEPRESSANTS
- E. NURSING INTERVENTIONS
  1. INSTRUCT THE CLIENT TO AVOID DRIVING OR OTHER ACTIVITIES REQUIRING ALERTNESS UNTIL THE RESPONSE TO MEDICATION IS KNOWN.
  2. IF USED FOR PROPHYLAXIS, TAKE AT LEAST 30 MINUTES BEFORE EXPOSURE TO CONDITIONS THAT ELICIT NAUSEA.
  3. ADVISE THE CLIENT OF THE IMPORTANCE OF THE USE OF SUNSCREEN TO PREVENT PHOTOSENSITIVITY REACTIONS.
  4. ENCOURAGE ORAL RINSES AND SUGARLESS GUM AND CANDY FOR DRY MOUTH.
- F. TYPES
  1. DIPHENHYDRAMINE (BENADRYL) FOR MOTION SICKNESS

XVII. DIURETIC EAR MEDICATIONS
- A. DESCRIPTION
  1. INCREASE URINARY OUTPUT OF SODIUM AND WATER FROM THE BODY
- B. USES
  1. TO REDUCE INNER EAR ENDOLYMPH SWELLING AS IN MÉNIÈRE'S DISEASE
  2. ENDOLYMPH EDEMA
- C. ADVERSE REACTIONS
  1. DEHYDRATION, HYPOTENSION
  2. HYPOKALEMIA, HYPOMAGNESEMIA, HYPONATREMIA, HYPERCALCEMIA
  3. ALKALOSIS
  4. IMPOTENCE
  5. PHOTOSENSITIVITY
- D. CONTRAINDICATIONS/PRECAUTIONS
  1. HYPERSENSITIVITY TO THIAZIDE DIURETICS
  2. HYPERSENSITIVITY TO SULFONAMIDE DERIVATIVES
- E. NURSING INTERVENTIONS
  1. INSTRUCT THE CLIENT TO TAKE THE MEDICATION EARLY IN THE DAY TO PREVENT NOCTURIA.
  2. ASSESS FOR A SENSITIVITY TO THIAZIDE DIURETICS OR SULFONAMIDE DERIVATIVES.
- F. TYPES
  1. CHLOROTHIAZIDE (DIURIL)
  2. FUROSEMIDE (LASIX)

XVIII. NASAL MEDICATIONS
- A. PRINCIPLES FOR ADMINISTRATION OF NASAL MEDICATIONS
  1. NASAL MEDICATIONS ARE USUALLY IN THE FORM OF DROPS OR SPRAYS.
  2. WASH THE HANDS BEFORE ADMINISTERING NASAL MEDICATIONS TO AVOID CONTAMINATION OF THE APPLICATOR.

3. WASH THE HANDS AFTER ADMINISTRATION TO RINSE OFF ANY RESIDUE ON THE HANDS.
4. WHEN SEVERAL NASAL MEDICATIONS ARE ADMINISTERED, WAIT AT LEAST 3 MINUTES BETWEEN MEDICATION DOSES.
5. USE A SEPARATE BOTTLE OF NASAL MEDICATION FOR EACH CLIENT TO AVOID CROSS CONTAMINATION.
6. INSTRUCT THE CLIENT WITH CARDIOVASCULAR DISEASE, HYPERTENSION, DIABETES, GLAUCOMA, PROSTATIC HYPERTROPHY, OR HEPATIC OR RENAL DISEASE TO AVOID THE USE OF DECONGESTANTS.
7. NASAL SPRAYS SHOULD BE USED FOR NO MORE THAN 2–3 DAYS OR MORE THAN 3–4 TIMES DAILY.
8. INSTRUCT THAT THE CLIENT MAY NEED TO INCREASE FLUID INTAKE TO RELIEVE ORAL DRYNESS.
9. SHAKE THE MEDICATION PRIOR TO ADMINISTRATION, IF DIRECTED.

B. PROCEDURE FOR THE ADMINISTRATION OF NASAL MEDICATIONS
1. ASSESS THE CLIENT'S NASAL AIRFLOW AND NASAL SECRETIONS.
2. ASSESS THE MUCOUS MEMBRANE OF THE NARES FOR SWELLING AND IRRITATION.
3. ASSESS FOR POTENTIAL CONTRAINDICATIONS WHEN ADMINISTERING IN THE PRESENCE OF CORONARY ARTERY DISEASE, DIABETES, GLAUCOMA, PROSTATIC HYPERTROPHY, OR HEPATIC OR RENAL DISEASE.
4. ASSESS FOR ACUTE ASTHMA OR OTHER RESPIRATORY DISEASE THAT MAY BE AGGRAVATED BY DRYING OF SECRETIONS.
5. INSTRUCT THE CLIENT TO BLOW THE NOSE BEFORE THE ADMINISTRATION OF NASAL MEDICATIONS.
6. INSTRUCT THE CLIENT TO TILT THE HEAD BACKWARD FOR ADMINISTRATION OF NASAL MEDICATION.
7. INSTRUCT THE CLIENT TO SNUFF THE MEDICATION AS IT IS ADMINISTERED.
8. INSTRUCT THE CLIENT NOT TO BLOW THE NOSE FOR 20–30 MINUTES FOR MEDICATION ABSORPTION.

XIX. **NASAL ANTIHISTAMINE MEDICATIONS**
A. DESCRIPTION
1. BIND WITH HISTAMINE RECEPTORS ON TARGET CELLS TO BLOCK HISTAMINE
2. RELIEVE ACUTE CLINICAL MANIFESTATIONS OF ALLERGIC RESPONSE
B. USES
1. ALLERGIC RHINITIS
2. SUPPRESSION OF RESPONSE TO REACTIVE ANTIGENS
C. ADVERSE REACTIONS
1. CENTRAL NERVOUS SYSTEM STIMULATION: INSOMNIA, EXCITATION, HEADACHE, AND IRRITABILITY
2. INCREASED BLOOD PRESSURE, PALPITATIONS, AND TACHYCARDIA
3. INCREASED INTRAOCULAR PRESSURE
4. DYSURIA
5. REBOUND NASAL CONGESTION WITH TOPICAL NASAL SPRAYS
D. CONTRAINDICATIONS/PRECAUTIONS
1. OPERATING HEAVY EQUIPMENT OR DRIVING
2. AVOID TAKING WITH A MONOAMINE OXIDASE INHIBITOR.
3. ALCOHOL
E. NURSING INTERVENTIONS
1. INFORM THE CLIENT THAT OPERATING MACHINERY OR DRIVING MAY BE DANGEROUS DUE TO SEDATIVE EFFECT.
2. DROWSINESS USUALLY PASSES AFTER 2 WEEKS OF TREATMENT.
3. INSTRUCT THE CLIENT TO REPORT PALPITATIONS, CHANGE IN HEART RATE, OR CHANGE IN BOWEL OR BLADDER HABITS.
4. INSTRUCT THE CLIENT TO AVOID ALCOHOL WITH ANTIHISTAMINES BECAUSE OF ADDITIVE DEPRESSANT EFFECT.
5. SECOND-GENERATION DRUGS HAVE FEWER ADVERSE REACTIONS.
6. SECOND-GENERATION DRUGS ARE MORE EXPENSIVE THAN FIRST-GENERATION DRUGS.
7. SECOND-GENERATION DRUGS HAVE A RAPID ONSET OF ACTION WITH NO DRUG TOLERANCE WITH PROLONGED USE.
8. INSTRUCT THE CLIENT TO AVOID TAKING WITH ANY MONOAMINE OXIDASE INHIBITOR.
F. TYPES (SEE TABLE 17-4)

Table 17-4 Nasal Antihistamine Medications

Generation	Type	Medication
First	Ethanolamines	Carbinoxamine (Clistin) Loratidine (Tavist) Diphenhydramine (Benadryl)
	Ethylenediamines	Pyrilamine (Nisaval) Tripelennamine (PBZ)
	Alkylamines	Brompheniramine (Dimetane) Chlorpheniramine (Chlor-Trimeton)
	Piperazines	Hydroxyzine (Atarax, Vistaril) Cyclizine (Marezine)
	Phenothiazines	Promethiazine (Phenergan)
Second		Loratidine (Claritin) Cetirizine (Zyrtec) Fexofenadine (Allegra)

© Cengage Learning 2015

XX. NASAL DECONGESTANT MEDICATIONS
A. DESCRIPTION
   1. STIMULATE ADRENERGIC RECEPTORS TO PROMOTE VASOCONSTRICTION
   2. REDUCE NASAL EDEMA AND RHINORRHEA
B. USES
   1. REDUCE INFLAMMATION AND EDEMA OF THE NASAL MUCOSA
C. ADVERSE REACTIONS
   1. CENTRAL NERVOUS SYSTEM STIMULATION, CAUSING INSOMNIA, EXCITATION
   2. HEADACHE, IRRITABILITY, INCREASED BLOOD AND OCULAR PRESSURE
   3. PALPITATIONS, TACHYCARDIA
   4. SPRAYS: REBOUND NASAL CONGESTION
D. CONTRAINDICATIONS/PRECAUTIONS
   1. CARDIOVASCULAR DISEASE
   2. HYPERTENSION
   3. DIABETES MELLITUS
   4. GLAUCOMA
   5. PROSTATIC HYPERTROPHY
   6. HEPATIC OR RENAL DISEASE
E. NURSING INTERVENTIONS
   1. INSTRUCT THE CLIENT OF THE ADVERSE REACTIONS.
   2. INFORM THE CLIENT THAT SOME PREPARATIONS ARE CONTRAINDICATED FOR CLIENTS WITH CARDIOVASCULAR DISEASE, HYPERTENSION, DIABETES, GLAUCOMA, PROSTATIC HYPERTROPHY, AND HEPATIC AND RENAL DISEASES.
   3. INSTRUCT THE CLIENT THAT THESE MEDICATIONS SHOULD NOT BE USED FOR MORE THAN 3 DAYS OR MORE THAN 3–4 TIMES PER DAY BECAUSE LONGER USE INCREASES RISK OF REBOUND CONGESTION.
   F. TYPES (SEE TABLE 17-5)

XXI. NASAL CORTICOSTEROID MEDICATIONS
A. DESCRIPTION
   1. INHIBIT INFLAMMATORY RESPONSE IN NASAL TISSUE
   2. PROPHYLACTIC USE DURING ALLERGY SEASON OR ANTIGEN EXPOSURE
B. USES
   1. INHIBIT ALLERGY AND INFLAMMATORY RESPONSES TO THE ENVIRONMENT
C. ADVERSE REACTIONS
   1. MILD TRANSIENT NASAL BURNING AND STINGING
   2. RARE: LOCALIZED FUNGAL INFECTION
D. NURSING INTERVENTIONS
   1. INSTRUCT THE CLIENT TO AVOID HOUSE DUST, DUST MITES, MOLD SPORES, POLLENS, PET ALLERGENS, AND SMOKE.
   2. INSTRUCT THE CLIENT TO USE ON REGULAR BASIS AND NOT P.R.N.
   3. INFORM THE CLIENT THAT SPRAYS ACT TO DECREASE INFLAMMATION ON A DAILY BASIS AND EFFECT IS NOT IMMEDIATE AS WITH DECONGESTANT SPRAYS.
   4. INSTRUCT THE CLIENT TO DISCONTINUE USE IF NASAL INFECTION DEVELOPS.
E. TYPES
   1. BECLOMETHASONE (VANCENASE)
   2. BUDESONIDE (RHINOCORT)
   3. FLUTICASONE (FLONASE)
   4. TRIAMCINOLONE (NASACORT)

XXII. MAST CELL STABILIZERS
A. DESCRIPTION
   1. INHIBIT DEGRANULATION OF SENSITIZED MAST CELLS, WHICH OCCURS AFTER EXPOSURE TO SPECIFIC ANTIGENS
B. USES
   1. DECREASE REACTION WHEN EXPOSED TO ANTIGENS
C. ADVERSE REACTIONS
   1. MINIMAL ADVERSE REACTIONS
   2. OCCASIONAL BURNING OR NASAL IRRITATION

Table 17-5 Nasal Decongestant Medication

Route	Medication
Oral	Pseudoephedrine (Sudafed) Phenylpropanolamine (Dura-Vent)
Topical nasal spray	Oxymetazoline (Dristan) Phenylephrine (Neo-Synephrine)

© Cengage Learning 2015

D. NURSING INTERVENTIONS
1. INSTRUCT THE CLIENT TO AVOID HOUSE DUST, DUST MITES, MOLD SPORES, POLLENS, PET ALLERGENS, AND SMOKE.
2. INFORM THE CLIENT THAT THE SPRAY WILL PREVENT CLINICAL MANIFESTATIONS.
3. INSTRUCT THE CLIENT TO BEGIN 2 WEEKS BEFORE POLLEN SEASON BEGINS AND USE THROUGHOUT THE SEASON.
4. IF AN ISOLATED ALLERGY, SUCH AS CAT, USE PROPHYLACTICALLY 10–15 MINUTES BEFORE EXPOSURE.
E. TYPES
1. CROMOLYN SPRAY (NASALCROM)
2. NEDOCROMIL SPRAY (TILADE)

XXIII. **ANTICHOLINERGIC NASAL MEDICATIONS**
A. DESCRIPTION
1. BLOCK HYPERSECRETORY EFFECTS BY COMPETING FOR BINDING SITES ON THE CELL
2. REDUCE RHINORRHEA IN THE COMMON COLD, ALLERGIC AND NONALLERGIC RHINITIS
B. USES
1. INHIBIT ALLERGY AND INFLAMMATORY RESPONSES TO THE ENVIRONMENT
C. ADVERSE REACTIONS
1. DRYNESS OF THE MOUTH AND NOSE
2. NO SYSTEMIC EFFECTS
D. NURSING INTERVENTIONS
1. INSTRUCT THE CLIENT TO SHAKE THE CANISTER WELL.
2. INSTRUCT THE CLIENT TO TILT THE HEAD BACK SLIGHTLY, INSERT THE TIP, AND HOLD THE OPPOSITE NOSTRIL CLOSED.
3. WHILE PRESSING ON THE CANISTER, INSTRUCT THE CLIENT TO INHALE GENTLY.
4. INSTRUCT THE CLIENT TO HOLD THE BREATH FOR A FEW SECONDS, THEN BREATHE THROUGH THE MOUTH.
5. REPEAT THE PROCESS IN THE OTHER NOSTRIL.
6. REINFORCE THAT THE EFFECT IS NOT IMMEDIATE AS WITH DECONGESTANTS.
7. INSTRUCT THE CLIENT THAT THE MEDICATION MUST BE USED ROUTINELY.
8. INSTRUCT THE CLIENT TO GARGLE AND RINSE THE MOUTH AFTER USE TO HELP DECREASE DRYNESS AND IRRITATION.
E. TYPES
1. IPRATROPIUM BROMIDE (ATROVENT)

XXIV. **ANTIBIOTIC MEDICATIONS FOR NASAL INFECTIONS**
A. DESCRIPTION
1. KILL OR INHIBIT MICROORGANISM INFECTION
B. USES
1. SINUSITIS INFECTIONS
2. PHARYNGEAL INFECTIONS
3. PERITONSILLAR ABSCESS
C. ADVERSE REACTIONS
1. NAUSEA AND VOMITING
2. ABDOMINAL PAIN, DIARRHEA
3. URTICARIA, RASHES
D. NURSING INTERVENTIONS
1. INSTRUCT THE CLIENT TO TAKE THE MEDICATION AROUND THE CLOCK AND TO TAKE THE ENTIRE BOTTLE.
2. INSTRUCT THE CLIENT NOT TO SHARE THE MEDICATION WITH ANYONE ELSE.
3. INFORM THE CLIENT TO OBSERVE FOR AND REPORT SUPERINFECTION, YEAST INFECTION, OR FOUL-SMELLING STOOLS.
4. INFORM THE CLIENT THAT SOME MEDICATIONS DECREASE THE EFFECT OF ORAL CONTRACEPTIVES.
5. INFORM THE CLIENT THAT ALTERNATE OR AN ADDITIONAL METHOD OF CONTRACEPTION SHOULD BE USED WHILE ON THE MEDICATION.

PRACTICE QUESTIONS

1. The nurse should question which of the following drugs for use in a client who has glaucoma?
    1. Acetazolamide (Diamox)
    2. Pilocarpine
    3. Atropine sulfate
    4. Mannitol

2. The nurse is administering an adrenergic blocking agent, such as a beta blocker, to a client with glaucoma. Which of the following

would the nurse interpret as indicative of a serious adverse reaction?
1. Photophobia
2. Blurred vision
3. Drop in blood pressure
4. Exacerbation of asthma

3. The nurse administers which of the following drugs to a client who has keratitis?
1. Acyclovir (Zovirax)
2. Acetazolamide (Diamox)
3. Scopolamine (Isopto Hyoscine)
4. Idoxuridine (Stoxil)

4. The nurse is to administer timolol (Timoptic) 1 drop in each eye. Which of the following comments by the client indicates the need for further teaching?
1. "I must wash my hand before putting in my drops."
2. "This drug will decrease the fluid in my eye."
3. "I'll need to take this until my eye pressure is normal."
4. "Adverse reactions include dizziness and double vision."

5. The nurse instructs the client that the best position for instilling nose spray is to
1. bend the head forward.
2. push one nare to the side.
3. tilt the head backward.
4. open the mouth to facilitate breathing.

6. The nurse is assigned to administer eyedrops to a client being prepared for cataract surgery. Which of the following types of eyedrop does the nurse expect to administer?
1. An osmotic diuretic
2. A miotic agent
3. A mydriatic agent
4. A thiazide diuretic

7. The nurse selects a topical anti-infective from which of the following?
Select all that apply:
[ ] 1. Amoxicillin
[ ] 2. Polymixin B
[ ] 3. Neomycin
[ ] 4. Cefaclor (Ceclor)
[ ] 5. Chloramphenicol Chloromycetin
[ ] 6. Clarithromycin (Biaxin)

8. A client with Ménière's disease asks the nurse why meclizine hydrochloride (Antivert) is being administered. The most appropriate response by the nurse is which of the following?
1. "It will control the vertigo."
2. "It will help you sleep."
3. "It will decrease your pain."
4. "It will alleviate your nausea."

9. When providing care to a client who is receiving phenylephrine HCl (Neo-Synephrine), the nurse should monitor the client for which of the following adverse reactions?
Select all that apply:
[ ] 1. Urinary retention
[ ] 2. Dry skin
[ ] 3. Hypertension
[ ] 4. Tachycardia
[ ] 5. Headache
[ ] 6. Decreased sensitivity to light

10. The nurse is caring for a client receiving a miotic topical drug for glaucoma. Which of the following adverse reactions would the nurse evaluate and report that systemic absorption has taken place?
Select all that apply:
[ ] 1. Abdominal cramps
[ ] 2. Blurred vision
[ ] 3. Diarrhea
[ ] 4. Increased salivation
[ ] 5. Eye ache
[ ] 6. Brow ache

11. The nurse is collecting a medication history from a client with herpes simplex 1 of the eye. The nurse should ask the client if which of the following drugs are taken?
1. Trifluridine (Viroptic)
2. Cromolyn
3. Idoxuridine (Stoxil)
4. Acetazolamide (Diamox)

12. The nurse should understand that a client is to receive which of the following drugs to paralyze the ciliary body muscles?
1. Phenylephrine HCl (Neo-Synephrine)
2. Homatropine
3. Hydroxyamphetamine-hydrobromide (Paredrine)
4. Cromolyn

13. Which of the following discharge instructions should the nurse include on diazepam (Valium) for a client going home after an acute exacerbation of Ménière's disease?
Select all that apply:
[ ] 1. Take on an empty stomach
[ ] 2. Use alcohol sparingly
[ ] 3. Avoid driving
[ ] 4. Report any urinary incontinence
[ ] 5. Drowsiness may occur at the beginning of treatment
[ ] 6. Get up slowly after lying down

14. The nurse should question which of the following drugs that is ordered to be given prior to an eye refraction?
1. Scopolamine
2. Pilocarpine (Pilocar)

3. Phenylephrine HCl (Neo-Synephrine)
4. Hydroxyamphetamine (Paredrine)

15. The nurse understands that a client is to receive prednisolone (Pred Forte) for which of the following purposes?
    1. Acts as an antiviral
    2. Decreases aqueous fluid
    3. Decreases intraocular pressure
    4. Is an anti-inflammatory

16. Which of the following interventions is a priority for the nurse to implement when a client with glaucoma receiving betaxolol (Betoptic) experiences bradycardia, headache, and depression?
    1. Report these adverse reactions as systemic
    2. Decrease the dose
    3. Take the vital signs prior to administering
    4. Refer the client for treatment of the depression

17. The nurse assesses a client receiving brinzolamide (Azopt) for which of the following adverse reactions?
    Select all that apply:
    [ ] 1. Urinary retention
    [ ] 2. Constipation
    [ ] 3. Blurred vision
    [ ] 4. Loss of appetite
    [ ] 5. Transient stinging
    [ ] 6. Redness

18. The nurse is caring for a client with allergic rhinitis and evaluates which of the following drugs to act as a mast cell stabilizer?
    1. Diphenhydramine (Benadryl)
    2. Brompheniramine (Dimetane)
    3. Loratidine (Claritin)
    4. Cromolyn (Nasalcrom)

19. Which of the following drugs should the nurse question in a client with cardiovascular disease and hypertension?
    1. Pseudoephedrine (Sudafed)
    2. Diphenhydramine (Benadryl)
    3. Loratidine (Claritin)
    4. Cetirizine (Zyrtec)

20. A client on diazepam (Valium) asks the nurse why the physician said to avoid drinking alcohol while taking this medication. Which of the following responses by the nurse appropriately explains what alcohol will do?
    1. Cause a decrease in vasoconstriction
    2. Increase the sedative effect
    3. Interfere with the absorption of Valium
    4. Promote a decreased sensitivity to Valium

21. When admitting a new client with glaucoma, the nurse notes an order for

atropine. The nurse should question this order because atropine
    1. causes a moistening effect.
    2. is likely to cause respiratory depression.
    3. causes an increase in intraocular pressure.
    4. may cause diuresis.

22. Prior to discharge, the nurse instructs the client who is receiving dipivefrin (Propine) to notify the physician if which of the following occurs?
    1. Fatigue
    2. Increase in urinary frequency
    3. Weight gain of five pounds in two weeks
    4. Tachycardia

23. The nurse should administer dipivefrin (Propine) at which of the following times?
    1. Every 12 hours
    2. Daily
    3. 1 hour after a meal
    4. With food 3 times per day

24. Which of the following is essential that the nurse include in the assessment of a client who works evenings and takes pilocarpine (Pilocar)?
    1. Hypotension
    2. Urinary retention
    3. Constipation
    4. Decreased dark adaptation

25. The nurse is collecting a health history from a client who is to begin taking acetazolamide (Diamox). Which of the following questions should the nurse ask to determine the safety of this drug?
    1. "Do you operate dangerous equipment?"
    2. "Have you ever had an allergy to sulfa?"
    3. "Have you had any chest pains or a heart attack?"
    4. "Have you had any frequent diarrhea?"

26. The nurse instructs a client who is prescribed a topical ear medication to
    1. use with earplugs to retain the drops.
    2. avoid using daily.
    3. report a sedative effect.
    4. administer at room temperature.

27. The registered nurse is planning to delegate nursing tasks for the day. Which of the following tasks may be delegated to a licensed practical nurse?
    1. Instruct a client taking antihistamines on the adverse reactions
    2. Assess a client for cardiovascular disease before administering a nasal decongestant
    3. Review an electrolyte panel of a client taking a diuretic ear medication
    4. Cleanse a client's eyelid with plain water to soften and remove crusting

ANSWERS AND RATIONALES

1. 3. Atropine sulfate is an anticholinergic drug that is used as a mydriatic to dilate the pupil. This blocks the drainage of aqueous humor. If used by a client who has glaucoma, it could cause an acute attack by increasing the intraocular pressure. Glaucoma is treated by drugs that constrict the pupil to allow for the escape of aqueous humor and that reduce intraocular pressure. Acetazolamide (Diamox) is a carbonic anhydrase inhibitor that decreases the aqueous fluid. Pilocarpine is a cholinergic agonist used in the treatment of glaucoma. Mannitol is an osmotic diuretic that draws the aqueous fluid from the eye by osmosis.

2. 4. Adrenergic blocking agents (beta blockers) are miotics used in the treatment of glaucoma. They decrease the aqueous production and intraocular pressure. Adverse reactions include stinging, photophobia, burning, tearing, and blurred vision. Although a decrease in blood pressure may occur, the most serious adverse reaction is an exacerbation in a client's asthma.

3. 4. Keratitis is inflammation of the cornea that is treated with topical idoxuridine (Stoxil), which is an anti-infective. Acyclovir (Zovirax) is an antiviral used in the treatment of herpes zoster ophthalmicus. Acetazolamide (Diamox) is a carbonic anhydrase inhibitor used for a client who has glaucoma to decrease the aqueous fluid. Scopolamine (Isopto Hyoscine) is a mydriatic that is used for cycloplegic refractions and uveitis.

4. 3. Timolol (Timoptic) is an antiglaucoma agent. This is required daily for the rest of the client's life unless surgical intervention is performed. It will decrease the aqueous fluid and decrease the intraocular pressure. Hand washing is an aseptic measure to prevent microorganism transfer. Adverse reactions include dizziness, double vision, and other visual changes.

5. 3. Tilting the head backward can facilitate movement of the drug into the nasal passages.

6. 3. A mydriatic agent produces dilation of the pupil. Mydriatic eyedrops are used preoperatively for cataract surgery. They not only dilate the pupil, but also constrict blood vessels. A miotic agent constricts the pupil. An osmotic diuretic will decrease intraocular pressure. A thiazide diuretic promotes the excretion of body fluid and is not prescribed for cataract surgery.

7. 2. 3. 5. Polymixin B, Neomycin, and chloramphenicol (Chloromycetin) are examples of topical anti-infective ear medications.

Amoxicillin, cefaclor (Ceclor), and clarithromycin (Biaxin) are examples of systemic anti-infective ear medications.

8. 4. Meclizine hydrochloride (Antivert) is an antiemetic used to alleviate the nausea that occurs in Ménière's disease from the violent vertigo. It does not directly stop the vertigo.

9. 3. 4. 5. Phenylephrine (Neo-Synephrine) is an adrenergic drug used for a variety of purposes, such as a topical ocular vasoconstrictor in uveitis, open-angle glaucoma, refraction without cycloplegia, and nasal congestion. Adverse reactions include hypertension, tachycardia, and headache.

10. 1. 3. 4. Miotic drugs are used in the treatment for glaucoma to constrict the pupil. Topical adverse reactions include blurred vision and eye and brow ache. Systemic adverse reactions include abdominal cramps, diarrhea, and increased salivation.

11. 1. Trifluridine (Viroptic) is an antiviral drug used to treat herpes simplex 1. Cromolyn is an antiallergic drug used to treat conjunctivitis by reducing the itching and redness. Idoxuridine (Stoxil) is an anti-infective used topically to treat keratitis. Acetazolamide (Diamox) is a carbonic anhydrase inhibitor used in the treatment of glaucoma to decrease aqueous fluid.

12. 2. Homatropine is a cycloplegic mydriatic administered for ciliary muscle paralysis. Phenylephrine HCl (Neo-Synephrine) and hydroxyamphetamine-hydrobromide (Paredrine) are mydriatics used to dilate the pupil. Cromolyn is used to treat conjunctivitis by reducing itching and redness.

13. 3. 5. 6. Diazepam (Valium) is an antianxiety, anticonvulsant, and a skeletal muscle relaxant that has been proven to be helpful in the treatment of Ménière's disease. Interventions that should be in the plan of care for a client taking diazepam (Valium) include taking the drug with food to alleviate gastrointestinal upset, being aware that drowsiness may occur at the beginning of treatment, getting up slowly after lying down, and avoiding alcohol and driving.

14. 2. Pilocarpine (Pilocar) is a cholinergic used in the treatment of glaucoma. It should be questioned because it stimulates the iris to contract. Scopolamine is a cycloplegic and phenylephrine HCl (Neo-Synephrine) is a mydriatic used for eye refraction. Hydroxyamphetamine (Paredrine) is a mydriatic used diagnostically to differentiate among postganglionic, central, or preganglionic Horner's syndrome.

15. 4. Prednisolone (Pred Forte) is a topical corticosteroid used to treat postoperative eye inflammation.

16. 1. Betaxolol (Betoptic) is a beta-adrenergic blocker given for glaucoma. The adverse reactions are generally considered as being transient discomfort. Adverse reactions, although rare, may include bradycardia, pulmonary distress, headache, depression, and heart block. These indicate a systemic reaction and must be reported.

17. 3. 5. 6. Brinzolamide (Azopt) is a topical carbonic anhydrase inhibitor that decreases the aqueous humor production. Adverse reactions include blurred vision, transient stinging, redness, and diarrhea.

18. 4. Cromolyn (Nasalcrom) is the only mast cell stabilizer. Diphenhydramine (Benadryl), brompheniramine (Dimetane), and loratidine (Claritin) are all antihistamines.

19. 1. Pseudoephedrine (Sudafed) is a nasal decongestant used for temporary relief of nasal congestion from the common cold, hay fever, or other respiratory allergies. Decongestants such as pseudoephedrine (Sudafed) are contraindicated in clients with cardiovascular disease and hypertension. Diphenhydramine (Benadryl), loratidine (Claritin), and cetirizine (Zyrtec) are all antihistamines and are not contraindicated.

20. 2. Alcohol is a central nervous system depressant and, when taken with Valium, will give an additive effect and increase the sedative value of the Valium. Alcohol causes vasoconstriction, not vasodilation. Alcohol will serve as an additive effect when taken with Valium, yielding an increased sensitivity to the Valium.

21. 3. Atropine is a cycloplegic mydriatic. It blocks the effects of acetylcholine on the sphincter muscle of the iris and the accommodative muscle of the ciliary body. Atropine causes an increase in intraocular pressure. In the treatment of glaucoma, the goal is to decrease intraocular pressure in order to avoid damage

to the optic nerve. Adverse reactions of atropine include a decrease in secretions and urinary hesitancy or retention, but not diuresis.

22. 4. Dipivefrin (Propine) is a sympathomimetic that can cause tachycardia. An increase in urinary frequency, fatigue, and weight gain are not adverse reactions.

23. 1. Dipivefrin (Propine) is a sympathomimetic drug used in the treatment of glaucoma. Treatment includes regular administration of the eyedrops every 12 hours. The objective of the treatment is to reduce the intraocular pressure.

24. 4. Pilocarpine (Pilocar) is a cholinergic agonist used in the treatment of glaucoma. Due to the contraction of the iris, it causes a decreased adaptation to dark. Other adverse reactions include hypertension, urinary frequency, and diarrhea.

25. 2. Acetazolamide (Diamox) is a carbonic anhydrase inhibitor used in the treatment of glaucoma. It should not be used if a prior history to a sulfa allergy is known. It inhibits carbonic anhydrase in the kidney, which decreases the formation of bicarbonate and hydrogen ions from carbon dioxide, thus decreasing the availability of the ions for transport.

26. 4. Topical ear medications should be administered at room temperature because the cold can cause dizziness. Earplugs are not used to retain drops. Treatment of a fungal infection requires application once or twice daily. Topical ear medication has no sedative effect.

27. 4. A registered nurse may delegate the cleansing of a client's eyelid with plain water to soften and remove crusting to a licensed practical nurse. A licensed practical nurse may not instruct a client taking antihistamines on the adverse reactions, assess a client for cardiovascular disease before administering a nasal decongestant, or review the electrolyte panel of a client taking a diuretic ear medication. These nursing tasks require the knowledge level of a registered nurse.

REFERENCES

Broyles, B., Reiss, B., & Evans, M. (2012). *Pharmacological aspects of nursing care* (8th ed.). Clifton Park, NY: Delmar Cengage Learning.

Kees, J., Hayes., E., & McCuistion, L. (2012). *Pharmacology: A nursing process approach* (7th ed.). St. Louis, MO: Saunders Elsevier.

Spratto, G. R., & Woods, A. L. (2012). *PDR nurse's drug handbook 2012.* Clifton Park, NY: Delmar Cengage Learning.

CHAPTER 18

DRUGS FOR THE RESPIRATORY SYSTEM

I. DRUGS FOR BRONCHODILATION

A. DESCRIPTION
1. AEROSOLIZED BRONCHODILATORS ACT AS BETA$_2$-ADRENERGIC RECEPTOR AGONISTS.
2. STIMULATION OF BETA$_2$ RECEPTORS CAUSES THE SMOOTH MUSCLE OF THE BRONCHI TO RELAX AND DILATE.
3. ALSO CALLED ADRENERGIC AGONISTS OR BETA STIMULANTS
4. ANTAGONIZE THE EFFECTS OF LEUKOTRIENES, WHICH ARE COMPONENTS OF A SLOW-REACTING SUBSTANCE OF ANAPHYLAXIS

B. SYMPATHOMIMETICS
1. USES
   a. These drugs are used to dilate bronchial smooth muscles in clients with asthma or chronic obstructive pulmonary disease (COPD) with bronchospasm.
   b. Pirbuterol (Maxair) prevents bronchospasm, including that caused by asthma.
2. ADVERSE REACTIONS
   a. Tachycardia and headache (most common)
   b. Nervousness
   c. Anxiety, tremors
   d. Palpitations, chest pain or tightness
   e. Nausea, diarrhea
   f. Dry mouth
3. CONTRAINDICATIONS AND PRECAUTIONS
   a. Salmeterol xinafoate (Serevent) should not be used for acute clinical manifestations. Recommended use is for long-term maintenance and prevention of bronchospasm and to prevent exercise-induced or nocturnal clinical manifestations.
   b. Tachycardia due to arrhythmias
   c. Hyperthyroidism
   d. Diabetes mellitus
   e. Prostatic hypertrophy
   f. Seizures
   g. Coronary artery disease
4. DRUG INTERACTIONS
   a. Anticholinergics: concomitant use aggravates glaucoma.
   b. Antidiabetics: hyperglycemic effect of epinephrine may increase need of insulin or hypoglycemic agents.
   c. Beta-adrenergic blocking agents: cause bronchial constriction
   d. Digitalis glycosides: may cause cardiac arrhythmias
5. NURSING INTERVENTIONS
   a. Instruct the client in the correct use of the inhaler or nebulizer.
   b. Instruct the client to use the bronchodilator inhaler before the steroid inhaler (if both are ordered).
   c. Monitor the client to adverse reactions.
   d. Assess vital signs.
   e. Instruct the client to stop smoking to preserve lung function.
6. TYPES
   a. Albuterol (Salbutamol, Proventil, Ventolin)
   b. Pirbuterol (Maxair)
   c. Metaproterenol (Alupent)
   d. Terbutaline (Brethine, Brethaire)
   e. Salmeterol xinafoate (Serevent)
   f. Atropine sulfate
   g. Ipratropium bromide (Atrovent)
   h. Isoetharine (Bronkosol)
   i. Epinephrine (Adrenalin, Primatene Mist)
   j. Isoproterenol (Isuprel, Medihaler-Iso)

C. XANTHINE DERIVATIVES
   (METHYLXANTHINES)
   1. USES
      a. These drugs produce bronchial smooth
         muscle relaxation, resulting in dilation,
         and are indicated for clients with
         asthma or COPD with bronchospasms.
      b. With chronic bronchitis, emphysema,
         and apnea, they increase the sensitivity
         of the brain's respiratory center to
         carbon dioxide and stimulate the
         respiratory drive.
      c. These drugs decrease diaphragm
         fatigue and may improve ventricular
         function with chronic bronchitis and
         emphysema.
   2. ADVERSE REACTIONS
      a. Gastrointestinal (GI) reactions
         such as nausea, vomiting, abdominal
         cramping, epigastric pain, anorexia,
         or diarrhea
      b. Because of the stimulant effect, the
         client may experience headache,
         irritability, restlessness, anxiety,
         insomnia, or dizziness.
      c. Cardiovascular reactions may include
         tachycardia, palpitations, or
         dysrhythmias.
   3. CONTRAINDICATIONS AND
      PRECAUTIONS
      a. Therapeutic range of theophylline is
         10–20 mcg/ml.
      b. Theophylline levels may be decreased
         in smokers.
      c. Lactation
      d. Infants, small children, older adult
         clients
   4. DRUG INTERACTIONS (SEE TABLE 18-1)
   5. NURSING INTERVENTIONS
      a. Carefully monitor blood levels for
         possible toxicity.
      b. Monitor closely for drug–drug,
         drug–disease interactions, and all
         adverse reactions.
   6. TYPES
      a. Aminophylline (Phyllocontin,
         Truphylline)
      b. Anhydrous theophylline
      c. Theophylline (Slo-Phyllin, Theo-Dur,
         Theobid, Theospan, Uniphyl,
         Theovent)
D. LEUKOTRIENE RECEPTOR ANTAGONISTS
   1. USES
      a. Chemical mediator that results in
         inflammatory changes in the lung
      b. Cysteinyl leukotrienes promote an
         increase in eosinophil migration,
         mucus production, and airway wall
         edema, which result in
         bronchoconstriction.

Table 18-1 Factors That Influence Theophylline Clearance

Decreased Clearance (Increased Drug Level)	Increased Clearance (Decreased Drug Level)
Diseases	**Diseases**
Renal failure	Hyperthyroidism
Cirrhosis or liver disease	
Alcoholism	
Upper respiratory tract infection	
Hypothyroidism	
Drugs	**Drugs**
Caffeine	Isoproterenol (Isuprel)
Allopurinol (Zyloprim)	Rifampin (Rifadin)
Erythromycin (E-Mycin)	Phenobarbital
Cimetidine (Tagamet)	Phenytoin (Dilantin)
Oral contraceptives	
Ciprofloxacin (Cipro)	
Calcium channel blockers	
Other Factors	**Other Factors**
Older age	Cigarette smoking

© Cengage Learning 2015

      c. Indicated as adjunct therapy for the
         prophylaxis and chronic treatment of
         asthma triggered by allergic and
         environmental stimuli
      d. These drugs either block the
         leukotrienes released in response
         to the allergen (zafirlukast), or
         inhibit leukotriene formation
         (zileuton).
   2. ADVERSE REACTIONS
      a. Headache, dizziness, weakness
      b. Churg-Strauss syndrome
      c. Elevated liver enzymes, drug-induced
         hepatitis
      d. Arthralgia, back pain, myalgia
   3. CONTRAINDICATIONS AND
      PRECAUTIONS
      a. They are not bronchodilators and
         are not to be used to treat acute
         asthma attacks.
      b. Lactation
   4. DRUG INTERACTIONS
      a. Warfarin (Coumadin): clients taking
         zafirlukast (Accolate) may need their
         dose of Coumadin adjusted.
   5. NURSING INTERVENTIONS
      a. Assess respiratory status.
      b. Monitor effectiveness of the
         medication.
      c. Monitor liver enzymes.
   6. TYPES
      a. Zafirlukast (Accolate)
      b. Zileuton (Zyflo)
      c. Montelukast sodium (Singulair)

II. DRUGS FOR CONGESTION
A. DESCRIPTION
1. THESE ARE SYMPATHOMIMETIC DRUGS AND CAN BE ADMINISTERED AS SYSTEMIC OR TOPICAL.
2. SYSTEMIC DECONGESTANTS STIMULATE THE SYMPATHETIC NERVOUS SYSTEM TO REDUCE SWELLING OF THE RESPIRATORY TRACT'S VASCULAR NETWORK.
3. TOPICAL DECONGESTANTS ACT DIRECTLY ON THE ALPHA RECEPTORS OF THE VASCULAR SMOOTH MUSCLE IN THE NOSE, CAUSING ARTERIOLES TO CONSTRICT.
4. BECAUSE OF THE ARTERIOLES CONSTRICTING, VERY LITTLE DRUG IS ABSORBED SYSTEMICALLY WHEN ADMINISTERED TOPICALLY.
B. DECONGESTANTS
1. USE
a. The combination of reduced blood flow to the nasal mucous membranes and decreased capillary permeability reduces swelling and improves respiration.
b. Help to drain sinuses, clear nasal passages, and open eustachian tubes
2. ADVERSE REACTIONS
a. Topical decongestants have few adverse reactions because of minimal absorption.
b. May include burning and stinging of the nasal mucosa, sneezing, mucosal dryness, or ulceration
c. Systemic decongestants may cause central nervous system stimulation and result in nervousness, restlessness, insomnia, nausea, palpitations, difficulty urinating, and elevated blood pressure.
d. The most common adverse reaction related to prolonged topic use of decongestants (more than 5 days) is rebound nasal congestion.
3. CONTRAINDICATIONS AND PRECAUTIONS
a. Monoamine oxidase inhibitor (MAOI)
b. Any drug that may produce hypertension
c. Cardiac arrhythmias
d. Ischemic heart disease
e. Diabetes mellitus
f. Hyperthyroidism
4. DRUG INTERACTIONS (SEE SYMPATHOMIMETICS ON PAGE 405.)
5. NURSING INTERVENTIONS
a. Instruct the client on the proper use of the medications (systemic or topical).
b. Monitor the client for effectiveness.
c. Assess for adverse reactions.

6. TYPES
a. Systemic:
1) Phenylpropanolamine
2) Pseudoephedrine (Afrin, Allermed, Drixoral, Sudafed)
b. Topical:
1) Sympathomimetic amines: ephedrine, epinephrine, phenylephrine. Imidazoline derivatives of sympathomimetic amines: naphazoline, oxymetazoline, tetrahydrozoline, and xylometazoline

III. DRUGS FOR BRONCHOSPASM
A. DESCRIPTION
1. INHIBITS CHOLINERGIC RECEPTORS IN BRONCHIAL SMOOTH MUSCLE, RESULTING IN BRONCHODILATION
B. ANTICHOLINERGICS
1. USES
a. These drugs are used to prevent or reverse bronchospasms in clients with asthma.
b. Used in maintenance therapy of reversible airway obstruction due to COPD
c. Management of rhinorrhea (allergic and nonallergic) (intranasal)
2. ADVERSE REACTIONS
a. Dizziness, headache, nervousness
b. Blurred vision, sore throat
c. Epistaxis, nasal dryness or irritation (nasal spray)
d. Bronchospasm, cough
e. Hypotension, palpitations
f. Gastric irritation, nausea
3. CONTRAINDICATIONS AND PRECAUTIONS
a. Acute bronchospasm
b. Glaucoma
c. Urinary retention
d. Pregnancy
e. Children under 5 years of age
4. DRUG INTERACTIONS
a. Potential toxicity to fluorocarbon if used with other inhalation bronchodilators having a fluorocarbon propellant
5. NURSING INTERVENTIONS
a. Assess for allergies.
b. Assess respiratory status.
c. Monitor for effectiveness of medications.
d. Instruct the client on the proper use of the inhaler, nebulizer, or nasal spray.
e. Instruct the client to rinse the mouth after inhaler use.
f. Encourage sugarless gum or candy to minimize dry mouth.

6. TYPES
  a. Atropine
  b. Ipratropium (Atrovent)

IV. DRUGS FOR INFLAMMATION
  A. DESCRIPTION
    1. CORTICOSTEROIDS HAVE A SIGNIFICANT ANTI-INFLAMMATORY EFFECT BECAUSE OF THEIR ABILITY TO INHIBIT PROSTAGLANDIN SYNTHESIS.
    2. THEY INHIBIT ACCUMULATION OF MACROPHAGES AND LEUKOCYTES AT THE SITES OF INFLAMMATION AND INHIBIT PHAGOCYTOSIS AND LYSOSOMAL ENZYME RELEASE.
  B. CORTICOSTEROIDS
    1. USES
      a. These drugs reduce immune or inflammatory reactions and are used as a follow-up treatment after other agents are administered for severe immune or inflammatory reactions.
      b. Decreasing the inflammatory response opens the airways and decreases resistance.
      c. Inhalation drugs are used for maintenance and prophylactic treatment of asthma. They are not used for severe asthmatic attacks, because they may take 1 to 4 weeks to achieve their full effect.
      d. Nasal drugs are used for seasonal allergic rhinitis and other chronic nasal inflammatory conditions, including nasal polyps.
      e. Systemic drugs are used in the treatment of asthma and other allergic or inflammatory respiratory conditions.
    2. ADVERSE REACTIONS
      a. Depression, euphoria, headache, mood swings, restlessness
      b. Cataracts, increased intraocular pressure
      c. Hypertension
      d. Anorexia, nausea, vomiting
      e. Peptic ulceration
      f. Acne, decreased wound healing, ecchymoses, capillary fragility, hirsutism, petechiae
      g. Adrenal suppression, hyperglycemia
      h. Thromboembolism, thrombophlebitis
      i. Weight gain or weight loss
      j. Muscle wasting, osteoporosis, aseptic necrosis of joints, muscle pain
      k. Cushingnoid appearance (moon face, buffalo hump)
      l. Increased susceptibility to infection, masked signs of infection
      m. Hoarseness, throat irritation, dysphonia, oral candidiasis (inhalation therapy)

    3. CONTRAINDICATIONS AND PRECAUTIONS
      a. Suspected infection because these drugs may mask infection
      b. Cardiac disease
      c. Hypertension
      d. Open-angle glaucoma
      e. Lactation with high doses
    4. DRUG INTERACTIONS
      a. Antacids: decrease effectiveness
      b. Antibiotics: concomitant use may result in resistance strain and severe infection.
      c. Antidiabetic drugs: concomitant use may necessitate increased dose of antidiabetic drug.
      d. Digitalis toxicity: increase risk of digitalis toxicity
      e. Furosemide (Lasix) and thiazide diuretics: there is loss of potassium with both drugs.
      f. Heparin: increase risk of hemorrhage
      g. Nonsteroidal anti-inflammatory drugs (NSAIDs) and salicylates: increase risk of stomach ulcers
    5. NURSING INTERVENTIONS
      a. Assess respiratory status.
      b. Monitor for adverse reactions of medications.
      c. Instruct the client on the proper use of medications and equipment (inhalers, nasal sprays, nebulizers, spacers).
      d. Monitor the effectiveness of medication regimen.
      e. Instruct a client using an inhaler to gargle and rinse the mouth out with water or mouthwash after each dose to reduce the risk of oral candidiasis and irritation.
      f. After initial therapy, taper down to the lowest inhaled dose possible to control clinical manifestations.
      g. Monitor growth and development in children.
      h. Monitor the client for severe adverse reactions with long-term high-dose systemic medication.
      i. Administer the steroid last when used with other inhalers.
    6. TYPES
      a. Inhalation drugs
        1) Beclomethasone (Becloforte, Beclovent, Vaanceril)
        2) Budesonide (Pulmicort)
        3) Flunisolide (AeroBid)
        4) Fluticasone (Flovent)
        5) Triamcinolone (Azmacort)
      b. Nasal drugs
        1) Beclomethasone (Beconase, Vancenase)
        2) Budesonide (Rhinocort)

    3) Dexamethasone (Decadron)
    4) Flunisolide (Nasalide)
    5) Fluticasone (Flonase)
    6) Mometasone (Nasonex)
    7) Triamcinolone (Nasacort)
  c. Systemic drugs
    1) Cortisone (Cortone)
    2) Hydrocortisone (Cortef, Hydrocortone, Solu-Cortef)
    3) Methylprednisolone (Solu-Medrol, Medrol)
    4) Prednisolone (Prednisol)
    5) Prednisone (Deltasone)
    6) Triamcinolone (Amcort, Kenacort, Kenaject, Tristoject)
    7) Betamethasone (Celestone)
    8) Budesonide (Entocort)
    9) Dexamethasone (Decadron, Dexasone, Solurex)

V. DRUGS FOR ASTHMA
  A. DESCRIPTION
    1. MAST CELL STABILIZERS (CROMOLYN SODIUM AND NEDOCROMIL)
    2. PREVENT THE RELEASE OF HISTAMINE AND SLOW-REACTING SUBSTANCE OF ANAPHYLAXIS FROM SENSITIZED MAST CELLS BY STABILIZING THE MAST CELL MEMBRANE
  B. CROMOLYN SODIUM/NEDOCROMIL
    1. USES
      a. Prophylactic treatment for asthma and not for acute attacks
      b. Does not have bronchodilator properties—it acts by inhibiting the release of histamine to prevent an asthma attack.
      c. Prevents exercise-induced bronchospasm
      d. Adjunct therapy in the prophylaxis of allergic disorders, including rhinitis and asthma
    2. ADVERSE REACTIONS
      a. Bronchospasm or severe coughing
      b. Sneezing, wheezing, cough, nasal congestion, and throat irritation
      c. Dizziness
      d. Painful or difficult urination
      e. Joint swelling and pain
      f. Nausea, headache
      g. Skin rash (maculopapular) and urticaria (itching) with cromolyn
    3. CONTRAINDICATIONS AND PRECAUTIONS
      a. Acute asthma attacks
      b. Status asthmaticus
      c. Hypersensitivity
      d. Children
    4. DRUG INTERACTIONS
      a. None noted

    5. NURSING INTERVENTIONS
      a. Monitor for adverse reactions.
      b. Instruct the client on the proper use of drugs.
      c. Instruct the client on adverse reactions that should be reported to the physician.
      d. Inform the client that optimal response to cromolyn may take 2 months of daily use.
      e. Instruct the client that the drug must be used even when free of clinical manifestations.
      f. Administer by inhalation because cromolyn is poorly absorbed when given orally.
      g. Hold the cromolyn and notify the physician if bronchospasm or severe cough occurs.
    6. TYPE
      a. Cromolyn sodium (Intal, Gastrocrom)
      b. Nedocromil (Tilade)

VI. DRUGS FOR MANAGING SECRETIONS
  A. DESCRIPTION
    1. REDUCE THE VISCOSITY AND SURFACE TENSION OF PURULENT AND NONPURULENT PULMONARY SECRETIONS AND FACILITATE THEIR REMOVAL BY SPLITTING DISULFIDE BONDS
  B. MUCOLYTIC AGENTS
    1. USES
      a. Mucolytic agents facilitate sputum expectoration.
      b. They act directly on mucus, breaking down sticky, thick secretions so they can more easily be expectorated.
      c. For clients with cystic fibrosis or those with thick secretions or with difficulty raising secretions
      d. Adjunct in the treatment of acute and chronic bronchopulmonary disease
      e. Acetylcysteine (Mucomyst) also restores glutathione, a substance that plays an important role in oxidation-reduction processes. Glutathione's enzymatic action in the liver reduces acetaminophen toxicity from overdose.
      f. May be used to prepare clients for bronchography and other bronchial studies
      g. An antidote for acetaminophen overdose or toxicity
    2. ADVERSE REACTIONS
      a. Nausea
      b. Bronchospasm
      c. Pharyngitis, voice alterations, laryngitis
      d. Conjunctivitis
      e. Rash, urticaria

3. CONTRAINDICATIONS AND PRECAUTIONS
  a. Hypersensitivity
4. DRUG INTERACTIONS
  a. Activated charcoal decreases effectiveness. Therefore, when using for acetaminophen overdose, remove activated charcoal from the stomach before administering.
  b. Acetylcysteine is incompatible with antibiotics and should be administered separately.
5. NURSING INTERVENTIONS
  a. Inform the client that the drug smells like "rotten eggs" and may cause nausea.
  b. When given orally, mix with juice and give with a straw to avoid liquid touching the tongue and taste buds.
  c. Inform the client that the drug can be inhaled or taken orally.
6. TYPES
  a. Acetylcysteine (Mucomyst) is the most commonly used agent.
  b. Dornase alfa (Pulmozyme)
C. EXPECTORANTS
  1. USES
    a. Increase production of respiratory tract fluids, reducing the thickness, adhesiveness, and surface tension of mucus, making it easier to clear from the airways.
    b. Soothe mucous membranes in the respiratory tract
  2. ADVERSE REACTIONS
    a. Rare
    b. Vomiting, diarrhea, drowsiness, nausea, or abdominal pain if taken in large doses
  3. CONTRAINDICATIONS AND PRECAUTIONS
    a. Chronic cough such as that experienced in asthma, emphysema, or smoking
  4. DRUG INTERACTIONS
    a. Anticoagulants—increase the risk of bleeding
  5. NURSING INTERVENTIONS
    a. Monitor sputum production and characteristics.
    b. Assess respiratory status.
    c. Instruct the client on proper coughing techniques.
  6. TYPES
    a. Guaifenesin (Humibid, Hytuss, Liquibid, Organidin, Robitussin, Tussin)

VII. **DRUGS FOR MANAGING COUGH**
  A. DESCRIPTION
    1. NARCOTIC AND NONNARCOTIC DRUGS THAT SELECTIVELY DEPRESS THE COUGH CENTER IN THE MEDULLA AND SUPPRESS OR INHIBIT COUGHING
  B. ANTITUSSIVES
    1. USES
      a. Typically used to treat dry, nonproductive coughs
      b. Benzonatate (Tessalon) acts by anesthetizing stretch receptors in the bronchi, alveoli, and pleura.
      c. Dextromethorphan (Benylin; the most widely used), codeine, and hydrocodone suppress the cough reflex by direct action on the cough center in the medulla of the brain.
      d. Codeine and hydrocodone are narcotics and reserved for treating intractable cough, usually associated with lung cancer.
    2. ADVERSE REACTIONS
      a. Dizziness, drowsiness
      b. Nausea, vomiting, stomach pain
    3. CONTRAINDICATIONS AND PRECAUTIONS
      a. MAO inhibitors
      b. Glaucoma
      c. Prostatic hypertrophy
      d. Obstructive pulmonary disease
    4. DRUG INTERACTIONS
      a. Central nervous system depressants: codeine and hydrocodone can cause central nervous system (CNS) depression and have addictive effects when taken with other CNS depressants.
    5. NURSING INTERVENTIONS
      a. Assess respiratory status.
      b. Document cough and sputum production.
      c. If cough persists beyond several weeks, stop the medication and reassess cause.
      d. Instruct the client to avoid driving or operating equipment while taking CNS depressants.
    6. TYPES
      a. Benzonatate (Tessalon)
      b. Codeine
      c. Dextromethorphan hydrobromide (Benylin, Pertussin, Robitussin, Sucrets)
      d. Hydrocodone bitartrate

VIII. **DRUGS FOR TUBERCULOSIS**
  A. DESCRIPTION
    1. A COMBINATION OF DRUGS IS USED TO KILL OR INHIBIT THE GROWTH OF MYCOBACTERIA RESPONSIBLE FOR TUBERCULOSIS.
    2. COMBINATION THERAPY WITH TWO OR MORE AGENTS IS REQUIRED, UNLESS USED AS PROPHYLAXIS (ISONIAZID [INH] ALONE).

B. ANTITUBERCULIN
   1. USES
      a. Chemotherapy to treat pulmonary or military tuberculosis
      b. All drugs are hepatotoxic.
   2. ADVERSE REACTIONS
      a. Optic neuritis
      b. Skin rash
      c. Red-orange color to urine, saliva, tears, and feces (rifampicin)
      d. Thrombocytopenia
      e. Peripheral neuritis
      f. Hepatotoxicity
      g. Gastrointestinal (GI) upset, nausea, vomiting
   3. CONTRAINDICATIONS AND PRECAUTIONS
      a. Renal disease
      b. Liver disease
   4. DRUG INTERACTIONS
      a. Anticoagulants: decrease anticoagulant effect
      b. Meperidine (Demerol): increase risk of hypotension or central nervous system depression
   5. NURSING INTERVENTIONS
      a. Obtain sputum sample before starting drugs.
      b. Instruct the client on the importance of adherence to the drug regimen for the entire time (6–12 months).
      c. Inform the client that a noninfectious state occurs after 1–2 weeks of continuous drug therapy.
      d. Administer on an empty stomach.
      e. Encourage the client to maintain an adequate nutritional status.
      f. Inform the client that yearly follow-up checkups are necessary.
      g. Monitor liver function.
      h. Instruct the client to wear glasses instead of contacts if on rifampin—contacts will become permanently discolored.
      i. Instruct the client to avoid alcohol while on therapy to reduce risk of hepatotoxicity.
      j. Instruct the client on the importance of hand washing and covering the nose and mouth when sneezing or coughing.
      k. Inform the client about droplet precautions and isolation when in the hospital.
      l. Place the client in a negative-pressure room.
      m. Provide the client with psychological support, stressing the need for long-term therapy.
      n. Instruct the client to use alternative birth control because these drugs negate the birth control pill.
      o. Monitor the client taking streptomycin for eighth cranial nerve damage.
      p. Administer vitamin B_6 (pyridoxine) in conjunction with INH to prevent peripheral neuritis.
   6. TYPES
      a. Ethambutol (Myambutol)
      b. Rifampin (Rifadin, Rimactane)
      c. INH
      d. Streptomycin
      e. Rifapentine (Priftin)

IX. OXYGEN
   A. DESCRIPTION
      1. OXYGEN (O_2) IS A POTENT DRUG PRESCRIBED BY PHYSICIANS FOR RELIEF OF HYPOXEMIA AND SYMPTOMS OF HYPOXIA.
      2. ROOM AIR IS APPROXIMATELY 21% FIO_2 (FRACTION OF INSPIRED OXYGEN).
   B. OXYGEN THERAPY
      1. USES
         a. Administered by prescription at low-flow and high-flow concentrations (see Table 18-2).
      2. TYPES
         a. Low flow
            1) Nasal cannula, nasal prongs
            2) Simple face mask
            3) Partial rebreather mask
            4) Nonrebreather mask
         b. High flow
            1) Venturi mask
            2) Aerosol mask, face tent, tracheostomy collar
            3) T-piece, T-tube, blowby
            4) Transtracheal
      3. CONTRAINDICATIONS AND PRECAUTIONS
         a. Combustion: oxygen itself does not burn, but it supports combustion.
         b. Sparks, flames, smoking, and flammable solutions are prohibited when oxygen is in use.
         c. Oxygen-induced hypoventilation: chemoreceptors in the brain (medulla) are normally sensitive to high $PaCO_2$ levels to stimulate breathing and increase respiratory rate. With chronic lung disease and increasing levels of $PaCO_2$ ($> 60–65$ mm Hg), peripheral chemoreceptors take over and the breathing stimulus is triggered by low PaO_2 levels ($PaO_2 < 55–60$). Giving higher concentrations of O_2 ($> 2–3$ L/min) can decrease respiratory rate and depth, leading to oxygen-induced hypoventilation, apnea, and respiratory arrest.

Table 18-2 Modes of Oxygen Delivery

System	FIO₂ Delivered	Nursing Interventions
Low Flow		
Nasal cannula, nasal prongs	24–40% at 1–6 L/min 1 L/min delivers 24% 2 L/min delivers 28% 3 L/min delivers 32% 4 L/min delivers 36% 5 L/min delivers 40% 6 L/min delivers 44%	Ensure proper fit for most effective O₂ delivery. Assess the nares and ears for breakdown. Assess patency of the nostrils. Apply water-soluble jelly to the nares. Provide humidity as necessary. Assess respirations. Monitor for mouth breathing; if so, the nasal cannula may not be effective.
Simple face mask	40–60% at 5–8 L/min 5 L/min delivers 40% 6 L/min delivers 45% 8 L/min delivers 55%	Set the flow rate to at least 5 L/min to flush carbon dioxide from the mask. Assess for snug fit of the mask for best oxygen delivery. Assess for pressure areas over the nose and ears. Consider order for the nasal cannula during meals.
Partial rebreather mask	60–75% at 6–11 L/min Need a liter flow rate high enough to maintain inspiration and expiration	Make sure the reservoir does not twist or kink, which results in a deflated bag. Adjust the flow rate to keep the reservoir bag inflated.
Nonrebreather mask	80–95% at liter flow to maintain reservoir bag 2/3 full	Monitor the client closely. Ensure that the valves and flaps of the nonrebreather mask are working properly. Remove mucus or saliva as necessary from the valves or flaps of the mask. Suffocation can occur if the reservoir bag kinks or if the oxygen source disconnects. The client may require intubation.
High Flow Venturi mask (Venti mask)	24–55% with flow rates usually 4–10 L/min; provides high humidity	Keep the orifice for the venturi adapter open and uncovered. Assess the mask for snug fit and tubing free of kinks. Assess for dry mucous membranes. Change to nasal cannula during meals. Assess for skin irritation or breakdown from the straps or mask.
Aerosol mask, face tent, tracheostomy collar	24–100%, with flow rates of at least 10 L/min; provides high humidity	Assess that aerosol mist escapes from the vents of the delivery system during inspiration and expiration. Empty condensation from the tubing. Change the aerosol water container as needed.
T-piece, T-tube, blowby	24–100%, with flow rates of at least 10 L/min; provides high humidity	Empty condensation from the tubing. Keep the exhalation port open and uncovered. Position the T-piece so that it does not pull on the tracheostomy or endotracheal tube.
Transtracheal oxygen therapy (TTO) (SCOOP is one brand of catheter made by TTO systems.)	Individual flow rates are prescribed for activity, for rest, and for the nasal cannula.	Make a surgical insertion site and insert special sterile oxygen tubing into the trachea. Tubing and site care performed much like tracheostomy care. This technique is sometimes found to be more effective and more cosmetically acceptable for clients on long-term oxygen.

© Cengage Learning 2015

FIO₂ = fraction of inspired oxygen
Room air = 21%

d. Oxygen toxicity: related to concentration of oxygen, duration of therapy, and degree of lung disease. Recommend FIO₂ levels of 50% or greater be limited to no more than 24–48 hours. Administer the lowest concentration of oxygen required to meet client needs. In newborns, high concentrations can cause damage to the retina and cause blindness.

e. Absorption atelectasis: room air is 79% nitrogen, an important element in preventing alveoli collapse. With high concentrations of oxygen, nitrogen is replaced in the alveoli and atelectasis occurs.

   f. Drying of the mucous membranes: oxygen flow rates > 2 L/min need humidification.

   g. Infection: organisms may be harbored in the moist humidification systems, and in delivery equipment (tubing, masks, and cannulas).

4. DRUG INTERACTIONS

   a. None

5. NURSING INTERVENTIONS

   a. Assess the client's need and appropriate delivery system.

   b. Administer the type of oxygen delivery system depending on:

      1) Oxygen concentration required by the client

      2) Oxygen concentration delivered by the system

      3) Client comfort

      4) Expense to the client

      5) Importance of humidity

      6) Client mobility

   c. Assess the effectiveness of the delivery system and concentration.

   d. Perform a respiratory assessment.

   e. Auscultate for breath sounds, crackles, or wheezes.

   f. Empty condensation from the tubing and check water levels of the humidifier (sterile water).

   g. Oxygen may also need to be warmed if the upper airways are bypassed by the system providing oxygen.

   h. Change equipment per policy.

   i. Keep delivery devices clean.

C. INHALERS, NASAL SPRAY, AND NEBULIZERS

1. USES

   a. Metered dose inhalers (MDIs) are frequently used to administer oral and topical medications.

   b. Doses vary, but generally, 2 puffs is standard for MDIs, with no more than 12 puffs in 24 hours.

   c. Nebulizers can deliver medication through a face mask or mouthpiece using compressed air or oxygen with a gas flow of 6–10 L/min.

2. ADVERSE REACTIONS

   a. Throat irritation and oral candidiasis with steroids (inhaler/nebulizer)

   b. Epistaxis and dry membranes (nasal spray)

   c. Note specific side effects of medication administered by these routes.

3. CONTRAINDICATIONS AND PRECAUTIONS

Table 18-3 Proper Use of Metered Dose Inhaler

Shake the inhaler.

Remove the cap.

Instruct the client to stand or sit erect.

Inhale deeply through the mouth.

Exhale forcefully (breathe out as much as possible).

Hold the metered dose inhaler 1–2 inches from the mouth (or use a spacer).

Activate the inhaler with the mouth open while inhaling deeply and consistently.

Close the mouth and hold the breath approximately 10 seconds (or as long as possible).

Exhale.

Wait 2–5 minutes between puffs and repeat as above.

If possible, follow with mouth care; must do mouth care after steroids.

Maximum air inhalers are placed in the mouth and activated automatically.

Spacers can be used for young children and older adults and are recommended for steroids.

Spacers (aerochamber) can significantly improve the delivery of medication to the lungs and should be used whenever possible.

Check canister fullness by placing the canister in a bowl of water. If it sinks, the canister is full. If it is empty, the canister will float.

© Cengage Learning 2015

   a. Contents of the MDI container are under pressure; do not store near heat or open flame and do not puncture the container.

   b. Do not put the lips around the inhaler; place two finger-breadths away before activating and inhaling or use a spacer for better inhalation deep in airways.

4. NURSING INTERVENTIONS

   a. Inform the client that nebulizer treatments will last from 5–15 minutes.

   b. Instruct the client on the proper use of an MDI (see Table 18-3).

   c. Monitor for adverse reactions of specific medications and routes of administration.

   d. Instruct the client on how to use a nasal spray (see Table 18-4).

Table 18-4 Proper Use of Nasal Spray

Clear the nasal passages gently before administration.

Do not inhale during administration (so medication remains in the nasal passages).

Prime the pump initially with 7 pumps.

If used regularly, no further priming is needed.

If not used in 24 hours, prime with 2 actuations.

If not used for > 7 days, prime with 7 actuations.

© Cengage Learning 2015

PRACTICE QUESTIONS

1. A client has been receiving intravenous theophylline and the physician writes new orders to discontinue the IV medication and begin an immediate-release oral form of the medication. When should the nurse schedule the first dose of the oral medication to be administered?
   1. Immediately after stopping the intravenous infusion of theophylline
   2. Begin 4 to 6 hours after stopping the intravenous infusion of theophylline
   3. Begin the initial dose at bedtime
   4. Start the oral dose with the morning medications and breakfast

2. A client with acute asthma is treated for inspiratory and expiratory wheezes and a decreased forced expiratory volume. Which class of prescribed drugs should the nurse administer first to this client?
   1. Oral steroids
   2. Bronchodilators
   3. Inhaled steroids
   4. Mucolytics

3. The nurse is admitting a client with asthma who is to be started on theophylline. Which of the following questions would be appropriate to ask this client?
   1. "Are you a diabetic and taking insulin?"
   2. "Do you take cimetidine (Tagamet)?"
   3. "Do you use aspirin on a daily basis?"
   4. "Do you exercise routinely?"

4. After instructing a client to use a beclomethasone (Vanceril) inhaler, which of the following statements by the client indicates to the nurse that the teaching has been successful?
   1. "I will limit myself to two cups of coffee per day."
   2. "I will take it before bed each night."
   3. "I will take it with meals to mask the taste."
   4. "I will rinse my mouth after each use."

5. Which of the following statements made by the client indicates to the nurse that the client does not understand how to use cromolyn sodium (Intal) and is in need of further instructions?
   1. "If I don't feel better in 2 to 3 weeks, I should stop taking the medication."
   2. "I will call my doctor if this medication causes severe coughing."
   3. "I have to take this medication routinely, even when I feel good."
   4. "I do not stop my other medications just because I'm taking this one."

6. When instructing a client to use a metered dose inhaler, it would be essential for the nurse to include which of the following aspects? Instruct the client to
   1. hold the breath for 3 seconds after using the inhaler.
   2. take a quick deep breath after activating the canister.
   3. activate the canister at the beginning of a slow deep breath.
   4. place the canister 6 inches in front of an open mouth.

7. The nurse selects which of the following inhalation drugs for inflammation? Select all that apply:
   [ ] 1. Cortisone (Cortone)
   [ ] 2. Belomethasone (Beclovent)
   [ ] 3. Dexamethasone (Decadron)
   [ ] 4. Flunisolide (Aero-Bid)
   [ ] 5. Prednisone (Deltasone)
   [ ] 6. Trriamcinolone (Azmacort)

8. A client who has asthma asks the nurse why the preferred route of administration for corticosteroids is inhalation. The appropriate response by the nurse is which of the following?
   1. "Inhaled medications are easier to take."
   2. "The systemic adverse reactions are reduced."
   3. "No weaning is required when stopping the drug."
   4. "Oral care is not required."

9. A client with asthma awakens in the middle of the night with an asthma attack. Which of the following inhaler medications should the nurse administer first?
   1. Albuterol (Proventil)
   2. Triamcinolone acetonide (Azmacort)
   3. Fluticasone propionate (Flovent)
   4. Cromolyn (Intal)

10. After a client diagnosed with pneumonia has an episode of respiratory distress, the client is intubated and placed on a ventilator. The breath sounds are diminished and the chest x-ray shows left lower lobe consolidation. The physician orders respiratory treatments with acetylcysteine (Mucomyst). The nurse should monitor the client for which of the following results from this treatment?
    1. Bronchodilation
    2. Increased sputum, removed with suctioning
    3. Decreased level of consciousness
    4. Hypotension

11. The nurse is caring for a client with lung cancer who has an intractable cough and is exhausted from the effort of coughing. Which of the following drugs should the nurse administer to this client?
    1. Rifampin (Rifadin)
    2. Acetylcysteine (Mucomyst)
    3. Fluticasone (Flovent)
    4. Codeine

12. Which of the following treatments is the priority for the nurse to administer to a client who has a positive tuberculosis (TB) skin test but has no other evidence of active disease?
    1. No treatment and repeat skin test in 6 months
    2. Isoniazid (INH) for 12 months
    3. Multidrug therapy for at least 12 months
    4. Streptomycin for 12 months

13. The nurse is developing a medication schedule for a client who is receiving isoniazid (INH). To promote the best absorption, this medication would be administered
    1. on an empty stomach.
    2. with antacids to relieve stomach upset.
    3. with food.
    4. 30 minutes after meals.

14. Which of the following is the priority for the nurse to monitor in a client who has been on a ventilator and on 70% FIO_2 for the past 72 hours?
    1. Atelectasis
    2. Pulmonary fibrosis
    3. Expense to client
    4. Oxygen dependence

15. The nurse is caring for a client who has chronic obstructive lung disease (COPD) and pneumonia. After being extubated, which of the following orders should the nurse question?
    1. Continuation of the current antibiotics
    2. O_2 per nasal cannula at 6 L/min
    3. Out of bed with assistance
    4. Continuation of current nebulizer treatments

16. It is essential that the nurse use humidifiction for an oxygen flow rate of greater than what flow per minute to prevent drying of the mucous membranes? _____

17. The nurse is preparing to teach a class on the appropriate use of nebulizers and metered dose inhalers. Which of the following should the nurse include in the class?
    1. Metered dose inhalers require a gas flow rate of 6 to 10 L/min
    2. Nebulizers deliver medication through a face mask or mouthpiece
    3. Nebulizers deliver doses in puffs
    4. Metered dose inhalers require refrigeration

18. The nurse selects which of the following types of low flow for oxygen therapy? Select all that apply:
    [ ] 1. Venturi mask
    [ ] 2. Aerosol mask
    [ ] 3. Nasal cannula
    [ ] 4. Nonrebreather mask
    [ ] 5. Transtracheal
    [ ] 6. Simple face mask

19. The nurse is instructing a client on the proper use of the pump for nasal spray administration. Which of the following statements by the client indicates a need for further instruction?
    1. "I should clear my nasal passages gently before using the pump."
    2. "I should inhale deeply during administration of the medication."
    3. "I should prime the pump if it hasn't been used for more than 24 hours."
    4. "I should not inhale during administration of the medication."

20. The nurse is admitting a client who was recently diagnosed with asthma and has been taking a long-acting theophylline (Theo-Dur). After reviewing the client's history, the nurse discovered that the client has a manic disorder controlled by lithium (Eskalith). Which of the following is a priority for the nurse to include in this client's treatment plan?
    1. Increase the dose of lithium
    2. Obtain a serum lithium level
    3. Increase the dose of theophylline
    4. Obtain a consult for a psychiatric consultation

21. A client questions a prescription for pyridoxine (B_6) after being started on the triple-drug therapy for tuberculosis (ethambutol, rifampin, and isoniazid). The nurse explains that pyridoxine will
    1. prevent skin rash from the ethambutol.
    2. reduce the time the other drugs must be taken.
    3. counter the peripheral neuritis of the isoniazid.
    4. prevent damage to the eighth cranial nerve from the streptomycin.

22. The nurse is collecting a medication history on a client admitted with asthma who has been taking theophylline. Which of the following drugs is a priority for the nurse to notify the physician that the client has also been taking for a urinary tract infection?
    1. Cephradine (Velosef)
    2. Cephapirin sodium (Cefadyl)
    3. Trimethoprim and sulfamethoxazole (Bactrim)
    4. Ciprofloxacin (Cipro)

23. A client arrives at the emergency room in status asthmaticus. Which of the following is the priority nursing action?
    1. Administer aminophylline intravenously as ordered
    2. Monitor the respiratory status and for signs of hypoxia
    3. Administer inhaled bronchodilator therapy as ordered
    4. Provide emotional support

24. The nurse evaluates which of the following as the appropriate method of improving oxygenation in a client with chronic airway limitation (CAL) who is lethargic, sleeps with the mouth open, is receiving 2 L/minute of oxygen per nasal cannula, and has a pulse oximetry check of 88%?
    1. Keep the client awake more so deeper breaths can be taken
    2. Turn the oxygen up to 4 L/minute
    3. Obtain an order for a face mask and use nasal cannula during meals
    4. Intubate the client and place the client on a ventilator

25. Which of the following are adverse reactions of drugs for bronchodilation?
    Select all that apply:
    [ ] 1. Headache
    [ ] 2. Tachycardia
    [ ] 3. Sneezing
    [ ] 4. Back pain
    [ ] 5. Palpitation
    [ ] 6. Depression

26. The nurse is preparing to delegate the nursing tasks for the day. Which of the following tasks should the nurse delegate to a licensed practical nurse?
    1. Monitor a client using a decongestant for the effectiveness of the drug
    2. Develop a teaching plan for effective coughing techniques for a client taking an expectorant
    3. Increase the oxygen flow rate to a client receiving oxygen by a simple face mask
    4. Administer a nasal spray to a client with rhinitis

ANSWERS AND RATIONALES

1. 2. After stopping IV therapy, a period of 4 to 6 hours should elapse before initiating oral therapy. The half-life of the drug is 3 to 15 hours in nonsmoking adults, and 4 to 5 hours in adult heavy smokers. If the oral dose is initiated too soon it could lead to adverse reactions, such as nausea, vomiting, diarrhea, irritability, insomnia, or headache. More serious theophylline toxicity is manifested by cardiac arrhythmias, hypotension and peripheral vascular collapse, tachycardia, hyperglycemia, or seizures. The therapeutic serum level for theophylline is 10 to 20 mcg/ml.

2. 2. The most immediate need of a client with inspiratory and expiratory wheezes and a decreased forced expiratory volume is to dilate the bronchioles and improve air exchange. Steroids (inhaled or oral) may follow the emergent treatment to reduce the inflammation, but would not be first-line drugs. Mucolytics are not appropriate for the client with asthma, as there is little mucus production associated with asthma.

3. 2. Cimetidine (Tagamet) will decrease theophylline clearance and may increase serum drug levels. The dose may have to be reduced for this client. Insulin and aspirin do not affect drug clearance.

4. 4. Inhaled steroids increase the risk of oral candidiasis and irritation. Clients should rinse the mouth out with water or mouthwash after each dose. If other drugs are taken by inhaler at the same time, the steroid should be the last drug given. Many may cause nausea, so should not be taken around mealtime. The client should be instructed to follow the schedule of dosing intervals. It is not a one-time-per-day drug. Caffeine is not limited and, in fact, has some bronchodilating effect. Inhaled steroids are used for maintenance and prophylactic treatment of asthma.

5. 1. Cromolyn sodium (Intal) is a drug used prophylactically for asthma to inhibit the degranulation of sensitized mast cells that occur after exposure to certain antigens and to prevent histamine release. This drug may take 4 to 8 weeks for optimal effect. It may cause bronchospasm in some individuals. Steroids and other drugs are continued along with the cromolyn. If cromolyn is effective, steroids can often be tapered down. Do not stop inhalation or nasal medication abruptly. Rapid withdrawal of the drug may precipitate an asthmatic attack.

6. 3.   Proper technique for using a metered dose inhaler is to have the client place the canister either in the mouth or 2 inches in front of an open mouth. The canister must be activated at the beginning of a slow deep inspiratory effort. The inhalation is followed by 5 to 10 seconds of breath holding. Sequence is then repeated if a second puff is ordered.

7. 2. 4. 6. Inhaled drugs for inflammation include beclomethasone (Beclovent), flunisolide (AeroBid), and triamcinolone (Azmacort). An example of a nasal drug for inflammation is dexamethasone (Decadron). Cortisone (Cortone) and prednisone (Deltasone) are examples of systemic drugs for inflammation.

8. 2.   The inhaled glucocorticoids are effective on topical administration, and systemic adverse reactions can be reduced when delivered by this route. Instruction is necessary for the client to properly learn the technique of using inhalers. Inhaled steroids should not be stopped suddenly, and oral care is necessary after every treatment to reduce oral candidiasis.

9. 1.   The initial treatment for acute asthma is a bronchodilator. Steroids such as triamcinolone acetonide (Azmacort) and fluticasone propionate (Flovent) may be given after initial bronchospasm is relieved. Cromolyn (Intal) has no immediate effect and is a prophylactic mast cell inhibitor.

10. 2.   Acetylcysteine (Mucomyst) is a mucolytic agent that breaks down thick secretions and facilitates sputum expectoration. Adverse reactions include nausea and bronchospasm. There is no effect on level of consciousness or vital signs.

11. 4.   Codeine is a narcotic drug that selectively depresses the cough center in the medulla and inhibits coughing. It is typically used in a dry, nonproductive, intractable cough. It is used with caution in combination with other central nervous system depressants. Rifampin (Rifadin) is a drug used to treat tuberculosis. Acetylcysteine (Mucomyst) is a mucolytic that decreases the viscosity of purulent and nonpurulent secretions and facilitates their removal. Fluticasone (Flovent) is an inhaled corticosteroid used in the treatment of asthma.

12. 2.   A positive skin test with no other evidence of disease indicates exposure to the disease. Isoniazid (INH) therapy for 12 months is the usual protocol. Once a client has a positive skin test, it will always be positive and there is no value in repeating a test. Multidrug therapy is used to treat active disease, and streptomycin or Amikacin is often added in the induction phase of treatment.

13. 1.   Isoniazid (INH) should be taken on an empty stomach, either 1 hour before or 2 hours after meals. Avoid antacids with the medication.

14. 2.   Clients on an FIO_2 of 50% or greater for 24 to 48 hours have a higher incidence of pulmonary fibrosis and oxygen toxicity. Atelectasis can occur but is generally reversible and therefore not the greatest concern. Expense is considered, but treatment requirements for the client take priority. Oxygen dependence is related to pulmonary disease.

15. 2.   For a client with chronic obstructive lung disease (COPD), there is an insensitivity to high levels of carbon dioxide and therefore an inspiratory drive that is now triggered by low oxygen levels. Giving higher concentrations of oxygen (greater than 2 to 3 L/min) can decrease the respiratory rate and depth, leading to oxygen-induced hypoventilation, apnea, and respiratory arrest.

16. 2.   It is important to use humidification of greater than a flow rate of 2 to prevent drying of the mucous membranes.

17. 2.   Nebulizers deliver medication through a face mask or mouthpiece, using compressed air or oxygen with a gas flow of 6 to 10 L/min. Metered dose inhalers deliver medication via puffs. Generally, the standard is 2 puffs per administration, a wait of 2 to 5 minutes between puffs, and no more than 12 puffs in 24 hours for most medications. Metered dose inhalers do not require refrigeration.

18. 3. 4. 6. Types of low-flow oxygen therapy include nasal cannula, nonrebreather mask, and simple face mask. Types of high-flow oxygen therapy include Venturi mask, aerosol mask, and transtracheal.

19. 2.   The client should not inhale during administration, so that the medication can remain in the nasal passages for best absorption. Initially, and if not used for more than 7 days, the pump needs to be primed with seven actuations; if not used within 24 hours, prime with two actuations.

20. 2.   Theophylline may reduce the effects of lithium by increasing its rate of excretion. The client may need to have the dose of lithium increased, but not before the client's current serum lithium level is known. There is no indication to increase the theophylline dose. Obtaining a serum theophylline level would also be appropriate.

21. 3.   Pyridoxine (B_6) helps counter the peripheral neuritis associated with isoniazid therapy. Skin rash is a possible adverse reaction of ethambutol, and clients on streptomycin should be monitored for hearing loss, particularly those with renal insufficiency. The duration of therapy is not shortened by pyridoxine.

22. 4. Ciprofloxacin (Cipro) causes a decrease in theophylline clearance and can elevate serum drug levels, causing theophylline toxicity.

23. 3. Administering aminophylline intravenously, monitoring the respiratory status and for signs of hypoxia, and providing emotional support are all appropriate interventions, but the initial action should be focused on improving oxygenation (airway, breathing, circulation). An inhalation bronchodilator will act quickly and should be followed by intravenous medications.

24. 3. Clients who are mouth breathers may not get the full benefit from nasal cannula administration of oxygen. A face mask may be more effective. Face masks are removed for meals and a nasal cannula would be appropriate at that time. The client's oxygenation may improve when awake, but one cannot be kept awake all the time. Clients with chronic airway limitation (CAL) should not receive oxygen greater than 2 to 3 L/minute because greater oxygen administration may suppress the respiratory drive.

25. 1. 2. 5. Adverse reactions of drugs for bronchodilation include headache, tachycardia, and palpitation. Insomnia is an adverse reaction of xanthine derivatives. Back pain is an example of leukotriene receptor antagonist adverse reaction. Sneezing is an example of adverse decongestant adverse reactions.

26. 4. A licensed practical nurse cannot monitor a drug for its effectiveness or develop a teaching plan. These are job functions reserved for a registered nurse. Neither a registered nurse nor a licensed practical nurse can increase the oxygen flow rate to a client without a physician's order. Once a physician's order is obtained, a registered nurse should increase the flow rate.

REFERENCES

Broyles, B., Reiss, B., & Evans, M. (2012). *Pharmacological aspects of nursing care* (8th ed.). Clifton Park, NY: Delmar Cengage Learning.

Daniels, R., & Nicoll, L. (2012). *Contemporary medical-surgical nursing.* Clifton Park, NY: Delmar Cengage Learning.

Kee, J., Hayes, E., & McCuistion, L. (2012). *Pharmacology: A nursing process approach* (7th ed.). St. Louis, MO: Saunders Elsevier.

Spratto, G. R., & Woods, A. L. (2012). *PDR nurse's drug handbook 2012.* Clifton Park, NY: Delmar Cengage Learning.

CHAPTER 19

DRUGS FOR THE CARDIOVASCULAR SYSTEM

I. **INOTROPIC AGENTS**
  A. DESCRIPTION
    1. INCREASE THE FORCE OF THE HEART'S CONTRACTIONS, POSITIVE INOTROPIC EFFECT
    2. THREE TYPES
      a. Cardiac glycosides
      b. Phosphodiesterase inhibitors
      c. Sympathomimetics
    3. USES
      a. Congestive heart failure (all types)
      b. Supraventricular dysrhythmias, such as atrial fibrillation or atrial flutter (cardiac glycosides)
  B. CARDIAC GLYCOSIDES
    1. DIGOXIN (LANOXIN)
      a. Uses
        1) In addition to positive inotropic effect, digoxin has a negative chronotropic effect, producing a reduced heart rate.
        2) Creates an increase in stroke volume
      b. Adverse reactions
        1) Decreasing renal function increases drug levels in the blood.
        2) Low potassium levels can increase its toxicity.
        3) Cardiovascular
          a) Any type of dysrhythmia, including bradycardia or tachycardia
        4) Central nervous system (CNS)
          a) Headache
          b) Fatigue
          c) Malaise
          d) Confusion
          e) Convulsions
        5) Gastrointestinal (GI)
          a) Anorexia
          b) Nausea
          c) Vomiting
          d) Diarrhea
        6) Visual
          a) Colored vision such as green, yellow, or purple
          b) Halo vision
          c) Flickering lights
      c. Contraindications and precautions
        1) Ventricular fibrillation or tachycardia
        2) Hypersensitivity to cardiac glycosides
        3) Digoxin toxicity
        4) Pregnancy
        5) Decreased renal function
      d. Drug interactions
        1) Antacids: decrease the effect of digoxin
        2) Diuretics: increase potassium and magnesium losses, increasing the risk of digitalis toxicity
        3) Hypoglycemic drugs: decrease the effect of digoxin
        4) Propranolol (Inderal): potentiates digitalis-induced bradycardia
      e. Nursing interventions
        1) Monitor serum digoxin levels. Therapeutic digoxin level is 0.5 to 2 ng/ml.
        2) Monitor serum electrolytes, especially potassium.
        3) Monitor renal function tests, blood urea nitrogen (BUN), and creatinine.
        4) Monitor the client for adverse reactions.
        5) Take the apical pulse for 1 full minute before administering.
        6) Notify the physician of anorexia, nausea, vomiting, or bradycardia (pulse below 60 beats per minute).

7) Treat drug toxicity.
  a) Discontinue the drug.
  b) Determine digoxin and electrolyte levels.
  c) Give potassium supplements for hypokalemia.
  d) Initiate supportive therapy for GI clinical manifestations (nausea, vomiting, or diarrhea).
  e) Start cardiac monitoring.
  f) Determine the severity of symptoms of toxicity. (For example, are there life-threatening cardiac dysrhythmias or heart block?)
  g) Antidote: Digibind for severe toxicity

C. PHOSPHODIESTERASE INHIBITORS
  1. MILRINONE (PRIMACOR)
    a. Uses
      1) Inodilator, exerts both a positive inotropic effect and a vasodilator effect, which in turn decreases the work of the heart
      2) Causes relaxation and compliance of the heart muscle
      3) Short-term management of congestive heart failure
      4) May be given before heart transplantation
    b. Adverse reactions
      1) Ventricular dysrhythmias
      2) Hypotension
      3) Angina
      4) Hypokalemia
      5) Tremor
      6) Thrombocytopenia
    c. Contraindications and precautions
      1) Hypersensitivity
      2) Lactation
    d. Nursing interventions
      1) Monitor for ventricular dysrhythmia.
      2) Treat drug toxicity.
        a) No specific antidote exists for an overdose.
        b) Hypotension is the primary effect seen with excessive doses. The dose is generally decreased or discontinued for excessive hypotension.
      3) Monitor complete blood count (CBC) and electrolytes.
      4) Monitor vital signs. Closely monitor the heart rate and blood pressure.

D. SYMPATHOMIMETIC DRUGS
  1. DOPAMINE (INTROPIN)
    a. Uses
      1) Cardiogenic shock due to myocardial infarction

      2) Trauma
      3) Open heart surgery
      4) Cardiac decompensation such as congestive heart failure
    b. Adverse reactions
      1) Tachycardia
      2) Dysrhythmias
      3) Angina
      4) Dyspnea
    c. Contraindications and precautions
      1) Lactation
      2) Tachycardia
    d. Drug interactions
      1) Anesthetics: increase the risk of dysrhythmias
      2) Diuretics: potentiate the effects of dopamine
      3) Monoamine oxidase inhibitors: increase the effect of dopamine
      4) Tricyclic antidepressant: increases the effect of dopamine
    e. Nursing interventions
      1) Administer by continuous IV infusion.
      2) Monitor the cardiovascular status continuously.
      3) Ensure that the client is on a cardiac monitor.
      4) Phentolamine infiltrated into extravasated tissue can limit the potential for necrosis from high doses of dopamine.

  2. DOBUTAMINE (DOBUTREX)
    a. Uses
      1) Heart failure
    b. Adverse reactions
      1) Tachycardia
      2) Ventricular ectopic activity
      3) Chest pain
      4) Hypertension or precipitous drop in blood pressure
    c. Contraindications and precautions
      1) Idiopathetic hypertrophic subaortic stenosis
    d. Drug interactions
      1) Anesthetics: increase the risk of dysrhythmias
      2) Diuretics: potentiate the effects of dopamine
      3) Monoamine oxidase inhibitors: increase the effect of dopamine
      4) Tricyclic antidepressant: increases the effect of dopamine
    e. Nursing interventions
      1) Administer by continuous IV infusion.
      2) Monitor the cardiovascular status continuously.

3) Ensure the client is on a cardiac monitor.

4) Monitor the blood pressure.

II. ADRENERGIC AGONISTS

A. DESCRIPTION

1. KEYS TO UNDERSTANDING ADRENERGIC AGONISTS

a. Knowledge of the receptors that the drug can activate

b. Knowledge of the therapeutic and adverse effects that receptor activation can elicit

2. CLINICAL CONSEQUENCES OF ALPHA$_1$ ACTIVATION

a. Description

1) Vasoconstriction in blood vessels of the skin, viscera, and mucous membranes

a) Hemostasis

b) Nasal decongestion

c) Delayed local anesthetic absorption

d) Blood pressure elevation

2) Mydriasis (pupil dilation)

a) Eye examination

b. Adverse reactions

1) Hypertension due to widespread vasoconstriction

2) Necrosis due to IV extravasation and localized vasoconstriction

3) Bradycardia due to vasoconstriction-mediated hypertension and stimulation of baroreceptors, causing the heart rate to decline

3. CLINICAL CONSEQUENCES OF ALPHA$_2$ ACTIVATION

a. Description: Reduction of sympathetic outflow to the heart and blood vessels, causing bradycardia, decreased cardiac output, and vasodilation

4. CLINICAL CONSEQUENCES OF BETA$_1$ ACTIVATION

a. Description (all the clinically relevant responses result from activating beta$_1$ receptors in the heart)

1) Cardiac arrest

a) Initiate contraction in a heart that has stopped beating

2) Heart failure

a) Improve cardiac performance by positive inotropic effect

3) Shock

a) Maintain blood flow to vital organs by increasing heart rate and force of contraction improving tissue perfusion

4) Atrioventricular (AV) heart block

a) Enhance impulse conduction through the AV node

b. Adverse reactions

1) Altered heart rate or rhythm, tachycardia (excessive heart rate), and dysrhythmias (irregular heartbeat)

2) Angina by increased cardiac oxygen demand (by increasing heart rate and force of contraction)

5. CLINICAL CONSEQUENCES OF BETA$_2$ ACTIVATION

a. Description: therapeutic applications of beta$_2$ activation are limited to the lung and uterus.

b. Adverse reactions

1) Hyperglycemia due to action on the liver to promote breakdown of glycogen into glucose

2) Tremor due to activation of receptors in the skeletal muscle, enhancing contraction

6. CLINICAL CONSEQUENCES OF DOPAMINE RECEPTOR ACTIVATION

a. Description

1) Peripheral dopamine receptor activation causes dilation of the vasculature of the kidneys; used to reduce the risk of renal failure in shock.

2) Enhances cardiac performance by activation of the beta$_1$ receptors in the heart

7. TYPES

a. Epinephrine (Adrenalin)

b. Norepinephrine

c. Isoproterenol (Isuprel)

III. BETA BLOCKERS

A. DESCRIPTION

1. COMPETE WITH AND BLOCK NOREPINEPHRINE AND EPINEPHRINE AT THE BETA-ADRENERGIC RECEPTORS LOCATED THROUGHOUT THE BODY

2. THE BETA-ADRENERGIC RECEPTOR SITES CAN THEN NO LONGER BE STIMULATED BY THE NEUROTRANSMITTERS, NOREPINEPHRINE AND EPINEPHRINE, AND SYMPATHETIC NERVOUS SYSTEM (SNS) STIMULATION IS BLOCKED.

3. TWO TYPES

a. Cardioselective beta$_1$ blockers, beta$_1$-adrenergic blockers

b. Nonspecific beta blockers, beta$_1$- and beta$_2$-adrenergic blockers

B. CARDIOSELECTIVE BETA$_1$ BLOCKERS, BETA$_1$-ADRENERGIC BLOCKERS

1. DESCRIPTION

a. Block the beta$_1$-adrenergic receptors on the surface of the heart

    b. Decrease heart rate and myocardial oxygen demand by decreasing myocardial contractility, reduce velocity of impulse conduction through the atrioventricular (AV) node

    c. Because their effects on beta$_2$ receptors are normally minimal, these drugs are preferred to the nonselective beta blockers for clients with asthma or diabetes. (See the side effects of nonspecific beta blockers on page 422.)

    d. At higher doses, will block beta$_2$ receptors as well as beta$_1$ receptors

2. USES

    a. Hypertension

    b. Dysrhythmias

    c. Angina

    d. Myocardial infarction

3. ADVERSE REACTIONS

    a. Bradycardia

    b. Reduced cardiac output due to decreasing heart rate and decreased force of myocardial contraction

    c. Precipitation of heart failure due to suppression of cardiac function

    d. AV heart block

    e. If beta blocker is stopped abruptly, anginal pain or ventricular dysrhythmias may develop; referred to as rebound excitation.

    f. Insomnia, depression

    g. Hypotension

4. CONTRAINDICATIONS AND PRECAUTIONS

    a. Sinus bradycardia

    b. Second- or third-degree AV block

    c. Cardiac failure

    d. Asthma

    e. Diabetes mellitus

5. DRUG INTERACTIONS

    a. Antihypertensive agents: increase hypotensive effect

    b. Insulin: increases hypoglycemic effect

    c. Rifampin: decreases effect of beta blockers

    d. Amiodarone: increases bradycardia effect

6. NURSING INTERVENTIONS

    a. Monitor heart rate, respirations, and blood pressure.

    b. Monitor the client for clinical manifestations of hypoglycemia.

    c. Monitor electrocardiogram (ECG) for IV administration.

    d. Instruct the client to rise from a lying position slowly.

    e. Monitor glucose level if appropriate.

7. TYPES

    a. Acebutolol (Sectral)

    b. Atenolol (Tenormin)

    c. Betaxolol (Kerlone)

    d. Bisoprolol (Zebeta)

    e. Esmolol (Brevibloc)

    f. Metoprolol tartrate (Lopressor)

    g. Metoprolol succinate (Toprol XL)

C. NONSPECIFIC BETA BLOCKERS, BETA$_1$ AND BETA$_2$-ADRENERGIC BLOCKERS

1. DESCRIPTION

    a. Same effects as the cardioselective beta$_1$ blockers

    b. Also block beta$_2$-adrenergic receptors on the smooth muscle of the bronchioles and blood vessels

    c. May constrict blood vessels by blocking beta$_2$-adrenergic receptors on the smooth muscle of blood vessels

    d. May impair the production of glucose from glycogen and mobilization of glucose in response to hypoglycemia, which can be detrimental to clients with diabetes

    e. Impair the secretion of insulin from the pancreas, causing an elevated blood glucose, which can be detrimental to clients with diabetes

2. USES

    a. Hypertension

    b. Heart failure

    c. Angina

3. ADVERSE REACTIONS

    a. Bronchiole constriction, narrowing of the airways that is insignificant in most clients but in clients with asthma may be life threatening

    b. Bradycardia

    c. Hypotension

    d. Insomnia, depression

4. CONTRAINDICATIONS AND PRECAUTIONS

    a. Sinus bradycardia

    b. Second- and third-degree heart block

    c. Cardiogenic shock

    d. Cardiac failure

    e. Asthma

    f. Chronic obstructive pulmonary disease (COPD)

    g. Diabetes mellitus

    h. Congestive heart failure (CHF)

5. DRUG INTERACTIONS

    a. Antihypertensives: increase hypotensive effect

    b. Diuretics: increase hypotensive effect

    c. Nonsteroidal anti-inflammatory drugs (NSAIDs): decrease effect of beta blockers

    d. Cimetidine (Tagamet): increases effect of beta blockers

       e. Insulin: increases hypoglycemic effect

  6. NURSING INTERVENTIONS

      a. Determine allergies to food or medication.

      b. Determine history of COPD, such as emphysema, asthma, or chronic bronchitis.

      c. Determine history of hypotension, cardiac dysrhythmias, bradycardia, CHF, or any other cardiovascular disease.

      d. Encourage the client to change positions slowly to prevent or minimize postural hypotension.

      e. Monitor the pulse apically for 1 full minute prior to drug administration and contact the physician if pulse is < 60 beats per minute.

      f. Monitor the blood pressure and contact the physician if blood pressure is less than 100 mm Hg.

      g. Notify the physician of weight gain, especially if more than 2 pounds in a week; weakness; shortness of breath; and edema.

      h. Notify the physician of confusion, depression, hallucinations, nightmares, palpitations, and dizziness.

  7. TYPES

      a. Carteolol (Cartrol)

      b. Carvedilol (Coreg)

      c. Labetalol (Normodyne, Trandate)

      d. Nadolol (Corgard)

      e. Penbutolol (Levatol)

      f. Pindolol (Visken)

      g. Propranolol (Inderal)

      h. Sotalol (Betapace)

      i. Timolol (Blocadren)

IV. CALCIUM-CHANNEL BLOCKERS (CCBs)

  A. DESCRIPTION

    1. PREVENT CALCIUM IONS FROM ENTERING CELLS, WITH THEIR GREATEST EFFECTS ON THE HEART AND BLOOD VESSELS

    2. AS AN ACTION POTENTIAL TRAVELS DOWN THE SURFACE OF A VASCULAR SMOOTH MUSCLE (VSM) CELL, CALCIUM CHANNELS OPEN AND CALCIUM IONS FLOW INWARD, INITIATING THE CONTRACTILE PROCESS. IF CALCIUM CHANNELS ARE BLOCKED, CONTRACTION WILL BE PREVENTED AND VASODILATION WILL RESULT. CCBs ACT SELECTIVELY ON PERIPHERAL ARTERIOLES AND ARTERIES AND ARTERIOLES OF THE HEART. CALCIUM CHANNELS HELP REGULATE THE FUNCTION OF THE MYOCARDIUM, THE SINOATRIAL (S-A) NODE, AND THE ATRIOVENTRICULAR (AV) NODE.

    3. IN CARDIAC MUSCLE (MYOCARDIUM), CALCIUM ENTRY HAS A POSITIVE INOTROPIC EFFECT. IF CALCIUM CHANNELS ARE BLOCKED, CONTRACTILE FORCE WILL DIMINISH (REDUCE FORCE OF CONTRACTION).

    4. THE PACEMAKER ACTIVITY OF THE S-A NODE IS REGULATED BY CALCIUM INFLUX. WHEN CALCIUM CHANNELS ARE OPEN, DISCHARGE OF THE S-A NODE INCREASES, WHEN CALCIUM CHANNELS CLOSE, ACTIVITY DECLINES. CALCIUM-CHANNEL BLOCKADE REDUCES HEART RATE (SLOWS HEART RATE).

    5. THE EXCITABILITY OF AV NODAL CELLS IS REGULATED BY CALCIUM ENTRY. WHEN CALCIUM CHANNELS ARE OPEN, CALCIUM ENTRY INCREASES AND CELLS OF THE AV NODE DISCHARGE MORE READILY. WHEN CALCIUM CHANNELS ARE CLOSED, DISCHARGE OF AV NODAL CELLS IS SUPPRESSED. CALCIUM-CHANNEL BLOCKADE DECREASES THE VELOCITY OF CONDUCTION THROUGH THE AV NODE (SUPPRESSES CONDUCTION THROUGH THE AV NODE).

    6. BELONG TO THREE CHEMICAL FAMILIES: DIHYDROPYRIDINES, PHENYLALKYLAMINE, AND BENZOTHIAZEPINE

  B. USES

    1. HYPERTENSION

    2. ANGINA

    3. CARDIAC DYSRHYTHMIAS

  C. ADVERSE REACTIONS

    1. REFLEX TACHYCARDIA

    2. FLUSHING

    3. DIZZINESS

    4. HEADACHE

    5. PERIPHERAL EDEMA

    6. GINGIVAL HYPERPLASIA

  D. CONTRAINDICATIONS AND PRECAUTIONS

    1. PREGNANCY

    2. LACTATION

    3. HYPOTENSION

    4. SICK SINUS SYNDROME

    5. SECOND- OR THIRD-DEGREE HEART BLOCK

  E. DRUG INTERACTIONS

    1. BETA-ADRENERGIC BLOCKING AGENTS: DEPRESS THE MYOCARDIAL CONTRACTILITY AND AV CONDUCTION

2. CIMETIDINE: INCREASES EFFECTS OF CALCIUM-CHANNEL BLOCKERS

3. FENTANYL: SEVERE HYPOTENSION

F. NURSING INTERVENTIONS

1. INSTRUCT THE CLIENT TO SWALLOW THE SUSTAINED-RELEASED DRUG WHOLE, WITHOUT CRUSHING OR CHEWING.

2. INSTRUCT THE CLIENT TO NOTIFY THE PHYSICIAN IF THE ANKLES AND FEET SWELL.

3. ADMINISTER THE PRESCRIBED DIURETIC FOR EDEMA.

4. MONITOR THE BLOOD PRESSURE.

5. REPORT SUSTAINED HYPOTENSION.

6. ASSESS FOR REFLEX TACHYCARDIA.

7. INSTRUCT THE CLIENT TO SIT UP FROM A RECLINING POSITION SLOWLY.

G. TYPES

1. DIHYDROPYRIDINES
   a. Nifedipine (Adalat, Procardia)
   b. Amlodipine (Norvasc)
   c. Felodipine (Plendil)
   d. Isradipine (DynaCirc)
   e. Nicardipine (Cardene, Cardene SR)
   f. Nisoldipine (Sular)

2. PHENYLALKYLAMINE
   a. Verapamil (Calan)

3. BENZOTHIAZEPINES
   a. Diltiazem (Cardizem)

V. **ANTIDYSRHYTHMIC DRUGS**

A. DESCRIPTION

1. EFFECT CHANGES IN THE S-A NODE AND ECTOPIC PACEMAKERS, AV NODE, CONDUCTION VELOCITY, AUTONOMIC NERVOUS SYSTEM INNERVATION, ABSOLUTE REFRACTORY PERIOD, AND VARIOUS SEGMENTS OF THE ELECTROCARDIOGRAM

2. EFFECTIVE IN TREATING A VARIETY OF CARDIAC DYSRHYTHMIAS

B. ADVERSE REACTIONS COMMON TO ANTIDYSRHYTHMIC DRUGS

1. HYPERSENSITIVITY

2. NAUSEA, VOMITING, AND DIARRHEA

3. DIZZINESS, HEADACHE, AND BLURRED VISION

4. PROARRHYTHMIC EFFECT (OCCURS MOST FREQUENTLY WITH QUINIDINE, AMIODARONE, MORICIZINE, OR PROPAFENONE THERAPY)

C. CLASS I (WITH SUBCLASSES IA, IB, IC): SODIUM-CHANNEL BLOCKERS

1. GENERAL DESCRIPTION CLASS I
   a. Block cardiac sodium channels
   b. Decrease conduction velocity in the atria, ventricles, and His-Purkinje system

2. CLASS IA ACTION (SEE TABLE 19-1)
   a. Delay repolarization

3. CLASS IB ACTION (SEE TABLE 19-2)
   a. Accelerate repolarization

4. CLASS IC ACTION (SEE TABLE 19-3)
   a. Can exacerbate existing dysrhythmias and create new ones

5. OTHER CLASS I (HAS CHARACTERISTICS OF ALL THREE SUBCLASSES): MORICIZINE (ETHMOZINE)
   a. Potential for adverse cardiac effects, reserved for use for life-threatening ventricular dysrhythmias that have not responded to safer drugs

D. CLASS II: BETA BLOCKERS

1. DESCRIPTION
   a. Reduce or block SNS stimulation to the heart and heart's conduction system
   b. Result in reduced heart rate, delayed AV node conduction, reduced myocardial contractility, and decreased myocardial automaticity
   c. These effects are particularly beneficial after myocardial infarction (MI) when the heart is hyperirritable and predisposed to many types of dysrhythmias.

2. USES
   a. Supraventricular tachyarrhythmias
   b. Hypertension
   c. Angina

3. ADVERSE REACTIONS
   a. Bradycardia
   b. Hypotension
   c. Heart failure
   d. Heart block

4. CONTRAINDICATIONS AND PRECAUTIONS
   a. Severe bradycardia
   b. Second- or third-degree heart block
   c. Cardiogenic shock
   d. Asthma

5. DRUG INTERACTIONS
   a. Antihypertensives: additive hypotensive effect
   b. Calcium-channel blockers: increase effect of beta blockers

6. NURSING INTERVENTIONS
   a. Assess apical pulse before administration—if below 60 beats per minute, withhold dose and consult the physician.
   b. Instruct the client to sit up from a recumbent position slowly.
   c. Discontinue if bradycardia, hypotension, CHF, tachycardia, respiratory depression, or bronchospasm (overdose clinical manifestation) develop.

Table 19-1 Class IA Antidysrhythmics

Drug	Action/Used For	Adverse Reactions	Contraindications/ Drug Interactions	Nursing Interventions
Disopyramide (Norpace, Norpace CR)	Action similar to quinidine Anticholinergic actions greater than those of quinidine Used primarily to treat ventricular dysrhythmias (ventricular tachycardia, ventricular fibrillation); reserved for those clients who cannot tolerate safer medications (e.g., quinidine, procainamide) Pronounced reduction in contractility	Anticholinergic responses (dry mouth, blurred vision, urinary retention) Severe hypotension Widening of the QRS interval Ventricular dysrhythmias Cardiovascular depression: pronounced reduction in contractility	Systemic lupus erythematosus (SLE) Second-degree, third-degree, or complete heart block CHF Beta blockers	Initiate supportive therapy in response to adverse reactions. Whenever used, pressor drugs should be immediately available.
Procainamide (Pronestyl, Procanbid, Pronestyl-SR, Procan SR)	Broad spectrum: action similar to quinidine, but toxicity makes it less desirable for long-term use Weakly anticholinergic; not likely to increase ventricular rate	Lupuslike syndrome Ventricular dysrhythmias Torsade de pointes resulting from prolonged Q-T interval GI clinical manifestations Hypotension Blood dyscrasias (agranulocytosis, thrombocytopenia, neutropenia)	Systemic lupus erythematosus (SLE) Second-degree, third-degree, or complete heart block without pacemaker Cautious use in renal or hepatic failure	Notify the physician immediately for widening of the QRS complex (by 50% or more) and excessive prolonged Q-T interval. Monitor clients on long-term therapy for clinical manifestations resembling those of SLE (joint pain and inflammation, hepatomegaly, unexplained fever, soreness of the mouth, throat, or gums). Monitor for signs of infection, bruising, and bleeding. Clients who receive quinidine for atrial fibrillation are at risk of arterial emboli. Observe for signs of thromboembolism (sudden chest pain, dyspnea).
Quinidine (Quinidex, Cardioquin, Quinaglute, Dura-Tab)	Broad spectrum: used for long-term suppression of ventricular and supraventricular dysrhythmias Slows impulse conduction and delays repolarization in the atria, ventricles, and His-Purkinje systems to suppress dysrhythmias Supraventricular tachycardia (SVT) Atrial fibrillation Atrial flutter Sustained ventricular tachycardia Strongly anticholinergic; blocks vagal input to the heart, causing increased S-A node automaticity and AV conduction. Clients should be pretreated with a drug that suppresses AV conduction.	Diarrhea, GI upset A natural source of quinidine is the bark of the South American cinchona tree. Cinchonism (ringing in the ears, headache, nausea, vertigo, and disturbed vision) can develop with one quinidine dose. Cardiotoxicity (sinus arrest, AV block, ventricular tachydysrhythmias, asystole) Hypotension Arterial embolization	Quinidine can double digoxin levels. Complete heart block (CHB) Digoxin toxicity Cautions: Partial AV block CHF Hypotensive states Hepatic dysfunction	Administer with food to reduce GI side effects. Discontinue the drug and notify the physician for clinical manifestations of cinchonism. Notify the physician immediately for widening of the QRS complex (by 50% or more) and excessive prolonged Q-T interval. Monitor drug levels of digoxin and for signs of digoxin toxicity. Clients who receive quinidine for atrial fibrillation are at risk of arterial emboli. Observe for signs of thromboembolism (sudden chest pain, dyspnea).

Table 19-2 Class IB Antidysrhythmics

Drug	Action/Used For	Adverse Reactions	Contraindications/ Drug Interactions	Drug Interactions
Lidocaine (Xylocaine)	Ventricular dysrhythmias Decreases cardiac cell automaticity (ability to depolarize on their own)	CNS effects: drowsiness, confusion, and paresthesias CV effects: hypotension, bradycardia, and dysrhythmias Toxic doses may produce convulsions and respiratory arrest.	Severe S-A or AV intraventricular block, or Stokes-Adams or Wolff-Parkinson-White syndrome Adjust dose accordingly for liver disease.	Ensure resuscitation equipment is available for severe adverse reactions. Convulsions from overdose can be managed with diazepam (Valium) or phenytoin (Dilantin). Administer by IV only due to extensive first-pass effect. (When taken orally, the liver metabolizes most of it to inactive metabolites.) IM can be used in an emergency.
Mexiletine (Mexitil)	Ventricular dysrhythmias Oral agent with action similar to IV lidocaine	GI: nausea, vomiting, diarrhea, constipation CNS: tremor, dizziness, sleep disturbances, psychosis Convulsions CV: can cause dysrhythmias	Hypersensitivity Cardiogenic shock Second- or third-degree AV block Use cautiously in liver failure.	Administer with food to reduce GI adverse reactions.
Phenytoin (Dilantin)	Digoxin-induced ventricular dysrhythmias Reduces automaticity, especially in the ventricles Reserved for severe, acute dysrhythmias produced by digoxin toxicity Increases AV node conduction to help counteract the decrease in AV node conduction caused by digoxin toxicity	Too rapid IV administration can cause hypotension, dysrhythmias, and cardiac arrest. CNS effects: sedation, ataxia, and nystagmus	Not to be used in atrial fibrillation or atrial flutter because enhanced AV conduction could increase atrial impulses reaching the ventricles and drive the ventricles at an excessive rate	Administer slowly by IV, no more than 50 mg/min. Monitor BP and ECG continuously during infusion.
Tocainide (Tonocard)	Life-threatening ventricular dysrhythmias Oral analog of lidocaine	GI: nausea CNS: tremor Pulmonary fibrosis Pneumonitis	Serious adverse effects; should be reserved for clients with severe ventricular dysrhythmias that have not responded to safer drugs Cautious use in renal or hepatic impairment	Administer with food to reduce GI adverse reactions.

      d. Monitor the blood pressure—withhold if systolic blood pressure is less than 90.
      e. Monitor intake and output.
      f. Monitor for cold manifestations, fatigue, or lightheadedness—may require a drug change.
    7. TYPES
      a. Atenolol (Tenormin)
      b. Esmolol (Brevibloc)
      c. Propranolol (Inderal)
  E. CLASS III: POTASSIUM-CHANNEL BLOCKERS (DRUGS THAT DELAY REPOLARIZATION)
    1. DESCRIPTION
      a. Prolong the effective refractory period (ERP), the time during which a cell is unable to respond to excitation and initiate a new action potential

      b. Prolong myocardial action potential (cardiac cells' ability to self-propagate waves of depolarization)
      c. Block both alpha- and beta-adrenergic cardiac stimulation
    2. USES
      a. Ventricular tachycardia or fibrillation
      b. Atrial dysrhythmias that are difficult to treat or resist treatment
    3. ADVERSE REACTIONS
      a. Hypotension
      b. Anorexia, nausea, and vomiting
      c. Visual impairment, photophobia, dry eyes
      d. Ataxia, dizziness, tremor
      e. Bradycardia, AV block, heart failure
      f. Hyperthyroidism or hypothyroidism

Table 19-3 Class IC Antidysrhythmics

Drug	Action/Used For	Adverse Reactions	Contraindications/ Drug Interactions	Nursing Interventions
Flecainide (Tambocor)	Life-threatening ventricular dysrhythmias	Prolonged PR and widening of QRS complex Decreased myocardial contractility Diminished cardiac conduction Increase absolute refractory period Prodysrhythmic	CHF Should not be combined with other agents that can decrease contractile force (e.g., beta blockers) Reserved for severe ventricular dysrhythmias that have not responded to safer drugs Cautious use in renal or hepatic impairment	Monitor for excessive QRS widening. Monitor for increasing dysrhythmias.
Propafenone (Rythmol)	Life-threatening ventricular dysrhythmias	Prolonged PR and widening of QRS complex Decreased myocardial contractility Diminished cardiac conduction Prodysrhythmic Beta-adrenergic blocking properties can decrease myocardial contractility and promote bronchospasm. Dizziness Altered taste Blurred vision GI: abdominal discomfort, anorexia, nausea, vomiting	Uncontrolled CHF Bradycardia Bronchial asthma Reserved for severe ventricular dysrhythmias that have not responded to safer drugs	Administer with food to reduce GI adverse reactions.

4. CONTRAINDICATIONS AND PRECAUTIONS
   a. Hypersensitivity
   b. Sinus bradycardia
   c. Second- or third-degree AV block
   d. Cardiogenic shock
5. DRUG INTERACTIONS
   a. Quinidine: increases quinidine toxicity
   b. Digoxin: increases digoxin level, leading to toxicity
   c. Procainamide: increases procainamide toxicity
   d. Phenytoin: increases phenytoin toxicity
6. NURSING INTERVENTIONS
   a. Monitor the blood pressure.
   b. Perform periodic assessments of the liver, lung, thyroid, neurologic, and GI functions.
   c. Assess the pulse.
7. TYPES
   a. Bretylium tosylate (Bretylol)
   b. Amiodarone (Cordarone)
   c. Sotalol (Betapace)
F. CLASS IV: CALCIUM-CHANNEL BLOCKERS
  1. DESCRIPTION
   a. Prolong AV node ERP
   b. Reduce AV node conduction
   c. Reduce rapid ventricular conduction caused by atrial flutter

2. USES
   a. Atrial flutter
   b. Atrial fibrillation
   c. Paroxysmal supraventricular tachycardia
3. ADVERSE REACTIONS
   a. Bradycardia
   b. AV block
   c. Hypotension
   d. Heart failure
   e. Edema
   f. Constipation
4. CONTRAINDICATIONS AND PRECAUTIONS
   a. Hypersensitivity
   b. Wolff-Parkinson-White (WPW) syndrome
   c. Severe hypotension
   d. Cardiogenic shock
   e. Sick sinus syndrome
   f. Second- or third-degree AV block
5. DRUG INTERACTIONS
   a. Digoxin: increases the risk of AV block
6. NURSING INTERVENTIONS
   a. Monitor the blood pressure (withhold the drug if the systolic blood pressure is less than 90 mm Hg or the diastolic blood pressure is less than 60 mm Hg).
   b. Instruct the client to sit up slowly from a recumbent position.
   c. Instruct the client to avoid caffeine-containing beverages.

Table 19-4 Unclassified Antidysrhythmics

Drug	Action/Used For	Adverse Reactions	Contraindications/ Drug Interactions	Nursing Interventions
Digoxin (Lanoxin)	• Supraventricular dysrhythmias • Decreases conduction through the AV node and decreases automaticity in the S-A node	• Dysrhythmias (risk increased with hypokalemia) • GI: anorexia, nausea, vomiting, abdominal discomfort • CNS: fatigue, visual disturbances	• See Inotropic Agents on page 419.	• See Inotropic Agents on page 419.
Adenosine (Adenocard)	• Used to terminate paroxysmal supraventricular tachycardia (SVT)	• Adverse effects are short lived, lasting less than 1 minute. • Bradycardia • Dyspnea from bronchoconstriction • Hypotension • Facial flushing from vasodilation • Chest discomfort	• Second- or third-degree heart block • Sick sinus syndrome • Atrial fibrillation or flutter • Ventricular tachycardia	• Bolus IV administration in a vessel close to the heart followed immediately by saline flush (half-life is less than 10 seconds)
Ibutilide (Corvert)	• Atrial fibrillation and atrial flutter	• Prodysrhythmic effect—ventricular tachycardia and Torsades de pointes		• Class IA antidysrhythmic drugs and other Class III drugs should not be given concomitantly with ibutilide. They should not be given within 4 hours after infusion of ibutilide.

© Cengage Learning 2015

7. TYPES
   a. Diltiazem (Cardizem)
   b. Verapamil (Calan, Isoptin, Verelan)
G. UNCLASSIFIED ANTIDYSRHYTHMICS (SEE TABLE 19-4)

VI. **ANTIANGINAL DRUGS**
   A. DESCRIPTION
      1. PREVENTION OF MYOCARDIAL INFARCTION (MI) AND DEATH
      2. PREVENTION OF MYOCARDIAL ISCHEMIA AND ANGINAL PAIN
      3. PHARMACOLOGIC CLASS: ANTIANGINAL NITRATE CORONARY VASODILATORS
      4. THREE FAMILIES
         a. Organic nitrates such as nitroglycerin
         b. Beta blockers such as propranolol (Inderal)
         c. Calcium-channel blockers such as verapamil (Calan)
   B. TYPES
      1. ORGANIC NITRATES (SEE TABLE 19-5)
         a. Description
            1) Decrease oxygen demand by dilating veins, which decreases preload
            2) Increase oxygen supply by relaxing coronary artery spasms (vasospastic angina)
            3) Dilation of both large and small coronary vessels, causing redistribution of blood and therefore oxygen delivery to ischemic myocardium

            4) Dilation of diseased, atherosclerotic arteries as long as there is smooth muscle surrounding the coronary artery

VII. **DRUGS ACTING ON THE RENIN-ANGIOTENSIN SYSTEM**
   A. DESCRIPTION
      1. DRUG EFFECTS RESULT FROM INTERFERENCE WITH THE RENIN-ANGIOTENSIN SYSTEM (RAS).
      2. ANGIOTENSIN II
         a. Potent vasoconstrictor acting directly on vascular smooth muscle (VSM), prominent in the arterioles and less prominent in the veins, causing blood pressure rise
         b. Indirect vasoconstrictor, acts in the CNS to increase sympathetic outflow to blood vessels, acts on the adrenal medulla to cause release of epinephrine
         c. Acts on the adrenal cortex to promote synthesis and secretion of aldosterone; aldosterone acts on the kidney to cause retention of sodium and water, thereby increasing plasma volume and blood pressure
         d. May cause pathologic structural changes in the heart and blood vessels, hypertrophy (increased mass of a structure), and remodeling (redistribution of mass within a structure)
         e. Formed through two sequential reactions: the first catalyzed by

Table 19-5 Nitroglycerin

Drug	Action/Used For	Adverse Reactions	Contraindications/ Drug Interactions	Nursing Interventions

• Sublingual tablets (Nitrostat, NitroQuick)
• Translingual sprays (Nitrolingual)
• Transmucosal tablets (Nitrogard)
• Oral tablets, SR (Nitrong)
• Oral capsules, SR (Nitro-Bid, Plateau Caps, Nitroglyn, Timecaps
• Transdermal patches (Deponit, Minitran, Nitrodisc, Nitro-Dur, Transderm-Nitro
• Topical ointment (Nitro-Bid, Nitrol) Intravenous (Nitro-Bid IV, Tridil)"
	• Act directly on vascular smooth muscle to promote vasodilation
	• Act primarily on veins; dilation of arterioles is only modest
	• By dilating veins, nitroglycerin decreases venous return to the heart, decreasing ventricular filling; the decrease in wall tension (preload) decreases oxygen demand.
	• Relaxes or prevents spasm in coronary arteries, increasing oxygen supply
	• Acute antianginal therapy: sublingual, transmucosal tablets, translingual spray
	• Sustained antianginal therapy: transdermal patches, topical ointment, transmucosal tablets, sustained-release oral tablets or capsules
	• Intravenous therapy: perioperative control of blood pressure, production of controlled hypotension during surgery, treatment of CHF associated with acute MI, and unstable and chronic angina when clinical manifestations cannot be controlled with preferred medications
		• Headache
		• Orthostatic hypotension
		• Reflex tachycardia (if nitrate-induced venodilation occurs too rapidly)
			• Hypotensive drugs (nitro can intensify the effect of other hypotensive drugs, e.g., beta blockers, calcium-channel blockers, diuretics, and other blood-pressure-lowering drugs).
			• Sildenafil (Viagra) can intensify nitro-induced vasodilation; can cause life-threatening hypotension.
			• Increased intercranial pressure
			• Inadequate cerebral perfusion
			• Constrictive pericarditis
			• Severe hypotension
			• Severe anemia
			• When given orally, a large percentage of nitroglycerin is removed from circulation by the liver, called a "large first-pass effect." This is the reason for the various delivery systems that can bypass that effect (e.g., sublingual, buccal, etc.).
				• Warn clients taking sildenafil (Viagra) not to take it within 24 hours of taking nitroglycerin.
				• Assess orthostatic BP, pulse.
				• Assess pain: duration, time started, activity being performed, character.
				• Assess tolerance: a "nitrate-free" period should be provided to prevent tolerance to the drug.
				• Assess for headache, light-headedness, decreased BP; may indicate a need for decreased dosage.
				• Protect the drug from light, moisture; place in a cool environment.
				• Administer sublingual nitro:
				  • Give as soon as pain begins, up to 3 doses, 5 minutes apart.
				  • Instruct the client to hold the dose under the tongue while it dissolves.
				  • Instruct the client to discard the bottle 6 months after opening.
				• Administer sustained-release oral tablets and capsules:
				  • Instruct the client to swallow sustained-release formulations intact.
				• Administer transdermal delivery systems:
				  • Apply to a hairless area of the skin.
				  • Rotate sites to avoid local irritation.
				• Administer translingual spray:
				  • As with sublingual tablets, administer no more than 3 doses in a 15-minute interval.
				  • Instruct the client not to inhale the spray.
				• Administer transmucosal (buccal) tablets:
				  • Place the tablet between the cheek and gum or the upper lip and gum.
				  • Instruct clients not to chew or swallow.
				• Administer topical ointment:
				  • Rotate sites to minimize irritation to the skin.
				• Administer IV infusion:
				  • Monitor heart rate and BP continuously.
				  • Avoid using polyvinyl chloride tubing (nitro absorbs into this type of tubing).

© Cengage Learning 2015

renin, the second by angiotensin-converting enzyme (ACE)

  1) Renin is produced by juxtaglomerular cells of the kidney and undergoes controlled release into the bloodstream, where it converts angiotensin into angiotensin I.

    a) Release of renin occurs in response to a decline in blood pressure, blood volume, plasma sodium content, or renal perfusion pressure.

    b) Release of renin is *suppressed* by elevation in blood pressure, blood volume, and plasma sodium content.

  2) ACE catalyzes the conversion of angiotensin I into angiotensin II. ACE is present in abundance, and conversion of angiotensin I into angiotensin II occurs almost instantaneously after angiotensin I has been formed.

B. ANGIOTENSIN-CONVERTING ENZYME (ACE) INHIBITORS

  1. DESCRIPTION

    a. Inhibit ACE

      1) Inhibit production of angiotensin II, causing vasodilation (primarily

in the arterioles and to a lesser
extent in the veins)

    2) Reduction in blood volume
(through effects on the kidney)

    3) Prevention or reversal of
possible angiotensin-II-
mediated pathologic changes
in the heart and blood vessels

2. USES

    a. Hypertension

    b. Heart failure

    c. Myocardial infarction (MI)

    d. Diabetic and nondiabetic
nephropathy

3. ADVERSE REACTIONS

    a. First-dose hypotension, caused by
widespread vasodilation secondary
to abrupt lowering of angiotensin II
levels

    b. Cough

    c. Hyperkalemia (inhibition of
aldosterone release can cause
potassium retention by the kidney)

    d. Renal failure

    e. Fetal injury (if used during the
second and third trimesters of
pregnancy)

    f. Angioedema

    g. Dysgeusia (impaired or distorted
sense of taste), can cause anorexia
and weight loss

    h. Rashes (maculopapular,
morbilliform, others)

    i. Neutropenia

    j. GI: nausea, vomiting, diarrhea,
abdominal pain

    k. CNS: headache, dizziness, fatigue,
paresthesias, and insomnia

4. CONTRAINDICATIONS AND
PRECAUTIONS

    a. Renal artery stenosis (If ACE is used
in the presence of renal artery
stenosis, it interferes with the
protective mechanisms in place in
the kidney that support glomerular
filtration and causes a drop in urine
production.)

    b. Pregnancy

    c. Hypersensitivity

5. DRUG INTERACTIONS

    a. Diuretics: may intensify first-dose
hypotension

    b. Antihypertensive drugs: hypotensive
effects of ACE inhibitors may have
additive effects with those of other
antihypertensive drugs

    c. Lithium: may result in accumulation
to toxic levels

6. NURSING INTERVENTIONS

    a. Determine blood pressure prior to
treatment.

    b. Begin with low doses and gradually
increase the dose.

    c. Administer captopril (Capoten) and
moexipril (Univasc) at least 1 hour
before meals.

    d. Monitor the blood pressure closely
for 2 hours after the first dose and
periodically thereafter. Instruct the
client to lie down if hypotension
develops.

    e. Inform the client about the
possibility of persistent, dry,
irritating, nonproductive cough.

    f. Instruct the client to avoid
potassium supplements and
potassium-containing salt substitutes
unless they are prescribed by the
physician. Potassium-sparing
diuretics must also be avoided.

    g. Discontinue ACE inhibitor and avoid
its use if angioedema characterized
by giant wheals and edema of the
tongue, glottis, and pharynx occurs.
It can be fatal. Treat severe reactions
with subcutaneous epinephrine.

    h. Avoid high doses to minimize rash
and dysgeusia (mainly seen with
captopril).

    i. Obtain a white blood cell (WBC)
count and differential prior to start of
treatment. Neutropenia (mainly seen
with captopril) poses a high risk of
infection. Inform clients about early
signs of infection (fever, sore throat,
mouth sores) and instruct them to
notify the physician if these occur.

7. TYPES

    a. Benazepril hydrochloride (Lotensin)

    b. Captopril (Capoten)

    c. Enalapril maleate (Vasotec)

    d. Enalaprilat (Vasotec I.V.)

    e. Fosinopril sodium (Monopril)

    f. Lisinopril (Prinivil, Zestril)

    g. Moexipril (Univasc)

    h. Perindopril erbumine (Aceon,
Coversyl)

    i. Quinapril hydrochloride (Accupril)

    j. Ramipril (Altace)

    k. Trandolapril (Mavik)

**VIII. DIURETIC DRUGS (SEE DIURETICS—
THIAZIDE, LOOP, AND POTASSIUM-
SPARING DIURETICS IN CHAPTER 25 AND
OSMOTIC DIURETICS IN CHAPTER 22.)**

IX. ANTIHYPERTENSIVE DRUGS

A. DESCRIPTION

    1. ARTERIAL PRESSURE IS THE
PRODUCT OF CARDIAC OUTPUT
AND PERIPHERAL RESISTANCE. AN
INCREASE IN EITHER WILL INCREASE
BLOOD PRESSURE.

2. CARDIAC OUTPUT IS INFLUENCED BY FOUR FACTORS. AN INCREASE IN ANY OF THESE FACTORS WILL INCREASE CARDIAC OUTPUT, CAUSING BLOOD PRESSURE TO RISE.
   a. Heart rate
   b. Myocardial contractility (force of contraction)
   c. Blood volume
   d. Venous return of blood to the heart
3. PERIPHERAL VASCULAR RESISTANCE IS REGULATED BY ARTERIOLAR CONSTRICTION.
4. BLOOD PRESSURE MAY BE REDUCED WITH DRUGS THAT AFFECT THESE FACTORS.
5. THREE REGULATORY SYSTEMS REGULATE THESE FACTORS:
   a. Sympathetic baroreceptor reflex
      1) Baroreceptors in the aortic arch and carotid sinus sense blood pressure and relay this information to the brainstem.
      2) When blood pressure is perceived as too low, the brainstem sends impulses along sympathetic nerves to stimulate the heart and blood vessels.
      3) Blood pressure is then elevated by stimulation of beta$_1$ receptors in the heart (increasing cardiac output) and stimulation of vascular alpha$_1$ receptors (causing vasoconstriction).
      4) When blood pressure is restored to an acceptable level, sympathetic stimulation subsides.

B. RENIN-ANGIOTENSIN SYSTEM (RAS)
   1. RENIN IS RELEASED FROM JUXTAGLOMERULAR CELLS OF THE KIDNEY IN RESPONSE TO REDUCED RENAL BLOOD FLOW, REDUCED BLOOD VOLUME, REDUCED BLOOD PRESSURE, AND STIMULATION OF BETA$_1$-ADRENERGIC RECEPTORS ON THE CELL SURFACE.
   2. RENIN PROMOTES THE CONVERSION OF ANGIOTENSINOGEN INTO ANGIOTENSIN I, A WEAK VASOCONSTRICTOR.
   3. ANGIOTENSIN-CONVERTING ENZYME (ACE) ACTS ON ANGIOTENSIN I TO FORM ANGIOTENSIN II, A COMPOUND THAT CONSTRICTS SYSTEMIC (ELEVATES BLOOD PRESSURE BY INCREASING PERIPHERAL RESISTANCE) AND RENAL BLOOD VESSELS (ELEVATES BLOOD PRESSURE BY REDUCING GLOMERULAR FILTRATION, CAUSING RETENTION OF SALT AND WATER, INCREASING BLOOD VOLUME).
   4. IN ADDITION TO VASOCONSTRICTION, ANGIOTENSIN II CAUSES RELEASE OF ALDOSTERONE FROM THE ADRENAL CORTEX. ALDOSTERONE ACTS ON THE KIDNEYS TO FURTHER INCREASE RETENTION OF SODIUM AND WATER.

C. KIDNEY
   1. WHEN BLOOD PRESSURE FALLS, SO DOES GLOMERULAR FILTRATION RATE (GFR), PROMOTING SODIUM, CHLORIDE, AND WATER RETENTION.
   2. INCREASED BLOOD VOLUME INCREASES VENOUS RETURN, CARDIAC OUTPUT, AND ARTERIAL PRESSURE.

D. USES
   1. HYPERTENSION

E. ADVERSE REACTIONS
   1. ORTHOSTATIC HYPOTENSION
   2. WEAKNESS
   3. SEDATION
   4. CONSTIPATION
   5. BRADYCARDIA
   6. DEPRESSION

F. CONTRAINDICATIONS AND PRECAUTIONS
   1. HYPOTENSION
   2. BRADYCARDIA
   3. AV HEART BLOCK
   4. HEART FAILURE
   5. ASTHMA
   6. PREGNANCY

G. DRUG INTERACTIONS
   1. TRICYCLIC ANTIDEPRESSANT: DECREASES ANTIHYPERTENSIVE EFFECT
   2. VASODILATOR DRUGS: INCREASE ANTIHYPOTENSIVE EFFECT
   3. THIAZIDE DIURETICS: INCREASE ANTIHYPOTENSIVE EFFECT
   4. LITHIUM: INCREASE RISK OF LITHIUM TOXICITY

H. NURSING INTERVENTIONS
   1. MONITOR BLOOD PRESSURE (STANDING AND SUPINE).
   2. ADMINISTER AT BEDTIME TO DECREASE SEDATIVE EFFECT.
   3. INSTRUCT THE CLIENT TO SIT OR STAND UP SLOWLY FROM A RECLINING POSITION.
   4. INSTRUCT THE CLIENT TO AVOID DRIVING OR OPERATING HAZARDOUS EQUIPMENT UNTIL THE EFFECT OF THE DRUG IS KNOWN.

I. TYPES
   1. AGENTS ACTING DIRECTLY ON
      VASCULAR SMOOTH MUSCLE
      a. Diazoxide IV (Hyperstat)
      b. Nitroprusside (Nitropress)
   2. ALPHA$_1$-ADRENERGIC BLOCKING
      AGENTS
      a. Doxazosin mesylate (Cardura)
      b. Prazosin hydrochloride (Minipress)
      c. Terazosin (Hytrin)
   3. ANGIOTENSIN II RECEPTOR
      BLOCKERS
      a. Candesartan cilexetil (Atacand)
      b. Eprosartan mesylate (Teveten)
      c. Irbesartan (Avapro)
      d. Losartan potassium (Cozaar)
      e. Olmesartan medoxomil (Benicar)
      f. Valsartan (Diovan)
   4. ANGIOTENSIN-CONVERTING
      ENZYME (ACE) INHIBITORS
      a. Benazepril hydrochloride (Lotensin)
      b. Captopril (Capoten)
      c. Enalapril maleate (Vasotec)
      d. Fosinopril sodium (Monopril)
      e. Lisinopril (Prinivil, Zestril)
      f. Perindopril erbumine (Aceon)
      g. Quinapril hydrochloride (Accupril)
      h. Ramipril (Altace)
      i. Trandolapril (Mavik)
   5. BETA-ADRENERGIC BLOCKING
      AGENTS
      a. Atenolol (Tenormin)
      b. Betaxolol hydrochloride (Betoptic)
      c. Bisoprolol fumarate (Zebeta)
      d. Metoprolol succinate (Toprol XL)
      e. Nadolol (Corgard)
      f. Penbutolol sulfate (Levatol)
      g. Propranolol hydrochloride (Inderal)
      h. Timolol (Blocadren)
   6. CALCIUM-CHANNEL BLOCKING
      AGENTS
      a. Amlodipine (Norvasc)
      b. Bepridil hydrochloride (Vascor)
      c. Diltiazem hydrochloride (Cardizem)
      d. Felodipine (Plendil)
      e. Isradipine (DynaCirc)
      f. Nicardipine hydrochloride (Cardene)
      g. Nifedipine (Procardia)
      h. Nimodipine (Nimotop)
      i. Nisoldipine (Sular)
      j. Verapamil (Calan)
   7. CENTRALLY ACTING AGENTS
      a. Clonidine hydrochloride (Catapres)
      b. Guanfacine hydrochloride (Tenex)
      c. Methyldopa
      d. Methylodopate hydrochloride
         (Aldomet)
   8. MISCELLANEOUS AGENTS
      a. Bosentan (Tracleer)
      b. Carvedilol (Coreg)
      c. Epoprostenol sodium (Flolan)

      d. Labetalol hydrochloride
         (Normodyne, Trandate)
      e. Minoxidil, oral (Loniten)
X. **COAGULATION MODIFIER AGENTS
    (ANTICOAGULANT, ANTIPLATELET, AND
    THROMBOLYTIC DRUGS)**
    A. DESCRIPTION
       1. DRUGS FALL INTO THREE MAJOR
          CATEGORIES:
          a. Anticoagulants: drugs that disrupt
             the coagulation cascade, and thereby
             suppress the production of fibrin
             1) Parenteral: heparin
                a) Decreases fibrin formation by
                   promoting inactivation of
                   clotting factors
             2) Oral: warfarin (Coumadin)
                a) Decreases fibrin formation by
                   decreasing synthesis of
                   clotting factors
          b. Antiplatelet drugs: inhibit platelet
             aggregation
          c. Thrombolytic drugs: promote the
             lysis of fibrin, and thereby cause
             dissolution of thrombi
    B. PARENTERAL ANTICOAGULANTS
       1. HEPARIN
          a. Description
             1) Rapid acting, administered only
                by injection
             2) Suppresses coagulation by helping
                antithrombin III inactivate
                thrombin, factor Xa, and other
                clotting factors. By doing so, it
                ultimately suppresses formation of
                fibrin.
             3) Action develops quickly, within
                minutes of IV administration.
          b. Uses
             1) Prevention of thrombosis in veins
             2) Pulmonary embolism
             3) Evolving stroke
             4) Massive deep vein thrombosis
                (DVT)
             5) In open heart surgery (prevent
                coagulation in heart-lung
                machine)
             6) Renal dialysis (prevent
                coagulation in dialyzers)
             7) Prevent postoperative venous
                thrombosis
             8) Disseminated intravascular
                coagulation (DIC)
             9) Adjunct to thrombolytic therapy
                of acute MI
          c. Adverse reactions
             1) Hemorrhage
             2) Heparin-induced
                thrombocytopenia: a state
                characterized by increased
                thrombosis despite a reduction in

circulating platelets (platelet count < 100,000/mm^3)

3) Hypersensitivity reactions (chills, fever, urticaria [itching]): a small test dose may be administered to minimize the risk prior to the full therapeutic dose.

4) Subcutaneous administration may produce local irritation and hematoma.

d. Contraindications and precautions

1) Use with extreme caution in all clients for whom there is a high likelihood of bleeding (hemophilia, increased capillary permeability, dissecting aneurysm, peptic ulcer disease, severe hypertension, or threatened abortion).

2) Use with caution in clients with severe liver or kidney disease.

3) Contraindicated for clients with thrombocytopenia and uncontrollable bleeding; during and immediately following surgery on the eye, brain, or spinal cord; following lumbar puncture; and following regional anesthesia

e. Drug interactions

1) Aspirin: increases risk of hemorrhage

2) Ibuprofen: increases risk of hemorrhage

f. Nursing interventions

1) Monitor for signs of blood loss such as reduced blood pressure, increased heart rate, bruises, petechiae, hematomas, red or black stools, cloudy or discolored urine, pelvic pain (suggestive of ovarian hemorrhage), headache or faintness (suggestive of cerebral hemorrhage), and lumbar pain (suggestive of adrenal hemorrhage).

2) Control dose according to an established protocol. Some institutions use the activated partial thromboplastin time (APTT) as a control value; others use heparin level.

3) Avoid concurrent use of antiplatelet drugs such as aspirin.

4) Administer by injection only: subcutaneous, intermittent IV administration, or continuous IV infusion.

a) Subcutaneous injection should be performed with a 1/2- to 5/8-inch, 25- or 26-gauge needle, into the fatty layer of the abdomen (but not within 2 inches of the umbilicus). Apply firm but gentle pressure to the injection site for 1–2 minutes following administration. Rotate and record injection sites.

b) Intermittent IV administration should be performed through a heparin (or saline) lock every 4–6 hours. APTT or heparin level should be determined before each dose during the early phase of treatment and daily thereafter. Rotate injection sites every 2–3 days.

c) Continuous IV infusion should be administered using a constant infusion pump or other approved volume control unit. Check the infusion rate every 30–60 minutes.

5) Obtain baseline values for blood pressure, heart rate, complete blood cell counts, platelet counts, hematocrit, and APTT or heparin level.

6) Check dosage with a second nurse.

g. Antidote: protamine

1) Bonds to heparin, forming a heparin-protamine complex that has no anticoagulant activity

2) Neutralization of heparin occurs immediately and lasts for 2 hours.

3) 1 mg of protamine will inactivate 100 units of heparin.

4) Administered by slow IV injection

h. Treatment of heparin-induced thrombocytopenia: lepirudin

1) Reduces thrombosis by inhibiting thrombin, the enzyme that converts fibrinogen into fibrin

2) Produces effective anticoagulation in about 80% of clients, reducing the risk of death and new thrombotic complications

3) Carries the same risk of bleeding

4) Dosing is by continuous IV infusion.

2. LOW-MOLECULAR-WEIGHT HEPARINS (LMWS): ENOXAPARIN

(LOVENOX), DALTEPARIN
(FRAGMIN), ARDEPARIN (NORMIFLO)
  a. Description
    1) Heparin preparations composed
      of molecules that are shorter than
      those found in standard heparin
    2) May be given on a fixed-dose
      schedule and do not require
      laboratory (APTT, heparin level)
      monitoring
    3) May be given at home, whereas
      standard heparin must be given
      in a hospital
    4) Less likely to cause
      thrombocytopenia
    5) Preferentially inactivate factor
      Xa, unlike standard heparin,
      which inactivates factor Xa and
      thrombin
  b. Uses
    1) Prevention of DVT
    2) Treatment of established DVT
    3) Ischemic stroke
    4) Pulmonary embolism
    5) Non-Q-wave MI
  c. Adverse reactions
    1) Bleeding (incidence of bleeding
      complications less than with
      standard heparin)
    2) Thrombocytopenia (incidence is
      less than with standard heparin)
  d. Contraindications and precautions
    (See Heparin on page 433.)
  e. Drug interactions (See Heparin on
    page 433.)
  f. Nursing interventions
    1) Similar to standard heparin,
      except without the need for
      laboratory monitoring of APTT or
      heparin level
  g. Antidote: protamine (See Heparin on
    page 433.)
  h. Treatment of heparin-induced
    thrombocytopenia: lepirudin
    (See Heparin on page 433.)
C. ORAL ANTICOAGULANTS
  1. WARFARIN (COUMADIN)
  a. Description
    1) Four clotting factors (factors VII,
      IX, X, and prothrombin) require
      vitamin K for their synthesis.
    2) Suppresses coagulation by acting
      as an antagonist of vitamin K
    3) Has no effect on clotting factors
      that already existed at the time of
      administration
    4) Decay of preexisting clotting
      factors occurs with a half-life of 6
      hours to 2.5 days.
    5) Initial responses to warfarin may
      not be evident until 8–12 hours
      after administration.

    6) Peak effects do not develop for
      several days.
    7) After discontinuing, coagulation
      remains inhibited for 2–5 days.
  b. Indications
    1) Prevention of thrombosis in the
      veins
    2) Long-term prophylaxis of
      thrombosis
      a) Prevention of venous
        thrombosis and associated
        pulmonary embolism
      b) Prevention of
        thromboembolism associated
        with prosthetic heart valves
      c) Prevention of thrombosis
        during atrial fibrillation
      d) Reduces the risk of recurrent
        transient ischemic attack (TIAs)
      e) Reduces the risk of
        recurrent MI
  c. Adverse reactions
    1) Hemorrhage
    2) Fetal hemorrhage and
      teratogenesis from use during
      pregnancy
    3) Adverse effects other than
      hemorrhage are uncommon.
  d. Contraindications and precautions
    1) Severe thrombocytopenia or
      uncontrollable bleeding
    2) Lumbar puncture
    3) Regional anesthesia
    4) Surgery of the eye, brain, or
      spinal cord
    5) High risk of bleeding, such as in
      hemophilia, increased capillary
      permeability, dissecting
      aneurysm, GI ulcers, and severe
      hypertension or women
      anticipating abortion
    6) Vitamin K deficiency
    7) Liver disease and alcoholism
    8) Pregnancy
    9) Lactation
  e. Drug interactions
    1) Many drugs interact with
      warfarin. Listed are those
      especially likely to produce
      interactions of clinical
      significance.
      a) Heparin: as an anticoagulant,
        it directly increases the
        bleeding tendencies brought
        on by warfarin. Concurrent
        therapy with heparin can
        influence PT values.
      b) Aspirin: inhibits platelet
        aggregation, acts directly on
        the GI tract to cause ulcers; in
        combination with warfarin,
        increases the potential for

hemorrhage. Drugs similar to aspirin such as indomethacin (ibuprofen) should be avoided as well.

    c) Vitamin K: may decrease anticoagulant effects by promoting clotting factor synthesis

  f. Nursing interventions

    1) Monitor prothrombin time (PT), a test especially sensitive to alterations in vitamin K dependent factors. PT test results used to be reported as a PT ratio, which is simply the ratio of the client's PT to a control PT, but test results can vary widely among laboratories. To ensure that test results from different laboratories are comparable, results are now reported in terms of an international normalized ratio (INR).

    2) Frequently determine PT-INR during therapy. In addition, PT-INR should be determined whenever a drug that interacts with warfarin is added to or deleted from the regimen.

    3) Draw blood for PT determinations no sooner than 5 hours after an IV injection of heparin and no sooner than 24 hours after a subcutaneous injection.

    4) Instruct the client to carry identification such as a Medic Alert bracelet to inform emergency personnel of warfarin use.

    5) Provide the client with detailed verbal and written instructions regarding signs of bleeding, dosage size and timing, and scheduling of PT tests.

    6) Instruct the client to notify surgeons and dentists of warfarin use.

    7) Encourage the use of a soft toothbrush to minimize gingival bleeding.

    8) Encourage the use of an electric razor to reduce the risk of bleeding while shaving.

    9) Avoid administering Coumadin to a pregnant woman. Warfarin enters breast milk. Women taking Coumadin should be advised against breastfeeding.

  g. Antidote: vitamin K_1 (phytonadione)

    1) Antagonizes warfarin's actions and can reverse warfarin-induced inhibition of clotting factor synthesis

    2) May be given orally, IV, or subcutaneously

    3) If levels of clotting factors need to be raised quickly, fresh whole blood, fresh frozen plasma, or plasma concentrates of vitamin K–dependent clotting factors may be infused.

2. DABIGATRAN ETEXILATE (PRADAXA)

  a. Description

    1) Direct thrombin inhibitor

    2) Prevents the development of a thrombus

  b. Uses

    1) Reduce the risk of stroke and systemic embolism in nonvascular atrial fibrillation

  c. Adverse reactions

    1) Bleeding

    2) Dyspepsia

    3) Uppper abdominal pain

    4) Diarrhea

  d. Contraindications

    1) Serious hypersensitivity (anaphylactoid reaction)

    2) Pathological bleeding

  e. Drug interactions

    1) Amiodarone increases renal clearance.

    2) Clopidogrel increases serious bleeding.

    3) Fibrinolytic therapy (alteplase) increases serious risk of bleeding.

    4) Heparin increases risk of severe bleeding.

    5) Ketoconazole increases renal clearance.

    6) NSAIDs increase risk of severe bleeding.

    7) Quinidine increases renal clearance.

    8) Rifamycin (rifampin) decreases efficacy of dabigatran.

    9) Verapamil increases renal clearance.

  f. Nursing interventions

    1) When converting from warfarin to dabigatran, stop warfarin and begin dabigatran when INR is below 2.

    2) Assess bleeding.

    3) Assess for GI upset, stomach pain, nausea, and heartburn.

    4) Swallow whole; do not break, chew, or empty capsule contents.

    5) Avoid surgical procedure or dental procedure without physician approval.

    6) Practice reliable contraception.

D. ANTIPLATELET DRUGS
  1. DESCRIPTION
  a. Suppress platelet aggregation
  b. Prevention of thrombosis in arteries
  c. Three major groups of antiplatelet drugs
    1) Aspirin
    2) ADP receptor antagonists
    3) GP IIb/IIIa receptor agonists
  2. ASPIRIN
  a. Description
    1) Prevention of arterial thrombosis
    2) Suppresses platelet aggregation
    3) Irreversible; therefore, effects persist for the life of the platelet (7–10 days)
  b. Uses
    1) Primary prophylaxis of MI
    2) Prevention of reinfarction in clients who have experienced an acute MI
    3) Prevention of stroke in clients with a history of TIAs
    4) Chronic stable angina
    5) Unstable angina
    6) Angioplasty and other revascularization procedures
  c. Adverse reactions
    1) Gastrointestinal effects: gastric distress, heartburn, and nausea; GI bleeding, ulceration, and perforation
    2) Bleeding
    3) Renal impairment
    4) Salicylism: characterized by tinnitus (ringing in the ears), sweating, headache and dizziness; begins to develop when aspirin levels climb just slightly above therapeutic
    5) Reye's syndrome
    6) Anemia in pregnant women (from GI blood loss) and postpartum hemorrhage
    7) Hypersensitivity reactions develop in 0.3% of aspirin users, most likely in adults who have asthma, hay fever, chronic urticaria, or nasal polyps.
  d. Contraindications and precautions
    1) Bleeding disorders such as hemophilia, vitamin K deficiency
    2) Children with chickenpox or influenza because of Reye's syndrome
  e. Drug interactions
    1) Aspirin: increases anticoagulant effects of warfarin
    2) Glucocorticoids: in combination, greatly increase the risk of gastric ulceration

    3) Alcohol: in combination, increases the risk for gastric bleeding
  f. Nursing interventions
    1) Instruct the client to discontinue the drug 1 week prior to elective surgery or anticipated date of delivery for pregnant women.
    2) Instruct the client to take with food, milk, or a glass of water to reduce gastric upset.
    3) Instruct the client not to crush or chew enteric-coated or sustained-release formulations.
    4) Instruct the client to discard aspirin preparations that smell of vinegar (decomposing aspirin smells of acetic acid).
    5) Clients with a recent history of peptic ulcer disease should avoid aspirin.
    6) Inform the client not to consume alcohol.
    7) Instruct the client to notify the physician if gastric irritation is severe or persistent.
    8) Avoid in a client with bleeding disorders.
    9) Administer a low dose in a client with renal impairment.
    10) Administer parenteral epinephrine to treat severe hypersensitivity reaction.
    11) Instruct the client about manifestations of salicylism.
    12) Discuss the risks to expectant mothers and infants against the benefits of therapy.
  3. ADP RECEPTOR BLOCKERS
  a. Description
    1) Oral antiplatelet that inhibits ADP-mediated aggregation
    2) Irreversible, so antiplatelet effects persist for the life of the platelet
  b. Uses
    1) Prevention of thrombotic stroke
    2) Prevention of thrombus formation in coronary artery stents after implantation
    3) Prevention of myocardial infarction
    4) Prevention of ischemic stroke
  c. Adverse reactions
    1) Neutropenia
    2) Agranulocytosis
    3) Thrombotic thrombocytopenia characterized by fever, anemia, renal dysfunction, and neurological disturbances—risk is lower with clopidogrel (Plavix)

4) Diarrhea, abdominal pain, flatulance, nausea, and dyspepsia
5) Rash, purpura, and pruritus

d. Contraindications and precautions
   1) Lactation
   2) Neutropenia
   3) Thrombocytopenia
   4) Active bleeding disorder such as with a peptic ulcer or intracranial hemorrhage

e. Drug interactions
   1) Heparin, warfarin, aspirin, and NSAIDs increase the risk of bleeding.

f. Nursing interventions
   1) Inform the client of the signs of TTP and to notify the physician if they occur.
   2) Perform a complete blood count and white cell differential every 2 weeks for the first 12 weeks of treatment or at any sign of an infection.
   3) Administer ticlopidine (Ticlid) with food.
   4) Administer clopidogrel (Plavix) without regard to food.
   5) Discontinue 7 days prior to elective surgery.
   6) Monitor for bleeding when taken with aspirin, heparin, NSAIDs, or warfarin.
   7) Avoid administering to a client with a bleeding disorder.

g. Types
   1) Ticlopidine (Ticlid)
   2) Clopidogrel (Plavix)

4. GLYCOPROTEIN IIB/IIIA RECEPTOR ANTAGONISTS
   a. Description
      1) Most effective antiplatelet drugs on the market
      2) Cause reversible blockade of platelet GP IIb/IIIa receptors and inhibit the final step in aggregation
   b. Uses
      1) Acute coronary syndrome: unstable angina and non-Q-wave MI
      2) Percutaneous coronary intervention (PCI): reduce the risk of rapid reocclusion following coronary artery revascularization with balloon or laser angioplasty, or atherectomy using an intra-arterial rotating blade. Reocclusion is common because PCI damages the arterial wall and encourages platelet aggregation.

c. Adverse reactions
   1) Bleeding
d. Contraindications and precautions
   1) Active bleeding
   2) Stroke
e. Drug interactions
   1) Aspirin, heparin, Coumadin, and NSAIDs: increase the risk of bleeding
f. Nursing interventions
   1) Inform the client that the antiplatelet effects persist for 24–48 hours after abciximab (ReoPro) and stopping an infusion.
   2) Inform the client that the antiplatelet effects persist for 4 hours after stopping an infusion of epitifibatide (Integrelin) and tirofiban (Aggrastat).
g. Types
   1) Abciximab (ReoPro)
   2) Eptifibatide (Integrelin)
   3) Tirofiban (Aggrastat)

E. OTHER ANTIPLATELET DRUGS
   1. DIPYRIDAMOLE (PERSANTINE)
   2. CILOSTAZOL (PLETAL)
F. THROMBOLYTIC DRUGS
   1. STREPTOKINASE (KABIKINASE, STREPTASE)
      a. Description
         1) First thrombolytic drug available
         2) First binds to plasminogen to form streptokinase-plasminogen complex, catalyzes the conversion of other plasminogen molecules into plasmin, an enzyme that digests the fibrin meshwork of clots
         3) Plasmin also degrades fibrinogen and other clotting factors, increasing the risk of hemorrhage.
      b. Uses
         1) Acute coronary thrombosis (acute MI)
         2) DVT
         3) Massive pulmonary emboli
      c. Adverse reactions
         1) Bleeding
         2) Intracranial hemorrhage (occurs in 1% of clients, the most serious concern)
         3) Antibody production: allergic reactions and neutralization of streptokinase (rendering the drug ineffective) due to the fact that it is a foreign protein extracted from cultures of streptococci
            a) If a repeat course of thrombolytic is needed, a different thrombolytic should be used.

4) Hypotension (unrelated to blood loss or allergic reaction, incidence is 1–10%)

5) Fever, temperature elevation of 1.5°F or more, develops in one-third of clients.

d. Contraindications and precautions

1) Clients at risk for bleeding

e. Drug interactions

1) Anticoagulants such as heparin or warfarin: increase the risk of severe bleeding

2) Antiplatelet drugs such as aspirin: increase the risk of severe bleeding

f. Nursing interventions

1) Manage oozing (bleeding) with pressure dressings.

2) Discontinue the drug for severe bleeding and:

a) Replace lost blood with whole blood or blood products (packed red blood cells, fresh frozen plasma).

b) Excessive fibrinolysis can be reversed with IV aminocaproic acid (Amicar), which prevents activation of plasminogen and directly inhibits plasmin.

3) Minimize physical manipulation of the client.

4) Avoid subcutaneous and IM injections.

5) Minimize invasive procedures.

6) Minimize concurrent use of anticoagulants such as heparin or warfarin.

7) Minimize concurrent use of antiplatelet drugs such as aspirin.

8) Obtain baseline values for blood pressure, heart rate, platelet counts, hematocrit, APTT, PT, and fibrinogen level.

9) Administration may be by IV infusion, slow IV injection, IV bolus, intracoronary infusion, or intracoronary bolus.

10) Do not administer heparin and streptokinase through the same IV line.

2. ALTEPLASE (tPA) (ACTIVASE)

a. Description

1) Also known as tissue plasminogen activator (tPA)

2) Produced commercially by recombinant DNA technology

3) Identical to naturally occurring human tPA, an enzyme that promotes conversion of

plasminogen to plasmin, an enzyme that digests the fibrin matrix of clots

b. Uses

1) Acute MI (slightly better than streptokinase for treating acute MI)

2) Pulmonary embolism

3) Ischemic stroke

c. Adverse reactions

1) Bleeding tendencies

2) Higher risk of intracranial hemorrhage than with streptokinase

d. Contraindications and precautions (See Streptokinase on page 438.)

e. Drug interactions (See Streptokinase on page 438.)

f. Nursing interventions (See Streptokinase on page 438.)

3. OTHER THROMBOLYTIC DRUGS

a. Types

1) Urokinase (Abbokinase)

2) Reteplase (Retavase)

XI. ANTILIPEMIC DRUGS

A. DESCRIPTION: LOW-DENSITY LIPOPROTEIN (LDL) CHOLESTEROL AND CORONARY ARTERY DISEASE (CAD)

1. RISK OF DEVELOPING CORONARY ARTERY DISEASE (CAD) DIRECTLY RELATED TO INCREASED LEVELS OF BLOOD CHOLESTEROL IN THE FORM OF LDLS

2. THE PRIMARY METHOD FOR LOWERING LDL CHOLESTEROL IS MODIFICATION OF DIET.

3. DRUGS SHOULD BE EMPLOYED ONLY IF DIET MODIFICATION AND AN EXERCISE PROGRAM FAIL TO REDUCE LDL CHOLESTEROL TO AN ACCEPTABLE LEVEL—AND THEN ONLY IF THE COMBINATION OF ELEVATED LDL CHOLESTEROL AND OTHER RISK FACTORS JUSTIFIES DRUG USE.

B. HMG COA REDUCTASE INHIBITORS ("STATINS")

1. DESCRIPTION

a. Most effective drugs for lowering LDL cholesterol (LDLs deliver cholesterol to peripheral tissue)

b. Because cholesterol synthesis normally increases during the night, statins are most effective when given in the evening.

c. If statins are withdrawn, serum cholesterol will return to pretreatment levels, so treatment must continue lifelong.

   d. Increase levels of high-density lipoprotein (HDL) cholesterol (HDLs carry cholesterol from peripheral tissues back to the liver)
   e. Promote plaque stability by decreasing plaque cholesterol content
   f. Reduce inflammation at the plaque site
   g. Improve abnormal endothelial function
   h. Enhance blood vessel dilation
   i. Reduce risk of thrombosis
2. THERAPEUTIC USES
   a. Prevent or retard CAD through lowering of LDL cholesterol, increasing HDL cholesterol, and lowering of very-low-density lipoproteins (VLDLs). The role of VLDLs (triglycerides) in CAD is unclear; the link between elevated levels of VLDLs and development of atherosclerosis is not firmly established.
3. ADVERSE REACTIONS
   a. Headache
   b. Rash
   c. GI disturbances (dyspepsia, cramps, flatulence, constipation, abdominal pain)
   d. Hepatotoxicity
   e. Myopathy
4. CONTRAINDICATIONS AND PRECAUTIONS
   a. Liver disease
   b. Alcohol
   c. Pregnancy
5. DRUG INTERACTIONS
   a. Inhibitors of CYP3A4 (itraconazole, ketoconazole, erythromycin, clarithromycin, HIV protease inhibitors, cyclosporine, nefazodone, and grapefruit juice): increase statin levels of atorvastatin, lovastatin, and simvastatin—most dramatically, lovastatin and simvastatin. When combined, caution should be exercised.
   b. Gemfibrozil or fenofibrate: increase the risk of statin-induced myopathy
6. NURSING INTERVENTIONS
   a. Liver function tests (LFTs) should be done before treatment and periodically thereafter.
   b. Instruct the client to notify the physician if unexplained muscle pain or tenderness is noted.
   c. Obtain baseline data values for total cholesterol, LDL cholesterol, HDL cholesterol, and triglycerides (VLDLs).

7. TYPES
   a. Atorvastatin (Lipitor)
   b. Fluvastatin (Lescol)
   c. Lovastatin (Mevacor)
   d. Pravastatin (Pravachol)
   e. Simvastatin (Zocor)
C. BILE-ACID-BINDING RESINS
   1. USES
      a. Reduce LDL cholesterol, usually combined with a statin
   2. ADVERSE REACTIONS
      a. Constipation
      b. Bloating, indigestion, nausea
      c. May decrease uptake of fat-soluble vitamins
   3. CONTRAINDICATIONS AND PRECAUTIONS
      a. Complete obstruction or atresia of the bile duct
   4. DRUG INTERACTIONS
      a. Thiazide diuretics: decrease effect of thiazide diuretics
      b. Digoxin: decrease effect of digoxin
      c. Lovastatin: effects may be cumulative
      d. Tetracycline: decrease effect of tetracycline
   4. NURSING INTERVENTIONS
      a. Encourage the client to increase dietary fiber and fluids to minimize constipation.
      b. Administer prescribed vitamin supplements.
      c. Administer oral drugs 1 hour before the resin or 4 hours after the resin.
      d. Mix with fluids or pulpy fruits such as applesauce before ingestion to reduce risk of impaction and esophageal irritation.
   5. TYPES
      a. Cholestyramine (Questran, Prevalite, LoCHOLEST)
      b. Colestipol (Colestid)
D. NICOTINIC ACID—NIACIN
   1. DESCRIPTION
      a. Vitamin B complex
      b. Adjunct therapy in a client with high serum triglycerides
   2. USES
      a. Reduces LDL and VLDL levels and increases HDL levels
   3. ADVERSE REACTIONS
      a. Skin: flushing, itching (intense flushing of the face, neck, and ears occurs in practically all clients)
      b. GI: gastric upset, nausea, vomiting, diarrhea
      c. Hepatotoxicity
      d. Can raise blood levels of homocysteine, a possible risk factor

in CAD (treatment with folic acid
can help lower homocysteine levels)

  e. Hyperglycemia

  f. Gouty arthritis

4. CONTRAINDICATIONS AND
  PRECAUTIONS

  a. Liver disease

  b. Diabetes mellitus

  c. Gout

5. DRUG INTERACTIONS

  a. HMG-CoA reductase inhibitors:
  increase risk of myopathy and
  rhabdomyolysis

6. NURSING INTERVENTIONS

  a. Administer aspirin 30 minutes
  before each dose to reduce the effect
  of intense flushing.

  b. Assess liver function before
  treatment and periodically
  thereafter.

E. FIBRIC ACID DERIVATIVES ("FIBRATES")

1. DESCRIPTION

  a. Most effective drugs available for
  lowering triglyceride levels

  b. Raise HDL cholesterol

  c. Little or no effect on LDL cholesterol

2. USES

  a. Reduce triglycerides

3. ADVERSE REACTIONS

  a. Cholelithiasis

  b. Myopathy

  c. Dizziness

  d. Anemia

  e. Urticaria

  f. Blurred vision

4. CONTRAINDICATIONS AND
  PRECAUTIONS

  a. Gallbladder disease

  b. Hepatic disease

  c. Renal disease

  d. Lactation

5. DRUG INTERACTIONS

  a. Anticoagulants: increase the
  anticoagulant effects

  b. Sulfonylureas: increase the
  hypoglycemic effect

6. NURSING INTERVENTIONS

  a. Instruct the client about the clinical
  manifestations of gallbladder disease
  and to notify the physician.

  b. Instruct the client to report clinical
  manifestations of muscle pain or
  weakness.

  c. Administer 30 minutes before meals.

  d. Use caution when driving or
  operating heavy equipment until
  effects of the drug are known.

  e. Instruct the client to report any
  manifestations of bruising or
  bleeding.

  f. Instruct the client to limit intake of
  alcohol.

7. TYPES

  a. Gemfibrozil (Lopid)

  b. Fenofibrate (Tricor)

F. EXETIMIBE (ZETIA)

1. DESCRIPTION

  a. Function at the border of the small
  intestine to inhibit the absorption
  of cholesterol, leading to a decrease
  in the delivery of cholesterol to the
  liver

  b. Compliments the action of HMG-
  CoA reductase inhibitors

  c. Reduces total cholesterol,
  LDL cholesterol, apo B, and
  triglycerides as well as HDL
  cholesterol

  d. Has no effect on fat-soluble vitamins

2. USES

  a. Primary hypercholesterolemia

  b. Uses with diet or HMG-CoA
  reductase inhibitors

3. ADVERSE REACTIONS

  a. Back pain

  b. Abdominal pain

  c. Diarrhea

  d. Arthralgia

  e. Sinusitis

  d. Coughing

4. CONTRAINDICATIONS

  a. Pregnancy

  b. Active liver disease

  c. Nursing women

  d. Children under the age of 10 years

5. DRUG INTERACTIONS

  a. Antacids decrease effectiveness.

  b. Cholestyramine decreases
  effectiveness.

  c. Cyclosporine increases AUC and
  C_{max}.

  d. Fenofibrate/Gemfibrozil increases
  total ezetimibe levels.

6. NURSING INTERVENTIONS

  a. Imolement cholesterol diet therapy
  before drug therapy

  b. May be given with a HMG-CoA
  reductase inhibitor

  c. Give at least 2 hours before or 4
  hours after bile sequestrant.

  d. Adhere to weight reduction

  e. Monitor CBC, lipid oanel, CK, renal,
  and LFTs.

PRACTICE QUESTIONS

1. Which of the following is the priority for the nurse to assess before administering digoxin (Lanoxin)?
   1. Auscultate the apical pulse for 1 full minute
   2. Palpate the radial pulse for 60 seconds
   3. Monitor the renal function tests
   4. Assess the serum potassium

2. Upon finding a client in cardiac arrest, the nurse should administer which of the following drugs first?
   1. Atropine
   2. Epinephrine
   3. Lidocaine
   4. Atenolol (Tenormin)

3. After medication teaching on atenolol (Tenormin), which of the following statements by a client with diabetes mellitus demonstrates an understanding of the atenolol?
   1. "It may cause hyperglycemia."
   2. "It may mask an early indication of hypoglycemia."
   3. "It may increase the action of insulin."
   4. "It may diminish the action of insulin."

4. The nurse is caring for a client with hypertension. Which of the following drugs should the nurse administer?
   1. Mexiletine (Mexitil)
   2. Triamterene and hydrochlorothiazide (Dyazide)
   3. Digoxin (Lanoxin)
   4. Warfarin

5. Based on an understanding of nitroglycerin, the nurse administers it for which of the following reasons to a client with angina?
   1. Increase afterload
   2. Increase preload
   3. Constrict the arteries
   4. Dilate the veins

6. The nurse is caring for a client with atrial fibrillation who is being treated with a variety of drugs. The nurse administers which of the following drugs in combination with quinidine that may result in an increased level of the drug?
   1. Furosemide (Lasix)
   2. Digoxin (Lanoxin)
   3. Propranolol (Inderal)
   4. Triamterene and hydrochlorothiazide (Dyazide)

7. The nurse should administer amiodarone (Cordarone) to treat which of the following arrhythmias?

   1. Sinus bradycardia
   2. Bundle branch block
   3. Ventricular tachycardia
   4. Junctional rhythm

8. Which of the following is the priority nursing intervention for a client who is receiving adenosine (Adenocard) for supraventricular tachycardia (SVT)?
   1. Document the presence of peripheral pulses
   2. Monitor the pulse oximetry
   3. Assure a patent IV in the antecubital vein
   4. Prepare for emergency defibrillation

9. A client has been taking Viagra and is now experiencing angina. The physician has prescribed nitroglycerin p.r.n. for the angina. Which of the following should the nurse include in the discharge instructions?
   1. Viagra should not be used within 24 hours of taking nitroglycerin
   2. Nitroglycerin and Viagra should be taken at the same time
   3. Viagra is not effective when used in combination with nitroglycerin
   4. The effect of nitroglycerin is impaired by concurrent use with Viagra

10. Which of the following adverse reactions should the nurse assess in a 70-year-old adult who is receiving a continuous infusion of lidocaine?
    1. Hypertension
    2. Osteoarthritis
    3. Confusion
    4. Decreased visual acuity

11. Based on an understanding of beta blockers used for unstable angina, the nurse administers a beta blocker because of which of the following actions?
    1. To increase myocardial contractility
    2. To decrease heart rate
    3. To promote cardiovascular fluid shift
    4. Coronary artery vasodilation

12. Which of the following interventions should the nurse include in the plan of care for a client taking an ACE inhibitor?
    1. Monitor the blood pressure closely for 2 hours after the first dose
    2. Begin with a high dose and gradually decrease the dose
    3. Administer potassium supplements to the client
    4. Begin with daily dosing followed by dosing every other day

13. The nurse selects from which of the following calcium-channel blockers to administer to a client with hypertension?
Select all that apply:
[ ] 1. Amlodipine (Norvasc)
[ ] 2. Enoxaparin (Lovenox)
[ ] 3. Dabigatran etexilate (Pradaxa)
[ ] 4. Verapamil (Calan)
[ ] 5. Diltiazem hydrochloride (Cardizem)
[ ] 6. Mexiletine (Mexitil)

14. A client's family member asks the nurse how to know if the client is improving while receiving furosemide (Lasix) for congestive heart failure. The nurse's response should be based on the understanding that improvement in the client's condition is characterized by
1. diminishing oxygen needs.
2. increased thirst.
3. weight gain.
4. intake greater than output.

15. A client with congestive heart disease returns to the clinic with muscle aching. The physician orders a potassium level, which shows hypokalemia. The drug regimen includes furosemide (Lasix) 80 mg b.i.d. In addition to treatment with a potassium supplement, the nurse administers which of the following prescribed drugs?
1. Bumetanide (Bumex)
2. Torsemide (Demadex)
3. Spironolactone (Aldactone)
4. Clonidine (Catapres)

16. While providing care to a client on cholestyramine (Questran), the nurse should monitor the client for which of the following?
Select all that apply:
[ ] 1. Urinary retention
[ ] 2. Abdominal pain
[ ] 3. Bradycardia
[ ] 4. Flatulence
[ ] 5. Constipation
[ ] 6. Confusion

17. The nurse is caring for a client on a heparin infusion when the client expresses concern over a progressively painful headache. Which of the following is the priority nursing action?
1. Stop the heparin infusion
2. Administer protamine
3. Notify the physician
4. Administer morphine

18. A client has been taking warfarin sodium (Coumadin) for the prevention of deep vein thrombosis. When the home care nurse arrives for a weekly visit, the client reports having been using aspirin (acetylsalicylic acid) daily for arthritic pain since hearing a commercial on television bolstering its benefits. Which of the following is the most appropriate response by the nurse, based on an understanding of the effect of combining Coumadin with aspirin?
1. "As long as you use aspirin only once a day, there will be no problems."
2. "Coumadin and aspirin used in combination increases the potential for bleeding."
3. "Aspirin and Coumadin may be used safely together."
4. "Coumadin may be used with aspirin without problem if vitamin K is taken with each dose."

19. The nurse is instructing a client on clopidogrel bisulfate (Plavix). Which of the following statements by the client indicates an understanding of the effect of this drug?
1. "I should ambulate slowly."
2. "I may experience hypotension."
3. "I should use caution taking other drugs that cause bleeding."
4. "I should take a stool softener while on this drug."

20. The nurse should monitor a client with an acute myocardial infarction who is receiving intravenous streptokinase (Streptase) for which of the following serious adverse reactions?
1. Intracranial hemorrhage
2. Intractable nausea
3. Extension of myocardial damage
4. Pulmonary embolus

21. The nurse is caring for a client taking atorvastatin (Lipitor). The client admits to consuming 6 to 12 beers daily. The nurse should monitor the client for what potentially serious adverse reaction to Lipitor?
1. Nephrotoxicity
2. Hypertension
3. Hepatotoxicity
4. Dyspepsia

22. The nurse is developing a medication schedule for a client receiving simvastatin (Zocor). To promote maximal effectiveness, the nurse should administer the drug
1. 30 minutes before a meal.
2. with meals.
3. at bedtime.
4. early in the morning.

23. The nurse assesses a client taking heparin for thrombocytopenia when the platelets drop below what level mm^3? _____

24. The nurse is caring for a client admitted with severe rectal bleeding who is receiving warfarin (Coumadin) therapy. Which of the following interventions should have priority in the plan of care?
1. Accurate intake and output

2. Discontinue the warfarin
3. Assure a patent 18-gauge IV
4. Administer vitamin K

25. The registered nurse is preparing to delegate assignments for the day. Which of the following assignments would be appropriate to delegate to a licensed practical nurse?
1. Contact a client's physician when the blood pressure is lower than 100 mm Hg

before administering a beta$_2$-adrenergic blocker
2. Monitor the heparin level daily before administering heparin
3. Question administration of streptokinase (Streptase) to a client admitted and suspected of an intracranial hemorrhage
4. Take the blood pressure before administering a dose of verapamil (Calan)

ANSWERS AND RATIONALES

1. 1. A long-standing hallmark in the nursing interventions of the plan of care for a client taking digoxin (Lanoxin) is to take the apical pulse for a full minute. This is the priority nursing action. Bradycardia, in which the pulse is less than 60 beats per minute for 1 full minute, is one potential sign of digoxin toxicity. Although monitoring the renal function tests and serum potassium are appropriate interventions in the plan of care for a client taking Lanoxin, they are not the priority.

2. 2. Epinephrine is the initial drug administered for cardiac arrest using the advanced cardiac life support (ACLS) algorithm. Atropine is used to restore cardiac rate in a client experiencing symptomatic sinus bradycardia. Lidocaine is used in the treatment of arrhythmias. Atenolol (Tenormin) is a beta-adrenergic blocking drug used for hypertension.

3. 2. Beta blockers, such as atenolol (Tenormin), depress the heart rate and prevent tachycardia, one of the early indications of hypoglycemia.

4. 2. Dyazide contains a combination of potassium-sparing diuretic and thiazide diuretic, triamterene and hydrochlorothiazide, to induce antihypertension by diminishing blood volume. Mexiletine (Mexitil) is an antiarrhythmic used in the treatment of ventricular arrhythmias. Digoxin (Lanoxin) is a cardiac glycoside used in the treatment of congestive heart failure and to slow the heart rate in a client with sinus tachycardia. Warfarin (Coumadin) is an anticoagulant.

5. 4. Nitroglycerin is a coronary vasodilator used in the treatment of angina. The venodilation decreases preload by decreasing blood return to the heart. Decreased preload diminishes the work of the heart, which reduces the oxygen needs and diminishes the anginal pain.

6. 2. Quinidine is an antiarrhythmic used in combination with digoxin and may potentially double digoxin levels. Furosemide (Lasix) is a loop diuretic. Digoxin (Lanoxin) is a cardiac glycoside used to control the rapid ventricular

contraction rate in atrial fibrillation or atrial flutter, slow the heart rate in sinus tachycardia, and in the treatment of recurrent paroxysmal atrial tachycardia with paroxysmal AV junctional rhythm. Propranolol (Inderal) is a beta-adrenergic blocking drug used in the treatment of hypertension. Triamterene and hydrochlorothiazide (Dyazide) is a combination antihypertensive drug.

7. 3. Amiodarone (Cordarone) is an antiarrhythmic that prolongs the duration of the action potential and refractory period, thus preventing life-threatening ventricular arrhythmias such as ventricular tachycardia by decreasing the sinus rate. Sinus bradycardia, bundle branch block, and junctional rhythm are all arrhythmias in which there is a slow heart rate.

8. 3. Adenosine (Adenocard) is an antiarrhythmic that must be given in a large vessel, closest to the heart, due to its extremely short half-life. Documenting the presence of peripheral pulses, monitoring the pulse oximetry, and preparing for emergency defibrillation are all appropriate interventions, but the drug cannot be administered without IV access, so this is the priority.

9. 1. When used in combination, Viagra and nitroglycerin may cause life-threatening hypotension. The manufacturer's recommendations state that Viagra should not be used within 24 hours of taking nitroglycerin.

10. 3. Lidocaine is an antiarrhythmic used in the treatment of ventricular arrhythmias. Confusion is a potential adverse reaction of a lidocaine infusion and is more common in the older adult.

11. 2. Beta blockers decrease the heart rate, diminishing the work of the heart and the oxygen needs, which results in a decrease in the anginal pain.

12. 1. ACE inhibitors used in the treatment of hypertension have a high potential for "first dose" hypotension, necessitating precautionary blood pressure monitoring.

13. 1. 5. 6. Amlodipine (Norvasc), diltiazem hydrochloride (Cardizem), and verapamil (Calan) are all calcium-channel blockers. Enoxaparin (Lovenox) is a low-molecular-weight heparin. Dabigatran etexilate (Pradaxa) is an oral anticoagulant. Mexiletine (Mexitil) is a Class B antidysrhythmic.

14. 1. With congestive heart failure (CHF), fluid accumulates in the lung tissue due to ineffective pump action by the heart. As a diuretic, furosemide (Lasix) works to remove excess bodily fluids via the kidneys. The fluid shifts out of the lung tissue and therefore diminishes oxygen needs.

15. 3. Spironolactone (Aldactone) is a potassium-sparing diuretic. Its diuretic action is scant and it works to retain potassium. It is very often used in combination with the more powerful loop diuretics, such as furosemide (Lasix), to counteract their potassium-wasting effects. Bumetanide (Bumex) and torsemide (Demadex) are loop diuretics, which deplete the body of potassium. Clonidine (Catapres) is an antihypertensive.

16. 2. 4. 5. Cholestyramine (Questran) is an antihyperlipidemic. It absorbs and combines with intestinal bile acids, forming an insoluble, nonabsorbable complex that is excreted in the feces. Adverse reactions include abdominal pain, flatulence, and constipation.

17. 3. The priority nursing action is to notify the physician. Headache, although rare, is an adverse reaction to a heparin hypersensitivity. The nurse may anticipate stopping the heparin infusion or administering protamine sulfate, a heparin antagonist, but the priority intervention is to notify the physician of a potential hypersensitivity.

18. 2. Aspirin inhibits platelet aggregation, diminishing the potential for clot formation. Warfarin (Coumadin) is an anticoagulant that interferes with blood clot formation by interfering with the synthesis of vitamin K clotting factors, resulting in depletion of the clotting factors. The combination of Coumadin and aspirin increases the potential for bleeding.

19. 3. Clopidogrel bisulfate (Plavix) is an antiplatelet drug that inhibits platelet aggregation, diminishing the potential for clot formation. Caution should be used when taking other drugs that may increase bleeding. Plavix may cause the adverse reactions of hypertension and diarrhea.

20. 1. Streptokinase (Streptase) is a thrombolytic enzyme used in the treatment of deep vein thrombosis, arterial thrombosis, acute evolving myocardial infarction, and pulmonary embolism, and to clear an occluded arteriovenous and IV cannula. It is a priority that the client is monitored for an intracranial hemorrhage that could potentially lead to coma and death.

21. 3. Atorvastatin (Lipitor) is an antihyperlipidemic and HMG-CoA reduction inhibitor. The risk for hepatotoxicity while using Lipitor is increased by excessive alcohol ingestion.

22. 3. Simvastatin (Zocor) is an antihyperlipidemic. Because cholesterol synthesis normally increases during the night, statins such as Zocor are most effective when given in the evening.

23. 100,000. Heparin-induced thrombocytopenia is a state characterized by increased thrombosis despite a reduction in circulating platelets less than $100,000/mm^3$.

24. 3. Although maintaining an accurate intake and output, discontinuing the Coumadin, and administering vitamin K may be anticipated, the priority intervention is to assure an 18-gauge IV needed for potential transfusion of blood, if bleeding causes hypovolemia and low hemoglobin.

25. 4. Contacting a client's physician, monitoring the heparin level, and questioning the administration of a drug are all nursing tasks that should be performed by a registered nurse. A licensed practical nurse (LPN) may take a blood pressure before administering a drug. LPNs are trained to take the blood pressure; if the blood pressure is too low or too high, it becomes the responsibility of the registered nurse to notify the physician.

REFERENCES

Broyles, B., Reiss, B., & Evans, M. (2012). *Pharmacological aspects of nursing care* (8th ed.). Clifton Park, NY: Delmar Cengage Learning.

Daniels, R., & Nicoll, L. (2012). *Contemporary medical-surgical nursing.* Clifton Park, NY: Delmar Cengage Learning.

Spratto, G. R., & Woods, A. L. (2012). *PDR nurse's drug handbook 2012.* Clifton Park, NY: Delmar Cengage Learning.

CHAPTER 20

DRUGS FOR THE GASTROINTESTINAL SYSTEM

I. **DRUGS FOR GASTROESOPHAGEAL REFLUX DISEASE (GERD)**

A. DESCRIPTION

  1. DRUGS THAT PROMOTE HEALING OF TISSUES AND PAIN REDUCTION BY DECREASING THE AMOUNT OF ACID BEING REGURGITATED INTO THE ESOPHAGUS (ANTISECRETORY)

  2. RELIEVE CLINICAL MANIFESTATIONS OF GERD—PYROSIS (HEARTBURN) AND DYSPEPSIA

  3. USED FOR GERD AND PEPTIC ULCER DISEASE

B. HISTAMINE 2-RECEPTOR ANTAGONISTS

  1. USES

    a. Suppress gastric acid secretion and pepsin production

    b. Selectively block histamine 2-receptor sites located on parietal cells

    c. Prevent gastrin from causing release of histamine and stimulation of hydrochloric acid production

    d. Decrease pepsin production from chief cells

  2. ADVERSE REACTIONS

    a. Rare, primarily cimetidine (Tagamet)

    b. Gastrointestinal (GI): diarrhea or constipation, nausea, vomiting

    c. Central nervous system (CNS): headache, confusion, hallucinations, lethargy, somnolence, or restlessness

    d. Cardiovascular (CV): dysrhythmias and hypotension with IV use

    e. Endocrine: gynecomastia, reduced libido, impotence

  3. CONTRAINDICATIONS AND PRECAUTIONS

    a. Known drug allergies to any histamine 2-receptor antagonists

    b. Impaired hepatic or renal function

    c. Pregnancy

    d. Lactation

  4. DRUG INTERACTIONS SPECIFICALLY FOR CIMETIDINE (TAGAMET)

    a. Benzodiazepine: increases effect of benzodiazepine

    b. Carbamazepine (Tegretol): increases effect of carbamazepine

    c. Lidocaine: increases effect of lidocaine

    d. Phenytoin: increases effect of phenytoin

    e. Theophylline: increases effect of theophylline

    f. Propranolol: increases effect of propranolol

    g. Warfarin (Coumadin): increases anticoagulant effects

    h. Antacids: decrease effect of cimetidine

    i. Calcium-channel blockers: increase effect of calcium-channel blockers

    j. Tricyclic antidepressants: increase effect of tricyclic antidepressants

  5. NURSING INTERVENTIONS

    a. Assess for history of drug allergies to histamine 2-receptor antagonists.

    b. Monitor liver and kidney function.

    c. Assess the client for headache, which may be a minor adverse reaction.

    d. Assess for drug interactions with cimetidine (Tagamet), other histamine 2-receptor antagonists; have no known drug interactions except antacids.

    e. Administer before meals and at bedtime.

  6. TYPES

    a. Cimetidine (Tagamet)

    b. Famotidine (Pepcid)

    c. Nizatidine (Axid)

    d. Ranitidine (Zantac)

C. PROTON PUMP INHIBITORS

  1. USES

    a. Suppress gastric acid secretion by inhibiting enzymes in the parietal cells

   b. Inhibit the hydrogen and potassium ATPase enzyme (proton pump)
   c. Primarily used for GERD and peptic ulcer disease
 2. ADVERSE REACTIONS
   a. GI: diarrhea, nausea, vomiting
   b. CNS: dizziness, headache
 3. CONTRAINDICATIONS AND PRECAUTIONS
   a. Known drug allergies to any proton pump inhibitor
   b. Pregnancy
   c. Lactation
   d. Impaired hepatic or renal function
 4. DRUG INTERACTIONS
   a. Warfarin (Coumadin): prolonged rate of warfarin elimination
   b. Phenytoin (Dilantin): increases effect of phenytoin
   c. Diazepam (Valium): increases effect of diazepam
 5. NURSING INTERVENTIONS
   a. Assess for history of drug allergies to proton pump inhibitors.
   b. Administer before meals.
   c. Avoid crushing.
   d. Monitor liver, kidney, and urinary function.
   e. Assess for adverse reactions.
 6. TYPES
   a. Omeprazole (Prilosec)
   b. Lansoprazole (Prevacid)
   c. Esomeprazole (Nexium)
   d. Pantoprazole (Protonix)
   e. Rabeprazole (Aciphex)
D. ANTACIDS
 1. DESCRIPTION
   a. Alkaline compounds that neutralize acids of the stomach
   b. May cause acid rebound with use over time
 2. USES
   a. Decrease destruction and enhance protection of the mucosal lining
   b. Acid neutralization above pH of 5 also decreases pepsin production.
   c. Choice of antacid depends on adverse effects and medical condition.
   d. Primarily used for GERD and peptic ulcer disease
 3. ADVERSE REACTIONS
   a. Sodium based: use cautiously with cardiac or renal dysfunction, severe electrolyte imbalances
   b. Calcium based: calcium imbalances, constipation
   c. Magnesium salts: neurological damage, diarrhea
   d. Aluminum salts: calcium and phosphorus imbalances, constipation

   e. Magnesium and aluminum combinations: may block adverse GI effects and electrolyte imbalances
 4. CONTRAINDICATIONS AND PRECAUTIONS
   a. Known drug allergies to any antacid
   b. Any condition affected by electrolyte and acid-base imbalances
   c. Impaired renal function
   d. Appendicitis
 5. DRUG INTERACTIONS
   a. Antacids will greatly affect absorption of other drugs.
   b. Must not be taken with other drugs
 6. NURSING INTERVENTIONS
   a. Administer antacid 1 hour before and 2 hours after other drugs.
   b. Administer 1 hour before and 3 hours after meals and at bedtime.
   c. Instruct the client to chew tablets and follow with glass of water or milk.
   d. Shake liquid suspensions well.
   e. Assess the client for electrolyte and acid-base imbalances.
   f. Avoid alcohol and other CNS depressants.
   g. Report CNS effects.
 7. TYPES (SEE TABLE 20-1)
E. PROKINETICS (CHOLINERGICS)
 1. USES
   a. Stimulate parasympathetic activity, mimicking effects of acetylcholine
   b. Increase rate of gastric emptying and motility, thus decreasing reflux symptoms
   c. Increase the resting tone of the esophageal sphincter and upper GI contractions
   d. Used for delayed gastric motility

Table 20-1 Common Antacids

Compound	Name	Bowel Effects
Sodium bicarbonate	Baking soda	Constipation
Calcium carbonate	Tums	Constipation
Aluminum hydroxide	Amphojel, ALternaGEL	Constipation
Aluminum carbonate	Basaljel	Constipation
Magnesium hydroxide	Milk of Magnesia (MOM)	Diarrhea
Magnesium and aluminum	Maalox, Mylanta, Gelusil, Di-Gel	Diarrhea
Magaldrate	Riopan	Diarrhea or constipation

© Cengage Learning 2015

2. ADVERSE REACTIONS
   a. GI: diarrhea, nausea, vomiting, cramping
   b. CNS: mild sedation, fatigue, restlessness, extrapyramidal manifestations, flushing, sweating
   c. GU: urgency
   d. CV: bradycardia, hypotension, cardiac arrhythmias
   e. Eyes, ears, nose, and throat (EENT): pupillary constriction
3. CONTRAINDICATIONS AND PRECAUTIONS
   a. Pregnancy
   b. Lactation
   c. Gastrointestinal hemorrhage
   d. Drugs such as phenothiazines are likely to cause extrapyramidal manifestations.
4. DRUG INTERACTIONS
   a. Alcohol and other CNS depressants: addictive sedative effect
   b. Acetaminophen: increases acetaminophen absorption
   c. Levodopa: decreases metoclopramide on gastric emptying
   d. Narcotic analgesics: decrease effect of metoclopramide
5. NURSING INTERVENTIONS
   a. Administer before meals and at bedtime.
   b. Assess for history of drug allergies to metoclorapramide.
   c. Instruct the client to avoid alcohol and other CNS depressants.
   d. Instruct the client to avoid driving until the effects of the drug are known.
   e. Report extrapyramidal manifestations such as trembling of the hands and grimacing.
   f. Assess bowel sounds to ensure motility.
6. TYPES
   a. Metoclopramide (Reglan)

II. DRUGS FOR PEPTIC ULCER DISEASE (PUD)
A. DESCRIPTION
   1. OVERALL GOALS INCLUDE ALLEVIATING CLINICAL MANIFESTATIONS, PROMOTING HEALING, PREVENTING COMPLICATION, AND RECURRENCES.
   2. PROMOTE HEALING OF ULCERS IN THE STOMACH, SMALL INTESTINE (DUODENUM), AND ESOPHAGUS AND REDUCE PAIN BY REDUCING ACID PRODUCTION
   3. IMPROVE MUCOSA AND PROTECT ERODED ULCERATIVE SITES AND LINING OF THE GI TRACT
   4. SOME ERADICATE A CAUSATIVE AGENT, *HELICOBACTER PYLORI* INFECTION.

B. ANTISECRETORY AGENTS HISTAMINE 2-RECEPTOR ANTAGONISTS AND PROTON PUMP INHIBITORS (SEE PAGES 445–446)
C. ANTACIDS (SEE PAGE 446)
D. ANTIPEPTIC AND CYTOPROTECTIVE—SUCRALFATE (CARAFATE)
   1. USES
      a. Protects eroded ulcer sites to prevent further acidic damage
      b. Forms a paste-like substance over damaged mucosa
      c. Used for acute treatment and maintenance
   2. ADVERSE REACTIONS
      a. Nausea
      b. Constipation
      c. Diarrhea
   3. CONTRAINDICATIONS AND PRECAUTIONS
      a. Pregnancy
      b. Lactation
   4. DRUG INTERACTIONS
      a. Quinolones: decrease quinolone bioavailability
      b. Phenytoin (Dilantin): decreases phenytoin absorption
      c. Digoxin (Lanoxin): decreases digoxin absorption
      d. Theophylline: decreases theophylline absorption
      e. Warfarin (Coumadin): decreases warfarin hypothrombinemic effect
   5. NURSING INTERVENTIONS
      a. Give 30 minutes before or after antacid.
      b. Encourage the client to increase fluids, exercise, and dietary bulk for constipation.
      c. Administer four times a day—1 hour before meals and at bedtime.
      d. Instruct the client to avoid alcohol.
E. PROSTAGLANDIN/CYTOPROTECTIVE—MISOPROSTOL (CYTOTEC)
   1. USES
      a. Protects the lining of the stomach to prevent further acidic damage
      b. Prostaglandin inhibits gastric acid secretion, increasing bicarbonate and mucus production.
      c. For prevention of ulcers caused by nonsteroidal anti-inflammatory drug (NSAID) use
   2. ADVERSE REACTIONS
      a. GI: diarrhea, abdominal pain, nausea
      b. Genitourinary (GU): excessive bleeding, miscarriages, and other menstrual problems
   3. CONTRAINDICATIONS AND PRECAUTIONS
      a. Pregnancy (causes abortion)
      b. Lactation
      c. Known allergy to prostaglandins

4. DRUG INTERACTIONS
   a. Magnesium-based antacids: increase diarrhea
5. NURSING INTERVENTIONS
   a. Administer at meals and bedtime.
   b. Instruct the client to ensure protection against pregnancy; will induce contractions.

F. ANTIBIOTICS WITH BISMUTH SALICYLATES OR ANTISECRETORY AGENTS, OR BOTH
   1. USES
      a. Prevent further ulcerative damage caused by *H. pylori*
      b. Used as a combination of different anti-infectives with or without an antisecretory agent (proton pump inhibitors or histamine H_2 antagonists)
      c. Provides anti-infective and antiulcer effects
      d. Bismuth subsalicylate (Pepto-Bismol) acts as an anti-infective, disrupting bacterial cell wall function causing cell death, and provides an antisecretory effect on gastrointestinal secretions and antidiarrheal effect.
   2. ADVERSE REACTIONS
      a. See specific anti-infective agents, particularly tetracycline.
      b. Bismuth: temporary darkening of stool and tongue
      c. See particular antisecretory agents.
   3. CONTRAINDICATIONS AND PRECAUTIONS
      a. Pregnancy
      b. Lactation
      c. Use of aspirin or other salicylates
   4. DRUG INTERACTIONS
      a. Tetracyclines: may decrease absorption
      b. See specific anti-infective agent.
      c. See specific antisecretory agent.
   5. NURSING INTERVENTIONS
      a. Monitor *H. pylori* breath test results.
      b. Assess stools and tongue for discoloration from bismuth.
      c. Assess over-the-counter use of many drugs that contain salicylates.
      d. Administer with full glass of water.
   6. TYPES (SEE TABLE 20-2)

G. ANTICHOLINERGICS/ PARASYMPATHOLYTICS (USED RARELY)
   1. USES
      a. Decrease motility and acid production caused by parasympathetic activity
      b. Block the effect of acetylcholine

Table 20-2 Two 14-Day Anti-Infective Combination Therapies for Treatment of PUD with Confirmed Infection by *H. pylori*

Therapy 1	Therapy 2
Triple Antibiotic with Antisecretory Agent (Proton Pump Inhibitor), Metronidazole (Flagyl), Tetracycline (Achromycin), Bismuth subsalicylate (Pepto-Bismol), Lansoprazole (Prevacid)	Triple Antibiotic with Antisecretory Agent (Histamine H_2-Receptor Antagonist), Metronidazole (Flagyl), Tetracycline (Achromycin), Bismuth subsalicylate (Pepto-Bismol), Famotidine (Pepcid)
Double Antibiotic with Antisecretory Agent (Proton Pump Inhibitor), Clarithromycin (Biaxin), Amoxicillin (Amoxil), Omeprazole (Prilosec)	Double Antibiotic with Antisecretory Agent (Histamine H_2-Receptor Antagonist), Clarithromycin (Biaxin), Amoxicillin (Amoxil), Ranitidine (Zantac)

© Cengage Learning 2015

2. ADVERSE REACTIONS
   a. GI: constipation, dry mouth, difficulty swallowing, paralytic ileus
   b. CNS: decreased sweating, mood changes, agitation, confusion
   c. CV: increased heart rate, flushing, palpitations
   d. GU: urinary retention
   e. EENT: blurred vision, light sensitivity, pupillary dilation
   f. Skin: rash, fever, heat intolerance
3. CONTRAINDICATIONS AND PRECAUTIONS
   a. Pregnancy
   b. Lactation
   c. Any medical condition that would be exacerbated by drug effect
   d. Known allergy to these drugs
   e. Impaired liver or kidney function
   f. Older adult clients
4. DRUG INTERACTIONS
   a. Antihistamines: increase antihistamine effect
5. NURSING INTERVENTIONS
   a. Instruct the client to avoid over-the-counter drugs.
   b. Instruct the client to use dark glasses with photophobia.
   c. Instruct the client to take lozenges for dry mouth and provide for adequate hydration.
   d. Instruct the client to include fluids and fiber to prevent constipation.
   e. Monitor for adverse reactions.
6. TYPES
   a. Propantheline (Pro-Banthine)
   b. Pirenzepine (Gastrozepine): causes fewer anticholinergic side effects

III. DRUGS FOR CONSTIPATION
A. DESCRIPTION
1. LAXATIVES ARE USED ONLY AFTER THE CLIENT DOES NOT ADEQUATELY RESPOND TO OTHER NONPHARMACOLOGIC INTERVENTIONS SUCH AS A HIGH-FIBER DIET AND INCREASED FLUIDS.
2. PREVENT CATHARTIC ABUSE AND DEPENDENCE.
3. MONITOR BOWEL MOVEMENTS AND PROVIDE ONGOING ABDOMINAL ASSESSMENT.
4. MILD LAXATIVES ARE GENERALLY ATTEMPTED BEFORE STRONGER LAXATIVE USE.
5. LAXATIVES MAY BE REQUIRED FOR DIAGNOSTIC EXAMINATIONS BEFORE OR AFTER THE PROCEDURE.
6. LAXATIVES ARE GENERALLY CONTRAINDICATED WITH INFLAMMATORY BOWEL CONDITIONS.
7. USUALLY GIVEN IN TABLET, LIQUID, SUPPOSITORY, OR ENEMA FORM
B. STOOL SOFTENERS OR SURFACTANT LAXATIVES
1. USES
a. Mildest form of cathartic
b. Detergent action lowers surface tension, allowing water and fats to enter and soften stool.
c. Used especially for clients who should avoid straining
2. ADVERSE EFFECTS
a. GI: diarrhea and mild cramps
3. CONTRAINDICATIONS AND PRECAUTIONS
a. Known gastrointestinal disorders
b. Renal dysfunction
4. DRUG INTERACTIONS
a. Avoid concomitant use of mineral oil—increase absorption of mineral oil from the GI tract.
5. NURSING INTERVENTIONS
a. Administer with a full glass of water.
b. Treat underlying causes.
6. TYPES
a. Docusate sodium (Colace)
b. Docusate calcium (Surfak)
c. Docusate with casanthranol (Peri-Colace) is a stool softener combined with a stimulant.
C. BULK LAXATIVES
1. USES
a. Promote peristalsis and natural evacuation
b. Stool increases in mass with the addition of fiber to promote evacuation.
2. ADVERSE REACTIONS
a. GI: diarrhea
3. CONTRAINDICATIONS AND PRECAUTIONS
a. Presence of other gastrointestinal manifestations
b. Known gastrointestinal disorders such as obstruction
c. Pregnancy
d. Lactation
4. DRUG INTERACTIONS
a. Digoxin (Lanoxin): decrease absorption of digitalis
b. Warfarin (Coumadin): increase risk of bleeding
c. Anti-infective: increase incidence of diarrhea
5. NURSING INTERVENTIONS
a. Mix with full 8 ounces of fluid and administer immediately.
b. Follow with full glass of water after administration.
c. Monitor for fecal impaction.
6. TYPES
a. Psyllium (Metamucil)
b. Methylcellulose (Citrucel)
c. Calcium polycarbophil (FiberCon)
D. STIMULANT LAXATIVES
1. USES
a. Stimulate movement of feces through the intestine
b. Direct chemical irritation of sensory nerve endings in the intestinal wall
2. ADVERSE EFFECTS
a. GI: diarrhea, abdominal cramps, nausea
b. Electrolyte imbalances such as potassium
3. CONTRAINDICATIONS AND PRECAUTIONS
a. Presence of other gastrointestinal manifestations
b. Known gastrointestinal disorders
c. Congestive heart failure (CHF)
d. Long-term use (results in loss of bowel tone)
e. Pregnancy
f. Lactation
4. DRUG INTERACTIONS
a. Warfarin (Coumadin): increases risk of bleeding
5. NURSING INTERVENTIONS
a. Administer with full glass of water on an empty stomach.
b. Avoid crushing or chewing tablets.
c. Avoid administering within 1 hour of antacids, cimetidine (Tagamet), milk, or other drugs.
d. Assess for laxative dependency.

6. TYPES
   a. Cascara sagrada, casanthrol (Cascara)
   b. Bisacodyl (Dulcolax, Fleets)
   c. Senna (Senokot)
   d. Castor oil
   e. Golytely liquid

E. LUBRICANT LAXATIVES
   1. USES
      a. Aid passage of stool through the intestine
      b. Lubricate stool and reduce water absorption
   2. ADVERSE REACTIONS
      a. GI: anorexia, nausea, vomiting
      b. Skin: rash
      c. Respiratory: with aspiration—lipid pneumonia
   3. CONTRAINDICATIONS AND PRECAUTIONS
      a. Presence of other gastrointestinal manifestations
      b. Known gastrointestinal disorders
      c. Oral administration to dysphagic older adult clients
      d. Lactation
      e. Pregnancy
   4. DRUG INTERACTIONS
      a. Warfarin (Coumadin): increases risk of bleeding
   5. NURSING INTERVENTIONS
      a. Instruct the client that prolonged use can interfere with absorption of fat-soluble vitamins (A, D, E, K) and electrolytes.
      b. Follow a retention enema with a cleansing enema.
   6. TYPES
      a. Liquid petroleum (mineral oil)

F. HYPEROSMOTIC LAXATIVES
   1. DESCRIPTION
      a. Synthetic disaccharide that contains the monosaccharides galactose and fructose
      b. Digestion and absorption do not occur in the stomach or small intestine.
      c. Compound reaches the colon unchanged.
      d. Digested in the colon by bacteria, resulting in acidic compounds
      e. Formation of acids expels ammonia from the body.
   2. USES
      a. Increases water content to stool
      b. Chronic constipation
      c. Portal systemic encephalopathy
   3. ADVERSE REACTIONS
      a. GI: diarrhea, abdominal cramping, nausea, vomiting
      b. Metabolic: hyperglycemia, dehydration, and hyperosmolar nonketotic coma, hypernatremia

   c. CNS: headache, dizziness
   d. CV: irregular heartbeat
   4. CONTRAINDICATIONS AND PRECAUTIONS
      a. Presence of other gastrointestinal manifestations
      b. Known gastrointestinal, cardiac, renal, hepatic, diabetic disorders
      c. Pregnancy
      d. Lactation
   5. DRUG INTERACTIONS
      a. Laxatives: increase incidence of adverse reactions
   6. NURSING INTERVENTIONS
      a. Administer with fruit juice, water, or milk to increase palatability.
      b. Encourage fluid intake.
      c. Monitor for hyperglycemia.
   7. TYPES
      a. Glycerin (Glycerol)
      b. Lactulose (Cephulac)

G. SALINE OR OSMOTIC LAXATIVES
   1. USES
      a. Cause mechanical stimulation of peristaltic activity
      b. Osmotic retention of fluid in the colon distends the colon.
   2. ADVERSE REACTIONS
      a. GI: diarrhea
      b. Electrolyte imbalance with prolonged use
   3. CONTRAINDICATIONS AND PRECAUTIONS
      a. Presence of other gastrointestinal manifestations
      b. Known gastrointestinal disorders
      c. Pregnancy
      d. Renal insufficiency
   4. DRUG INTERACTIONS
      a. Digoxin (Lanoxin): decreases absorption of digitalis
      b. Tetracyclines: decrease effect of tetracycline
   5. NURSING INTERVENTIONS
      a. Shake the bottle to ensure that suspension is mixed (milk of magnesia).
      b. Follow with full glass of water after administration.
      c. Administer at bedtime or in the morning on an empty stomach.
      d. Chill the solution and give on an empty stomach and at a time to avoid interference with sleep (citrate of magnesia).
      e. Citrate of magnesia is used for bowel prep but not routinely for constipation.
   6. TYPES
      a. Magnesium hydroxide (Milk of Magnesia [MOM])
      b. Magnesium citrate (Citrate of Magnesia)

H. LUBIPROSTONE (AMITIZA)
1. DESCRIPTION
   a. Locally acting calcium-channel blocker activator that enhances a chloride-rich intestinal fluid secretion without changing sodium and potassium serum levels
   b. Through increasing intestinal fluid secretion, lubiprotone increases intestinal motility.
   c. The main site of action appears to be the luminal portion of the GI epithelium.
2. USES
   a. Chronic idiopatheic constipation
   b. Irritable bowel syndrome
3. ADVERSE REACTIONS
   a. Fatigue
   b. Dizziness
   c. Headache
   d. Diarrhea
   e. Flatulence
   f. Nausea
   g. Vomiting
4. CONTRAINDICATIONS AND PRECAUTIONS
   a. History of mechanical GI obstruction
   b Severe diarrhea
5. NURSING INTERVENTIONS
   a. Monitor bowel sounds.
   b. Inform client to take with food and water to reduce incidence of nausea.
   c. May cause dizziness
   d. Review importance of diet, increased fluid intake and regular daily exercise.

IV. **DRUGS FOR DIARRHEA**
A. DESCRIPTION
1. FOR SYMPTOMATIC MANAGEMENT OF DIARRHEA BY BLOCKING STIMULATION OF THE GI TRACT AND REDUCING GI MOTILITY
2. IF ACUTE CLINICAL MANIFESTATIONS ARE NOT RELIEVED IN 2 DAYS, DISCONTINUE USE AND SEEK MEDICAL ATTENTION FOR UNDERLYING CONDITION.
3. IMPLEMENT MEASURES TO ENSURE CLIENT SAFETY AND COMFORT, ESPECIALLY FOR CHRONIC DIARRHEA.
4. ADMINISTER CAREFULLY SO AS NOT TO EXCEED RECOMMENDED DOSING.
B. ANTIDIARRHEALS
1. USES
   a. Inhibit peristaltic activity by direct action on intestinal muscles (loperamide [Imodium])
   b. Kaolin has adsorbent effect; pectin helps consolidate stool (Kaopectate).
   c. Inhibit receptors responsible for peristalsis (diphenoxylate [Lomotil] and paregoric)
   d. Direct antimicrobial and antisecretory effect (bismuth)

2. ADVERSE REACTIONS
   a. GI: nausea, vomiting, anorexia, abdominal cramping, diarrhea, mild cramps, toxic megacolon
   b. CNS: headache, dizziness, drowsiness
   c. Skin: pruritus, rash
3. CONTRAINDICATIONS AND PRECAUTIONS
   a. Known gastrointestinal disorders and delayed gastric motility
   b. Pregnancy
   c. Lactation
   d. Hepatic and renal dysfunction
   e. Diarrhea caused by anti-infectives or microorganisms that have invaded the intestinal mucosa or poisons
4. DRUG INTERACTIONS
   a. MAO inhibitors: increase risk of hypertensive crisis
   b. Alcohol and other CNS depressants: result in CNS depression
5. NURSING INTERVENTIONS
   a. Perform thorough abdominal assessment.
   b. Monitor for electrolyte imbalances and dehydration (potassium, blood urea nitrogen [BUN]).
   c. Caution against driving or performing hazardous activities.
   d. Assess for underlying disorders.
6. TYPES
   a. Kaolin and subsalicylate (Kaopectate)
   b. Loperamide (Imodium)
   c. Diphenoxylate hydrochloride with atropine sulfate (Lomotil)
   d. Paregoric (camphorated opium tincture)
   e. Bismuth subsalicylate (Pepto-Bismol)
   f. Difenoxin (Motofen)

V. **DRUGS FOR NAUSEA AND VOMITING**
A. DESCRIPTION
1. ALL ANTIEMETICS REDUCE THE STIMULATION OF THE VOMITING REFLEX LOCATED IN THE MEDULLA BY EITHER INTERFERING WITH THE LOCAL RESPONSE SENT TO THE BRAIN OR THE CENTRAL RESPONSE AT THE VOMITING CENTER ITSELF.
2. DRUGS TO BE CONSIDERED FOR TREATMENT OF MILD NAUSEA MAY INCLUDE ANTACIDS OR CYTOPROTECTIVE DRUGS.
3. GENERALLY GIVEN IN IV, IM, TRANSDERMAL PATCH, OR RECTAL SUPPOSITORY FORM IN THE PRESENCE OF NAUSEA AND VOMITING; ORAL FORM CAN BE GIVEN FOR EMESIS PREVENTION.
4. GENERALLY GIVE ½ HOUR BEFORE ANTICIPATED NAUSEA OR VOMITING.

5. FOR CLIENTS TAKING HIGHLY
   EMETOGENIC DRUGS, ANTIEMETIC
   DRUG COMBINATIONS MAY BE MORE
   EFFECTIVE.
B. DOPAMINE RECEPTOR ANTAGONIST
   (PHENOTHIAZINE-TYPE) ANTIEMETICS
   1. USES
      a. These drugs treat nausea and
         vomiting, specifically severe
         vomiting and vomiting associated
         with anesthesia, toxins, and
         chemotherapy.
      b. Centrally suppress the chemoreceptor
         trigger zone (CTZ) by blocking
         dopamine receptors.
   2. ADVERSE REACTIONS
      a. CNS: sedation, drowsiness,
         extrapyramidal symptoms
         (akathisia and acute dystonia),
         persistent tardive dyskinesia,
         neuroleptic malignant syndrome,
         hypothermia
      b. Skin: photosensitivity reaction
      c. Hematology: agranulocytosis,
         pancytopenia
      d. CV: hypotension
      e. Sensory: blurred vision, dry mouth
      f. Respiratory: respiratory depression
   3. CONTRAINDICATIONS AND
      PRECAUTIONS
      a. Hypersensitivity to phenothiazine
         derivatives
      b. Alcohol withdrawal
      c. Comatose states and brain damage
      d. Bone marrow depression
      e. Pregnancy
      f. Lactation
      g. Hepatic, renal, and cardiovascular
         dysfunction
      h. Prediagnosed breast cancer
   4. DRUG INTERACTIONS
      a. CNS depressants: decrease effect of
         antiemetic
      b. Tricyclic antidepressants: additive
         anticholinergic effects
      c. Phenytoin (Dilantin): may decrease
         or increase phenytoin effects
      d. Alcohol: additive CNS depressant
         effects
      e. Antacids: decrease effect of
         antiemetic
   5. NURSING INTERVENTIONS
      a. Assess blood pressure (BP) and
         cardiac status.
      b. Assess fluid status; may cause pink
         or reddish brown discoloration of
         urine.
      c. Assess visual changes.
      d. Instruct the client to avoid activities
         requiring mental alertness.
      e. Instruct the client to avoid abruptly
         stopping the drug.

f. Monitor serum electrolytes, liver
   function, urinalysis, and complete
   blood count.
g. Instruct the client to protect the skin
   with sunscreen and protective clothing.
h. Administer parenterally deep IM by
   Z-track.
i. Administer tablets whole.
j. Dilute liquid form before use.
   6. TYPES
      a. Chlorpromazine (Thorazine)
      b. Prochlorperazine (Compazine)
      c. Promethazine (Phenergan)
      d. Perphenazine (Triaflon)
      e. Thiethylperazine (Torecan)
      f. Triflupromazine (Vesprin)
C. SEROTONIN (5-HT$_3$) RECEPTOR
   ANTAGONIST ANTIEMETICS
   1. USES
      a. These drugs treat nausea and
         vomiting, specifically vomiting
         associated with cancer chemotherapy,
         radiation therapy, and anesthesia.
      b. Inhibit serotonin receptors (5-HT$_3$),
         which initiate the vomiting reflex
   2. ADVERSE REACTIONS
      a. CNS: headache, dizziness, sedation
      b. GI: diarrhea
   3. CONTRAINDICATIONS AND
      PRECAUTIONS
      a. Pregnancy
      b. Lactation
      c. Liver dysfunction
   4. DRUG INTERACTIONS
      a. Rifampin (Rifadin): decreases plasma
         level
   5. NURSING INTERVENTIONS
      a. Assess fluid, electrolyte, and
         cardiovascular status.
      b. Oral and intravenous dilution
         amounts vary.
      c. Headache generally requires an
         analgesic.
   6. TYPES
      a. Dolasetron (Anzemet)
      b. Granisetron (Kytril)
      c. Ondansetron (Zofran)
D. ANTICHOLINERGICS/ANTIHISTAMINE
   ANTIEMETICS
   1. USES
      a. These drugs treat nausea and
         vomiting, specifically vomiting
         associated with anesthesia, motion
         sickness, and vertigo.
      b. Depress labyrinthine activity and the
         vestibular-cerebellar pathways,
         which treat motion sickness, vertigo,
         and emesis
   2. ADVERSE REACTIONS
      a. GI: dry mouth
      b. CNS: drowsiness
      c. CV: hypotension

3. CONTRAINDICATIONS AND PRECAUTIONS
   a. Narrow-angle glaucoma
   b. Pregnancy
   c. Lactation
   d. Prostate, GU and GI obstructions
4. DRUG INTERACTIONS
   a. Alcohol: increases CNS depressant effects
   b. Barbiturates: increase CNS depressant effects
   c. CNS depressants: additive CNS depressant effects
5. NURSING INTERVENTIONS
   a. Administer with food, milk, or water to minimize gastrointestinal irritation.
   b. Instruct the client to avoid activities requiring mental alertness.
   c. Instruct the client that there may be an interference with allergic skin tests.
6. TYPES
   a. Cyclizine (Marezine)
   b. Dimenhydrinate (Dramamine)
   c. Hydroxyzine (Vistaril, Atarax)
   d. Meclizine (Antivert)
   e. Scopolamine (Hyoscine): this drug comes in transdermal patch form.

E. OTHER TYPES—TRIMETHOBENZAMIDE (TIGAN)
   1. USES
      a. Less effective than phenothiazine types and with less adverse effects
      b. Blocks the chemoreceptor trigger zone in the medulla, which acts on the vomiting center
   2. ADVERSE REACTIONS
      a. Hypotension
      b. Hypersensitivity reaction
   3. CONTRAINDICATIONS AND PRECAUTIONS
      a. Pregnancy
      b. Lactation
      c. Known sensitivity to local anesthetics in rectal form
      d. Hypersensitivity to narcotics
      e. High fever
   4. DRUG INTERACTIONS
      a. Alcohol: increases CNS depressant effects
      b. CNS depressants: increase CNS depressant effects
   5. NURSING INTERVENTIONS
      a. Instruct the client to avoid activities requiring mental alertness.
      b. Give the drug deep IM by Z-track method.
      c. Wash hands carefully after applying the scopolamine patch behind the ear.

F. OTHER TYPES
   1. METOCLOPRAMIDE (REGLAN): (SEE PROKINETICS ON PAGES 446–447.)
   2. DEXAMETHASONE (DECADRON): (SEE CORTICOSTEROIDS IN CHAPTER 18.)
   3. LORAZEPAM (ATIVAN): (SEE ANTIANXIETY DRUGS IN CHAPTER 28.)
   4. DRONABINOL (MARINOL) AND TWO CANNABINOIDS APPROVED FOR CHEMOTHERAPY-INDUCED EMESIS AND AVAILABLE IN CAPSULE FORM FOR CHEMOTHERAPY-INDUCED NAUSEA AND VOMITING.

VI. **EMETICS**
A. DESCRIPTION
   1. ACTIVE INGREDIENT IS EMETINE, WHICH STIMULATES THE VOMITING REFLEX LOCATED IN THE MEDULLA BY STIMULATING THE CHEMORECEPTOR TRIGGER ZONE AND IRRITATING GASTRIC MUCOSA.
   2. USE OF SYRUP OF IPECAC WAS ONCE MOST COMMON IN THE UNITED STATES, ALTHOUGH THE POISON CONTROL CENTER NO LONGER RECOMMENDS IT WITH FREQUENCY.
   3. SYRUP OF IPECAC IS NOT TO BE CONFUSED WITH ACTIVATED CHARCOAL.
B. SYRUP OF IPECAC
   1. USES
      a. Accidental poisoning
      b. Currently being abused by clients with bulimia nervosa
      c. Fatal dose is 10–25 mg (each dose contains 21 mg of emetine).
      d. Emetine is excreted slowly, so a daily dose of 30 ml is toxic and fatal after several months.
      e. Recommended dose:
         1) Children less than 1 year of age: 5–10 ml followed by ½ to 1 glass of water
         2) Children over 1 year of age: 15 ml followed by 1–2 glasses of water
         3) Adults: 30 ml followed by 3–4 glasses of water
         4) Vomiting generally occurs within 20 minutes or dose may be repeated.
   2. ADVERSE REACTIONS
      a. GI: bloody diarrhea
      b. CNS: depression, convulsions, coma
      c. CV: cardiotoxicity; cardiomyopathy; dysrhythmias, particularly atrial fibrillation
      d. Musculoskeletal: myopathy, muscle aching, hypoflexia

3. CONTRAINDICATIONS AND
   PRECAUTIONS
   a. Unconscious client
   b. Pregnancy
   c. Lactation
   d. Poisoning from caustic substances
      such as gasoline, kerosene, drain
      opener or petroleum products
      because the vomiting would reexpose
      the mucosa to the irritation
4. DRUG INTERACTIONS
   a. Activated charcoal: potentiates
      emetic effect
   b. Carbonated products: cause gastric
      distention
   c. Milk products: decrease absorption
5. NURSING INTERVENTIONS
   a. Call the poison control center before
      administering to determine if syrup
      of ipecac is appropriate.
   b. Obtain electrocardiogram (ECG)
      before administration.
   c. Assess vital signs before
      administration.
   d. Avoid giving with milk products
      because they delay the emesis.
   e. Avoid giving with carbonated
      beverages because they increase
      abdominal distention.
   f. Assess for ipecac abuse in clients
      suspected of having bulimia
      nervosa.
   g. Abusing ipecac of potentially fatal
      results from cardiotoxicity.

C. ACTIVATED CHARCOAL
   1. USES
      a. Binds and inactivates the poison
         until excreted
      b. Healthcare provider may to give as
         soon as possible after ingestion of
         poisoning but not within 1–2 hours
         of syrup of ipecac
      c. Given as a powder prepared in
         an aqueous slurry to absorb the
         poison
      d. Recommended dose:
         1) Children: not more than 1 dose
         2) Adults: 30–100 mg
   2. ADVERSE REACTIONS
      a. GI: black tarry stools, diarrhea,
         constipation
   3. CONTRAINDICATIONS AND
      PRECAUTIONS
      a. Unconscious client
      b. Pregnancy
      c. Lactation
      d. Poisoning from caustic substances
         such as cyanide

4. DRUG INTERACTIONS
   a. Syrup of ipecac: potentiates emetic
      effect
5. NURSING INTERVENTIONS
   a. Avoid giving within 1–2 hours after
      ingestion of syrup of ipecac.
   b. Assess vital signs before administration.
   c. May give with a laxative to promote
      elimination
   d. Assess for bulimina, a binge–purge
      disorder in which the clients
      commonly abuse ipecac.

VII. DRUGS FOR DIVERTICULITIS
   A. DESCRIPTION
      1. DRUGS ARE GIVEN TO INCREASE
         COMFORT (ANALGESICS).
      2. DRUGS ARE ALSO GIVEN TO ADD
         SUBSTANCE TO STOOL FORMATION
         (SEE BULK LAXATIVES ON PAGE 449).
      3. DRUGS MAY ALSO BE GIVEN AS
         ANTISPASMOTICS (SEE SELECTIVE
         ANTICHOLINERGIC—
         PROPANTHELINE [PRO-BANTHINE]
         ON PAGE 455).

VIII. DRUGS FOR INFLAMMATORY BOWEL
      DISEASE (CROHN'S DISEASE—REGIONAL
      ILEITIS AND ULCERATIVE COLITIS)
   A. DESCRIPTION
      1. DRUGS ARE GIVEN TO REDUCE
         GASTROINTESTINAL MOTILITY
         AND SPASM (SEE SELECTIVE
         ANTICHOLINERGIC—PROPANTHELINE
         [PRO-BANTHINE] ON PAGE 455).
      2. DRUGS ARE ALSO GIVEN TO REDUCE
         INFLAMMATION (SEE
         GLUCOCORTICOIDS IN CHAPTER 23).
      3. DRUGS ARE ALSO GIVEN TO REDUCE
         BACTERIAL COUNT ALONG WITH
         ANTI-INFLAMMATORY EFFECT (SEE
         SELECTIVE SULFONAMIDE IN
         CHAPTER 25).
   B. AMINOSALICYLATES
      1. USES
         a. Reduce bacterial count, namely
            E. coli and Clostridium in stool
         b. Act locally on the intestinal flora
         c. Produce an anti-inflammatory effect
         d. Inhibit prostaglandins, which can
            cause diarrhea and interfere with fluid
            and electrolyte absorption in the colon
      2. ADVERSE REACTIONS
         a. GI: nausea, vomiting, bloody
            diarrhea, abdominal pain, anorexia,
            flatulence, and dyspepsia
         b. Skin: allergic reactions, rash, arthralgia
         c. Hematology: hematologic disorders
            (anemias, agranulocytosis)

3. CONTRAINDICATIONS AND
   PRECAUTIONS
   a. Hepatic or renal dysfunction
   b. Pregnancy
   c. Lactation
   d. Known sensitivity to sulfasalazine
      (Azulfidine) and other sulfonamides
   e. Salicylates
   f. Intestinal obstruction
   g. Blood dyscrasias
4. DRUG INTERACTIONS
   a. Sulfonylureas: impairment of
      sulfonylurea metabolism
5. NURSING INTERVENTIONS
   a. Monitor blood counts and folate
      levels—a supplement may be needed.
   b. Instruct the client that the skin and
      urine may turn orange.
   c. Administer after eating.
   d. Instruct the client to swallow whole.
   e. Schedule doses evenly over 24 hours
      to help avoid gastrointestinal effects.
6. TYPES
   a. Sulfasalazine (Azulfidine)
   b. Mesalamine (5-ASA)
   c. Olsalazine (Dipentum)
C. SELECTIVE ANTICHOLINERGIC—
   PROPANTHELINE (PRO-BANTHINE)
   1. USES
      a. Decreases the smooth muscle tone of
         the intestinal muscle, which will reduce
         gastrointestinal motility and spasms
      b. Decreases the smooth muscle in
         biliary and urinary tracts
      c. Used in pancreatitis, ureteral and
         urinary bladder spasms
   2. ADVERSE REACTIONS
      a. GI: constipation, dry mouth
      b. Sensory: blurred vision, mydriasis,
         increased ocular pressure
      c. CNS: drowsiness
      d. Urogenital: difficult urination,
         decreased sexual activity
   3. CONTRAINDICATIONS AND
      PRECAUTIONS
      a. Narrow-angle glaucoma
      b. Pregnancy
      c. Lactation
      d. Tachycardia, myocardial infarction (MI),
         and other cardiac problems
      e. Intestinal obstruction and ileus
      f. Myasthenia gravis
      g. Hepatic and renal dysfunction
      h. CNS damage
   4. DRUG INTERACTIONS
      a. Ketoconazole (Nizoral): decreases
         anticholinergic effect
      b. Potassium: increases GI lesions

5. NURSING INTERVENTIONS
   a. Assess gastrointestinal, central
      nervous, and cardiac systems for
      adverse reactions.
   b. Instruct the client to relieve dry
      mouth with sucking hard candy,
      chewing gum, and rinsing with
      water frequently.
   c. Instruct the client to change positions
      slowly.
   d. Instruct the client to avoid activities
      requiring mental alertness.
   e. Administer 1 hour before or after
      antacids.
   f. Give 30–60 minutes before meals and
      at bedtime.
IX. **DRUGS FOR ANORECTAL PROBLEMS**
   A. DESCRIPTION
      1. ANORECTAL PREPARATIONS
         PROVIDE TREATMENT FOR
         HEMORRHOIDS AND OTHER
         ANORECTAL CONDITIONS.
      2. DRUGS RELIEVE MANIFESTATIONS
         SUCH AS INFLAMMATION,
         IRRITATION, PAIN, ITCHING,
         SWELLING.
      3. THEIR INGREDIENTS VARY WIDELY:
         a. Local anesthetics (benzocaine,
            dibucaine)
         b. Anti-inflammatory (hydrocortisone)
         c. Emollients (mineral oil, lanolin)
         d. Astringents (witch hazel, zinc oxide)
      4. AVAILABLE IN MANY FORMS:
         SUPPOSITORIES, CREAMS, FOAMS,
         OINTMENTS, AND MEDICATED PADS
X. **DRUGS FOR DISSOLVING GALLSTONES**
   A. DESCRIPTION
      1. DISSOLVE GALLSTONES BY
         SUPPRESSING CHOLESTEROL, A
         COMPONENT OF BILE, WHICH CAN
         PRECIPITATE INTO CRYSTALS AND
         STONES WHEN CONCENTRATED
      2. PREVENT STONES FROM FORMING
      3. ADMINISTERED OVER WEEKS OR
         MONTHS FOR THERAPEUTIC EFFECT
      4. GIVEN IN ORAL FORM OR VIA
         CATHETER INSERTED INTO THE
         COMMON BILE DUCT
      5. NOT EFFECTIVE IF STONES HAVE
         CALCIFIED
      6. TOXICITY OF DRUGS WEIGHED
         AGAINST THERAPEUTIC EFFECTS
   B. GALLSTONE DISSOLVERS
      1. USES
         a. Utilized as a conservative intervention
            for dissolving cholesterol-type
            gallstones (cholelithiasis)

    b. Utilized as an alternative to surgical removal of gallstones when surgery may be contraindicated

    c. Dissolvers are bile acids that reduce cholesterol content in bile, thus allowing for dissolving of cholesterol stones.

    d. Dissolvers dissolve radiolucent stones only, which describe cholesterol stones.

    e. Ineffective against radiopaque stones, such as calcium stones.

2. ADVERSE REACTIONS

    a. Hepatic: liver enzyme changes, hepatitis, elevated cholesterol and triglyceride levels

    b. GI: nausea, vomiting, diarrhea, abdominal pain, anorexia, flatulence, and dyspepsia

3. CONTRAINDICATIONS AND PRECAUTIONS

    a. Hepatic dysfunction

    b. Biliary obstruction

    c. Pregnancy (known to cause teratogenesis)

    d. Lactation

    e. Known allergic reactions

4. DRUG INTERACTIONS

    a. Aluminum-based antacids: decrease effect of gallbladder dissolver

    b. Antilipemic agents such as cholestyramine (Questran) and colestipol (Colestid): decrease effect of gallbladder dissolver

5. NURSING INTERVENTIONS

    a. Administer drugs at least 2 hours apart to avoid drug interactions.

    b. Monitor liver function.

    c. Offer small frequent meals, which may help with gastrointestinal manifestations.

    d. Avoid crushing capsules for maximum effect.

6. TYPES

    a. Chenodiol (Chenix)

    b. Monoctanoin (Moctanin)

    c. Ursodiol (Actigall)

XI. **BILE ACID SEQUESTRANTS**

A. DESCRIPTION

    1. ACT BY COMBINING BILE ACIDS IN THE INTESTINE TO FORM AN INSOLUBLE COMPLEX ELIMINATED IN THE FECES

    2. RESULT IS A PARTIAL REMOVAL OF THE BILE ACIDS FROM THE ENTEROHEPATIC CIRCULATION.

B. CHOLESTYRAMINE (QUESTRAN) AND COLESTIPOL HCL (COLESTID) (SEE CHAPTER 19, DRUGS FOR THE CARDIOVASCULAR SYSTEM)

C. HMG-COA REDUCTASE INHIBITORS (STATINS) (SEE CHAPTER 19, DRUGS FOR THE CARDIOVASCULAR SYSTEM).

XII. **DRUGS FOR HEPATITIS**

A. DESCRIPTION

    1. DRUGS ARE GIVEN TO PROVIDE IMMUNITY AGAINST EXPOSURE TO HEPATITIS A AND B.

    2. DRUGS ARE ALSO GIVEN AS IMMUNOMODULATORS AND ANTIVIRALS TO FIGHT FOREIGN INVASION OF ANTIGENS AND VIRUSES (SEE GENERAL DISCUSSION OF ANTIVIRALS IN CHAPTER 26).

    3. INTERFERONS HAVE ANTIVIRAL, IMMUNOMODULATORY, AND ANTINEOPLASTIC ACTIONS AND MAY BE GIVEN FOR TREATMENT OF HEPATITIS.

    4. INTERFERONS HAVE THREE FAMILIES: ALPHA, BETA, AND GAMMA.

    5. ALL INTERFERONS USED TO TREAT HEPATITIS ARE FROM THE ALPHA FAMILY—INTERFERON ALFA.

    6. DRUGS USED TO TREAT HEPATITIS GENERALLY HAVE MODEST THERAPEUTIC RESPONSES.

B. INTERFERON ALFA

    1. USES

        a. Used to treat chronic hepatitis B (lamividine is another drug used to treat chronic hepatitis B)

        b. Used to treat chronic hepatitis C in combination with oral ribavirin

    2. ADVERSE REACTIONS

        a. Immune: flulike symptoms such as fever, myalgia, headache, chills

        b. CNS: depression, including suicide ideation, fatigue

        c. GI: anorexia, diarrhea, abdominal pain, weight loss

        d. Other: cough, alopecia, bone marrow depression, thyroid dysfunction, heart damage

    3. CONTRAINDICATIONS AND PRECAUTIONS

        a. Cardiac and pulmonary dysfunction

        b. Pregnancy, lactation

        c. Psychiatric disorders

      d. Allergy to other interferons and history of anaphylaxis to immunoglobulins

      e. Hepatic dysfunction

  4. DRUG INTERACTIONS

      a. None established

  5. NURSING INTERVENTIONS

      a. Administer IM or subcut only.

      b. Assess for manifestations of depression.

      c. Provide for adequate hydration.

      d. Assess cardiac and thyroid status and liver studies.

  6. TYPES

      a. Interferon alfa-2a (Roferon): chronic hepatitis C

      b. Interferon alfa-2b (Intron A): chronic hepatitis B or C

      c. Interferon alfa-n1 (Wellferon): chronic hepatitis C

      d. Interferon alfacon-1 (Infergen): chronic hepatitis C

C. ANTIVIRAL—LAMIVUDINE (EPIVIR)

  1. USES

      a. In the treatment of hepatitis B and HIV

  2. ADVERSE REACTIONS

      a. CNS: neuropathy, insomnia, dizziness, headache, fever, chills

      b. GI: nausea, diarrhea, abdominal pain, weight loss

      c. Other: lactic acidosis, hepatomegaly with steatosis

  3. CONTRAINDICATIONS AND PRECAUTIONS

      a. Pregnancy

      b. Lactation

      c. Hypersensitivity to lamivudine

      d. Renal dysfunction

  4. DRUG INTERACTIONS

      a. Trimethoprim-sulfamethoxazole (Bactrim, Septra): increase in lamivudine levels

  5. NURSING INTERVENTIONS

      a. Assess for adverse reactions.

      b. Monitor hematologic, liver, and renal studies, especially amylase.

D. ANTIVIRAL—RIBAVIRIN (VIRAZOLE)

  1. USES

      a. Used to treat chronic hepatitis C

      b. Used in combination with interferon alfa only

  2. ADVERSE REACTIONS

      a. CV: hypotension, MI, cardiac arrest

      b. Sensory: conjunctivitis

      c. GI: increases in liver enzymes

      d. Respiratory: dyspnea, apnea, ventilator dependence

      e. Hematology: hemolytic anemia

  3. CONTRAINDICATIONS AND PRECAUTIONS

      a. Cardiac and pulmonary dysfunction

      b. Pregnancy

      c. Lactation

  4. DRUG INTERACTIONS

      a. Antivirals: decrease antiretroviral activity

  5. NURSING INTERVENTIONS

      a. Assess cardiac and respiratory systems.

      b. Monitor fluid status.

      c. Instruct the client to avoid pregnancy because the drug causes teratogenic effects.

XIII. DRUGS FOR PANCREATIC ENZYME REPLACEMENT

A. DESCRIPTION

  1. DRUGS ARE GIVEN TO REPLACE PANCREATIC ENZYMES—LIPASE, AMYLASE, CHYMOTRYPSIN, AND TRYPSIN.

  2. ANTACIDS AND HISTAMINE 2-RECEPTOR ANTAGONISTS ARE GIVEN IN ADDITION TO REDUCE GASTRIC PH SO ENZYMES WILL NOT BE DEACTIVATED, IF GASTRIC ACID IS EXCESSIVE.

B. PANCREATIC ENZYMES

  1. USES

      a. Used to replace pancreatic enzyme deficiencies caused by pancreatic disorders (pancreatitis, pancreatic surgery, pancreatic duct obstruction) and cystic fibrosis

  2. ADVERSE REACTIONS

      a. GI: nausea, vomiting, diarrhea, abdominal cramping

      b. Allergic reactions

  3. CONTRAINDICATIONS AND PRECAUTIONS

      a. Rare

  4. DRUG INTERACTIONS

      a. Rare

  5. NURSING INTERVENTIONS

      a. Enteric-coated microsphere capsules are preferred over tablets because they are more likely to dissolve in the duodenum and jejunum.

      b. Administer enzymes with meals and snacks.

      c. Monitor for stools that are less fatty and decreased in frequency.

  6. TYPES

      a. Pancrelipase (Viokase, Cotazym, Pancrease MT, Pancrecarb MS-8)

      b. Pancreatin

PRACTICE QUESTIONS

1. The nurse evaluates that medication teaching has been effective when the client states that ranitidine (Zantac)
   1. decreases gastric acid levels.
   2. changes hormonal levels.
   3. increases pepsin levels.
   4. decreases pH levels.

2. Which of the following should the nurse include in the teaching plan the nurse is preparing for a client taking sucralfate (Carafate)?
   1. Sucralfate reduces gastric acid production
   2. Administer sucralfate with breakfast
   3. Separate administration of sucralfate with other drugs by 2 hours
   4. Sucralfate works against *H. pylori*

3. Which of the following is a priority for the nurse to administer to a client with gastroesophageal reflux disease (GERD)?
   1. Cytoprotectors
   2. Antibiotics
   3. Proton pump inhibitors
   4. Anticholinergics

4. The nurse should assess which of the following body systems while administering intravenous cimetidine (Tagamet) to a client?
   1. Urinary
   2. Immune
   3. Respiratory
   4. Cardiovascular

5. The nurse should monitor a client taking lansoprazole (Prevacid) for which of the following adverse reactions?
   Select all that apply:
   [ ] 1. Headache
   [ ] 2. Oliguria
   [ ] 3. Anxiety
   [ ] 4. Dry mouth
   [ ] 5. Diarrhea
   [ ] 6. Decreased appetite

6. A client is experiencing peptic ulcer disease caused by *H. pylori*. The nurse should plan to administer which of the following oral drug combinations? Clarithromycin (Biaxin) with
   1. tetracycline (Achromycin) with sodium bicarbonate (baking soda).
   2. metronidazole (Flagyl) and aluminum hydroxide (Amphogel).
   3. amoxicillin (Amoxil) and omeprazole (Prilosec).
   4. penicillin (Pen-G) and nizatidine (Axid).

7. The nurse should instruct which of the following clients that taking which antacid may result in constipation? A client taking
   1. magaldrate (Riopan).
   2. magnesium and aluminum (Maalox).
   3. aluminum carbonate (Basaljel).
   4. magnesium hydroxide (milk of magnesia).

8. The nurse is caring for a client who admits to a 15-year history of gastric ulcers. The nurse instructs this client to take which of the following drugs for minor aches and pains?
   1. Acetaminophen (Tylenol)
   2. Buffered aspirin
   3. Plain aspirin
   4. Ibuprofen (Motrin)

9. Which of the following antacids should the nurse question administering to the client with a gastric ulcer and congestive heart failure?
   1. Magaldrate (Riopan)
   2. Calcium carbonate (Tums)
   3. Magnesium hydroxide (milk of magnesia)
   4. Sodium bicarbonate (baking soda)

10. The nurse is developing a medication schedule for a client who is receiving magnesium and aluminum (Mylanta) for gastritis. To promote the best absorption, this drug should be administered Select all that apply:
    [ ] 1. at bedtime
    [ ] 2. 1 hour before meals
    [ ] 3. immediately after meals
    [ ] 4. upon arising in the morning
    [ ] 5. 1 hour after meals
    [ ] 6. 30 minutes after meals

11. After obtaining a medication history from a client who informs the nurse of her early pregnancy, which of the following drugs is a priority for the nurse to obtain an order to discontinue?
    1. Misoprostol (Cytotec)
    2. Docusate (Surfak)
    3. Magnesium hydroxide (Milk of Magnesia)
    4. Bismuth subsalicylate (Pepto-Bismol)

12. When administering cimetidine (Tagamet), the nurse assesses the client for which of the following adverse reactions?
    Select all that apply:
    [ ] 1. Tinnitus
    [ ] 2. Alopecia
    [ ] 3. Diarrhea
    [ ] 4. Mental confusion
    [ ] 5. Dizziness
    [ ] 6. Dyspepsia

13. The client is to begin taking methylcellulose (Citrucel) daily. The nurse will include which of the following instructions in the teaching plan?
    1. Administer with at least 8 ounces of liquid
    2. Administer at hour of sleep
    3. Discontinue if no bowel movement in 5 days
    4. Discontinue if taking docusate (Colace)

14. The nurse should include which of the following in the medication instructions given to a client who is being started on antiemetics?
    1. Take the antiemetic within 1 hour after activity that promotes nausea
    2. Stop taking the antiemetic when the activity that induces the nausea ceases
    3. The urine may turn an orangish color
    4. Avoid activities that require mental alertness

15. The nurse informs a student nurse that the loperamide (Imodium) prescribed for a client who is experiencing diarrhea has which of the following actions?
    1. Inhibits the peristaltic activity of intestinal muscles
    2. Consolidates the stool in the intestine
    3. Lowers the surface tension, allowing more water into stool
    4. Distends the intestine by osmotic retention of fluid

16. Which of the following is a priority for the nurse to include in the plan of care for a client taking ondansetron (Zofran) for chemotherapy?
    1. Monitor the client for fluid and electrolyte imbalance
    2. Instruct the client to take the Zofran 30 minutes before the chemotherapy
    3. Instruct the client to take an analgesic for the adverse reaction to a headache
    4. Encourage the client to avoid activities that may cause drowsiness

17. Which of the following is the priority for the nurse to include in the plan of care for a client receiving metoclopramide (Reglan) with chemotherapy in a clinic?
    1. Instruct the client to avoid driving home
    2. Offer gum or hard candy for dry mouth
    3. Administer ½ to 1 hour before the chemotherapy treatment
    4. Assess the client for extrapyramidal clinical manifestations

18. The nurse should question which of the following medication administration orders?
    1. Cimetidine (Tagamet) 300 mg orally four times a day to an 86-year-old client with gastroesophageal reflux disease
    2. Famotidine (Pepcid) 20 mg and Maalox 30 ml orally at bedtime to a 23-year-old client with a peptic ulcer
    3. Lansoprazole (Prevacid) 15 mg orally daily to a 51-year-old client with a duodenal ulcer
    4. Omeprazole (Prilosec) 20 mg orally three times a day to a client with a pathological hypersecretion condition

19. The nurse selects the ideal antacid for a client because of which of the following characteristics?
    1. Sweet to taste, cathartic in nature, and effective for a prolonged period of time
    2. Short acting and readily absorbed
    3. Not absorbed by the body and acts as a laxative
    4. Decreases acidity without constipating or cathartic properties

20. After administering ursodiol (Actigall) to the client with gallbladder disease, the nurse evaluates the priority outcome to be
    1. decreased vomiting.
    2. increased comfort.
    3. reduced stone formation.
    4. decreased bile production.

21. The nurse has administered prochlorperazine (Compazine) on several occasions over the past week to the client experiencing severe vomiting. The nurse should assess this client for which of the following adverse reactions? Select all that apply:
    [ ] 1. Bradycardia
    [ ] 2. Weight loss
    [ ] 3. Akathisia
    [ ] 4. Orthostatic hypotension
    [ ] 5. Acute dystonia
    [ ] 6. Oliguria

22. The nurse is collecting a nursing history from a client admitted on pancreatin. Which of the following diseases should the nurse question in the client's medical history?
    1. Hepatitis
    2. Cirrhosis
    3. Gallbladder cancer
    4. Cystic fibrosis

23. When providing care to a client who is on propantheline (Pro-Banthine), the nurse should assess the client for
    Select all that apply:
    [ ] 1. dry mouth
    [ ] 2. diarrhea
    [ ] 3. blurred vision
    [ ] 4. hypertension
    [ ] 5. urinary frequency
    [ ] 6. tachycardia

24. The nurse has instructed the client about sulfasalazine (Azulfidine), which was prescribed for her ulcerative colitis. The nurse evaluates which of the following statements by the client to indicate that the client understood the instructions?
    1. "Nausea, vomiting, and abdominal pain are adverse reactions of Azulfidine."
    2. "I should chew the tablets thoroughly and follow with a sip of water."
    3. "I may notice that my urine turns blue."
    4. "Azulfidine will decrease intestinal gas production."

25. The client was recently diagnosed with chronic hepatitis C. The nurse plans to instruct the client about which of the following drugs that is used in combination with oral ribavirin?

1. Lamivudine (Epivir HBV)
2. Interferon alfa
3. Interferon gamma
4. Ganciclovir (Cytovene)

26. The nurse is preparing to delegate which of the following nursing tasks to a licensed practical nurse?
    1. Administer IV ondansetron (Zofran) to a client experiencing nausea from chemotherapy
    2. Instruct a client on the adverse reactions of propantheline (Pro-Banthine)
    3. Administer trimethobenzamide (Tigan) Z-track to a client prior to chemotherapy
    4. Develop a medication schedule for a client taking an antacid and several other drugs

ANSWERS AND RATIONALES

1. 1. Ranitidine (Zantac) is a histamine 2-receptor antagonist, which suppresses gastric acid secretion. Changing hormonal levels is not a primary action of ranitidine. Cimetidine (Tagamet) suppresses pepsin production. Zantac also reduces hydrogen ion concentration, which will increase pH levels.

2. 3. The administration of sucralfate (Carafate) should be separated from other drug administration by 2 hours to protect those drugs from binding to the protective adhesive that forms. Sucralfate is an antipeptic/cytoprotective gastrointestinal drug used to protect eroded ulcer sites from further acidic damage. Sucralfate should be administered 1 hour before meals. Antibiotics are used in peptic ulcer disease to fight against *H. pylori.*

3. 3. Drugs used to promote healing the tissues damaged by acid reflux include antacids and antisecretory drugs, such as proton pump inhibitors and histamine 2-receptor antagonists. Cytoprotective/antipeptics and antibiotics (and anticholinergics) are primarily used for peptic ulcer disease. Cholinergics are used on rare occasion for gastroesophageal reflux to increase the rate of gastric emptying.

4. 4. Cimetidine (Tagamet) is a histamine 2-receptor blocking drug used in the treatment of ulcers and gastroesophageal reflux disease. The cardiovascular system needs to be assessed. Intravenous cimetidine (Tagamet) can cause dysrhythmias and hypotension. Other body systems that need to be assessed include the gastrointestinal, hematologic, metabolic, central nervous system, and genital systems. Tagamet does not affect the urinary, immune, or respiratory systems.

5. 1. 3. 4. 5. Lansoprazole (Prevacid) is a proton pump inhibitor used in the treatment of ulcers and gastroesophageal reflux disease. Adverse reactions associated with Prevacid include headache, anxiety, dry mouth, and diarrhea.

6. 3. Clarithromycin (Biaxin) is used in combination with amoxicillin (Amoxil) and omeprazole (Prilosec) as an effective combination to combat *H. pylori.*

7. 3. Most antacids affect the bowel. Some promote constipation, such as aluminum carbonate (Basaljel), and others promote diarrhea, such as magnesium. Effects can be minimized by combining aluminum and magnesium.

8. 1. Acetaminophen (Tylenol) has no adverse effect on the gastric mucosa and produces no ulcerative effects when administered for pain. Buffered aspirin does not reduce the incidence of gastric ulcers, although enteric-coated aspirin dissolves in the intestine rather than the stomach. Plain aspirin is associated with development of gastric ulcers. Nonsteroidal anti-inflammatory drugs, such as ibuprofen (Motrin), may cause gastric ulceration.

9. 4. Sodium bicarbonate has higher sodium levels than other antacids and is contraindicated for clients with ulcerative disease and heart failure. Magnesium-based and calcium-based antacids, such as magaldrate (Riopan), calcium carbonate (Tums), and magnesium hydroxide (Milk of Magnesia), are often chosen for clients

with heart failure because of their low sodium content.

10. 1. 2. 5. Ideally antacids should be administered 1 hour before meals, 1 hour after meals, and at bedtime to reduce gastric acid secretion and promote ulcer healing. Administering an antacid first thing in the morning is not appropriate because the neutralizing action lasts only approximately 30 minutes and there is nothing in the stomach to slow its emptying.

11. 1. Although all drug use needs to be questioned in the first trimester of pregnancy, misoprostol (Cytotec), which may be used in peptic ulcer prevention as a prostaglandin and cytoprotective agent, is known to cause miscarriages. Docusate (Surfak) is a mild surfactant laxative, which has no adverse effects. Magnesium hydroxide (Milk of Magnesia) and bismuth subsalicylate are mild antacids with no teratogenic effects.

12. 3. 4. 5. Cimetidine (Tagamet) is a histamine 2-receptor blocking drug used in the treatment of ulcers and gastroesophageal reflux disease. Adverse reactions include diarrhea, mental confusion (especially in the older adult), and dizziness.

13. 1. Methylcellulose is a bulk laxative. Bulk laxatives must be given with at least 8 ounces of liquid to provide enough water to increase the size of the stool mass and stretch the intestinal wall, promoting peristalsis. Bulk laxatives should be taken when the client is most active. The therapeutic effect occurs within 2 to 3 days. Stool softeners are not contraindicated with bulk laxative use.

14. 4. A client taking an antiemetic should be instructed to avoid activities that require mental alertness because all antiemetics cause varying degrees of drowsiness that will affect the ability to perform a task.

15. 1. Loperamide (Imodium) directly inhibits peristaltic activity of the intestinal muscles, which results in decreased gastrointestinal motility. Consolidating stool in the intestine describes pectin, which is a component of the antidiarrheal Kaopectate. Lowering the surface tension allows more water into the stool, which describes surfactant laxatives or stool softeners. Distending the intestine by osmotic retention of fluid describes the action of saline or osmotic laxatives.

16. 1. Ondansetron (Zofran) is a serotonin receptor antagonist, which suppresses the vomiting reflex and chemotherapy-induced emesis. Because diarrhea is the most common adverse reaction of Zofran and the client may be experiencing vomiting from the chemotherapy, the client may become dehydrated. The client should be monitored for fluid and electrolyte imbalances. Although it is appropriate to tell the client to take the Zofran 30 minutes before the chemotherapy, to avoid activities that may cause drowsiness, and to take an analgesic if a headache occurs, they are not the priority interventions.

17. 1. Although it is appropriate to offer a client receiving metoclopramide (Reglan) gum or hard candy, administer the Reglan ½ to 1 hour before the chemotherapy, and assess the client for extrapyramidal clinical manifestations, the priority nursing intervention is to instruct the client to avoid driving home.

18. 1. Cimetidine (Tagamet), a histamine 2-receptor blocking agent, should be avoided in the older adult because it causes confusion.

19. 4. The ideal antacid would decrease the acidity of the gastric secretions without either constipating or cathartic effects.

20. 3. Gallstone dissolvers, such as ursodiol, are bile acids that reduce the cholesterol content in bile and allow for the dissolution of cholesterol-type gallstones. Decreased vomiting may result from a decrease in pain, which more likely will occur with analgesic use. Increased comfort will primarily occur with analgesic use and may be a secondary effect of stone dissolution. Ursodiol reduces the cholesterol content of bile, but hepatic production of bile is not affected.

21. 3. 4. 5. Prochlorperazine (Compazine) is a phenothiazine-type antiemetic that results in extrapyramidal effects, such as akathisia and acute dystonia. Other adverse reactions include tachycardia, weight gain, orthostatic hypotension, and urinary difficulties such as loss of bladder control.

22. 4. Pancreatin is a pancreatic enzyme used to replace enzyme deficiencies caused by disorders such as cystic fibrosis. Hepatitis and cirrhosis may cause vitamin and other hepatic deficiencies, but not pancreatic enzyme deficiencies. Enzyme replacement is generally not indicated for gallbladder cancer.

23. 1. 3. 6. Anticholinergic agents, such as propantheline (Pro-Banthine), cause dry mouth, constipation, urinary retention, blurred vision, tachycardia, and orthostatic hypotension.

24. 1. Sulfasalazine (Azulfidine) is an anti-inflammatory agent and sulfonamide, which reduces gastrointestinal motility, inflammation, and microbial flora such as *E. coli*. Nausea, vomiting, and abdominal pain are adverse reactions. Decreasing gas formation is the action of simethicone. The tablets are not chewed, and Azulfidine

should be administered with a full glass of water. The skin and urine may turn yellow-orange.

25. 2.   In clients with chronic hepatitis C, modest responses have occurred with combining ribavirin with interferon alfa. All interferons of the alfa class are used to treat hepatitis. Lamivudine is used only in the treatment of hepatitis B virus. Interferons of the gamma class are not utilized for hepatitis. Ganciclovir is utilized to treat herpes viruses.

26. 3.   A licensed practical nurse may administer a drug by Z-track. Administering a drug IV, instructing a client on the adverse reactions of a drug, and developing a medication schedule for a client taking an antacid and several other drugs are nursing tasks reserved for a registered nurse.

REFERENCES

Broyles, B., Reiss, B., & Evans, M. (2012). *Pharmacological aspects of nursing care* (8th ed.). Clifton Park, NY: Delmar Cengage Learning.

Daniels, R., & Nicoll, L. (2012). *Contemporary medical-surgical nursing.* Clifton Park, NY: Delmar Cengage Learning.

Spratto, G. R., & Woods, A. L. (2012). *PDR nurse's drug handbook 2012.* Clifton Park, NY: Thomson Delmar Learning.

CHAPTER 2

DRUGS FOR THE ENDOCRINE SYSTEM

I. DRUGS FOR ANTERIOR PITUITARY DISORDERS
  A. DESCRIPTION
   1. THE ANTERIOR PITUITARY GLAND SECRETES ADRENOCORTICOTROPIC HORMONE (ACTH), THYROID-STIMULATING HORMONE (TSH), GROWTH HORMONE (GH), FOLLICLE-STIMULATING HORMONE (FSH), LUTEINIZING HORMONE (LH), AND PROLACTIN.
   2. SECRETION OF THE ANTERIOR PITUITARY HORMONES IS UNDER THE CONTROL OF RELEASING FACTORS AND INHIBITING FACTORS SECRETED BY THE HYPOTHALAMUS.
   3. THE MOST COMMON CONDITIONS OF HYPERSECRETION OF ANTERIOR PITUITARY DISORDERS ARE CUSHING'S SYNDROME (INCREASED ACTH) AND ACROMEGALY (INCREASED GROWTH HORMONE).
   4. THE MOST COMMON CONDITION OF HYPOSECRETION IS GROWTH FAILURE.
  B. GROWTH HORMONE
   1. USES
     a. Growth hormone is given when failure is due to growth hormone deficiency.
     b. Drugs that inhibit the production or release of growth hormone are given in acromegaly where there is a hypersecretion of growth hormone.
   2. ADVERSE REACTIONS
     a. Allergic reactions
     b. Circulating GH antibodies
     c. Hyperglycemia
     d. Pain and swelling at the injection site
     e. Myalgia
   3. CONTRAINDICATIONS AND PRECAUTIONS
     a. In client whose epiphyses have closed
     b. Active intracranial lesions
     c. Severe respiratory impairment
     d. Lactation

   4. DRUG INTERACTIONS
     a. Glucocorticoids: decrease response to growth hormone
   5. NURSING INTERVENTIONS
     a. Document the client's growth rate for the past 6–12 months prior to treatment.
     b. Instruct the client for the need for annual bone age assessments.
     c. Maintain regular blood or urine glucose monitoring.
     d. Instruct the parents to record height measurements at regular intervals and to notify the physician if expected results are not achieved.
   6. TYPES
     a. Somatrem (Protropin): for growth failure
     b. Somatropin (Humatrope): for growth failure
     c. Brompheniramine maleate (Bromphen): for acromegaly
     d. Octreotide acetate (Sandostatin): for acromegaly

II. DRUGS FOR POSTERIOR PITUITARY DISORDERS
  A. DESCRIPTION
   1. THE POSTERIOR PITUITARY GLAND HORMONES ARE VASOPRESSIN (ANTIDIURETIC HORMONE [ADH]) AND OXYTOCIN.
   2. VASOPRESSIN INCREASES WATER REABSORPTION FROM THE RENAL TUBULES.
   3. OXYTOCIN FACILITATES MILK PRODUCTION DURING LACTATION AND PROMOTES CONTRACTION OF THE UTERUS DURING LABOR AND DELIVERY.
   4. THE MOST COMMON CONDITION OF HYPOSECRETION OF ADH IS DIABETES INSIPIDUS.
  B. VASOPRESSIN (ANTIDIURETIC HORMONE)
   1. USES
     a. Antidiuretic to treat diabetes insipidus
     b. Also given to treat transient ADH deficiency in neurological injuries

c. Vasopressin tannate in oil is preferred for use in chronic cases because of its longer duration of action (24–96 hours).
   1) Given intramuscularly (IM)
   2) Vial must be warmed or shaken vigorously before administration.
   3) Sites must be rotated to prevent lipodystrophy.
   4) Adverse reaction of abdominal cramps
d. Desmopressin, a synthetic vasopressin without the vascular effects of natural ADH, has longer action and fewer side effects; administered intranasally or intravenously (IV)
e. Lypressin administered intranasally; short-acting

2. ADVERSE REACTIONS
   a. Hypersensitivity, anaphylaxis, cardiac arrest
   b. Intranasal congestion, rhinopharyngitis, irritation
   c. Headache, drowsiness, listlessness
   d. Hypertension
   e. Water intoxication, hyponatremia
   f. Myocardial infarction (MI), coronary insufficiency, cardiac arrhythmias

3. CONTRAINDICATIONS AND PRECAUTIONS
   a. Chronic nephritis
   b. Ischemic heart disease

4. DRUG INTERACTIONS
   a. Alcohol: decreases antidiuretic effect
   b. Epinephrine: decreases antidiuretic effect
   c. Lithium: decreases antidiuretic effect
   d. Guanethidine: increases vasopressor action
   e. Neostigmine: increases vasopressor action
   f. Chlorpropamide: increases diuretic activity
   g. Clofibrate: increases diuretic activity
   h. Carbamazepine: increases diuretic activity

5. NURSING INTERVENTIONS
   a. Administer vasopressin tannate in oil IM—never give IV (can form an emboli).
   b. Instruct the client to warm the vial to body temperature prior to drawing up and not to shake the vial or mix vigorously.
   c. Instruct the client to rotate injection sites to prevent lipodystrophy.
   d. Monitor the client for abdominal cramps.
   e. Assess weight daily and edema.
   f. Monitor blood pressure (BP), weight, urine specific gravity, serum osmolality, and intake and output (I & O) throughout treatment. Report sudden changes in pattern.
   g. Monitor the older adult client for cardiac problem that may be precipitated by even a small dose.

h. Assess the client frequently for alertness and orientation because lethargy, confusion, and headache may indicate onset of water intoxication.
i. Measure and record specific gravity and output.
j. Instruct the client to avoid hypertonic fluids such as undiluted syrups, which increase urine output.
k. Instruct the client regarding intranasal or IM administration.
l. Inform the client that rhinitis or upper respiratory infection may decrease the effectiveness of therapy by the intranasal route.
m. Inform the client that if urine output increases, the physician should be notified to adjust the dosage.
n. Instruct the client how to use intranasal sprays if ordered.

6. TYPES
   a. Desmopressin (DDAVP, Stimate)
   b. Lypressin (Diapid)
   c. Vasopressin injection (Pitressin)
   d. Vasopressin tannate in oil (Pitressin Tannate)

III. DRUGS FOR THYROID DISORDERS

A. DESCRIPTION
   1. THYROID GLAND SECRETES T_4 AND T_3.
   2. THE RATE OF SECRETION OF THYROID HORMONES IS UNDER CONTROL OF THE THYROID-STIMULATING HORMONE (TSH), THYROTROPIN, FROM THE ANTERIOR PITUITARY GLAND.
   3. INCREASED SECRETION OF THYROID HORMONES CAUSES HYPERTHYROIDISM (GRAVES' DISEASE).
   4. DECREASED SECRETION OF THYROID HORMONES CAUSES HYPOTHYROIDISM (MYXEDEMA).

B. THYROID HORMONES
   1. USES
      a. Thyroid hormones increase the metabolic rate of all body tissues and have an important role in cell replication and normal growth.
      b. They regulate oxygen consumption and body heat production.
      c. Hormones are given as replacement for deficiency of hormones in hypothyroidism, myxedema, and cretinism.
      d. Dosage is based on serum TSH concentration.
      e. Liothyronine sodium (Cytomel) acts more rapidly than the other drugs but its action is of shorter duration.
      f. Bone loss may occur with treatment.
      g. Dosages are highly individualized. Combination drugs of T_4 and T_3 contain various ratios of the hormones.

2. ADVERSE REACTIONS
   a. Irritability, nervousness, tremors
   b. Insomnia
   c. Headache
   d. Palpitations, tachycardia, arrhythmias
   e. Hypertension
   f. Nausea, diarrhea, change in appetite
   g. Weight loss
   h. Leg cramps
   i. Heat intolerance
   j. Menstrual irregularities
   k. Hyperthyroidism
3. CONTRAINDICATIONS AND PRECAUTIONS
   a. Aspirin hypersensitivity
   b. Severe cardiovascular conditions
   c. Adrenal insufficiency
   d. Pregnancy
   e. Diabetes mellitus
   f. Addison's disease
   g. Diabetes insipidus
4. DRUG INTERACTIONS
   a. Phenytoin (Dilantin): increases effect of thyroid hormone
   b. Tricyclic antidepressants: increase effect of thyroid hormone
   c. Digitalis glycosides: increase effect of digitalis
   d. Anticoagulants: increase effect of anticoagulant, may cause hypoprothrombinemia
   e. Indomethacin (Indocin): increases effect of indomethacin
   f. Cholestyramine (Questran), colestipol (Colestid): decrease absorption of thyroid hormones
   g. Epinephrine, norepinephrine: increase the risk of cardiac insufficiency
5. NURSING INTERVENTIONS
   a. Assess the client for the effectiveness of the drug, such as diuresis, loss of weight, decreased puffiness, increased sense of well-being, increase in activity, and increased serum T_4 and T_3 levels.
   b. Assess the pulse rate prior to each dose. Notify the physician if it is greater than 100 beats per minute.
   c. Monitor for clinical manifestations of hyperthyroidism.
   d. Monitor prothrombin time and assess for bleeding if the client is also receiving anticoagulant therapy.
   e. Instruct the client to take the drug at the same time each day, preferably before breakfast because food interferes with the absorption of the drug.
   f. Instruct the client that the drug is a lifelong replacement therapy.
   g. Instruct the client how to monitor the pulse and to report rate or rhythm changes to the physician.

   h. Instruct the client to immediately report signs of thyrotoxicosis such as palpitations, chest pain, tachycardia, excessive sweating, and increased temperature.
   i. Inform the client not to change brands of the drug because differences in formulations exist.
6. TYPES
   a. Levothyroxine sodium T_4 (Eltroxin, Levothroid, Synthroid)
   b. Liothyronine (Cytomel)
   c. Liotrix (Euthroid, Thyrolar), T_4/T_3
   d. Thyroglobulin (Proloid), T_4/T_3
   e. Thyroid (Armour Thyroid, Thyrar), T_4T_3
C. ANTITHYROID MEDICATIONS
   1. DESCRIPTION
      a. Antithyroid drugs inhibit thyroid hormone synthesis or release.
      b. Antithyroid drugs do not interfere with release or activity of previously formed thyroid hormones; thus, a period of time is necessary before maintenance doses can be established.
      c. Action of antithyroid drugs is slow, taking 2–4 weeks before noticeable improvement.
      d. Initial dosage is large, then reduced to maintenance dose—takes 6–18 months or longer.
      e. Important to space doses at regular intervals as blood levels are reduced in about 8 hours.
      f. Methimazole (Tapazole) is 10 times as potent as propylthiouracil (Propyl-Thyracil). Actions are less consistent than with propylthiouracil (Propyl-Thyracil) but effects appear more promptly.
      g. Methimozole (Tapazole) is given when the client is allergic to propylthiouracil (Propyl-Thyracil).
   2. USES
      a. Hyperthyroidism (Graves' disease)
      b. Iodine-induced thyrotoxicosis
      c. Hyperthyroidism or thyroiditis
      d. To achieve a state of euthyroidism prior to surgery or radioactive iodine therapy
      e. In palliative treatment of toxic nodular goiter
   3. ADVERSE REACTIONS
      a. Nausea and vomiting
      b. Rash, urticaria
      c. Agranulocytosis
      d. Drowsiness
      e. Hypothyroidism
      f. Sensitivity
   4. CONTRAINDICATIONS AND PRECAUTIONS
      a. Pregnancy
      b. Lactation
      c. Concurrent administration of sulfonamides or coal tar derivatives

   d. Infection
   e. Bone marrow depression
   f. Impaired liver function
5. DRUG INTERACTIONS
   a. Anticoagulants: increase effect of
      anticoagulants
   b. Antineoplastic agents: additive bone
      marrow depression
   c. Lithium: additive antithyroid effects
   d. Potassium iodide: additive antithyroid
      effects
   e. Sodium iodide: additive antithyroid
      effects
6. NURSING INTERVENTIONS
   a. Assess the client for improvement in
      weight gain, reduced pulse rate, and
      reduced serum T_4 levels.
   b. Instruct the client to report any
      unexplained bleeding.
   c. Instruct the client to observe for signs
      of hypothyroidism and report them to
      the physician.
   d. Instruct the client that therapy may last
      from 6 months to several years.
   e. Instruct the client to take the drug at
      the same time each day with relation to
      meals because food may affect
      absorption rate.
   f. Instruct the client to immediately report
      sore throat, fever, skin rash, and swelling
      of cervical lymph nodes to the physician
      (potential for agranulocytosis).
   g. Instruct the client not to use over-the-
      counter (OTC) drugs for asthma, coryza,
      and cough because these drugs contain
      iodine, which is contraindicated.
   h. Instruct the client to take the pulse daily.
7. TYPES
   a. Propylthiouracil (Propyl-Thyracil; PTU)
   b. Methimazole (Tapazole)
D. IODINE AND IODIDE COMPOUNDS
   1. USES
      a. Iodine or iodide compounds are often
         given in conjunction with antithyroid
         drugs to decrease the release and
         syntheses of thyroid hormones and
         reduce the vascularity and size of the
         thyroid gland prior to a thyroidectomy.
      b. Iodine or iodide compounds cause
         thyroid hormones to be stored in the
         thyroid gland rather than being
         released into the circulation.
      c. Radioactive iodine I^{123} and I^{131} destroy
         overactive thyroid cells and are used
         primarily in treating hyperthyroidism
         in older adult clients.
      d. Iodine and iodide compounds reduce
         the metabolic rate more quickly than
         antithyroid medications but their
         action is not as sustained.

   e. Iodine and iodide compounds are
      usually given after a course of
      prophythiouracil (Propyl-Thyracil) to
      prepare the client for surgery. If given
      before treatment with PTU, the client
      may have an exacerbation of
      hyperthyroidism.
   2. ADVERSE REACTIONS
      a. Diarrhea
      b. Hypothyroidism
      c. Hypersensitivity
      d. Iodine poisoning (iodism)
   3. CONTRADICTIONS AND PRECAUTIONS
      a. Hypersensitivity to iodine
      b. Additive hypothyroidism with lithium
      c. Increases the antithyroid effect of
         antithyroid agents
   4. DRUG INTERACTIONS
      a. Lithium: additive hypothyroidism
      b. Antithyroid drugs: increase antithyroid
         effects
      c. Potassium iodide combined with
         potassium-sparing diuretics,
         angiotensin-converting-enzyme (ACE)
         inhibitors, or potassium supplements:
         increase hyperkalemia
   5. NURSING INTERVENTIONS
      a. Instruct the client to take with meals in
         water or fruit juice or at bedtime with
         food or juice.
      b. Instruct the client to always drink the
         medication through a straw to prevent
         staining the teeth.
      c. Avoid giving with milk because dairy
         products decrease absorption.
      d. Instruct the client to report any
         gastrointestinal (GI) bleeding,
         abdominal pain, distention, nausea,
         or vomiting.
      e. Instruct the client to avoid use of OTC
         drugs such as cough syrups, gargles,
         expectorants, bronchodilators, salt
         substitutes, cod liver oil, and multiple
         vitamins because they often contain
         iodide solutions.
      f. Instruct the client to report a metallic
         taste, stomatitis, swollen and tender
         salivary glands, skin lesions, and
         headache because they indicate iodism.
      g. Monitor for hypersensitivity reaction,
         including rash, pruritus, laryngeal
         edema, and wheezing.
      h. Monitor for clinical manifestations of
         hyperthyroidism, including
         tachycardia, palpitations, nervousness,
         insomnia, diaphoresis, heat
         intolerance, tremors, and weight loss.
   6. TYPES
      a. Potassium iodide (Pima, SSKI)
      b. Lugol's solution

IV. DRUGS FOR PARATHYROID DISORDERS

A. DESCRIPTION

1. THE PARATHYROID GLANDS SECRETE THE HORMONE PARATHORMONE, WHICH REGULATES CALCIUM AND PHOSPHORUS METABOLISM.
2. INCREASED SECRETIONS OF PARATHORMONE INCREASE SERUM CALCIUM LEVELS BY INCREASING THE ABSORPTION OF CALCIUM FROM THE KIDNEYS, INTESTINES, AND BONES.
3. LOW SERUM CALCIUM LEVELS STIMULATE THE RELEASE OF PARATHORMONE.
4. VITAMIN D ENHANCES THE ACTION OF PARATHORMONE.
5. INCREASED SECRETIONS OF PARATHORMONE DECREASE SERUM PHOSPHORUS LEVELS.
6. THE MOST COMMON CONDITION IS A DEFICIENCY OF PARATHORMONE (HYPOPARATHYROIDISM), WHICH OCCURS AS A RESULT OF INTERRUPTED BLOOD SUPPLY TO THE GLANDS OR SURGICAL REMOVAL OF GLAND TISSUE DURING A THYROIDECTOMY, PARATHYROIDECTOMY, OR RADICAL NECK DISSECTION.
7. PARENTERAL PARATHORMONE CAN BE ADMINISTERED TO TREAT ACUTE HYPOPARATHYROIDISM WITH TETANY, BUT THERE IS A HIGH INCIDENCE OF ALLERGIC REACTION TO PARATHORMONE.

B. CALCIUM SUPPLEMENTS

1. USES
   a. Calcium gluconate IV is the first choice for increasing serum calcium levels in tetany.
   b. Calcium salts are given orally in chronic conditions to supplement a high-calcium/low-phosphorus diet.
   c. Aluminum hydroxide gel or aluminum carbonate (Gelusil, Amphojel) is given with calcium salts to bind phosphate and promote its elimination by the GI tract.
   d. Vitamin D is given to enhance absorption of calcium from the GI tract.
2. ADVERSE REACTIONS
   a. Hypotension
   b. Syncope
   c. Bradycardia, arrhythmias, cardiac arrest
   d. Hypercalciuria, calculi
3. CONTRAINDICATIONS AND PRECAUTIONS
   a. Hypercalcemia
   b. Renal calculi
   c. Ventricular fibrillation
   d. Hypercalcemia increases the risk of cardiac glycoside toxicity.
4. DRUG INTERACTIONS
   a. Thiazide diuretics: increase risk of hypercalcemia
5. NURSING INTERVENTIONS
   a. Administer IV calcium at a slow rate through a small-bore needle into a large vein to avoid extravasation.
   b. Assess the IV site for patency. Extravasation may cause cellulitis, necrosis, and sloughing.
   c. Slow the rate of IV calcium to avoid a drop in BP and cardiac arrest.
   d. Instruct the client to remain recumbent for 30–60 minutes following IV administration.
   e. Monitor for clinical manifestations of hypercalcemia and hypocalcemia.
   f. Monitor the BP, pulse, and electrocardiogram (ECG) at frequent intervals during therapy.
   g. Monitor the client on cardiac glycosides for signs of toxicity.
   h. Monitor calcium, chloride, sodium, potassium, magnesium, and albumin periodically.
   i. Instruct the client in clinical manifestations of hypocalcemia—such as paresthesia, muscle twitching, laryngospasm, and cardiac arrhythmia—and hypercalcemia—such as nausea, vomiting, anorexia, thirst, severe constipation, paralytic ileus, and bradycardia—and to report any changes to the physician promptly.
   j. Instruct the client in calcium-rich food sources such as milk, milk products, dark green vegetables, soybeans, and tofu.
   k. Instruct the client that calcium absorption may be inhibited by foods high in zinc, such as nuts, seeds, sprouts, and legumes.
   l. Instruct the client to take oral calcium at least 1 hour after meals.
6. TYPES
   a. Calcium salts
   b. Calcium acetate
   c. Calcium carbonate
   d. Calcium chloride
   e. Calcium citrate
   f. Calcium glubionate
   g. Calcium gluceptate
   h. Calcium gluconate
   i. Calcium lactate
   j. Tricalcium phosphate

V. DRUGS FOR ADRENAL DISORDERS

A. DESCRIPTION

1. THE ADRENAL CORTEX SECRETES CORTICOSTEROIDS AND THE ADRENAL MEDULLA SECRETES CATECHOLAMINES.
2. THE PITUITARY GLAND SECRETES ACTH, WHICH ACTS ON THE ADRENAL CORTEX

TO SECRETE THE GLUCOCORTICOID HORMONE (CORTISOL).

3. HORMONES PRODUCED BY THE ADRENAL CORTEX INCLUDE GLUCOCORTICOIDS (MAINLY HYDROCORTISONE), MINERALOCORTICOIDS (MAINLY ALDOSTERONE), AND ANDROGENS (MALE SEX HORMONES).

4. GLUCOCORTICOIDS INFLUENCE GLUCOSE METABOLISM, THEREBY HAVING A WIDESPREAD EFFECT ON THE BODY.

5. MINERALOCORTICOIDS HAVE A MAJOR EFFECT ON FLUID AND ELECTROLYTE BALANCE.

6. ANDROGENS AFFECT THE SECONDARY SEX CHARACTERISTICS (MASCULINIZATION) WHEN SECRETED IN EXCESS.

7. THE MAJOR CONDITION OF HYPERSECRETION OF ADRENAL CORTEX HORMONES IS CUSHING'S SYNDROME.

8. THE MAJOR CONDITION OF HYPERSECRETION OF ADRENAL CORTEX MINERALOCORTICOIDS IS PRIMARY ALDOSTERONISM.

9. THE MAJOR CONDITION OF HYPOSECRETION OF ADRENAL CORTEX GLUCOCORTICOIDS AND MINERALOCORTICOID IS ADDISON'S DISEASE.

B. USES

1. GLUCOCORTICOIDS ARE USED TO SUPPLY ADRENAL CORTEX HORMONES WHEN THERE IS ADRENOCORTICAL INSUFFICIENCY IN CONDITIONS SUCH AS ADRENAL ATROPHY, AUTOIMMUNE RESPONSE, INFECTION, OR SURGICAL REMOVAL OF THE ADRENAL GLANDS.

2. GLUCOCORTICOIDS IN THE FORM OF CORTICOSTEROIDS ARE GIVEN TO INHIBIT THE INFLAMMATORY RESPONSE WHEN THERE IS TISSUE INJURY AND TO SUPPRESS ALLERGIC RESPONSES.

3. MINERALOCORTICOIDS PROMOTE SODIUM ION ABSORPTION AND POTASSIUM OR HYDROGEN ION EXCRETION BY THE KIDNEYS AND GI TRACT, THUS RESTORING NORMAL BLOOD PRESSURE.

C. ADVERSE REACTIONS OF GLUCOCORTICOIDS

1. HYPERGLYCEMIA
2. HYPOKALEMIA
3. OSTEOPOROSIS
4. PEPTIC ULCERATION
5. MUSCLE WASTING
6. POOR WOUND HEALING
7. REDISTRIBUTION OF BODY FAT
8. MOOD SWINGS
9. HIRSUTISM, ACNE
10. HYPERTENSION
11. NAUSEA, VOMITING, ANOREXIA
12. ECCHYMOSIS, FRAGILITY, PETECHIAE

D. CONTRAINDICATIONS AND PRECAUTIONS OF GLUCOCORTICOIDS

1. ACTIVE UNTREATED INFECTIONS (MASKS SIGNS OF INFECTION SUCH AS FEVER OR INFLAMMATION)

2. HYPOKALEMIA MAY INCREASE THE RISK OF CARDIAC GLYCOSIDE TOXICITY.

E. DRUG INTERACTIONS

1. INSULIN OR HYPOGLYCEMIC AGENT: MAY INCREASE NEED FOR INSULIN OR HYPOGLYCEMIC AGENT

2. DIURETICS, AMPHOTERICIN B, TICARCILLIN (TICAR): MAY RESULT IN ADDITIVE HYPOKALEMIA

3. NONSTEROIDAL ANTI-INFLAMMATORY DRUGS (NSAIDs), ASPIRIN, OR ALCOHOL: INCREASE RISK OF GASTROINTESTINAL EFFECTS

F. NURSING INTERVENTIONS

1. INSTRUCT THE CLIENT TO TAKE WITH FOOD OR FLUID TO REDUCE GASTRIC IRRITATION.

2. MONITOR FOR CLINICAL MANIFESTATIONS OF CUSHING'S SYNDROME, ESPECIALLY WHEN ON LONG-TERM THERAPY.

3. ASSESS VITAL SIGNS, INTAKE AND OUTPUT, WEIGHT, AND SLEEP PATTERNS.

4. MONITOR BLOOD GLUCOSE LEVEL FOR HYPERGLYCEMIA.

5. INSTRUCT THE CLIENT TO AVOID ALTERING THE DOSE OR STOPPING THERAPY ABRUPTLY.

6. MONITOR FOR THE POSSIBILITY OF MASKED INFECTION AND DELAYED HEALING.

7. ASSESS THE CLIENT FOR SIGNS OF INFECTION.

8. INFORM THE CLIENT THAT SLIGHT WEIGHT GAIN AND INCREASE IN APPETITE ARE EXPECTED AT THE BEGINNING OF THERAPY, BUT IF THE CLIENT GAINS 5 LB OR MORE AFTER WEIGHT IS STABILIZED, THE PHYSICIAN SHOULD BE NOTIFIED.

9. INSTRUCT THE CLIENT TO AVOID ALCOHOL AND CAFFEINE, WHICH MAY CONTRIBUTE TO STEROID ULCER DEVELOPMENT IN LONG-TERM THERAPY.

10. INSTRUCT THE CLIENT TO EAT FOODS HIGH IN POTASSIUM.
11. INFORM THE CLIENT NOT TO USE ASPIRIN OR OTHER OTC DRUGS UNLESS PRESCRIBED BY THE PHYSICIAN.
12. INSTRUCT THE CLIENT TO CARRY MEDICAL IDENTIFICATION INFORMATION AT ALL TIMES.
13. INSTRUCT THE CLIENT THAT LONG-ACTING GLUCOCORTICOIDS SHOULD NEVER BE ABRUPTLY DISCONTINUED.
14. ADMINISTERING SUPPLEMENTAL DOSES MAY BE NECESSARY FOR STRESS, SURGERY, INFECTION, OR INJURY.

G. ADVERSE REACTIONS OF MINERALOCORTICOIDS
1. THROMBOEMBOLISM OR FAT EMBOLISM
2. HYPERGLYCEMIA
3. SODIUM AND FLUID RETENTION
4. HYPOKALEMIA
5. HYPOCALCEMIA
6. HYPERSENSITIVITY
7. OSTEOPOROSIS
8. IMPAIRED WOUND HEALING
9. WEIGHT GAIN, INCREASED APPETITE
10. MOOD SWINGS

H. CONTRAINDICATIONS AND PRECAUTIONS OF MINERALOCORTICOIDS
1. HYPERSENSITIVITY TO GLUCOCORTICOIDS
2. ACUTE GLOMERULONEPHRITIS
3. VIRAL OR BACTERIAL DISEASES OF SKIN INFECTIONS NOT CONTROLLED BY ANTIBIOTICS
4. SMALLPOX VACCINATION OR OTHER IMMUNOLOGIC PROCEDURES

I. DRUG INTERACTIONS
1. INSULIN AND SULFONYLUREAS: MAY DIMINISH THE ANTIDIABETIC EFFECTS OF INSULIN AND SULFONYLUREAS
2. DIURETICS: INCREASE POTASSIUM LOSS
3. WARFARIN (COUMADIN): CONCURRENT USE WITH WARFARIN MAY DECREASE PROTHROMBIN TIME.

J. NURSING INTERVENTIONS
1. MONITOR FOR SIGNS OF HYPOKALEMIA AND HYPERKALEMIC METABOLIC ALKALOSIS.
2. MONITOR BP, I & O, AND WEIGHT.
3. INSTRUCT THE CLIENT TO BE ALERT FOR SIGNS OF POTASSIUM LOSS ASSOCIATED WITH HIGH-SODIUM INTAKE, SUCH AS MUSCLE WEAKNESS, PARESTHESIA, POLYURIA, DIMINISHED REFLEXES, ARRHYTHMIAS, CARDIAC FAILURE, NAUSEA, AND ANOREXIA.
4. INSTRUCT THE CLIENT THAT SODIUM INTAKE MAY REQUIRE RESTRICTIONS AND THAT ANY SIGNS OF FLUID RETENTION SHOULD BE REPORTED TO THE PHYSICIAN.
5. INSTRUCT THE CLIENT TO WEIGH DAILY AND REPORT ANY GAIN OF 5 LB OR MORE PER WEEK.
6. INFORM THE CLIENT THAT POTASSIUM MAY BE INCREASED IN THE DIET, OR SUPPLEMENTAL POTASSIUM MAY BE NEEDED DURING TREATMENT.
7. INSTRUCT THE CLIENT TO NOTIFY THE PHYSICIAN OF INFECTION, TRAUMA, OR STRESS.

K. TYPES OF ADRENOCORTICOSTEROIDS
1. BETAMETHASONE
2. CORTISONE
3. DEXAMETHASONE
4. FLUDROCORTISONE—POTENT MINERALOCORTICOID
5. HYDROCORTISONE
6. METHYLPREDNISOLONE
7. PREDNISOLONE
8. PREDNISONE
9. TRIAMCINOLONE

L. ADVERSE REACTIONS OF ANDROGENS
1. HYPERCALCEMIA
2. HYPERCHOLESTEROLEMIA
3. SODIUM AND WATER RETENTION WITH EDEMA
4. RENAL CALCULI
5. INCREASED LIBIDO
6. HYPERSENSITIVITY
7. PRIAPISM
8. GYNECOMASTIA
9. MENSTRUAL IRREGULARITIES
10. FEMALE VIRILIZATION
11. HEPATIC TOXICITY

M. CONTRAINDICATIONS AND PRECAUTIONS
1. HYPERSENSITIVITY
2. CARDIAC, HEPATIC, OR RENAL DISEASE
3. PROSTATE OR BREAST CANCER IN MEN
4. BENIGN PROSTATIC HYPERTROPHY WITH OBSTRUCTION
5. PREPUBERTAL MALES OR OLDER ADULT CLIENTS

N. DRUG INTERACTIONS
1. ORAL ANTICOAGULANTS: MAY CAUSE BLEEDING
2. INSULIN: MAY DECREASE INSULIN DOSAGE IN CLIENTS WITH DIABETES MELLITUS

O. NURSING INTERVENTIONS
1. ASSESS I & O AND WEIGHT DAILY DURING THE DOSE STABILIZATION PERIOD.
2. ONCE STABILIZED, INSTRUCT THE CLIENT TO CHECK WEIGHT AT LEAST TWO TIMES PER WEEK AND NOTIFY THE PHYSICIAN OF AN INCREASE OF MORE THAN 5 LB PER WEEK.

3. INSTRUCT THE CLIENT TO ASSESS FOR EDEMA, ESPECIALLY DEPENDENT EDEMA.
4. INFORM THE CLIENT OF THE IMPORTANCE OF PERIODIC LAB WORK TO MONITOR SERUM CHOLESTEROL AND CALCIUM AND CARDIAC AND LIVER FUNCTION.
5. INSTRUCT THE CLIENT TO TAKE THE DRUG WITH FOOD.
6. MONITOR THE CLIENT FOR HYPERCALCEMIA, HYPOGLYCEMIA, OR BLEEDING TENDENCIES AND NOTIFY THE PHYSICIAN IF THEY DEVELOP.
7. INSTRUCT A MALE CLIENT TO REPORT PRIAPISM (SUSTAINED AND POSSIBLY PAINFUL ERECTIONS), REDUCED EJACULATORY VOLUME, AND GYNECOMASTIA.
8. INSTRUCT THE FEMALE CLIENT TO REPORT IF SHE IS PREGNANT OR PLANNING A PREGNANCY BECAUSE MASCULINIZATION OF THE FETUS IS POSSIBLE DURING THE FIRST TRIMESTER.
9. INSTRUCT A FEMALE CLIENT RECEIVING HIGH DOSES IN BREAST CANCER TREATMENT TO REPORT ANY MANIFESTATIONS OF VIRILIZATION.
10. INSTRUCT THE FEMALE CLIENT TO USE NONHORMONAL CONTRACEPTIVE DEVICES DURING TREATMENT PERIOD.
11. DISCONTINUE THERAPY IF SERUM CALCIUM RISES ABOVE 14 MG/DL.

P. TYPES
1. FLUOXYMESTERONE
2. TESTOSTERONE

VI. DRUGS FOR DIABETES MELLITUS
A. DESCRIPTION
1. INSULIN IS PRODUCED BY THE BETA CELLS IN THE ISLETS OF LANGERHANS IN THE PANCREAS AND HAS A KEY ROLE IN THE METABOLISM OF CARBOHYDRATES, FAT, AND PROTEIN BY:
   a. Stimulating the active transport of glucose into muscle and adipose tissue cells
   b. Regulating the rate at which carbohydrates are burned by the cells for energy
   c. Promoting the conversion of glucose to glycogen for storage in the liver
   d. Promoting the conversion of fatty acids into fat, which can be stored as adipose tissue
   e. Promoting conversion of amino acids to proteins in muscle
   f. Promoting intracellular shifts of potassium and magnesium
2. THE RATE OF INSULIN SECRETION IS REGULATED BY BLOOD GLUCOSE LEVELS.
3. ORAL ANTIDIABETIC AGENTS INCLUDE THE SULFONYLUREAS, BIGUANIDES, ALPHA GLUCOSIDASE INHIBITORS, THIAZOLIDINEDIONES, AND MEGLITINIDES.
4. ORAL ANTIDIABETIC AGENTS ARE CATEGORIZED AS FIRST- AND SECOND-GENERATION DRUGS AND NONSULFONYLUREAS (SEE TABLE 21-1).
5. GLUCAGON IS SECRETED BY THE ALPHA CELLS FROM THE ISLETS OF LANGERHANS IN THE PANCREAS AND STIMULATES HEPATIC PRODUCTION OF GLUCOSE FROM GLYCOGEN STORES.

B. USES
1. INSULIN IS USED AS A HORMONE REPLACEMENT IN THE TREATMENT OF CLIENTS WITH TYPE 1 DIABETES MELLITUS WHO ARE UNABLE TO PRODUCE INSULIN.
2. ANTIDIABETIC AGENTS ARE USED IN THE TREATMENT OF CLIENTS WITH TYPE 2 DIABETES MELLITUS WHO PRODUCE AN INSUFFICIENT AMOUNT OF INSULIN.
3. ANTIDIABETIC AGENTS IMPROVE INSULIN ACTION AT THE CELLULAR LEVEL.
4. GLUCAGON, A HYPERGLYCEMIA AGENT, IS USED IN THE ACUTE MANAGEMENT OF SEVERE HYPOGLYCEMIA WHEN ADMINISTRATION OF GLUCOSE IS NOT FEASIBLE.

C. ADVERSE REACTIONS OF INSULIN
1. HYPOGLYCEMIA
2. COMA
3. LIPOATROPHY AND LIPOHYPERTROPHY OF THE INJECTION SITE
4. LOCAL ALLERGIC REACTION AT THE INJECTION SITE
5. INSULIN RESISTANCE
6. ALLERGIC REACTION, INCLUDING ANAPHYLAXIS

D. CONTRAINDICATIONS AND PRECAUTIONS OF INSULIN
1. HYPERSENSITIVITY TO A PARTICULAR TYPE OF INSULIN

E. DRUG INTERACTIONS
1. ALCOHOL: HYPOGLYCEMIC EFFECTS
2. SALICYLATES: HYPOGLYCEMIC EFFECTS
3. EPINEPHRINE: DECREASES THE EFFECTIVENESS OF INSULIN AS A RESULT OF EPINEPHRINE-INDUCED HYPERGLYCEMIA
4. FUROSEMIDE (LASIX) AND THIAZIDE DIURETICS: HYPOGLYCEMIC EFFECTS
5. PROPRANOLOL (INDERAL): INHIBITS REBOUND OF BLOOD GLUCOSE AFTER INSULIN-INDUCED HYPOGLYCEMIA
6. CORTICOSTEROIDS: DECREASE EFFECT OF INSULIN AS A RESULT OF CORTICOSTEROID-INDUCED HYPERGLYCEMIA

Table 21-1 Types of Oral Hypoglycemic Drugs

Generic Name (Trade Name)	Usual Daily Dose	Action	Major Adverse Reactions, Precautions, Contraindications
First-generation sulfonylureas		First- and second-generation sulfonylureas act by directly stimulating the pancreas to secrete insulin. They also improve the action of the insulin at the cellular level. Second-generation sulfonylureas are preferred for the older adult because they have a shorter half-life and are excreted more rapidly, preventing prolonged hypoglycemia.	First- and second-generation sulfonylureas can cause gastrointestinal manifestations, dermatologic reactions, and prolonged hypoglycemia.
Short-acting Tolbutamide (Orinase)	500–2,000 mg		
Intermediate-acting Acetohexamide (Dymelor)	250–1,500 mg		
Tolazamide (Tolinase)	100–750 mg		
Long-acting Chlorpropamide (Diabenese)	100–500 mg		An additional adverse reaction of chlorpropamide (Diabenese) is an Antabuse-type reaction when alcohol is ingested.
Second-generation sulfonylureas			
Glipizide (Glucotrol)	5–25 mg		
Glipizide XL (Glucotrol XL)	5 mg		
Glyburide (Micronase)	2.5–10 mg		
Glimepride (Amaryl)	1–2 mg		
Nonsulfonylureas			
Biguanides		Biguanides facilitate the action of insulin on peripheral receptor sites.	Lactic acidosis. May interact with anticoagulants, corticosteroids, diuretics, and contraceptives. Should not be administered when severe renal impairment is present.
Metformin (Glucophage)	1,500 mg		
Alpha glucosidase inhibitors		Alpha glucosidase inhibitors delay the absorption of glucose in the GI tract, lowering the postprandial blood glucose level.	Diarrhea and flatulence. Must be taken immediately before a meal. If hypoglycemia occurs, the client must take glucose.
Acarbose (Precose)	1,500 mg		May affect liver function. May cause ovulation in perimenopausal anovulatory women.
Thiazolininediones			
Troglitazone (Rezulin)	200–400 mg	Thiazolininediones in conjunction with insulin at the receptor sites without increasing the secretion of insulin from the beta cells.	
Rosiglitazone (Avandia)	4–8 mg		Cardiac effects. Carries Black Box Warning that increases the risk of heart attack.
Meglitinides			Hypoglycemia. Dose must be followed by a meal.
Repaglinide (Prandin)	0.5–4 mg	Meglitinides lower the blood glucose level by stimulating beta cells to release insulin.	

7. GUANETHIDINE: HYPOGLYCEMIC EFFECT
8. MONAMINE OXIDASE (MAO) INHIBITORS: HYPOGLYCEMIC EFFECT
9. FENFLURAMINE: ADDITIVE HYPOGLYCEMIC EFFECT
10. TETRACYCLINES: HYPOGLYCEMIC EFFECT
11. THYROID PREPARATIONS: DECREASE EFFECT OF ANTIDIABETIC DUE TO THYROID-INDUCED HYPERGLYCEMIA
12. ESTROGENS: DECREASE EFFECT OF INSULIN DUE TO IMPAIRMENT OF GLUCOSE TOLERANCE
13. DOBUTAMINE: DECREASES EFFECT OF INSULIN

F. TYPES (SEE TABLE 21-2)
G. NURSING INTERVENTIONS
1. MONITOR BLOOD GLUCOSE FREQUENTLY WHEN THERAPY IS INITIATED AND ROUTINELY WHEN STABILIZED.
2. MONITOR FOR SIGNS OF HYPOGLYCEMIA AT PEAK TIME OF INSULIN, SUCH AS APPREHENSION, CHILLS, PERSPIRATION, CONFUSION, DOUBLE VISION, DROWSINESS, INABILITY TO CONCENTRATE, NAUSEA, RAPID PULSE, AND SHAKINESS.
3. MONITOR FOR SIGNS OF HYPERGLYCEMIA, SUCH AS DROWSINESS, FLUSHED SKIN, ACETONE BREATH (FRUITY ODOR), POLYURIA, POLYDIPSIA, AND ANOREXIA.
4. MONITOR WEIGHT AT FREQUENT INTERVALS. AN INCREASE OR DECREASE IN WEIGHT MAY AFFECT INSULIN REQUIREMENTS.
5. CHECK THE TYPE, SOURCE, DOSE, AND EXPIRATION DATE OF THE INSULIN WITH ANOTHER NURSE PRIOR TO ADMINISTRATION.
6. GIVE ONLY THE ORDERED TYPE OF INSULIN. DO NOT INTERCHANGE INSULINS, WITHOUT A PHYSICIAN'S ORDER.
7. USE ONLY INSULIN SYRINGES THAT ARE CALIBRATED IN UNITS.
8. BEFORE WITHDRAWING THE INSULIN, ROTATE THE VIAL BETWEEN THE PALMS OF THE HANDS TO ENSURE THE MEDICATION IS MIXED INTO THE SOLUTION. DO NOT SHAKE THE VIAL.

Table 21-2 Types of Insulin

Type	Agent	Onset	Peak	Duration	Comments
Rapid acting	Humalog	10–15 minutes	1 hour	3 hours	Given for rapid reduction of glucose level Also given to aid nocturnal hypoglycemia
Short acting	Humulin R Novolin R Iletin I Semilente	½–1 hour	2–3 hours	4–6 hours	Usually administered 30 minutes before a meal Requires multiple injections per day when used alone Often used in combination with intermediate-acting or long-acting insulin
Intermediate acting	Humulin N Iletin II NPH NPH Lente Novolin L	3–4 hours	4–12 hours	16–24 hours	Important that food be taken near peak time
Long acting	Humulin U Ultralente Ultralente Iletin	6–8 hours	12–16 hours	20–30 hours	Important to have a snack prior to retiring These insulins have a long, slow, sustained action rather than sharp peaks.
Insulin mixtures	30% regular plus 70% NPH Humulin 70/30 Novolin 70/30	½–1 hour	2–12 hours	18–24 hours	Premixed insulins with a combination of short-acting and long-acting insulins
	25% regular lispro 75% insulin lispro protamine Humalog Mix 75/25 50% regular and 50% NPH	15–30 minutes	1–1.65 hours	Up to 24 hours	
	Humulin 50/50	30–60 minutes	2–5.5 hours	18–24 hours	

9. WHEN MIXING TWO INSULINS, DRAW UP THE REGULAR INSULIN DOSE FIRST. THIS PREVENTS CONTAMINATION OF THE REGULAR INSULIN.

10. INSULIN SHOULD BE KEPT IN A COOL PLACE AND DOES NOT NEED REFRIGERATION. OPENED VIALS SHOULD NOT BE USED AFTER 30 DAYS.

11. REGULAR INSULIN IS THE ONLY INSULIN THAT CAN BE ADMINISTERED IV. THE SOLUTION IN THE VIAL SHOULD BE CLEAR, NOT CLOUDY.

12. REGULAR INSULIN MAY BE ADMINISTERED DIRECT IV UNDILUTED OR DILUTED IN COMMONLY USED IV SOLUTIONS; HOWEVER, INSULIN POTENCY MAY BE REDUCED BY PLASTIC OR GLASS ADMINISTRATION SYSTEMS.

13. REGULAR INSULIN MAY BE ADMINISTERED UP TO 50 UNITS OVER 1 MINUTE. WHEN THE BLOOD GLUCOSE LEVEL REACHES 250 MG/ 100 ML, THE RATE SHOULD BE DECREASED.

14. MONITOR BP, INTAKE AND OUTPUT, BLOOD GLUCOSE, AND URINE KETONES EVERY HOUR WHEN ADMINISTERING IV INSULIN IN TREATMENT OF KETOACIDOSIS.

15. ADMINISTER GLUCAGON, EPINEPHRINE, OR IV GLUCOSE 10–50% IF THE CLIENT IS UNRESPONSIVE DURING HYPOGLYCEMIA REACTION.

16. INSTRUCT THE CLIENT AND FAMILY ON TECHNIQUES OF INSULIN ADMINISTRATION. INCLUDE THE TYPE OF INSULIN; EQUIPMENT; ROTATION OF THE VIAL, IF NECESSARY, PRIOR TO DRAWING UP; INJECTION SITES (ABDOMEN, POSTERIOR ARMS, ANTERIOR THIGHS, AND HIPS); ROTATION OF SITES TO PREVENT LIPODYSTROPHY; INJECTION INTO SUBCUTANEOUS TISSUE AT 45° OR 90° ANGLE; AND STORAGE OF VIALS.

17. INSTRUCT THE CLIENT AND FAMILY THAT ROTATION OF SITES SHOULD BE SYSTEMATIC AND THE SITE SHOULD NOT BE USED AGAIN FOR A 2- TO 3-WEEK PERIOD.

18. INSTRUCT THE CLIENT AND FAMILY THAT INJECTIONS SHOULD BE 1.5 INCHES APART.

19. INSTRUCT THE CLIENT AND FAMILY ON THE CLINICAL MANIFESTATIONS OF HYPOGLYCEMIA AND HYPERGLYCEMIA AND HOW TO TREAT THESE CONDITIONS SHOULD THEY OCCUR. ADVISE THE CLIENT TO CARRY A SOURCE OF SUGAR AND IDENTIFICATION AT ALL TIMES.

20. INSTRUCT THE CLIENT AND FAMILY THAT HEAT, MASSAGE, AND EXERCISE MAY INCREASE THE ABSORPTION RATE OF INSULIN, RESULTING IN A HYPOGLYCEMIC REACTION.

21. INSTRUCT THE CLIENT NOT TO CHANGE BRANDS OF INSULIN OR SYRINGES ONCE STABILIZED.

22. INSTRUCT THE CLIENT IN THE TECHNIQUE OF BLOOD GLUCOSE MONITORING AND THAT IF THE CLIENT IS EXPERIENCING STRESS OR AN ILLNESS, BLOOD GLUCOSE MONITORING SHOULD BE DONE MORE FREQUENTLY AND THE PHYSICIAN SHOULD BE NOTIFIED OF ANY DEVIATIONS FROM THE USUAL RESULTS.

23. INSTRUCT THE CLIENT OF THE NEED TO STRICTLY ADHERE TO THE DIET AND EXERCISE PROGRAM AS DIRECTED BY THE PHYSICIAN.

24. INSTRUCT THE CLIENT AND FAMILY IN THE CORRECT TECHNIQUE TO PREPARE, DRAW UP, AND ADMINISTER GLUCAGON BY SUBCUTANEOUS INJECTION SHOULD THE CLIENT BE UNRESPONSIVE IF HYPOGLYCEMIA OCCURS.

25. INSTRUCT THE CLIENT AND FAMILY THAT BLOOD GLUCOSE SHOULD RISE APPROXIMATELY 5 MINUTES AFTER THE ADMINISTRATION OF GLUCAGON. IF THERE IS NO RESPONSE IN 20 MINUTES, THEY SHOULD SEEK EMERGENCY ASSISTANCE.

26. INFORM THE FAMILY THAT THE CLIENT SHOULD RECEIVE A FORM OF ORAL GLUCOSE WHEN CONSCIOUSNESS RETURNS.

27. INFORM THE CLIENT AND FAMILY THAT THE MOST IMPORTANT KEYS TO SUCCESS IN MANAGING DIABETES ARE COMPLIANCE IN TAKING THE MEDICATION AS PRESCRIBED AND STRICTLY ADHERING TO A DIET AND EXERCISE PROGRAM.

PRACTICE QUESTIONS

1. Which of the following should the nurse include in the instructions given to a client receiving somatropin (Humatrope)?
   1. Get an annual bone age assessment
   2. Schedule a fasting blood sugar once a year if there is a family history of diabetes mellitus
   3. Record height weekly and report linear growth of 7 to 15 cm in the first year
   4. Notify the physician if urine output increases

2. Which of the following assessment findings is an anticipated outcome for a client with diabetes insipidus who is receiving vasopressin (Pitressin) injections?
   1. Urine output of 2500 ml/day
   2. Weight loss of 4 pounds in one week
   3. Urine specific gravity of 1.005
   4. Oral intake of 4500 ml/day

3. The nurse instructs a client in the use of lypressin (Diapid) for the treatment of diabetes insipidus. Which of the following adverse reactions are appropriate to include in the instructions? Select all that apply:
   [ ] 1. Pain at injection site
   [ ] 2. Syncope
   [ ] 3. Hypertension
   [ ] 4. Rhinopharyngitis
   [ ] 5. Headache
   [ ] 6. Drowsiness

4. The client starting on vasopressin asks the nurse, "Why did the physician say to avoid drinking alcohol while taking this medication?" Which of the following responses by the nurse is appropriate? "Alcohol will
   1. cause an increase in vasoconstriction."
   2. decrease the antidiuretic effect."
   3. interfere with the absorption of vasopressin in the stomach."
   4. promote a hypersensitivity to vasopressin."

5. The nurse reviews a list of which of the following first-generation sulfonylureas? Select all that apply:
   [ ] 1. Glipizide (Glucotrol)
   [ ] 2. Tolbutamide (Orinase)
   [ ] 3. Acarbose (Precose)
   [ ] 4. Tolazamide (Tolinase)
   [ ] 5. Chlorpropamide (Diabenese)
   [ ] 6. Rosiglitazone (Avandia)

6. Prior to discharge, the nurse instructs a client who is receiving liothyronine (Cytomel) to notify the physician if which of the following occurs?
   1. A pulse rate of more than 100 beats per minute

2. A weight loss of 5 pounds in 2 weeks
   3. More frequent urination
   4. Excessive sleepiness

7. The nurse instructs a client who is started on levothyroxine sodium (Synthroid) that the best time to take the medication is
   1. 1 hour after a meal.
   2. with a bedtime snack.
   3. 30 minutes before breakfast.
   4. once a day with any meal.

8. Which of the following is essential that the nurse include in the assessment of a client receiving methimazole (Tapazole)?
   1. Serum sodium levels
   2. White blood cell count and differential
   3. Platelet count
   4. Serum lipid levels

9. The nurse instructs a client who has been prescribed Lugol's solution to notify the physician if which of the following occurs?
   1. Blurred vision
   2. Weight gain
   3. Increased urinary output
   4. Brassy taste in mouth

10. When a client experiencing thyrotoxicosis arrives at the emergency room, the nurse should administer which of the following drugs intravenously?
    1. 50% dextrose
    2. Saturated solution of potassium iodide
    3. Calcium gluconate
    4. Theophylline

11. The nurse is caring for a client who developed tetany postoperatively. The client is to receive aluminum hydroxide gel (Gelusil) and calcium gluconate (Kalcinate). The nurse should understand that the client is to receive aluminum hydroxide gel (Gelusil) for which of the following purposes?
    1. To neutralize the hydrochloric acid in the stomach so that the calcium can be absorbed
    2. To coat the esophagus and stomach linings from the irritation of the calcium salts
    3. To bind dietary phosphorus and promote the elimination of insoluble aluminum phosphate by the GI tract
    4. To increase the rate of gastric emptying to enhance absorption of calcium in the small intestine

12. The nurse is collecting a health history from a client who is to begin taking calcium lactate. Which of the following questions should the

nurse ask to determine the safety of taking calcium supplements?
1. "Have you had any kidney stones within the past year?"
2. "Have you ever been told that you have high blood pressure?"
3. "Have you had any chest pains or a heart attack?"
4. "Have you had any problems with frequent diarrhea?"

13. A client with Addison's disease is scheduled for hernia surgery in the morning. Which of the following drugs should the nurse expect to give with a sip of water the morning of surgery?
1. Micronase
2. Prednisone
3. Synthroid
4. Furosemide (Lasix)

14. The nurse is caring for a client taking prednisone. The nurse should instruct the client that the best time to take the drug to promote absorption is
1. at bedtime with a full glass of water.
2. on an empty stomach.
3. in the morning with breakfast.
4. 2 hours after a meal.

15. The nurse should monitor which of the following laboratory reports for a client receiving long-term corticosteroid therapy?
1. Magnesium and calcium
2. Cholesterol and sodium
3. Hemoglobin and hematocrit
4. Glucose and potassium

16. The nurse should monitor a client who has been taking fludrocortisone acetate for several months for which of the following adverse reactions of this drug?
1. Pedal edema
2. Hyperkalemia
3. Episodes of hypoglycemia
4. Weight loss

17. The nurse should instruct a female client who has been prescribed testosterone to notify the physician if which of the following is experienced?
1. Irregular menses
2. Decreased libido
3. Engorged breasts
4. Low-pitched voice

18. The nurse should assess a client who received Humulin N insulin at 0730 for hypoglycemia at
1. 2000 hours.
2. 1600 hours.
3. 2400 hours.
4. 1000 hours.

19. Which of the following should the nurse include in the medication instructions for a client taking chlorpropamide (Diabinese)?
1. Avoid drinking alcohol
2. Take on an empty stomach each morning
3. Take once a day at bedtime with milk or juice
4. Avoid food products that contain aspartame (NutraSweet)

20. Which of the following should the nurse include in the insulin administration instructions for a client being discharged on insulin?
1. Inject into the extremity to be exercised to enhance absorption
2. The muscles in the abdomen and thigh are the easiest to use for self-administration
3. Insert the needle and then aspirate prior to injecting
4. Sites should be rotated systematically and not used again for 2 to 3 weeks

21. After administering 5 units of regular insulin per minute to a client in diabetic ketoacidosis, the nurse should add dextrose to the intravenous fluids when the blood glucose reaches which of the following levels?
1. 350 mg/dl
2. 300 mg/dl
3. 400 mg/dl
4. 450 mg/dl

22. After receiving blood glucose monitoring instructions from the nurse, which of the following client statements indicates an understanding of when more frequent monitoring is necessary?
1. "I should check my glucose level after each additional period of exercise."
2. "I will need to take more insulin and monitor my glucose more often when I go to the dentist."
3. "I should monitor my glucose more often when I am under stress."
4. "I will need to check my glucose level more frequently when I go on vacation."

23. The nurse instructs a type 1 diabetic client to avoid which of the following while taking insulin?
1. Furosemide (Lasix)
2. Dicumarol (Bishydroxycoumarin)
3. Reserpine (Serpasil)
4. Cimetidine (Tagamet)

24. The nurse should instruct the family of a diabetic client to administer glucagon by which of the following routes?
1. Sublingually
2. Rectally
3. Intravenously
4. Subcutaneously

25. The nurse instructs the family that after the administration of the drug glucagon, the client's blood sugar should begin to rise and the client should regain consciousness. The nurse should tell the family members to wait for how long for the client to respond before summoning emergency assistance?
    1. 4 minutes
    2. 20 minutes
    3. 30 minutes
    4. 40 minutes

26. The registered nurse is preparing to delegate the nursing tasks for the day. Which of the following nursing tasks should the nurse delegate to a licensed practical nurse?
    1. Administer intravenous insulin to a client in diabetic ketoacidosis
    2. Administer an oral calcium supplement 1 hour after meals
    3. Develop a medication schedule for a client with diabetes mellitus and congestive heart failure
    4. Assess a client taking iodine for signs of iodine poisoning

ANSWERS AND RATIONALES

1. 1. Somatropin (growth hormone) is given when there is growth failure prior to epiphyseal closure. Annual bone assessment is necessary to make certain that epiphyseal closure has not occurred. Growth hormone increases the glucose level in the blood, so that those with a family history of diabetes are likely to develop diabetes mellitus. Fasting blood sugars should be done more frequently than once a year to detect development of diabetes mellitus. Linear growth of 7 to 20 cm in the first year is normal and not necessary to report. Growth hormone does not affect urinary output.

2. 1. The client with diabetes insipidus who is receiving vasopressin injections should have an improvement in the clinical manifestations of diabetes insipidus (polyuria and polydipsia). The client should notice an increase in weight and a decrease in urine output. The urine output of 2500 ml is in the normal range. Urine specific gravity of 1.005 and an oral intake of 4500 ml/day are characteristic of untreated diabetes insipidus.

3. 3. 4. 5. 6. Lypressin (Diapid) is an antidiuretic hormone used to treat diabetes insipidus. It is only administered intranasally, not by injection. Adverse reactions include intranasal congestion, rhinorrhea, irritation, hypertension, headache, and drowsiness.

4. 2. Alcohol causes vasodilatation, not vasoconstriction, in a client taking vasopressin. Alcohol does decrease the antidiuretic effect of vasopressin from its action on the kidneys. Vasopressin is injected and absorbed intramuscularly. Hypersensitivity reactions occur with vasopressin, but are not related to the ingestion of alcohol.

5. 2. 4. 5. First-generation sulfonylureas include tolbutamide (Orinase), tolazamide (Tolinase), and chlorpropamide (Diabenese). Glipizide

(Glucotrol) is a second-generation. Acarbose (Precose) and rosiglitazone (Avandia) are nonsulfonylureas.

6. 1. Liothyronine (Cytomel) is a thyroid drug used in the treatment of hypothyroidism. It increases the metabolic rate, but a rate of more than 100 beats per minute is an indication that the dosage needs to be decreased. Weight loss and diuresis would be expected therapy outcomes. A client with hypothyroidism would be very lethargic and sleep most of the day. The activity level should increase as a response to the drug, and a nap during the day would improve the condition.

7. 3. Food interferes with the absorption of levothyroxine (Synthroid). The client should take the drug at the same time of day, preferably before breakfast.

8. 2. A serious adverse reaction to antithyroid drugs is agranulocytosis, a severe reduction in the number of granulocytes (basophils, eosinophils, and neutrophils). Antithyroid drugs do not affect serum sodium and lipid levels or platelet count.

9. 4. Clients receiving iodine preparations, such as Lugol's solution, are advised to notify the physician if they experience a brassy taste in the mouth, which may be significant for iodism (excessive amounts of iodine in the body). Blurred vision, weight gain, and increased urinary output are clinical manifestations of endocrine disorders, but are not attributed to iodine preparations.

10. 2. The client with thyrotoxicosis (thyroid storm) is experiencing severe hyperthyroidism. Saturated solution of potassium iodide is given IV, because it acts quickly to reduce the metabolic rate. Dextrose 50% is an emergency drug for the treatment of hypoglycemia. Calcium gluconate is used for hypoparathyroidism in clients who are

experiencing tetany. Theophylline is an emergency drug for clients experiencing breathing difficulties.

11. 3. Aluminum hydroxide gel (Gelusil) is given in conjunction with calcium gluconate to bind dietary phosphorus and promote the elimination of insoluble aluminum phosphate in the feces in a client who is experiencing tetany. The client with tetany has decreased serum calcium and an increase in serum phosphate levels. The neutralization of hydrochloric acid in the stomach does not affect the absorption of calcium. Calcium gluconate is not irritating to the mucosa of the esophagus and stomach. Aluminum hydroxide gel decreases, rather than increases, the rate of gastric emptying.

12. 1. Calcium salts cause an increase in serum calcium, which can lead to calcium deposits in the kidneys; therefore, calcium salts are contraindicated for the client with a history of renal calculi. A history of hypertension and myocardial infarction are not cardiovascular changes that would be contraindications. Calcium salts may cause constipation.

13. 2. The client with Addison's disease has a deficiency in glucocorticoids and mineralocorticoids. The treatment is lifelong replacement therapy with prednisone. Glucocorticoids must never be withdrawn abruptly and are therefore given the morning of surgery. A client receiving Micronase would have type 2 diabetes mellitus and the drug could be administered later in the day. A client receiving Synthroid for the treatment of hypothyroidism could also miss the morning dose without consequence. Furosemide (Lasix), a loop diuretic, would not be given to a client with Addison's disease because clients with Addison's disease have low sodium levels.

14. 3. Prednisone is irritating to the gastric mucosa and should be given with food or fluid in the morning with breakfast. The client needs the higher cortisol levels in the daytime, when one is more active. It should not be given on an empty stomach or 2 hours after a meal.

15. 4. Corticosteroids increase glucose metabolism (effect of glucocorticoids) and the absorption of sodium and elimination of potassium (effect of mineralocorticoids). Thus, clients receiving long-term corticosteroid therapy need to be monitored for increased blood glucose levels and low serum potassium. Corticosteroids do not affect calcium, magnesium, cholesterol levels, or hemoglobin and hematocrit levels.

16. 1. Fludrocortisone acetate, a mineralocorticoid, promotes sodium ion absorption and potassium ion excretion by the kidneys. A major side effect of the drug is sodium retention, which

would contribute to the development of pedal edema. Other adverse reactions are hypokalemia, hyperglycemia, and weight gain.

17. 4. Females receiving testosterone should notify the physician if any signs of virilism appear. Testosterone antagonizes the effects of estrogen on the endometrium, so that it is expected that menstruation will become irregular. It is also expected that libido will decrease. Testosterone is given to treat engorged breasts.

18. 2. Hypoglycemia occurs during the peak action time of specific insulin. Humulin N insulin peaks in 4 to 12 hours after administration. The peak time is too early at 1000 hours and too late at 2000 hours and 2400 hours.

19. 1. When clients take chlorpropamide (Diabinese), an antidiabetic agent, there is an additional adverse reaction, which is an Antabuse-type reaction, when alcohol is ingested. To prevent gastrointestinal adverse reactions, the drug should be taken with breakfast. Antidiabetic agents are given daily each morning and aspartame is not contraindicated for this category of antidiabetic drugs.

20. 4. The client needs to develop a systematic plan for rotating injection sites. Once a site is injected, it should not be used again for 2 to 3 weeks. If an injection were to be given into an extremity to be exercised, it would cause rapid absorption of the insulin and cause hypoglycemia. Insulin injections are given into subcutaneous tissue, not into muscles. It is not recommended that clients aspirate prior to injecting insulin.

21. 2. Dextrose is added to the intravenous fluids when the blood glucose level reaches 250 to 300 mg/dl, so that the blood sugar doesn't drop too rapidly and put the client at risk for hypoglycemia. The values of 350 mg/dl, 400 mg/dl, and 450 mg/dl are not low enough to add dextrose.

22. 3. Stressful situations, whether they be physiological or emotional, precipitate the release of hormones, which elevate the blood sugar levels and alter the body's need for insulin. Exercising should be part of the daily routine and would not be an indication for more frequent blood glucose monitoring. A dental examination would not normally cause a significant rise in blood glucose level. Vacationing should not impact the blood sugar level, unless the daily routines of insulin injections or oral antidiabetic agents, nutrition, and exercise were changed substantially.

23. 1. Furosemide (Lasix), a loop diuretic, is one of several drugs that increases serum glucose levels and is therefore contraindicated if one is taking insulin. Dicumarol, an anticoagulant; reserpine, an antihypertensive agent; and cimetidine, an H_2-receptor antagonist, do not affect blood sugar levels.

24. 4. Family members are taught to give glucagon either subcutaneously or intramuscularly to clients in hypoglycemia who are unresponsive. It is only available in injectable form, so it cannot be given sublingually or rectally. Family members would not routinely be taught to administer a drug intravenously.

25. 2. The blood glucose level should begin to rise in approximately 5 to 20 minutes after an injection of glucagon. It would take more than 4 minutes for the client to respond. If the client doesn't respond in 20 to 30 minutes, emergency personnel need to be summoned to administer dextrose intravenously.

26. 2. A licensed practical nurse may administer a calcium supplement 1 hour after meals. Developing a medication schedule, administering intravenous insulin, and assessing a client taking iodine for signs of iodine poisoning are tasks that should be performed by a registered nurse.

REFERENCES

Broyles, B., Reiss, B., & Evans, M. (2012). *Pharmacological aspects of nursing care* (8th ed.). Clifton Park, NY: Delmar Cengage Learning.

Daniels, R., & Nicoll, L. (2012). *Contemporary medical-surgical Nursing.* Clifton Park, NY: Delmar Cengage Learning.

Spratto, G. R., & Woods, A. L. (2012). *PDR nurse's drug handbook 2012.* Clifton Park, NY: Delmar Cengage Learning.

CHAPTER 22

DRUGS FOR THE NEUROLOGICAL SYSTEM

I. **DRUGS FOR TREATING SEIZURE DISORDERS (ANTICONVULSANTS) (SEE TABLE 22-1)**
   A. DESCRIPTION
      1. USED TO CONTROL SEIZURE ACTIVITY, NOT TO "CURE" THE DISORDER
      2. CHOICE OF DRUG SELECTED IS DETERMINED BY THE TYPE OF SEIZURE DISORDER, CLIENT PREFERENCE, AND ADVERSE REACTION PROFILE.
      3. USUALLY AN INITIAL DRUG IS SELECTED. IF INEFFECTIVE, THE DOSAGE MAY BE INCREASED. IF SEIZURE CONTROL IS STILL NOT ACHIEVED, ADDITIONAL DRUGS MAY BE ADDED OR CHANGED.
      4. ANTICONVULSANTS ARE POSTULATED TO CONTROL SEIZURES BY:
         a. Decreasing the ability of sodium ions to enter cells, thereby decreasing excitability of cell membranes
         b. Potentiating the ability of gamma-aminobutyric acid, a neurotransmitter that causes inhibition of cell membranes
      5. THE HERB GINKGO MAY DECREASE THE EFFECTIVENESS OF ANTICONVULSANTS.
   B. PHENYTOIN (DILANTIN)
      1. USES
         a. Drug of initial choice for seizure disorders
         b. Utilized to treat any seizure type except absence seizures
         c. Used to both treat and prevent seizures
         d. Inhibits seizures by affecting synaptic transmission
      2. ADVERSE REACTIONS
         a. Central nervous system (CNS) effects (ataxia, sleepiness, lethargy)
         b. Gastrointestinal (GI) distress (nausea and vomiting)
         c. Gingival hyperplasia
         d. Uncommon adverse reactions include allergic reactions, hepatitis, and bone marrow depression.
         e. Dilantin toxicity may develop. Client exhibits increased CNS effects.

Table 22-1 Commonly Used Drugs of Choice for Specific Types of Seizures

Type of Seizure	Drugs of Choice
Tonic-clonic	Phenytoin (Dilantin)
	Valproic acid (Depakene)
	Carbamazepine (Tegretol)
	Primidone (Mysoline)
	Phenobarbital (Luminal)
Absence	Ethosuximide (Zarontin)
	Valproic acid (Depakene)
	Divalproex sodium (Depakote)
Myoclonic	Clonazepam (Klonopin)
Atonic	Clonazepam (Klonopin)
Partial	Carbamazepine (Tegretol)
	Phenytoin (Dilantin)
	Valproic acid (Depakene)
	Lamotrigine (Lamictal)
	Gabapentin (Neurontin)
	Felbamate (Felbatol)
	Phenobarbital (Luminal)
	Primidone (Mysoline)
	Tiagabine (Gabitril)
	Topiramate (Topamax)
Status epilepticus	Diazepam (Valium)
	Fosphenytoin (Cerebyx)
	Lorazepam (Ativan)
	Phenobarbital (Dilantin)

© Cengage Learning 2015

3. CONTRAINDICATIONS AND
PRECAUTIONS
   a. CNS depression
   b. History of allergic reaction
   c. Hepatic or renal disease
   d. Bradycardia or heart block
4. DRUG INTERACTIONS
   a. Antacids: decrease phenytoin effect related to decrease GI absorption
   b. Alcohol: decreases phenytoin effect
   c. Warfarin (Coumadin): increases phenytoin effect
   d. Oral contraceptive pills: decrease effect of the oral contraceptive, and estrogen-induced fluid retention may precipitate seizures
   e. Corticosteroids: decrease corticosteroid effect
5. NURSING INTERVENTIONS
   a. Administer the drug on the prescribed schedule in order to maintain a therapeutic drug level.
   b. Administer the drug with meals in order to decrease gastric irritation.
   c. When administering oral suspension of phenytoin, shake the bottle well in order to adequately mix the drug.
   d. Administer diluted intravenous (IV) phenytoin slowly in order to decrease irritation to the venous system. Flush the IV line with saline following administration of the drug in order to prevent venous irritation.
   e. Administration of phenytoin too rapidly by IV push can cause cardiac arrhythmias and hypotension.
   f. Monitor for narrow therapeutic serum level at 5–20 mcg/mL. After initiation of therapy, it takes 7–10 days for level to stabilize.
   e. Monitor for therapeutic effects of the drug. Therapeutic effects of phenytoin are optimized within 7–10 days.
   f. Monitor for CNS effects, which are most common during initiation of the drug.
   g. Monitor liver function studies to assess for liver damage.
   h. Encourage meticulous oral hygiene to prevent gingival hyperplasia.
   i. Closely monitor the client when the drug is being initiated or discontinued.
   j. Instruct the client to avoid alcohol, stimulants, and drugs that may alter the effects of phenytoin.
   k. Monitor for phenytoin toxicity as evidenced by increased CNS effects.
   l. Monitor serum Dilantin levels (normal = 5–20 mcg/mL).
   m. Never add it to any other drug solution.
   n. Administer Dilantin once or twice a day as a result of longer average half-life (18–24 hours).
   o. Dilantin may be given orally in capsule, liquid, or chewable forms or intravenously. It is not recommended for intramuscular administration.
      1) IV administration
      2) Is irritating to vessels—flush IV liberally with saline before and after administration
6. TYPES
   a. Phenytoin (Dilantin): one of most commonly used antiseizure medications
   b. Fosphenytoin (Cerebyx): a medication that is a precursor to phenytoin; Fosphenytoin is converted to phenytoin in the body.
C. VALPROIC ACID (DEPAKENE)
1. USES
   a. Tonic-clonic seizures
   b. Absence seizures
   c. Partial seizures
   d. Bipolar disorder
   e. Prophylaxis for migraine headaches
2. ADVERSE REACTIONS
   a. Nausea, vomiting
   b. Dyspepsia
   c. Sedation
   d. Drowsiness
   e. Prolonged bleeding time
   f. Hepatotoxicity
   g. Pancreatitis
3. CONTRAINDICATIONS AND PRECAUTIONS
   a. Hepatic dysfunction
   b. Bleeding disorders
   c. Allergic to the drug
4. DRUG INTERACTIONS
   a. Phenobarbital: increases phenobarbital and may cause increased risk of phenobarbital toxicity
   b. Antacids: increase risk of valproic acid toxicity
   c. Alcohol: increases risk of CNS depression
5. NURSING INTERVENTIONS
   a. Administer in gelatin capsule, tablet form, syrup, IV, or a powder form that may be sprinkled on foods.
   b. Avoid use in young children because it can cause fatal liver disease.
   c. Take with or after meals to decrease GI upset.
   d. Avoid suddenly stopping the drug.

D. CARBAMAZEPINE (TEGRETOL)
   1. USES
      a. Tonic-clonic (grand mal) seizures
      b. Partial seizures
      c. Occasionally used to treat bipolar depression
      d. Trigeminal neuralgia (tic douloureux)
   2. ADVERSE REACTIONS
      a. Relatively few adverse reactions compared to phenytoin and phenobarbital
      b. Adverse reactions most prominent when initiating therapy
      c. Central nervous system reactions are the most common.
      d. Leukopenia
      e. May trigger condition similar to syndrome of inappropriate antidiuretic hormone (SIADH) that leads to hyponatremia
      f. Bone marrow suppression (rare)
   3. CONTRAINDICATIONS AND PRECAUTIONS
      a. History of allergic response
      b. History of bone marrow depression
      c. Lactation
   4. DRUG INTERACTIONS
      a. Erythromycin, cimetidine and valproic acid: increase effects of carbamazepine
      b. Alcohol, phenytoin, phenobarbital: decrease effects of carbamazepine
   5. NURSING INTERVENTIONS
      a. Monitor complete blood count (CBC) and sodium levels.
      b. Administer with meals to reduce GI distress.
      c. Do not crush sustained-release tablets.
      d. Administer at bedtime to decrease CNS effects and GI adverse reactions.
      e. Instruct a client taking monoamine oxidase (MAO) inhibitors to discontinue them 2 weeks prior to initiating carbamazepine.

E. ETHOSUXIMIDE (ZARONTIN)
   1. USES
      a. Drug of choice for absence seizures
   2. ADVERSE REACTIONS
      a. Nausea and vomiting
      b. Drowsiness
      c. Anorexia
      d. Weight loss
   3. CONTRAINDICATIONS AND PRECAUTIONS
      a. Sensitivity to drug
   4. DRUG INTERACTIONS
      a. Valproic acid: causes decreased metabolism of ethosuximide and increased incidence of adverse reactions

   5. NURSING INTERVENTIONS
      a. Assess for nausea and vomiting (take with food if GI upset occurs).
      b. Monitor CBC every 3 months and liver function studies.
      c. Monitor weekly weight.
F. GABAPENTIN (NEURONTIN)
   1. USES
      a. Added to drug regimen for partial seizures if monotherapy is ineffective
   2. ADVERSE REACTIONS
      a. Dizziness
      b. Fatigue
      c. Irritability
      d. Ataxia
      e. Increased appetite
      f. Weight gain
   3. CONTRAINDICATIONS AND PRECAUTIONS
      a. Renal impairment
      b. Lactation
   4. DRUG INTERACTIONS
      a. Alcohol: increases effect of gabapentin
      b. Antacids: decrease bioavailability of gabapentin
      c. Cimetidine: decreases renal excretion of gabapentin
   5. NURSING INTERVENTIONS
      a. Monitor renal function studies.
      b. Monitor for drowsiness and dizziness.
      c. Instruct the client to avoid driving or other hazardous behavior.
      d. Avoid letting 12 hours pass between any two doses—administer three times a day.
      e. Instruct the client to avoid antacids because they decrease the bioavailability of the drug.
G. FELBAMATE (FELBATOL)
   1. USES
      a. Used as second-line drug for intractable atonic or partial seizures
      b. Used as an adjunct treatment of seizures associated with Lennox-Gastaut syndrome, which is characterized by a combination of frequent myoclonic and tonic seizures with intericatal slow spike waves on the electroencephalogram (EEG).
   2. ADVERSE REACTIONS
      a. Nausea, vomiting
      b. Dizziness
      c. Hyponatremia
      d. Hypokalemia
      e. Photosensitivity
      f. Aplastic anemia
      g. Liver toxicity

3. CONTRAINDICATIONS AND PRECAUTIONS
   a. History of bone marrow suppression
   b. Liver dysfunction
   c. Aplastic anemia
4. DRUG INTERACTIONS
   a. Carbamazepine: increases serum carbamazepine level
   b. Phenytoin: increases phenytoin level
   c. Valproic acid: increases valproic acid levels
5. NURSING INTERVENTIONS
   a. Monitor CBC and liver function studies.
   b. Client may sign a consent form acknowledging the increased risk of aplastic anemia and liver failure; therefore, its use is discouraged except when safer drugs have not been tolerated or effective.
   c. Monitor for weight loss and decreased appetite.
   d. Instruct the client to avoid ultraviolet light or sunlight because exposure causes photosensitivity.

H. BENZODIAZEPINES
1. USES
   a. Myoclonic seizures
   b. Status epilepticus
   c. Atonic seizures
2. ADVERSE REACTIONS
   a. Respiratory depression and decreased level of consciousness
   b. Drowsiness, fatigue, confusion
   c. Increased appetite, weight gain, constipation
   d. Difficulty with urination, urinary retention
3. CONTRAINDICATIONS AND PRECAUTIONS
   a. Central nervous system depressants
   b. Narrow-angle glaucoma
   c. Impaired hepatic or renal function
4. DRUG INTERACTIONS
   a. Other central nervous system depressants, narcotics/opiates, barbiturates, and tranquilizers/hypnotics: increase CNS effects
   b. Antacids: decrease absorption of benzodiazepine
   c. Digoxin: increases digoxin level
   d. Valproic acid: increases effect of benzodiazepine
5. NURSING INTERVENTIONS
   a. Monitor for respiratory depression.
   b. Monitor vital signs frequently.
   c. Instruct the client that an abrupt withdrawal may cause withdrawal reactions, seizures, and status epilepticus.
   d. The drug may be given in IV form.

   e. Do not mix with any other drug solutions.
   f. Administer according to schedule IV controlled drug.
   g. Instruct the client that tolerance may develop with long-term use.
   h. Instruct the client to avoid abrupt discontinuation of the drug because it may precipitate seizures.
6. TYPES
   a. Clonazepam (Klonopin)
   b. Clorazepate (Tranxene)
   c. Diazepam (Valium)
      1) Short half-life: must be given in repeated dosages or followed by longer-acting antiseizure medication
      2) Rectal gel form available (Diastat)
   d. Lorazepam (Ativan)
      1) Drug of choice for status epilepticus
      2) Short acting and should be followed with a long-acting anticonvulsant

II. **DRUGS FOR TREATING PARKINSON'S DISEASE (ANTIPARKINSONIAN DRUGS)**
A. USES
   1. USED TO BALANCE LEVELS OF NEUROTRANSMITTERS IN THE BRAIN BY EITHER INCREASING THE AMOUNT OF AVAILABLE DOPAMINE OR DECREASING THE AMOUNT OF ACETYLCHOLINE
   2. CHOICE OF WHICH DRUG TO BE INITIATED DEPENDS ON WHETHER PARKINSON'S DISEASE IS IDIOPATHIC OR CAUSED BY A DRUG.
B. ADVERSE REACTIONS
   1. ANOREXIA, NAUSEA, OR VOMITING
   2. "WEARING OFF" OF MEDICATION
   3. DYSKINESIAS (INVOLUNTARY CHOREIFORM MOVEMENTS)
   4. POSTURAL HYPOTENSION
   5. SEDATION
   6. SLEEPINESS
   7. CONFUSION
   8. DRY MOUTH
C. CONTRAINDICATIONS AND PRECAUTIONS
   1. NARROW-ANGLE GLAUCOMA
   2. ANGINA
   3. TRANSIENT ISCHEMIC ATTACKS (TIAS)
   4. HISTORY OF MELANOMA OR UNDIAGNOSED SKIN LESIONS
   5. RENAL DISEASE (AMANTADINE)
D. DRUG INTERACTIONS
   1. TRICYCLIC ANTIDEPRESSANTS: DECREASE EFFECT OF ANTIPARKINSONIAN DRUG

2. MAO INHIBITORS: CONCOMITANT ADMINISTRATION MAY RESULT IN HYPERTENSION
3. ANTACIDS: INCREASE EFFECT OF ANTIPARKINSONIAN DRUG
4. ANTICHOLINERGICS: DECREASE EFFECT OF ANTIPARKINSONIAN DRUG

E. NURSING INTERVENTIONS
1. ENCOURAGE THE CLIENT TO CONTINUE THE DRUG EVEN WHEN AN IMMEDIATE IMPROVEMENT IS NOT NOTICED.
2. MONITOR FOR IMPROVEMENT IN CLINICAL MANIFESTATIONS.
3. INSTRUCT THE CLIENT TO CONTACT THE PHYSICIAN PRIOR TO TAKING OTHER PRESCRIPTION AND OVER-THE-COUNTER (OTC) OR HERBAL REMEDIES.
4. INSTRUCT THE CLIENT TO AVOID DRIVING OR OTHER HAZARDOUS ACTIVITIES IF DIZZINESS OR DROWSINESS IS EXPERIENCED.
5. WITH THE EXCEPTION OF LEVODOPA, ADMINISTER DRUGS WITH FOOD TO DECREASE THE RISK OF NAUSEA AND VOMITING.

F. TYPES
1. LEVODOPA (TO REPLACE DOPAMINE)
2. CARBIDOPA (LODOSYN): USUALLY GIVEN WITH LEVODOPA IN COMBINATION PRODUCT CALLED SINEMET
3. AMANTADINE (SYMMETREL) INCREASES DOPAMINE LEVELS AND ALSO IS USED TO TREAT INFLUENZA.
4. BROMOCRIPTINE (PARLODEL), PERGOLIDE (PERMAX), PRAMIPEXOLE (MIRAPEX) AND ROPINIROLE (REQUIP) ACT BY STIMULATING THE BRAIN'S DOPAMINE RECEPTORS.
5. SELEGILINE (ELDEPRYL) ACTS BY INHIBITING BREAKDOWN OF MAO.
6. TOLCAPONE (TASMAR), CATECHOL-O-METHYLTRANSFERASE (COMT) INHIBITOR

III. **ANTICHOLINERGIC MEDICATIONS (CHOLINERGIC BLOCKING DRUGS)**
A. USES
1. PARKINSON'S DISEASE TO DECREASE TREMORS AND SPASTIC MOVEMENTS
2. ADJUNCT USE TO DECREASE ADVERSE REACTIONS OF SOME ANTIPSYCHOTIC DRUGS
3. ANTIDOTE FOR SOME TYPES OF POISONS, INCLUDING TOXIC MUSHROOM INGESTION, INSECTICIDES, CHOLINERGIC

AGONIST DRUGS, AND CHOLINESTERASE INHIBITOR DRUGS

B. ADVERSE REACTIONS
1. TACHYCARDIA
2. CNS STIMULATION FOLLOWED BY CNS DEPRESSION
3. CONSTIPATION
4. DRY MOUTH
5. URINARY RETENTION
6. DECREASED SWEATING (WHICH MAY LEAD TO HEAT STROKE)
7. VISUAL EFFECTS (BLURRED VISION, PHOTOPHOBIA, MYDRIASIS)
8. HALLUCINATION
9. CONFUSION

C. CONTRAINDICATIONS AND PRECAUTIONS
1. BENIGN PROSTATIC HYPERTROPHY (BPH)
2. MYASTHENIA GRAVIS
3. HYPERTHYROIDISM
4. NARROW-ANGLE GLAUCOMA
5. TACHYARRHYTHMIAS
6. HEART FAILURE
7. GASTROESOPHAGEAL REFLUX DISEASE (GERD)

D. DRUG INTERACTIONS
1. ANTIHISTAMINES: INCREASE ANTICHOLINERGIC REACTIONS
2. ANTIPSYCHOTIC DRUGS: INCREASE REACTIONS
3. TRICYCLIC ANTIDEPRESSANTS: ADDITIVE ANTICHOLINERGIC ADVERSE REACTIONS
4. OTC SLEEPING AIDS: INCREASE ANTICHOLINERGIC REACTIONS
5. CHOLINERGIC DRUGS: DECREASE EFFECTS OF ANTICHOLINERGIC DRUGS

E. NURSING INTERVENTIONS
1. INSTRUCT THE CLIENT TO AVOID HEAT STROKE.
2. ENCOURAGE THE CLIENT TO CHEW GUM AND HARD CANDY TO MINIMIZE DRY MOUTH.
3. ENCOURAGE THE CLIENT TO USE GOOD ORAL HYGIENE TO PREVENT TOOTH DECAY RELATED TO LACK OF SALIVA.
4. INSTRUCT THE CLIENT TO NOTIFY THE PHYSICIAN IF URINARY RETENTION DEVELOPS.
5. ENCOURAGE THE CLIENT TO INCREASE FIBER AND FLUIDS TO REDUCE RISK OF CONSTIPATION.
6. PREVENT ACCIDENTAL POISONING IN CHILDREN.
7. THE ANTIDOTE IS PHYSOSTIGMINE SALICYLATE (ANTILIRIUM) AND IS GIVEN SLOWLY INTRAVENOUSLY.

8. CAREFULLY MONITOR OLDER
ADULTS BECAUSE THEY ARE MORE
LIKELY TO DEVELOP ADVERSE
EFFECTS.

F. TYPES
   1. ATROPINE
   2. TRIHEXYPHENIDYL (ARTANE)
   3. BIPERIDEN (AKINETON)
   4. PROCYCLIDINE (KEMADRIN)
   5. BENZTROPINE (COGENTIN)—DRUG
      THAT HAS BOTH ANTIHISTAMINE
      AND ANTICHOLINERGIC REACTIONS;
      MAY BE ADDED TO OTHER
      ANTIPARKINSONIAN DRUGS TO
      INCREASE REACTIONS

IV. **SKELETAL MUSCLE RELAXANTS**
A. USES
   1. ACUTE MUSCLE SPASMS AND PAIN
   2. SPASTICITY
   3. MALIGNANT HYPERTHERMIA
   4. ARTHRITIS
   5. SPONDYLITIS
   6. CEREBRAL PALSY
B. ADVERSE REACTIONS
   1. SEDATION
   2. CONFUSION
   3. DIZZINESS
   4. NAUSEA AND VOMITING
   5. RESPIRATORY DEPRESSION
   6. HYPOTENSION
C. CONTRAINDICATIONS AND
   PRECAUTIONS
   1. DECREASED RENAL FUNCTION
   2. DECREASED HEPATIC FUNCTION
   3. RESPIRATORY DEPRESSION
   4. ORPHENADRINE (NORFLEX) AND
      CYCLOBENZAPRINE (FLEXERIL) ARE
      CONTRAINDICATED IN CLIENTS
      WITH GLAUCOMA, URINARY
      RETENTION, OR
      TACHYARRHYTHMIAS DUE
      TO ANTICHOLINERGIC
      REACTIONS.
   5. PSYCHOLOGICAL OR PHYSICAL
      DEPENDENCE
D. DRUG INTERACTIONS
   1. ALCOHOL: INCREASES SEDATIVE
      EFFECT
   2. SLEEPING AIDS: INCREASE SEDATIVE
      EFFECT
   3. ANTIANXIETY AGENTS: INCREASE
      SEDATIVE EFFECT
   4. MAO INHIBITORS: INCREASE
      CENTRAL NERVOUS SYSTEM
      DEPRESSION
E. NURSING INTERVENTIONS
   1. ASSESS FOR DECREASED MUSCLE
      SPASM OR SPASTICITY.
   2. ASSESS FOR PAIN.

3. INSTRUCT THE CLIENT TO AVOID
   DRIVING OR PERFORMING OTHER
   HAZARDOUS ACTIVITIES.
4. ADMINISTER DIAZEPAM (VALIUM)
   SLOWLY IV.
5. MONITOR FOR RESPIRATORY
   DEPRESSION.

F. TYPES
   1. BACLOFEN (LIORESAL)
   2. CYCLOBENZAPRINE (FLEXERIL)
   3. DANTROLENE (DANTRIUM)
   4. DIAZEPAM (VALIUM)
   5. METAXALONE (SKELAXIN)
   6. ORPHENADRINE CITRATE (NORFLEX)
   7. CARISOPRODOL (SOMA)
   8. CHLORZOXAZONE (PARAFON FORTE)
   9. METHOCARBAMOL (ROBAXIN)

V. **DIRECT-ACTING SKELETAL MUSCLE
   RELAXANTS**
A. USES
   1. SKELETAL MUSCLE SPASMS
   2. MULTIPLE SCLEROSIS
   3. CEREBRAL PALSY
   4. SPINAL CORD INJURY
   5. STROKE
B. ADVERSE REACTIONS
   1. MUSCLE WEAKNESS
   2. DIARRHEA
   3. PHOTOSENSITIVITY
   4. CHANGES IN SENSORY PERCEPTION
   5. INSOMNIA
   6. DEPRESSION
C. CONTRAINDICATIONS AND
   PRECAUTIONS
   1. SEVERE HEPATIC DYSFUNCTION
   2. BLACK BOX WARNING: OBTAIN
      LIVER FUNCTION TESTS AT START
      OF THERAPY, INCLUDING AST AND
      ALT
D. DRUG INTERACTIONS
   1. WARFAIN: MAY DECREASE PROTEIN
      BINDING OF DANTROLENE
   2. CNS DEPRESSANTS: MAY INCREASE
      CNS DEPRESSION
   3. ESTROGEN: MAY INCREASE RISK OF
      HEPATOTOCITY
E. NURSING INTERVENTIONS
   1. ADVISE CLIENT TO AVOID EXCESSIVE
      SUN EXPOSURE.
   2. INSTRUCT CLIENT TO TAKE WITH
      MEALS OR MILK IN FOUR DIVIDED
      DOSES.
   3. INSTRUCT CLIENT TO AVOID
      DRIVING UNTIL CNS EFFECTS ARE
      KNOWN.
   4. MONITOR SWALLOWING DURING
      THERAPY—CLIENT MAY HAVE
      DIFFICULTY SWALLOWING DURING
      THERAPY.

VI. CENTRAL NERVOUS SYSTEM STIMULANTS

A. USES
1. NARCOLEPSY
2. ATTENTION-DEFICIT HYPERACTIVITY DISORDER (ADHD)
3. OBESITY

B. ADVERSE REACTIONS
1. ENHANCED MOOD, EUPHORIA
2. EXCESSIVE CNS STIMULATION (AGITATION, RESTLESSNESS, ANXIETY, INSOMNIA)
3. HYPERACTIVITY
4. TACHYCARDIA, PALPITATIONS
5. HYPERTENSION
6. PSYCHOLOGICAL OR PHYSICAL DEPENDENCE
7. WEIGHT LOSS

C. CONTRAINDICATIONS AND PRECAUTIONS
1. ANXIETY
2. GLAUCOMA
3. HYPERTHYROIDISM
4. HISTORY OF SUBSTANCE ABUSE

D. DRUG INTERACTIONS
1. CAFFEINE: INCREASES CNS REACTIONS
2. STIMULANTS (OTC OR ILLEGAL DRUGS): INCREASE CNS REACTIONS
3. MAO INHIBITORS: INCREASE REACTIONS

E. NURSING INTERVENTIONS
1. MONITOR FOR SIGNS OF PSYCHOLOGICAL DEPENDENCE.
2. MONITOR FOR THERAPEUTIC RESULTS.
3. MONITOR WEIGHT.
4. INSTRUCT THE CLIENT TO NOTIFY THE PHYSICIAN IF ADVERSE REACTIONS OCCUR.
5. INSTRUCT THE CLIENT ABOUT ADDITIVE EFFECTS OF CAFFEINE.
6. ADMINISTER DRUGS EARLY IN THE DAY TO PREVENT INSOMNIA.

F. TYPES
1. AMPHETAMINE
2. DEXTROAMPHETAMINE (DEXEDRINE)
3. METHAMPHETAMINE (DESOXYN)
4. METHYLPHENIDATE (RITALIN)
5. XANTHINES (CAFFEINE)

VII. CHOLINERGIC MEDICATIONS

A. USES
1. DIAGNOSIS AND TREATMENT OF MYASTHENIA GRAVIS
2. TREATMENT OF ALZHEIMER'S DISEASE

B. ADVERSE REACTIONS
1. CNS REACTIONS (DIZZINESS, SEIZURES, DECREASED LEVEL OF CONSCIOUSNESS)
2. RESPIRATORY FAILURE
3. ARRHYTHMIAS, CARDIAC ARREST
4. NAUSEA AND VOMITING

C. CONTRAINDICATIONS AND PRECAUTIONS
1. URINARY TRACT OBSTRUCTION
2. ASTHMA
3. CORONARY ARTERY DISEASE
4. HEPATIC DYSFUNCTION (TACRINE)

D. DRUG INTERACTIONS
1. CIMETIDINE: INCREASES EFFECTS OF TACRINE
2. ANTICHOLINERGIC DRUGS: DECREASE THE EFFECTS OF CHOLINERGIC DRUGS
3. ANTIHISTAMINES: DECREASE THE EFFECTS OF CHOLINERGIC AGENTS

E. NURSING INTERVENTIONS
1. ASSESS THE CLIENT WITH MYASTHENIA GRAVIS FOR MUSCLE WEAKNESS.
2. MONITOR FOR THERAPEUTIC RESULTS.
3. WHEN USING TENSILON TO DIFFERENTIATE BETWEEN MYASTHENIC CRISIS AND CHOLINERGIC CRISIS, THE PHYSICIAN IS IN ATTENDANCE. HAVE INTUBATION AND RESUSCITATION EQUIPMENT IMMEDIATELY AVAILABLE. DRUG IS GIVEN IV OR INTRAMUSCULARLY (IM).
4. INSTRUCT THE CLIENT NOT TO DISCONTINUE THE DRUG WITHOUT CHECKING WITH THE PHYSICIAN.
5. ATROPINE IV IS THE ANTIDOTE FOR OVERDOSE WITH CHOLINERGIC DRUGS.
6. MONITOR LIVER FUNCTION STUDIES IF THE CLIENT IS TAKING TACRINE.
7. ADMINISTER THE DRUGS ON A TIMELY SCHEDULE.
8. DRUG OVERDOSE MAY PRECIPITATE CHOLINERGIC CRISIS. MONITOR FOR HYPOTENSION AND RESPIRATORY FAILURE. TREATMENT OF CHOLINERGIC CRISIS IS THE ADMINISTRATION OF IV ATROPINE.
9. UNDERMEDICATION MAY RESULT IN MYASTHENIC CRISIS. TREATMENT OF MYASTHENIC CRISIS INVOLVES ADMINISTRATION OF MORE OF THE DRUG.
10. MONITOR FOR URINARY RETENTION AND BLADDER DISTENTION.
11. ADMINISTER NEOSTIGMINE PER OS (PO), IM, OR SUBCUT.

F. TYPES
1. NEOSTIGMINE (PROSTIGMIN): USED FOR LONG-TERM TREATMENT OF MYASTHENIA GRAVIS
2. DONEPEZIL (ARICEPT): USED FOR TREATMENT OF ALZHEIMER'S DISEASE
3. EDROPHONIUM (TENSILON): SHORT-ACTING CHOLINERGIC DRUG USED PRIMARILY FOR DIAGNOSIS OF MYASTHENIA GRAVIS OR TO DIFFERENTIATE BETWEEN MYASTHENIC AND CHOLINERGIC CRISES
4. AMBENONIUM (MYTELASE): LONGER-ACTING DRUG USED FOR TREATMENT OF MYASTHENIA GRAVIS
5. PYRIDOSTIGMINE (MESTINON): OFTEN THE DRUG OF CHOICE FOR LONG-TERM TREATMENT OF MYASTHENIA GRAVIS
6. TACRINE (COGNEX): USED TO TREAT ALZHEIMER'S DISEASE

VIII. CORTICOSTEROIDS
A. USES
1. CEREBRAL EDEMA ASSOCIATED WITH BRAIN TUMORS, POSTOPERATIVE CEREBRAL EDEMA FROM CRANIOTOMY, OR TRAUMATIC HEAD INJURIES
B. ADVERSE REACTIONS
1. GI UPSET
2. CUSHING'S SYNDROME WITH LONG-TERM USE
3. CNS SYSTEM REACTIONS: (ELEVATED MOOD, DEPRESSION, PSYCHOLOGICAL DEPENDENCE)
C. CONTRAINDICATIONS AND PRECAUTIONS
1. SYSTEMIC FUNGAL INFECTIONS
2. SYSTEMIC BACTERIAL INFECTIONS
3. DIABETES MELLITUS
4. PEPTIC ULCER DISEASE
5. RENAL DYSFUNCTION
6. CONGESTIVE HEART FAILURE
7. HYPERTENSION
D. DRUG INTERACTIONS
1. DIURETICS: POTENTIATE HYPOKALEMIA
2. ANTIHISTAMINES: DECREASE THE EFFECTS OF CORTICOSTEROIDS
3. ANTACIDS: DECREASE EFFECT OF CORTICOSTEROIDS
4. BARBITURATES: DECREASE EFFECT OF CORTICOSTEROIDS
E. NURSING INTERVENTIONS
1. INSTRUCT THE CLIENT NOT TO ABRUPTLY DISCONTINUE THE DRUG.

2. INSTRUCT THE CLIENT ON METHODS TO PREVENT INFECTION SUCH AS HAND WASHING.
3. ADMINISTER WITH MEALS OR MILK TO DECREASE NAUSEA.
4. INSTRUCT THE CLIENT TO NOTIFY THE PHYSICIAN WHEN MAJOR STRESS OR SEVERE ILLNESS IS EXPERIENCED (MAY NEED INCREASED DOSE OF CORTICOSTEROID).
5. MONITOR FOR THERAPEUTIC EFFECTS.
F. TYPES
1. DEXAMETHASONE IS USUALLY THE CORTICOSTEROID OF CHOICE FOR CEREBRAL EDEMA.

IX. OSMOTIC DIURETICS
A. USES
1. REDUCE INTRACRANIAL PRESSURE (ICP)
B. ADVERSE REACTIONS
1. HYPOTENSION OR HYPERTENSION
2. FLUID AND ELECTROLYTE IMBALANCES (SUCH AS THIRST, MUSCLE CRAMPS, WEAKNESS)
3. ACUTE RENAL INSUFFICIENCY
C. CONTRAINDICATIONS AND PRECAUTIONS
1. ANURIA
2. CONGESTIVE HEART FAILURE
3. PULMONARY CONGESTION
D. DRUG INTERACTIONS
1. LITHIUM
2. IMIPRAMINE
3. POTASSIUM
E. NURSING INTERVENTIONS
1. INFUSE THROUGH AN IV LINE WITH A FILTER.
2. MONITOR THE IV SITE FOR INFILTRATION (INFILTRATION RESULTS IN TISSUE NECROSIS).
3. MONITOR THE VITAL SIGNS FREQUENTLY.
4. MAINTAIN A STRICT INTAKE AND OUTPUT (I & O).
F. TYPES
1. MANNITOL (OSMITROL)

X. MEDICATIONS TO TREAT MIGRAINE HEADACHES
A. USES
1. MIGRAINE HEADACHES
B. ADVERSE REACTIONS
1. CHEST TIGHTNESS
2. HYPERTENSION
3. NAUSEA
4. PARESTHESIAS
5. IMPAIRED PERIPHERAL CIRCULATION (ERGOTAMINES)
6. NAUSEA AND VOMITING (ERGOTAMINES)

C. CONTRAINDICATIONS AND PRECAUTIONS
  1. ANGINA
  2. MYOCARDIAL INFARCTION (MI)
  3. HYPERTENSION
  4. ERGOTAMINES CONTRAINDICATED DURING PREGNANCY
D. DRUG INTERACTIONS
  1. MAO INHIBITORS: MAY CAUSE CARDIAC ARRHYTHMIAS AND MI
  2. ERGOTAMINES AND TRIPTANS CANNOT BE TAKEN CONCURRENTLY DUE TO RISK OF SEVERE HYPERTENSION AND CEREBROVASCULAR ACCIDENT.
E. NURSING INTERVENTIONS
  1. SUMATRIPTAN (IMITREX) MAY BE ADMINISTERED SUBCUTANEOUSLY, ORALLY, OR BY NASAL SPRAY BUT NOT INTRAVENOUSLY (POTENTIAL LETHAL REACTIONS MAY OCCUR).
  2. ERGOTAMINES (ERGOMAR) MAY BE GIVEN SUBLINGUALLY OR BY INHALATION AT THE ONSET OF A MIGRAINE HEADACHE.
  3. INSTRUCT THE CLIENT TO TAKE THE ANTIMIGRAINE DRUG AT THE ONSET OF CLINICAL MANIFESTATIONS.
  4. INFORM THE CLIENT OF THE ADMINISTRATION PROTOCOL. TRIPTANS MAY BE REPEATED IF THE MIGRAINE PERSISTS. HOWEVER, ADMINISTER NO MORE THAN 300 MG OF SUMATRIPTAN, 5 MG OF NARATRIPTAN, OR 10 MG OF ZOLMITRIPTAN WITHIN 24 HOURS.
  5. INFORM THE CLIENT THAT WHEN FREQUENT MIGRAINE HEADACHES ARE EXPERIENCED, PROPHYLAXIS MAY BE REQUIRED. DRUGS COMMONLY USED FOR MIGRAINE PROPHYLAXIS INCLUDE ASPIRIN, NSAIDS, AND BETA-ADRENERGIC BLOCKERS (PROPRANOLOL).
F. TYPES
  1. NARATRIPTAN (AMERGE)
  2. RIZATRIPTAN (MAXALT)
  3. SUMATRIPTAN (IMITREX)
  4. ZOLMITRIPTAN (ZOMIG)
  5. ERGOTAMINE TARTRATE (ERGOMAR)
  6. ERGOTAMINE TARTRATE AND CAFFEINE (CAFERGOT)

PRACTICE QUESTIONS

1. The nurse should monitor a client receiving pyridostigmine (Mestinon) for which of the following adverse reactions?
   1. Constipation
   2. Decreased heart rate
   3. Hypertension
   4. Increased intraocular pressure

2. The nurse should assess for which of the following after slowly administering lorazepam (Ativan) intravenously to a client who has been experiencing seizures in rapid succession?
   1. Tachycardia
   2. Hypertension
   3. Tissue hypoxia
   4. Respiratory depression

3. A client is taking phenytoin (Dilantin) 200 mg daily. The nurse monitors the client for which of the following adverse reactions?
   1. Diarrhea
   2. Pruritus
   3. Sedation
   4. Hypertension

4. The nurse infuses phenytoin (Dilantin) with which of the following solutions to control seizures?
   1. Normal saline
   2. D_5W
   3. Lactated Ringer's
   4. D_5W 0.5 normal saline

5. Phenytoin (Dilantin) has been prescribed for a client. Based on an understanding of medication, the nurse caring for the client should
   1. maintain a Dilantin level of 30 to 50 µg/ml.
   2. dilute IV Dilantin with 5% dextrose.
   3. administer good oral hygiene.
   4. give intramuscularly.

6. The nurse is caring for a client who is receiving phenobarbital for epilepsy. The nurse identifies the nursing diagnosis "High risk for injury related to unpredictable intermittent neurological dysfunction." Which of the following is a priority to include in this client's plan of care?

1. Consume alcohol in moderation
2. Drive a car only during the day
3. Lie down at the first sign of an aura
4. Increase fiber in the diet and fluids

7. The nurse obtains a subtherapeutic serum level for a client who is receiving phenytoin (Dilantin) with seizure activity under control. Based on the results of the Dilantin level, the appropriate nursing action is to
   1. change the medication to carbamazepine (Tegretol).
   2. increase the dose of the phenytoin (Dilantin).
   3. add phenobarbital to the drug regimen.
   4. continue the phenytoin (Dilantin) as ordered.

8. The nurse is caring for a client who has cerebral edema following a cerebrovascular accident. The nurse should understand that the client is to receive mannitol IV for which of the following purposes?
   1. Inhibit prothrombin formation
   2. Prevent platelet aggregation
   3. Decrease intracranial pressure
   4. Perfusion of occluded intracranial arteries

9. Which of the following would the nurse recognize as the appropriate rationale for the administration of the drug levodopa (L-dopa) to a client with Parkinson's disease?
   1. The drug activates enzymes to degrade dopamine
   2. The drug blocks the release of dopamine
   3. The drug provides the precursor of dopamine
   4. The drug inhibits the synthesis of dopamine

10. The nurse is caring for a client who has tetanus and is experiencing seizures unrelieved by sedation. Which of the following drugs should the nurse administer?
    1. Diazepam (Valium)
    2. D-tubocurarine (Curate)
    3. Chlorpromazine (Thorazine)
    4. Phenytoin (Dilantin)

11. The nurse is caring for a client who is receiving dexamethasone (Decadron) for a spinal cord tumor. The nurse should assess for which of the following adverse reactions?
    1. Hypoglycemia
    2. Nausea
    3. Constipation
    4. Hypotension

12. The nurse is caring for a client who is experiencing an overdose of atropine. The nurse should prepare to administer which of the following drugs?
    1. Diazepam (Valium)
    2. Dexamethasone (Decadron)

3. Physostigmine salicylate (Antilirium)
4. Epinephrine

13. Benztropine (Cogentin) has been prescribed for a client. Based on an understanding of the adverse reactions, the nurse caring for the client should do which of the following?
    1. Inform the client that diarrhea is a common adverse reaction
    2. Instruct the client to drink alcohol in moderation
    3. Turn and position the client frequently
    4. Monitor the client for urinary retention

14. The nurse is caring for a client with myasthenia gravis who has become progressively weaker. Edrophonium (Tensilon) has been prescribed for which of the following purposes?
    1. Treat the client's muscle weakness
    2. Differentiate between a cholinergic crisis and myasthenic crisis
    3. Increase skeletal muscle relaxation
    4. Decrease difficulty breathing

15. When providing care for a client who is receiving methylphenidate (Ritalin), the nurse should monitor the client for
    Select all that apply:
    [ ] 1. Constipation
    [ ] 2. Weight gain
    [ ] 3. Tachycardia
    [ ] 4. Nervousness
    [ ] 5. Gingival hyperplasia
    [ ] 6. Palpitation

16. The nurse reviews which of the following type of drugs used for partial seizures?
    Select all that apply:
    [ ] 1. Clonazepam (Klonopin)
    [ ] 2. Ethosuximide (Zanrontin)
    [ ] 3. Fosphenytoin (Cerebyx)
    [ ] 4. Phenytoin (Dilantin)
    [ ] 5. Phenobarbital (Luminal)
    [ ] 6. Primidone (Mysoline)

17. The nurse should monitor which of the following laboratory tests in a client receiving ethosuximide (Zarontin)?
    1. Thyroid profile and follicle-stimulating hormone
    2. Calcium and magnesium
    3. Potassium and sodium
    4. Complete blood count and liver function studies

18. The nurse is teaching a class on drugs used in the treatment of neurological disorders. Which of the following should the nurse include in the class?
    1. Allergic reactions, hepatitis, and bone marrow depression are common adverse reactions to anticonvulsants

2. Antihistamines and antipsychotic drugs decrease the effect of anticholinergic drugs
3. Narrow-angle glaucoma is a contraindication in the use of antiparkinsonian drugs
4. Cushing's syndrome occurs with short-term corticosteroid use

19. The nurse should assess a client receiving ergotamine tartrate (Ergomar) for which of the following adverse reactions?
    Select all that apply:
    [ ] 1. Nausea
    [ ] 2. Urinary retention
    [ ] 3. Hypertension
    [ ] 4. Constipation
    [ ] 5. Dry mouth
    [ ] 6. Tachycardia

20. Methysergide maleate (Sansert) has been prescribed for a client experiencing cluster headaches. Which of the following should the nurse include in the medication instructions?
    1. Sansert may be safely used in the management of acute migraine attacks
    2. Administer the medication sublingually
    3. Discontinue the medication for 1 month after every 4 months
    4. One additional tablet may be taken after 30 minutes if the headache has not subsided

21. The nurse questions an order to administer rizatriptan (Maxalt) to which of the following clients? A client with
    1. gastroesophageal reflux disease.
    2. Parkinson's disease.
    3. hypertension.
    4. osteoarthritis.

22. The registered nurse is preparing to delegate nursing tasks for the day. Which of the following tasks should the nurse delegate to a licensed practical nurse?
    1. Administration of intravenous phenytoin (Dilantin) to a client with partial seizures
    2. Develop a nutritional plan for a client experiencing migraine headaches
    3. Monitor a client taking carbidopa (Lodosyn) for adverse reactions
    4. Offer a client taking trihexyphenidyl (Artane) increased fluids

23. The nurse monitors a client taking phenytoin (Dilantin) for therapeutic effects between how many days after treatment begins?

    _____

24. The nurse is caring for a client taking felbamate (Felbatol) for partial seizures. Which of the following actions should the nurse include in the plan of care for this client?
    1. Monitor the client for an increased appetite and weight gain
    2. Instruct the client that hyperkalemia and hypernatremia are adverse reactions
    3. Have the client sign a consent form acknowledging the increased risk of aplastic anemia and liver failure
    4. Monitor the serum sodium level

25. The nurse should monitor a client carefully and use extreme caution when administering phenobarbital with what additional drug?
    1. Valproic acid (Depakene)
    2. Phenytoin (Dilantin)
    3. Carbamazepine (Tegretol)
    4. Ethosuximide (Zarontin)

ANSWERS AND RATIONALES

1. 2. Pyridostigmine (Mestinon) is a cholinergic drug used in the treatment of myasthenia gravis. Adverse reactions include bradycardia, diarrhea, and hypotension.

2. 4. Lorazepam (Ativan) is given intravenously in the treatment of status epilepticus. A client receiving Ativan for status epilepticus must be closely monitored for respiratory depression.

3. 3. Phenytoin (Dilantin) is an anticonvulsant used in the treatment of seizures. Adverse reactions include sedation, hypotension, and constipation.

4. 1. Phenytoin (Dilantin) should not be used intravenously with dextrose because it forms a

precipitate. Dilantin should only be infused intravenously with normal saline.

5. 3. Gingival hyperplasia is an adverse reaction to phenytoin (Dilantin). Administering good oral hygiene is the appropriate intervention. The normal therapeutic Dilantin level is 7.5 to 20 μg/ml. Dilantin should not be administered with dextrose because it forms precipitates. It should only be infused with normal saline. Dilantin is not administered intramuscularly.

6. 3. The priority nursing intervention for a client with epilepsy and a nursing diagnosis of "High risk for injury related to unpredictable intermittent neurological dysfunction" is to lie

down at the first sign of an aura. Safety is always the priority. The client should be advised to avoid alcohol with phenobarbital because of the combined sedative effect. Because of this client's neurological nursing diagnosis, the client should not be driving at a time of unpredictability. Increasing fiber and fluids in the diet have no impact on safety.

7. 4. Therapeutic ranges for drugs serve only as a guide. The therapeutic drug range excludes a serum level lower than where the client continues to have seizures and higher than where the client experiences toxic effects. If a client's seizures are well controlled at a subtherapeutic level, the dose does not need to be increased because it appears to be stabilizing the client's seizures, which is the goal of therapy.

8. 3. Mannitol is an osmotic diuretic used to promote systemic diuresis in cerebral edema and to decrease intracranial pressure.

9. 3. Levodopa (L-dopa) is an antiparkinsonian drug. When L-dopa enters the bloodstream, it is converted to dopamine by the enzyme dopadecarboxylase and increases the dopamine available to the brain.

10. 2. When seizures are not controlled by sedation, d-tubocurarine (Curate) is a skeletal-muscle-paralyzing drug that is used.

11. 2. Adverse reactions to dexamethasone (Decadron) include hypertension, hyperglycemia, nausea, and diarrhea.

12. 3. Physostigmine salicylate (Antilirium) is a specific antidote for atropine overdose. A client exhibiting an atropine overdose would present with flushing, warm and dry skin, decreased salivation, tachycardia, and urinary retention.

13. 4. Urinary retention is a common adverse reaction to benztropine (Cogentin), which is an anticholinergic drug used in the treatment of Parkinson's disease. Other common adverse reactions include constipation, dry mouth, blurry vision, and tachycardia. The client should be instructed to avoid driving or operating heavy machinery.

14. 2. Edrophonium (Tensilon) is used to differentiate between a cholinergic crisis and a myasthenic crisis. If a client is experiencing a cholinergic crisis, edrophonium (Tensilon) will result in an increase in the muscle weakness. If a client is experiencing a myasthenic crisis, edrophonium (Tensilon) will result in an improvement of the client's clinical manifestations.

15. 3. 4. 6. Methylphenidate hydrochloride (Ritalin) is a central nervous system stimulant used in the treatment of an attention-deficit disorder. Adverse reactions to Ritalin include tachycardia, palpitations, nervousness, agitation, hyperexcitability, insomnia, dizziness, and weight loss.

16. 4. 5. 6. Phenytoin (Dilantin), Phenobarbital (Luminal), and Primidone (Mysoline) are drugs used to treat partial seizures. Ethosuximide (Zarontin) is used to treat absence seizures. Fosphenytoin (Cerebyx) is used to treat status epilepticus.

17. 4. Ethosuximide (Zarontin) is an anticonvulsant drug used to treat absence seizures. Complete blood count and liver function studies should be monitored. Anticonvulsants are contraindicated in hepatic dysfunction and bleeding disorders.

18. 3. Narrow-angle glaucoma is a contraindication in the use of antiparkinsonian drugs. Allergic reactions, hepatitis, and bone marrow depression are uncommon adverse reactions to anticonvulsants. Common adverse reactions include central nervous system effects such as drowsiness, nervousness, ataxia, and dizziness. Common gastrointestinal adverse reactions include gingival hyperplasia, nausea, vomiting, and epigastric discomfort. Antihistamines and antipsychotic drugs increase the effects of antiparkinsonian drugs. Clinical manifestations of Cushing's syndrome include buffalo hump, moon face, abdominal distention, ecchymosis, hypertension, weakness, osteoporosis, amenorrhea, and impotence, and are the result of long-term corticosteroid use.

19. 1. 3. 6. Ergotamine tartrate (Ergomar) is an alpha-adrenergic blocking agent used in the treatment of migraine, cluster, and other vascular headaches. Adverse reactions include nausea, vomiting, diarrhea, abdominal pain, tachycardia, hypertension or hypotension, paresthesia, weakness, and itching.

20. 3. Methysergide maleate (Sansert) is a synthetic ergot derivative used to prevent but not manage acute migraine attacks because of the serious adverse reactions. It is recommended to discontinue Sansert for 1 month after every 4 to 6 months. This too is part of the prescription protocol to prevent serious adverse reactions. The client should never take an additional tablet if the first does not provide relief. This is likely an indication that the drug is not effective for this client. Sansert is taken orally, not sublingually. Ergotamine tartrate (Ergomar) is administered sublingually in the treatment of vascular headaches.

21. 3. Rizatriptan (Maxalt) is used in the treatment of migraine headaches. It is contraindicated for a client with hypertension because hypertension is also an adverse reaction to the drug.

22. 4. It would be appropriate to delegate increasing fluids to a client taking trihexyphenidyl (Artane) to a licensed practical nurse. Artane is an anticholinergic drug that causes constipation. A licensed practical nurse may not administer intravenous drugs, develop a nutritional plan, or monitor a client for adverse reactions.

23. 7–10. Therapeutic effects of phenytoin are optimized within 7–10 days.

24. 3. Felbamate (Felbatol) is a second-line drug used for intractable atonic or partial seizures. It may be appropriate to have a client sign a consent form acknowledging the increased risk of aplastic anemia and liver failure. Weight loss, decreased appetite, hypokalemia, and hyponatremia are adverse reactions. Complete blood count and liver function studies should be monitored. The serum sodium level would be monitored with carbamazepine (Tegretol).

25. 1. The combination of phenobarbital and valproic acid (Depakene) may increase the risk of phenobarbital toxicity.

REFERENCES

Broyles, B., Reiss, B., & Evans, M. (2012). *Pharmacological aspects of nursing care* (8th ed.). Clifton Park, NY: Thomson Delmar Learning.

Daniels, R., & Nicoll, L. (2012). *Contemporary medical-surgical nursing.* Clifton Park, NY: Delmar Cengage Learning.

Spratto, G. R., & Woods, A. L. (2012). *PDR nurse's drug handbook 2012.* Clifton Park, NY: Delmar Cengage Learning.

CHAPTER 23

DRUGS FOR THE INTEGUMENTARY SYSTEM

I. **DRUGS FOR INFLAMMATION—TOPICAL GLUCOCORTICOIDS**
   A. DESCRIPTION
      1. AVAILABLE IN CREAM, OINTMENT, AND GEL DEPENDING ON THE NEED TO PENETRATE
      2. POTENCY VARIES FROM LOW TO SUPERHIGH.
      3. INTENSITY OF RESPONSE DEPENDS ON POTENCY, VEHICLE, AND METHOD OF APPLICATION.
      4. OCCLUSIVE DRESSINGS ENHANCE ABSORPTION BY AS MUCH AS 10 TIMES.
      5. TOPICAL STEROIDS MAY BE ABSORBED IN SYSTEMIC CIRCULATION BASED ON THE LENGTH OF USE AND SURFACE AREA COVERED.
      6. SCALP, AXILLA, FACE, EYELIDS, NECK, PERINEUM, AND GENITALIA ARE ESPECIALLY PERMEABLE. THE BACK, PALMS, AND SOLES ARE MUCH LESS PERMEABLE.
   B. USES
      1. RELIEVE INFLAMMATION AND ITCHING
      2. USED FOR INSECT BITES, MINOR BURNS, SEBORRHEIC DERMATITIS, PSORIASIS, ECZEMA, AND PEMPHIGUS (AUTOIMMUNE DISORDER IN WHICH THERE IS A BLISTERING OF THE EPIDERMIS OF THE SKIN AND MUCOUS MEMBRANES)
   C. ADVERSE REACTIONS
      1. LOCAL
         a. Atrophy of the dermis and epidermis, leading to thinning of the skin and striae formation (stretch marks)
         b. Purpura (red spots) from local hemorrhage
         c. Telangiectasia (red, wartlike lesions) caused by capillary dilation
         d. Acne
         e. Hypertrichosis (excessive hair growth on the face)
         f. Risk of infection and irritation

      2. SYSTEMIC
         a. Growth retardation in children
         b. Adrenal suppression in all age groups
         c. Systemic toxicity is more likely with long-term therapy on extensive areas of skin surface using high-potency agents and occlusive dressings.
   D. CONTRAINDICATIONS AND PRECAUTIONS
      1. REPLACEMENT THERAPY IN ANY ACUTE OR CHRONIC ADRENAL CORTICAL INSUFFICIENCY
      2. PREGNANCY
      3. LACTATION
   E. DRUG INTERACTIONS (SEE CHAPTER 21, DRUGS FOR THE ENDOCRINE SYSTEM)
   F. NURSING INTERVENTIONS
      1. CLEANSE THE AREA BEFORE APPLYING THE DRUG.
      2. WASH HANDS, WEAR GLOVES, APPLY SPARINGLY, AND RUB INTO THE AREA.
      3. APPLY AN OCCLUSIVE DRESSING.
      4. DOCUMENT THE SITE OF THERAPY, INCLUDING SIZE, COLOR, LOCATION, DEPTH, ODOR, SWELLING, DRAINAGE, AND NATURE OF INFECTION.
      5. MONITOR THE CLIENT FOR SIGNS OF INFECTION.
      6. ASSESS THE CLIENT FOR SYSTEMIC ABSORPTION.
      7. NOTIFY THE PHYSICIAN OF REDNESS, DILATED BLOOD VESSELS, PURPLE DISCOLORATION, BRUISING, PUSTULES, OR DEPRESSED SHINY WRINKLED SKIN.
   G. TYPES
      1. SUPERHIGH POTENCY
         a. Betamethasone dipropionate (Diprolene)
         b. Clobetasol propionate (Temovate)
         c. Diflorasone diacetate (Psorcon, Maxiflor, Florone)
      2. HIGH POTENCY
         a. Amcinonide (Cyclocort)
         b. Desoximetasone (Topicort)

c. Fluocinolone acetonide (Synalar-HP)
d. Triamcinolone acetonide (Aristocort)
e. Fluocinonide (Lidex)
3. MEDIUM POTENCY
   a. Betamethasone valerate (Valisone, Betatrex)
   b. Flurandrenolide (Cordran)
4. LOW POTENCY
   a. Desonide (DesOwen, Tridesilon)
   b. Dexamethasone sodium phosphate (Decadron Phosphate)
   c. Hydrocortisone (Cortizone-10, Hycort)

II. **DRUGS USED TO REMOVE KERATIN-CONTAINING LESIONS**
   A. DESCRIPTION: KERATOLYTIC AGENTS PROMOTE SHEDDING OF THE HORNY LAYER OF THE SKIN (STRATUM CORNEUM).
   B. USES
      1. WARTS, CORNS, AND CALLUSES
   C. ADVERSE EFFECTS
      1. LOCAL
         a. Irritation and excessive drying are common with both salicylic acid and sulfur.
      2. SYSTEMIC
         a. Salicylism is possible because salicylic acid is readily absorbed through the skin. Observe for ringing of the ears, hyperpnea, psychological disturbances, drowsiness, and impaired hearing.
   D. CONTRAINDICATIONS AND PRECAUTIONS
      1. LOCAL SKIN IRRITATION
   E. NURSING INTERVENTIONS
      1. MONITOR THE SKIN WHERE THE SALICYLIC ACID OR SULFUR IS APPLIED FOR LOCAL SKIN IRRITATION.
      2. APPLY THE SMALLEST AMOUNT OF MEDICATION AS POSSIBLE TO REDUCE THE RISK OF ADVERSE EFFECTS.
      3. MONITOR THE CLIENT FOR SALICYLISM.
   F. TYPES
      1. SALICYLIC ACID
         a. Promotes desquamation by dissolving intracellular cement that binds scales to the stratum corneum.
         b. Comes in concentrations of 3–6% (low) to 40% (high)
         c. Low concentrations used to treat dandruff, seborrheic dermatitis, acne, and psoriasis
         d. High concentrations used to remove warts, corns, and calluses
      2. SULFUR
         a. Promotes drying and peeling
         b. Treats acne, dandruff, psoriasis, and seborrheic dermatitis
         c. Available in lotion, gel, and shampoo
         d. Concentration ranges from 2–10%.

III. **DRUGS TO TREAT PSORIASIS**
   A. USES
      1. SELECTION OF DRUG IS BASED ON THE SEVERITY OF CLINICAL MANIFESTATIONS.
      2. MILD PSORIASIS IS TREATED WITH TOPICAL STEROIDS AND KERATOLYTIC AGENTS.
      3. MODERATE PSORIASIS IS TREATED WITH COAL TAR OR ANTHRALIN (ANTHRA-DERM, MICANOL). EXPOSING SKIN TO ULTRAVIOLET B LIGHT CAN ENHANCE EFFECTIVENESS OF THESE DRUGS.
      4. SEVERE PSORIASIS MAY BE TREATED WITH METHOTREXATE (RHEUMATREX) OR ETRETINATE (TEGISON) AND UVB LIGHT.
      5. ALEFACEPT (AMEVIVE) IS THE FIRST BIOLOGICAL THERAPY FOR MODERATE TO SEVERE CHRONIC PLAQUE PSORIASIS.
      6. EFALIZUMAB (RAPTIVA) IS THE SECOND IMMUNOSUPPRESSIVE RECOMBINANT MONOCLONAL ANTIBODY INDICATED IN THE TREATMENT OF PLAQUE PSORIASIS.
   B. ADVERSE EFFECTS
      1. TAZAROTENE (TAZORAC)
         a. Itching, burning, stinging, dry skin, and redness
         b. Less commonly, rash, inflammation, or bleeding
         c. Sensitizes skin to sunlight, so protection against exposure is advised
      2. ANTHRALIN (ANTHRA-DERM, MICANOL)
         a. Redness, irritation of the skin
         b. Conjunctivitis if used near the eyes
      3. COAL TAR
         a. Irritation, stinging, burning
         b. No systemic toxicity
      4. CALCIPOTRIENE (DOVONEX)
         a. Irritation
         b. Hypercalcemia if used in very high doses
      5. METHOTREXATE (RHEUMATREX)
         a. Severe toxicity risk, including diarrhea, ulcerative stomatitis, anemia, leucopenia, thrombocytopenia
         b. Liver function must be monitored.
         c. Causes congenital malformations, so prevent pregnancy
      6. ETRETINATE (TEGISON)
         a. Hair loss, peeling of palms, soles, and fingertips are very common.
         b. Dry nose, thirst, sore mouth, and bone and joint pain frequently occur.
         c. Headache, muscle cramps, and eye irritation also are common.
      7. ACITRETIN (SORIATANE)
         a. Hair loss, skin peeling, dry skin, mouth, nosebleeds, and gingivitis are common.
         b. Like etretinate, it causes bone and joint pain, muscle cramps, and dry eyes.

8. ALEFACEPT (AMEVIVE)
   a. Serious infections, injection site pain, dizziness, cough, and pruritus
9. EFALIZUMAB (RAPTIVA)
   a. Thrombocytopenia
   b. Hypersensitivity reaction
   c. Headache
   d. Fever
   e. Chills
   f. Nausea
   g. Myalgia
C. CONTRAINDICATIONS AND PRECAUTIONS
   1. PREGNANCY
   2. ECZEMATOUS SKIN
   3. LACTATION
D. DRUG INTERACTIONS
   1. FLUOROQUINOLONES, PHENOTHIAZINES, SULFONAMIDES, TETRACYCLINES, AND THIAZIDES: INCREASE PHOTOSENSITIVITY
   2. ALCOHOL: INCREASES RISK OF TETRAGENIC EFFECTS ON THE FETUS
   3. ORAL CONTRACEPTIVES: DECREASE THE EFFECTIVENESS OF PROGESTIN
E. NURSING INTERVENTIONS
   1. APPLY THE GEL FORM OF TAZORAC ONCE A DAY IN THE EVENING.
   2. AVOID COVERING MORE THAN 20% OF BODY SURFACE AREA WITH TAZORAC.
   3. DRY SKIN CAREFULLY BEFORE APPLYING.
   4. WEAR OLD CLOTHES OR COVER THE AREA WITH DRESSINGS AFTER APPLYING ANTHRALIN.
   5. APPLY ANTHRALIN AT BEDTIME AND LEAVE ON OVERNIGHT.
   6. INFORM THE CLIENT THAT COAL TAR HAS AN UNPLEASANT SMELL AND MAY STAIN THE HAIR AND SKIN.
   7. ADMINISTER SORIATANE WITH ORAL DOSING WITH MEALS.
   8. INSTRUCT THE CLIENT TO USE AN ALTERNATIVE BIRTH CONTROL.
F. TYPES
   1. TOPICAL DRUGS
      a. Corticosteroids
      b. Tazarotene (Tazorac)
         1) Retinoid that is applied to skin and converts to tazarotenic acid
         2) Stays on skin long after application of drug has stopped
         3) Benefits persist for several months
      c. Anthralin (Anthra-Derm, Micanol)
         1) Inhibits DNA synthesis to suppress overgrowth of epidermal cells
         2) Comes in ointment and cream forms with concentration of 0.1–1%
         3) Stains clothing, skin, and hair
      d. Coal tar
         1) Suppresses DNA synthesis, mitosis, and cell proliferation
         2) Comes as shampoo, lotion, and cream
         3) Made from juniper, birch, or pine tar as well as coal
      e. Calcipotriene (Dovonex)
         1) Analog of vitamin D that suppresses cell differentiation and proliferation
         2) Takes 1–2 months to work
   2. SYSTEMIC DRUGS
      a. Methotrexate (Rheumatrex)
         1) Cytotoxic, especially in tissues that are actively dividing
         2) Slows growth of epidermal cells in psoriasis
         3) Highly toxic drug that is used in severe, debilitating psoriasis that has not responded to any other therapy
         4) Oral, intramuscular (IM), intravenous (IV) administration with various dosing schedules based on the individual
      b. Etretinate (Tegison)
         1) Highly toxic drug that is being phased out of use
         2) Acts on epithelial cells to inhibit formation of keratin, proliferation, and differentiation; also has some anti-inflammatory effects
         3) Reserved for those who have not responded to any other therapies
         4) Takes up to 6 months to see a clinical response
         5) Oral dosing with half-life of 120 days due to storage of drug in fat
      c. Acitretin (Soriatane)
         1) Retinoid that is the principal active metabolite of etretinate with shorter half-life (49 hours)
         2) Inhibits keratinization, differentiation, and proliferation of epidermal cells; also anti-inflammatory
         3) Used in severe psoriasis after other drugs have been ineffective
      d. Alefacept (Amevive)
         1) Produces longer remissions
         2) Administered by IM route
      e. Efalizumab (Raptiva)
         1) Stimulates body's immune system to fight disease
         2) Administered subcutaneously

IV. **DRUGS USED TO TREAT ACNE**
   A. DESCRIPTION
      1. ACNE VULGARIS TREATMENT IS BASED ON THE SEVERITY OF CLINICAL MANIFESTATIONS.
      2. NONDRUG MEASURES TO REDUCE OILINESS OF SKIN ARE TRIED FIRST.
      3. THE GOAL IS TO PREVENT SCARRING AND LIMIT THE DURATION OF CLINICAL MANIFESTATIONS.
   B. ADVERSE EFFECTS
      1. BENZOYL PEROXIDE
         a. Dry, peeling skin
         b. If burning, blistering, or scaling occur, reduce frequency of use.

2. ANTIMICROBIALS
   a. Systemic drugs reduce the effectiveness of oral contraceptives, so counsel clients to use an alternate form of birth control.
   b. Those taking systemic antimicrobials may have sensitivity to the sun.
   c. Azelaic acid may cause loss of pigment in those with dark complexions.
3. RETINOIDS
   a. Topical: blistering, peeling, burning
   b. Systemic: adverse reactions limit usefulness
      1) Nosebleeds, inflammation of the lips, eyes; dry and itching skin of the face; pain and stiff muscles, bones, and joints
      2) Depression and suicide have also been reported (rare).

C. CONTRAINDICATIONS AND PRECAUTIONS
   1. PREGNANCY
   2. ECZEMA
   3. SUNBURN
D. DRUG INTERACTIONS
   1. CONCOMITANT USE OF TOPICAL TRETINOIN PRODUCTS: INCREASES SKIN IRRITATION
   2. FLUOROQUINOLONES, PHENOTHIAZINES, SULFONAMIDE TETRACYCLINE, AND THIAZIDES: INCREASE PHOTOSENSITIVITY WITH TOPICAL TRETINOIN PRODUCTS
   3. ORAL CONTRACEPTIVES: POSSIBLE INADEQUATE PREGNANCY PROTECTION
   4. VITAMIN A: INCREASES ADVERSE REACTIONS WHEN GIVEN WITH RETINOIDS
E. NURSING INTERVENTIONS
   1. INFORM THE CLIENT TAKING ISOTRETINOIN (ACCUTANE) OF THE ASSOCIATED RISKS.
   2. INSTRUCT THE CLIENT TAKING ISOTRETINOIN (ACCUTANE) TO PRACTICE A RELIABLE METHOD OF BIRTH CONTROL 1 MONTH BEFORE AND 1 MONTH AFTER THERAPY TO PREVENT SERIOUS FETAL COMPLICATIONS.
   3. INSTRUCT THE CLIENT TO WEAR PROTECTIVE CLOTHING AND EYEWEAR FOR PROTECTION FROM PHOTOSENSIVITY THAT MAY OCCUR WITH ISOTRETINOIN (ACCUTANE).
   4. INSTRUCT THE CLIENT TO AVOID WASHING THE FACE FOR 1 HOUR AFTER APPLYING TOPICAL TRETINOIN.
   5. INSTRUCT THE CLIENT TO AVOID ANOTHER SKIN CARE PRODUCT OR COSMETICS FOR 1 HOUR AFTER APPLYING TOPICAL TRETINOIN.

6. INSTRUCT THE CLIENT TO AVOID ALCOHOL-BASED FACIAL PREPARATIONS SUCH AS SHAVING LOTION, PERFUMES, MEDICATED SOAPS, AND SKIN CLEANERS WITH USE OF TOPICAL TRETINOIN.
F. TYPES
   1. BENZOYL PEROXIDE
      a. Topical used to suppress growth of *P. acnes* by releasing active oxygen
      b. Promotes peeling of the horny layer of the epidermis
      c. Available in lotion, cream, gel in concentrations from 2.5% to 10%
   2. ANTIMICROBIALS
      a. Topical
         1) For mild to moderate acne, clindamycin (Cleocin) and erythromycin (Eryderm) are used alone or in combination with benzoyl peroxide.
         2) Combined drug Benzamycin contains 3% erythromycin and 5% benzoyl peroxide.
         3) Suppress growth of *P. acnes* without systemic effects
         4) Azaleic acid (Azelex) may be used instead of benzoyl peroxide because of fewer adverse reactions.
      b. Oral
         1) Moderate to severe acne is treated with tetracycline, minocycline, erythromycin, and azithromycin.
         2) Suppress growth of *P. acnes* and reduce inflammation
         3) Tetracycline is drug of choice because of low cost and low toxicity.
         4) Azithromycin is reserved for clients intolerant of or unresponsive to tetracycline; more expensive and longer half-life.
   3. RETINOIDS—DERIVATIVES OF VITAMIN A
      a. Topical
         1) Tretinoin (Retin-A, Renova, Avita) and tazarotene (Tazorac) used for mild to moderate acne; may combine with benzoyl peroxide and systemic antibiotics
         2) Increase turnover of epithelial cells, which promotes the removal of comedones and suppresses formation of new plugs; reduce thickness of stratum corneum to allow other anti-acne drugs to penetrate more effectively
         3) Adapalene (Differin) takes 8–12 weeks to work and may seem to exacerbate acne initially.
         4) Increased risk of sunburn with all topical retinoids—use sunscreen and protective clothing.

b. Systemic
  1) Isotretinoin (Accutane), oral therapy for severe acne in those who have not responded to other therapies; usual treatment is 15–20 weeks.
  2) Reduce sebum production, size of sebaceous glands, inflammation, and lower population of *P. acnes*
  3) Cause sensitivity to the sun

V. DRUGS USED TO TREAT SUPERFICIAL FUNGAL INFECTIONS

A. DESCRIPTION
  1. SUPERFICIAL FUNGAL INFECTIONS ARE CAUSED BY TWO GROUPS OF ORGANISMS: *CANDIDA* AND DERMATOPHYTES. BOTH ARE TREATED WITH EITHER TOPICAL OR ORAL MEDICATIONS.
  2. *CANDIDA* INFECTIONS USUALLY OCCUR IN MOIST MUCOUS MEMBRANES AND SKIN.
  3. DERMATOPHYTE INFECTIONS, THE MORE COMMON OF THE TWO, AFFECT THE SKIN, HAIR, AND NAILS. MOST COMMON ARE:
    a. Tinea pedis (athlete's foot)—ringworm of foot
    b. Tinea corporis—ringworm of the body
    c. Tinea cruris (jock itch)—ringworm of the groin
    d. Tinea capitis—ringworm of the scalp

B. ADVERSE EFFECTS
  1. AZOLES
    a. Stinging, redness, itching, and peeling with topical application
    b. Stomach upset with oral dosing
  2. ALLYLAMINES
    a. Stinging, redness, itching, and peeling with topical application
    b. Diarrhea, dyspepsia, and liver injury with oral dosing
  3. OTHERS
    a. Irritation, burning

C. CONTRAINDICATIONS AND PRECAUTIONS
  1. HYPERSENSITIVITY
  2. PREGNANCY
  3. LACTATION

D. DRUG INTERACTIONS
  1. ORAL CONTRACEPTIVES: MAY DECREASE PROTECTION WITH KETOCONAXOLE
  2. CORTICOSTEROIDS: INCREASE RISK OF TOXICITY WITH KETOCONAXOLE AND FLUCONAZOLE
  3. PROTON PUMP INHIBITORS: DECREASE EFFECT OF KETOCONAXOLE
  4. CIMETIDINE: DECREASES TERBINAFINE CLEARANCE

E. NURSING INTERVENTIONS
  1. AVOID LETTING TROPICAL PRODUCTS COME IN CONTACT WITH THE EYES.
  2. APPLY NIZORAL SHAMPOO TO WET HAIR IN AN AMOUNT SUFFICIENT TO COVER THE ENTIRE SCALP FOR 1 MINUTE, FOLLOWED BY RINSING AND REPEATING, LEAVING THE SHAMPOO ON THE SCALP FOR 3 MINUTES.
  3. WHEN MONISTAT IS USED FOR VAGINAL INFECTION, REFRAIN FROM SEXUAL INTERCOURSE OR USE A CONDOM TO PREVENT REINFECTION.
  4. AVOID OCCLUSIVE DRESSINGS.

F. TYPES
  1. AZOLES: WORK BY INHIBITING SYNTHESIS OF ERGOSTEROL, AN ESSENTIAL PART OF THE FUNGAL CYTOPLASMIC MEMBRANE
    a. Clotrimazole (Gyne-Lotrimin, Mycelex)
      1) Topical: troche, cream, intravaginal application
      2) For ringworm and *Candida* infections of the skin and mouth
    b. Ketoconazole (Nizoral)
      1) Oral for ringworm and *Candida* infection of the mouth or fungal infection of the nails
      2) Topical for ringworm and *Candida* infection of the skin—cream and shampoo
    c. Miconazole (Micatin, Monistat)
      1) Topical for ringworm and *Candida* infection of the skin—cream, liquid, suppository, and powder
    d. Fluconazole (Diflucan)
      1) Oral for *Candida* infection of the mouth or fungal infection of the nails
  2. ALLYLAMINES: WORK BY INHIBITING SQUALENE EPOXIDASE THAT INHIBITS THE SYNTHESIS OF ERGOSTEROL, A COMPONENT OF THE FUNGAL CELL MEMBRANE
    a. Naftifine (Naftin)
      1) Topical for ringworm—cream and gel
    b. Terbinafine (Lamisil)
      1) Topical for ringworm
      2) Oral for fungal infection of the nails
    c. Butenafine (Mentax)
      1) Topical for athlete's foot
  3. OTHERS
    a. Tolnaftate (Tinactin, Aftate)
    b. Haloprogin (Halotex)
    c. Undecylenic acid (Desenex, Cruex)
    d. Ciclopirox olamine (Loprox)
    e. Griseofulvin (Fulvicin, Grisactin)—oral for tinea capitis

VI. ANTIVIRAL DRUGS

A. DESCRIPTION
  1. ANTIVIRAL DRUGS IN TOPICAL, ORAL, OR IV FORMS TREAT HERPES SIMPLEX

(ORAL OR GENITAL), ZOSTER (SHINGLES), OR VARICELLA (CHICKENPOX).

   2. REDUCE THE DURATION AND SEVERITY OF LESIONS

B. ADVERSE REACTIONS

   1. ACYCLOVIR

     a. Oral—nausea, vomiting, diarrhea, headache, vertigo

     b. Topical—stinging, burning

   2. VALACYCLOVIR

     a. Oral—nausea, vomiting, diarrhea, headache, vertigo

C. CONTRAINDICATIONS AND PRECAUTIONS

   1. HYPERSENSITIVITY

   2. IMMUNOCOMPROMISED CLIENTS

   3. RENAL IMPAIRMENT

D. DRUG INTERACTIONS

   1. CIMETIDINE (TAGAMET) AND PROBENECID (BENEMID): DECREASE THE RENAL CLEARANCE

E. NURSING INTERVENTIONS

   1. INSTRUCT THE CLIENT THAT DRUG TREATMENT IS NOT A CURE BUT MANAGES THE DISEASE.

   2. INSTRUCT THE CLIENT TO TAKE THE DRUG AS PRESCRIBED.

   3. MAINTAIN THE FLUID AND NUTRITIONAL INTAKE TO PREVENT CRYSTALLURIA.

   4. APPLY TOPICAL ZOVIRAX EVERY 3 HOURS UP TO SIX TIMES A DAY USING A FINGER COT OR GLOVE TO AVOID TRANSMISSION TO OTHER BODY SITES.

   5. ADJUST ORAL OR IV ZOVIRAX IN ACUTE RENAL IMPAIRMENT.

   6. ADMINISTER VALTREX COMBINED WITH ZOVIRAX TO REDUCE POSTHERPETIC NEURALGIA.

   7. INSTRUCT THE CLIENT WITH GENITAL HERPES TO USE A CONDOM EVEN WHEN LESIONS ARE ABSENT.

F. TYPES

   1. ACYCLOVIR (ZOVIRAX): SUPPRESSES SYNTHESIS OF VIRAL DNA

   2. VALACYCLOVIR (VALTREX)

VII. DRUGS USED TO TREAT BURNS

A. DESCRIPTION

   1. TOPICAL SULFONAMIDES ARE USED TO PREVENT BACTERIAL COLONIZATION ON THE SKIN OF CLIENTS WITH SECOND- OR THIRD-DEGREE BURNS.

   2. ABSORPTION THROUGH THE SKIN CAN CAUSE SYSTEMIC EFFECTS.

   3. APPLIED IN WATER-BASED CREAM OR SOLUTION

B. ADVERSE EFFECTS

   1. ACIDOSIS, PAIN AND BURNING, MACULOPAPULAR RASH: MAFENIDE ACETATE (SULFAMYLON)

   2. TRANSIENT LEUKOPENIA, MACULAR RASH: SILVER SULFADIAZINE (SILVADENE)

   3. ELECTROLYTE IMBALANCES (LOW SODIUM, CHLORIDE, POTASSIUM, AND CALCIUM): SILVER NITRATE SOLUTION

C. CONTRAINDICATIONS AND PRECAUTIONS

   1. HYPERSENSITIVITY TO SULFONAMIDES

   2. IMPAIRED LIVER OR RENAL FAILURE

   3. INTESTINAL OR URINARY OBSTRUCTIONS

   4. PREGNANCY

   5. BLOOD DYSCRASIAS

D. DRUG INTERACTIONS

   1. ANTICOAGULANTS: INCREASE DRUG EFFECTS

   2. ANTIDIABETICS: INCREASE HYPOGLYCEMIC EFFECT

E. NURSING INTERVENTIONS

   1. APPLY TOPICAL CREAM WITH GLOVES OVER THE ENTIRE SURFACE OF THE BURN.

   2. CONTINUE TREATMENT UNTIL HEALING IS PROGRESSING WELL OR UNTIL THE BURN SITE IS READY FOR GRAFTING.

   3. COVER TREATED BURNS WITH A THIN DRESSING.

   4. ADMINISTER ANALGESICS TO AVOID PAIN ON APPLICATION WITH SULFAMYLON.

   5. REPORT ANY ABNORMAL ODOR, DRAINAGE, OR FEVER, AS WELL AS RASHES, BRUISING, BLEEDING, SWELLING, OR DIFFICULTY BREATHING.

   6. APPLY SILVADENE AS A NONPAINFUL APPLICATION ONE TO TWO TIMES A DAY USING STERILE TECHNIQUE.

   7. DISCONTINUE SULFAMYLON FOR 1–2 DAYS TO RESTORE ACID-BASE BALANCE BECAUSE IT MAY CAUSE ACIDOSIS.

   8. APPLY SILVER NITRATE TO THE GAUZE DRESSING EVERY 2 HOURS.

   9. INSTRUCT THE CLIENT THAT SILVER NITRATE STAINS EVERYTHING BLACK OR BROWN.

F. TYPES

   1. SILVER SULFADIAZINE (SILVADENE)

     a. Acts by releasing free silver that inhibits synthesis of folic acid needed for DNA, RNA, and proteins; effective against most bacteria, some fungi, and *Candida*

     b. Especially effective against *Pseudomonas*

   2. MAFENIDE ACETATE (SULFAMYLON)

     a. Acts by suppressing the synthesis of folic acid; effective against most bacteria but not *Candida*

   3. SILVER NITRATE SOLUTION

     a. Broad-spectrum antimicrobial, effective against *Candida*

     b. Penetrates eschar poorly

PRACTICE QUESTIONS

1. Which of the following should the nurse include in the plan of care for a client taking isotretinoin (Accutane)?
   Select all that apply:
   [ ] 1. Avoid letting cream come in contact with eyes
   [ ] 2. Inform the client about the risks of taking Accutane
   [ ] 3. Instruct the client to wear protective clothing and eyewear for protection from photosensitivity
   [ ] 4. Cover treated area with a thin dressing
   [ ] 5. Monitor for salicylism
   [ ] 6. Instruct the client to practice reliable method of birth control for 1 month before and 1 month after treatment

2. The nurse should instruct a client taking an oral retinoid to avoid which of the following?
   1. Dairy products
   2. Carbonated drinks
   3. Extremely cold air
   4. Vitamin A supplements

3. The nurse is caring for a client who has been taking isotretinoin (Accutane) for the past 2 months. Which of the following is a priority for the nurse to report?
   1. Pruritus
   2. Depression
   3. Dry skin
   4. Headache

4. The nurse instructs a client with pruritus to take an oral antihistamine to relieve the itching. Which of the following should be included in this instruction?
   1. "The effects will be best if you take the medication around the clock."
   2. "Take the medication only when the itching is at its worst."
   3. "Use the oral medication in combination with a topical antihistamine."
   4. "Increase the dosage of the oral medication as needed if the itching is severe."

5. The nurse is discharging a client who has second-degree burns on the hands and arms. Treatment includes application of silver sulfadiazine (Silvadene) to the burn area twice a day. Which of the following must be included in wound care instructions for this client?
   1. "Wash the area with warm water before the application of Silvadene."
   2. "Apply salve after the Silvadene to seal the medication into the burned area."

3. "Apply the Silvadene using sterile technique."
   4. "Apply the medication only at bedtime."

6. A 22-year-old has been diagnosed with acne vulgaris and is to start on tetracycline. Which of the following is a priority question to ask this client before therapy is started?
   1. "How long have you had the cystlike nodules on your face?"
   2. "When was your last menstrual period?"
   3. "How many times a day do you scrub your face?"
   4. "Have you been taking any oral medication for acne?"

7. The nurse is instructing a client about use of benzoyl peroxide to treat acne. Which of the following should be included?
   1. Overuse can cause extreme dryness of the skin
   2. Use caution when driving or operating heavy machinery
   3. Nausea and vomiting may occur
   4. A decrease in appetite may occur

8. The nurse is providing instruction to a client about use of lindane (Kwell) shampoo for treatment of *Pediculus humanus capitis* (head lice). Which of the following should be included in the teaching?
   1. Apply the shampoo to dry hair and leave on for 4 to 5 minutes
   2. Wet the hair first and massage the shampoo in for 1 minute
   3. Use the shampoo on dry hair, rinse, then shampoo with regular shampoo
   4. Apply the shampoo to wet hair and rinse thoroughly

9. The nurse is instructing the mother of four children on how to treat all of the children for *Pediculus humanus capitis* (head lice) with Kwell shampoo. The ages of the children are 8 years, 5 years, 2 years, and a premature infant who now weighs 6 pounds. Which one of the following is the priority to include in the instructions given to this mother?
   1. The cost associated with purchasing shampoo for four children may lead to undertreatment
   2. Lindane (Kwell) may cause seizures in premature babies
   3. There is an increased incidence of reinfection from one child to another
   4. Help will be needed to apply the shampoo

10. The physician prescribes ketoconazole (Nizoral) to treat systemic candidiasis. The client asks, "What are the main advantages of this drug?" The nurse's best response is which of the following?
    1. "It can be given orally and is safer than amphotericin B."
    2. "It is less expensive than other medications."
    3. "It is the physician's choice."
    4. "It can be used once a week instead of daily."

11. The nurse should monitor a client taking a drug to remove keratin-containing lesions for which of the following adverse reactions of salicylism? Select all that apply:
    [ ] 1. Leukopenia
    [ ] 2. Ulcerative stomatitis
    [ ] 3. Dizziness
    [ ] 4. Impaired hearing
    [ ] 5. Drowsiness
    [ ] 6. Hair loss

12. When teaching a client about using salicylic acid as a drug to promote shedding of the horny layer of skin, the nurse should explain which of the following about salicylic acid?
    1. It is not absorbed through the skin
    2. It may burn the skin
    3. It is not advised for dandruff
    4. It may cause acne

13. The nurse is caring for a pressure ulcer using a topical debriding agent. Another nurse asks the nurse the type of drug typically used for this purpose. Which of the following is the best response?
    1. An enzyme ointment
    2. A corticosteroid cream
    3. An antipsoriatic lotion
    4. A topical antihistamine

14. The nurse should monitor a client taking betamethasone for which of the following adverse reactions? Select all that apply:
    [ ] 1. Weight loss
    [ ] 2. Decreased appetite
    [ ] 3. Hypotension
    [ ] 4. Muscle wasting
    [ ] 5. Edema
    [ ] 6. Skin thinning

15. The registered nurse is preparing to make out the clinical assignments for the day. Which of the following nursing tasks may the nurse delegate to a licensed practical nurse?
    1. Inform a client taking etretinate (Tegison) to use birth control when taking the drug
    2. Instruct a client using isotretinoin (Accutane)
    3. Administer acyclovir (Zovirax) intravenously to a client
    4. Ask the client if stinging occurs when applying topical acyclovir (Zovirax)

16. The nurse is teaching the client about using tretinoin (Retin-A) for treatment of acne vulgaris. Which of the following indicates that the teaching has been successful?
    1. The client avoids washing the skin with drying soap
    2. The client limits exposure to sunlight
    3. The client reduces the intake of caffeine-containing foods
    4. The client stops using the medication if a stinging feeling occurs

17. The nurse should inform a client taking fluconazole (Diflucan) to be aware of which of the following adverse reactions? Select all that apply:
    [ ] 1. Tremors
    [ ] 2. Headache
    [ ] 3. Constipation
    [ ] 4. Skin rash
    [ ] 5. Pruritus
    [ ] 6. Abdominal pain

18. After instructing a client on the application of anthralin, the client states, "I want to apply the medication to the nonaffected areas to prevent other lesions from developing." Which of the following responses by the nurse is most appropriate?
    1. "The medication can cause chemical burns, so it should be used on the psoriatic lesions only."
    2. "Anthralin is very expensive, so limit its use to the psoriatic lesions."
    3. "As long as you leave it on for a maximum of 2 hours, it should be all right."
    4. "Because anthralin promotes fluid and electrolyte loss, you should limit the areas that are treated."

19. The client is being treated with haloprogin (Halotex) for tinea pedis (athlete's foot). Which of the following statements by the client indicates the client understands the teaching about the medication?
    1. "I will apply the ointment daily for 6 weeks."
    2. "I will use the powder three times a day."
    3. "I will soak my feet in cold water before each application."
    4. "I will apply the medication every morning and evening for 2 to 4 weeks."

20. The client with a rash in the axilla is prescribed amcinonide (Cyclocort) topical. For which of the following adverse reactions should the nurse monitor the client?
    1. Gastrointestinal manifestations
    2. Cracking and splitting of the skin
    3. Thinning of the skin
    4. Loss of pigmentation

21. A female client with herpes genitalis is receiving education about the medication regimen. Which of the following would be most appropriate to include in the teaching?
    1. Use one applicator of terconazole intravaginally at bedtime for 7 days
    2. Use topical acyclovir every 4 hours five times a day for 10 days
    3. Use sulconazole nitrate twice a day and massage in
    4. Use one applicator of tioconazole intravaginally at bedtime for 7 days

22. During the early emergent phase of a burn injury, clients are at risk for infection. Which of the following prescribed drugs would the nurse anticipate administering to prevent infection?
    1. Mafenide acetate (Sulfamylon)
    2. Lindane (Kwell)
    3. Acitretin (Soriatane)
    4. Azelaic acid (Azelex)

23. The nurse should monitor a client receiving mafenide acetate (Sulfamylon) for which of the following adverse reactions?
    Select all that apply:
    [ ] 1. Petechiae
    [ ] 2. Constipation
    [ ] 3. Pain
    [ ] 4. Acidosis
    [ ] 5. Rash
    [ ] 6. Erythema

24. A client with sebhorrheic dermatitis of the face is being treated with topical ketoconazole (Nizoral). Which of the following behaviors by the client indicates that teaching has been effective?
    1. Application of a thick layer of cream; washing the area once a week
    2. Removal of any dry scales prior to application of the cream to aid absorption
    3. Applying an emollient before applying the ketoconazole
    4. Applying moisturizing cream sparingly after applying the ketoconazole

ANSWERS AND RATIONALES

1. 2. 3. 6. Nursing interventions for isotretinoin (Accutane) include informing the client of the associated risks, practicing protective clothing and eyewear for protection from photosensitivity, and instructing the client to practice a reliable method of birth control for 1 month before and 1 month after treatment with Accutane. Superficial fungal infections should not come in contact with the eyes. After applying a drug to a burn site it is covered with a thin dressing. A client taking a drug for keratin-containing lesions should be monitored for salicylism.

2. 4. Oral retinoids are derived from vitamin A; hence, taking supplemental vitamin A could cause an overdose of this fat-soluble vitamin.

3. 2. Isotretinoin (Accutane) is a retinoid used in the treatment of acne. Adverse reactions include pruritus, dry skin, and headache and should be reported, but the priority adverse reaction to report is depression. There have been reports of depression and possibly suicidal ideation associated with the use of isotretinoin.

4. 1. Oral antihistamines have their maximal effect when taken regularly around the clock.

Drowsiness is an adverse reaction that is also minimized by this dosing.

5. 1. Burn wounds should be cleansed prior to application of Silvadene cream. This helps remove dead tissue and old cream. There is no need to apply salve over the Silvadene. Silvadene provides a protective cover by itself. The client should use a clean technique at home rather than a sterile technique. The treatment must be twice a day, generally in the morning and evening.

6. 2. Because tetracycline is teratogenic, it is a priority to establish that the client is not pregnant before starting the drug. Tetracycline is not the drug of choice for a cystlike type of acne. Scrubbing of the face has no impact on the use of tetracycline systemically. Although asking a client if an oral medication for acne has been taken is appropriate, it is not the priority because of the teratogenic effects of the tetracycline.

7. 1. Benzoyl is an effective drying agent that can cause too much drying if overused. Benzoyl peroxide is topical and does not have systemic adverse reactions. Benzoyl peroxide is not associated with the adverse reactions of nausea, vomiting, or a decrease in appetite.

8. 1. The Kwell shampoo should be applied to dry hair and left on the scalp for 4 to 5 minutes to allow for maximal effect. Treatment should be repeated in a week.

9. 2. It is a priority to inform the parent that applying Kwell shampoo to premature infants may cause seizures. Purchasing Kwell shampoo for three children may be costly, but it is essential to prevent the spread of *Pediculus humanus capitis* (head lice). Although an increased incidence of reinfection of the children from one child to another is a minor concern, it is not the priority. Securing help to apply the shampoo may be beneficial, but it is not the priority.

10. 1. Ketoconazole (Nizoral) is just as effective to treat systemic candidiasis and not as dangerous as amphotericin B. Amphotericin B is highly toxic and used for progressive and potentially fatal infections. Although expense is a consideration, safety is the most important factor.

11. 3. 4. 5. Dizziness, impaired hearing, and drowsiness are adverse reactions of salicylism. Leukopenia and ulcerative stomatitis are adverse reactions of methotrexate (Rheumatrex). Hair loss is n adverse reaction to etretinate (Tegison).

12. 1. Salicylic acid has its effect on the keratin layer of the skin. The acid is too mild to burn the skin. It can be used for dandruff. It may also be used to treat acne, because it causes drying and sloughing.

13. 1. An enzyme ointment best describes the classification of agents used for debriding pressure ulcers. Corticosteroids do not have debridement properties. Drugs used for psoriasis do not debride. Topical antihistamines are used for itching and inflammation rather than debridement.

14. 4. 5. 6. Betamethasone (Diprolene) is a superhigh-potency corticosteroid that causes weight gain, increased appetite, hypertension, muscle wasting, edema, and skin thinning.

15. 4. A licensed practical nurse may ask a client if stinging occurs when a topical drug is applied. Informing or instructing a client about certain effects of a drug are nursing tasks that should be performed by a registered nurse. Administering a drug intravenously is also a task that belongs to a registered nurse.

16. 2. Tretinoin (Retin-A) is a retinoid that causes sensitivity to sunlight and susceptibility to sunburn, so limiting exposure and using sunscreen of at least 15 SPF are advised. The use of a drying soap assists the client in treating the acne. Although the use of caffeine has no relationship to the medication itself, some clients find that certain foods aggravate their acne and are advised to avoid them or reduce the amount consumed. A stinging sensation is normal for clients with sensitive skin. Avoiding abrasive soaps and keratolytic agents, like benzoyl peroxide and salicylic acid, can reduce this sensation.

17. 2. 4. 6. Fluconazole (Diflucan) is an antifungal used in the treatment of candidiasis. Adverse reactions include diarrhea, headache, skin rash, and abdominal pain.

18. 1. Anthralin may be used in the treatment of psoriasis. It inhibits DNA synthesis to suppress the overgrowth of epidermal cells. It is a strong irritant and should be applied only to affected skin. It may be very irritating to unaffected skin. It also stains clothing, skin, and hair.

19. 4. Haloprogin (Halotex) is an antifungal. Treatment for tinea pedis (athlete's foot) requires twice-a-day application of Halotex. Soaking the feet in cold water will not improve absorption of the medication.

20. 3. Amcinonide (Cyclocort) is a topical steroid. Regular use of topical steroids is associated with the adverse effect of thinning of the skin and appearance of "stretch marks."

21. 2. Acyclovir (Zovirax) is an antiviral used in the treatment of genital herpes. It is used every 4 hours five times a day for 10 days. Terconazole, sulconazole nitrate, and tioconazole are all antifungal drugs.

22. 1. Sulfamylon is a topical anti-infective that is used to prevent infections in burn wounds. Lindane (Kwell) is used to treat pediculosis. Acitretin (Soriatane) is a retinoid used in the treatment of psoriasis. Azelaic acid (Azelex) is used in the treatment of acne.

23. 3. 4. 5. 6. Mafenide acetate (Sulfamylon) is a sulfonamide used in the treatment of burns. The topical application is painful and may result in acidosis. Rash and erythema are other adverse reactions.

24. 2. Topical ketoconazole (Nizoral) is best absorbed through skin that is free of scales. Gentle washing with soap and water to remove scales will aid in absorption of the topical antifungal. A thin layer that is rubbed in will be more effectively absorbed. The old cream and dead skin must be removed daily. Application of an emollient prior to application of the antifungal will reduce absorption of the antifungal. Moisturizing creams are of no value in treating the fungal infection that caused the dermatitis to begin with.

REFERENCES

Broyles, B., Reiss, B., & Evans, M. (2012). *Pharmacological aspects of nursing care* (8th ed.). Clifton Park, NY: Delmar Cengage Learning.

Daniels, R., & Nicoll, L. (2012). *Contemporary medical-surgical nursing.* Clifton Park, NY: Delmar Cengage Learning.

Spratto, G. R., & Woods, A. L. (2012). *PDR nurse's drug handbook 2012.* Clifton Park, NY: Delmar Cengage Learning.

DRUGS FOR THE MUSCULOSKELETAL SYSTEM

I. **ANALGESICS**
  A. DESCRIPTION
    1. MEDICATION USED TO TREAT MILD, MODERATE, AND SEVERE MUSCULOSKELETAL PAIN
    2. THIS GROUP INCLUDES MANY TYPES OF MEDICATIONS.
  B. USES (SEE TABLE 24-1)
    1. BLOCK PROSTAGLANDIN PRODUCTION, INHIBITING TRANSDUCTION AT THE NOCICEPTORS (FREE NERVE ENDINGS): SALICYLATES AND NONSTEROIDAL ANTI-INFLAMMATORY DRUGS (NSAIDS)
    2. BLOCK ACTION POTENTIAL INITIATION, INHIBITING TRANSDUCTION AT THE NOCICEPTORS: TOPICAL ANESTHETICS AND CORTICOSTEROIDS
    3. ELEVATE PAIN THRESHOLD: NONOPIOID ANALGESICS
    4. BLOCK RELEASE OF SUBSTANCE P FROM NERVE ENDINGS, INTERRUPTING PAIN SIGNALS TO THE BRAIN (TRANSMISSION): OPIOIDS
    5. DECREASE CONSCIOUS EXPERIENCE OF PAIN (PERCEPTION): OPIOIDS, NSAIDS
  C. ADVERSE REACTIONS
    1. ALL SALICYLATES
      a. Abdominal (cramps, pain, discomfort, heartburn or indigestion, nausea or vomiting)
      b. Edema
      c. Diarrhea
      d. Dizziness
      e. Drowsiness
      f. Headache
    2. ACETYLATED SALICYLATES
      a. Ulcers
      b. Internal bleeding
      c. Confusion
      d. Deafness
      e. Tinnitus (ringing in the ear)

    3. NONACETYLATED SALICYLATES
      a. Deafness
      b. Tinnitus
    4. NSAIDS
      a. Tinnitus
      b. Gastrointestinal (GI) irritation (dyspepsia, nausea, ulcer, hemorrhage)
      c. Prolonged bleeding time
      d. Headache
      e. Skin rashes
      f. Renal insufficiency or other renal changes
      g. Exacerbation with asthma (cross-reactivity with aspirin)
      h. Allergy (rapid or irregular pulse, hives, wheezing, or tightness of the chest)
    5. NONOPIOID ANALGESICS
      a. Acetaminophen
        1) Skin rashes
        2) Hepatotoxicity (especially with alcohol use)
        3) Leukopenia
      b. Capsaicin cream
        1) Local burning
        2) Erythema
      c. Tramadol
        1) GI irritation (dyspepsia, nausea, ulcer, hemorrhage)
        2) Dizziness
        3) Headache
        4) Sleep disturbances
        5) Pruritus
    6. OPIOID ANALGESICS
      a. GI irritation (dyspepsia, nausea, vomiting, ulcer, hemorrhage)
      b. Constipation
      c. Dizziness
      d. Headache
      e. Orthostatic hypotension
      f. Sedation
      g. Respiratory depression
      h. Shortness of breath

Table 24-1 Matching Drugs and Diagnoses

Diagnosis or Surgical Intervention	Analgesics					Biologic Agents	DMARDs	Corticosteroids	Bisphosphonates	Other Drugs
	Salicylates	NSAIDs	Nonopioids	Opioids	Other					
Soft tissue injury	X		X	X						X
Carpal tunnel syndrome	X		X							
Dislocation/subluxation	X		X	X						X
Fracture	X		X	X					X	X
Osteomyelitis			X	X	X			X		X
Osteoporosis									X	X
Amputation	X		X	X						X
Osteomalacia									X	X
Paget's disease									X	
Rheumatoid arthritis	X	X	X	X	X	X	X	X	X	X
Osteoarthritis	X	X	X		X			X		X
Lupus	X	X	X	X	X	X	X	X	X	X
Gout		X	X				X	X		X
Reactive arthritis	X	X	X			X	X	X		X
Fibromyalgia	X	X	X		X					X
Arthroplasty	X	X	X	X	X					X

NSAIDs = nonsteroidal anti-inflammatory drugs, Other = other types of analgesic

DMARDs = disease-modifying antirheumatic drugs

    i. Urinary retention
    j. Mood changes
    k. Dry mouth
    l. Increased sweating
    m. Itching
    n. Weakness
  D. CONTRAINDICATIONS AND PRECAUTIONS
    1. ACETYLATED SALICYLATES: HEAVY USE OF ALCOHOL, USE OF BLOOD THINNERS, SENSITIVITY OR ALLERGY TO ASPIRIN, KIDNEY DISEASE, LIVER DISEASE, HEART DISEASE, HIGH BLOOD PRESSURE, ASTHMA, PEPTIC ULCERS
    2. NONACETYLATED SALICYLATES: HEAVY ALCOHOL USE, USE OF NSAIDS, ALLERGY TO NONACETYLATED DRUGS, HEART DISEASE, KIDNEY DISEASE
    3. TRADITIONAL NSAIDS: CHRONIC DISEASES SUCH AS KIDNEY DISEASE, LIVER DISEASE, AND HEART DISEASE; HYPERTENSION; ASTHMA; STOMACH ULCERS; OR IMMEDIATELY AFTER SURGERY
    4. COX-2 NSAIDS: HISTORY OF HEART ATTACK, STROKE, ANGINA, BLOOD CLOTS, HYPERTENSION, SENSITIVITY TO ASPIRIN AND OTHER NSAIDS

  5. NONOPIOID ANALGESICS: ACETAMINOPHEN AND ALCOHOL CONSUMPTION OF THREE OR MORE DRINKS A DAY IS CONTRAINDICATED.
  6. OPIOID ANALGESICS: PHYSICAL AND PSYCHOLOGICAL DEPENDENCE, CENTRAL NERVOUS SYSTEM (CNS) DEPRESSANTS (ANTIHISTAMINES, TRANQUILIZERS, SLEEPING AIDS, MUSCLE RELAXANTS), LIVER DISEASE, HISTORY OF ALCOHOL OR DRUG ABUSE
E. DRUG INTERACTIONS
  1. SALICYLATES
    a. Anticoagulants: increase effect of anticoagulant
    b. Corticosteroids: both are ulcerogenic.
    c. Furosemide: increases risk of salicylate toxicity
    d. NSAIDs: additive ulcerogenic effects
  2. NSAIDS
    a. Acetaminophen: increases risk of hypertension
    b. Aspirin: decreases effect of NSAIDs and increases risk of GI effects
    c. Selective serotonin reuptake inhibitors (SSRIs): increase risk of GI effects

Table 24-2 Protection for Stomach Problems with NSAIDs

Protection	Explanation/Drug
Add an acid-reducing drug.	Histamine blockers such as cimetidine (Tagamet) and ranitidine hydrochloride (Zantac) or proton pump inhibitors such as omeprazole (Prilosec) and lansoprazole (Prevacid)
Take a combination drug therapy to reduce risk of ulcers and promote healing of ulcers.	Misoprostol (Cytotec) replaces prostaglandins, which NSAIDs block. Arthrotec contains both misoprostol and an NSAID diclofenac sodium. Prevacid NapraPac contains prevacid and naproxen together.
Take COX-2 NSAIDs.	These have a protective effect and do not produce stomach upset as traditional NSAIDs.
Switch NSAIDs.	Some NSAIDs bother clients more than others.
Reduce dosage with physician approval.	Starting with a low dose and increasing sometimes helps with stomach upset.
Avoid alcohol.	Alcohol and NSAID combinations increase risks of ulcers.
Take with food.	Food helps to relieve stomach upset when taking NSAIDs.
Watch other drugs the client is taking.	NSAIDs, taken in combination with other drugs, increase the risk of stomach ulcers (particularly with corticosteroids and blood thinners).
Avoid doubling NSAIDs.	Some over-the-counter (OTC) drugs contain NSAIDs and when taken with prescribed NSAIDs increase the risk of stomach ulcers.
Alter the timing of NSAIDs.	Taking the NSAID later in the day may avoid stomach upset (always check with the physician before allowing the client to use this strategy).
Do not take too much.	If the pain continues, have the client speak to the physician about changing the dose or drug (never increase the dose without the physician's approval).

© Cengage Learning 2015

F. NURSING INTERVENTIONS
1. ALL SALICYLATES
   a. Administer with food, milk, or antacids as indicated or with full glass of water.
   b. Report signs of bleeding (tarry stools, bruising, petechiae, nosebleeds).
   c. Instruct the client to avoid chewing the tablets.
   d. Avoid crushing or mixing enteric-coated and time-released forms.
   e. Avoid combining with NSAIDs.
   f. Administer in continuous large doses for pain in arthritis.
   g. Discard aspirin by the expiration date (when expired, some drugs are not as effective; aspirin breaks down into products that can damage the kidneys).
   h. Monitor the client for confusion, deafness, or ringing in the ears, which indicate an overdose.
2. ALL NSAIDS
   a. Administer with food, milk, or antacids as indicated or with full glass of water (see Table 24-2).
   b. Report signs of bleeding (tarry stools, bruising, petechiae, nosebleeds), edema, skin rashes, headaches that persist for days, or visual disturbances.
   c. Monitor for fluid retention (daily weights, blood pressure [BP]).
   d. Instruct the client that maximum effect is only achieved with regular use.
   e. Notify the physician if the client drinks alcohol or uses blood thinners, angiotensin-converting-enzyme (ACE) inhibitors, lithium, warfarin, or furosemide, or has allergy to aspirin.

   f. Instruct the client to avoid taking with other NSAIDs.
   g. Instruct the client that the NSAID may be taken with low-dose aspirin.
   h. Instruct the client to take as directed at the same time each day.
3. COX-2 NSAIDS
   a. Instruct the client to avoid taking with other NSAIDs.
   b. Notify the physician if the client is sensitive to aspirin or other NSAIDs.
   c. Notify the physician if the client is sensitive to sulfonamides or has a history of cardiovascular disease or hypertension and is taking celecoxib (Celebrex).
4. NONOPIOID ANALGESICS
   a. Instruct the client to avoid the use of alcohol, which can cause liver damage.
   b. Monitor for overuse in clients (maximum dose in 24 hours should not be exceeded).
   c. Instruct the client that the maximum effect is only achieved with regular use.
   d. Instruct the client to avoid using acetaminophen with other products containing acetaminophen.
   e. Instruct the client to avoid using for more then 10 days for pain without a physician's order.
5. OPIOID ANALGESICS
   a. Encourage fluids and fiber if not contraindicated to prevent constipation.
   b. Administer with an antiemetic if nausea occurs.

c. Report signs of bleeding with types that include aspirin (tarry stools, bruising, petechiae, nosebleeds).

d. Monitor complete blood count (CBC) and liver function tests.

e. Instruct the client and family to report any CNS or respiratory changes.

f. Instruct the client that sedation results in decreased reaction time.

g. Have an awareness that clients may attempt to sell these drugs illegally, and, if suspected, this should be reported.

h. Instruct the client to avoid taking more than the physician has prescribed.

i. Instruct the client that the drug may be taken with or without food and at the same time each day.

j. Instruct the client to avoid operating heavy machinery.

k. Instruct the client to avoid stopping the drug abruptly unless the physician has ordered to do so.

l. Instruct the client when taking combination-type opioids mixed with acetaminophen such as Vicodin that other drugs containing acetaminophen should be avoided.

G. TYPES
  1. TWO TYPES OF SALICYLATES
     a. Acetylated, also known as aspirin, are over-the-counter (OTC) drugs such as Anacin, Ascriptin, Bayer, Bufferin, Ecotrin, and Excedrin.
     b. Nonacetylated can be OTC or prescription drugs.
        1) OTC drugs include:
           a) Choline and magnesium salicylates such as Tricosal and Trilisate
           b) Choline salicylate in liquid form only such as Arthropan
           c) Magnesium salicylates such as Bayer Select, Doan's Pills
        2) Prescription drugs include:
           a) Magnesium salicylates such as Magan, Mobidin, Mobigesic
           b) Salicylates such as Amigesic, Disalcid, Marthritic, Mono-Gesic, Salflex, Salsitab
           c) Sodium salicylate (generic form only)
  2. NSAIDS ARE THE MOST USED AND LARGEST CLASS OF ARTHRITIS DRUGS IN BOTH OTC AND PRESCRIPTION PREPARATIONS.
     a. OTC choices such as ibuprofens, ketoprofens, and naproxen sodium (Aleve)
     b. Prescription choices of traditional NSAIDs

1) Diclofenac potassium (Cataflam)
2) Diclofenac sodium (Voltaren, Voltaren XR)
3) Diclofenac sodium with misoprostol (Arthrotec)
4) Diflunisal (Dolobid)
5) Etodolac (Lodine, Lodine XL)
6) Fenoprofen calcium (Nalfon)
7) Flurbiprofen (Ansaid)
8) Ibuprofen (Motrin)
9) Indomethacin (Indocin, Indocin SR)
10) Ketoprofen (Orudis, Oruvail)
11) Meclofenamate sodium (Meclomen)
12) Mefenamic acid (Ponstel)
13) Meloxicam (Mobic)
14) Nabumetone (Relafen)
15) Naproxen (Naprosyn, Naprelan)
16) Naproxen sodium (Anaprox)
17) Oxaprozin (Daypro)
18) Piroxicam (Feldene)
19) Sulindac (Clinoril)
20) Tolmetin sodium (Tolectin)
21) Ketorolac tromethamine (Toradol)
c. Prescription choices cyclooxgenase-2 (COX-2) inhibitors, which are safer to the stomach
   1) Celecoxib (Celebrex)
3. NONOPIOID ANALGESICS: ACETAMINOPHEN IS THE FIRST CHOICE OF PAIN RELIEF FOR OSTEOARTHRITIS PAIN, ACCORDING TO THE AMERICAN COLLEGE OF RHEUMATOLOGY GUIDELINES.
   a. OTC choices such as Anacin, Excedrin caplets, Panadol, Tylenol
   b. Do not relieve inflammation but do relieve arthritis pain
4. OPIOID ANALGESICS ARE PRESCRIBED FOR ACUTE MUSCULOSKELETAL PROBLEMS BUT ARE NOT TRADITIONALLY PRESCRIBED FOR CLIENTS WITH ARTHRITIS; HOWEVER, THAT IS CHANGING.
   a. Hydrocodone with acetaminophen (Dolacet, Hydrocet, Lorcet, Lortab, Vicodin)
   b. Oxycodone (OxyContin, Roxicodone)
   c. Propoxyphene hydrochloride (Darvon)
   d. Tramadol (Ultram)
   e. Ultracet (a combination of tramadol and acetaminophen used for acute pain)
5. TOPICAL ANESTHETICS FOR MILD PAIN
   a. Available as creams, gels, salves
   b. Usually have one of three ingredients
      1) Capsaicin: a natural ingredient found in cayenne peppers; agent names include Zostrix, Zostrix HP, Capzasin-P.

      2) Counterirritants such as menthol, oil of wintergreen, camphor, and eucalyptus oil; turpentine oil brands such as ArthriCare, Eucalyptamint, Icy Hot, Therapeutic Mineral Ice

      3) Salicylates: compounds that inhibit pain and inflammation by seeping through the skin. Brand names include Aspercreme, BenGay, Flexall, Mobisyl, Sportscreme.

  6. CORTICOSTEROIDS (SEE CHAPTER 21— DRUGS FOR THE ENDOCRINE SYSTEM)

II. BIOLOGIC RESPONSE MODIFIERS (BRMS)

A. DESCRIPTION
1. UP TO TWO-THIRDS OF CLIENTS WITH RHEUMATOID ARTHRITIS RESPOND TO BRMS WHEN OTHER THERAPY HAS FAILED.
2. THESE DRUGS ARE VERY EXPENSIVE.

B. USES
1. INHIBIT CYTOKINES (PROTEINS THAT CONTRIBUTE TO INFLAMMATION)
2. BLOCK THE CYTOKINE KNOWN AS TUMOR NECROSIS FACTOR ALPHA: MONOCLONAL ANTIBODIES
3. BLOCK THE CYTOKINE INTERLEUKIN-1
4. FOR RHEUMATOID ARTHRITIS AND LUPUS WHEN DISEASE-MODIFYING ANTIRHEUMATIC DRUG (DMARD) THERAPY FAILS

C. ADVERSE REACTIONS
1. FLULIKE CLINICAL MANIFESTATIONS (CHILLS, FEVER, MUSCLE ACHES, WEAKNESS, LOSS OF APPETITE, NAUSEA, VOMITING, DIARRHEA)
2. RASH
3. BLEEDING
4. BRUISING
5. SWELLING
6. INFUSION REACTIONS SUCH AS CHEST PAIN, BP CHANGES, DIFFICULTY BREATHING, HIVES, REDNESS AND PAIN, ITCHING AT THE INFUSION SITE
7. UPPER RESPIRATORY INFECTIONS SUCH AS SINUS INFECTIONS, SORE THROAT, COUGHING, ABDOMINAL PAIN
8. ANAKINRA CAN CAUSE LOW WHITE BLOOD CELL (WBC) COUNT OR LOW PLATELET COUNT.

D. CONTRAINDICATIONS AND PRECAUTIONS
1. RECURRENT INFECTIONS SUCH AS PNEUMONIA
2. ACTIVE INFECTION, EXPOSURE TO TUBERCULOSIS, OR NERVOUS SYSTEM DISORDERS SUCH AS MULTIPLE SCLEROSIS, SEIZURES, MYELITIS, OPTIC NEURITIS
3. CLIENTS WITH HEART FAILURE SHOULD NOT RECEIVE ANY MONOCLONAL ANTIBODY.

E. DRUG INTERACTIONS
1. IMMUNOSUPPRESSANTS: FEWER INFUSION REACTIONS COMPARED TO CLIENTS TAKING NO IMMUNOSUPPRESSANTS

F. NURSING INTERVENTIONS
1. ALL BMRS
   a. Avoid giving live vaccines.
   b. Pneumonia and flu vaccine may be given if injected.
   c. Drugs must be infused or injected through IV.
   d. All except infliximab (Remicade) must be refrigerated prior to use.
2. ETANERCEPT (ENBREL)
   a. Mix by injecting liquid into the vial of powder.
   b. Do not shake; instead swirl to mix.
   c. It may be injected into the thigh, abdomen, or upper arm.
3. INFLIXIMAB (REMICADE)
   a. IV infusion over 2 hours
   b. Client should also be taking methotrexate once a week.
4. ADALIMUMAB (HUMIRA) AND ANAKINRA (KINERET)
   a. Comes in prefilled syringes
   b. May be injected into the thigh, abdomen, or upper arm
   c. Do not shake.

G. TYPES
1. MONOCLONAL ANTIBODIES
   a. Etanercept (Enbrel)
   b. Infliximab (Remicade)
   c. Adalimumab (Humira)
2. INTERLEUKIN-1: ANAKINRA (KINERET)

III. DISEASE-MODIFYING ANTIRHEUMATIC DRUGS (DMARDS)

A. DESCRIPTION
1. DRUGS TO CONTROL THE DISEASE SYMPTOMS FOR CERTAIN TYPES OF ARTHRITIS
2. ALL THE MECHANISMS OF ACTION ARE NOT COMPLETELY UNDERSTOOD.
3. USED EARLY IN THE DISEASE TO PREVENT DEFORMITY AND DISABILITY LATER IN THE DISEASE PROCESS
4. GENERALLY, THESE DRUGS ARE EFFECTIVE BUT THEY TAKE TIME TO SHOW RESULTS.
5. INCLUDE DRUGS FROM MANY CLASSES
6. ALL DMARD DOSING MUST TAKE INTO ACCOUNT DISEASE SEVERITY, AGE, BODY WEIGHT, AND OTHER DRUGS THE CLIENT IS TAKING.

B. USES
1. MOST COMMONLY USED FOR RHEUMATOID ARTHRITIS
2. LESS FREQUENTLY USED FOR JUVENILE ARTHRITIS, ANKYLOSING

SPONDYLITIS, PSORIATIC ARTHRITIS, AND LUPUS,
3. SUPPRESS THE IMMUNE SYSTEM
4. INHIBIT T-CELL FUNCTION

C. ADVERSE REACTIONS
1. GI EFFECTS (DIARRHEA, LOSS OF APPETITE, NAUSEA, VOMITING, CRAMPS, PAIN, HEARTBURN)
2. LOW LABS (WBC COUNT, RED BLOOD CELL [RBC] COUNT)
3. MOUTH (METALLIC TASTE IN THE MOUTH, ULCERS, ENLARGED GUMS, TONGUE IRRITATION AND SORENESS, WHITE SPOTS)
4. URINE (BLOOD IN URINE, PROTEIN)
5. SKIN (RASH, ITCHING, DARKENING, FLUSHING)
6. FEVER, CHILLS, BLURRED VISION, HEADACHE, INCREASED SENSITIVITY TO SUNLIGHT
7. LIVER, KIDNEY FAILURE
8. TIREDNESS, WEAKNESS, DIZZINESS
9. HAIR LOSS OR GROWTH
10. MISSING MENSTRUAL PERIODS, INFERTILITY
11. HYPERTENSION, SHORTNESS OF BREATH
12. TREMBLING AND SHAKING HANDS
13. JOINT PAIN

D. CONTRAINDICATIONS AND PRECAUTIONS
1. HISTORY OF DISEASES SUCH AS BLOOD, INFLAMMATORY BOWEL, LIVER, OR KIDNEY DISEASE; HYPERTENSION; LUPUS; COLITIS; OR RECURRENT INFECTIONS
2. METHOTREXATE: NOT USED IN LIVER OR LUNG DISEASE, ALCOHOLISM, ACTIVE INFECTION, OR HEPATITIS
3. MINOCYCLINE: HYPERSENSITIVITY TO TETRACYCLINES
4. PENICILLAMINE: HYPERSENSITIVITY TO PENICILLIN
5. SULFASALAZINE: HYPERSENSITIVITY TO SULFA OR ASPIRIN

E. DRUG INTERACTIONS
1. ALLOPURINOL: INCREASE EFFECTS OF AZATHIOPRINE
2. AURANOFIN, GOLD SODIUM THIOMALATE: ALLERGY TO GOLD-CONTAINING DRUGS
3. MINOCYCLINE: DO NOT TAKE WITH ALLERGY TO TETRACYCLINES.
4. PENICILLAMINE: DO NOT TAKE WITH PENICILLIN ALLERGY.
5. SULFASALAZINE: DO NOT TAKE WITH ALLERGY TO SULFA DRUGS OR ASPIRIN.

F. NURSING INTERVENTIONS
1. INSTRUCT THE CLIENT TO MINIMIZE EXPOSURE TO SUNLIGHT AND WEAR SUNSCREEN.
2. MONITOR BLOOD, LIVER FUNCTION, AND URINE STUDIES.
3. AZATHIOPRINE (IMURAN) CAN CAUSE CANCER SUCH AS LYMPHOMAS.
4. MONITOR THE CLIENT FOR AN INCREASED SUSCEPTIBILITY TO INFECTIONS.
5. INFORM THE CLIENT THAT JOINT PAIN MAY BE EXPERIENCED FOR 1–2 DAYS AFTER AN INJECTION OF GOLD SODIUM THIOMALATE (MYOCHRYSINE).
6. ENCOURAGE THE CLIENT TO HAVE A BASELINE EYE EXAM BECAUSE VISION CAN BE DAMAGED WITH LONG-TERM THERAPY OF HYDROXYCHLOROQUINE SULFATE (PLAQUENIL).
7. INFORM THE CLIENT THAT LEFLUNOMIDE (ARAVA) MUST BE STOPPED PRIOR TO CONCEPTION, AND AN ELIMINATION PROCESS WITH THE DRUG CHOLESTYRAMINE (QUESTRAN) SHOULD BE DONE PRIOR TO CONCEPTION.
8. ADMINISTER METHOTREXATE (RHEUMATREX)
   a. Perform a baseline chest x-ray and monitor periodically.
   b. Monitor liver function and blood counts for adverse reactions.
   c. Report dry cough, fever, and difficulty breathing immediately to the physician.
   d. Monitor the client for an increased risk for blood diseases such as lymphomas.
   e. Encourage the client to restrict alcohol consumption.
9. SULFASALAZINE (AZULFIDINE)
   a. Encourage the client to drink adequate fluids to prevent urine crystals.
   b. Inform the client that the sperm count may be lower and may interfere with conception.
10. ADMINISTER AURANOFIN (RIDAURA) AND AZATHIOPRINE (IMURAN) WITH WATER, MILK, OR FOOD.
11. ADMINISTER MINOCYCLINE (MINOCIN) AND PENICILLAMINE (CUPRIMINE) WITH WATER ON AN EMPTY STOMACH.
12. ADMINISTER CYCLOPHOSPHAMIDE (CYTOXAN) WITH BREAKFAST, DRINK 2000 ML OR MORE OF FLUIDS THROUGHOUT THE DAY, AND EMPTY THE BLADDER BEFORE GOING TO BED.

G. TYPES
  1. GENERAL USE FOR RHEUMATOID ARTHRITIS, JUVENILE ARTHRITIS, ANKYLOSING SPONDYLITIS, PSORIATIC ARTHRITIS, LUPUS
     a. Auranofin—oral gold (Ridaura)
     b. Azathioprine (Imuran)
     c. Cyclosporine (Neoral, Sandimmune)
     d. Gold sodium thiomalate—injectable gold (Myochrysine)
     e. Hydroxychloroquine sulfate (Plaquenil)
     f. Leflunomide (Arava)
     g. Methotrexate (Rheumatrex, Trexall)
     h. Minocycline (Minocin)—not FDA approved for arthritis
     i. Penicillamine (Cuprimine, Depen)
     j. Sulfasalazine (Azulfidine, Azulfidine EN-Tabs)
  2. USED TO TREAT SEVERE ORGAN DISEASE OR VASCULITIS
     a. Chlorambucil (Leukeran)
     b. Cyclophosphamide (Cytoxan)

IV. **CORTICOSTEROIDS**
  A. DESCRIPTION
    1. EFFECTIVE IN THE CONTROL OF INFLAMMATION BUT HAVE MANY SERIOUS ADVERSE REACTIONS WHEN TAKEN IN LONG DURATIONS
    2. MAY CAUSE PROFOUND AND VARIED METABOLIC EFFECTS
    3. MODIFY THE BODY'S IMMUNE RESPONSES TO STIMULI
    4. DOSES VARY ACCORDING TO THE DISEASE.
  B. USES
    1. USED IN MANY DISEASES TO REDUCE INFLAMMATION, SUCH AS MUSCULOSKELETAL, GI, GENITOURINARY (GU), OR LUNG DISEASES
  C. ADVERSE REACTIONS
    1. BRUISING
    2. CATARACTS
    3. HYPERGLYCEMIA
    4. HYPERLIPIDEMIA
    5. ATHEROSCLEROSIS
    6. HYPERTENSION
    7. INCREASED APPETITE
    8. INDIGESTION
    9. INSOMNIA
    10. MOOD SWINGS
    11. MUSCLE WEAKNESS
    12. NERVOUSNESS OR RESTLESSNESS
    13. OSTEOPOROSIS
    14. INFECTION
    15. THINNING SKIN
  D. CONTRAINDICATIONS AND PRECAUTIONS
    1. FUNGAL INFECTIONS
    2. TUBERCULOSIS
    3. ACTIVE THYROID DISEASE
    4. DIABETES
    5. ULCERS
    6. HYPERTENSION
    7. OSTEOPOROSIS
  E. DRUG INTERACTIONS
    1. MEDROL: DO NOT TAKE IF ALLERGIC TO YELLOW NO. 5 DYE.
    2. ANTACIDS: DECREASE EFFECT OF CORTICOSTEROIDS
    3. ANTIDIABETICS: HYPERGLYCEMIC EFFECT
    4. BARBITURATES: DECREASE EFFECT OF CORTICOSTEROIDS
    5. ESTROGENS: INCREASE ANTI-INFLAMMATORY EFFECT
    6. FUROSEMIDE: INCREASES POTASSIUM LOSS
    7. HEPARIN: INCREASES ULCEROGENIC EFFECTS
    8. IMMUNOSUPPRESSANTS: INCREASE RISK OF INFECTION
    9. NSAIDS: INCREASE ULCEROGENIC EFFECTS
  F. NURSING INTERVENTIONS
    1. MONITOR THE CLIENT FOR ADVERSE REACTIONS BY HAVING YEARLY EYE EXAMS, BONE DENSITY TESTS, AND BLOOD TESTS.
    2. INSTRUCT THE CLIENT ON THE SIGNS OF INFECTION AND PROVIDE INSTRUCTIONS TO NOTIFY THE PHYSICIAN IF ANY SIGNS PRESENT.
    3. INSTRUCT THE CLIENT ON DIET AND EXERCISE AND THE IMPORTANCE OF AVOIDING WEIGHT GAIN.
    4. INSTRUCT THE CLIENT TO TAPER OFF AND TO AVOID DISCONTINUING ABRUPTLY.
    5. INSTRUCT THE CLIENT TO TAKE AS ORDERED AND THAT TAKING TOO MUCH OR TOO LITTLE CAN BE DANGEROUS.
    6. ADMINISTER WITH FOOD.
    7. MONITOR THE CLIENT'S BLOOD PRESSURE.
    8. MONITOR SERUM SODIUM, GLUCOSE, ELECTROLYTES, AND PLATELETS WITH LONG-TERM THERAPY.
    9. MONITOR FOR DEPRESSION.
    10. ENCOURAGE THE CLIENT TO EAT A HIGH-PROTEIN DIET DUE TO THE BREAKDOWN OF GLUCONEOGENESIS AND TO INCREASE POTASSIUM IN THE DIET.
    11. ENCOURAGE THE CLIENT TO EAT A DIET HIGH IN CALCIUM TO AVOID OSTEOPOROSIS.
    12. INFORM THE CLIENT THAT WOUNDS MAY HEAL MORE SLOWLY.

G. TYPES
1. BETAMETHASONE (CELESTONE)
2. CORTISONE ACETATE (CORTONE)
3. DEXAMETHASONE (DECADRON, HEXADROL)
4. HYDROCORTISONE (CORTEF, HYDROCORTONE)
5. METHYLPREDNISOLONE (MEDROL)
6. PREDNISOLONE (PRELONE)
7. PREDNISOLONE SODIUM PHOSPHATE (PEDIAPRED)
8. PREDNISONE (DELTASONE, ORASONE, PREDNICEN-M, STERAPRED)

V. **GOUT MEDICATIONS**
A. DESCRIPTION: IN CHRONIC GOUT, NEED TO TARGET THE CAUSE (BUILDUP OF URIC ACID), SO MANY DRUGS MIGHT BE UTILIZED.
B. USES
1. REDUCE PAIN AND INFLAMMATION IN ACUTE GOUT
2. SLOW URIC ACID PRODUCTION: ALLOPURINOL (ZYLOPRIM), FEBUXOSSTAT (ULORIC)
3. ASSIST WITH URIC ACID EXCRETION: PROBENECID (BENEMID)
4. REDUCE PAIN AND INFLAMMATION: COLCHICINE
C. ADVERSE REACTIONS
1. SKIN (RASH, HIVES, ITCHING)
2. GI (DIARRHEA, NAUSEA, VOMITING, STOMACH PAIN, LOSS OF APPETITE)
3. HEADACHE
4. WORSENING OF GOUT
D. CONTRAINDICATIONS AND PRECAUTIONS
1. KIDNEY OR LIVER DISEASE
2. INFECTIONS OR IN CLIENTS WHO ARE IMMUNOSUPPRESSED AND TAKE IMMUNOSUPPRESSIVE DRUGS
3. LACTATION
E. DRUG INTERACTIONS
1. PROBENECID (BENEMID)
   a. Aspirin: inhibits uricosuric activity
   b. NSAIDs: increase effect of NSAIDs
   c. Allopurinol: additive effects to decrease uric acid levels
   d. Zidovudine (AZT): increases bioavailability of AZT
2. COLCHICINE
   a. CNS depressants: increase depressant effect
F. NURSING INTERVENTIONS
1. ADMINISTER WITH FOOD OR IMMEDIATELY AFTER A MEAL.
2. ENCOURAGE THE CLIENT TO INCREASE FLUIDS TO 2000 ML OR MORE PER DAY.
3. INSTRUCT THE CLIENT TO STOP TAKING IF A RASH APPEARS BECAUSE THIS MAY INDICATE ALLERGY.
4. INSTRUCT THE CLIENT TO AVOID TAKING WITH ASPIRIN OR OTHER NSAIDS.
5. INSTRUCT THE CLIENT TO AVOID ALCOHOL.
6. INFORM THE CLIENT THAT ACUTE GOUT ATTACKS ARE COMMON WHEN BEGINNING ALLOPURINOL THERAPY BUT CAN BE MINIMIZED BY TAKING LOW DOSES AND COMBINING WITH COLCHICINES.
7. MONITOR THE URINE GLUCOSE BECAUSE THESE DRUGS MAY INTERFERE WITH URINE GLUCOSE TESTS, LEADING TO FALSE POSITIVES.
8. STOP THE DRUG AND REPORT NAUSEA, VOMITING, AND DIARRHEA BECAUSE THESE ARE SIGNS OF TOXICITY.
G. TYPES
1. ACUTE GOUT (NSAIDS, CORTICOSTEROIDS, OR COLCHICINES [ANTI-INFLAMMATORY AGENTS])
2. CHRONIC GOUT
   a. Allopurinol (Lopurin, Zyloprim)
   b. Probenecid (Benemid)
   c. Losartan (Cozaar, Hyzaar) and fenofibrate (Tricor) help with excretion of uric acid.
   d. Febuxostat (Uloric)

VI. **FIBROMYALGIA MEDICATIONS**
A. DESCRIPTION
1. MANY DRUGS FROM VARIOUS CLASSES HAVE BEEN PROVEN TO BE EFFECTIVE IN TREATING FIBROMYALGIA.
2. THESE DRUGS FOCUS ON PAIN AND SLEEP DISTURBANCES.
B. USES
1. THOUGHT TO ACT ON INHIBITING SEROTONIN REUPTAKE AND ANTIHISTAMINE EFFECT: TRICYCLIC ANTIDEPRESSANTS
2. PRECISE MECHANISM UNKNOWN: MAY REDUCE THE CALCIUM-DEPENDENT RELEASE OF SEVERAL NEUROTRANSMITTERS: MISCELLANEOUS ANTICONVULSANT (LYRICA)
3. ACT INDIRECTLY TO HELP WITH PAIN: SSRI ANTIDEPRESSANTS
4. ACT ON PAIN BY DECREASING THE CONSCIOUS EXPERIENCE OF PAIN (PERCEPTION): OTHER ANTIDEPRESSANTS
5. ACT TO INHIBIT PERIODIC LIMB MOVEMENT THAT AFFECTS SLEEP QUALITY: BENZODIAZEPINES
6. BLOCK THE ACTION POTENTIAL INITIATION INHIBITING

TRANSDUCTION: OTHER TYPES OF DRUGS SUCH AS MUSCLE RELAXANTS AND ANTISEIZURE MEDICATIONS

C. ADVERSE REACTIONS
1. ALL ANTIDEPRESSANTS
   a. Constipation
   b. Dizziness
   c. Drowsiness
   d. Dry mouth
   e. Headache
   f. Tiredness
   g. Weight gain
2. SSRI ANTIDEPRESSANTS AND OTHER ANTIDEPRESSANTS HAVE ADDITIONAL ADVERSE REACTIONS.
   a. Decreased sexual desire or ability
   b. Difficulty sleeping
   c. Sedation
   d. GI (nausea, vomiting, decreased appetite, diarrhea, cramps, gas, pain)
   e. Nervous (anxiety, nervousness, restlessness, trembling, shaking)
   f. Urinary retention
   g. Skin (rash, itching, rash)
3. BENZODIAZEPINES
   a. Depression
   b. Clumsiness, dizziness
   c. Slurred speech
   d. Sedation
4. OTHER DRUGS FOR PAIN
   a. Cyclobenzaprine (Flexeril): blurred vision, dizziness, drowsiness, dry mouth
   b. Carisoprodol (Soma): dry eyes and mouth, restlessness, sedation
   c. Gabapentin (Neurontin): dizziness, drowsiness, clumsiness, nausea
   d. Modafinil (Provigil): headache, nausea
   e. Orphenadrine (Norflex): dry eyes and mouth, restlessness, sedation
   f. Tizanidine (Zanaflex): drowsiness
   g. Zaleplon (Sonata): headache
   h. Zolpidem (Ambien): drowsiness, hangover effect

D. CONTRAINDICATIONS AND PRECAUTIONS
1. ANTIDEPRESSANTS
   a. Seizures
   b. Urinary retention
   c. Glaucoma
   d. Other chronic eye problems
   e. Heart problems

E. DRUG INTERACTIONS
1. SSRI ANTIDEPRESSANTS, COMBINED WITH ALCOHOL OR OTHER ANTIDEPRESSANTS, CAN INCREASE THE DRUGS' EFFECT AND INCREASE THE RISK FOR ADVERSE REACTIONS.
2. BUPROPION (WELLBUTRIN)
   a. Do not take within 14 days of a monamine oxidase (MAO) inhibitor: increased acute toxicity to bupropion.
   b. Alcohol: decreases seizure threshold

F. NURSING INTERVENTIONS
1. HAVE AN AWARENESS THAT A CLIENT MAY ATTEMPT TO SELL THESE DRUGS ILLEGALLY, AND, IF SUSPECTED, THIS SHOULD BE REPORTED.
2. ENCOURAGE CLIENTS TO RESTRICT ALCOHOL CONSUMPTION.
3. ANTIDEPRESSANTS:
   a. Instruct the client to avoid stopping these drugs abruptly.
   b. Instruct the client that adverse reactions may occur unless withdrawal is gradual.
4. INSTRUCT THE CLIENT ON THE PROPER WITHDRAWAL TECHNIQUE FOR BENZODIAZEPINES BECAUSE IN RARE CASES THEY ARE ADDICTIVE AND WITHDRAWAL CAN BE DIFFICULT.
5. INSTRUCT THE CLIENT THAT ZALEPLON AND ZOLPIDEM SHOULD ONLY BE TAKEN WHEN A FULL 8 HOURS IS AVAILABLE TO RECOVER BECAUSE THEY CAN CAUSE SHORT-TERM MEMORY LOSS.
6. ADMINISTER THE DOSE AT BEDTIME TO AVOID MORNING DROWSINESS.
7. INSTRUCT THE CLIENT TO AVOID DRIVING OR OPERATING HEAVY EQUIPMENT DUE TO DROWSINESS.
8. INFORM THE CLIENT THAT DRUGS MAY BE PRESCRIBED TO COUNTERACT THE EFFECTS OF DRY EYES AND MOUTH.

G. TYPES
1. TRICYCLIC ANTIDEPRESSANTS TO IMPROVE SLEEP QUALITY
   a. Amitriptyline hydrochloride (Elavil, Endep)
   b. Doxepin (Adapin, Sinequan)
   c. Nortriptyline (Aventyl, Pamelor)
2. SSRI ANTIDEPRESSANTS TO HELP WITH PAIN
   a. Citalopram (Celexa)
   b. Fluoxetine (Prozac)
   c. Paroxetine (Paxil)
   d. Sertraline (Zoloft)
3. OTHER ANTIDEPRESSANTS FOR PAIN CONTROL
   a. Bupropion (Wellbutrin, Zyban)
   b. Trazodone (Desyrel)
   c. Venlafaxine (Effexor)
   d. Nefazodone (Serzone)
   e. Mirtazapine (Remeron)
4. BENZODIAZEPINES TO IMPROVE SLEEP QUALITY
   a. Temazepam (Restoril)
   b. Aprazolam (Xanax)
   c. Clonazepam (Klonopin)
   d. Lorazepam (Ativan)

5. OTHER TYPES OF DRUGS FOR PAIN
   a. Cyclobenzaprine (Cycloflex, Flexeril)
   b. Carisoprodol (Soma)
   c. Gabapentin (Neurontin)
   d. Modafinil (Provigil)
   e. Orphenadrine (Norflex)
   f. Tizanidine (Zanaflex)
   g. Zaleplon (Sonata)
   h. Zolpidem (Ambien)
6. ANTICONVULSANTS
   a. Pregablin (Lyrica): dizziness, somnolence, weight gain

VII. OSTEOPOROSIS MEDICATIONS
A. DESCRIPTION
   1. THESE DRUGS PREVENT FURTHER LOSS OF BONE AND MINIMIZE INCIDENCE OF FRACTURES.
   2. SOME OF THESE DRUGS HAVE PROVEN TO ADD BONE AFTER BONE LOSS HAS BEGUN.
   3. THE CHALLENGES ARE TO IDENTIFY THE CLIENTS WHO WOULD BENEFIT MOST FROM THESE DRUGS AND TO IDENTIFY THE CORRECT TYPE OF DRUG FOR THEIR TREATMENT.
B. USES
   1. TREAT OSTEOPOROSIS FROM BOTH PRIMARY AND SECONDARY CAUSES
   2. REPLACE LOST ESTROGEN AFTER MENOPAUSE: ESTROGEN REPLACEMENT THERAPIES (ERTS)
   3. TISSUE-SPECIFIC AGONIST AND ANTAGONIST ACTIONS: SELECTIVE ESTROGEN RECEPTOR MODULATORS (SERMS)
   4. SUPPRESSES OSTEOCLAST ACTIVITY: CALCITONIN
   5. BIND TO BONE SURFACES AND INHIBIT OSTEOCLASTS: BISPHOSPHONATES
   6. ALLOW NEW BONE TO FORM: BONE FORMATION AGENTS
C. ADVERSE REACTIONS
   1. ESTROGEN REPLACEMENT THERAPY
      a. Breast: increased size, pain, possible increased risk of cancer
      b. GI: bloating, nausea, weight gain
      c. Swelling: lower extremities
      d. Heart disease
   2. SERMS—RALOXIFENE HYDROCHLORIDE (EVISTA): HOT FLASHES, LEG CRAMPS
   3. CALCITONIN (NASAL SPRAY): NASAL IRRITATIONS AND BLEEDS
   4. BISPHOSPHONATES: ABDOMINAL PAIN, HEARTBURN
   5. BONE FORMATION AGENT: CALCIUM ELEVATION, DIZZINESS, LEG CRAMPS
D. CONTRAINDICATIONS AND PRECAUTIONS
   1. ERT
      a. History of breast cancer
      b. Pregnancy
      c. Lactation

2. SERMS (DO NOT USE PRIOR TO MENOPAUSE OR IN CLIENTS WITH A HISTORY OF BLOOD CLOTS)
3. CALCITONIN: PROTEIN ALLERGY
4. BISPHOSPHONATES
   a. Esophagus, stomach, or kidney problems
   b. Aspirin and aspirin-containing drugs
5. MONOCLONAL ANTIBODY
   a. Hypocalcemia
6. BONE FRAGMENT AGENT
   a. History of any cancer
   b. Radiation therapy
   c. Children or growing adult
   d. Hypercalcemia
   e. Any metabolic bone disease other than osteoporosis
E. DRUG INTERACTIONS
   1. ESTROGENS
      a. Anticoagulants: decrease anticoagulant response
      b. Antidiabetics: impair glucose tolerance
      c. Anticonvulsants: estrogen-induced fluid retention may precipitate seizures
   2. BISPHOSPHONATES
      a. Antacids: decrease absorption
      b. Aspirin: increases risk of upper GI effects
      c. Calcium supplements: decrease absorption
      d. NSAIDs: increase risk of upper GI effects
F. NURSING INTERVENTIONS
   1. ESTROGENS
      a. Instruct the client to take with food to minimize the GI effects.
      b. Instruct the client to report leg pain, chest pain, dizziness, and weakness of the arms and legs or numbness (thromboembolic problems).
      c. Instruct the client to avoid smoking.
   2. BISPHOSPHONATES
      a. Instruct the client to get adequate intake of vitamins C and D.
      b. Administer in the morning with a full glass of water on an empty stomach.
      c. Instruct the client to avoid eating for 30 minutes and not to lie down or bend over for 30 minutes.
      d. Administer Reclast IV annually
   3. MONOCLONAL ANTIBODY
      a. Take subcutaneously in the upper arm, upper thigh, or abdomen every 6 months.
      b. Administer 1000 mg calcium every day.
      c. Administer 400 units of vitamin D daily.
G. TYPES
   1. ERT
      a. Conjugated estrogens with progesterone: Premphase, Prempro, Activella
      b. Conjugated estrogens without progesterone: Premarin
      c. Esterified estrogen: Estratab, Estrace

2. SERMS: RALOXIFENE HYDROCHLORIDE
   (EVISTA)
3. CALCITONIN (NASAL SPRAY)
4. BISPHOSPHONATES
   a. Alendronate (Fosamax)
   b. Risedronate (Actonel)

   c. Ibandronate (Boniva)
   d. Zoledronic acid (Reclast)
5. MONOCLONAL ANTIBODY
   a. Denosumab (Prolia)
6. BONE FORMATION AGENT:
   TERIPARATIDE (FORTEO)

PRACTICE QUESTIONS

1. The nurse explains to the client that which of the following drugs is the drug of choice in Raynaud's phenomenon?
   1. Nonsteroidal anti-inflammatories
   2. Corticosteroids
   3. Aspirin
   4. Calcium-channel blockers

2. Allopurinol (Zyloprim) and colchicine have been prescribed for a client with gout and diabetes mellitus. Which of the following instructions should be given to this client?
   1. Blood glucose tests may not be valid
   2. Urine sugar tests may not be valid
   3. Protein restrictions can cause diabetic ketoacidosis
   4. Protein cannot be restricted so increased dosing of allopurinol may be required

3. The nurse should administer which of the following prescribed drugs to a client with rheumatoid arthritis who has severe joint involvement and a positive rheumatoid factor?
   1. Methotrexate
   2. Naproxen (Naprosyn)
   3. Acetylsalicylic acid (aspirin)
   4. Hydroxychloroquine sulfate (Plaquenil)

4. Which of the following should the nurse consider before administering an opioid analgesic to a child?
   1. The child's age, weight, height, and respiratory status
   2. Children are less susceptible to adverse reactions
   3. Addiction is increased in children
   4. Sedation is increased in children

5. The nurse instructs a client who has salsalate (Disalcid) prescribed for a sprained ankle. Which of the following statements by the client indicates the client understood the instructions?
   1. "It may cause me to have a headache and I should report this to my physician."

   2. "It can be purchased at the drug store without a prescription, because there are few adverse reactions."
   3. "There are some adverse reactions associated with Disalcid, but none that I need report to the doctor."
   4. "If I get dizzy after taking Disalcid, I should lie down and let the drug wear off before I resume my activities."

6. The nurse is collecting a medication history for a client who has meloxicam (Mobic) prescribed. Which of the following drugs that the client is taking should the nurse question?
   1. Atorvastatin calcium (Lipitor)
   2. Alendronate sodium (Fosamax)
   3. Omeprazole (Prilosec)
   4. Diclofenac potassium (Cataflam)

7. A client who has osteoarthritis and is taking acetaminophen (Tylenol) orally and applying capsaicin cream topically to the knees develops a rash. Based on an understanding of the action of the drugs, which of the following is most likely the cause of the rash?
   1. The rash is an allergic reaction to acetaminophen (Tylenol) but not to the capsaicin
   2. The rash is an allergic reaction to capsaicin but not to the acetaminophen (Tylenol)
   3. A rash is not an adverse reaction to either the acetaminophen (Tylenol) or the capsaicin
   4. A rash is an adverse reaction to both the acetaminophen (Tylenol) and capsaicin

8. The nurse is admitting a client with fibromyalgia and a fractured hip who is taking sertraline (Zoloft) and diazepam (Valium). The physician orders morphine 10 mg IV push for the acute pain. Which of the following adverse reactions is a priority for the nurse to consider before administering the morphine?
   1. Sedation
   2. Gastrointestinal upset

3. Constipation
4. Dizziness

9. The nurse is caring for a client who is receiving salicylate (Disalcid) to manage arthritis pain. Which statement would indicate the client has a good understanding of this drug?
   1. "I should take this drug on an empty stomach and not eat for 30 minutes."
   2. "To work well on my pain, I should make sure to take all the doses every day."
   3. "I only need to take this drug when I am in pain."
   4. "I can take this drug and Naprosyn together to help my pain."

10. Which of the following adverse reactions of infliximab (Remicade) should the nurse include in the medication instructions given to a client? Select all that apply:
    [ ] 1. Hypertension
    [ ] 2. Headache
    [ ] 3. Urinary retention
    [ ] 4. Fever
    [ ] 5. Rash
    [ ] 6. Hearing loss

11. When the first class of drugs prescribed for rheumatoid arthritis fails, the nurse anticipates which category of drugs will be prescribed?
    1. Nonsteroidal anti-inflammatory
    2. Disease-modifying antirheumatic
    3. Salicylates
    4. Biologic response modulators

12. Which of the following would be the best indicators to the nurse that a client receiving Naprosyn for rheumatoid arthritis is experiencing adverse reactions from this drug? Select all that apply:
    [ ] 1. Tinnitus
    [ ] 2. Blurred vision
    [ ] 3. Confusion
    [ ] 4. Headache
    [ ] 5. Vasoconstriction
    [ ] 6. Hypokalemia

13. A client who had an osteoarthritic knee replacement has been receiving ibuprofen (Motrin) and experiencing excellent pain relief with this drug. Recently the client has been experiencing amblyopia, heartburn, nausea, and diarrhea. Which of the following would be the best nursing action for the nurse to include in this client's plan of care?
    1. Administer the Motrin with milk
    2. Give the Motrin 2 hours before meals
    3. Administer the Motrin with prescribed misoprostol (Cytotec)
    4. Give the Motrin with aspirin 2 hours after meals

14. A client with rheumatoid arthritis is being treated with etanercept (Enbrel). Which of the following statements by the nurse indicates the nurse understands the proper handling of this medication?
    1. "I will mix the drug by injecting liquid into the vial of powder, swirl it, and inject the drug into the client's upper arm."
    2. "I will take the prefilled syringe and warm it before injecting it into the client's upper arm."
    3. "I will infuse the drug through a peripheral IV over a period of 2 hours."
    4. "I will shake the prefilled syringe and inject it into the client's thigh."

15. The nurse is caring for a client with systemic scleroderma. The nurse understands that the client is to receive penicillamine (Cuprimine) for which of the following purposes?
    1. Inhibits the accumulation of collagen
    2. Prevents infection
    3. Causes thinning of the skin
    4. Decreases inflammation

16. Which of the following should the nurse consider before administering anakinra (Kineret) to a client with rheumatoid arthritis?
    1. Live vaccines should never be given to this client
    2. Oral doses must be taken with a full glass of water on an empty stomach
    3. Flu vaccines should be given annually to avoid complications from the flu
    4. Biologic response modifiers must be infused in the physician's office

17. The nurse is admitting a client with fibromyalgia who is tearful and states, "I am in so much pain that I can't sleep. I just don't know what can be done for me." Which of the following should the nurse include in the instructions given to this client?
    1. The Food and Drug Administration has approved many drugs for the treatment of fibromyalgia
    2. Anticholinergics have been proven to be beneficial with painful muscles and tissues
    3. Treatment will focus on relieving both pain and sleep disturbances
    4. Medications that are used in the treatment of fibromyalgia do not relieve sleep disturbances

18. The nurse should instruct a client to drink how many ml of fluid daily when taking allopurinol (Zyloprim)?_____

19. The nurse is caring for a client with fibromyalgia who is experiencing pain and insomnia. Which of the following prescribed

drugs should the nurse administer to relieve pain and insomnia?
1. Cyclobenzaprine (Flexeril)
2. Acetaminophen (Tylenol)
3. Trazodone (Desyrel)
4. Clonazepam (Klonopin)

20. The nurse should include which of the following in the plan of care for a client who has rheumatoid arthritis for which methotrexate (Rheumatrex) has been prescribed?
1. Instruct the client to avoid sunlight
2. Instruct the client to avoid engaging in strenuous exercise
3. Monitor the client for respiratory depression
4. Restrict the client's fluid intake

21. When providing care to a client who is on dexamethasone (Decadron), the nurse should monitor the client for which of the following adverse reactions?
Select all that apply:
[ ] 1. Hyperglycemia
[ ] 2. Acne
[ ] 3. Hypotension
[ ] 4. Dehydration
[ ] 5. Menstrual irregularities
[ ] 6. Depression

22. Which of the following interventions should the nurse include in the plan of care for a client taking denosumab (Prolia)?
Select all that apply:
[ ] 1. Administer subcutaneously in the upper arm, upper thigh, or abdomen every 6 months
[ ] 2. Administer 1000 mg calcium a day
[ ] 3. Instruct the client to take with food
[ ] 4. Instruct the client to avoid lying down for 30 minutes after receiving drug
[ ] 5. Administer 400 units of vitamin D every day
[ ] 6. Instruct the client to report chest pain, dizziness, and weakness of the arms or legs

23. The nurse is caring for a client with a history of chronic gout. The nurse should understand that the client is to receive probenecid (Benemid) for which of the following purposes?
1. Slows uric acid production
2. Decreases inflammation
3. Increases uric acid excretion
4. Reduces pain

24. The nurse tells a client that which of the following adverse reactions may be experienced when taking pregablin (Lyrica)?
Select all that apply:
[ ] 1. Headache
[ ] 2. Dry eyes
[ ] 3. Dizziness
[ ] 4. Somnolence
[ ] 5. Slurred speech
[ ] 6. Weight gain

25. The nurse is discharging a client with osteoporosis who is to begin on alendronate (Fosamax). Which of the following should the nurse include in the medication instructions?
1. Take with food or within 30 minutes of eating
2. Notify the physician if urinary retention develops
3. Avoid taking within 2 hours of eating calcium-rich foods
4. Avoid driving while taking the medication

26. The nurse is preparing to delegate clinical assignments to a licensed practical nurse. Which of the following assignments may the nurse delegate?
1. Instruct a client taking an opioid analgesic on the effects of sedation on reactive time
2. Monitor the white blood count and platelets in a client receiving interleukin-1 anakinra (Kineret)
3. Evaluate a client with rheumatoid arthritis on compliance with drug therapy
4. Administer prednisolone (Prelone) with food to a client with rheumatoid arthritis

ANSWERS AND RATIONALES

1. 4. The drugs of choice to treat Raynaud's phenomenon are calcium-channel blockers, such as diltiazem (Cardizem) and nifedipine (Procardia). They are particularly useful in treating acute episodes, but are also used in chronic episodes. They relieve vasospastic attacks by relaxing the smooth muscles of the arterioles.

2. 2. Urine sugar tests may indicate false positives when taking gout medications. Blood glucose testing is still accurate. Protein restrictions do not cause diabetic ketoacidosis, and protein is not restricted for diabetic clients.

3. 1. Because of the serious adverse reactions, such as hepatotoxicity and bone marrow depression, methotrexate is reserved for severe rheumatoid arthritis with severe systemic involvement and a positive rheumatoid factor. Laboratory monitoring must be obtained periodically

throughout treatment. Methotrexate acts by facilitating a rapid anti-inflammatory response within days to weeks.

4. 1.   Age, weight, height, and respiratory status must be considered before administering an opioid analgesic to children. There is no evidence to support that addiction or sedation are increased risks in children.

5. 1.   Salsalate (Disalcid) is a nonacetylated salicylate prescription drug. All adverse reactions should be reported to the physician. If the client becomes dizzy, lying down is appropriate, but the physician should be notified before resuming normal activities.

6. 4.   Diclofenac potassium (Cataflam) is a nonsteroidal anti-inflammatory. Because the client is already taking meloxicam (Mobic), taking two anti-inflammatories at the same time is contraindicated. Taking two anti-inflammatory drugs increases the incidence of adverse reactions. Atorvastatin calcium (Lipitor) is an antihyperlipidemic. Alendronate sodium (Fosamax) is a bone growth regulator used in the treatment of osteoporosis. Omeprazole (Prilosec) is a proton pump inhibitor used in the treatment of ulcers and gastroesophageal reflux disease.

7. 4.   Both acetaminophen (Tylenol) and capsaicin may cause a rash.

8. 1.   Sedation is an adverse reaction to sertraline (Zoloft), diazepam (Valium), and morphine.

9. 2.   Salicylate (Disalcid) should be taken with food and on a regular schedule. Disalcid should not be taken with an anti-inflammatory drug such as Naprosyn.

10. 2. 4. 5.   Infliximab (Remicade) may be used with methotrexate for inhibition of the progression of the structural damage in clients with rheumatoid arthritis who have been unsuccessfully treated with methotrexate alone. Adverse reactions include fever, fatigue, headache, dizziness, depression, rash, and urticaria.

11. 4.   Disease-modifying antirheumatic drugs (DMARDs) are the first drugs used to try to reduce joint clinical manifestations in rheumatoid arthritis. Biologic response modulators have a 66% success rate after failure with DMARDs.

12. 1. 2. 3. 4.   Naprosyn is a nonsteroidal anti-inflammatory drug used in the treatment of musculoskeletal and soft tissue inflammatory disorders, such as rheumatoid arthritis. Adverse reactions include headache, dizziness, blurred vision, confusion, tinnitus, and gastrointestinal upset. Naprosyn results in vasodilation and hyperkalemia.

13. 3.   The most appropriate nursing action for a client who verbalizes effective pain relief from a nonsteroidal anti-inflammatory (NSAID) medication such as ibuprofen (Motrin) for osteoarthritis but is now complaining of gastrointestinal upset is to administer misoprostol (Cytotec) in conjunction with the Motrin. Cytotec is frequently given in conjunction with an NSAID drug that is causing gastrointestinal upset. Cytotec inhibits gastric acid secretion, has mucosal protective properties, and does not interfere with the efficacy of the Motrin. It is given for the duration that the NSAID drug is taken. Amblyopia (blurred vision) has no impact on the gastrointestinal upset. If a client experiences heartburn, nausea, and diarrhea, the NSAID may be administered with food and milk. If no gastrointestinal upset is experienced, the NSAID is given on an empty stomach.

14. 1.   Etanercept (Enbrel) is an immunomodulator used in the treatment of moderate to severe rheumatoid arthritis for clients who have been unsuccessfully treated with one or more antirheumatic drugs. It comes in a vial as a powder. It must be liquefied by adding liquid and swirling to mix. It should not be shaken. It is injected into the upper arm, abdomen, or thigh.

15. 3.   Systemic sclerosis or scleroderma is a connective tissue disorder that results in degenerative, fibrotic, and inflammatory changes of the skin, blood vessels, skeletal muscles, and internal organs. Penicillamine (Cuprimine) is an antirheumatic drug that is investigationally used. It acts by thinning the skin.

16. 1.   Anakinra (Kineret) is a biologic response modifier that acts by inhibiting cytokines. Administering a live vaccine will manifest the disease process. Flu vaccines should be given each year, but not in the live virus form such as FluMist. Currently, there is no oral dosing of these medications. All biologic response modifiers are expensive, but only infliximab (Remicade) is infused through an IV.

17. 3.   The Food and Drug Administration has approved no drugs specifically for the treatment of fibromyalgia. However, many classes of drugs have proven to be beneficial in relieving pain and sleep disturbances for these clients. Treatment will focus on relieving the pain and facilitating sleep. Anticholinergics are not used to treat clinical manifestations of fibromyalgia.

18.   Allopurinol (Zyloprim) is an anti-gout medication and the nurse should encourage the client to drink 2000 ml of fluids a day to flush out the system.

19. 1.   Cyclobenzaprine (Flexeril) is a skeletal muscle relaxant that is administered to a client with fibromyalgia who is experiencing both pain and insomnia (sleeplessness). Acetaminophen (Tylenol) is a nonopioid analgesic and is

administered for pain. Trazodone (Desyrel) is an antidepressant prescribed for depression with or without anxiety. Clonazepam (Klonopin) is a benzodiazepine used in the treatment of depression.

20. 1. Methotrexate (Rheumatrex) is a disease-modifying antirheumatic drug (DMARD). Exposure to the sunlight makes the skin more susceptible to adverse reactions of the sun, such as damage to the eye and sunburn, so the client should be advised to avoid sunlight and wear sunscreen and sunglasses. There are no indications that aerobic exercise causes any adverse events to occur with DMARD therapy. Respiratory depression is not an adverse reaction to DMARDs. Fluids should be encouraged to at least 2000 ml daily to ensure adequate hydration and prevent nephrotoxicity.

21. 1. 2. 5. Adverse reactions to corticosteroids, such as dexamethasone (Decadron), include hyperglycemia, acne, menstrual irregularities, hypertension, edema, and euphoria.

22. 1. 2. 5. Nursing interventions for denosumab (Prolia) include administering it subcutaneously in the upper arm, upper thigh, or abdomen; administering 1000 mg of calcium daily; and administering 400 units of vitamin D daily. Instructing the client to take the drug with food is an intervention for estrogen. Avoiding lie down after administration of the drug for 30 minutes is an intervention for a bisphosphate. Instructing the client to report leg pain, chest pain, dizziness, and weakness of the arms and legs is an intervention for estrogen.

23. 3. Probenecid (Benemid) is an antigout drug that acts by inhibiting renal tubular reabsorption of uric acid, promoting uric acid excretion, and decreasing serum urate levels. Allopurinol (Zyloprim) slows uric acid production. Colchicine acts by reducing the pain and inflammation.

24. 3. 4. 6. Adverse reactions of pregablin (Lyrica) include dizziness, somnolence, and weight gain. Headache is an adverse reaction of modafinil (Provigil), a drug given for pain. An adverse reaction of orphenadrine (Norflex) is headache. Slurred speech is an adverse reaction of a benzodiazepine.

25. 3. Alendronate (Fosamax) should not be taken with food or within 2 hours of calcium-rich foods. It is best if it is taken 30 minutes before food. Urinary retention and sedation are not adverse reactions to Fosamax.

26. 4. It is within the job description of a licensed practical nurse to administer prednisolone (Prelone) with food. Instructing a client taking an opioid analgesic on the effects of sedation, monitoring the white blood count and platelets of a client receiving interleukin-1 anakinra (Kineret), and evaluating compliance with drug therapy are all clinical assignments that require the expertise of a registered nurse.

REFERENCES

Broyles, B., Reiss, B., & Evans, M. (2012). *Pharmacological aspects of nursing care* (8th ed.). Clifton Park, NY: Delmar Cengage Learning.

Daniels, R., & Nicolls, L. (2012). *Contemporary medical-surgical nursing.* Clifton Park, NY: Delmar Cengage Learning.

Spratto, G. R., & Woods, A. L. (2012). *PDR nurse's drug handbook 2012.* Clifton Park, NY: Delmar Cengage Learning.

CHAPTER 25

DRUGS FOR THE GENITOURINARY SYSTEM

I. URINARY TRACT ANTI-INFECTIVES

A. DESCRIPTION

1. USED TO TREAT ACUTE, RECURRENT, AND CHRONIC URINARY TRACT INFECTIONS
2. POTENT ANTIMICROBIALS SUCH AS PENICILLINS, CEPHALOSPORINS, FLUOROQUINOLONES, AMINOGLYCOSIDES, AND SULFONAMIDES USED PRIMARILY IN THE SHORT-TERM TREATMENT OF URINARY TRACT INFECTIONS
   a. Result in systemic adverse reactions
   b. Increased incidence of bacterial resistance

B. PENICILLINS

1. USES
   a. Broad-spectrum antibiotic used in the treatment of urinary tract infection caused by enteric bacteria
   b. Increasing resistance to *E. Coli* developing
   c. Interfere with cell wall replication
2. ADVERSE REACTIONS
   a. Gastrointestinal (GI): nausea, vomiting, diarrhea
   b. Integumentary: rash, urticaria
   c. Hematology: anemia, increased bleeding time
3. CONTRAINDICATIONS AND PRECAUTIONS
   a. Hypersensitivity to penicillins
   b. Pregnancy or lactation
4. DRUG INTERACTIONS
   a. Probenecid (Benemid): increases effects and decreases renal elimination
   b. Oral contraceptives: decrease effectiveness of oral contraceptive
   c. Anticoagulants: increase anticoagulant effects
5. NURSING INTERVENTIONS
   a. Assess the client with impaired renal failure for toxicity.
   b. Monitor blood and liver function tests.
   c. Perform culture and sensitivity before initiating drug therapy.
   d. Assess the client for allergies before initiating therapy.
6. TYPES
   a. Amoxicillin
      1) Has better absorption and less adverse reactions
   b. Amoxicillin-clavulanate (Augmentin)
      1) May be more effective with resistance problems
   c. Ampicillin

C. SULFONAMIDES

1. USES
   a. Used in the treatment of acute urinary tract infections
   b. Bacteriostatic action that blocks the bacterial synthesis of essential nucleic acid
   c. Inexpensive classifications of drugs
2. ADVERSE REACTIONS
   a. GI: nausea, vomiting, abdominal pain
   b. Central nervous system (CNS): headache, dizziness, insomnia
3. CONTRAINDICATIONS AND PRECAUTIONS
   a. Hypersensitivity to sulfonamides
   b. Pregnancy or lactation
4. DRUG INTERACTIONS
   a. Anticoagulants: increased effects
   b. Sulfonylurea agents in diabetes mellitus: increased incidence of hypoglycemia
   c. Thiazide diuretics: thrombocytopenia
5. NURSING INTERVENTIONS
   a. Monitor blood and kidney tests.
   b. Assess the client for allergy before initiating drug therapy.
   c. Monitor intake, output, and pH of urine.
   d. Obtain culture and sensitivity before initiating therapy.

6. TYPES
   a. Trimethoprim-sulfamethoxazole (Bactrim, Septra)
      1) Effective against aerobic enteric bacteria, except *Pseudomonas*
      2) Used in the treatment of recurrent and complicated urinary tract infections
      3) Combination of trimethoprim and sulfamethoxazole decreases the incidence of bacterial resistance.

D. CEPHALOSPORINS
   1. USES
      a. Four different generations of cephalosporins chemically and pharmacologically related to penicillin
      b. May be bacteriostatic or bactericidal by interfering with the bacterial cell wall synthesis and altering the osmotic stability of the growing bacterial cell wall, which results in the cell's death
      c. Used to treat urinary tract infections caused by gram-positive or gram-negative organisms
      d. Initially were advantageous over penicillins because of their resistance to enzymatic degradation by penicillinase (beta lactamase). As a result of the overuse of cephalosporins, bacterial resistance has developed.
      e. May be used in urinary tract infections resistant to amoxicillin and trimethoprim-sulfamethoxazole (Bactrim)
   2. ADVERSE REACTIONS
      a. GI: diarrhea, nausea, vomiting, abdominal pain
      b. CNS: headache, dizziness, weakness
      c. Hematology: leukopenia, thrombocytopenia, agranulocytosis, anemia
      d. Integumentary: rash, urticaria, dermatitis
      e. Genitourinary (GU): proteinuria, vaginitis, candidiasis, nephrotoxicity
   3. CONTRAINDICATIONS
      a. Hypersensitivity to cephalosporins
      b. Similar chemical property to penicillin may result in cross-sensitivity to clients with known allergy to penicillin.
      c. Pregnancy or lactation
   4. DRUG INTERACTIONS
      a. Aminoglycosides: increase risk of toxicity
      b. Loop diuretics: increase risk of toxicity
      c. Probenecid (Benemid): decreases renal elimination and increases blood levels
   5. NURSING INTERVENTIONS
      a. Administer with extreme caution to clients with sensitivity to penicillin.

   b. Monitor for superinfection, especially in older adults.
   c. Monitor bleeding and prothrombin time.
   d. Monitor blood urea nitrogen (BUN) and creatinine levels in clients with a renal impairment.
   e. Maintain accurate intake and output—may indicate nephrotoxicity.
   f. Instruct the client to take all prescribed medication.
   g. Monitor blood studies.
   h. Assess for ecchymosis or bleeding.
   i. Instruct the client with diabetes mellitus to test urine with Clinistix or Keto-Diastix to avoid false positive results.
   j. Oral absorption increases when taken with food.
   k. Obtain stool specimen for *C. difficile* with persistent diarrhea.
   6. TYPES
      a. First generation: cefadroxil (Duricef), cefazolin (Ancef), cephalexin (Keflex), cephradine (Velosef)
      b. Second generation: cefaclor (Ceclor), cefamandole (Mandol), cefotetan (Cefotan), cefoxitin (Mefoxin), cefuroxime (Zinacef, Ceftin)
      c. Third generation: cefdinir (Omnicef), cefixime (Suprax), cefoperazone (Cefobid), ceftazidime (Fortaz), ceftriaxone (Rocephin)
      d. Fourth generation: cefepime (Maxipime)

E. FLUOROQUINOLONES
   1. USES
      a. Broad-spectrum antibiotics used in the treatment of urinary tract infections caused by most organisms
      b. Exhibit bactericidal properties by interfering with the duplication of DNA
   2. ADVERSE REACTIONS
      a. GI: nausea, vomiting, diarrhea
      b. CNS: dizziness, drowsiness, headache, restlessness
      c. Integumentary: rash, pruritus, urticaria, photosensitivity
   3. CONTRAINDICATIONS AND PRECAUTIONS
      a. Hypersensitivity to quinolones
      b. Pregnancy or lactation
      c. Renal disease
   4. DRUG INTERACTIONS
      a. Antacids: decrease absorption
      b. Caffeine: increases effects of caffeine
      c. Didanosine (Videx): decreases effectiveness of fluoroquinolone
      d. Dairy products: decrease absorption
      e. Glyburide (Diaβeta, Micronase): hypoglycemia

f. Theophylline: may cause toxicity
g. Anticoagulants: increase effectiveness of anticoagulants

5. NURSING INTERVENTIONS
a. Avoid administering 2 hours before or after antacids or ferrous sulfate.
b. Increase fluids to 3 liters daily to prevent crystalluria.
c. Monitor urine pH, white blood cell (WBC) count, culture, and sensitivity.
d. All fluoroquinolones may be administered with or without food, but enoxacin (Penetrex) and norfloxacin (Noroxin) should be administered on an empty stomach.
e. Instruct the client to take all prescribed medication.
f. Monitor for dizziness and assist with ambulation.
g. Instruct the client to avoid direct sunlight because of photosensitivity.

6. TYPES
a. Ciprofloxacin (Cipro)
b. Enoxacin (Penetrex)
c. Gatifloxacin (Tequin)
d. Levofloxacin (Levaquin)
e. Norfloxacin (Noroxin)
f. Ofloxacin (Floxin)

II. MISCELLANEOUS URINARY TRACT ANTI-INFECTIVES

A. DESCRIPTION
1. USED TO TREAT RECURRENT OR CHRONIC URINARY TRACT INFECTIONS
2. EXERT AN ANTISEPTIC ACTION ON THE URINARY TRACT
3. LESS POTENT ANTI-INFECTIVES
a. Less systemic adverse reactions
b. Decreased incidence of bacterial resistance

B. METHENAMINE MANDELATE (MANDELAMINE) AND METHENAMINE HIPPURATE (HIPREX)
1. USES
a. Combined action of methenamine and mandelic acid or hippurate acid with the release of formaldehyde in an acidic environment alters the pH of the urine.
b. In the presence of acidic urine (pH less than 5.5), formaldehyde is released to produce a bactericidal action in the urinary tract.
c. Frequently used prophylactically or suppressive therapy between infections

2. ADVERSE REACTIONS
a. GI: gastric upset
b. GU: crystalluria

3. CONTRAINDICATIONS AND PRECAUTIONS
a. Impaired renal failure

4. DRUG INTERACTIONS
a. Antacids: decrease effectiveness
b. Sulfonamides: precipitate formed in acid urine
c. Thiazide diuretics: decrease effectiveness

5. NURSING INTERACTIONS
a. Increase fluids to 3 liters daily to prevent crystalluria.
b. Instruct the client to take with or immediately after meals to decrease GI upset.
c. Inform the client that it is normal for the urine to turn blue.

C. NALIDIXIC ACID (NEGGRAM)
1. USES
a. Bactericidal action effective against *E. coli, Proteus, Klebsiella,* and *Enterobacter*
b. Effective against acute and chronic urinary tract infections

2. ADVERSE REACTIONS
a. GI: nausea, vomiting, diarrhea, abdominal pain
b. CNS: dizziness, headache, drowsiness
c. Integumentary: pruritus, urticaria, rash, and photosensitivity
d. Eyes, ears, nose, and throat (EENT): sensitivity to light

3. CONTRAINDICATIONS AND PRECAUTIONS
a. Hypersensitivity
b. CNS damage
c. Liver failure
d. Renal disease
e. Pregnancy or lactation
f. Infants under 3 months of age

4. DRUG INTERACTIONS
a. Antacids: decrease effects

5. NURSING INTERVENTIONS
a. Instruct the client to avoid sunlight and use sunscreen for photosensitivity.
b. Administer with food.
c. Instruct the client to avoid taking 2 hours before or 2 hours after antacids.
d. Instruct the client to avoid driving and to seek assistance with ambulation.

D. NITROFURANTOIN (FURADANTIN), NITROFURANTOIN MACROCRYSTALS (MACRODANTIN)
1. USES
a. Bactericidal action effective against *E. coli, Klebsiella, Staphylococcus aureus, Proteus, Enterobacter*

2. ADVERSE REACTIONS
a. GI: nausea, vomiting, diarrhea, abdominal pain
b. CNS: dizziness, headache, drowsiness
c. Integumentary: pruritus, rash, urticaria

3. CONTRAINDICATIONS AND PRECAUTIONS
   a. Hypersensitivity
   b. Renal disease
   c. Infants under 1 month of age
4. DRUG INTERACTIONS
   a. Probenecid (Benemid): increases toxicity
5. NURSING INTERVENTIONS
   a. Instruct the client to take with food.
   b. Instruct the client that urine may turn a yellowish-brown color.
   c. Avoid crushing the tablets.
   d. Instruct the client to seek assistance with ambulation if dizziness occurs and to avoid driving.

III. ANTIMUSCARINICS
A. DESCRIPTION
   1. ALSO REFERRED TO AS ANTICHOLINERGICS OR ANTISPASMODICS
   2. USED TO TREAT NEUROGENIC BLADDER, BLADDER SPASMS, AND URINARY INCONTINENCE
   3. RELAXES THE URINARY TRACT SMOOTH MUSCLE BY INHIBITING ACETYLCHOLINE
   4. USED WITH CAUTION IN OLDER ADULTS
B. USES
   1. NEUROGENIC BLADDER
   2. BLADDER SPASMS
C. ADVERSE REACTIONS
   1. GI: NAUSEA, VOMITING, ABDOMINAL PAIN, CONSTIPATION, DRY MOUTH
   2. CNS: DROWSINESS, DIZZINESS, RESTLESSNESS, ANXIETY
   3. CARDIOVASCULAR: TACHYCARDIA, PALPITATIONS, HYPERTENSION, FLUSHING
   4. EENT: BLURRED VISION, INCREASED OCULAR TENSION
   5. GU: URINARY HESITANCY, RETENTION, DYSURIA
   6. INTEGUMENTARY: RASH, URTICARIA, DECREASED PERSPIRATION
D. CONTRAINDICATIONS AND PRECAUTIONS
   1. GLAUCOMA
   2. MYASTHENIA GRAVIS
   3. INTESTINAL OBSTRUCTION
   4. SEVERE COLITIS
   5. UNSTABLE CARDIOVASCULAR SYSTEM
   6. PREGNANCY OR LACTATION
E. DRUG INTERACTIONS
   1. ACETAMINOPHEN: DECREASES EFFECTS OF ACETAMINOPHEN
   2. LEVODOPA (L-DOPA): DECREASES EFFECTS OF LEVODOPA
   3. DIGOXIN: INCREASES DIGOXIN LEVEL

4. ANTIDEPRESSANTS: INCREASE EFFECTS
5. ANTIHISTAMINES: INCREASE EFFECTS
6. HYPNOTIC/SEDATIVES: INCREASE EFFECTS
7. OPIATES: INCREASE EFFECTS
8. PHENOTHIAZINES: INCREASE EFFECTS
F. NURSING INTERVENTIONS
   1. MONITOR THE CLIENT WITH ABDOMINAL DISTENTION, COLOSTOMY, OR ILEOSTOMY FOR CLINICAL MANIFESTATIONS OF INTESTINAL OBSTRUCTION.
   2. MAINTAIN AN ACCURATE INTAKE AND OUTPUT (I & O).
   3. INSTRUCT THE CLIENT TO AVOID DRIVING OR HAZARDOUS ACTIVITIES UNTIL DRUG EFFECTS ARE KNOWN.
   4. INSTRUCT THE CLIENT TO AVOID STRENUOUS AND HOT WEATHER ACTIVITIES.
   5. INSTRUCT THE CLIENT TO CHEW GUM OR SUCK ON HARD CANDY.
   6. INSTRUCT THE CLIENT TO REPORT CHANGES IN VISION.
G. TYPES
   1. OXYBUTYNIN CHLORIDE (DITROPAN)
   2. PROPANTHELINE BROMIDE (PRO-BANTHINE)
   3. TOLTERODINE (DETROL)

IV. URINARY ANALGESIC
A. DESCRIPTION
   1. EXERTS A TOPICAL ANALGESIC EFFECT ON THE MUCOSA LINING OF THE URINARY TRACT
   2. GENERALLY GIVEN IN CONJUNCTION WITH A URINARY ANTI-INFECTIVE
B. PHENAZOPYRIDINE HCL (PYRIDIUM)
   1. USES
      a. Pain associated with urinary frequency, urgency, dysuria, itching
   2. ADVERSE REACTIONS
      a. GI: nausea, vomiting, diarrhea
      b. CNS: headache, dizziness
      c. Hematology: thrombocytopenia, agranulocytosis, hemolytic anemia, leukopenia, neutropenia, methemoglobinemia
      d. Integumentary: pruritus, rash
      e. GU: reddish-orange-colored urine
   3. CONTRAINDICATIONS AND PRECAUTIONS
      a. Hypersensitivity
      b. Glomerulonephritis
      c. Pyelonephritis
      d. Renal insufficiency
   4. DRUG INTERACTIONS
      a. None established
   5. NURSING INTERVENTIONS
      a. Inform the client that urine will turn reddish orange.

    b. Monitor client complaints of urinary frequency, urgency, dysuria, or itching.

    c. Monitor complete blood count (CBC) and liver function studies.

    d. Inform the client to take the drug until the course of the anti-infective is completed.

    e. Administer with food to decrease GI effects.

V. CHOLINERGICS

A. DESCRIPTION

  1. PRIMARILY ACT DIRECTLY ON MUSCARINIC ACETYLCHOLINE RECEPTORS

  2. FACILITATE CONTRACTION OF DETRUSOR MUSCLE OF THE URINARY BLADDER

B. USES

  1. POSTOPERATIVE OR POSTPARTUM URINARY RETENTION

  2. NEUROGENIC ATONY OF THE BLADDER WITH RETENTION

C. ADVERSE REACTIONS

  1. GI: NAUSEA, VOMITING, DIARRHEA, ABDOMINAL CRAMPS, ERUCTATION, FECAL INCONTINENCE, BORBORYGMI

  2. CARDIOVASCULAR: HYPOTENSION, BRADYCARDIA, REFLEX TACHYCARDIA, FLUSHING

  3. CNS: DIZZINESS

  4. INTEGUMENTARY: RASH, URTICARIA, INCREASED PERSPIRATION

  5. RESPIRATORY: ACUTE ASTHMA, DYSPNEA

  6. GU: URINARY URGENCY

D. CONTRAINDICATIONS AND PRECAUTIONS

  1. ASTHMA

  2. CHRONIC OBSTRUCTIVE PULMONARY DISEASE

  3. CORONARY ARTERY DISEASE

  4. BRADYCARDIA

  5. HYPOTENSION

E. DRUG INTERACTIONS

  1. GANGLIONIC BLOCKERS: INCREASE EFFECTS, PARTICULARLY HYPOTENSION

  2. CHOLINERGIC AGONISTS: INCREASE EFFECTS

F. NURSING INTERVENTIONS

  1. MONITOR VITAL SIGNS.

  2. MAINTAIN AN ACCURATE I & O.

  3. INSTRUCT THE CLIENT TO SLOWLY ARISE TO A SITTING POSITION AND MAKE POSITION CHANGES.

  4. INSTRUCT THE CLIENT TO TAKE THE DRUG ON AN EMPTY STOMACH, 1 HOUR BEFORE OR 2 HOURS AFTER MEALS, TO DECREASE INCIDENCE OF NAUSEA.

  5. INSTRUCT THE CLIENT TO AVOID OPERATING POTENTIALLY HAZARDOUS EQUIPMENT UNTIL THE EFFECTS OF THE DRUG ARE KNOWN.

G. TYPES

  1. BETHANECHOL (DUVOID, URECHOLINE)

VI. DIURETICS

A. DESCRIPTION

  1. USED TO PROMOTE THE EXCRETION OF SODIUM AND WATER FROM THE BODY AND PREVENT THE REABSORPTION OF SODIUM

  2. USED IN THE TREATMENT OF EDEMA, HYPERTENSION, AND CONGESTIVE HEART FAILURE

B. THIAZIDE DIURETICS

  1. USES

    a. Inhibit sodium and chloride reabsorption in the distal tubule while blocking chloride reabsorption in the ascending loop of Henle, which may result in metabolic alkalosis

    b. A greater-than-normal exchange of sodium-potassium takes place, leading to hypokalemia.

  2. ADVERSE REACTIONS

    a. Fluid and electrolyte imbalances: hypokalemia, hyponatremia, hypochloremia, hypomagnesium, hypercalcemia

    b. GI: nausea, vomiting, constipation, diarrhea

    c. CNS: drowsiness, dizziness, fatigue, weakness

    d. GU: frequency, polyuria

    e. Integumentary: rash, photosensitivity

    f. Hematology: leukopenia, thrombocytopenia, aplastic anemia, hemolytic anemia

    g. Cardiovascular: orthostatic hypotension, irregular pulse, dehydration

    h. Metabolic: hyperlipidemia, hyperglycemia

  3. CONTRAINDICATIONS AND PRECAUTIONS

    a. Renal disease

    b. Hypokalemia

    c. Older adults

    d. Diabetes mellitus

    e. Gout

  4. DRUG INTERACTIONS

    a. Antihypertensives: increase antihypertensive effects

    b. Anticoagulants: decrease effects

    c. Glucocorticoids: increase hypokalemia effects

    d. Nonsteroidal anti-inflammatories (NSAIDs): decrease the diuretic action

    e. Cardiac glycosides: increase the risk of cardiac glycoside toxicity

    f. Lithium: increases risk of toxicity

5. NURSING INTERVENTIONS
   a. Monitor blood pressure.
   b. Monitor the client for orthostatic hypotension.
   c. Monitor the laboratory results.
   d. Maintain accurate I & O.
   e. Monitor weight.
   f. Instruct the client to avoid strenuous activity or extended periods of time in the sun.
   g. Instruct the client on foods rich in potassium such as citrus fruits, bananas, apricots, and potatoes.
   h. Instruct the client to avoid standing in one position for a prolonged period of time or changing positions quickly.

6. TYPES
   a. Bendroflumethiazide (Naturetin)
   b. Chlorothiazide (Diuril)
   c. Chlorthalidone (Hygroton)
   d. Hydrochlorothiazide (HydroDIURIL, Esidrex)
   e. Hydroflumethiazide (Diucardin, Saluron)
   f. Indapamide (Lozol)
   g. Methyclothiazide (Aquatensen, Enduron)
   h. Metolazone (Zaroxolyn)
   i. Polythiazide (Renese)
   j. Quinethazone (Hydromox)
   k. Trichlormethiazide (Naqua)

C. LOOP DIURETICS
   1. USES
      a. Inhibit the reabsorption of sodium and chloride in the ascending loop of Henle, resulting in a decreased concentration of urine
      b. More potent than thiazide diuretics, resulting in severe hypokalemia
   2. ADVERSE REACTIONS
      a. GI: nausea, vomiting, diarrhea, abdominal cramps
      b. CNS: headache, fatigue, weakness
      c. Cardiovascular: orthostatic hypotension
      d. EENT: hearing loss
      e. Fluid and electrolyte imbalances: hypokalemia, hyponatremia, hypochloremia, hypomagnesemia, hyperuricemia, hypocalcemia
      f. Hematology: leukopenia, thrombocytopenia, neutropenia, anemia
      g. Integumentary: rash, pruritus
      h. GU: polyuria
   3. CONTRAINDICATIONS AND PRECAUTIONS
      a. Hypovolemia
      b. Renal disease
      c. Hypersensitivity to sulfonamides
      d. Diabetes mellitus

4. DRUG INTERACTIONS
   a. Antihypertensives: increase antihypertensive effects
   b. Aminoglycerides: increase ototoxicity
   c. Cardiac glycosides: increase potassium and magnesium loss
   d. Corticosteroids: increase potassium loss
   e. Cephalosporins: increase nephrotoxicity
   f. Opiates: increase orthostatic hypotension
   g. Salicylates: decrease diuretic effects

5. NURSING INTERVENTIONS
   a. Monitor blood pressure.
   b. Maintain an accurate I & O.
   c. Monitor weight.
   d. Assess the client for hearing loss.
   e. Monitor the laboratory tests.
   f. Administer in the morning to prevent nocturia.
   g. Administer with food to decrease GI effects.
   h. Instruct the client to avoid activities that promote fluid loss, such as strenuous and hot weather activities.
   i. Instruct the client to change positions slowly to prevent orthostatic hypotension.
   j. Administer prescribed potassium supplement.

6. TYPES
   a. Bumetanide (Bumex)
   b. Ethacrynic acid (Edecrin)
   c. Furosemide (Lasix)
   d. Torsemide (Demadex)

D. POTASSIUM-SPARING DIURETICS
   1. USES
      a. Compete with aldosterone in the distal renal tubule, promoting the excretion of water, sodium, chloride, and bicarbonate while sparing potassium
      b. Not considered potent diuretics and may be used in conjunction with a thiazide or loop diuretic
   2. ADVERSE REACTIONS
      a. GI: nausea, vomiting, diarrhea
      b. CNS: dizziness, headache
      c. Fluid and electrolyte imbalances: hyperkalemia, hyponatremia
      d. Cardiovascular: hypertension
      e. Endocrine: gynecomastia
   3. CONTRAINDICATIONS AND PRECAUTIONS
      a. Hyperkalemia
      b. Severe renal disease
   4. DRUG INTERACTIONS
      a. Ace inhibitors: increase hyperkalemia
      b. Antihypertensives: hypertension
      c. Anticoagulants: decrease effects
      d. Lithium: increases toxicity

5. NURSING INTERVENTIONS
   a. Monitor the client for indications of hyperkalemia and hyponatremia.
   b. Monitor blood pressure.
   c. Maintain an accurate I & O.
   d. Instruct the client to avoid potassium supplements and salt substitutes.
6. TYPES
   a. Spironolactone (Aldactone)
   b. Triamterene (Dyrenium)
   c. Amiloride HCl (Midamor)

E. CARBONIC ANHYDRASE INHIBITORS
   1. USES
      a. Use as diuretics greatly reduced as a result of the development of newer more effective diuretics
      b. Carbonic anhydrase is an enzyme acting in the renal tubule to decrease the reabsorption of water, sodium, and potassium.
      c. Used primarily in the treatment of glaucoma by decreasing intraocular pressure
   2. ADVERSE REACTIONS
      a. GI: nausea, vomiting, anorexia, constipation, diarrhea
      b. CNS: drowsiness
      c. GU: frequency, hypokalemia, polyuria
      d. Hematology: aplastic anemia, leukopenia, hemolytic anemia
      e. Integumentary: rash, pruritus
      f. EENT: myopia, tinnitus
      g. Fluid and electrolyte imbalances: hypokalemia, hyperglycemia, hypocalcemia, hyperchloremia, hyponatremia
   3. CONTRAINDICATIONS AND PRECAUTIONS
      a. Electrolyte imbalances
      b. Severe renal disease
   4. DRUG INTERACTIONS
      a. Amphetamines: increase action
      b. Salicylates: increase toxicity
      c. Anticholinergics: increase anticholinergic effects

5. NURSING INTERVENTIONS
   a. Assess the client for tinnitus.
   b. Monitor the client for hypokalemia.
   c. Instruct the client to take the drug early because of polyuria.
   d. Maintain an accurate intake and output.
6. TYPES
   a. Acetazolamide (Diamox)
   b. Dichlorphenamide (Daranide)
   c. Methazolamide (Neptazane)

F. COMBINATION POTASSIUM-SPARING HYDROCHLOROTHIAZIDE DIURETIC
   1. USES
      a. Combine a potassium-sparing and thiazide diuretic for the purpose of decreasing the adverse reactions of each (hypokalemia with thiazide diuretic and hyperkalemia with potassium-sparing diuretic)
      b. Increase the antihypertensive effect
   2. ADVERSE REACTIONS
      a. Similar to both potassium-sparing and thiazide diuretics but with less intensity
   3. CONTRAINDICATIONS AND PRECAUTIONS
      a. Renal disease
   4. DRUG INTERACTIONS
      a. Antihypertensives: increase antihypertensive effects
   5. NURSING INTERACTIONS
      a. Monitor the client for hyperkalemia or hypokalemia.
      b. Maintain an accurate I & O.
      c. Monitor blood pressure.
   6. TYPES
      a. Spironolactone and hydrochlorothiazide (Aldactone)
      b. Triamterene and hydrochlorothiazide (Dyazide, Maxzide)
      c. Amiloride and hydrochlorothiazide (Moduretic)

PRACTICE QUESTIONS

1. When providing care to a client who is on amoxicillin and potassium clavulanate (Augmentin), the nurse should monitor the client for
   1. constipation.
   2. polyuria.
   3. decreased temperature.
   4. increased bleeding.

2. Which of the following should the nurse consider before administering glyburide (Micronase) and chlorthalidone (Hygroton) to a client with diabetes mellitus, hypertension, and edema?
   1. The combination of an oral hypoglycemic agent and a diuretic increases the adverse reactions

2. A thiazide diuretic decreases the action of glyburide
3. There is no drug interaction between Hygroton and Micronase
4. A second-generation oral hypoglycemic agent increases the action of diuretics

3. The nurse is teaching a class on anti-infectives used to treat urinary tract infections. Which of the following should the nurse include in the class?
   1. *E. coli* has developed a resistance to penicillin anti-infectives
   2. Sulfonamides are frequently prescribed for *Pseudomonas* infections
   3. Fluoroquinolones have a limited use in the treatment of urinary tract infections
   4. Cephalosporins are the anti-infective of choice for clients sensitive to penicillin

4. Which of the following should the nurse include in the plan of care for a client with diabetes mellitus and congestive heart failure who is receiving NPH insulin, cefuroxime (Zinacef), and triamterene (Dyrenium)?
   1. Encourage the client to choose foods high in potassium
   2. Monitor the client for clinical manifestations of hypernatremia
   3. Test the client's urine with a Clinistix or Ketodiastix
   4. Notify the physician that the client has a hypersensitivity to quinolones

5. Phenazopyridine hydrochloride (Pyridium) is prescribed for a client with acute cystitis. Which of the following should the nurse explain to the client?
   1. Dry mouth is a common anticipated adverse reaction
   2. Gastrointestinal adverse reactions are eliminated when taken on an empty stomach
   3. The urine will turn a reddish-orange color
   4. Exposure to sunlight enhances the effects of the drug

6. Ciprofloxacin (Cipro) has been prescribed for a client with a urinary tract infection who is also receiving theophylline. Based on an understanding of the effects of the two drugs, the nurse should monitor the client for which of the following?
   Select all that apply:
   [ ] 1. Visual disturbances
   [ ] 2. Tachycardia
   [ ] 3. Seizures
   [ ] 4. Oliguria
   [ ] 5. Nausea
   [ ] 6. Flaccid paralysis

7. The nurse reviews the fluoroquinolones from which of the following lists?
   Select all that apply:
   [ ] 1. Ciprofloxacin (Cipro)
   [ ] 2. Nitrofurantoin (Furadantin)
   [ ] 3. Enoxacin (Penetrex)
   [ ] 4. Cefadroxil (Duricef)
   [ ] 5. Trimethoprim-sulfamethoxazole (Bactrim)
   [ ] 6. Norofloxacin (Noroxin)

8. The nurse is caring for a client who has sustained a traumatic brain injury and is experiencing a neurogenic bladder. The nurse should understand that the client is to receive which of the following drugs in the treatment of neurogenic bladder?
   1. Phenazopyridine HCL (Pyridium)
   2. Nalidixic acid (NegGram)
   3. Methenamine, phenylsalicylate, atropine, and hyoscyamine (Urised)
   4. Probanthine bromide (Pro-Banthine)

9. The nurse is caring for a client with congestive heart failure. The nurse should understand that the client is to receive furosemide (Lasix) for which of the following purposes?
   1. Acts in the renal tubule to decrease the reabsorption of water, sodium, and potassium
   2. Inhibits sodium and chloride reabsorption in the distal tubule while blocking chloride reabsorption in the ascending loop of Henle
   3. Competes with aldosterone in the distal renal tubule, promoting the excretion of water, sodium, chloride, and bicarbonate while sparing potassium
   4. Inhibits the reabsorption of sodium and chloride in the ascending loop of Henle

10. The nurse should monitor a client receiving nalidixic acid (NegGram) for which of the following adverse reactions?
    Select all that apply:
    [ ] 1. Drowsiness
    [ ] 2. Sensitivity to light
    [ ] 3. Headache
    [ ] 4. Urinary frequency
    [ ] 5. Bradycardia
    [ ] 6. Constipation

11. Tolterodine (Detrol) has been prescribed for an older adult client who has dementia and is experiencing incontinence. The client's medical history reveals congestive heart failure, edema, and hypertension. Which of the following adverse reactions is a priority to report for this client?
    1. Dry mouth
    2. Restlessness
    3. Urinary retention
    4. Nausea

12. The nurse assists a client receiving furosemide (Lasix) to make which of the following dietary selections that are high in potassium?
Select all that apply:
[ ] 1. Raisins
[ ] 2. Spinach
[ ] 3. White bread
[ ] 4. Corn flakes cereal
[ ] 5. Salmon
[ ] 6. Avocado

13. The nurse is caring for a client who is receiving chlorothiazide (Diuril) who is complaining of forgetfulness, lethargy, weakness, nausea, and vomiting. The nurse assesses the client to have decreased reflexes and polyuria. The nurse should report this as
1. hypercalcemia.
2. hypermagnesemia.
3. hyperkalemia.
4. hypernatremia.

14. A client with a urinary tract infection has received medication instructions on Levofloxacin (Levaquin). Which of the following statements by the client indicates a need for further instructions?
1. "I will increase my daily intake of fluids."
2. "I will take my medication with an antacid to decrease stomach upset."
3. "I will stay out of the direct sunlight."
4. "I will ask for assistance with walking if I get dizzy."

15. The nurse should administer which of the following prescribed diuretics for the purpose of decreasing the adverse effects of hypokalemia and hyperkalemia?
1. Quinethazone (Hydromox)
2. Ethacrynic acid (Edecrin)
3. Triameterene and hydrochlorothiazide (Dyazide)
4. Acetazolamide (Diamox)

16. Which of the following questions is a priority for the nurse to ask a client before administering ceftriaxone (Rocephin)?
1. "Do you have an allergy to penicillin?"
2. "Are you sensitive to the sunlight?"
3. "Do you have a known bleeding disorder?"
4. "Are you prone to gastrointestinal upset?"

17. The nurse is developing a medication schedule for a client who is to receive cefadroxil (Duricef) orally. Based on an understanding of the drug, which of the following administration methods would promote the best absorption?
1. On an empty stomach
2. At bedtime
3. With food
4. Duricef cannot be administered orally

18. Which of the following would be the best indication to the nurse that an antimicrobial given repeatedly in the treatment of chronic urinary tract infections has resulted in a superinfection?
Select all that apply:
[ ] 1. Stomatitis
[ ] 2. Urinary retention
[ ] 3. Loose, foul-smelling stools
[ ] 4. Ecchymosis
[ ] 5. Vaginal itching
[ ] 6. Fever

19. The nurse should monitor a client taking dichlorphenamide (Daranide) for which of the following adverse reactions?
Select all that apply:
[ ] 1. Tinnitus
[ ] 2. Hyperglycemia
[ ] 3. Hypercalcemia
[ ] 4. Myopia
[ ] 5. Urinary retention
[ ] 6. Anxiety

20. Which of the following is a priority to include in the plan of care for starting antimicrobial therapy?
1. Encourage the client to increase fluids
2. Stay with the client for 30 minutes after the initial dose
3. Maintain an accurate intake and output
4. Monitor the client's blood and liver function tests

21. The registered nurse making out clinical assignments for the day may delegate which of the following nursing skills to a licensed practical nurse?
1. Assess a client taking trimethoprim-sulfamethoxazole (Bactrim) for an allergy before initiating therapy
2. Notify the physician that a client taking ciprofloxacin (Cipro) is taking theophylline
3. Assess the BUN and creatinine in a client taking cefadroxil (Duricef)
4. Maintain an accurate intake and output in a client taking spironolactone (Aldactone)

22. The nurse is reviewing the medical history of a client taking dichlorphenamide (Daranide). For which of the following conditions is Daranide contraindicated or to be used with extreme caution?
1. Hyperkalemia
2. Osteoporosis
3. Diabetes mellitus
4. Scleroderma

23. Based on an understanding of the drug interactions for a client taking a loop diuretic and an aminoglyceride, for which of the

following should the nurse monitor the client?
1. Hypokalemia
2. Orthostatic hypotension
3. Ototoxicity
4. Decreased diuretic effects

24. The nurse should monitor a client taking bumetanide (Bumex) for which of the following adverse reactions?
Select all that apply:
[ ] 1. Hypertension
[ ] 2. Polyuria

[ ] 3. Hypokalemia
[ ] 4. Weakness
[ ] 5. Constipation
[ ] 6. Hyponatremia

25. Which of the following nursing actions should the nurse include in the plan of care for a client taking nalidixic acid (NegGram)?
1. Administer on an empty stomach
2. Instruct the client to take with an antacid
3. Instruct the client to avoid activities that promote fluid loss
4. Monitor blood pressure

ANSWERS AND RATIONALES

1. 4. Amoxicillin and potassium clavulanate (Augmentin) is a penicillin anti-infective. Diarrhea, fever, and increased bleeding time are adverse reactions.

2. 2. Glyburide (Micronase) is a sulfonylurea (second-generation) oral hypoglycemic agent. Chlorthalidone (Hygroton) is a thiazide diuretic. The thiazide diuretic decreases the action of the oral hypoglycemic agent and should be administered with caution to a client with diabetes mellitus.

3. 1. There is an increasing resistance to *E. coli* infections with penicillin anti-infectives. Sulfonamides are effective against aerobic bacteria, except *Pseudomonas*. Fluoroquinolones are effective broad-spectrum antibiotics used in the treatment of urinary tract infections caused by most organisms. Cephalosporins are chemically similar to penicillin and may result in a cross-sensitivity in clients with a known allergy to penicillin.

4. 3. It is appropriate to test the urine of a client with diabetes mellitus with a Clinistix or Ketodiastix to avoid a false positive when administering cefuroxime (Zinacef), a cephalosporin. Triamterene is a potassium-sparing diuretic, and foods high in potassium do not need to be encouraged. Encouraging foods high in potassium could lead to hyperkalemia. Triamterene results in hyponatremia, not hypernatremia.

5. 3. Phenazopyridine hydrochloride (Pyridium) is a urinary analgesic that exerts a topical analgesic effect on the mucosa lining of the urinary tract. It is normal for the urine to turn a reddish-orange color. Gastrointestinal adverse reactions are decreased by taking the drug with food.

6. 2. 3. 5. Ciprofloxacin (Cipro) and theophylline result in increased plasma theophylline

concentrations, prolonged theophylline half-life, and decreased hepatic clearance of the theophylline. The onset of toxicity may be sudden and severe, with arrhythmia and seizures as the first signs. Other indications of toxicity include nausea, vomiting, and irritability. Extreme caution must be used when administered Cipro and theophylline together. The theophylline levels should be closely monitored and the dose adjusted accordingly.

7. 1. 3. 6. Ciprofloxacin (Cipro), enoxcin (Penetrex), and norfloxacin (Noroxin) are all examples of fluroquinolones. Nitrofurantoin (Furadantin) is an example of a miscellaneous anti-infective. Cefadroxil (Duricef) is a cephalosporin. Trimethoprim-sulfamethoxazole (Bactrim) is a sulfonamide.

8. 4. Probanthine bromide (Pro-Banthine) is an antimuscarinic, also know as an anticholinergic or antispasmodic. It is used to relax the urinary tract smooth muscles by inhibiting acetylcholine in the treatment of bladder spasms or a neurogenic bladder. With a neurogenic bladder, urgency, frequency, incontinence, inability to void, and reflux are common clinical manifestations. Phenazopyridine HCL (Pyridium) is a urinary analgesic used for dysuria. Nalidixic acid (NegGram) and methenamine, phenylsalicylate, atropine, and hyoscyamine (Urised) are urinary anti-infectives used in the treatment of urinary tract infections.

9. 4. Furosemide (Lasix) is a loop diuretic that inhibits the reabsorption of sodium and chloride in the ascending loop of Henle. A carbonic anhydrase inhibitor acts in the renal tubule to decrease water, sodium, and potassium. A thiazide diuretic inhibits sodium and chloride reabsorption in the distal tubule while blocking chloride reabsorption in the ascending loop of Henle. A potassium-sparing

diuretic competes with aldosterone in the distal renal tubule, promoting the excretion of water, sodium, chloride, and bicarbonate while sparing potassium.

10. 1. 2. 3.   Nalidixic acid (NegGram) is a urinary tract anti-infective with a bactericidal action used in the treatment of urinary tract infections. Adverse reactions include drowsiness, headache, sensitivity to light, and diarrhea.

11. 3.   Although dry mouth, restlessness, urinary retention, and nausea are all adverse reactions to tolterodine (Detrol), urinary retention is the priority to report for a client with congestive heart failure and edema. Urinary retention is a potentially serious adverse reaction for a client already experiencing fluid retention with congestive heart failure.

12. 1. 2. 5. 6.   Furosemide (Lasix) is a potent loop diuretic that often causes a low potassium level. Clients should be instructed to choose foods high in potassium to make appropriate food choices. Raisins, spinach, salmon, and avocado are all foods high in potassium. White bread and corn flakes are low in potassium. Wheat bread and oatmeal, although still low, are better selections.

13. 1.   Hypercalcemia may be an adverse reaction of a client taking a thiazide diuretic such as chlorothiazide. Normal serum calcium is 9 to 11 mg/dl. Clinical manifestations of hypercalcemia include lethargy, weakness, anorexia, nausea, vomiting, confusion, personality changes, polyuria, dehydration, stupor, and coma.

14. 2.   Levofloxacin (Levaquin) is a fluoroquinolone. It may or may not be administered with food but should never be administered with an antacid. An antacid decreases the absorption of Levaquin. Fluids should be increased to prevent crystalluria. Direct sunlight should be avoided because of a photosensitivity. Dizziness is an adverse reaction and assistance with ambulation may be required.

15. 3.   Triameterene and hydrochlorothiazide (Dyazide) is an antihypertensive combination drug used for the purpose of decreasing the effects of both hypokalemia and hyperkalemia. Quinethazone (Hydromox) is a thiazide diuretic, ethacrynic acid (Edecrin) is a loop diuretic, and acetazolamide (Diamox) is a carbonic anhydrase inhibitor. All of these diuretics cause hypokalemia.

16. 1.   Ceftriaxone (Rocephin) is a cephalosporin that is chemically and pharmacologically related to penicillin. Because of this chemical similarity, there may be a cross-sensitivity in clients with a known allergy to penicillin.

17. 3.   Cefadroxil (Duricef) is a cephalosporin given in the treatment of acute urinary tract infections. The usual oral dose is 1–2 grams twice a day.

Oral absorption is increased when taken with food.

18. 1. 3. 5. 6.   A superinfection is the development of a new infection by an organism different from the organism causing the initial infection. The risk of a superinfection may increase with repeated antimicrobial therapy. Indications of a superinfection include a black hairy tongue, glossitis, stomatitis, loose and foul-smelling stools, anal itching, vaginal itching, cough, and fever.

19. 1. 2. 4.   Dichlorphenamide (Daranide) is a carbonic anhydrase inhibitor that acts in the renal tubule to decrease the reabsorption of water, sodium, and potassium. Adverse reactions include tinnitus, hyperglycemia, hypocalcemia, myopia, polyuria, and drowsiness.

20. 2.   It is a priority to stay with the client for the first 30 minutes when initiating antimicrobial therapy to monitor the client for a severe reaction, such as anaphylactoid reaction. Encouraging an increased fluid intake, monitoring the liver and blood studies, and maintaining an accurate intake and output are all appropriate interventions, but not the priority.

21. 4.   Nursing skills that involve assessment, monitoring, or notifying are skills that must be performed by a registered nurse. A licensed practical nurse does have the skill to maintain an accurate intake and output.

22. 1.   Dichlorphenamide (Daranide) is a potassium-sparing diuretic that is contraindicated or should be used only with extreme caution for a client with renal disease or with an electrolyte imbalance such as hyperkalemia.

23. 3.   There is a drug interaction between a loop diuretic and an aminoglyceride that may result in ototoxicity. If it is a medical necessity to have the client on both, it is essential that the client be monitored for manifestations of ototoxicity. A loop diuretic and corticosteroid interaction may result in hypokalemia. A drug interaction between a loop diuretic and an opiate may result in orthostatic hypotension. A drug interaction between a loop diuretic and a salicylate may decrease the diuretic effects.

24. 2. 3. 4. 6.   Bumetanide (Bumex) is a potent loop diuretic that may result in severe hypokalemia. Other adverse reactions include weakness, orthostatic hypotension, hyponatremia, polyuria, diarrhea, and abdominal cramps.

25. 4.   Nalidixic acid (NegGram) is a urinary anti-infective with bacteriocidal action used in the treatment of urinary tract infections. It should be administered with food to decrease the gastrointestinal effects. NegGram should not be administered with an antacid. An antacid should be administered 2 hours before or 2 hours after an antacid. NegGram has no bearing on fluid loss or blood pressure.

REFERENCES

Broyles, B., Reiss, B., & Evans, M. (2012). *Pharmacological aspects of nursing care* (8th ed.). Clifton Park, NY: Delmar Cengage Learning.

Daniels, R., & Nicoll, L. (2012). *Contemporary medical-surgical nursing.* Clifton Park, NY: Delmar Cengage Learning.

Spratto, G. R., & Woods, A. L. (2012). *PDR nurse's drug handbook 2012.* Clifton Park, NY: Delmar Cengage Learning.

CHAPTER 26

DRUGS FOR THE REPRODUCTIVE SYSTEM

I. DRUGS FOR THE NORMAL PHYSIOLOGICAL PROCESS OF AGING (MENOPAUSE)

A. DESCRIPTION

1. IN MENOPAUSE, OVARIAN SECRETION OF THE HORMONES ESTROGEN AND PROGESTERONE IS HALTED, RESULTING IN CHANGES IN TISSUES DEPENDENT ON THESE HORMONES.

2. ESTROGEN-RESPONSIVE TISSUES ARE FOUND IN THE FEMALE GENITAL ORGANS, BREAST TISSUE, THE PITUITARY GLAND, AND THE HYPOTHALAMUS.

3. CHANGES INCLUDE DECREASE IN THICKNESS OF THE VAGINAL WALL, DECREASE IN VAGINAL SECRETIONS, VAGINAL AND URETHRAL ATROPHY, LOSS OF BONE DENSITY, AND VASOMOTOR CLINICAL MANIFESTATION SUCH AS HOT FLASHES.

4. SOME WOMEN CHOOSE TO GO THROUGH MENOPAUSE WITHOUT HORMONE REPLACEMENT THERAPY (HRT) AND WILL USE NONHORMONAL DRUGS TO RELIEVE THE CLINICAL MANIFESTATIONS OF MENOPAUSE SUCH AS OSTEOPOROSIS (FOSAMAX), VAGINAL DRYNESS (WATER-SOLUBLE LUBRICANTS), AND HOT FLASHES (VITAMIN E).

5. SOME WOMEN CHOOSE TO USE HERBAL THERAPY WITH BLACK COHOSH, GINSENG, AND DONG QUAI FOR RELIEF OF CLINICAL MANIFESTATIONS.

6. SOME WOMEN CHOOSE TO TAKE HRT (ESTROGEN OR A COMBINATION OF ESTROGEN AND PROGESTERONE) OVER AN EXTENDED PERIOD OF TIME.

B. ESTROGEN

1. USES

a. Estrogen is given as an HRT when menopause occurs either naturally or surgically with removal of the ovaries.

b. Conjugated estrogens are most commonly prescribed.

c. When used as HRT in menopause, it reduces the risk of atherosclerosis, angina, coronary artery disease, and osteoporosis.

d. Estrogen HRT increases risk for breast cancer and dysfunctional uterine bleeding.

e. When used alone without progesterone, there is an increased incidence of uterine cancer.

f. When used in combination with progesterone, the client may have menstrual periods.

g. Progestin, usually prescribed as medroxyprogesterone acetate (Depo-Provera), is added to the monthly schedule the last 10–13 days of the cycle if the uterus is intact.

h. Calcium supplements are added to the monthly schedule to decrease the risk of osteoporosis.

i. Estrogen may be given for treatment of ovarian failure, female hypogonadism, postmenopausal osteoporosis, inoperable breast and prostate cancers, atropic vaginitis, and uterine conditions resulting from hormonal imbalance.

j. Estrogen is supplied as natural or synthetic hormone in forms of pills, injections, vaginal creams, and transdermal patches.

2. ADVERSE REACTIONS

a. Edema

b. Thromboembolism

c. Hypertension

d. Increase in weight
e. Spotting between menstrual periods
f. Breast tenderness
g. Dark skin patches that darken when exposed to the sun

3. CONTRAINDICATIONS AND PRECAUTIONS
   a. Contraindicated in clients with history of breast cancer, except in cases when cancer is not dependent on estrogen
   b. History of thromboembolitic disorders, hepatic or renal disorders, and undiagnosed vaginal bleeding (may increase risk of endometrial cancer)
   c. Pregnancy
   d. Hypersensitivity

4. DRUG INTERACTIONS
   a. Anticoagulants: decrease anticoagulant
   b. Antidiabetics: impair glucose tolerance that may change antidiabetic drug requirements
   c. Anticonvulsants: estrogen-induced fluid retention may precipitate seizures
   d. Barbiturates: decrease effect of estrogen
   e. Corticosteroids: increase risk of toxicological effect of corticosteroids
   f. Rifampin: decreases effect of estrogen

5. NURSING INTERVENTIONS
   a. Instruct the client of need for periodic physical examination, including blood pressure; weight; examination of breasts, abdomen, and pelvis; and Pap smears.
   b. Assess for alleviation of menopausal clinical manifestations such as hot flashes and vaginal dryness.
   c. Instruct the client to report any intermittent vaginal bleeding but explain that discontinuance of the drug will cause withdrawal bleeding.
   d. Instruct the client to weigh one to two times per week and report any sudden weight gain or fluid retention in the ankles and feet.
   e. Instruct the client in the procedure for performing Homans' sign and to report any pain, swelling, or tenderness with the procedure.
   f. Instruct the client to stop taking the estrogen and notify the physician immediately if pregnant.
   g. Inform the client that the use of caffeine products and smoking increase the risk of adverse reactions.
   h. Instruct the client to use a sunscreen or protective clothing when exposed to the sun.
   i. Inform the client of the dosage schedule and route of administration, stressing close adherence to the maintenance program.
   j. Instruct the client taking the pill form of estrogen to take it with meals or immediately after eating to reduce nausea.
   k. Instruct the client taking the pill form to take it daily as directed by the physician and if a dose is missed, the drug should be taken as soon as possible, but the missed dose should not be taken with the next day's dose.
   l. Instruct the client using vaginal cream to remain recumbent for 30 minutes after insertion of the drug and to wash the applicator with soap and water after each use.
   m. Instruct the client using vaginal cream to use sanitary napkins instead of tampons to protect clothing.
   n. Instruct the client using transdermal applications to apply to the trunk of the body in an area without body oil and to rotate sites.

6. TYPES
   a. Estradiol (Estrace, Estraderm)
   b. Estrogens conjugated (Premarin)
   c. Proprem (combination of Premarin and progestin)

II. DRUGS FOR MENSTRUAL DISORDERS

A. DESCRIPTION
   1. MENSTRUAL DISORDERS INCLUDE CONDITIONS OF AMENORRHEA, DYSMENORRHEA, PREMENSTRUAL SYNDROME, AND DYSFUNCTIONAL UTERINE BLEEDING.
   2. AMENORRHEA IS TREATED WITH DRUGS SUCH AS ESTROGEN TO STIMULATE OVULATION.
   3. DYSMENORRHEA IS TREATED WITH NONSTEROIDAL ANTI-INFLAMMATORY DRUGS (NSAIDs)/PROSTAGLANDIN INHIBITORS, HORMONAL THERAPY, ANALGESICS, AND NARCOTIC ANALGESICS.
   4. PREMENSTRUAL SYNDROME IS TREATED WITH OVULATORY SUPPRESSION DRUGS, PROGESTERONE, PROSTAGLANDIN INHIBITORS, VITAMINS B_6 AND E, DIURETICS, AND ANTIANXIETY AND ANTIDEPRESSANT DRUGS.
   5. DYSFUNCTIONAL UTERINE BLEEDING IS TREATED WITH NSAIDs/PROSTAGLANDIN INHIBITORS AND ORAL CONTRACEPTIVES (ESTROGEN AND PROGESTERONE).

B. NSAIDs/PROSTAGLANDIN INHIBITORS
   1. DESCRIPTION: A GROUP OF DRUGS THAT ARE NOT STEROIDS BUT HAVE ANTI-INFLAMMATORY PROPERTIES AND BLOCK THE FORMATION OF

PROSTAGLANDINS TO ALLEVIATE
INFLAMMATION, PAIN, AND FEVER
2. USES
   a. Mild to moderate pain and reduction of
      fever
   b. Joint pain in chronic rheumatoid
      arthritis and osteoarthritis
3. ADVERSE REACTIONS
   a. Heartburn
   b. Nausea and vomiting
   c. Gastrointestinal (GI) ulceration
   d. Nephrotoxicity
   e. Skin eruptions
   f. Hypersensitivity
4. CONTRAINDICATIONS AND
   PRECAUTIONS
   a. Urticaria
   b. Bronchospasm
   c. Active peptic ulcer
   d. Bleeding abnormalities
   e. Cardiac decompensation
   f. Impaired hepatic or renal function
   g. Hypersensitivity
5. DRUG INTERACTIONS
   a. Anticoagulants: increase prothrombin
      time
   b. Lithium: increases risk of lithium
      toxicity
6. NURSING INTERVENTIONS
   a. Question the client about a history of
      an allergic reaction to any NSAID.
   b. Instruct the client to take with meals,
      food, or milk to minimize gastric
      irritation.
   c. Monitor the client with a history of
      cardiac decompensation for fluid
      retention and edema.
   d. Monitor the hemoglobulin and renal
      and hepatic function studies.
   e. Monitor the client for masked
      inflammatory and pyretic conditions.
   f. Instruct the client to report any
      bleeding episodes, including dark, tarry
      stools or coffee-ground emesis.
   g. Instruct the client to report any skin
      rash, pruritus, or jaundice.
   h. Inform the client to avoid the use of
      alcohol with NSAIDs to decrease the
      risk of GI bleeding and bleeding
      disorders.
   i. Inform the client to begin to take the
      drug 1 to 2 days before menses to
      reduce uterine contractions from the
      prostaglandin.
7. TYPES OF NSAIDs AND
   PROSTAGLANDIN INHIBITORS
   a. Ibuprofen (Motrin)
   b. Naproxen (Naprosyn)
   c. Mefenamic acid (Ponstel)
   d. Acetylsalicylic acid (aspirin)

C. OVULATORY SUPPRESSION DRUGS
   1. DESCRIPTION
      a. Derivatives of testosterone with no
         estrogen or progesterone action
      b. They suppress pituitary secretion of
         follicle-stimulating hormone and
         luteinizing hormone, resulting in
         anovulation and amenorrhea.
   2. USES
      a. Interrupt progression of endometriosis
         and accompanying pain
      b. Use limited to 9 months for treatment of
         endometriosis and cannot be repeated
      c. Create anovulation and amenorrhea in
         the treatment of menorrhagia and
         premenstrual syndrome
   3. ADVERSE REACTIONS
      a. Virilization
      b. Gastroenteritis
      c. Decreased libido
      d. Hypersensitivity
      e. Hot flashes and sweating
      f. Vaginitis
      g. Irregular menstrual cycle
      h. Oily skin and hair
      i. Edema
      j. Decrease in breast size
   4. CONTRAINDICATIONS AND
      PRECAUTIONS
      a. Pregnancy
      b. Lactation
      c. Undiagnosed bleeding disorders of the
         female reproductive system
      d. Renal, cardiac, or hepatic dysfunction
   5. NURSING INTERVENTIONS
      a. Administration of the drug should be
         started during menstruation or after a
         negative pregnancy test.
      b. Monitor the client for weight gain and
         edema because the drug may cause
         fluid retention.
      c. Monitor periodic laboratory studies of
         renal, cardiac, and hepatic function.
      d. Instruct the client that amenorrhea
         caused by the drug is reversible and
         that bleeding may return in 2–3 months
         when administration is stopped.
      e. Inform the client that conception may
         occur when menses returns.
      f. Instruct the client to use a
         nonhormonal method of contraception
         for at least 2 months after beginning
         drug therapy to prevent an accidental
         pregnancy.
      g. Instruct the client to report
         immediately any signs of voice change
         to prevent permanent damage to voice.
   6. TYPES OF OVULATORY SUPPRESSION
      DRUGS
      a. Danazol (Cyclomen)

III. DRUGS FOR REPRODUCTIVE INFECTIOUS DISORDERS

   A. DESCRIPTION

      1. INFECTIONS OF THE FEMALE REPRODUCTIVE SYSTEM CAN BE CAUSED BY FUNGUS, BACTERIA, PROTOZOA, OR VIRUSES.

      2. INFECTIONS USUALLY ARE MANIFESTED BY INFLAMMATION OF TISSUES, ABNORMAL DISCHARGE, AND ITCHING (PRURITUS).

      3. RESISTANCE TO INFECTION IS REDUCED BY DOUCHING; ORAL CONTRACEPTIVES; BROAD-SPECTRUM ANTIBIOTICS; AGING; DISEASE PROCESSES; ORAL, ANAL, OR VAGINAL SEX WITH AN INFECTED PARTNER; AND POOR HYGIENIC PRACTICES.

      4. MAJOR INFECTIOUS DISEASES AFFECTING THE FEMALE REPRODUCTIVE SYSTEM ARE CANDIDIASIS (FUNGAL), BACTERIAL VAGINOSIS (BACTERIAL), TRICHOMONIASIS (PROTOZOAN), HERPESVIRUS TYPE 2 (VIRAL), CHLAMYDIA (BACTERIAL), GONORRHEA (BACTERIAL), PELVIC INFLAMMATORY DISEASE (BACTERIAL), AND TOXIC SHOCK SYNDROME (BACTERIAL).

   B. USES

      1. ANTIFUNGAL DRUGS ALTER THE PERMEABILITY OF THE FUNGAL CELL MEMBRANE AND ALTER THE FUNCTION OF FUNGAL ENZYMES.

      2. ANTIBIOTICS INHIBIT BACTERIAL PROTEIN SYNTHESIS AND HAVE A BACTERIOSTATIC ACTION AGAINST SUSCEPTIBLE BACTERIA.

      3. PROTOZOAN INFECTIONS ARE TREATED WITH ANTI-INFECTIVE DRUGS THAT HAVE AN AMEBICIDAL ACTION.

      4. ANTIVIRAL DRUGS INHIBIT VIRAL REPLICATION AND REDUCE THE TIME OF LESIONS TO HEAL.

   C. ADVERSE REACTIONS OF ANTIFUNGAL DRUGS

      1. ARRHYTHMIAS

      2. VULVOVAGINAL BURNING, ITCHING, IRRITATION

      3. BITTER TASTE

      4. INCREASED LIBIDO

      5. HIVES, SKIN RASH

      6. ALLERGIC REACTIONS, INCLUDING ANAPHYLAXIS

   D. CONTRAINDICATIONS AND PRECAUTIONS

      1. HYPERSENSITIVITY

   E. DRUG INTERACTIONS

      1. RIFAMPIN: DECREASES BLOOD LEVELS AND EFFECTIVENESS OF MICONAZOLE NITRATE

      2. ISONIAZID: DECREASES BLOOD LEVELS AND EFFECTIVENESS OF MICONAZOLE NITRATE

   F. NURSING INTERVENTIONS

      1. OBTAIN CULTURE AND SENSITIVITY PRIOR TO STARTING DRUG THERAPY. FIRST DOSE MAY BE GIVEN BEFORE RECEIVING RESULTS.

      2. INSTRUCT THE CLIENT TO AVOID GETTING THE DRUG ON THE HANDS OR IN THE EYES.

      3. INSTRUCT THE CLIENT USING TOPICAL APPLICATIONS THAT IMPROVEMENT SHOULD BE NOTED IN 1–2 WEEKS.

      4. INSTRUCT THE CLIENT TO INSERT THE APPLICATOR HIGH IN THE VAGINA AND TO USE A SANITARY NAPKIN RATHER THAN A TAMPON TO PREVENT SOILING OF CLOTHING.

      5. INFORM THE CLIENT TO REFRAIN FROM SEXUAL INTERCOURSE DURING TREATMENT TO AVOID REINFECTION.

      6. INFORM THE CLIENT THAT IF PLANNING SEXUAL INTERCOURSE, INTRAVAGINAL FOAMS AND CERTAIN LATEX PRODUCTS LIKE VAGINAL DIAPHRAGMS SHOULD NOT BE USED BECAUSE OF POSSIBLE INTERACTION.

      7. INSTRUCT THE CLIENT THAT OVER-THE-COUNTER (OTC) PREPARATIONS CAN BE PURCHASED FOR MINOR INFECTIONS, BUT TO SEEK MEDICAL ATTENTION IF INFECTION PERSISTS.

      8. INFORM THE CLIENT THAT THE DRUG IS AVAILABLE IN CREAM, LOTION, TOPICAL POWDER, SPRAY, VAGINAL SUPPOSITORIES, AND VAGINAL CREAMS.

      9. INFORM THE CLIENT THAT THE VAGINAL SUPPOSITORY FORM IS THE PREFERRED APPLICATION AND SHOULD BE INSERTED AT BEDTIME FOR 3 DAYS (MONISTAT 3) OR FOR 7 DAYS (MONISTAT 7).

   G. TYPES OF ANTIFUNGAL DRUGS

      1. MICONAZOLE NITRATE (MICATIN, MONISTAT)

      2. NYSTATIN (MYCOSTATIN)

      3. BUTOCONAZOLE (FEMSTAT)

      4. CLOTRIMAZOLE (GYNE-LOTRIMIN)

      5. TERCONAZOLE (TERAZOL)

   H. ADVERSE REACTIONS OF ANTI-INFECTIVES AND ANTIBIOTICS

      1. NAUSEA AND VOMITING

      2. DIARRHEA

      3. RASHES

      4. HYPERSENSITIVITY

      5. PHOTOSENSITIVITY

I. CONTRAINDICATIONS AND PRECAUTIONS
  1. HYPERSENSITIVITY
  2. TETRACYCLINE HYDROCHLORIDE SHOULD NOT BE GIVEN TO PREGNANT WOMEN IN THE LAST HALF OF THEIR PREGNANCY (OR NOT AT ALL) BECAUSE IT MAY PERMANENTLY DISCOLOR THE TEETH, CAUSE ENAMEL DEFECTS, OR RETARD BONE GROWTH OF THE FETUS.
J. DRUG INTERACTIONS
  1. ORAL ANTICOAGULANTS: INCREASE EFFECT OF ORAL ANTICOAGULANTS
  2. ALCOHOL: A DISULFIRAM-LIKE REACTION (ANTABUSE) MAY OCCUR WHEN ALCOHOL IS INGESTED WHILE ON METRONIDAZOLE (FLAGYL).
  3. DOXYCYCLINE MAY DECREASE THE EFFECTIVENESS OF ORAL CONTRACEPTIVES.
  4. CALCIUM, IRON, OR MAGNESIUM FORM CHELATES AND DECREASE ABSORPTION OF TETRACYCLINE GROUP OF DRUGS (INCLUDES DOXYCYCLINE).
K. NURSING INTERVENTIONS
  1. QUESTION THE CLIENT IF SHE HAS A KNOWN HYPERSENSITIVITY TO ANTI-INFECTIVES OR ANTIBIOTICS.
  2. OBTAIN CULTURE AND SENSITIVITY (C & S) PRIOR TO BEGINNING THE DRUG. FIRST DOSE MAY BE GIVEN BEFORE RECEIVING RESULTS OF THE C & S.
  3. INSTRUCT THE CLIENT TO TAKE THE DRUG AROUND THE CLOCK AND THAT IT MAY BE TAKEN WITH FOOD (EXCEPT AZITHROMYCIN).
  4. INSTRUCT THE CLIENT TO TAKE ALL OF THE DRUG EVEN IF THE CLINICAL MANIFESTATIONS DISAPPEAR AND SHE FEELS BETTER.
  5. INSTRUCT THE CLIENT TAKING ERYTHROMYCIN THAT THE DRUG SHOULD BE TAKEN 1 HOUR BEFORE OR 2 HOURS AFTER A MEAL WITH A FULL GLASS OF WATER (NOT WITH FRUIT JUICE BECAUSE THE ACIDITY MAY DECREASE DRUG EFFECTIVENESS).
  6. INSTRUCT THE CLIENT TO WEAR SUN PROTECTION IF GOING OUTDOORS.
  7. INSTRUCT THE CLIENT TO NOTIFY THE PHYSICIAN IF A BLACK, FURRY OVERGROWTH APPEARS ON THE TONGUE; VAGINAL ITCHING OR DISCHARGE OCCUR; OR LOOSE, FOUL-SMELLING STOOLS (SIGNS OF SUPERINFECTION) OCCUR.
  8. INSTRUCT THE CLIENT NOT TO USE ALCOHOL WHILE ON METRONIDAZOLE AND FOR 48 HOURS AFTER COMPLETING THE DRUG. ALSO ADVISE THAT DRUG MAY HAVE A METALLIC TASTE, AND DARK OR RED-BROWN URINE MAY OCCUR.
  9. INSTRUCT THE CLIENT ON AZITHROMYCIN TO TAKE ON AN EMPTY STOMACH BECAUSE FOOD OR ANTACIDS DECREASE ABSORPTION.
  10. INFORM THE CLIENT TAKING CIPROFLOXACIN TO TAKE 2 HOURS AFTER A MEAL OR 2 HOURS BEFORE OR AFTER TAKING ANTACIDS, SUCRALFATE, OR VITAMINS THAT CONTAIN IRON SO THAT PEAK SERUM LEVELS ARE NOT AFFECTED.
  11. INSTRUCT THE CLIENT TAKING TETRACYCLINE TO TAKE WITH A FULL GLASS OF WATER OR ON AN EMPTY STOMACH AT LEAST 1 HOUR BEFORE OR 2 HOURS AFTER MEALS. TETRACYCLINE WILL NOT BE EFFECTIVE IF TAKEN WITH MILK OR DAIRY PRODUCTS, FOOD, ANTACIDS, OR IRON.
  12. INSTRUCT THE CLIENT TAKING TETRACYCLINE TO USE A NONHORMONAL FORM OF CONTRACEPTION BECAUSE TETRACYCLINE DECREASES THE EFFECTIVENESS OF HORMONAL CONTRACEPTIVES AND THERE IS INCREASED RISK OF BREAKTHROUGH BLEEDING.
  13. INSTRUCT THE CLIENT WITH RECURRENT INFECTION OF THE NEED TO RETURN FOR A CULTURE 2 WEEKS AFTER COMPLETING ANTIBIOTIC THERAPY.
  14. INSTRUCT THE CLIENT TO AVOID SEXUAL INTERCOURSE UNTIL SHE AND HER PARTNER(S) HAVE COMPLETED THE COURSE OF THE DRUG AND FOLLOW-UP CULTURES OR SMEARS ARE DONE AND REPORTED AS NEGATIVE. WEEKLY CULTURE IS NEEDED UNTIL TWO ARE NEGATIVE.
L. TYPES OF ANTI-INFECTIVES OR ANTIBIOTICS
  1. AZITHROMYCIN (ZITHROMAX)—CHLAMYDIA
  2. CIPROFLOXACIN HYDROCHLORIDE (CIPRO) (SINGLE DOSE)—GONORRHEA
  3. CEFTRIAXONE SODIUM (ROCEPHIN) (IM)—IF PREGNANT WITH GONORRHEA
  4. DOXYCYCLINE (VIBRAMYCIN)—CHLAMYDIA, GONORRHEA
  5. TETRACYCLINE HYDROCHLORIDE (ACHROMYCIN V)—CHLAMYDIA, GONORRHEA
  6. ERYTHROMYCIN (ERYTHROMYCIN BASE, ESTOLATE, STEARATE)—IF

ALLERGIC TO DOXYCYCLINE OR TETRACYCLINE OR PREGNANT WITH CHLAMYDIA

7. METRONIDAZOLE (FLAGYL)—BACTERIAL VAGINOSIS, TRICHOMONIASIS

8. CEFOXITIN SODIUM (MEFOXIN)—RECOMMENDED FOR GONORRHEA AND TOXIC SHOCK SYNDROME

9. ROCEPHIN IM PLUS DOXYCYCLINE—PELVIC INFLAMMATORY DISEASE (PID)

M. ADVERSE REACTIONS OF ANTIVIRAL DRUGS

1. HEADACHE
2. SEIZURES
3. NAUSEA AND VOMITING
4. DIARRHEA
5. RASH, HIVES
6. RENAL FAILURE
7. CHANGES IN MENSTRUAL CYCLE

N. CONTRAINDICATIONS AND PRECAUTIONS

1. HYPERSENSITIVITY
2. IMMUNOCOMPROMISED CLIENTS
3. RENAL IMPAIRMENT
4. LACTATION

O. DRUG INTERACTIONS

1. PROBENECID: INCREASES BLOOD LEVELS OF ACYCLOVIR
2. ACYCLOVIR SHOULD NOT BE USED IN CONJUNCTION WITH OTHER NEPHROTOXIC DRUGS TO PREVENT RENAL DAMAGE.

P. NURSING INTERVENTIONS

1. MONITOR RENAL STUDIES (BLOOD UREA NITROGEN [BUN], SERUM CREATININE, AND CREATININE CLEARANCE) TO DETECT CHANGES IN RENAL FUNCTION.
2. INSTRUCT THE CLIENT TO START TAKING THE DRUG AS SOON AS HERPES CLINICAL MANIFESTATIONS APPEAR.
3. INSTRUCT THE CLIENT TO TAKE THE DRUG AS PRESCRIBED FOR THE ENTIRE COURSE OF THERAPY. ANY MISSED DOSES SHOULD BE TAKEN AS SOON AS REMEMBERED, BUT DOSES SHOULD NOT BE DOUBLED.
4. INFORM THE CLIENT THAT DRUGS ARE FOR TREATING CLINICAL MANIFESTATIONS AND DO NOT PROVIDE A CURE.
5. INSTRUCT THE CLIENT TO CLEAN LESIONS THREE TO FOUR TIMES A DAY WITH SOAP AND WATER AND TO DRY THOROUGHLY BEFORE APPLYING OINTMENT.
6. INSTRUCT THE CLIENT TO APPLY OINTMENT THREE TO SIX TIMES A DAY WITH FINGER PROTECTION USING A FINGER COT OR GLOVES TO PREVENT AUTOINOCULATION OF BODY PARTS OR SPREADING THE VIRUS TO OTHER INDIVIDUALS.
7. INSTRUCT THE CLIENT TO REFRAIN FROM SEXUAL INTERCOURSE IF EITHER PARTNER HAS CLINICAL MANIFESTATIONS OF HERPES.
8. INSTRUCT THE CLIENT TO USE CONDOMS WHEN HAVING INTERCOURSE TO PROTECT THE PARTNER.
9. INSTRUCT THE CLIENT TO HAVE YEARLY PAP SMEARS BECAUSE THERE IS RISK FOR DEVELOPING CERVICAL CANCER.
10. INSTRUCT THE CLIENT TO AVOID GETTING THE DRUG IN OR NEAR THE EYES.
11. INSTRUCT THE CLIENT NOT TO USE OTC CREAMS OR OINTMENTS UNLESS ADVISED BY THE PHYSICIAN.
12. INSTRUCT THE CLIENT THAT ORAL ACYCLOVIR IS NOT USUALLY GIVEN LONGER THAN 6 MONTHS BECAUSE RESISTANCE TO THE DRUG IS POSSIBLE.

Q. TYPES OF ANTIVIRAL DRUGS

1. ACYCLOVIR (ZOVIRAX)—HERPESVIRUS TYPE 2—IV, PO, AND TOPICAL OINTMENTS/CREAMS
2. VALACYCLOVIR (VALTREX)
3. FAMCICLOVIR (FAMVIR)
4. TRIFLURIDINE (VIROPTIC)—OPHTHALMIC SOLUTION

IV. DRUGS FOR TREATMENT OF ENDOMETRIOSIS

A. DESCRIPTION

1. ENDOMETRIOSIS OCCURS WHEN ENDOMETRIAL CELLS ARE IMPLANTED OUTSIDE THE UTERUS IN THE PELVIS, CAUSING BLEEDING, INFLAMMATION, AND ADHESIONS.
2. ENDOMETRIAL CELLS ARE STIMULATED BY OVARIAN HORMONES.

B. USES

1. ORAL CONTRACEPTIVES ARE GIVEN TO SUPPRESS STIMULATION OF ENDOMETRIAL CELLS AND RELIEVE THE CLINICAL MANIFESTATIONS OF DYSMENORRHEA.
2. SYNTHETIC ANDROGENS MAY BE USED TO CAUSE ATROPHY OF THE ENDOMETRIUM, RESULTING IN AMENORRHEA.
3. GONADOTROPIN-RELEASING HORMONE AGONISTS DECREASE ESTROGEN PRODUCTION, RESULTING IN AMENORRHEA.

C. ADVERSE REACTIONS, CONTRAINDICATIONS AND PRECAUTIONS, DRUG INTERACTIONS, AND NURSING INTERVENTIONS (SEE SECTION II, DRUGS FOR MENSTRUAL

DISORDERS [NSAIDs/PROSTAGLANDIN INHIBITORS AND OVULATORY SUPPRESSION DRUGS])

D. TYPES
1. IBUPROFEN (MOTRIN)—NSAID
2. NAPROXEN (NAPROSYN)—NSAID
3. ESTROGEN/PROGESTIN COMBINATION DRUGS FOR ORAL CONTRACEPTIVES
4. DEPO-PROVERA (IM)—PROGESTERONE CONTRACEPTIVE
5. DANAZOL (CYCLOMEN)—SYNTHETIC ANDROGEN
6. NAFARELIN ACETATE (SYNAREL)— GONADOTROPIN-RELEASING HORMONE AGONIST
7. LEUPROLIDE ACETATE (LUPRON)— GONADOTROPIN-RELEASING HORMONE AGONIST

V. **DRUGS FOR INFERTILITY, CONTRACEPTION, AND ELECTIVE ABORTION**
A. DESCRIPTION
1. INFERTILITY IS A COUPLE'S INABILITY TO ACHIEVE PREGNANCY AFTER 1 YEAR OF UNPROTECTED INTERCOURSE.
2. CONTRACEPTION IS THE PREVENTION OF FERTILIZATION OR IMPLANTATION OF A FERTILIZED OVUM IN THE UTERUS.
3. AN ELECTIVE ABORTION IS THE TERMINATION OF A PREGNANCY WITH THE EXPULSION OF THE PRODUCTS OF CONCEPTION.
B. USES
1. INFERTILITY IS TREATED WITH DRUGS THAT INDUCE OVULATION BECAUSE THE WOMAN IS NOT ABLE TO OVULATE OR SHE OVULATES IRREGULARLY.
2. CHEMICAL CONTRACEPTION IS PROVIDED IN THE FORM OF DRUGS THAT CONTAIN A COMBINATION OF ESTROGEN AND PROGESTIN OR PROGESTIN ONLY.
3. COMBINATION DRUGS INHIBIT OVULATION.
4. A PROGESTIN-ONLY DRUG IMPLANTED SUBDERMALLY IN THE UPPER ARM INHIBITS OVULATION AND CAUSES THE CERVICAL MUCUS TO BECOME THICK, THUS PREVENTING SPERM FROM REACHING THE UTERUS. DRUG EFFECT LASTS FOR UP TO 5 YEARS.
5. ELECTIVE ABORTIONS UTILIZE DRUGS THAT KILL THE FETUS, CAUSING EXPULSION; DRUGS THAT CAUSE UTERINE CONTRACTIONS AND EXPULSION; OR DRUGS THAT ARE PROGESTERONE ANTAGONISTS THAT PREVENT IMPLANTATION OF THE OVUM.

C. ADVERSE REACTIONS OF DRUGS TO TREAT INFERTILITY
1. NAUSEA AND VOMITING
2. WEIGHT GAIN
3. SPONTANEOUS ABORTION
4. MULTIPLE BIRTHS
5. ABDOMINAL DISTENTION AND PAIN
6. VISUAL DISTURBANCES
D. CONTRAINDICATIONS AND PRECAUTIONS
1. PREGNANCY
2. OVARIAN CYSTS
3. NEOPLASTIC LESIONS
E. NURSING INTERVENTIONS
1. INSTRUCT THE CLIENT THAT MULTIPLE BIRTHS ARE POSSIBLE WITH DRUG THERAPY.
2. INSTRUCT THE CLIENT TO WEIGH DAILY OR EVERY OTHER DAY AND REPORT SUDDEN WEIGHT GAINS.
3. INSTRUCT THE CLIENT THAT IF MENSES OCCURS, START THE NEXT CYCLE OF DRUG THERAPY ON THE FIFTH DAY ONCE OVULATION HAS BEEN DETERMINED (CLOMIPHENE CITRATE).
4. INSTRUCT THE CLIENT TO TAKE THE DRUG AT THE SAME TIME EACH DAY TO MAINTAIN LEVELS OF CLOMIPHENE CITRATE.
5. INSTRUCT THE CLIENT TO STRICTLY FOLLOW THE PHYSICIAN'S INSTRUCTIONS FOR SEXUAL INTERCOURSE IN RELATION TO DRUG THERAPY.
F. TYPES OF DRUGS TO TREAT INFERTILITY
1. CLOMIPHENE CITRATE (CLOMID)— ORAL NONSTEROIDAL ESTROGEN AGONIST OR ANTAGONIST
2. MENOTROPINS (MENOPUR) IM— COMBINATION OF FOLLICLE-STIMULATING HORMONE (FSH) AND LUTEINIZING HORMONE (LH) USED WITH HUMAN CHORIONIC GONADOTROPIN (HCG) TO INDUCE OVULATION AND PREGNANCY
3. CHORIONIC GONADOTROPIN (CHORON-10) IM—HCG
G. ADVERSE REACTIONS OF DRUGS FOR CONTRACEPTION
1. NAUSEA AND VOMITING
2. BREAKTHROUGH BLEEDING
3. BREAST TENDERNESS
4. HEADACHE
5. DEPRESSION
6. HIRSUTISM
H. CONTRAINDICATIONS AND PRECAUTIONS
1. PREGNANCY
2. LACTATION
3. ESTROGEN-DEPENDENT NEOPLASMS

4. HISTORY OF CARDIOVASCULAR DISORDERS
5. GALLBLADDER DISEASE
6. THROMBOTIC OR THROMBOEMBOLIC DISORDERS

I. NURSING INTERVENTIONS
1. ASSESS THE CLIENT FOR A HISTORY OF CARDIOVASCULAR AND GALLBLADDER DISEASE.
2. INSTRUCT THE CLIENT THAT THERAPY CANNOT BE STARTED UNTIL THE CLIENT STARTS MENSES OR HAS A NEGATIVE PREGNANCY TEST.
3. INSTRUCT THE CLIENT TO USE OTHER FORMS OF CONTRACEPTION DURING THE FIRST WEEK (ESTROGEN/PROGESTIN COMBINATION) AND FOR 3 WEEKS (PROGESTIN ONLY) WHEN CONTRACEPTIVES ARE STARTED.
4. INSTRUCT THE CLIENT TO TAKE ORAL DRUGS AS PRESCRIBED AND IF A DOSE IS MISSED, IT SHOULD BE TAKEN AS SOON AS REMEMBERED. TWO DOSES MAY BE TAKEN TOGETHER THE NEXT DAY.
5. INFORM THE CLIENT OF THE RISK FOR CARDIOVASCULAR DISEASE IF THE CLIENT SMOKES AND TAKES CONTRACEPTIVES.
6. INSTRUCT THE CLIENT TO WEIGH FREQUENTLY TO DETECT EARLY FLUID RETENTION.
7. INSTRUCT THE CLIENT IN THE TECHNIQUE OF CHECKING FOR HOMANS' SIGN TO DETECT EARLY DEVELOPMENT OF THROMBOPHLEBITIS.
8. INFORM THE CLIENT TO WAIT AT LEAST 3 MONTHS AFTER STOPPING PROGESTIN-ONLY DRUGS BEFORE GETTING PREGNANT TO AVOID BIRTH DEFECTS.
9. INFORM THE CLIENT OF THE NEED FOR PERIODIC FOLLOW-UP OF BREAST EXAMINATION, PELVIC EXAMINATION WITH PAP SMEAR, AND LABORATORY TESTS FOR CARDIAC AND HEPATIC FUNCTION.

J. TYPES OF DRUGS FOR CONTRACEPTION
1. NORETHINDRONE (BREVICON, OVCON, ORTHO-NOVUM 10/11 OR 7/7/7)—ESTROGEN/PROGESTERONE COMBINATION; USUALLY TAKEN FOR 21 DAYS OF CYCLE, OFF 7 DAYS
2. NORETHINDRONE (MICRONOR)—ORAL PROGESTIN, ALSO KNOWN AS THE "MINIPILL"; TAKEN DAILY WITHOUT A REST PERIOD
3. LEVONORGESTREL/ETHINYL ESTRADIOL (LYBREL)—91-DAY REGIMEN IN WHICH WOMEN HAVE A MENSTRUAL CYCLE EVERY 3 MONTHS RATHER THAN MONTHLY
4. MEDROXYPROGESTERONE ACETATE (DEPO-PROVERA) IM—PROGESTIN; PREVENTS PREGNANCY FOR 3 MONTHS
5. DIENOGEST (NATAZIA)—PROGESTIN USED WITH ESTRADIOL IN A COMBINATION ORAL FORMULATION. FIRST CONTRACEPTIVE THAT INVOLVES A FOUR-PHASE DOSE REGIMEN, WHICH DECREASES THE ESTROGEN DOSE AND INCREASES THE PROGESTIN DOSE IN A 28-DAY CYCLE. PREVENTS BREAKTHROUGH BLEEDING AND PREVENTS PREGNANCY BY SUPPRESSING OVULATION.
6. PLAN B OR PREVEN—KIT AVAILABLE FOR EMERGENCY CONTRACEPTION; USED AFTER UNPROTECTED INTERCOURSE OR SUSPECTED CONTRACEPTIVE FAILURE. CONTAINS FOUR TABLETS OF ETHINYL ESTRADIOL AND LEVONORGESTREL (PREVEN) OR TWO TABLETS OF LEVONORGESTREL (PLAN B). TAKE AS SOON AS POSSIBLE BUT WITHIN 72 HOURS OF UNPROTECTED SEX.

K. ADVERSE REACTIONS OF DRUGS FOR ELECTIVE ABORTION
1. HEADACHE
2. NAUSEA AND VOMITING
3. DIARRHEA
4. ABDOMINAL PAIN
5. UTERINE PAIN SIMILAR TO MENSES

L. CONTRAINDICATIONS AND PRECAUTIONS
1. HYPERSENSITIVITY
2. PREGNANT WOMEN WITH 55 OR MORE DAYS OF AMENORRHEA HAVE GREATER INCIDENCE OF ADVERSE REACTIONS (MIFEPRISTONE).

M. NURSING INTERVENTIONS
1. DISCUSS WITH THE CLIENT THE ADVERSE REACTIONS AND RISK FACTORS OF THE DRUGS.
2. ASSESS POSTPROCEDURE FOR EXCESSIVE BLEEDING AND CLINICAL MANIFESTATIONS OF INFECTION.
3. REPORT ANY COMPLAINTS OF SEVERE ABDOMINAL PAIN.

N. TYPE OF DRUGS FOR ELECTIVE ABORTION
1. MIFEPRISTONE (KNOWN PREVIOUSLY AS RU-486)—PROGESTERONE ANTAGONIST
2. METHOTREXATE (AMETHOPTERIN)—IV OR IM TO KILL THE FETUS
3. MISOPROSTOL (CYTOTEC)—SYNTHETIC PROSTAGLANDIN ANALOG

PRACTICE QUESTIONS

1. Which of the following is a priority for the nurse to include in the instructions for a client starting estrogen hormone replacement therapy for menopause?
   1. Report an increase in weight of 3 pounds or more to your doctor
   2. Take extra safety precautions to protect yourself from injury and falls
   3. You may have greater frequency and urgency in urination
   4. Remember to do a breast self-examination every month

2. After receiving instructions from the nurse regarding the drug alendronate (Fosamax), which of the following statements from a postmenopausal client indicates an understanding of the purpose of the drug?
   1. "This drug should help my mood swings."
   2. "This drug should eliminate my stress incontinence."
   3. "This drug should make my bones stronger."
   4. "This drug should relieve my hot flashes."

3. The nurse monitors a client receiving hormone replacement therapy for which of the following adverse reactions?
   Select all that apply:
   [ ] 1. Increase in weight
   [ ] 2. Menorrhagia
   [ ] 3. Hypertension
   [ ] 4. Virilization
   [ ] 5. Breast tenderness
   [ ] 6. Decreased libido

4. The nurse instructs the perimenopausal client that it is a priority to stop taking the prescribed estrogen if which of the following occurs?
   1. Spotting between menstrual periods
   2. Painful intercourse
   3. Breast tenderness
   4. Nausea and vomiting

5. Which of the following should the nurse include in the administration instructions for a client using estrogen vaginal cream?
   1. Insert a tampon afterward to protect your clothing
   2. Remain in bed for 30 minutes after inserting the drug
   3. Apply the drug topically every 10 days throughout the month
   4. Soak the applicator in bleach after each use

6. Based on an understanding of drugs, the nurse plans to instruct a client with amenorrhea to use which of the following drugs?

   1. Danazol (Danocrine)
   2. Progesterone (Progestin)
   3. Estrogen (Premarin)
   4. Naproxen (Naprosyn)

7. Which of the following should the nurse include in the instructions to a client receiving a nonsteroidal anti-inflammatory drug?
   1. Do not take with the drug lithium
   2. Avoid the use of products with caffeine
   3. Notify your physician if you become pregnant
   4. Take on an empty stomach

8. Which of the following allergies should the nurse assess for a client who is taking naproxen (Naprosyn) for the treatment of dysmenorrhea?
   1. Morphine
   2. Penicillin
   3. Aspirin
   4. Tylenol

9. Which of the following assessment findings is expected in a client with premenstrual syndrome (PMS) who is receiving danazol (Danocrine)?
   1. Breast tenderness
   2. Hirsutism
   3. Increased libido
   4. Amenorrhea

10. The nurse should instruct a client who is prescribed danazol (Danocrine) for the treatment of premenstrual syndrome (PMS) to take the first dose
    1. 2 weeks after the next menstrual period.
    2. during the next menstrual period.
    3. the next time thick vaginal mucus is discharged.
    4. 1 week prior to the beginning of the next menses.

11. The nurse instructs a client taking Premarin that which of the following adverse reactions may occur?
    Select all that apply:
    [ ] 1. Increase in weight
    [ ] 2. Heartburn
    [ ] 3. Bitter taste
    [ ] 4. Breast pain
    [ ] 5. Leg pain
    [ ] 6. Diarrhea

12. The nurse instructs the client taking miconazole nitrate (Monistat) to avoid which of the following drugs?
    1. Coumadin
    2. Isoniazid (Nydrazid)

3. Probenecid (Benemid)
4. Hydrochlorothiazide (Hydrodiuril)

13. Which of the following should the nurse include in the teaching plan for a client who has a recurrent gonorrheal infection and is treated with ciprofloxacin hydrochloride (Cipro)?
    1. The drug should be taken with meals or with a glass of milk
    2. Weekly cultures are necessary until two are negative
    3. The drug should not be discontinued until all the pills have been taken
    4. The drug will be started when the diagnostic culture and sensitivity results are obtained

14. Which of the following should the nurse include in the medication instructions for a client with gonorrhea who is prescribed tetracycline hydrochloride (Achromycin V)?
    1. Continue taking birth control pills
    2. Take two or three times during the day as prescribed
    3. Start the first dose after the results of the culture and sensitivity are determined
    4. Use sun protection and cover your body if going outdoors

15. The nurse informs a client that danazol (Dancrine) may be given for how many months in the treatment of endometriosis?_____

16. The nurse should notify the physician if which of the following occurs when treating a client receiving antibiotics for gonorrhea?
    1. Perineal lesions fail to clear in 2 to 3 days
    2. Sexual intercourse is painful
    3. A black furry growth appears on the tongue
    4. Spotting occurs between periods

17. The nurse is creating a medication schedule for erythromycin prescribed for a client with pelvic inflammatory disease. Which of the following times for administration should the nurse include in the schedule? Administer with
    1. a full glass of water between meals.
    2. fruit juice prior to each meal.
    3. an antacid 30 minutes before each meal.
    4. a glass of milk at each meal.

18. The nurse informs a client with bacterial vaginosis who has been taking metronidazole (Flagyl) that which of the following would indicate an expected response to the drug?
    1. Weight gain
    2. Metallic taste
    3. Reddish-brown urine
    4. Diarrhea

19. The nurse instructs a client who has trichomoniasis to avoid which of the following while taking metronidazole (Flagyl)?
    1. Lithium

2. Alcohol
3. Caffeine
4. Diazepam

20. Which of the following is correct to include in the procedure for a client with herpesvirus type 2 who is being treated with acyclovir (Zovirax)?
    1. Wash the lesions with bar soap and water and dry well
    2. Apply ointment to the lesions with a nonsterile glove
    3. Apply the medicated patch over a cluster of lesions
    4. Cover the lesions with an occlusive dressing

21. Which of the following laboratory tests would be most important for the nurse to monitor in a client with herpesvirus type 2 who has been taking acyclovir (Zovirax)?
    1. Alkaline phosphatase
    2. White blood cell count
    3. Prothrombin time
    4. Serum creatinine

22. The nurse instructs a client with a history of herpesvirus type 2 to take the prescribed acyclovir (Zovirax)
    1. for up to 1 year whenever the lesions return.
    2. at the first sign of clinical manifestations returning.
    3. when over-the-counter ointments fail to control itching.
    4. daily for 2 weeks to prevent reinfection.

23. A client who is prescribed danazol (Danocrine) for endometriosis asks the nurse, "What happens when I stop taking this drug?" The best response of the nurse would be
    1. "You will be cured of your endometriosis."
    2. "You will no longer have dysmenorrhea with your periods."
    3. "You will ovulate and start menstruating in 2 to 3 months."
    4. "You will have more regular periods."

24. The nurse should inform a client taking oral contraceptives for birth control that which of the following is a priority to immediately report?
    1. Spotting between periods
    2. Breast enlargement
    3. Increase in growth of body hair
    4. Calf pain with dorsiflexion of the foot

25. The nurse instructs a client who is prescribed a progestin-only contraceptive for birth control to
    1. take the drug the 5th to 30th day of each monthly menstrual cycle.
    2. use a barrier method of contraception for 4 months after starting the drug.
    3. wait 3 months to get pregnant after she stops taking the drug.
    4. stop taking the drug if she experiences a menstrual period.

26. Which of the following nursing tasks may the registered nurse safely delegate to a licensed practical nurse?
    1. Inform a client who is going through menopause on the pros and cons of using hormonal replacement therapy
    2. Advise a client taking estrogen to weigh one to two times per week and report any sudden weight gain or fluid retention in the ankles and feet
    3. Instruct a client on the purpose of ovulation suppression drugs
    4. Question a client taking a nonsteroidal anti-inflammatory drug about the presence of dark, tarry stools or a coffee-ground emesis.

ANSWERS AND RATIONALES

1. 4. Menopausal women who take estrogen hormone replacement therapy (HRT) are at risk for developing breast cancer; thus, monthly breast self-examinations are very important. It is normal for women who start HRT to gain weight. Menopausal women who do not start HRT will be at risk for osteoporosis and prone to fractures and will have greater frequency and urgency in urination.

2. 3. Alendronate (Fosamax) is a drug that decreases the rate of bone resorption and is used to prevent or treat osteoporosis in postmenopausal women. Fosamax is not helpful for other clinical manifestations of menopause, which include mood swings, stress incontinence, and hot flashes.

3. 1. 3. 5. The adverse reactions of hormone replacement therapy (HRT) include increase in weight, fluid retention, hypertension, breast tenderness, spotting between periods, and dark skin patches that darken when exposed to sunlight. Women on HRT who do menstruate have normal menstrual cycles without excessive bleeding. Virilization and decreased libido do not normally occur with HRT.

4. 4. Hormone replacement therapy (HRT) should not be taken if one is pregnant; if a woman begins to experience nausea and vomiting, it could indicate morning sickness accompanying a pregnancy. Spotting between menstrual periods and breast tenderness are adverse reactions to HRT. Painful intercourse may be due to vaginal dryness, which commonly occurs in menopause with the absence of estrogen.

5. 2. For proper absorption of the vaginal cream, the client should remain in bed for 30 minutes after insertion. A tampon would absorb the cream and reduce its effectiveness. Application schedules vary, but the cream should be applied at least one to three times per week. The applicator should be cleaned with soap and water after use.

6. 3. Amenorrhea is treated with drugs such as estrogen (Premarin) to stimulate ovulation. Danazol (Danocrine) is used to suppress ovulation. Progesterone (Progestin) causes the uterine lining to shed with menses. Naproxen (Naprosyn) is a nonsteroidal anti-inflammatory drug used in the treatment of dysmenorrhea.

7. 1. Nonsteroidal anti-inflammatory drugs (NSAIDs) interact with lithium to increase lithium toxicity. Caffeine is not contraindicated with the use of NSAIDs. NSAIDs are not hormones and would not affect pregnancy. NSAIDs should be taken with food or milk to minimize gastric irritation.

8. 3. Naproxen (Naprosyn) and acetylsalicylic acid (aspirin) are both nonsteroidal anti-inflammatory drugs (NSAIDs), and a hypersensitivity to any NSAID creates a hypersensitivity to all of the others in the group. Allergies to morphine and penicillin would not affect the use of NSAIDs. Tylenol is a nonnarcotic analgesic that does not cause the same bleeding tendencies as aspirin and is often used as a substitute for aspirin when aspirin is contraindicated.

9. 4. Danazol (Danocrine) is an ovulatory suppression drug used to create anovulation and amenorrhea in the treatment of premenstrual syndrome (PMS). It does not cause breast tenderness or hirsutism. Danazol is known to decrease libido rather than increase it.

10. 2. Danazol (Danocrine) is started during the menses to ensure that the client is not pregnant. The client could be pregnant 2 weeks after her menstrual period and 1 week prior to the start of the next menses. Thick mucus discharge could indicate that the client has ovulated and possibly conceived.

11. 1. 4. 5. Adverse reactions for Premarin include an increase in weight, leg pain, and breast tenderness. Bitter taste is an adverse reaction of an antifungal drug. Diarrhea is an adverse

reaction of an antibiotic. Heartburn is an adverse reaction of a nonsteroidal drug.

12. 2. Isoniazid (Nydrazid) is an antitubercular drug that decreases the effectiveness and blood levels of the antifungal drug miconazole nitrate (Monistat). Coumadin, probenecid (Benemid), and hydrochlorothiazide (Hydrodiuril) are not contraindicated when Monistat is prescribed.

13. 2. The effectiveness of antibiotic therapy in the treatment of recurrent gonorrhea is determined by vaginal cultures done weekly and is considered successful when two cultures are negative. Ciprofloxacin hydrochloride (Cipro) should be taken on an empty stomach, as food affects peak serum levels. Cipro is given as a single dose for the treatment of gonorrhea. When the clinical manifestations are obvious for a diagnosis of a specific infectious disease, the drug is started once the culture has been obtained but before the results are available.

14. 4. A major adverse reaction of most antibiotics, including tetracycline hydrochloride (Achromycin V), is photosensitivity; thus, clients should use sun protection and cover their bodies when going outdoors. Clients taking Achromycin V should use a nonhormonal type of contraceptive, as there is decreased effectiveness of hormonal contraceptives and a possibility of breakthrough bleeding. This drug should be taken around the clock to maintain blood levels. The first dose of any antibiotic can be started after the specimen for culture and sensitivity has been obtained but before the results are known.

15. 9 Use is limited to 9 months for treatment of endometriosis and may not be repeated.

16. 3. A black furry growth that appears on the tongue is an indication of the presence of a superinfection. Herpesvirus type 2 has lesions on the perineal area but gonorrhea does not. Clients with gonorrhea may have painful sexual intercourse and spotting between periods as part of the disease process.

17. 1. Erythromycin is an antibiotic used in the treatment of pelvic inflammatory disease. It should be taken with a full glass of water 1 hour before or 2 hours after a meal. It should not be taken with fruit juices. It is not necessary to take it with an antacid, and taking it 30 minutes prior to a meal would interfere with absorption. Erythromycin should be taken on an empty stomach; milk and meals would both interfere with absorption.

18. 3. Metronidazole (Flagyl) is an antifungal drug used to treat bacterial vaginosis. It may cause reddish-brown urine, which is of no clinical significance. Weight gain, a metallic taste, and diarrhea are adverse reactions that are not considered to be normal.

19. 2. A disulfiram-like reaction may occur when alcohol is ingested while one is taking metronidazole (Flagyl). Lithium, caffeine, and diazepam are not known to be contraindicated with Flagyl.

20. 2. Acyclovir (Zovirax) is supplied as an ointment, which is applied topically to the lesions of a client with herpesvirus type 2. A nonsterile glove or finger cot should be used in applying the ointment to prevent cross-contamination. Liquid soap should be used rather than bar soap, as the bar soap would become contaminated for use by others. Acyclovir is not supplied as a transdermal patch and the lesions should be left open to air.

21. 4. Acyclovir (Zovirax) is an antiviral used in the treatment of herpes. Clients receiving acyclovir (Zovirax) for herpesvirus type 2 need to be assessed frequently to detect changes in renal function, as the drug can be nephrotoxic. Serum creatinine is a good laboratory test to monitor renal function. Zovirax is not known to affect liver function, white cell count, or bleeding and clotting time.

22. 2. Acyclovir (Zovirax) should be taken as soon as the client notices the clinical manifestations are reappearing. Acyclovir is not recommended to be taken for longer than a 6-month period. Over-the-counter ointment and creams should not be used, as they may delay healing and spread infection. Acyclovir should not be taken before clinical manifestations appear, and it does not prevent reinfection.

23. 3. Danazol (Danocrine) is a synthetic androgen that is used to cause atrophy of the endometrium, resulting in amenorrhea. When the drug is stopped, the reactions are reversible and ovulation and menses will return in 2 to 3 months. These drugs do not cure endometriosis, but alleviate the clinical manifestations during drug therapy. A client taking this drug may still have some endometrial cells, which are stimulated by estrogen, so the dysmenorrhea may return. Danazol does not affect the regularity of menstrual periods.

24. 4. Clients taking oral contraceptives are at risk for developing thrombophlebitis as evidenced by calf pain with dorsiflexion of the foot. Spotting between periods, breast enlargement, and an increase in growth of body hair are adverse reactions that occur with the use of oral contraceptives.

25. 3. Clients taking progestin-only drugs for birth control are instructed to wait 3 months to get pregnant once the drug is stopped, to avoid the risk of birth defects to the fetus. Progestin-only drugs are taken daily throughout the month. A barrier method of contraception is needed only

for the first 3 weeks after starting the drug. Progestin-only contraceptives inhibit ovulation, but the menstrual cycle is not usually disrupted.

26. 4.   It is not appropriate for either a licensed practical nurse or a registered nurse to inform a client on the pros and cons of hormone replacement therapy. This is the responsibility of the physician. Giving a client information or instruction on how to take a drug is a nursing task reserved for the registered nurse. Instructing a client on the purpose of a drug is a responsibility of the physician that may be reinforced by the registered nurse. A licensed practical nurse may question a client taking a nonsteroidal anti-inflammatory drug about experiencing dark, tarry stools or coffee-ground emesis. The licensed practical nurse should in turn notify the registered nurse if they are present. The registered nurse in turn notifies the physician.

REFERENCES

Broyles, B., Reiss, B., & Evans, M. (2012). *Pharmacological aspects of nursing care* (8th ed.). Clifton Park, NY: Delmar Cengage Learning.

Daniels, R., & Nicoll, L. (2012). *Contemporary medical-surgical nursing.* Clifton Park, NY: Delmar Cengage Learning.

Spratto, G. R., & Woods, A. L. (2012). *PDR nurse's drug handbook 2012.* Clifton Park, NY: Delmar Cengage Learning.

CHAPTER 27

ANTINEOPLASTIC DRUGS

I. CHEMOTHERAPY
A. DESCRIPTION
1. SYSTEMIC ADMINISTRATION OF DRUGS TO KILL CANCER CELLS
2. TWO MAJOR CATEGORIES OF DRUGS
   a. Cell-cycle specific: cell must be in a certain phase of division; not effective during G_0 phase
   b. Cell-cycle nonspecific: effective in all phases of cell division
3. ACTION
   a. Affects metabolism and reproduction of normal cells as well as cancer cells
   b. Tumor cell growth and response to chemotherapy defined by the Gompertzian curve (see Figure 27-1)
   c. Tumor response to chemotherapy based on the client's:
      1) Health status
      2) Ability to tolerate the dose, regimen, adverse reactions
      3) Previous experience with chemotherapy (toxicities or tumor resistance may preclude using the same drug again)
      4) Tumor characteristics
         a) Greater effect with higher mitotic rate (more often in nonresting phases)
         b) Smaller tumors more affected
         c) Adequate blood supply to deliver chemotherapy (e.g., most chemotherapy does not cross the blood–brain barrier)
         d) Drug resistance
   d. Results of chemotherapy administration
      1) Complete remission: no evidence of cancer
      2) Partial remission: regression of at least 50% or greater
      3) Improvement: regression of 25–50%
      4) Nonresponsive: less than 25% regression
      5) Progression: tumor growth despite drug
4. ADMINISTRATION
   a. Primarily by IV or oral routes depending on accepted regimen
   b. Direct administration to the tumor site may also be used depending on tumor location
   c. Care must be given when administering certain chemotherapy agents IV because some (vesicants) may cause severe tissue damage if extravasation occurs; others (irritants) will also cause tissue inflammation.
   d. May be administered centrally (PICC line, central venous catheters, implanted ports) or through a peripheral IV line depending on the planned length of the regimen, drug, institutional guidelines, and status of client's veins
   e. Given for both solid and hematologic malignancies
   f. Various types often used in combination to:
      1) Decrease adverse reactions
      2) Decrease drug resistance
      3) Attain greatest tumor cell kill
   g. Combinations are administered on a regular schedule, multiple consecutive times over several months or years based on the type of cancer (i.e., regimen).
   h. The time between each administration is called a cycle.
   i. The cycle length is determined by the type of chemotherapy and cancer being treated.
   j. Cycle length must be long enough for recuperation of normal cells (including white blood cells [WBCs]) but not

Figure 27-1 Gompertzian curve

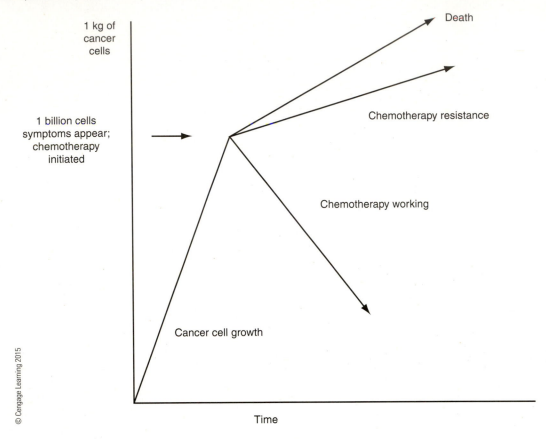

1 kg of
cancer
cells

1 billion cells
symptoms appear;
chemotherapy
initiated

Death

Chemotherapy resistance

Chemotherapy working

Cancer cell growth

© Cengage Learning 2015

Time

sufficiently long for cancer cells to
replenish.

B. ADVERSE REACTIONS
   1. CHEMOTHERAPY AGENTS PRODUCE
   ADVERSE REACTIONS RELATED TO
   THEIR EFFECTS ON NORMAL CELLS
   THAT DIVIDE MOST OFTEN, SUCH AS
   EPITHELIAL AND BONE MARROW
   CELLS, AS WELL AS THEIR TOXIC
   NATURE.
   2. ADVERSE REACTIONS ASSOCIATED
   WITH CHEMOTHERAPY (TO A MORE
   OR LESSER DEGREE DEPENDING ON
   THE AGENT) INCLUDE:
      a. Alopecia ranging from thinning hair to
      total loss of all body hair
      b. Nausea and vomiting
      c. Fatigue
      d. Neutropenia, anemia,
      thrombocytopenia
      e. Constipation, diarrhea
      f. Mucositis, stomatitis, alterations in
      taste
      g. Skin, eye, vaginal dryness, and nail
      changes
      h. Loss of fertility
      i. Alterations in body image, coping, fear
      of death

   3. POSSIBLE LONG-TERM ADVERSE
   REACTIONS
      a. Leukemias and other secondary
      malignancies
      b. Various organ toxicities
      c. Infertility
      d. Alterations in memory or learning ability
C. NURSING INTERVENTIONS (SEE
   CHAPTER 11, ONCOLOGY DISORDERS)
D. CELL-CYCLE-SPECIFIC CHEMOTHERAPY
   AGENTS (SEE TABLE 27-1)
   1. ANTIMETABOLITES
      a. Drugs (examples): capecitabine
      (Xeloda), clofarabine (Clolar),
      cytarabine (Cytosar-u), cytosine
      arabinoside (Cytosar-U), 5-fluorouracil
      (Adrucil), fludarabine (Fludara),
      gemcitabine (Gemzar), hydroxyurea
      (Hydrea), mercaptopurine (Purinethol),
      methotrexate, 6-thioguanine (6-TG)
      b. Action
         1) Work primarily during the S phase
         2) Interfere with DNA and
         RNA synthesis
   2. VINCA ALKALOIDS
      a. Drugs (examples): vinblastine (Velban),
      vincristine (Oncovin), vinorelbine
      (Navelbine)

Table 27-1 Selected Cell-Cycle-Specific Chemotherapy Agents

Class/Drug	Potential Indications	Routes	Vesicant/ Irritant	Specific Toxicities	Nursing Interventions
Antimetabolites					
• Methotrexate	Multiple cancers	IV, IM, IT, p.o.	No	Nephrotoxicity	Administer leucovorin as ordered to minimize toxicities; assess renal function.
• 5-fluorouracil (Adrucil)	Stomach, colon, breast, pancreas	IV, topical	No	Photosensitivity; diarrhea	Instruct the client to avoid sun exposure.
Vinca alkaloids					
• Vincristine (Oncovin)	Multiple cancers	IV	Vesicant	Neurotoxicity	Assess for numbness and constipation.
Taxanes					
• Paclitaxel (Taxol)	Breast, ovarian	IV over 3 hours	Vesicant	Hypersensitivity	Premedicate as ordered with antihistamine or corticosteroid.
Camptothecins					
• Topotecan (Hycamtin)	Ovarian	IV	No	Myelosuppression	Monitor complete blood count (CBC).
Epipodophyllotoxins					
• Etoposide (VePesid)	Testicular, small-cell lung	IV, p.o.	Irritant	Hypotension and bronchospasm	Administer over 30–60 minutes to minimize these effects.
Miscellaneous					
• Bleomycin (Blenoxane)	Squamous cell at various sites, Hodgkin's, testicular	IV, IM, subcut	Irritant	Pulmonary; hypersensitivity	Assess for cough, dyspnea, rales; administer test dose of the drug as ordered.

© Cengage Learning 2015

b. Action
  1) Work primarily during the M phase
  2) Prevent cell division by affecting microtubules
3. TAXANES
  a. Drugs (examples): paclitaxel (Taxol), docetaxel (Taxotere)
  b. Action
    1) Work during the M phase
    2) Strengthen microtubules, preventing pulling apart of replicated strands of DNA during mitosis
4. CAMPTOTHECINS
  a. Drugs (examples): topotecan (Hycamtin), irinotecan (Camptosar)
  b. Action
    1) Work in the S phase
    2) Inhibit topoisomerase I used in DNA synthesis and replication
5. OTHER MISCELLANEOUS DRUGS
  a. L-asparaginase (Elspar): causes cell death in G_1
  b. Prednisone: causes cell death in G_1
  c. Bleomycin (Blenoxane): causes cell death in G_2
  d. Etoposide (VePesid): interferes with synthesis of DNA in the S and G_2 phases

E. CELL-CYCLE-NONSPECIFIC CHEMOTHERAPY AGENTS (SEE TABLE 27-2)
  1. ALKYLATING AGENTS
    a. Drugs (examples): cyclophosphamide (Cytoxan), carboplatin (Paraplatin), cisplatin (Platinol), nitrogen mustard
    b. Action
      1) Create breaks and links in DNA chains, making replication at the time of synthesis impossible
  2. ANTITUMOR ANTIBIOTICS
    a. Drugs (examples): doxorubicin hydrochloride (Adriamycin), mitomycin C (Mutamycin), mitoxantrone (Novantrone)
    b. Action
      1) Variety of mechanisms to prevent DNA and RNA synthesis (breaks in chains, links, etc.) when time comes for the cell to enter the cycle
  3. NITROSUREAS
    a. Drug (example): carmustine (BiCNU)
    b. Action
      1) Similar to alkylating agents
      2) Able to cross the blood–brain barrier

Table 27-2 Selected Cell-Cycle-Nonspecific Chemotherapy Agents

Class/Drug	Potential Indications	Routes	Vesicant/ Irritant	Specific Toxicities	Nursing Interventions
Alkylating					
• Cisplatin (Platinol)	Testicular, ovarian, bladder	IV	Irritant/vesicant	Renal; ototoxicity	Vigorous IV hydration and diuretic as ordered; monitor blood urea nitrogen (BUN), creatinine; instruct the client to report tinnitus, refer for hearing test.
• Ifosfamide (Ifex)	Testicular	IV	Irritant	Hemorrhagic cystitis	IV or oral hydration with frequent voiding; assess and instruct the client to report frequency, hematuria; administer mesna or bladder irrigation as ordered.
• Cyclophosphamide (Cytoxan)	Breast, lymphoma, various others	IV, p.o.	No	Hemorrhagic cystitis	(See ifosfamide.)
Antitumor Antibiotics					
• Doxorubicin (Adriamycin)	Multiple cancers	IV	Vesicant	Cardiotoxicity	Monitor cumulative dose; assess Electrocardiogram (ECG) and for shortness of breath (SOB), hypertension, and edema.
• Mitoxantrone (Novantrone)	Leukemia, lymphoma	IV	Irritant/vesicant	Cardiotoxicity	(See doxorubicin.)

© Cengage Learning 2015

F. ADMINISTRATION OF CHEMOTHERAPY AGENTS

1. SAFE HANDLING

a. Preparation

1) By the pharmacist is ideal
2) Under vented, laminar-flow cabinet with the blower operated around the clock
3) Wash hands before and after preparation.
4) Do not eat, drink, or attend to personal hygiene in the area.
5) Wear disposable, protective gown and nonpowdered gloves (latex or equivalent).
6) Use a plastic-backed absorbent pad on the work area.
7) Use Luer-Lock attachments (instead of needles) as possible.
8) Open ampules away from self and with gauze around their necks.
9) Add diluents slowly and cautiously; aspirate air from the vial before adding the diluent and wait for pressure equalization before withdrawing the needle to avoid spray of contents.
10) Dispose of waste in approved containers.
11) Prime the tubing before adding chemotherapy to the IV bag.

b. Administration

1) Chemotherapy should only be administered by trained nurses.
2) Wash hands thoroughly before and after administration.
3) Prevent contact with chemotherapy agents (pregnant or lactating nurses should use particular caution).
4) Institute universal body fluid precautions (especially within 48 hours of administration).
5) Wear a disposable gown with cuffs, a mask, and nonpowdered gloves (latex or equivalent) for administration, and clean up any spills.
6) Do not prime the tubing with the chemotherapy agent under nonvented conditions.
7) Do not expel air from the syringe into the air under nonvented conditions (see the pharmacist and expel air into the gauze, disposing of it properly).
8) Dispose of waste in approved, appropriately marked containers.
9) Double-bag contaminated client gowns or linens; mark and send for appropriate washing.
10) Have an approved spill kit available in the area where chemotherapy is given.
11) Wash self or other contaminated objects several times with generous amounts of soap and water.
12) Seek medical attention if contamination occurs.

2. CLIENT SAFETY (PERIPHERAL IV)

a. Select a distal site on the extremity, utilizing the side of the body opposite that of prior surgery, radiation, or injury.
b. Examine the extremity for proximal venipuncture sites and move proximal to that site.
c. Choose sites between the antecubital space and wrist.

d. Check for blood return before starting infusion.

e. Secure the IV site with clear tape to promote visualization.

f. Begin infusion with fluids and antiemetics as ordered.

g. Instruct the client to inform the nurse of pain or burning sensation during chemotherapy infusion; stop infusion immediately if this occurs.

h. If more than one agent is to be given, infuse the vesicant first when venous flow is optimal.

i. Infuse agents via an infusion pump if ordered; vesicants should be monitored directly and not allowed to infuse unobserved by the nurse.

j. Flush the IV with up to 10 ml of normal saline on completion.

3. MANAGEMENT OF EXTRAVASATION

a. Pain is the primary symptom, although swelling, redness, and vesicles may appear without pain.

b. Treat as extravasation if it is suspected.

c. Follow institutional policy or procedures.

d. Stop infusion.

e. Inform the physician immediately.

f. Leave the needle or IV catheter in the client's arm.

g. Aspirate the remaining chemotherapy agent from the IV catheter.

h. Infuse the antidote (if one exists) into the catheter as ordered or according to standing order.

i. Antidote may also be injected into the skin around the IV site as ordered.

j. Apply topical corticosteroid cream to the site as ordered and cover.

k. Apply warmth or cold to the site based on the agent that infiltrated.

l. Elevate the arm.

m. Instruct the client to notify the nurse or physician of worsening changes.

n. Thoroughly document the date, time, site of infiltration, needle size, drug being administered, amount believed to be extravasated, appearance of site, nursing interventions used, and physician notification.

II. HORMONAL AGENTS

A. DESCRIPTION

1. KILL HORMONALLY SENSITIVE CANCER CELLS SUCH AS IN PROSTATE, BREAST, AND OVARIAN TUMORS

2. DRUG EXAMPLES: ADRENOCORTICOIDS, ANDROGENS, ESTROGENS, ANTIESTROGENS, PROGESTERONES, ANTITESTOSTERONES

3. ACTION

a. Kill lymphoid cells and promote cells entering the cell cycle, making them vulnerable to chemotherapy (e.g., prednisone)

b. Compete with the body's natural hormones for receptors such as an antiestrogen-like tamoxifen (Tamofen)

c. Act on the feedback mechanism within the pituitary to stop hormone production by the end organ such as an antitestosterone like leuprolide acetate (Lupron)

B. ADVERSE REACTIONS

1. ADVERSE REACTIONS VARY AND ARE ASSOCIATED WITH THE CHANGE IN THE HORMONAL ENVIRONMENT.

2. ADVERSE REACTIONS ASSOCIATED WITH ADRENOCORTICOIDS:

a. Increased appetite, weight gain

b. Gastric irritation, ulcer

c. Hyperglycemia

d. Fluid retention

e. Moon face

f. Immunosuppression

3. ADVERSE REACTIONS ASSOCIATED WITH SEX HORMONES:

a. Hot flashes

b. Loss of libido

c. Weight gain

d. Thrombolytic events

e. Nausea, vomiting

C. NURSING INTERVENTIONS

1. INSTRUCT THE CLIENT ABOUT POTENTIAL ADVERSE REACTIONS AND WHICH TO REPORT IMMEDIATELY.

2. REFER TO SEXUAL DYSFUNCTION COUNSELING AS NEEDED.

3. MONITOR GLUCOSE AND ELECTROLYTES WHEN ADMINISTERING ADRENOCORTICOSTEROIDS.

III. BIOLOGIC RESPONSE MODIFIERS

A. DESCRIPTION

1. LESS COMMONLY USED THAN CHEMOTHERAPY

2. MAY BE USED ALONE OR IN ADDITION TO CHEMOTHERAPY AND RADIATION

3. BASED ON ENHANCING IMMUNE SYSTEM TO RECOGNIZE AND DESTROY CANCER CELLS

4. MODIFIERS ARE CYTOKINES USUALLY RELEASED FROM CELLS OF THE IMMUNE SYSTEM SUCH AS LEUKOCYTES, LYMPHOCYTES, MACROPHAGES.

5. MANY ARE STILL IN CLINICAL TRIALS.

6. EXAMPLES: INTERFERONS, INTERLEUKINS, TUMOR NECROSIS FACTOR, AND COLONY-STIMULATING

FACTORS; FILGRASTIM (NEUPOGEN), EPOETIN ALPHA (EPOGEN), AND MONOCLONAL ANTIBODIES SUCH AS RITUXIMAB (RITUXAN), AND TRASTUZUMAB (HERCEPTIN)

7. ACTION
   a. Not all are thoroughly understood but they may:
      1) Change the client's immune response
      2) Kill tumor cells directly
      3) Affect the tumor cell's ability to grow or spread
8. MAY BE ADMINISTERED BY MULTIPLE ROUTES, INCLUDING CLIENT SELF-INJECTION AT HOME OVER SEVERAL DAYS OR WEEKS

B. ADVERSE REACTIONS
   1. FLULIKE CLINICAL MANIFESTATIONS
      a. Fever
      b. Chills
      c. Body aches
      d. Headache
      e. Malaise or fatigue
      f. Hypotension
      g. Tachycardia
      h. Capillary leak syndrome and pulmonary edema (high dose IL-2)
      i. Nausea, vomiting, diarrhea
      j. Rash, hives, pruritus

C. NURSING INTERVENTIONS
   1. NURSING INTERVENTIONS WILL VARY BASED ON THE AGENT USED.
   2. ADMINISTER ACETAMINOPHEN PRETREATMENT AND EVERY 4 HOURS AFTER, AS ORDERED, IF FLULIKE CLINICAL MANIFESTATIONS APPEAR.
   3. ADMINISTER PRESCRIBED MEPERIDINE (DEMEROL) IF RIGORS OCCUR DURING DRUG ADMINISTRATION.
   4. MONITOR VITAL SIGNS AND BLOOD COUNTS.
   5. INSTRUCT THE CLIENT TO REPORT CLINICAL MANIFESTATIONS OF SHORTNESS OF BREATH, PAIN, EDEMA.
   6. OBTAIN DAILY WEIGHTS IF THE CLIENT IS HOSPITALIZED AND RECEIVING A MODIFIER LIKELY TO CAUSE EDEMA.
   7. PACE THE CLIENT'S ACTIVITIES DUE TO WHAT MAY BE SEVERE FATIGUE.
   8. INFORM THE CLIENT ON SELF-INJECTION AS ORDERED.

PRACTICE QUESTIONS

1. A client asks the nurse if the chemotherapy will only affect the cancer cells in the body. Which of the following is the appropriate response by the nurse?
   1. "The chemotherapy affects only the cancer cells."
   2. "The chemotherapy affects both the normal as well as the cancer cells."
   3. "It depends on the type of chemotherapy."
   4. "The effect on cells is different in every client."

2. The nurse evaluates chemotherapy to be most effective in which of the following clients?
   1. A client who is well nourished
   2. A client who has had chemotherapy before
   3. A 40-year-old male with lung cancer
   4. A 30-year-old woman with breast cancer

3. The nurse is preparing a class on chemotherapy administration for a group of student nurses. Which of the following routes of administration should the nurse include in the class?
   Select all that apply:
   [ ] 1. Intramuscularly
   [ ] 2. Intravenous
   [ ] 3. Rectal
   [ ] 4. Intrathecal
   [ ] 5. Oral
   [ ] 6. Directly into the tumor

4. A client asks the nurse what was meant when the physician stated, "There has been a partial remission of the cancer." Which of the following is the appropriate response by the nurse?
   1. "The cancer has regressed 50% or more."
   2. "The cancer has progressed by 25%."
   3. "The cancer has spread to lymph nodes."
   4. "The cancer has disappeared."

5. The client asks, "Why do I need to receive all these chemotherapy medicines on the same day?" The nurse's response is based on the understanding that chemotherapy given in combination
   1. is the only way that it will be paid for by insurance.
   2. achieves the greatest tumor cell kill.
   3. shortens the length of administration.
   4. decreases the chance of allergic reaction.

6. A client asks, "Why will I lose my hair from chemotherapy?" The appropriate response by the nurse is based on which of the following?
   1. It is difficult to predict
   2. Chemotherapy affects normal cells that divide often

3. All chemotherapy causes total alopecia
4. Special shampoos can be used to prevent alopecia

7. The nurse is planning to care for the adverse reactions in a client receiving chemotherapy. Which adverse reaction should take priority in this plan of care?
   1. Depression
   2. Headache
   3. Fatigue
   4. Rash

8. A client's family asks the nurse, "Why can't the chemotherapy be given once instead of in multiple cycles?" The nurse's response is based on which of the following?
   1. Certain chemotherapy works best during certain phases of the cell cycle
   2. No one could tolerate the entire dose in one administration
   3. Chemotherapy is only covered by insurance if given in small doses
   4. Most clients prefer several doses over one dose

9. The nurse is teaching a class on the various types of chemotherapy agents. Which of the following examples of chemotherapy agents should the nurse include in the cell-cycle-specific group?
   1. Cyclophosphamide (Cytoxan)
   2. Methotrexate
   3. Doxorubicin (Doxil)
   4. Nitrogen mustard

10. The nurse should administer which of the following cell-cycle-nonspecific chemotherapy agents to a client?
    1. Paclitaxel (Taxol)
    2. 5-fluorouracil (Adrucil)
    3. Cisplatin (Platinol)
    4. Vincristine (Oncovin)

11. Which of the following should the nurse consider before preparing to administer chemotherapy to a client?
    1. Wear disposable gown, mask, and gloves
    2. Wait for the chemotherapy agent to be prepared by the physician
    3. Do not assign a nurse who is pregnant to this client
    4. Prime the IV tubing with the chemotherapy agent

12. The nurse should include which of the following when preparing to select the client's IV site for chemotherapy administration? Choose an IV site
    1. distal to other venipuncture sites on the extremity.
    2. on the same side as the cancer surgery.
    3. between the antecubital space and wrist.
    4. with a large-diameter vein.

13. Prior to initiating chemotherapy administration for a client, the nurse should consider which of the following principles?
    1. All chemotherapy drugs must be administered by an infusion pump
    2. Vesicant drugs should be infused before nonvesicant drugs
    3. The client's arm should be elevated throughout administration
    4. The IV line should be flushed with 20 ml of D_5W between drugs

14. Which of the following is the priority nursing action when a client states, "My IV site hurts!" during chemotherapy administration?
    1. Reposition the needle
    2. Notify the physician
    3. Stop the infusion
    4. Apply a cold pack to the IV site

15. The nurse suspects that the vesicant IV chemotherapy being administered to the client has extravasated. Based on this assessment, which of the following is the priority intervention?
    1. Continue administration until extravasation is confirmed by the physician
    2. Stop the infusion and notify the physician
    3. Remove the IV needle immediately and reinsert the needle in another area
    4. Slow down the infusion and continue to observe the area

16. Which of the following client assignments is an appropriate assignment for a licensed practical nurse?
    1. Administer methotrexate orally to a client with lung cancer
    2. Develop a plan of care for a client receiving bleomycin (Blenoxane)
    3. Administer cisplatin (Platinol) intravenously to a client with bladder cancer
    4. Assist a client receiving ifosfamide (Ifex) to mark a bland diet

17. The nurse should administer which of the following prescribed drugs to a client receiving chemotherapy who has developed neutropenia?
    1. Leuprolide acetate (Lupron)
    2. Tamoxifen (Tamofen)
    3. Filgrastim (Neupogen)
    4. Trastuzumab (Herceptin)

18. The nurse is caring for a 30-year-old female with ovarian cancer who is receiving cisplatin (Platinol). Which of the following is a priority to include in this client's plan of care?
    1. Monitor the BUN and creatinine
    2. Instruct the client to report tinnitus
    3. Maintain IV hydration
    4. Instruct the client to use a reliable method of birth control

19. Which of the following is a priority for the nurse to monitor for a client receiving ifosfamide (Ifex) for testicular cancer?
    1. Hemorrhagic cystitis
    2. Alopecia
    3. Phlebitis
    4. Liver dysfunction

20. Which of the following is a priority for the nurse to monitor in a client who is receiving mitoxantrone (Novantrone) for leukemia?
    1. Congestive heart failure
    2. Amenorrhea
    3. Mucositis
    4. Pneumonia

ANSWERS AND RATIONALES

1. 2. Chemotherapy is a systemic treatment that affects normal as well as cancer cells. Cells of any tissue that are actively dividing will be more susceptible to its effects. Although the adverse reactions experienced by any one client may vary somewhat, cancer cells and normal cells are still both affected by the treatment.

2. 1. Chemotherapy is equally effective in both men and women. The type of cancer a client has does not affect the potential of the chemotherapy. Chemotherapy may actually be somewhat less effective in those who have been exposed to chemotherapy previously, due to cancer cell resistance. Clients who are overall in better health will be able to tolerate the prescribed dose and regimen of chemotherapy better than those who are not, rendering it as effective as possible. Age does not directly affect the chemotherapy or type of cancer. Age directly relates to the client's overall condition of health.

3. 2. 4. 5. 6. The intravenous and oral routes are the most common routes for chemotherapy administration for the majority of cancers. The intrathecal route may be used to circumvent the blood–brain barrier when cancer involves the central nervous system. Administering chemotherapy directly into the tumor is rare, and primarily used in clinical trials. The rectal route is not used for chemotherapy administration.

4. 1. A partial remission of a client's cancer indicates that it is not spreading further to the lymph nodes or growing (progressing), but rather that it has regressed (decreased) 50% or more. A complete remission would be characterized as the cancer appearing to have disappeared.

5. 2. Chemotherapy drugs are frequently used in combination because this helps to decrease cellular resistance and increase tumor cell kill. Insurance typically covers FDA-approved chemotherapy drugs given alone or in various combinations. Giving more than one chemotherapeutic drug usually increases the amount of time clients spend receiving these drugs. Combination chemotherapy is not used to decrease the incidence of allergic reaction; test dosages and premedication are used for this purpose.

6. 2. Chemotherapy drugs affect all cells of the body that divide often, such as the hair follicle cells, thus causing hair loss. Many chemotherapy drugs cause total alopecia, but some do not. There is no known, accepted method of preventing chemotherapy-related alopecia.

7. 3. Fatigue is the most common adverse reaction to chemotherapy. Clients receiving chemotherapy may experience depression and headache, but these are very individual to the client. Rash is more associated with an allergic reaction, a skin reaction to immunosuppression, or to specific types of chemotherapy, but is not common overall.

8. 1. Chemotherapy is given in multiple cycles to allow for recuperation of normal cells between doses and to catch cancer cells in various phases of the cell cycle when the chemotherapy would have the most effect. It is true that giving too large a dose of chemotherapy could be lethal to a client, but this is not the primary reason that chemotherapy is administered in cycles. The number of cycles has been established through clinical trials and is not dependent on insurance payment.

9. 2. Methotrexate is an antimetabolite and a cell-cycle-specific drug. Cyclophosphamide (Cytoxan), doxorubicin (Doxil), and nitrogen mustard are cell-cycle-nonspecific drugs.

10. 3. Cisplatin (Platinol) is an alkylating agent and a cell-cycle-nonspecific chemotherapy drug. Paclitaxel (Taxol), 5-fluorouracil (Adrucil), and vincristine (Oncovin) are all cell-cycle-specific chemotherapy drugs.

11. 1. Nurses should always wear protective clothing such as a disposable gown, mask, and gloves when administering chemotherapy. Chemotherapy drugs are usually prepared by a pharmacist or the nurse under a vented, laminar-flow cabinet. Pregnant nurses may administer chemotherapy using the usual precautions. The IV tubing should not be primed with the chemotherapy agent.

12. 3. The appropriate site for chemotherapy administration is between the antecubital space and wrist, proximal to any recent venipuncture site. Chemotherapy should be administered to a site with excellent blood return to assure the vessel is competent to receive chemotherapy without leakage. Leakage of the chemotherapy agent through the vein can occur if it is administered distal to a recent venipuncture site. Chemotherapy is usually not administered on the arm associated with the cancer surgery, if applicable (e.g., given right mastectomy, chemotherapy will be administered to the left arm).

13. 2. Vesicant chemotherapy agents should be administered before nonvesicant drugs if two such drugs are ordered in combination. This is due to the fact that the best blood flow, condition of vein, and site are desired for administration of a potentially tissue-damaging drug (vesicant). Because these factors could deteriorate during drug administration, the nurse should start with the vesicant. Some chemotherapy agents should be administered with an infusion pump, but others should not. The client's arm should be in a natural, relaxed position during administration. The IV line should be flushed with approximately 10 ml of normal saline between administrations of chemotherapy drugs.

14. 3. The priority nursing action that should be taken by the nurse if the client complains of a painful IV site during chemotherapy administration is to stop the infusion. The nurse would then assess the situation to determine the cause of the pain. Caution should be used regarding repositioning of the needle so as not to damage the vein. If extravasation is suspected, the needle should be left in place, and the physician notified. Applying heat or cold to the IV site may be ordered, based on the chemotherapy being administered. All of these interventions are performed only after stopping the infusion.

15. 2. The first action taken when extravasation is suspected is to stop the infusion and notify the physician. The nurse should not wait to stop the IV until confirmation of extravasation by

the physician. The needle should not be removed, as it will be used to aspirate drug from the site to treat the extravasation. The drug should not be restarted until the extravasation has been properly treated according to the physician's orders.

16. 4. Only specially trained registered nurses may administer chemotherapy drugs, regardless of the route. Developing a plan of care is a job task reserved for the registered nurse. A licensed practical nurse may assist a client receiving chemotherapy to mark a bland diet after the initial instruction has taken place.

17. 3. Filgrastim (Neupogen) is a colony-stimulating factor used in the treatment of neutropenia for a client receiving chemotherapy. Leuprolide acetate (Lupron) is an antineoplastic hormone used in the treatment of prostate cancer. Tamoxifen (Tamofen) is an antiestrogen used in breast cancer. Trastuzumab (Herceptin) is an antineoplastic used in the treatment of breast cancer.

18. 4. It is a priority to instruct a client who is of childbearing age and receiving cisplatin (Platinol) to use a reliable method of birth control. Monitoring the BUN and creatinine, maintaining IV hydration, and instructing the client to report tinnitus are all appropriate interventions but not the priority intervention.

19. 1. Ifosfamide (Ifex) is an alkylating antineoplastic drug used in the treatment of testicular cancer, generally as a third-line therapy. It must always be administered with mesna (Mesnex), the antidote for ifosfamide toxicity. Ifex is metabolized to products that cause hemorrhagic cystitis. At least 2 liters of oral or IV fluids should be given with mesna (Mesnex) to prevent bladder toxicity. Other less serious adverse reactions include alopecia, phlebitis, and liver dysfunction.

20. 1. Mitoxantrone (Novantrone) is an antineoplastic used in the treatment of leukemia. It can cause a potentially fatal congestive heart failure. Other less serious adverse reactions include amenorrhea, mucositis, and pneumonia.

REFERENCES

American Cancer Society. (2011). *Cancer facts and figures.* Atlanta, GA: Author.

Broyles, B., Reiss, B., & Evans, M. (2012). *Pharmacological aspects of nursing care* (8th ed.). Clifton Park, NY: Delmar Cengage Learning.

Daniels, R., & Nicoll, L. (2012). *Contemporary medical-surgical nursing.* Clifton Park, NY: Delmar Cengage Learning.

Spratto, G. R., & Woods, A. L. (2012). *PDR nurse's drug handbook 2012.* Clifton Park, NY: Delmar Cengage Learning.

CHAPTER 28

PSYCHOTROPIC DRUGS

I. **ANTIPSYCHOTICS**
  A. DESCRIPTION
    1. MEDICATIONS USED TO TREAT PSYCHOTIC SYMPTOMS
    2. THIS GROUP INCLUDES TWO DISTINCT TYPES OF MEDICATIONS.
    3. THE EXACT MECHANISM OF ACTION IS UNKNOWN IN MANY OF THESE MEDICATIONS.
    4. IT IS POSTULATED THAT A DYSREGULATION OF NEUROTRANSMITTERS OCCURS IN SCHIZOPHRENIA AND RELATED DISORDERS.
    5. THE ANTIPSYCHOTIC MEDICATIONS HELP REGULATE THESE NEUROTRANSMITTER SYSTEMS.
    6. THE NEUROTRANSMITTERS MOST OFTEN THOUGHT TO BE INVOLVED IN PSYCHOTIC DISORDERS INCLUDE DOPAMINE, SEROTONIN, NOREPINEPHRINE, GAMMA AMINOBUTYRIC ACID (GABA), AND ACETYLCHOLINE.
  B. USES
    1. PSYCHOTIC MANIFESTATIONS SUCH AS SCHIZOAFFECTIVE DISORDER, BRIEF REACTIVE PSYCHOSIS, AND PARANOID DELUSIONAL DISORDER
      a. Positive manifestations
      b. Negative manifestations
    2. THE POSITIVE MANIFESTATIONS ARE THOUGHT OF AS AN EXCESS OR DISTORTION OF NORMAL FUNCTION, WHEREAS THE NEGATIVE MANIFESTATIONS CAN BE THOUGHT OF AS A LOSS OF NORMAL FUNCTION.
    3. THE POSITIVE MANIFESTATIONS INCLUDE HALLUCINATIONS, DELUSIONAL THINKING, BIZARRE BEHAVIOR, AGGRESSION, AND PARANOIA.
    4. THE NEGATIVE MANIFESTATIONS INCLUDE AMOTIVATION, ANHEDONIA, BLUNTED AFFECT, ASOCIAL BEHAVIOR, AND AVOLITION.
    5. THE GENERAL TERM *THOUGHT DISORDER* REFERS TO THE POSITIVE MANIFESTATIONS.
    6. PSYCHOSIS OCCURS IN A SPECTRUM OF ILLNESSES, INCLUDING SCHIZOPHRENIA, SCHIZOAFFECTIVE DISORDER, BRIEF REACTIVE PSYCHOSIS, PARANOID DELUSIONAL DISORDER, DRUG-INDUCED PSYCHOSIS, AND SCHIZOID PERSONALITY DISORDER.
    7. THE ANTIPSYCHOTIC DRUGS MAY ALSO BE USED TO TREAT CLIENTS WITH BIPOLAR DISORDER, MAJOR DEPRESSION WITH PSYCHOTIC FEATURES, AND BORDERLINE PERSONALITY DISORDER IN WHICH THERE ARE PSYCHOTIC CLINICAL MANIFESTATIONS.
  C. ADVERSE REACTIONS
    1. THE TYPICAL ANTIPSYCHOTIC MEDICATIONS MAY RESULT IN EXTRAPYRAMIDAL ADVERSE REACTIONS (EPS). EPS IS COMPRISED OF THREE CATEGORIES OF ADVERSE REACTIONS:
      a. Akathisia, which is characterized by motor restlessness, apprehension, and irritability
      b. Dystonia, an acute reaction requiring immediate medical attention
        1) Signs of dystonia consist of facial grimaces; exaggerated posturing of the head, neck, or jaw; and oculogyric crisis.
        2) Younger male clients are at particular risk for dystonic reactions.

c. Drug-induced parkinsonism, in which the client presents with a shuffling gait, excessive drooling, tremors, and muscle rigidity. Older females are at greater risk for developing this effect.

2. TARDIVE DYSKINESIA IS A LONG-TERM SIDE EFFECT.

   a. Results from the extended use of antipsychotic drugs, particularly the older or conventional antipsychotics

   b. Clinical manifestations include abnormal involuntary muscle movements around the mouth, lip smacking, tongue darting, constant chewing movements, and involuntary movements of the arms or legs.

   c. There is no proven treatment for tardive dyskinesia.

   d. Older female clients are at greater risk for developing this disorder.

   e. Many of the typical antipsychotic medications, in particular chlorpromazine (Thorazine), cause photosensitivity.

f. Anticholinergic adverse reactions are common.

   1) Dry mouth, urinary retention

   2) Blurred vision, constipation

   3) Confusion and decreased memory

g. Orthostatic hypotension is a common side effect (see Table 28-1).

h. Agranulocytosis is a rare, serious side effect that can occur with clozapine (Clozaril), require weekly or biweekly monitoring of white blood cell (WBC) counts (see Table 28-2).

D. CONTRAINDICATIONS AND PRECAUTIONS

   1. HYPERSENSITIVITY

   2. CENTRAL NERVOUS SYSTEM (CNS) DEPRESSION

   3. BONE MARROW DEPRESSION

   4. LACTATION

   5. HEPATIC OR RENAL DISEASE

   6. OLDER ADULT CLIENTS

E. DRUG INTERACTIONS

   1. ALCOHOL: INCREASES CNS DEPRESSION

   2. ANTACIDS: DECREASE EFFECTS

Table 28-1 Adverse Reactions of Typical Antipsychotics

	Sedation	Anticholinergic Effects	Orthostatic Hypotension	Extrapyramidal Symptoms
Chlorpromazine (Thorazine)	++++	++++	++++	++
Fluphenazine (Prolixin Deconote)	+	+	+	++++
Haloperidol (Haldol)	+	+	+	++++
Mesoridazine (Serentil)	++	++++	++	+
Perphenazine (Apo-Perphenazine)	++	++	+++++	
Thioridazine (Mellaril)	+++	+++	+++	+
Thiothixine (Navane)	+	+	+	++++

Key: ++++ = Most effect; + = Least effect

© Cengage Learning 2015

Table 28-2 Adverse Reactions of Atypical Antipsychotics

	Clozapine (Clozaril)	Olanzapine (Zyprexa)	Risperidone (Risperdal)	Quetiapine (Seroquel)	Ziprasidone (Geodon)
Sedation	+++	++	+	+++	+
Weight gain	+++	+++	+	+	0
Excessive salivation	++	+++	0	0	0
Extrapyramidal	0	0	*	0	0
Anticholinergic	+++	++	+	++	+

Key: +++ Most common; 0 = Not present

*Occurs with high doses

© Cengage Learning 2015

3. ANTICHOLINERGICS: INCREASE ANTICHOLINERGIC EFFECTS
4. ANTIDEPRESSANTS: ADDITIVE ANTICHOLINERGIC EFFECTS
5. LITHIUM CARBONATE: INCREASES EXTRAPYRAMIDAL EFFECTS
6. NARCOTICS: INCREASE CNS DEPRESSION

F. NURSING INTERVENTIONS
1. MONITOR THE CLIENT FOR EPS.
2. NOTIFY THE PHYSICIAN OF EPS MANIFESTATIONS.
3. INSTRUCT THE CLIENT WHO IS TAKING A TYPICAL ANTIPSYCHOTIC TO USE SUNBLOCK AND PROTECTIVE CLOTHING WHEN OUTSIDE IN THE SUN FOR PHOTOSENSITIVITY.
4. INSTRUCT A CLIENT WITH ORTHOSTATIC HYPOTENSION TO STAND UP SLOWLY FROM A SITTING OR RECLINING POSITION.
5. INSTRUCT A CLIENT WITH DRY MOUTH TO CHEW SUGAR-FREE GUM, SUCK ON SUGARLESS CANDY, OR TAKE ICE CHIPS AND COOL SUGAR-FREE DRINKS.
6. INSTRUCT THE CLIENT TO AVOID EXTREMES IN TEMPERATURES.
7. INSTRUCT THE CLIENT TO AVOID DRIVING A CAR OR OPERATING MACHINERY UNTIL THE EFFECTS OF THE DRUG ARE KNOWN.
8. ADMINISTER WITH FOOD OR MILK.
9. MONITOR THE CLIENT FOR MANIFESTATIONS OF BLOOD DYSCRASIAS.
10. INFORM THE CLIENT THAT THE URINE MAY TURN PINK OR REDDISH BROWN.
11. INSTRUCT THE CLIENT ON LONG-TERM THERAPY TO HAVE ROUTINE OPHTHALMIC EXAMS BECAUSE LONG-TERM THERAPY MAY AFFECT VISION.
12. MONITOR THE CLIENT FOR TARDIVE DYSKINESIA.

G. TYPES
1. TYPICAL ANTIPSYCHOTICS ARE ALSO KNOWN AS CONVENTIONAL, TRADITIONAL, OR OLD. THESE DRUGS TREAT THE POSITIVE MANIFESTATIONS BUT ARE NOT VERY EFFECTIVE WITH NEGATIVE MANIFESTATIONS. INCLUDED ARE THE FOLLOWING DRUGS:
   a. Phenothiazine derivates, which include chlorpromazine (Thorazine), mesoridazine (Serentil), thioridazine (Mellaril), and perphenazine (Trilafon)
   b. Thioxanthenes, which include thiothixene (Navane)
   c. Butyrophenone derivatives such as haloperidol (Haldol)
2. ATYPICAL ANTIPSYCHOTICS ARE ALSO REFERRED TO AS NEW OR NOVEL. THESE DRUGS EFFECTIVELY TREAT BOTH POSITIVE AND NEGATIVE MANIFESTATIONS. EXAMPLES INCLUDE THE FOLLOWING DRUGS:
   a. Clozapine (Clozaril)
   b. Risperidone (Risperdal): now used in the treatment of schizophrenia in adolescents ages 13 to 17 years and for management of manic or mixed episodes of bipolar disorders in adolescents ages 10 to 17. Previously, only lithium was FDA approved for use in adolescents.
   c. Olanzapine (Zyprexa)
   d. Quetiapine (Seroquel)
   e. Ziprasidone (Geodon)

II. **ANTIDEPRESSANTS**
A. DESCRIPTION
1. ANTIDEPRESSANT DRUGS ARE WIDELY USED TO TREAT A VARIETY OF MOOD DISORDERS.
2. ANTIDEPRESSANT MEDICATIONS TARGET SPECIFIC NEUROTRANSMITTERS IN THE BRAIN, SUCH AS SEROTONIN AND NOREPINEPHRINE.
3. DIFFERENT TYPES OF ANTIDEPRESSANT MEDICATIONS TARGET DIFFERENT NEUROTRANSMITTERS.

B. INDICATIONS
1. MAJOR DEPRESSIVE EPISODES
2. DYSTHYMIA
3. CLIENTS WITH BIPOLAR DISORDER WHO ARE IN A DEPRESSED STATE
4. ANXIETY DISORDERS AND ANXIETY THAT MAY BE ASSOCIATED WITH AN AGITATED DEPRESSION
5. POSTTRAUMATIC STRESS DISORDER
6. RESIDUAL ATTENTION-DEFICIT DISORDER: BUPROPION (WELLBUTRIN)

C. ADVERSE REACTIONS
1. THE NEWER ANTIDEPRESSANTS HAVE FEWER ADVERSE REACTIONS, WHICH INCREASES COMPLIANCE.
2. PRIMARY ADVERSE REACTIONS OF THE TRICYCLIC ANTIDEPRESSANTS ARE ANTICHOLINERGIC IN NATURE, INCLUDING DRY MOUTH, URINARY RETENTION, MEMORY LOSS, AND BLURRED VISION.

3. ADVERSE REACTIONS IN THE SELECTIVE SEROTONIN REUPTAKE INHIBITOR (SSRI) CLASS ARE RELATED TO SEROTONIN UPTAKE BLOCKADE AND THE SUBSEQUENT EFFECT ON THE GASTROINTESTINAL (GI) SYSTEM.
   a. Diarrhea and nausea due to serotonin uptake blockade
   b. Blockage of norepinephrine uptake may result in anxiety and sweating.
   c. Other adverse reactions include sexual dysfunction, insomnia, and headaches.
4. BUPROPION (WELLBUTRIN) LOWERS THE SEIZURE THRESHOLD; ADVERSE REACTIONS INCLUDE DECREASED APPETITE AND INSOMNIA.
5. MIRTAZAPINE (REMERON) CAUSES SOMNOLENCE AND INCREASED APPETITE.

D. CONTRAINDICATIONS AND PRECAUTIONS
   1. SEVERELY IMPAIRED LIVER FUNCTION
   2. ACUTE RECOVERY PHASE FROM MYOCARDIAL INFARCTION
   3. CONCOMITANT USE OF MONOAMINE OXIDASE (MAO) INHIBITORS
   4. LACTATION
   5. SEIZURES

E. DRUG INTERACTIONS
   1. ANTIDEPRESSANTS
      a. Alcohol: increases GI complications
      b. Anticholinergics: additive anticholinergic effects
      c. Diazepam: additive sedative effects
      d. MAO inhibitors: hyperpyretic crisis, delirium, tremors, tachycardia, tachypnea, mydriasis, convulsions, disseminated intravascular coagulation (DIC), and even death
      e. SSRIs: increase toxic effects of tricyclic antidepressants
      f. Vasodilators: additive hypotensive effect
   2. SELECTIVE SEROTONIN REUPTAKE INHIBITORS
      a. Aspirin: increases GI bleeding
      b. MAO inhibitors: hyperthermia, myoclonus, autonomic instability, mental status change, and even death
      c. Nonsteroidal anti-inflammatory drugs (NSAIDs): increase GI bleeding
      d. Tricyclic antidepressants: increase effects of tricyclic antidepressants

F. NURSING INTERVENTIONS
   1. MONITOR THE CLIENT TAKING TRICYCLIC ANTIDEPRESSANT (TCA) FOR AN OVERDOSE THAT CAN BE LIFE THREATENING, RESULTING IN HEART BLOCK, CARDIAC ARRHYTHMIAS, HYPOTENSION, SEIZURES, COMA, AND FATALITIES.
   2. MONITOR A SEVERELY DEPRESSED CLIENT FOR POSSIBLE "CHEEKING" OR HOARDING OF THE DRUG AS A POSSIBLE OVERDOSE SUICIDE ATTEMPT.
   3. INSTRUCT THE CLIENT REGARDING POTENTIAL ADVERSE REACTIONS.
   4. INSTRUCT THE CLIENT TO CHEW SUGARLESS GUM, SUCK ON HARD CANDY, OR TAKE ICE CHIPS OR SUGAR-FREE SODA FOR DRY MOUTH.
   5. MONITOR THE CLIENT FOR POTENTIAL WEIGHT GAIN DUE TO INCREASED APPETITE.
   6. INSTRUCT THE CLIENT ON A HIGH-FIBER DIET FOR CONSTIPATION.

G. TYPES
   1. TRICYCLIC ANTIDEPRESSANTS ARE AN OLDER CLASS OF DRUGS.
      a. They include amitriptyline (Elavil), clomipramine (Anafranil), desipramine (Norpramin), doxepin (Sinequan), imipramine (Tofranil), and nortriptyline (Pamelor).
      b. These drugs are used less with the advent of the newer antidepressants, which have a more tolerable adverse reaction profile.
   2. SSRIs ARE A POPULAR CLASS OF ANTIDEPRESSANT MEDICATIONS.
      a. Include duloxetine (Cymbalta), fluoxetine (Prozac), sertraline (Zoloft), paroxetine (Paxil), fluvoxamine (Luvox), and citalopram (Celexa)
      b. More tolerable adverse reaction profile
   3. SECOND-GENERATION ANTIDEPRESSANTS ALL WORK ON NEUROTRANSMITTER MECHANISMS THAT ARE DIFFERENT THAN THE SSRIS, TRICYCLICS, AND MAO INHIBITORS.
      a. Included in the group are venlafaxine (Effexor), bupropion (Wellbutrin), mirtazapine (Remeron), trazodone (Desyrel), and nefazodone (Serzone).
      b. They also have more tolerable adverse reaction profiles.

III. LITHIUM
   A. DESCRIPTION
      1. LITHIUM IS A SALT THAT IS EXCRETED BY THE KIDNEYS.
      2. IT IS NOT METABOLIZED IN THE LIVER.

3. THE EXACT MECHANISM OF ACTION IS UNKNOWN.
4. IT IS BELIEVED THAT LITHIUM WORKS VIA AN ANTIKINDLING EFFECT.
5. *KINDLING* IS A PROCESS IN WHICH REPEATED STIMULATION OF A NEURON RESULTS IN AN ACTION POTENTIAL WITHIN THAT NEURON.

B. USES
1. MOOD STABILIZER FOR CLIENTS WITH BIPOLAR DISORDERS
2. BOTH MANIA AND THE DEPRESSIVE EPISODES CHARACTERISTIC OF BIPOLAR DISORDERS
3. TREATMENT-RESISTANT DEPRESSIONS AS AN ADJUNCT MEDICATION

C. ADVERSE REACTIONS
1. NAUSEA
2. DIARRHEA
3. A FINE HAND TREMOR
4. WEIGHT GAIN
5. EDEMA
6. CONFUSION AND MEMORY IMPAIRMENT
7. LITHIUM TOXICITY MAY INCLUDE VOMITING, ABDOMINAL PAIN, PROFUSE DIARRHEA, SEVERE TREMOR, COMA, AND SEIZURES.

D. CONTRAINDICATIONS AND PRECAUTIONS
1. RENAL DISEASE
2. BRAIN DAMAGE
3. LACTATION
4. CHILDREN
5. OLDER ADULTS
6. DEHYDRATION

E. DRUG INTERACTIONS
1. FUROSEMIDE: INCREASES LITHIUM TOXICITY
2. TRICYCLIC ANTIDEPRESSANTS: INCREASE TRICYCLIC ANTIDEPRESSANTS
3. PHENOTHIAZINES: DECREASE PHENOTHIAZINES OR INCREASE LITHIUM
4. DIAZEPAM: INCREASES RISK OF HYPOTHERMIA

F. NURSING INTERVENTIONS
1. INFORM THE CLIENT OF THE IMPORTANCE OF MEASURING THE LEVEL OF LITHIUM IN THE BLOOD TO ENSURE THAT AN ADEQUATE AMOUNT OF THE DRUG IS IN THE BODY.
2. MONITOR LITHIUM BLOOD LEVELS ONE TO TWO TIMES A WEEK DURING INITIATION OF THERAPY AND MONTHLY BECAUSE IT CAN BE TOXIC AT HIGH LEVELS.
3. OBTAIN THE SERUM LITHIUM LEVEL 8–12 HOURS AFTER THE LATEST DOSE OF LITHIUM.
4. ENCOURAGE THE CLIENT TO DRINK 10–12 GLASSES OF WATER EACH DAY TO AVOID DEHYDRATION. (LITHIUM IS A SALT THAT IS EXCRETED BY THE KIDNEYS AND ALTERS THE LEVEL OF THE DRUG IN THE BODY BY THE INTAKE OF FLUID.)
5. INSTRUCT THE CLIENT TO AVOID EXCESSIVE SWEATING DUE TO EXERCISING ON A HOT DAY AND INCREASING CONCENTRATIONS OF LITHIUM IN THE URINE.
6. ADMINISTER LITHIUM TWO OR THREE TIMES A DAY.
7. AVOID ADMINISTERING LITHIUM TO A CLIENT WITH A HISTORY OF POOR COMPLIANCE.
8. INSTRUCT THE CLIENT TO AVOID BEVERAGES WITH CAFFEINE BECAUSE THEY MAY AGGRAVATE EPISODES OF MANIA.
9. INSTRUCT THE CLIENT TO AVOID ALL OVER-THE-COUNTER (OTC) DRUGS UNLESS PRESCRIBED.
10. MAINTAIN A CONSTANT LEVEL OF SALT INTAKE TO AVOID WEIGHT GAIN AND EDEMA, CAUSED BY SODIUM RETENTION.

G. TYPES
1. LITHIUM CARBONATE (ESKALITH) IS THE MOST COMMON FORM OF LITHIUM.
2. LITHIUM IS ALSO AVAILABLE IN A SLOW-RELEASE FORM.

IV. **ANTICONVULSANTS**
A. DESCRIPTION: THE ANTICONVULSANT DRUGS, WHICH ARE PRIMARILY USED TO TREAT EPILEPSY, HAVE ALSO BEEN FOUND TO BE EFFECTIVE IN TREATING MOOD DISORDERS. (SEE CHAPTER 22, DRUGS FOR THE NEUROLOGICAL SYSTEM.)

B. USES
1. BIPOLAR DISORDERS
2. PREVENT MOOD SWINGS SEEN IN BIPOLAR DISORDERS
3. PARTICULARLY USEFUL FOR MANIC EPISODES
4. AGGRESSION
5. ANXIETY DISORDERS: GABAPENTIN (NEURONTIN)

C. ADVERSE REACTIONS
1. GASTROINTESTINAL ADVERSE REACTIONS, INCLUDING NAUSEA, DIARRHEA, AND DYSPEPSIA

2. SEDATION
3. TREMORS: VALPROIC ACID (DEPAKOTE)
4. DIZZINESS, LIGHTHEADEDNESS, OR BLURRED VISION WITH CARBAMAZEPINE (TEGRETOL)
5. RASHES, WHICH MAY LEAD TO STEVENS-JOHNSON SYNDROME, A POTENTIALLY LIFE-THREATENING CONDITION WITH LAMOTRIGINE (LAMICTAL)

D. CONTRAINDICATIONS AND PRECAUTIONS
1. IMPAIRED LIVER FUNCTIONS: CARBAMAZEPINE (TEGRETOL) AND VALPROIC ACID (DEPAKOTE)
2. HYPERSENSITIVITY
3. PREGNANCY
4. UREA CYCLE DISORDERS
5. LACTATION

E. DRUG INTERACTIONS
1. ALCOHOL: INCREASES CNS DEPRESSION
2. CNS DEPRESSANTS: INCREASE CNS DEPRESSION
3. CIMETIDINE: INCREASES EFFECT

F. NURSING INTERVENTIONS
1. INSTRUCT THE CLIENT ABOUT THE POTENTIAL ADVERSE REACTIONS.
2. INSTRUCT THE CLIENT THAT A DECREASE IN MENTAL ALERTNESS MAY OCCUR WITH THE INITIATION OF THERAPY, WHICH MAY RESOLVE WITH CONTINUED THERAPY.
3. MONITOR CLIENTS TAKING LAMOTRIGINE (LAMICTAL) FOR RASHES BECAUSE THIS CAN LEAD TO STEVENS-JOHNSON SYNDROME.
4. INSTRUCT THE CLIENT TO AVOID TAKING AN ANTICONVULSANT DRUG ABRUPTLY BECAUSE SEIZURES MAY RESULT.
5. INSTRUCT THE CLIENT TO TAKE AS PRESCRIBED.

G. TYPES
1. CARBAMAZEPINE (TEGRETOL) ACTS THROUGH AN ANTIKINDLING PROCESS, IS METABOLIZED IN THE LIVER, AND HAS THE POTENTIAL FOR SEVERAL DRUG INTERACTIONS.
2. VALPROIC ACID (DEPAKOTE) ALSO ACTS THROUGH AN ANTIKINDLING EFFECT AND IS ALSO METABOLIZED IN THE LIVER.
3. LAMOTRIGINE (LAMICTAL) IS AN ANTIEPILEPTIC DRUG USED FREQUENTLY TO TREAT BIPOLAR DISORDERS. IT ACTS BY STABILIZING NEURONAL MEMBRANES.
4. GABAPENTIN (NEURONTIN) IS AN ANTIEPILEPTIC DRUG USED FOR BIPOLAR DISORDERS WITH AN UNKNOWN MECHANISM OF ACTION.
5. TOPIRAMATE (TOPAMAX) IS A NEWER ANTIEPILEPTIC DRUG USED IN BIPOLAR DISORDERS; THE EXACT MECHANISM OF ACTION IS UNKNOWN.

V. **MONOAMINE OXIDASE (MAO) INHIBITORS**
A. DESCRIPTION
1. THE MONOAMINE OXIDASE INHIBITORS (MAOIS) ARE USED PRIMARILY TO TREAT DEPRESSIVE DISORDERS.
2. USED LESS COMMONLY THAN OTHER ANTIDEPRESSANTS DUE TO THE DIET RESTRICTIONS INDICATED WITH THEIR USE
3. THE MAOIS ACT BY IRREVERSIBLY INHIBITING MONOAMINE OXIDASE.
4. THIS DRUG IS METABOLIZED IN THE LIVER.
5. THE MAOIS INHIBIT TWO DIFFERENT TYPES OF MAOS:
   a. The first type is MAO-A. It oxidizes norepinephrine and serotonin and is found primarily in the brain.
   b. The second type is MAO-B. It oxidizes tyramine, dopamine, and phenylethyamine and is found throughout the body.

B. USES
1. MAJOR DEPRESSION
2. ATYPICAL DEPRESSION
3. TREATMENT-RESISTANT DEPRESSION

C. ADVERSE REACTIONS
1. DIZZINESS
2. HEADACHE
3. INSOMNIA

D. CONTRAINDICATIONS AND PRECAUTIONS
1. HYPERSENSITIVITY
2. CONGESTIVE HEART FAILURE
3. CEREBROVASCULAR DISEASE
4. LIVER DISEASE

E. DRUG INTERACTIONS
1. TRICYCLIC ANTIDEPRESSANT MEDICATION OR A SEROTONIN REUPTAKE INHIBITOR: SERATONERGIC CRISIS, HYPERTHERMIC CRISIS, NORADRENERGIC CRISIS OR HYPERTENSIVE REACTION; MAY BE LIFE THREATENING
2. OTC DRUGS: INCREASE EFFECTS
3. ALCOHOL: CNS DEPRESSION

Table 28-3 Foods High in Tyramine

Aged cheese (English Stilton, blue cheese, Danish blue, mozzarella, Gruyère)
Microbrewery beers
Chianti wine
Fava green beans
Concentrated yeast extracts
Pickled herring in brine
Sauerkraut
Salami, mortadella, air-dried sausage, chicken liver
Oriental soup stocks (e.g., miso)

© Cengage Learning 2015

F. NURSING INTERVENTIONS
   1. INSTRUCT THE CLIENT TO AVOID DRIVING OR OPERATING EQUIPMENT REQUIRING ALERTNESS UNTIL THE EFFECTS OF THE DRUG ARE KNOWN.
   2. INSTRUCT THE CLIENT TO AVOID ALCOHOL.
   3. INSTRUCT THE CLIENT NOT TO DISCONTINUE THE DRUG ABRUPTLY AFTER LONG-TERM THERAPY.
   4. INSTRUCT THE CLIENT TO CHEW SUGAR-FREE GUM, SUCK ON HARD CANDY, OR TAKE ICE CHIPS OR DIET SODA TO REDUCE DRY MOUTH.
   5. INFORM THE CLIENT ABOUT INTERACTIONS WITH OTC MEDICATIONS, IN PARTICULAR DEXTROMETHORPHAN, EPHEDRINE, AND PSEUDOEPHEDRINE (ROBITUSSIN, SUDAFED).
   6. INSTRUCT THE CLIENT TO AVOID FOODS HIGH IN TYRAMINE SUCH AS AGED CHEESE, AGED WINE, AND BEER, WHICH CAN PRECIPITATE A HYPERTENSIVE CRISIS (SEE TABLE 28-3).
   7. MONITOR THE CLIENT TAKING AN MAOI FOR "HOARDING" OR "CHEEKING" THE MEDICATIONS TO PREVENT ANY SUICIDE ATTEMPT.
G. TYPES
   1. PHENELZINE (NARDIL)
   2. TRANYLCYPROMINE (PARNATE)
   3. SELGILINE (ELDEPRYL)

VI. ANTIANXIETY AGENTS
A. DESCRIPTION
   1. THE SEDATIVE-HYPNOTICS INCLUDE A VARIETY OF DRUGS.
   2. THESE CLASSES OF AGENTS TREAT ANXIETY AND DAYTIME TENSION.
   3. MANY OF THE DRUGS MEDIATE THE ACTIONS OF GABA, WHICH IS AN INHIBITORY NEUROTRANSMITTER.

   4. SOME OF THE ANTIANXIETY DRUGS MAY ACT THROUGH ANTICHOLINGERIC ACTIONS.
B. USES
   1. ANXIETY
   2. PANIC DISORDERS
   3. SOCIAL ANXIETY DISORDERS
   4. ANGER AND AGGRESSION
   5. POSTTRAUMATIC STRESS DISORDER
   6. ALCOHOL WITHDRAWAL: BENZODIAZAPINES
C. ADVERSE REACTIONS
   1. CNS EFFECTS SUCH AS SEDATION, CONFUSION, AND DISORIENTATION
   2. ORTHOSTATIC HYPOTENSION
   3. DRY MOUTH
   4. BLURRED VISION
D. CONTRAINDICATIONS AND PRECAUTIONS
   1. HISTORY OF SUBSTANCE ABUSE OR DEPENDENCE
   2. HYPERSENSITIVITY
   3. ACUTE NARROW-ANGLE GLAUCOMA
   4. LIVER DISEASE
   5. LACTATION
E. DRUG INTERACTIONS
   1. CNS DEPRESSANTS: INCREASE CNS DEPRESSANT EFFECT
   2. ALCOHOL: POTENTIATES EFFECTS
   3. DIGOXIN: INCREASES RISK OF DIGOXIN TOXICITY
F. NURSING INTERVENTIONS
   1. MONITOR THE CLIENT FOR TOLERANCE AND PHYSICAL DEPENDENCE.
   2. INSTRUCT THE CLIENT TO AVOID STOPPING THESE DRUGS ABRUPTLY AFTER LONG-TERM USE.
   3. INSTRUCT THE CLIENT TO AVOID ALCOHOL OR BARBITURATES, WHICH COULD BE FATAL DUE TO CNS DEPRESSION.
   4. INSTRUCT THE CLIENT TO AVOID DRIVING OR OPERATING HEAVY EQUIPMENT WHILE TAKING THESE DRUGS BECAUSE THEY CAUSE DROWSINESS.
G. TYPES
   1. *BENZODIAZEPINES* REFER TO A FAMILY OF MEDICATIONS, INCLUDING ALPRAZOLAM (XANAX), CHLORDIAZEPOXIDE (LIBRIUM), DIAZEPAM (VALIUM), LORAZEPAM (ATIVAN), CLONAZEPAM (KLONOPIN), AND OXAZEPAM (SERAX).
   2. BETA BLOCKERS, SUCH AS PROPRANOLOL (INDERAL), MAY BE USED TO TREAT CERTAIN FORMS OF ANXIETY.
   3. BUSPIRONE (BUSPAR) IS A NONBENZODIAZEPINE ANTIANXIETY DRUG.

VII. HYPNOTICS
- A. DESCRIPTION
  1. HYPNOTICS TREAT INSOMNIA.
  2. THEY MAY ALSO BE USED AT TIMES TO TREAT ANXIETY.
  3. BENZODIAZEPINE DRUGS AFFECT THE GABA SYSTEM.
  4. THE MECHANISM OF ACTION FOR THE BARBITURATES ALSO INVOLVES THE GABA SYSTEM.
  5. NONBENZODIAZEPINE HYPNOTICS ACT BY REDUCING ELECTRICAL ACTIVITY IN THE BRAIN.
  6. HYPNOTICS MAY BECOME HABIT FORMING.
  7. THEY ARE INTENDED FOR SHORT-TERM USE.
- B. USES
  1. INSOMNIA
  2. SLEEP MOVEMENT DISORDER
  3. RESTLESS LEG SYNDROME
- C. ADVERSE REACTIONS
  1. DRY MOUTH, CONSTIPATION, AND URINARY RETENTION: ANTIHISTAMINES
  2. CLUMSINESS, DIZZINESS, AND MORNING HANGOVER: BARBITURATES
  3. NAUSEA, VOMITING, HEADACHE, AND DIZZINESS: CHLORAL HYDRATE (NOCTEC)
  4. DROWSINESS, DIZZINESS, AND DIARRHEA: ZOLPIDEM (AMBIEN)
- D. CONTRAINDICATIONS AND PRECAUTIONS
  1. HISTORY OF SUBSTANCE ABUSE
  2. ALCOHOL
  3. HYPERSENSITIVITY
- E. DRUG INTERACTIONS
  1. CNS DEPRESSANTS: INCREASE CNS DEPRESSANT EFFECT
  2. ALCOHOL: INCREASES CNS DEPRESSANT EFFECT
  3. FLUOXETINE: INCREASES EFFECTS OF HYPNOTIC
- F. NURSING INTERVENTIONS
  1. INSTRUCT THE CLIENT ABOUT THE RISK FOR POTENTIAL FALLS AND FRACTURES RELATED TO ATAXIA AND CONFUSION.
  2. MONITOR THE CLIENT FOR A "HANGOVER."
  3. INSTRUCT THE CLIENT TO AVOID THE USE OF ALCOHOL.
  4. INSTRUCT THE CLIENT TO AVOID DRIVING OR OPERATING HEAVY EQUIPMENT.
  5. INSTRUCT THE CLIENT TO AVOID ABRUPTLY DISCONTINUING THE USE OF HYPNOTICS AFTER LONG-TERM USE.
  6. ADMINISTER ½–1 HOUR BEFORE BEDTIME.
- G. TYPES
  1. BARBITURATES ARE USED TO TREAT INSOMNIA.
  2. CHLORAL HYDRATE (NOCTEC) IS ONE TYPE OF BARBITURATE.
  3. ANTIHISTAMINES, WHICH ARE SEDATING, MAY BE USED TO TREAT INSOMNIA.
  4. ZOLPIDEN (AMBIEN) IS A NONBENZODIAZEPINE HYPNOTIC.
  5. RAMELTEN (ROZEREM) IS THE FIRST INSOMNIA DRUG THAT ACTS BY A MECHANISM OTHER THAN CENTRAL NERVOUS SYSTEM DEPRESSION. IT IS A MELATONIN RECEPTOR ANTAGONIST THAT HELPS TO MAINTAIN THE CIRCADIAN RHYTHM.
  6. BENZODIAZEPINES MAY ALSO BE CONSIDERED HYPNOTICS AND MAY BE USED TO TREAT INSOMNIA. (SEE PAGE 558 FOR TYPES OF ANTIANXIETY DRUGS.)

VIII. STIMULANTS
- A. DESCRIPTION
  1. DRUGS THAT RESULT IN INCREASED ALERTNESS AND A FEELING OF INCREASED ENERGY
  2. USED FOR A NUMBER OF DISORDERS IN MENTAL HEALTH
  3. THERE IS A HIGH POTENTIAL FOR ABUSE.
  4. ACT ON THE CATECHOLAMINES AT POSTSYNAPTIC RECEPTOR SITES IN THE BRAIN
  5. BLOCK THE REUPTAKE OF CATECHOLAMINES, WHICH PROLONGS THEIR ACTION
  6. INCREASE ATTENTION AND CONCENTRATION IN ANYONE WHO TAKES THEM, INCREASING THE POTENTIAL FOR ABUSE
  7. MAY BE USED WITHOUT A PRESCRIPTION OR ILLEGALLY FOR WEIGHT LOSS
- B. USES
  1. ATTENTION-DEFICIT HYPERACTIVITY DISORDER IN CHILDREN
  2. ADULTS WHO HAVE RESIDUAL ATTENTION-DEFICIT DISORDER
  3. NARCOLEPSY AND DAYTIME SLEEPINESS
  4. TREATMENT-RESISTANT DEPRESSION
  5. CHRONIC MEDICAL CONDITIONS THAT ARE DEBILITATING, SUCH AS CANCER AND CHRONIC FATIGUE SYNDROME

C. ADVERSE REACTIONS
1. ANOREXIA OR APPETITE SUPPRESSION
2. WEIGHT LOSS
3. IRRITABILITY
4. ABDOMINAL PAIN
5. HEADACHES
6. INSOMNIA
7. PALPITATIONS AND TACHYCARDIA

D. CONTRAINDICATIONS AND PRECAUTIONS
1. TOURETTE'S SYNDROME
2. HISTORY OF DRUG ABUSE
3. ANXIETY AND AGITATION
4. HISTORY OF CARDIAC DISEASE
5. HYPERTENSION

E. DRUG INTERACTIONS
1. ANTICONVULSANTS: INCREASE EFFECTS
2. ANTIDEPRESSANTS: INCREASE EFFECTS
3. MAOIS: HYPERTENSIVE CRISIS
4. ORAL ANTICOAGULANTS: DECREASE EFFECTS

F. NURSING INTERVENTIONS
1. INSTRUCT THE CLIENT ABOUT THE POTENTIAL OF ABUSE.
2. MONITOR THE BLOOD PRESSURE.
3. MONITOR THE HEIGHT AND WEIGHT OF A CHILD BECAUSE THE GROWTH RATE MAY BE DECREASED AND APPETITE DEPRESSED.
4. INSTRUCT THE CLIENT THAT DRUG TOLERANCE DEVELOPS AFTER LONG-TERM USE.
5. INSTRUCT THE CLIENT TO AVOID CAFFEINE, WHICH INCREASES THE STIMULANT EFFECT.

G. TYPES
1. DEXTROAMPHETAMINE (DEXEDRINE)
2. METHYLPHENIDATE (RITALIN): COMMONLY USED WITH CHILDREN
3. PEMOLINE (CYLERT): COMMONLY USED WITH CHILDREN
4. MODAFINIL (PROVIGIL): USED PARTICULARLY IN TREATING NARCOLEPSY

PRACTICE QUESTIONS

1. The nurse reviews which of the following contraindications and precautions before administering a stimulant to an adult client with attention-deficit disorder?
Select all that apply:
[ ] 1. Anxiety
[ ] 2. Liver disease
[ ] 3. Urea cycle disorders
[ ] 4. Seizures
[ ] 5. History of cardiac disease
[ ] 6. Hypertension

2. The nurse should instruct a client to drink how many glasses of water a day when taking lithium? _____

3. The nurse is admitting a client with a diagnosis of suspected schizophrenia. Which of the following clinical manifestations should the nurse assess as a positive clinical manifestation of schizophrenia?
1. Anhedonia and blunted affect
2. Hallucinations and delusional thinking
3. Lack of motivation
4. Abnormal movements of the mouth

4. The nurse is caring for a client with Alzheimer's disease who is taking quetiapine (Seroquel) for paranoid ideations. Which of the following adverse reactions should the nurse assess this client for?
Select all that apply:
[ ] 1. Hypertension
[ ] 2. Headache
[ ] 3. Bradycardia
[ ] 4. Diarrhea
[ ] 5. Dry mouth
[ ] 6. Tardive dyskinesia

5. Which of the following should the nurse include in the plan of care for a client taking an antidepressant drug?
1. Encourage the client to drink low-calorie beverages
2. Instruct the client to take the drug on an empty stomach
3. Inform the client that urinary frequency is an adverse reaction
4. Monitor the client for bradycardia prior to administration

6. The nurse should include which of the following adverse reactions to Olanzapine (Zyprexa) in the drug instructions given to a client?
Select all that apply:
[ ] 1. Constipation
[ ] 2. Weight loss

[   ] 3. Loss of taste
[   ] 4. Hypotonia
[   ] 5. Insomnia
[   ] 6. Urinary retention

7. The nurse caring for a client administers sertraline (Zoloft) for which of the following disorders?
    1. Abnormal movement disorder
    2. Brief reactive psychosis
    3. Major depressive disorder
    4. Schizophrenia

8. The client is instructed to take mirtazapine (Remeron) for depression. Which of the following would best indicate that the client is complying with the prescribed regimen? The client
    1. places the tablet on the tongue and waits 30 seconds for it to dissolve.
    2. waits 2 hours after administration before driving or operating dangerous equipment.
    3. avoids caffeine and irritating foods in the diet.
    4. reports adverse reactions of bloody diarrhea.

9. Which of the following is a priority to include in the plan of care for a client taking fluoxetine (Prozac)?
    1. Monitor the client for orthostatic hypotension
    2. Avoid giving on an empty stomach
    3. Wait 14 days after taking a monoamine oxidase inhibitor before starting Prozac
    4. Administer simultaneously with thioridazine (Mellaril)

10. A client complains of having a dry mouth. Which of the following instructions should the nurse give to the client?
    1. "Try chewing sugar-free gum and drinking cool, sugar-free sodas."
    2. "You need to drink more milk products, especially with your drugs."
    3. "Avoid drinking fluids in the evenings."
    4. "Drink more fluids early in the day."

11. The nurse should question an order for bupropion (Wellbutrin) for which of the following clients?
    1. A client with a closed head injury
    2. A client with liver failure
    3. A client with kidney failure
    4. A client with chronic gastrointestinal upset

12. The priority nursing action for the nurse administering an antidepressant drug to a client is which of the following?
    1. Check the client's mouth for possible hoarding of the drug

2. Instruct the client that the therapeutic effects of the drug may take 2 weeks
3. Administer the drug with food
4. Monitor the blood pressure

13. A nurse is instructing a client about getting blood drawn the following day for a lithium carbonate (Eskalith) level. Which of the following instructions is important?
    1. "Do not take your morning dose of lithium until your blood has been drawn."
    2. "Do not eat anything in the morning before having your blood drawn."
    3. "Do not take your evening dose of lithium tonight."
    4. "Take your morning dose of lithium carbonate with a sip of water."

14. The nurse evaluates which of the following lab results as within the normal range for a client who is receiving lithium carbonate (Eskalith)?
    1. 1.5 to 2.0 mEq/L
    2. 0.1 to 0.5 mEq/L
    3. 1.8 to 2.5 mEq/L
    4. 0.6 to 1.2 mEq/L

15. A nurse educating a client about possible signs of lithium carbonate (Eskalith) toxicity should instruct the client to report which of the following adverse reactions?
    Select all that apply:
    [   ] 1. Weight gain
    [   ] 2. Vomiting
    [   ] 3. Diarrhea
    [   ] 4. Tremor
    [   ] 5. Salty taste
    [   ] 6. Abdominal pain

16. The nurse is caring for a client with a psychotic disorder who is receiving thioridazine (Mellaril). The nurse should monitor this client for which of the following abnormal laboratory results?
    1. Hyperkalemia
    2. Decreased alkaline phosphatase
    3. Agranulocytosis
    4. Hypocalcemia

17. The nurse is conducting a class on the adverse reactions to a variety of drugs such as lithium carbonate (Eskalith), carbamazepine (Tegretol), gabapentin (Neurontin), and valproic acid (Depakene). Which of the following common adverse reactions should the nurse include in the class?
    Select all that apply:
    [   ] 1. Nausea
    [   ] 2. Restlessness
    [   ] 3. Diarrhea

[ ] 4. Insomnia
[ ] 5. Dyspepsia
[ ] 6. Irritability

18. The nurse reads on the initial history and physical that anticonvulsant drugs are prescribed, but there is no diagnosis of a seizure disorder, and no report of treatment in a mental health clinic. The nurse concludes that the client is taking the anticonvulsant drugs to treat which of the following?
Select all that apply:
[ ] 1. Major depression
[ ] 2. Bipolar disorders
[ ] 3. Anxiety disorders
[ ] 4. Aggression
[ ] 5. Cognitive disorders
[ ] 6. Brief reactive psychosis

19. A client has been treated for depression with phenelzine (Nardil). The nurse recognizes that the drug was difficult to take for which of the following reasons?
   1. It requires dosing several times a day, thus decreasing compliance
   2. It has the potential for serious interactions with other medications
   3. It requires adherence to a strict diet
   4. It has been found to be ineffective in treating psychiatric disorders

20. The nurse is caring for a client who is taking phenelzine (Nardil). Which of the following should the nurse include in the medication instructions?
   1. "Common adverse reactions include sleepiness and agitation."
   2. "You may experience a decrease in appetite."
   3. "Tell your physician all of the other drugs you are taking."
   4. "If you have a history of low blood sugar, you should not take this drug."

21. The nurse is discharging a client taking flurazepam (Dalmane). Which of the following instructions should be given?
   1. Drink a small glass of wine at bedtime to enhance sleep
   2. Drive cautiously after taking the drug
   3. Drink low-calorie fluids for a dry mouth
   4. A "hangover effect" may be experienced in the morning

22. The nurse is instructing an older adult client who has been prescribed a hypnotic for insomnia. Which of the following instructions should be given?
   1. "Ask for help getting out of bed."
   2. "You may feel more hungry when you are taking this drug."
   3. "You may notice that you're feeling more irritable and moody when you take this drug."
   4. "This drug may cause movements of your mouth that you can't control."

23. The nurse should administer which of the following drugs to a client who is severely ill with schizophrenia, does not respond to conventional antipsychotic drugs, and has suicidal ideations?
   1. Haloperidol (Haldol)
   2. Chlorpromazine (Thorazine)
   3. Risperidone (Risperdal)
   4. Clozapine (Clozaril)

24. Which of the following interventions is a priority and will help the older adult client comply with the drug regimen?
   1. Educate the family members about drug administration
   2. Contact the client frequently as a reminder to take drugs
   3. Educate the client on ways to manage adverse reactions
   4. Count the number of pills left in the bottle at each visit

25. The nurse reads in the record that the client is receiving a stimulant drug. The nurse reviews the medical record and administers which of the following drugs?
   1. Buspirone (BuSpar)
   2. Alprazolam (Xanax)
   3. Modafinil (Provigil)
   4. Amitriptyline (Elavil)

26. The nurse is preparing to delegate nursing tasks to a licensed practical nurse. Which of the following may be delegated to a licensed practical nurse?
   1. Assist a client taking a monoamine oxidase inhibitor to select a menu with foods low in tyramine
   2. Inform a client taking a hypnotic about the risk of falls and fractures
   3. Assess for abuse the parents of a child taking a stimulant
   4. Instruct the client and the family on the adverse reactions to an antipsychotic drug

ANSWERS AND RATIONALES

1. 1. 5. 6. Contraindications to stimulants include anxiety, history of cardiac disease, and hypertension. Liver disease is a contraindication for monoamine oxidase inhibitors. Urea cycle disorders are a contraindication for an anticonvulsant. A contraindication for antidepressants is seizures.

2. 10–12. Drinking 10–12 glasses of water a day will prevent dehydration. Lithium is a salt that is excreted by the kidneys and alters the level of the drug in the body by the intake of fluid.

3. 2. Positive clinical manifestations of schizophrenia include hallucinations and delusional thinking. Anhedonia, blunted affect, and lack of motivation are negative clinical manifestations of schizophrenia. Abnormal movements of the mouth indicate tardive dyskinesia.

4. 2. 5. 6. Quetiapine (Seroquel) is an antipsychotic drug that is used for psychotic disorders. Adverse reactions include orthostatic hypotension, headache, tachycardia, constipation, dry mouth, and tardive dyskinesia.

5. 1. Antidepressants are used to treat depression. Adverse reactions include weight gain, gastrointestinal upset, urinary retention, and tachycardia. Clients must be cautioned to avoid high-caloric drinks to avoid weight gain.

6. 1. 5. 6. Olanzapine (Zyprexa) is an antipsychotic drug used to treat schizophrenia and the acute mania associated with bipolar disorders. Adverse reactions include weight gain, constipation, hypertonia, insomnia, and urinary retention.

7. 3. Sertraline (Zoloft) is a selective serotonin reuptake inhibitor (SSRI) antidepressant used in the treatment of major depression, obsessive-compulsive disorder, posttraumatic stress disorder, and panic disorders.

8. 1. Mirtazapine (Remeron) is a tetracyclic antidepressant used in the treatment of depression. The tablets come as oral disintegrating tablets and should be administered initially in the evening, before sleep, until the drug effects are known. The tablet should be placed on the tongue for 30 seconds until dissolved. The client should not engage in activities that require mental alertness until the drug effects are known. Although nausea and vomiting may occur, there are no food restrictions. Fluids may be encouraged for the adverse reaction to constipation.

9. 3. Fluoxetine (Prozac) is a selective serotonin reuptake inhibitor (SSRI) antidepressant. The client should be monitored for orthostatic hypotension and instructed to change positions with caution. Prozac may be administered with food to decrease gastrointestinal upset. It is a priority to wait 14 days after discontinuing a monoamine oxidase inhibitor (MAOI) and administering Prozac. Five weeks should pass between stopping Prozac and starting a MAOI. Prozac should not be administered with Mellaril.

10. 1. Clients who take antidepressants and antipsychotic drugs may experience dry mouth as an adverse reaction. The client should avoid high-calorie fluids, which may promote weight gain. Drinking low-calorie fluids and chewing sugarless gum are encouraged to avoid gaining weight.

11. 1. Bupropion (Wellbutrin) is an antidepressant that is known to lower the seizure threshold and is contraindicated for clients with known seizure disorders or closed head injuries.

12. 1. Clients who are suicidal may attempt to hoard their drugs by "cheeking" them to be used later for a suicide attempt. Extreme caution should be used with suicidal clients.

13. 2. Lithium carbonate (Eskalith) is an antimanic drug used in the treatment of bipolar disorders (manic phase) and in the prevention of bipolar manic-depressive psychosis. The lithium blood level is most accurate if the blood is drawn 12 hours after the last dose of drug. The client should avoid eating prior to having a lithium level drawn to avoid a food–lithium interaction and an inaccurate result.

14. 4. Lithium carbonate (Eskalith) is an antimanic drug. The client's lithium carbonate level should be monitored. The normal range is 0.6 to 1.2 mEq/L.

15. 2. 3. 4. 6. Lithium carbonate (Eskalith) is an antimanic drug. Usual adverse reactions include headache, drowsiness, dizziness, hypotension, dry mouth, salty taste, and fatigue. Toxic adverse reactions include vomiting, diarrhea, tremors, abdominal pain, muscle weakness, lassitude, severe thirst, tinnitus, and dilute urine.

16. 3. Thioridazine (Mellaril) is an antipsychotic and atypical neuroleptic used in the treatment of psychotic disorders, schizophrenia, major depressive disorders, and organic brain syndrome. Mellaril may cause agranulocytosis (reduction in the number of white blood cells).

17. 1. 3. 5. Lithium carbonate (Eskalith) is an antimanic and antipsychotic drug used in the treatment of bipolar disorders. Carbamazepine (Tegretol) is an anticonvulsant used to treat absence seizures. It is also used investigationally in the treatment of bipolar

disorders, schizophrenia, and psychotic behavior with dementia. Gabapentin (Neurontin) is an anticonvulsant used in the adjunct treatment of partial seizures. It also is used investigationally for bipolar disorders. Valproic acid (Depakene) is an anticonvulsant used in the treatment of seizures. Common adverse reactions for all of these drugs include nausea, diarrhea, and dyspepsia.

18. 2. 3. 4. Anticonvulsant drugs are being used investigationally in the treatment of bipolar disorders, anxiety disorders, and aggression.

19. 3. Monoamine oxidase inhibitors (MAOIs), such as phenelzine (Nardil), interact with the tyramine found in many foods, thus requiring the individuals using these drugs to follow a strict diet. Compliance becomes an issue. Foods high in tyramine include aged cheese, salami, sauerkraut, avocados, chocolate, coffee, fava beans, and beer and wine containing yeast.

20. 3. Monoamine oxidase inhibitors (MAOIs), such as phenelzine (Nardil), have interactions with many different drugs, including over-the-counter drugs.

21. 4. Flurazepam (Dalmane) is a sedative and hypnotic that is used for insomnia. Clients are advised to avoid alcohol because alcohol taken in combination with hypnotics can have a lethal effect. Clients should not drive after taking hypnotics for safety reasons. Their reflexes would be dulled. Low-calorie fluids are not necessary because dry mouth is not an adverse reaction and Dalmane has no effect on appetite.

22. 1. Hypnotics may cause ataxia and confusion, increasing the risk of falls and fractures. Hypnotics will not increase the appetite, result in irritability, or cause extrapyramidal adverse reactions.

23. 4. Haloperidol (Haldol) is an antipsychotic used to treat manic states, drug-induced psychoses, and schizophrenia. Chlorpromazine (Thorazine) is an antipsychotic used to treat

acute and chronic psychoses, schizophrenia, and the manic phase of manic-depression. Risperidone (Risperdal) is an antipsychotic used in the treatment of schizophrenia. Clozapine (Clozaril) is an antipsychotic used to treat severely ill schizophrenic clients who do not respond to conventional antipsychotic therapy and have suicidal ideations. It carries a risk of life-threatening agranulocytosis.

24. 3. The priority intervention is to educate the client on how to manage the adverse reactions of the drugs. Unpleasant adverse reactions are often the reason for noncompliance with drugs. Educating the family members reinforces the education given the client. It should not be the priority intervention because it takes away the control from the client. Counting the number of pills left in the bottle at each appointment with the physician and calling the client as a reminder to take the pills as prescribed also take away the control from the client and display a sense of distrust.

25. 3. Modafinil (Provigil) is an analeptic drug administered to improve wakefulness in clients with excessive daytime sleepiness associated with narcolepsy. Buspirone (BuSpar) and alprazolam (Xanax) are antianxiety drugs. Amitriptyline (Elavil) is an antidepressant drug.

26. 1. A licensed practical nurse may assist a client taking a monoamine oxidase inhibitor to select a low-tyramine diet. The instructional teaching that must be performed by a registered nurse has already taken place and now the focus changes to assisting a client to select appropriate foods. It would not be appropriate to assess the parents of a child taking a stimulant for abuse unless there is an indication of potential abuse. Providing the family and client information on the adverse reactions to a drug and informing the client of potential complications should be performed by a registered nurse.

REFERENCES

Antai-Otong, D. (2008). *Psychiatric nursing, biological and behavioral concepts.* Clifton Park, NY: Delmar Cengage Learning.

Broyles, B., Reiss, B., & Evans, M. (2012). *Pharmacological aspects of nursing care* (8th ed.). Clifton Park, NY: Delmar Cengage Learning.

Frisch, N. C., & Frisch, L. E. (2006). *Psychiatric mental health nursing* (3rd ed.). Clifton Park, NY: Thomson Delmar Learning.

Spratto, G. R., & Woods, A. L. (2012). *PDR nurse's drug handbook 2012.* Clifton Park, NY: Delmar Cengage Learning.

PEDIATRIC NURSING

CHAPTER 29

GROWTH AND DEVELOPMENT

I. **DEFINITIONS**
   A. GROWTH: PHYSIOLOGIC INCREASE IN SIZE THROUGH CELL MULTIPLICATION AND DIFFERENTIATION
   B. MATURATION: PHYSIOLOGICAL CHANGES DUE TO GENETIC INHERITANCE
   C. DEVELOPMENT: PHYSIOLOGICAL, PSYCHOSOCIAL, AND COGNITIVE CHANGES OCCURRING OVER ONE'S LIFE SPAN DUE TO GROWTH, MATURATION, AND LEARNING

II. **PRINCIPLES OF GROWTH AND DEVELOPMENT**
   A. DEVELOPMENT IS ORDERLY AND SEQUENTIAL
      1. MATURATION FOLLOWS A PREDICTABLE, UNIVERSAL TIMETABLE.
      2. DEVELOPMENTAL CHANGES OCCUR RAPIDLY DURING THE FIRST YEAR OF LIFE AND SLOW DURING MIDDLE AND LATE CHILDHOOD.
   B. DEVELOPMENT IS DIRECTIONAL
      1. CEPHALOCAUDAL: FROM HEAD DOWNWARD (AREAS CLOSEST TO THE BRAIN/HEAD DEVELOP FIRST, FOLLOWED BY THE TRUNK THEN THE LEGS AND FEET).
      2. PROXIMODISTAL: FROM THE INSIDE OUT (CONTROLLED MOVEMENTS CLOSEST TO THE BODY'S CENTER [TRUNK, ARMS] DEVELOP BEFORE CONTROLLED MOVEMENTS DISTANT TO THE BODY [FINGERS]).
   C. DEVELOPMENT IS UNIQUE
      1. EVERY CHILD HAS A UNIQUE TIMETABLE FOR PHYSIOLOGICAL, PSYCHOSOCIAL, COGNITIVE, AND MORAL DEVELOPMENT.
   D. DEVELOPMENT IS INTERRELATED
      1. PHYSIOLOGICAL, PSYCHOSOCIAL, COGNITIVE, AND MORAL ASPECTS OF DEVELOPMENT AFFECT AND ARE AFFECTED BY ONE ANOTHER.

   E. DEVELOPMENT BECOMES INCREASINGLY DIFFERENTIATED
      1. RESPONSES BECOME MORE SPECIFIC AND SKILLFUL AS THE CHILD GETS OLDER.
   F. DEVELOPMENT BECOMES INCREASINGLY INTEGRATED AND COMPLEX
      1. AS NEW SKILLS ARE GAINED, MORE COMPLEX TASKS ARE LEARNED.
   G. CHILDREN ARE COMPETENT
      1. THEY POSSESS QUALITIES AND ABILITIES ENSURING THEIR SURVIVAL AND PROMOTING THEIR DEVELOPMENT.
   H. NEW SKILLS PREDOMINATE
      1. CHILDREN HAVE A STRONG DRIVE TO PRACTICE AND PERFECT NEW ABILITIES, ESPECIALLY WHEN THEY ARE YOUNG AND NOT CAPABLE OF COPING WITH SEVERAL NEW SKILLS SIMULTANEOUSLY.

III. **ISSUES OF HUMAN DEVELOPMENT**
   A. NATURE VERSUS NURTURE: WHAT INFLUENCE DO BIOLOGY (NATURE) AND THE ENVIRONMENT (NURTURE) HAVE ON AN INDIVIDUAL?
   B. CONTINUITY VERSUS DISCONTINUITY: WHAT IS THE NATURE OF DEVELOPMENTAL CHANGE ACROSS DEVELOPMENT?
   C. PASSIVITY VERSUS ACTIVITY: ARE CHILDREN PASSIVELY SHAPED BY THE EXTERNAL ENVIRONMENT OR INTERNALLY DRIVEN AND ACTIVE PARTICIPANTS IN THEIR DEVELOPMENT?
   D. CRITICAL VERSUS SENSITIVE PERIOD: HOW IMPORTANT ARE DIFFERENT TIME PERIODS IN DEVELOPMENT? ARE SOME PHASES MORE IMPORTANT THAN OTHERS IN DEVELOPING PARTICULAR ABILITIES, KNOWLEDGE, OR SKILLS?

E. UNIVERSALITY VERSUS CONTEXT SPECIFICITY: DOES CULTURE INFLUENCE DEVELOPMENT? ARE THERE SOME ASPECTS OF DEVELOPMENT THAT APPLY TO ALL CHILDREN IN ALL CULTURES?

F. ASSUMPTIONS ABOUT HUMAN NATURE: ARE CHILDREN INHERENTLY GOOD OR EVIL, OR NEITHER?

G. BEHAVIORAL CONSISTENCY: DO A CHILD'S BASIC BEHAVIORAL TRAITS CHANGE ACCORDING TO THE SETTING?

IV. THEORIES OF HUMAN DEVELOPMENT

A. PSYCHOANALYTIC PERSPECTIVE

  1. FREUD AND PSYCHOSEXUAL DEVELOPMENT: EMPHASIZES THE IMPORTANCE OF UNCONSCIOUS MOTIVATION AND EARLY CHILDHOOD EXPERIENCES IN INFLUENCING BEHAVIOR

    a. Three components of personality:
      1) Id: pleasure seeking
      2) Ego: reality
      3) Superego: conscience

    b. Stages of psychosexual development
      1) Oral (birth to 1 year)
        a) Receives satisfaction from oral needs being met
        b) Attachment to the mother is important because she usually meets the infant's needs.
      2) Anal (1 to 3 years)
        a) Learning to control body functions, especially toileting
      3) Phallic (3 to 6 years)
        a) Fascinated with gender differences, childbirth
        b) Oedipus/Electra complex
      4) Latency (6 to 11 years)
        a) Sexual drives submerged
        b) Appropriate gender roles adopted
        c) Learning about society
      5) Genital (12 years and older)
        a) Sexual desires directed toward opposite gender
        b) Learns how to form loving relationships and manage sexual urges in societally appropriate ways

  2. ERIKSON AND PSYCHOSOCIAL DEVELOPMENT: ACKNOWLEDGED CONTRIBUTION OF BIOLOGY, CULTURE, ENVIRONMENT, AND SOCIETY ON HUMAN DEVELOPMENT

    a. Stages of psychosocial development
      1) Trust versus mistrust (1 month to 1½ years)
        a) Learns world is good and can be trusted as basic needs are met

      2) Autonomy versus shame and doubt (1½ to 3 years)
        a) Learns independent behaviors regarding toileting, bathing, feeding, dressing
        b) Exerts self
        c) Exercises choices
      3) Initiative versus guilt (3 to 6 years)
        a) Goal directed
        b) Competitive, exploratory behavior
        c) Imaginative play
      4) Industry versus inferiority (6 to 11 years)
        a) Learns self-worth as the child gains mastery of psychosocial, physiological, and cognitive skills
        b) Becomes society/peer focused
      5) Identity versus role confusion (12 to 18 years)
        a) Develops sense of who I am
        b) Gains independence from parents
        c) Peers are important

B. BEHAVIORAL PERSPECTIVE

  1. SKINNER AND OPERANT CONDITIONING
    a. If behavior is rewarded, behavior will reoccur.
    b. If behavior is punished, behavior will be extinguished.

  2. BANDURA AND SOCIAL LEARNING
    a. Children learn by imitating and observing others.

C. COGNITIVE-STRUCTURAL PERSPECTIVE

  1. PIAGET AND COGNITIVE DEVELOPMENT: INTELLECTUAL GROWTH FOLLOWS AN ORDERLY PROGRESSION BASED ON MATURATIONAL LEVEL, EXPERIENCES, AND INTERNAL SELF-REGULATING MECHANISMS

    a. Terminology
      1) Schema: patterns of thought used to make sense of their experiences
      2) Assimilation: interpreting new information in terms of existing information
      3) Accommodation: revising, readjusting, realigning existing schema to accept new information
      4) Equilibrium: harmonious relationships between thought processes and the environment

    b. Stages of cognitive development
      1) Sensorimotor (birth to 2 years)
        a) Reflexive (birth to 1 month): predictable, innate survival reflexes

      b) Primary circular reactions (1 to 4 months): responds purposefully to stimuli; initiates, repeats satisfying behaviors

      c) Secondary circular reactions (4 to 8 months): learns from intentional behavior; motor skills/vision coordinated; recognizes familiar objects

      d) Coordination of secondary schemes (8 to 12 months): develops object permanence; anticipates others' actions; differentiates familiar/ unfamiliar

      e) Tertiary circular reactions (12 to 18 months): interested in novelty, repetition; understands causality; solicits help from others

      f) Mental combinations (18 to 24 months): simple problem solving; imitates

    2) Preoperational (2 to 7 years)

      a) Preconceptual (2 to 4 years)
        1. Egocentric thought
        2. Mental imagery
        3. Increasing language

      b) Intuitive (4 to 7 years)
        1. Sophisticated language
        2. Decreasing egocentric thought
        3. Reality-based play

    3) Concrete operations (7 to 11 years)

      a) Understands relationships, classification, conservation, seriation, reversibility
      b) Logical reasoning limited
      c) Less egocentric thought

    4) Formal operations (11 years and older)

      a) Capable of systematic, abstract thought

  2. KOHLBERG AND MORAL DEVELOPMENT

    a. Describes changes in thinking about moral judgments that reflect societal norms and values

    b. Influenced by internal and external factors

    c. Stages of moral development

      1) Preconventional level (birth to 7 years)
        a) Cannot differentiate right from wrong
        b) Conforming behavior based on fear of punishment and rewards

      2) Conventional level (7 to 12 years)
        a) Behavior evaluated on intent and others' reactions
        b) Obeys out of respect for laws, authority

      3) Postconventional level (12 years and older)
        a) Believes laws should further human values and express majority views
        b) Right and wrong defined on universal, comprehensive, and consistent, yet personal, ethical principles

D. CONTEXTUAL PERSPECTIVE

  1. HUMAN DEVELOPMENT IS A LIFELONG PROCESS AFFECTED BY OTHER INDIVIDUALS/ GROUPS AND THE HISTORICAL, CULTURAL, POLITICAL, AND ECONOMIC CONTEXT ONE LIVES IN.

    a. Human development is affected by relationships between the individual and a variety of environmental systems

V.   **NEWBORN (BIRTH TO 1 MONTH)**

A. PHYSIOLOGICAL DEVELOPMENT

  1. GENERAL APPEARANCE

    a. Head

      1) One-fourth of total body size
      2) Molding: misshapen head due to labor and delivery process
      3) Caput succedaneum
        a) Swelling of soft tissues of the scalp
        b) Develops within 24 hours of birth
        c) May extend over suture lines
        d) Resolves within a few days
      4) Cephalhematoma:
        a) Bruising of soft tissues of the scalp
        b) Develops within 24–48 hours of birth
        c) Does not cross suture lines
        d) May take 2–3 weeks to resolve
      5) Fontanels
        a) Occur at skull bone junctions
        b) Allow head to adapt to pelvis shape during delivery
        c) Two different fontanels: posterior: closes by 3 months; anterior: closes by 18 months
      6) Eyes
        a) Lids: may be puffy
        b) Eye color: indistinguishable

    b. Abdomen
      1) Large
      2) Round

    c. Extremities
      1) Short in comparison to the body
      2) Legs may be bowed.

d. Skin
   1) Mottled
   2) Acrocyanosis often seen in extremities
2. NEONATAL REFLEXES
   a. Rooting
      1) Stroke or touch cheek
      2) Head turns toward stimuli
      3) Disappears by 4 months
   b. Sucking
      1) Object touching lips or placed in mouth
      2) Disappears by 7 months
   c. Babinski
      1) Lateral aspect of the sole is stroked from the heel upward and across the ball of the foot.
      2) Hypertension of the toes
      3) Disappears by 1 year
   d. Grasp
      1) Palms of the hands or soles of the feet are touched near the base of the digits.
      2) Flexion of hands and toes
   e. Dance or step
      1) Newborn is held upright, one foot is allowed to touch a flat surface.
      2) Alternate stepping movements
      3) Disappears by 4 months
   f. Moro
      1) Elicited by sudden changes in position or jarring
      2) Arms extend, head moves back, fingers spread apart with the thumb and forefinger forming a "c," followed by arms being brought back to the center with the hands clenched, spine and lower extremities extended
      3) Disappears by 3–4 months
   g. Startle
      1) Elicited by sudden loud noise
      2) Abduction of the arms with flexion of the elbows, hands remain clenched
      3) Disappears by 4 months
   h. Tonic neck
      1) Arm and leg extend on the side, head is turned toward side; arm and leg flexed on opposite side
3. CARDIORESPIRATORY SYSTEM
   a. Respiration
      1) Rate: 30–60 breaths per minute
      2) Abdominal, shallow, irregular
   b. Heart rate
      1) 180 beats per minute for up to 4 hours of age
      2) 100–150 beats per minute after 4 hours of life

4. GASTROINTESTINAL SYSTEM
   a. Stomach
      1) Capacity: 60 ml
      2) Emptying time: 2½ to 3 hours
   b. Liver: immature, resulting in jaundice
      1) Two types of jaundice
         a) Physiological or normal jaundice; bilirubin = 8 mg/dl at 3–5 days after birth
         b) Abnormal jaundice: extreme elevation within the first 24 hours of life (greater than 14 mg/dl if breastfed, or if it persists, past 2 weeks)
         c) Treatment: phototherapy (high-intensity fluorescent lights)
         d) Nursing care: cover eyes with special patches to prevent damage to the retina during phototherapy.
   c. Stools
      1) Meconium
         a) First stool
         b) Black and tarry
         c) Usually passed within 24–48 hours of birth
      2) Transitional
         a) Usually occurs by the third day
         b) Green brown-yellow brown in color
      3) Breastfed
         a) Yellow to golden
         b) Pasty, sour milk odor
      4) Formula fed
         a) Pale to light yellow
         b) Firmer; strong odor
5. GENITOURINARY SYSTEM
   a. Urine
      1) 1–3 ml/kg/hr
      2) 2–6 voidings per day
   b. Male genitals
      1) Assess for presence of testes and appearance of rugae on the scrotal sac
      2) Circumcision: family choice, if carried out
         a) Anesthesia not typically used
         b) If plastibell used: it is left on the penis; do not pull ring off because it will fall off in 7–10 days.
         c) If plastibell is not used: gauze may be used; gauze may or may not be replaced if it falls off
6. MUSCULOSKELETAL SYSTEM
   a. Hypertonic flexion of extremities common
   b. Muscles not well defined

    c. Muscle tone not fully developed (head lag seen related to inability to support the head)

7. INTEGUMENTARY SYSTEM
    a. Delicate and often mottled
    b. Milia often seen
      1) Small white papules on the nose, face, forehead, upper torso
      2) Caused by plugged sebaceous gland
    c. Mongolian spot sometimes observed
      1) Irregularly dark pigmented area on the posterior lumbar region of African Americans, Asians, Native Americans
      2) No clinical significance
    d. Desquamation (peeling of skin)
      1) Related to maturity
        a) Preterm less seen
        b) Postterm more seen
    e. Telangiectatic nevi (capillary hemangiomas [stork bites])
      1) Seen at the nape of the neck, bridge of the nose
      2) Disappear with time

8. THERMOREGULATION: AT RISK FOR HEAT LOSS RELATED TO A LARGE BODY SURFACE AREA AND THIN SUBCUTANEOUS FAT

B. PSYCHOSOCIAL DEVELOPMENT
  1. ERIKSON: TRUST VERSUS MISTRUST
    a. Development of trust and attachment requires caregivers meet physiological and emotional needs.
    b. Supportive, nurturing, and loving environment is important.

C. COGNITIVE DEVELOPMENT
  1. CAN INTERACT WITH THE ENVIRONMENT AND SIGNAL NEEDS AND GRATITUDE WHEN NEEDS ARE MET
  2. CAN RESPOND TO AUDITORY STIMULI
  3. IS SENSITIVE TO TOUCH AND HANDLING
  4. CAN DECREASE RESPONSES TO DISTURBING STIMULI (HABITUATION)

D. HEALTH PROMOTION
  1. OPHTHALMIC DROPS OR OINTMENT REQUIRED BY MOST STATES AFTER DELIVERY
  2. VITAMIN K REQUIRED BY MOST STATES AFTER DELIVERY
    a. 1 mg IM for term newborn
    b. 0.5 mg IM for preterm newborn
  3. SCREENINGS
    a. Phenylketonuria (PKU)
    b. Hypothyroidism

4. IMMUNIZATIONS
    a. Promote disease resistance and prevention
    b. May begin at 2 weeks of age

5. NUTRITION: REQUIRES 120 CAL/KG/DAY
    a. Breast milk
      1) Advantages
        a) No mixing
        b) Correct temperature
        c) No sterilization needed
        d) Easily digested
        e) Fats well absorbed
        f) Contains antibodies and immunoglobulins
        g) Cost effective
    b. Formula
      1) Several formula options available
      2) Provides 20 kcal/oz
    c. On-demand feeds
      1) Breast-fed infants may nurse every 1½–3 hours.
      2) Formula-fed infants may feed every 3–4 hours.

6. HYGIENE
    a. Bathe every other day.
    b. In female infants, wipe from front to back.
    c. Keep the diaper area clean and dry to help prevent diaper rash.

7. REST AND SLEEP
    a. Newborn sleeps between 16 and 19 hours per day.
    b. AAP recommends supine or side-lying position, unless contraindicated (GER), to help prevent sudden infant death syndrome (SIDS).

8. ACTIVITY AND PLAY
    a. Newborns attend to sounds, sights, tastes, and smells
    b. Prefer to look at faces over objects
    c. Alert, interested, and sensitive to the environment

9. SAFETY AND INJURY PREVENTION
    a. Do not leave the newborn unattended unless in a crib with the side rails up.
    b. Risks
      1) Drowning
      2) Suffocation
      3) Burns
      4) Falls
      5) Motor vehicle accidents: use a car seat and avoid placing the newborn in the front seat.

E. NURSE'S ROLE IN FOSTERING HEALTHY NEWBORNS
  1. EDUCATE ABOUT CARE OF THE NEWBORN WITH FREQUENT REINFORCEMENT (SEE HEALTH PROMOTION).

2. PROVIDE INFORMATION ABOUT THE IMPORTANCE OF WELL-BABY CHECKUPS AND IMMUNIZATIONS.
3. EDUCATE ABOUT PREVENTING SHAKEN BABY SYNDROME.

VI. INFANT: (1 MONTH TO 1 YEAR)
   A. PHYSIOLOGICAL DEVELOPMENT
      1. ORDERLY, RAPID CHANGES
      2. INFLUENCED BY GENETICS, ENVIRONMENT, ETHNIC BACKGROUND, BIOLOGY
      3. WEIGHT
         a. Doubles within the first 6 months (gain is approximately 1.5 pounds per month)
         b. During the second 6 months, gain is less than 1 pound per month.
         c. By 12 months, birth weight will have tripled.
      4. HEIGHT
         a. Increases about 1 inch per month during the first 6 months
         b. By 12 months, there is almost a 50% increase in height from birth height.
      5. HEAD GROWTH
         a. By 12 months, infant brain will be two-thirds the size of an adult brain.
         b. Head circumference
            1) During the first 6 months, head circumference will increase by 0.5 inch per month.
            2) During the second 6 months of life, head circumference will grow approximately 0.25 inch per month.
         c. Fontanels
            1) Posterior fontanel closes by 2 months.
            2) Anterior fontanel closes by 12–18 months.
      6. MOTOR DEVELOPMENT
         a. Occurs in cephalocaudal and proximal-distal fashion
         b. Gross motor abilities develop before fine motor abilities.
            1) Gross motor
               a) Ability to use large muscle groups to maintain balance and postural control or locomotion
            2) Fine motor
               a) Ability to coordinate hand–eye movement in an orderly and progressive manner
   B. PSYCHOSEXUAL DEVELOPMENT
      1. FREUD
         a. Oral stage of development
            1) Need for pleasure dominates life
            2) Oral stimulation is central focus

            3) Learns to delay gratification as anticipates needs being met
            4) Nonnutritive sucking common and helps meet needs for oral gratification
   C. PSYCHOSOCIAL DEVELOPMENT
      1. ERIKSON
         a. Trust versus mistrust (See Section V, Newborn [Birth to 1 month], p. 570.)
   D. COGNITIVE DEVELOPMENT
      1. PIAGET
         a. Sensorimotor stage
            1) Birth to 24 months
            2) Knowledge acquired about an object through interaction with that object and the use of senses
   E. HEALTH PROMOTION
      1. HEALTH SCREENING VISITS (DEVELOPMENTAL ASSESSMENT, PHYSICAL EXAM, ANTICIPATORY GUIDANCE, SCREENINGS)
         a. Provide opportunity to assess and detect any problems
         b. Often scheduled every 2 months
      2. IMMUNIZATIONS
         a. DTaP, Hib, IPV, PCV, HepB given during the first 12 months of life
      3. NUTRITION
         a. Caloric requirements
            1) 100 kcal/kg/day by the time infant is 12 months
         b. Fluid requirements
            1) 1–1.5 ml/kcal expended/day
         c. Solid foods
            1) Provide semisolid single grain infant cereal and applesauce when the infant can sit well with support, tongue thrust has decreased, and the hunger seems unsatisfied after nursing or bottle feeding.
            2) Usually begins between 4 and 6 months
            3) Different solids introduced one at a time and about 1 week apart
         d. Weaning
            1) Process of giving up one method of feeding for another
            2) Behaviors consistent with weaning
               a) Eating from a spoon
               b) Holding the bottle
               c) Feeding self with fingers or a spoon
               d) Eating foods that require chewing
               e) Decreasing desire to be held during feeding
               f) Should be done gradually

4. HYGIENE
   a. Minimal bathing needed during the first year
   b. Gather all supplies before beginning.
   c. While giving a sponge bath, only expose those areas currently being washed.
   d. Use a mild baby shampoo to wash hair every other day to prevent cradle cap; scrub hair with a soft toothbrush.
   e. Avoid using baby powder because of possible aspiration pneumonia.
   f. Clip fingernails and toenails after bathing.

5. DENTAL HEALTH
   a. Tooth eruption
      1) Begins around 3–4 months
      2) First teeth to erupt are lower central incisors.
   b. Tooth hygiene
      1) Gently cleanse teeth and gums with a wet cloth.
      2) Fluoride supplement is needed if water does not contain 0.3 ppm of fluoride.
      3) Prevent bottle mouth syndrome by not offering a bottle when the infant is placed in bed for a nap or at night.
   c. Teething
      1) Periodontal membrane becomes swollen, red, and tender.
      2) Clinical manifestations
         a) Drooling
         b) Fussiness
         c) Low-grade fever
      3) Care
         a) Offer frozen teething ring.
         b) Offer ice cube wrapped in a washcloth.
         c) Offer a zwieback cracker.
         d) Offer a hard rubber toy.
         e) Apply a topical oral anesthetic (Orajel).
         f) If a fever is present, offer acetaminophen according to recommended dosage.

6. REST AND SLEEP
   a. Needs
      1) Newborn: 8 hours daytime; 8½ hours nighttime
      2) 1 month: 6¾ hours daytime; 8¾ hours nighttime
      3) 4 months: 4½ hours daytime; 10½ hours nighttime
      4) 6 months: 3–4 hours daytime; 11 hours nighttime
      5) 1 year: 2½ hours daytime; 11½ hours nighttime
   b. If infant awakens at night, provide:
      1) Soft music
      2) Rocking
      3) Pacifier
      4) Dim light
   c. To prevent sleep problems:
      1) Assist the caregiver in understanding individual needs.
      2) Provide information relative to healthy sleep patterns and signs of maturation.
   d. Position on the back or side rather than on the stomach.

7. ACTIVITY AND PLAY
   a. By 6 months to 1 year of age, toys should enhance language and sensorimotor skills.
   b. Encourage the caregiver to interact with the infant rather than just provide toys.
   c. Toys and activities appropriate for infants
      1) Birth–3 months
         a) Black-and-white or red-colored pattern cards
         b) Soft, cuddly toys
         c) Nonbreakable mirror
         d) Rattles
         e) Mobiles
         f) Music boxes
         g) Talking and singing
         h) Rocking and holding
         i) Gentle massage
         j) Interaction with other people
      2) 3–6 months
         a) Crib gyms
         b) Squeaky toys
         c) Teething rings
         d) Different textured toys
         e) Noise-making toys
         f) Talking and singing
         g) Play pat-a-cake, play peek-a-boo
         h) Social interaction with other people
      3) 6–9 months
         a) Safe place to creep/crawl
         b) Bathtub toys
         c) Jack-in-the-box
         d) Nested toys
         e) Big, soft blocks
         f) Drinking cup
         g) Toys to bang together
         h) Talking and singing
         i) Playing hide and seek
         j) Social interaction with other people

4. 9–12 MONTHS
   a. Continue with toys for 6–9 months of age
   b. Safe place for exploration
   c. Push-pull and motion toys

d. Colorful cloth books
e. Paper for tearing
f. Building blocks
g. Metal pots and pans
h. Different shaped and colored toys
i. Social interaction with other people
8. SAFETY AND INJURY PREVENTION
a. Accidental injury is the leading cause of infant death between 6 and 12 months of age.
b. Falls, drowning, burns, strangulation, motor vehicle accident, choking, and ingestion are the greatest dangers.
c. Due to developmental immaturity

F. ANTICIPATORY GUIDANCE
1. PACIFIERS
a. Help satisfy nonnutritive need to suck
b. Should not be used in place of general caregiving
2. FEEDING PROBLEMS
a. Improper feeding techniques
1) Feeding too much or too little
2) Feeding infrequently or too frequently
3) Selecting improper foods for the infant's motor and physiological development
4) Not being aware of infant cues to be burped or being satiated
5) Holding the bottle at an inappropriate angle
b. Spitting up
1) Common
2) Prevention strategies
a) Frequent burping
b) Position the child on the right side with the head slightly elevated.
c) Minimal handling after feeding
3. COMMUNICATION
a. Enables the infant to express needs, emotions, attitudes
b. Infant language development
1) Birth–2 months
a) Crying
b) Comfort sound with feeding
c) Coos
d) Vocalizes to familiar voice
2) 3–6 months
a) Vocalizes during play and pleasure
b) Squeals
c) Laughs aloud
d) Less crying
e) Uses vowels and consonant sounds that resemble syllables (ma, mu, ba, ga, ah, da)
3) 7–9 months
a) Increases vowel and consonant sounds

b) Uses two-syllable sounds (baba, dada)
c) Talks along with others
4) 10–12 months
a) Says "mama" and "dada" to identify caregivers
b) Repeats sounds made by others
c) Makes intentional gestures
d) Learns three to five words
4. TEMPERAMENT: THE WAY A CHILD BEHAVIORALLY INTERACTS WITH THE SURROUNDING ENVIRONMENT
a. Easy
1) Easygoing and adapts rapidly to stimuli
2) Has an overall positive mood
3) Likes to be around people
4) Sleeps and eats well
5) Has regular and predictable behavior
b. Difficult
1) Adapts slowly to stimuli
2) Has an overall negative mood
3) Requires a structured environment
4) Likes people but can do well alone
5) Seems to be in constant motion
6) Has irregular patterns of behavior
c. Slow to warm up
1) Adapts slowly to stimuli but is watchful
2) Quietly withdraws and usually moody
3) Primarily a loner and socially shy
4) Oversensitive and slow to mature
5) Primarily inactive
6) Reacts passively to changes in routine
5. COLIC
a. Recurrent episodes of unexplained crying and inability to be consoled
b. Occurs around 1–2 weeks of age; subsides spontaneously by 16 weeks
c. Caregiver teaching information
1) Feedings
a) Feed slowly.
b) Burp frequently.
c) Keep in upright position during feeding.
d) Do not overfeed.
e) If breastfeeding, avoid eating foods that may contribute to gas formation such as onions, cabbage, collards, dry beans.
2) Swaddle to decrease self-stimulation by jerky or sudden movements.
3) Take the infant for a car ride.
4) Use a swing for at least 20 minutes.

5) Walk or rock the infant while applying gentle pressure to his abdomen.
6) Gently massage the infant's back while he is lying down.
7) Supply background or "white" noise (hair dryer, vacuum cleaner, fan) or play a womb sound tape (known as a "souffle" toy) or some soft music.
8) Place the infant in a quiet, darkened room to reduce environment stimulus.

6. STRANGER AND SEPARATION ANXIETY
   a. Emerge at 8–12 months; peak at 12–15 months, disappear by 24 months
   b. Indicate object permanence
   c. Separation anxiety: demonstrated when the infant is separated from the caregiver
   d. Stranger anxiety: demonstrated when a stranger appears

7. ALTERNATIVE CHILDCARE
   a. Types of alternate childcare
      1) Center-based care
         a) Group care for two or more children
         b) Located usually in a home, school, church, or building designed for group care
         c) Licensed by local or state agencies
         d) Staff usually trained in childcare and development
         e) Structured program of activities
         f) Reliable hours of operation
      2) Family childcare
         a) Small group care
         b) Located in the provider's home
         c) Special arrangements possible
      3) In-home care
         a) Home care provided by a sitter or nanny
         b) Individualized care
         c) Easier to meet special needs (e.g., physical, mental, emotional problem)
         d) Provider may do light home tasks.

VII. TODDLER (12–36 MONTHS)
   A. PHYSIOLOGICAL DEVELOPMENT: PREDICTABLE BUT INDIVIDUAL VARIATION SEEN
      1. PHYSICAL GROWTH
         a. Slower than at earlier ages
         b. Average weight gain = 5 pounds per year
         c. Average height gain = 3 inches per year
         d. Head becomes more proportional in comparison to other parts of the body.
         e. Chest circumference increases.
         f. Most walk by 12–15 months.
         g. Most climb stairs by 18 months.
      2. NEUROLOGICAL SYSTEM
         a. Increased eye–hand coordination, manual dexterity, walking/running skills
      3. MUSCULOSKELETAL SYSTEM
         a. Increased bone length, muscle maturation, and muscle strength assist in autonomy development.
      4. GASTROINTESTINAL/ GENITOURINARY SYSTEM
         a. Stomach enlarges, all deciduous teeth erupt by 30 months, improved eye–hand coordination enable self-feeding.
         b. Physiologic anorexia is common, with ritualistic interest in certain foods.
         c. Caloric needs diminish but protein requirements remain higher than for other age groups.
         d. Bladder and bowel control has begun and for some is achieved.
      5. CARDIORESPIRATORY SYSTEM
         a. Becomes more mature
         b. Vital signs more stable and are similar to adult norms
         c. Respiratory and cardiac rates slow; blood pressure (BP) rises
      6. SENSORY SYSTEM
         a. Hearing, smell, taste, touch, and vision develop
         b. Baseline hearing and vision screening should be conducted.
   B. PSYCHOSEXUAL DEVELOPMENT
      1. FREUD'S ANAL STAGE OF DEVELOPMENT
      2. MASTURBATION IS COMMON AND SHOULD BE HANDLED MATTER-OF-FACTLY.
      3. TOILET TRAINING SHOULD NOT BE MANAGED RIGIDLY.
      4. DOMESTIC MIMICRY (IMITATION OF DOMESTIC AND ROLE ACTIVITY) HELPS TODDLERS UNDERSTAND GENDER ROLES.
      5. GENDER IDENTITY IS REINFORCED BY OBSERVING SAME- AND OPPOSITE-SEX CAREGIVERS ENACT THEIR GENDER ROLES, ATTITUDES, AND VALUES.
   C. PSYCHOSOCIAL DEVELOPMENT
      1. THREE MAJOR TASKS
         a. Gaining self-control
         b. Developing autonomy
         c. Increasing independence

2. ERIKSON: AUTONOMY VERSUS SHAME AND DOUBT
   a. 15 months
      1) Fears being alone, being abandoned, strangers, objects, and places
      2) Expresses independence by trying to feed and undress self
   b. 18 months
      1) Negativism predominates
      2) Fears water
      3) Temper tantrums
      4) Awareness of own gender begins
   c. 24 months
      1) May resist bedtime and naps
      2) Fears the dark and animals
      3) Temper tantrums, negativism, and dawdling continue
      4) Bedtime rituals important
      5) Explores genitalia
      6) Shows readiness for bowel and bladder control
   d. 36 months
      1) Temper tantrums, negativism, and dawdling behaviors subside.
      2) Self-esteem increases due to increased independence in eating, elimination, and dressing.
      3) Explores many emotions in pretend play
      4) Separation fears generally subside.
      5) May develop a fear of monsters

D. COGNITIVE DEVELOPMENT
   1. PIAGET'S SENSORIMOTOR AND PREOPERATIONAL PHASES OF COGNITIVE DEVELOPMENT
      a. Tertiary circular reactions (15–18 months)
         1) Experiences as many new situations as possible to achieve new skills/abilities
         2) Combines new and old knowledge to experiment and begin early reasoning
         3) Enhanced understanding of object permanence
         4) Learns to differentiate self from objects
         5) Develops awareness of spatial and causal concepts
      b. Mental combinations (18–24 months)
         1) Can infer a cause even if only experiencing the effect (threw a toy, child disciplined, toy put out of reach)
         2) Beginning to think before acting
         3) Imitation becomes more symbolic.
         4) Beginning sense of memory in early problem solving (better sense of time relationships)
         5) Egocentric in actions and thinking
      c. Preconceptual (2–4 years)
         1) Egocentric thoughts, play, and actions
         2) Improved sense of time, space, and causality
         3) Uses languages as mental representation increases
         4) Develops cognitive connection between new experience and things that occurred in the past (refuses to eat food because something before did not taste good)
         5) Begins trial-and-error learning
   2. LANGUAGE
      a. Dependent on physical maturity and caregiver encouragement and participation
      b. Normal milestones
         1) 12 months to 18 months
            a) Starts to combine two words
            b) 18- to 22-word vocabulary
         2) 18 months to 2 years
            a) Articulation lags behind
            b) 270- to 300-word vocabulary
         3) 2 years to 3 years
            a) Uses consonants and pronouns
            b) Begins to use word endings
            c) 900-word vocabulary

E. MORAL DEVELOPMENT
   1. HAS LITTLE CONCEPT OF RIGHT AND WRONG

F. HEALTH SCREENING
   1. ROUTINE WELL CHILD VISITS SHOULD BE MADE AT 15, 18, 24, AND 36 MONTHS OF AGE.
   2. INCLUDES:
      a. Physical examination
      b. Hemoglobin evaluation
      c. Dental evaluation
      d. Vision and hearing assessment
      e. Serum lead levels if poor growth patterns are noted
      f. Developmental assessment

G. HEALTH PROMOTION
   1. IMMUNIZATIONS: HEPB, DTAP, HIB, IPV, MMR, PCV, VARICELLA, AND INFLUENZA DURING THIS PERIOD
   2. NUTRITION
      a. Ability to chew, swallow, and use utensils improves.
      b. Offer 1 tablespoon of each food group for each year of age and meal.
   3. ELIMINATION
      a. Most ready to toilet train between 18 and 24 months
      b. Bladder control often more difficult to achieve than bowel control
      c. Needs to show signs of readiness for toilet training
         1) Awareness of wet diaper
         2) Able to follow directions

    3) Able to communicate elimination needs to the caregiver
    4) Able to remain dry for longer period
    5) Able to independently dress and undress
    6) Able to sit, squat, walk well

4. ACCIDENTS AND REGRESSION ARE COMMON AND SHOULD BE HANDLED NONCHALANTLY.

5. HYGIENE
  a. Bathed every other day unless needed more frequently
  b. Consistent bath time and ritual important

6. DENTAL HEALTH
  a. First visit to the dentist should be at 1 year of age or soon after first tooth erupts.
  b. If fluoride toothpaste is used, it should only be the size of a pea.
  c. Toothbrush should have soft bristles.

7. REST AND SLEEP
  a. Needs bedtime rituals
  b. Sleep requirement is 12–14 hours per day.
  c. Naps may not be needed.
  d. Nightmares are common.

8. ACTIVITY AND PLAY
  a. Purpose of play
    1) Facilitates cognitive development
      a) Permits exploration of the environment
      b) Learns about objects
      c) Learns problem solving
    2) Advances social development
    3) Vents frustrations
    4) Uses excess energy
    5) Assists in coping with inner conflicts and anxieties in nonthreatening ways
    6) Toddler play activities
      a) Pull toys
      b) Picture books
      c) Cars/trucks
      d) Stuffed toys
      e) Take apart toys
      f) Blocks
      g) Puzzles
      h) Wagons

9. SAFETY PROMOTION AND INJURY PREVENTION
  a. Toddlers are at risk for:
    1) Falls
    2) Motor vehicle accidents
    3) Aspiration
    4) Burns
    5) Ingestions

H. ANTICIPATORY GUIDANCE
  1. NEGATIVISM
    a. An expression of the toddler's constant search for autonomy
    b. Typically passes by 30 months of age
    c. Best to ignore behavior

  2. RITUALISM AND REGRESSION
    a. Best to ignore regression (often the result of changes in routine) and allow for ritualism

  3. DISCIPLINE
    a. Limit setting (letting the child know what he is able to do and not do) important
    b. Components of successful discipline
      1) Encourage supportive and loving relationship between caregivers and the child.
      2) Use positive reinforcement to promote desired behaviors.
      3) Remove reinforcement to reduce and eliminate undesired behaviors.

  4. SIBLING RIVALRY
    a. Intense feelings of jealousy between siblings
    b. Tips on handling sibling rivalry
      1) Have the toddler sleep over at the grandparents' home or others' who the child will stay with during time of sibling birth.
      2) Encourage visitors to spend time with the toddler as well as the new baby.
      3) Plan to spend time with the toddler apart from the new baby.
      4) Encourage the toddler to help with care of the new baby.

  5. TEMPER TANTRUMS
    a. Outward explosive reactions to inward stress or frustrating situations
    b. Best to ignore unless the child is at risk for being hurt

VIII. PRESCHOOLER (3–6 YEARS)
A. PHYSIOLOGIC DEVELOPMENT
  1. WEIGHT INCREASES 4–6 POUNDS PER YEAR.
  2. GROSS MOTOR DEVELOPMENT
    a. Walks well
    b. Runs well
    c. Jumps rope
    d. Hops on one foot
  3. FINE MOTOR DEVELOPMENT
    a. Dresses/undresses self
    b. Uses scissors
    c. Learning to draw figures
    d. Shows hand preference

B. PSYCHOSEXUAL DEVELOPMENT
  1. SEXUAL CURIOSITY IS PRESENT.
  2. FREUD'S OEDIPAL STAGE

C. PSYCHOSOCIAL DEVELOPMENT
  1. ERIKSON'S STAGE OF INITIATIVE VERSUS GUILT

D. COGNITIVE DEVELOPMENT
1. COGNITIVE ABILITY INCREASES.
2. PIAGET'S PREOPERATIONAL STAGE
a. Egocentrism: understands experiences only from his own perspective
b. Animism: believes objects have human qualities
c. Idiosyncratic: uses a personal system for organizing objects and events in his mind
d. Uses language to communicate needs with increasing number of words and phrases

E. MORAL DEVELOPMENT
1. KOHLBERG'S PREMORAL STAGE
a. Believes right and wrong are determined by rewards and punishments
b. May not understand why something is right or wrong
c. May have difficulty applying rules from one situation to another similar situation
d. Develops a concrete awareness of justice and fairness

F. SPIRITUAL DEVELOPMENT
1. BELIEVES GOD HAS PHYSICAL CHARACTERISTICS
2. UNDERSTANDS SIMPLE RELIGIOUS STORIES
3. PARTICIPATES IN SOME RELIGIOUS RITUALS, BUT MAY NOT UNDERSTAND THEIR SIGNIFICANCE
4. ACCEPTS RELIGION OF PARENTS

G. HEALTH SCREENING
1. YEARLY VISITS ARE IMPORTANT.
2. NEEDS TO INCLUDE:
a. Hearing and vision screening
b. Physical examination
c. Vital signs
d. Tuberculosis (TB) test
e. Assessment for risk of hyperlipidemia and high-dose exposure to lead
f. Developmental assessment

H. HEALTH PROMOTION
1. IMMUNIZATIONS: HEPB, DTAP, IPV, MMP#2, VARICELLA
2. NUTRITION
a. Should be eating table foods
b. Needs 6–11 servings of bread/cereal, 3–5 servings of vegetables, 2–4 servings of fruit, 3 servings of milk products, 2–3 servings of meat, sparse use of sweets/fats per day
c. Serving size should be 1 tablespoon of food per year of age, food group, or meal.
d. May be picky eaters
e. Can help in food preparation

3. ELIMINATION
a. Nighttime control is achieved.
b. Accidents may occur related to interest in activities.
c. Assume matter-of-fact attitude if there are accidents.
4. HYGIENE
a. Needs bath every day or two, depending on activity
b. Supervise baths even though the child is able to sit up in the tub.
c. Avoid use of bubble bath, as there is a relationship with its use and urinary tract infections (UTIs).
5. DENTAL HEALTH
a. Eruption of deciduous teeth is complete.
b. Prevention of dental caries is important.
1) Daily brushing and flossing
2) If toothpaste contains fluoride, use an amount equal to the size of a pea.
3) Visit the dentist every 6 months.
4) Avoid sugary snacks.
6. REST AND SLEEP
a. Needs 12 hours of sleep every day
b. Establish bedtime rituals.
1) Bath
2) Bedtime story
3) Listen to soothing music
4) Have chat with the caregiver
7. ACTIVITY AND PLAY
a. Refining gross and fine motor coordination and skill (crayons, scissors, tricycle, balls)
b. Encourage a variety of physical activities in a noncompetitive environment.
1) T-ball
2) Karate
3) Gymnastics
4) Bicycling
5) Dance
6) Encourage group play.
8. SAFETY AND INJURY PREVENTION
a. Needs close supervision related to increased mobility and skills
b. Is aware of potential dangers in the environment (hot objects, sharp instruments, dangerous heights)
c. Playgrounds, water, and cars are potential injury sites.

I. ANTICIPATORY GUIDANCE
1. PREPARATION FOR SCHOOL IS IMPORTANT.
2. DISCIPLINE AND LIMIT SETTING
a. Limit setting helps the child learn acceptable behavior.
b. Time-outs are helpful but need to be no longer than 1 minute per year of the child's age.
c. It is important to divert aggressive behaviors.

3. CHILDHOOD OBESITY
   a. Physical effects
      1) Hyperlipidemia
      2) Obstructive apnea
      3) Gallbladder disease
      4) Pancreatitis
      5) Hypertension
      6) Diabetes
   b. Psychological effects
      1) Lower self-esteem
      2) May find it hard to "fit in"
   c. Prevention/treatment
      1) Nutritional diets
      2) Increased amount of physical activity
      3) Teach appropriate ways to lead a healthy life.
4. SLEEP DISTURBANCES
   a. Usually resolve as the child gets older
   b. Bedtime fears
      1) Common
      2) Interventions for parents
         a) Use a night-light.
         b) Have an open discussion.
   c. Nightmares
      1) Fairly common
      2) Interventions for parents
         a) Parents need to comfort and reassure the child that nightmares are not real.
         b) Help the child remain in bed until he falls back to sleep.
   d. Sleep terrors, talking in sleep, sleepwalking
      1) Uncommon
      2) If occur frequently, needs to see health care provider
5. TELEVISION AND THE MEDIA
   a. Not a substitute for play
   b. Some programs are inappropriate for preschoolers.
   c. Limit TV to 1–2 hours/day.
   d. Avoid putting TV in the child's bedroom.
6. FEARS
   a. Real or imagined things
      1) Dark
      2) Bugs
      3) Animals
   b. Interventions for parents
      1) Talk to the child about fears.
      2) Use a night-light.
      3) Careful exposure to stimulus may diminish the fear.

IX. **SCHOOL AGE (6–12 YEARS)**
A. PHYSIOLOGIC DEVELOPMENT
   1. WEIGHT INCREASES 5–6 POUNDS PER YEAR.
   2. HEIGHT INCREASES 2 INCHES PER YEAR.
   3. MUSCLE STRENGTH AND SIZE INCREASE GRADUALLY, ALLOWING FOR DEVELOPMENT OF GROSS MOTOR SKILLS INCLUDING:
      a. Balancing
      b. Catching
      c. Throwing
      d. Running
      e. Jumping
      f. Climbing
   4. FINE MOTOR DEVELOPMENT IMPROVES, AND INCLUDES:
      a. Writing
      b. Tying shoes
      c. Dressing independently
   5. CARDIORESPIRATORY SYSTEM
      a. Increased efficiency
      b. Decreased pulse rate and heart rate (heart rate = 90–95/minute; respiratory rate = 20/minute)
      c. Tidal volume increases.
   6. DENTAL
      a. Deciduous teeth shed.
      b. Permanent teeth appear by 6 years.
         1) Four teeth erupt per year.
   7. IMMUNE SYSTEM
      a. Antibody production peaks by age 7.
      b. Similar to adults
   8. PREPUBESCENCE (LAST 2 YEARS OF SCHOOL-AGE PERIOD)
      a. Body changes (breast tissue development) may begin by age 9.
      b. Body odor may begin by age 9.
B. PSYCHOSEXUAL DEVELOPMENT
   1. FREUD'S LATENCY PERIOD (CALM)
   2. IDENTIFICATION WITH SAME SEX PEERS AND PARENT IMPORTANT
C. PSYCHOSOCIAL DEVELOPMENT
   1. DEVELOPS REALISTIC VIEW OF SELF AND PLACE IN THE WORLD
   2. ERIKSON'S INDUSTRY VERSUS INFERIORITY
   3. POSITIVE RELATIONSHIP WITH AFFIRMING ADULT IMPORTANT
D. COGNITIVE DEVELOPMENT
   1. PIAGET
      a. Child is able to imagine the world without having to experience it.
      b. Concrete operations
         1) Conservation: acknowledges a change in shape does not mean a change in amount
         2) Classification: ability to group items according to common characteristics
         3) Reversibility: ability to recognize that actions can move in reverse order

2. LANGUAGE IMPROVES.
  a. Vocabulary expands from 2000 to 50,000 words.
  b. Understands literal and nonliteral meaning of words
  c. Understands metaphors
  d. Becomes less egocentric
3. READING
  a. Learns to read
  b. Enjoys being read to
E. MORAL DEVELOPMENT
  1. KOHLBERG: CONVENTIONAL LEVEL
    a. Develops a conscience
    b. Avoids disapproval of others and maintains a positive relationship with others
    c. Accidents the result of punishment for disobeying
    d. Concerned about doing the "right" thing
     1) Understands the need to treat others as he would like to be treated as the child approaches adolescence
F. SPIRITUAL DEVELOPMENT
  1. BELIEVES IN A SUPREME BEING WHO LOVES AND GIVES TO OTHERS
  2. BEGINS TO THINK OF GOD AS A HUMAN BEING
  3. DEVELOPS A RELIGIOUS PHILOSOPHY THAT IS USED TO INTERPRET AND UNDERSTAND THE WORLD
  4. MAY PRAY FOR RECOVERY FROM ILLNESS AND PROTECTION FROM DANGER
G. HEALTH SCREENING
  1. AVERAGES TWO HEALTH CARE VISITS PER YEAR, SOME FOR MINOR ILLNESSES
  2. AAP RECOMMENDS ROUTINE MEDICAL EXAMS (EVERY 2 YEARS) NEED TO INCLUDE:
    a. Height
    b. Weight
    c. Physical exam
    d. Vision and hearing screening
    e. Vital signs
    f. Assessment of dietary intake and use of tobacco, alcohol, drugs
H. HEALTH PROMOTION
  1. IMMUNIZATIONS: DTAP, IPV, MMR, VARICELLA, HEPB, TD
  2. NUTRITION
    a. Nutritional needs remain steady.
    b. Encourage the avoidance of fast foods.
    c. Needs
     1) 2–3 servings of milk
     2) 2 servings of meat
     3) 6–9 servings of bread
     4) 3–4 servings of vegetables
     5) 2–3 servings of fruit

    d. Preventing obesity
     1) Offer a variety of healthy foods.
     2) Encourage the child to help with food preparation.
     3) Respect the child's ability to decide how much to eat.
     4) Consult the physician if the caregiver is concerned about the child's weight.
     5) Encourage physical activity and discourage sedentary activity such as television.
3. ELIMINATION
  a. Should be independent in toileting
  b. Encourage the child to use the bathroom when needed instead of ignoring urges.
4. HYGIENE
  a. Children over 7 should be able to carry out personal hygiene practices independently.
  b. May prefer showers over baths
  c. May need help cleaning hard-to-reach places
5. DENTAL HEALTH
  a. Encourage to brush with fluoride toothpaste at least 2 times a day and floss before bedtime.
  b. Encourage to see a pediatric dentist every 6 months.
  c. May develop malocclusion (abnormality of teeth so upper and lower teeth do not approximate, leaving them crowded or uneven)
    1) May need referral to an orthodontist for braces
6. REST AND SLEEP
  a. Needs 8–10 hours of sleep per day depending on age and activity
  b. Nightmares and night terrors are less common.
  c. Somnambulism (sleepwalking) is seen in 15% of children.
  d. Somniloquy (sleep talking) may occur but should not be a concern.
7. ACTIVITY AND PLAY
  a. Prefers games and sports with rules
  b. Provides opportunity to learn physically what the body is capable of
  c. Stimulates gross and fine motor development
  d. Discourage sedentary activities (watching TV, playing video/computer games).
8. SAFETY AND INJURY PREVENTION
  a. Factors contributing to injury and accidents
    1) Increased independence
    2) Desire for peer approval
    3) Increased involvement in physically challenging activities

b. Safety concerns
1) Motor vehicles
2) Bike/skateboard
3) Firearms
4) Pedestrian
5) Water hazards

I. ANTICIPATORY GUIDANCE
1. SCHOOL
a. Important for intellectual and social development
b. Cooperative learning (one child helps another learn) is important and encourages intellectual development.
2. HOMEWORK
a. Provides a positive atmosphere without chance for distraction
b. Interventions for parents
1) Show interest in the child's work.
2) Check and help if necessary.
3) Reevaluate after-school activities if the child has no time for homework.
3. PEERS
a. Important for social development (self-esteem, self-confidence, cooperation, competition, aggression, disagreement, and negotiation)
b. Help learn about the world and relationships with others
4. SELF-CONCEPT
a. Develops during this time
b. Influenced by
1) Physical appearance
2) Athletic ability
3) Academic achievement
4) Approval from caregivers
5) Peers
5. BULLYING (INFLICTING VERBAL OR PHYSICAL HARM ON OTHERS)
a. More common in boys
b. Reactions include:
1) Sadness
2) Reduced self-esteem
3) Having fewer friends
4) Being less popular
5) School absences
6) Physical complaints (headache, sleep disturbances, stomachache)
6. STRESS
a. Occurs when there is a discrepancy between demands placed on the child and the child's perceived ability to meet those demands
b. Signs
1) Frequent fatigue
2) Irritability
3) Changes in sleep or eating patterns
4) Substance abuse
5) Drop in academic performance
6) Headache
7) Stomachache

7. LATCH-KEY CHILDREN
a. Definition: home alone without adult supervision
b. Teach latch-key children:
1) Not to open the door to anyone not known
2) Not to tell a telephone caller that the caregiver is not home
3) Know where emergency numbers and neighbor's numbers are
4) Become involved in after-school routines
8. DISHONESTY
a. Not uncommon
b. Often just a phase/related to immature development
J. NURSING ROLE IN FOSTERING HEALTHY SCHOOL-AGE CHILDREN
1. ENCOURAGE INDEPENDENCE.
2. SET LIMITS.
3. EDUCATE CAREGIVERS ABOUT:
a. Nutrition
b. Exercise
c. Rest
d. Activity
e. Safety

X. **ADOLESCENT**
A. PHYSIOLOGICAL DEVELOPMENT
1. MUSCULOSKELETAL
a. Adolescent growth spurt (AGS)
1) Lasts about 4½ years
2) Body assumes an adult appearance.
3) Girls
a) Begins as early as 7½ years and as late as 12 years
b) Gain 8–10 pounds
c) Grow 2½–5 inches
4) Boys
a) Begins by age 13 years
b) Gain 12–14 pounds
c) Grow 3–6 inches
b. Peak height velocity (PHV): maximum annual rate of growth in height
c. Peak weight velocity (PWV): maximum annual rate of growth in height
2. GENITOURINARY SYSTEM
a. Reproductive hormones
1) Responsible for primary and secondary sexual characteristics
2) Boys
a) Follicle-stimulating hormone (FSH) is responsible for sperm production and maturation of seminiferous tubules.
b) Luteinizing hormone (LH) promotes testicular maturation and testosterone production.

3) Girls
  a) FSH stimulates ovarian follicle growth and estrogen production.
  b) LH initiates ovulation and formation of corpus luteum.
b. Tanner stages
  1) Five sequences of secondary sexual characteristics
    a) Females: breast development; pubic hair growth
    b) Males: growth of testes; growth of penis; growth of scrotum; growth of pubic hair
c. Menarche (first menstrual period)
  1) Indicates puberty and sexual maturity
  2) Occurs 2 years after breast development starts and after the AGS peaks
  3) Females can become pregnant after the first menstrual period.
d. Spermatogenesis
  1) Indicates puberty and sexual maturity
  2) First ejaculate usually does not contain mature sperm
  3) Occurs 1 year after penis begins AGS
3. CARDIORESPIRATORY SYSTEM
  a. Heart doubles in weight and increases in size by ½.
    1) BP = 100–120/50–70
    2) Pulse = 60–70 beats per minute
  b. Lungs increase in length and diameter.
    1) Respiratory rate: 16–20 breaths per minute
    2) Males: greater increase in vital capacity, volume, and rate than females
4. NEUROLOGICAL SYSTEM
  a. Brain growth continues.
  b. Myelin sheath growth allows faster neural processing and abstract thinking.
5. GASTROINTESTINAL SYSTEM
  a. Eruption of 32 teeth occurs by the 21st birthday.
  b. Approximates adult functioning and capacity
B. PSYCHOSEXUAL DEVELOPMENT
  1. FREUD
    a. Physical changes of puberty reawaken the sexual and aggressive energies felt toward parents during early childhood and repressed during late childhood.
    b. Adolescents need to redirect these urges from parental relationships to nonfamilial relationships and career endeavors.
    c. Separation/detachment from parents is necessary.

C. PSYCHOSOCIAL DEVELOPMENT
  1. MAJOR QUESTIONS TO BE ANSWERED ARE "WHO AM I?" AND "WHAT IS THE UNIQUE PLACE I HAVE IN THE WORLD?"
  2. ERIKSON'S IDENTITY VERSUS ROLE CONFUSION
D. COGNITIVE DEVELOPMENT
  1. PIAGET (FORMAL OPERATIONS)
    a. Abstract thinking
      1) Able to think about the possibilities in the world
      2) Becomes aware of differences between real and ideal world
  2. LANGUAGE DEVELOPMENT
    a. Becomes sophisticated in ability to understand words and abstract concepts
    b. Enjoys puns, satire, metaphors, parodies
  3. SOCIAL PERSPECTIVE TAKING: OCCURS WHEN THE CHILD CAN ASSUME ANOTHER PERSON'S PERSPECTIVE OR VIEWPOINT
  4. ADOLESCENT EGOCENTRISM (UNABLE TO APPROPRIATELY DIFFERENTIATE BETWEEN ONESELF AND THE OBJECTS OF ONE'S ATTENTION)
    a. Imaginary audience (belief of always being on stage)
    b. Personal fable (an exaggerated notion of own uniqueness)
E. MORAL DEVELOPMENT
  1. KOHLBERG'S CONVENTIONAL LEVEL
    a. Acceptance of norms and rules are defined either by close social networks or by more formal governmental system of culture/society.
      1) "Good" boy morality (maintaining good relationships)
      2) Authority-maintaining morality (upholding the law)
F. SPIRITUAL DEVELOPMENT
  1. MAY EXAMINE PARENTAL RELIGIOUS STANDARDS TO DECIDE IF THEY WILL BE INCORPORATED INTO HIS OWN LIFE
  2. EMPHASIZE INTERNAL ASPECTS OF RELIGIOUS COMMITMENT (WHAT IS BELIEVED) RATHER THAN ON ATTENDING CHURCH
G. HEALTH SCREENING
  1. ANNUAL VISITS INCLUDE DEVELOPMENTAL, PSYCHOLOGICAL, AND PHYSIOLOGICAL ASPECTS, AND SHOULD INCLUDE:
    a. Screening
      1) Eating disorders
      2) Sexual activity

3) Alcohol and other drug use
4) Depression
5) Risk for suicide
6) Vision
7) Hearing
   b. Examination of:
      1) Diet
      2) Physical activity
      3) School performance
      4) Vital signs
      5) Height
      6) Weight
      7) UA, HCT, HGB
   c. Testing for:
      1) TB
      2) Cholesterol
      3) HPV
      4) HIV
      5) GC
      6) Chlamydia
      7) Syphilis if sexually active

H. HEALTH PROMOTION
   1. GENERAL NURSING
      INTERACTIONS
      a. Caring, positive relationships
      b. Treat with dignity.
      c. Assess for improving health.
      d. Develop and maintain relationships
         with families.
      e. Know and understand adolescent
         development.
      f. Individualize communication.
      g. Discuss and explain common issues
         (see below).
      h. Be aware of biases impacting care.
   2. IMMUNIZATIONS: HEPB SERIES, MMP,
      TD, VARICELLA
   3. NUTRITION
      a. Increased needs for calories, proteins,
         minerals
         1) Females need 2000 cal/day
         2) Males need 2500–3000 cal/day
      b. Encourage healthy foods, rather than
         snack foods (easy to prepare, faddish,
         full of empty calories).
   4. ELIMINATION: SIMILAR TO ADULTS
   5. HYGIENE
      a. Should be independent
      b. Skin care important related to activity
         of sebaceous and sweat glands
   6. DENTAL HEALTH
      a. Should visit dentist two times
         a year
      b. Most permanent teeth have
         erupted.
      c. Braces may be needed to correct
         malocclusion.
      d. Should brush after eating and floss at
         bedtime
   7. REST AND SLEEP
      a. Needs about 8 hours per night

8. ACTIVITY AND PLAY
   a. Daily exercise
      1) Provides outlet for tension and
         anxiety
      2) Maintains muscle tone and
         development
   b. Contact sports
      1) May be dangerous
      2) Participate in sports according to
         size and ability
9. SAFETY AND INJURY PROMOTION
   a. Leading cause of death and injury
      1) Motor vehicles
      2) Sports
      3) Violence
      4) Suicide

I. ANTICIPATORY GUIDANCE
   1. BODY IMAGE
      a. Few adolescent females satisfied with
         appearance
      b. If unsatisfied with how one looks,
         may be at risk for potentially
         dangerous and life-threatening
         behaviors
   2. NUTRITIONAL ISSUES
      a. Obesity
         1) 11–22% obese or overweight
         2) Causes
            a) Decreased physical activities
            b) High-fat diets
            c) Home environment: parental
               obesity; low family income;
               lower levels of cognitive
               development
            d) May not want to master
               psychosocial and psychosexual
               tasks of adolescence
      b. Anorexia: restricting food intake
      c. Bulimia: eating then purging
   3. CAREGIVER–ADOLESCENT CONFLICT
      a. Rarely about hot topics (sex, drugs,
         religion, politics)
      b. Commonly about everyday family
         matters
         1) School work
         2) Social life
         3) Friends
         4) Home chores
         5) Disagreements with siblings
         6) Disobedience
         7) Personal hygiene
   4. SEXUAL ACTIVITY
      a. Of high school students, 45.6% have
         engaged in sexual activity.
      b. Reasons
         1) Feel grown-up
         2) Enhance self-esteem
         3) Experiment
         4) Be accepted
         5) Have someone care about them
         6) Gain control over life

7) Seek revenge
8) Prove they are "normal"
c. Risks
1) Sexually transmitted diseases (STDs)
2) Pregnancy
5. VIOLENCE
a. Second leading cause of death between 15 and 19 years of age is homicide, with most due to handguns.
b. Adolescents often feel unsafe at school or going to school.
6. SUICIDE
a. Third leading cause of death between 15 and 19 years of age
b. Females more likely to attempt suicide; males more likely to be successful
c. Signs
1) Depression
2) Mood swings

3) Increasing drug and alcohol use
4) Truancy
5) Writing and talking about death
7. DRUG AND ALCOHOL ABUSE
a. Sixteen percent of adolescents between 12 and 17 report illicit drug use.
b. Majority of high school students have tried alcohol.
8. TELEVISION AND MEDIA
a. Relationship between media violence, real-life aggression, and acceptance of aggressive attitudes
b. Relationship between involvement in the Internet and ability to form interpersonal relationships

PRACTICE QUESTIONS

1. Based on an understanding of Erikson's stages of psychosocial development, which of the following is a priority to communicate to the parents of an infant to assist them in meeting the basic needs of infancy?
1. Provide the infant with entertainment and stimulation for psychological growth
2. Talk with the infant during the times when the infant is awake
3. Hold the infant in a way the infant prefers
4. Attend to the infant's need for comfort, security, predictability, food, and warmth

2. The nurse is assessing a toddler's psychosocial developmental level using Erikson's eight stages. Which of the following behaviors would the nurse most likely find if the child were demonstrating being in shame and doubt instead of having mastered autonomy?
1. Dependency and constantly looking to others for approval
2. Sleep disturbance, crying, and vomiting
3. Always imitating others rather than using imagination
4. Frequent crying, emotional outbursts, and whining

3. A nurse is assessing the play of a 4-year-old child. Which of the following best describes what the nurse would observe in the play of a preschooler of this age?
1. Plays alongside but not with playmates, taking toys away from others, using a pounding bench, and playing with a musical toy
2. Interactive play, obeying limits, creating an imaginary friend, and engaging in fantasy play

3. Engaging in group sports and games and playing with puppets
4. Playing alone in the corner, engaged in putting a puzzle together

4. A preschooler knows ramming a tricycle into the garage door at home is not an acceptable behavior but does this at a friend's house. Which of the following statements by the nurse is the most appropriate reason for this difference in behavior at home and at the friend's house?
1. "Preschoolers value their own house more than they value the house of a playmate."
2. "The child's mother is much stricter and supervises children much more closely than does the playmate's mother."
3. "A young preschool child may have difficulty applying known rules to a different situation."
4. "There is a higher level of frustration when outside their own home and play territory."

5. The nurse should instruct the parents of an infant to start feeding solid food at how many months of age? _____

6. The nurse evaluates which of the following gross motor skills in an infant as normal? Select all that apply:
[ ] 1. At 4 months of age, the infant holds the head, chest, and abdomen up with the hands
[ ] 2. At 6 months of age, the infant can sit alone and use the hands for support

[ ] 3. At 8 months of age, the infant begins
          creeping by moving on the hands and
          knees with the abdomen off the floor
[ ] 4. At 1 month of age, the infant turns the
          head to the side while in a prone position
[ ] 5. At 7 months of age, the infant begins to
          roll from the back to the abdomen
[ ] 6. At 4 months of age, the infant can hold
          the head erect with minimal head
          bobbing while sitting

7. The nurse is assessing four newborns and
   evaluates which of the following findings to be
   consistent with physiologic or normal jaundice?
   1. A gradual rise in bilirubin to 8 mg/dl on day
      3 to 5 after birth
   2. A sudden elevation of unconjugated
      bilirubin within the first 24 hours
   3. Unconjugated bilirubin of 14 mg/dl in the
      breastfeeding baby
   4. Jaundice in a 2-week-old, small-weight infant

8. Which of the following should the nurse
   include in the immediate care instructions
   given to the parents of a newborn circumcised
   with a plastic bell?
   1. Gently lift the ring and squeeze warm water
      from a cotton ball onto the tip of the penis
      when changing the diaper
   2. Remove the bell when the baby is awake
      and active and likely to pull on the bell and
      dislodge it
   3. Remove the ring in 5 to 7 days when the
      circumcision is nearly or completely healed
   4. Wash the bell and the penis with hydrogen
      peroxide several times a day

9. The mother of a breast-fed newborn tells the
   nurse that the baby's stool is golden yellow,
   pasty instead of firm, and has a sour milk odor.
   Which of the following would be the best
   response by the nurse?
   1. "You probably need to feed this baby some
      cereal to firm up the stool."
   2. "Cut back on your fluid intake and be
      careful what you eat, as you pass this on to
      the baby."
   3. "I need to check your temperature and your
      breasts to determine if you have a breast
      abscess."
   4. "This is a normal stool for a newborn who is
      breast-fed."

10. A mother tells the nurse that her 6-month-old
    child is grasping things such as a spoon in the
    palms and asks when the child will be able to
    grasp a spoon between the thumb and fingers.
    The appropriate response by the nurse would
    be which of the following?
    1. "This is normal for this age. The pincer
       grasp isn't mastered until 8 months."

    2. "Encourage your child to play with an older
       child who uses the pincer grasp and your child
       will pick up the skill from the other child."
    3. "Begin teaching your baby to use the pincer
       grasp. It will take time."
    4. "I will ask your physician about doing
       developmental testing to evaluate your
       baby's level of development."

11. A mother expresses concern because her infant
    is walking sideways while holding onto
    furniture. Which of the following is the
    appropriate statement the nurse should make
    to this mother?
    1. "You may want to consider a neurological
       evaluation to rule out a pathological cause
       for this behavior."
    2. "If you will hold the baby's hands while
       the baby walks, you can break the baby of
       this habit."
    3. "Infants start walking sideways while
       holding onto furniture before walking or
       standing alone."
    4. "You need to make an appointment with
       your pediatrician and have this problem
       checked out."

12. Which of the following should the nurse
    include when preparing to teach a class on
    the introduction of new foods during the first
    year of life?
    1. Place up to three foods on the spoon at one
       time with an old favorite on the front of the
       spoon
    2. Introduce fruits first; introduce one new
       fruit per day until all fruits are introduced
    3. Alternate between offering one spoonful of
       fruits and one spoonful of vegetables
    4. Introduce one new food at a time at 7-day
       intervals

13. The nurse evaluates which of the following four
    infants to have an abnormal language
    development?
    1. A 9-month-old who uses two-syllable
       sounds such as "dada"
    2. A 7-month-old who is beginning to vocalize
       during play and pleasure
    3. A 2-month-old who begins vocalizing in the
       presence of familiar sounds
    4. An 11-month-old who uses intentional
       gestures

14. The nurse is instructing the parents of a toddler
    on the development of depth perception. Which
    of the following should the nurse instruct the
    parents to watch for?
    1. An increased fear of heights and of falling
       out of bed at night
    2. An unusual sense of dizziness that is
       experienced at times

3. A difficulty in learning to swim
4. An increased fall risk when the toddler is learning to walk, run, and climb stairs

15. Which of the following is the most age-appropriate explanation the nurse should give a toddler who is to take medication every morning for 7 days?
    1. "Your mommy will give you the medicine between 8:00 and 9:00 a.m. each morning until it is gone."
    2. "You will be taking your medicine every morning after breakfast until it is gone."
    3. "For a week you will be taking your medicine in the early morning."
    4. "Your mommy will give you your medicine every day by 9:00 a.m. until it is gone."

16. A mother tells the nurse about being frustrated by the toddler saying "no" to everything said. Which of the following statements by the nurse would be most helpful to the mother?
    1. "Reword every question so your child will eventually say 'yes.'"
    2. "This is an expression of your child's search for autonomy that will disappear at 30 months of age."
    3. "Walk away from your child when 'no' is said and pay attention when 'yes' is said so the behavior can be modified."
    4. "Start telling your child 'no' whenever something is asked for so your child will understand that negativity is not rewarding."

17. A couple is expecting their new baby any day and both are concerned their 2-year-old will have problems accepting a new sister or brother. Which of the following statements by the parents would indicate they have acted on the teaching the nurse offered to help the toddler to deal with the birth of the sibling?
    1. "We started toilet training this week and, hopefully, will have our 2-year-old trained by the time the baby is born."
    2. "We told the 2-year-old that a brother or sister will be a new playmate."
    3. "The grandparents have been keeping our 2-year-old frequently."
    4. "The 2-year-old was moved out of the nursery this week so we could prepare for the baby."

18. A mother is expressing concern to the nurse that her 5-year-old occasionally is urinating in the underwear instead of going to the bathroom. Which of the following questions is the priority for the nurse to ask to determine if this is a normal occurrence?
    1. "Do you remind your child to go to the bathroom every 2 hours?"

2. "Is this your firstborn child?"
3. "Has your child started school already?"
4. "Does this behavior occur when your child is engaged in some activity?"

19. A mother is concerned about her preschool-age child running into the street without looking. Which of the following instructions would be the priority for the nurse to give this mother?
    1. Offer verbal reminders to look before crossing the street
    2. Punishment is essential to prevent this behavior
    3. Prevent the child from crossing the street without the parent
    4. Children this age seldom run into the street without looking, unless distracted

20. Which of the following should the nurse include when instructing a mother to administer vitamins to a preschooler?
    1. Give the vitamins with sips of milk
    2. Give preschoolers half a vitamin
    3. Store the vitamins in a locked cabinet that the child cannot access
    4. Allow the child to be independent by self-administering the vitamins

21. Which of the following statements by the parents of a preschooler would indicate that the parents had implemented the nurse's instructions on dental hygiene practices?
    1. "Our child brushes the teeth without any help from us."
    2. "We give our child a pea-sized amount of fluoride toothpaste."
    3. "When our child is 6 years old, we will make an appointment to see the dentist."
    4. "When our child does a good job brushing, we offer a lollipop."

22. The nurse caring for preschoolers in a day care center will find which of the following problems to be more common at this age than at any other?
    1. Appendicitis and tonsillitis requiring day surgeries or 1-day hospitalization
    2. Accidents, cuts, bruises, and major traumas requiring emergency room care
    3. Poisoning with lead, plants, household chemicals, and other sources
    4. Minor illnesses such as colds, otitis media, and GI disturbances

23. Based on the growth and development of adolescent girls, the school nurse understands which of the following is the priority regarding body image?
    1. Most girls are satisfied with their physical appearance
    2. Few girls are satisfied with their physical appearance

3. The majority of girls think they are too thin
4. Girls are only concerned with the abdomen and hips

24. An adolescent tells the parents that refusing to go to school on a particular day doesn't have anything to do with not having anything appropriate to wear and having a "zit" (skin eruption) on the face. The nurse explains to the parents that this behavior exemplifies which of the following concepts?
    1. Imaginary audience
    2. Extreme and diagnosable narcissism
    3. Adolescent instability of emotions
    4. Disrespect for the school system

25. The nurse is teaching a class of adolescents to improve their diets. Which of the following approaches would be most helpful in achieving this goal?
    1. Send dietary information to the parents of the adolescents
    2. Have the adolescents get involved in meal planning after receiving information on dietary needs
    3. Show a film on dietary needs and what happens to the body if those needs are not met
    4. Conduct a series of lectures by a variety of health specialists on dietary needs of the adolescent

26. The registered nurse is preparing the clinical assignments for a pediatric unit. Which of the following assignments may the nurse delegate to a licensed practical nurse?
    1. Evaluate the growth and development of a preschooler
    2. Monitor the play activity of a toddler
    3. Assist a toddler in walking
    4. Instruct the parents on the dietary requirements of a school-age child

27. The nurse identifies which of the following as a characteristic of defecation in toddlers?
    1. Control of defecation normally begins after 3 years of age
    2. Toddlers frequently delay defecation because of play
    3. Constipation is a common problem among toddlers
    4. Control of defecation starts between 1 and 2 years of age

ANSWERS AND RATIONALES

1. 4. During infancy, trust is developing, which means that the infant's basic needs must consistently be met by reliable, nurturing caregivers, usually the parents. If these needs are not met, there is a danger that mistrust will occur.

2. 1. Autonomy versus shame and doubt is Erikson's stage for toddlers. Autonomy develops as children discover their new mental and physical abilities while improving language and motor skills and learning competencies related to independence (bathing, eating, toileting). Doubt occurs if children learn to mistrust not only themselves but also the immediate environment. Children demonstrating dependency and constantly needing approval for their actions have not resolved this conflict.

3. 2. Preschool age is an age group that follows toddlerhood and includes children between 3 and 6 years of age. Preschoolers enjoy group play and engage in imitative, dramatic, and imaginative play. They are becoming more tolerant of playmates, may have an imaginary friend, and enjoy activities that include memory games, construction toys, puzzles, books, art, and fantasy play.

4. 3. Preschool children are in the preconventional level of moral development. They are learning to conform their behavior to the expectations of others, but are not able to transfer reasons for their behavior to a different situation or environment, especially when the person rewarding them for good behavior is not always around.

5. 4–6. Semisolid single-grain infant cereal and applesauce should be introduced between 4 and 6 months of age.

6. 2. 3. 4. It is normal for an infant at 6 months of age to sit alone and use the hands for support. It is also normal for an 8-month-old infant to begin creeping, and a 1-month-old infant in the prone position to turn the head from side to side. It is not until 5 or 6 months of age that the infant begins to hold the head, chest, and abdomen up by bearing weight with the hands. It is also abnormal for an infant 7 months of age to just start to roll from the back to the abdomen. This is a skill that starts at 2 to 3 months. A 2-month-old infant begins to hold the head with minimal head bobbing.

7. 1. Physiologic or normal jaundice shows a gradual rise in bilirubin of 8 mg/dl at 3 to 5 days after

birth. The level falls to normal the second week of life. If the unconjugated level is greater than 12 mg/dl when the baby is formula-fed, greater than 14 mg/dl if the baby is breast-fed, or if the jaundice is persistent past 2 weeks of age, further evaluation is warranted.

8. 1. The immediate care of the circumcised newborn is dependent on the procedure performed. If the plastic bell was utilized, it is left on the penis. Gently lift the ring and squeeze warm water from a cotton ball onto the tip of the penis when changing the diaper. The ring will fall off in 7 to 10 days when the circumcision has healed.

9. 4. Transition stools of the newborn are green-brown to yellow-brown in color. They occur by the third day. Breast-fed infants' stool is yellow to golden, pasty, and has a sour milk odor. Formula-fed newborns' stool is pale to light yellow, firmer than the stool of a breast-fed infant, and has a strong odor.

10. 1. During the first month of life, a primitive grasp reflex enables the infant to hold objects with a tightly clenched fist. By the end of 2 months, this primitive reflex fades and the infant begins to actively grasp and momentarily hold an object before dropping it. At 3 months of age, the infant has the ability to hold the hand open, look at the fingers, and place them in the mouth. By 5 months, the infant can voluntarily grasp an object with the whole hand (palmar grasp) and can actively manipulate all grasped objects and place them in the mouth. Between 6 and 7 months, the infant can hold a bottle securely and willingly drop any grasped object. The palmar grasp is replaced with a thumb-and-finger pincer grasp at approximately 8 months.

11. 3. From 10 to 12 months, infant locomotion progresses rapidly. During this time, infants will take deliberate steps while holding onto something and will walk sideways while holding onto furniture before walking or standing alone. Once infants can stand alone, they will attempt to take a few steps alone.

12. 4. Due to the potential for an allergic reaction during the infant's first year of life, new foods should be introduced one at a time at 7-day intervals between each new food, so if the infant is allergic to the new food, it will be apparent. Generally, rice cereal is introduced first because it is least likely to cause allergies. Vegetables are offered next, followed by fruits. Vegetables are started before fruits to avoid getting the infant accustomed to the sweet taste.

13. 2. It is abnormal for a 7-month-old infant to start vocalizing during play and pleasure. This is a language skill that normally develops between 3 and 6 months.

14. 4. Before depth perception is fully developed, toddlers will have no sense of distance and may not realize how far away the floor is when learning to walk, run, and climb.

15. 2. Children of this age do not have the cognitive ability to understand explanations and are better able to understand time when it is associated with a familiar activity.

16. 2. Toddlers often resent being given directions or not being allowed to explore what they desire in an expanding environment. Often toddlers will delight in doing the opposite of what is asked and frequently respond "no" to requests.

17. 3. Sibling rivalry often arises when an infant is born into a family with a toddler. The arrival of the new baby can be devastating to toddlers because they now must compete for a caregiver's attention. One way to help toddlers is to have them stay with other family members who will be caring for them when the mother is in the hospital having the new baby. Grandparents are often these family members.

18. 4. It is not uncommon for preschoolers to become so engaged in their play or other interesting activities that they do not realize they need to go to the bathroom.

19. 1. Preschoolers have the cognitive ability to understand directions and the consequences of their behavior. However, to help them remember to behave in a certain way, they often need to be reminded.

20. 3. Multivitamins for children often taste like candy. Because preschoolers like the taste of these vitamins, they may be tempted to take more pills than needed unless the pills are stored in a locked cabinet the child has difficulty accessing.

21. 2. Toothpaste often contains fluoride, and young children are in danger of receiving too much.

22. 4. Common illnesses of the preschool years include mostly minor illnesses, such as otitis media, colds, or gastrointestinal disturbances. In fact, minor illnesses are more common during this time than at any other time in life because this is the age at which children start playing together more frequently, attend child care, or start preschool activities and thus have greater exposure to illness.

23. 2. Body image, or the mental conception of one's physical appearance, varies with maturation and changes across time, situations, and experiences one has with others. Adolescent females are more dissatisfied with their appearance and more likely to be concerned about particular parts of their bodies than are their male counterparts.

24. 1. The imaginary audience refers to the adolescent's belief of always being on stage and that others are always aware of the adolescent's physical appearance.

25. 2. Adolescents always seem hungry but often do not eat appropriately. Instead they prefer snack foods that are easy to prepare, faddish, and full of empty calories. Adolescent food habits are influenced by concerns about body image, peer pressure, emotional problems, busy schedules, and unsupervised meal preparation or purchase. They also may skip meals, eat fast foods, or snack frequently. The best way to help adolescents improve their nutrition is to explain the importance of a good diet and encourage adolescents to become involved in meal planning.

26. 3. Clinical assignments such as skills that involve evaluation, monitoring, and instructing are activities of the registered nurse. A licensed practical nurse may assist a toddler in walking.

27. 4. Control of defecation generally starts in toddlers between 1 and 2 years of age. Preschoolers, between 3 and 6 years of age, frequently delay defecation because of play and may experience constipation.

REFERENCES

Potts, N., & Mandleco, B. (2012). *Pediatric nursing: Caring for children and their families* (3rd ed.). Clifton Park, NY: Delmar Cengage Learning.

Spratto, G. R., & Woods, A. L. (2012). *PDR nurse's drug handbook 2012*. Clifton Park: NY: Delmar Cengage Learning.

CHAPTER 30

EYES, EARS, NOSE, AND THROAT DISORDERS

I. ANATOMY AND PHYSIOLOGY (SEE CHAPTER 2)

A. DIFFERENCES IN THE EYE AND EAR BETWEEN THE CHILD AND ADULT
  1. NYSTAGMUS IS COMMON IN THE INFANT.
  2. BINOCULAR VISION OCCURS AT 4 MONTHS OF AGE.
  3. STRABISMUS MAY OCCUR UP TO 6 MONTHS OF AGE (CONSIDERED ABNORMAL AFTER 6 MONTHS OF AGE).
  4. EYE MUSCLES DO NOT MATURE AT 1 YEAR OF AGE.
  5. VISUAL ACUITY THROUGH THE FIRST 4 YEARS OF LIFE:
     a. 16 weeks: 20/50 to 20/100
     b. 1 year: 20/50 or more
     c. 2 years: 20/40
     d. 3 years: 20/30
     e. 4 years: reaches adulthood level of 20/20
  6. HEARING IS COMPLETELY DEVELOPED AT BIRTH.
  7. EAR STRUCTURES THAT ARE ABNORMAL AT BIRTH MAY BE DUE TO A GENETIC DEFECT.

II. ASSESSMENT

A. HEALTH HISTORY
  1. PAST HEALTH HISTORY
     a. Eye specific: conjunctivitis, congenital problems, visual defects, headaches, difficulty reading
     b. Ear specific: acute otitis media, serous otitis media, acute otitis externa, hearing deficit, speech development
     c. Nose specific: polyps, sinus infection, septal deviation, allergic rhinitis
     d. Mouth and throat specific: tonsillitis, herpes simplex virus, strep throat, tonsillar abscess, caries, *Candida*

infections, frequent upper respiratory infection (URI), tooth eruption, baby bottle tooth decay
     e. Chronic illness: asthma, cystic fibrosis, congenital heart disease, eczema
  2. SURGICAL: TONSILLECTOMY, ADENOIDECTOMY, REPAIR OF SEPTAL DEVIATION, TYMPANOSTOMY TUBE PLACEMENT, NEUROSURGERY, TUMOR REMOVAL, FOREIGN BODY REMOVAL, EYE SURGERY
  3. ALLERGIES
     a. Pollen: sneezing; nasal congestion; watery or itchy eyes, or both; cough
     b. Insect stings: swelling of the throat and around the eyes
     c. Animal dander: sneezing; nasal congestion; watery or itchy eyes, or both
  4. SOCIAL HISTORY
     a. Smoke exposure
     b. Day care

B. PHYSICAL EXAM
  1. INSPECTION
     a. Head
        1) Symmetry
        2) Shape
        3) Size
     b. Scalp
        1) Hair distribution
        2) Lesions
        3) Suture ridging
        4) Fontanels
     c. Eye
        1) External structures: alignment, lesions, discharge, color, edema
        2) Internal structures
           a) Ophthalmoscopic exam
        3) Visual fields (extraocular muscle movements)
        4) Corneal light reflex
        5) Pupillary light response

6) Red reflex
7) Cross-uncover test
8) Vision screen
   a) Snellen eye charts
d. Ear
   1) External structures: alignment, lesions
   2) Internal structures
      a) Otoscopic exam
      b) Tympanic membrane: color, mobility, landmarks, and light reflex
   3) Hearing (see Table 30-1)
      a) Voice-whisper test
      b) Startle reflex test (in infants)
      c) Weber test
      d) Rinne test
      e) Audiogram
e. Nose
   1) External structures
      a) Patency of nares
   2) Internal structures: color, discharge, quantity and characteristics of discharge, edema, position of structures, lesions, polyps
f. Sinuses
   1) Observe for facial swelling.
g. Mouth
   1) Lips: color, lesions, moisture, swelling
   2) Oral mucosa: color, hydration, amount and characteristics of

saliva, lesions, dentition, breath odor, inflammation, Stenson's ducts
   3) Tongue: color, hydration, texture, symmetry, lesions, fasciculations, position in the mouth, frenulum, movement
   4) Teeth: number, position, malocclusion, caries
   5) Palate: lesions, color, petechiae
h. Throat: position, size, color and general appearance of the tonsils and adenoids
2. PERCUSSION
   a. Sinuses: dullness indicative of sinuses filled with fluid/cells resulting from infection, allergic process, or congenital absence of sinus
3. PALPATION
   a. Head: suture lines, fontanels, lesions
   b. Eye: check lacrimal sac for obstruction.
   c. Ear: auricle, mastoid tip, tragus: check for tenderness with movement.
   d. Sinuses: apply gentle pressure over the sinuses under the bony ridges of the orbit to assess for pain.
   e. Mouth: lips and palate: check for lesions, tone, intact structures.

III. **DIAGNOSTIC STUDIES**
   A. VISION TESTING
      1. SNELLEN ALPHABET CHART
         a. Description: visual acuity is checked at 20 feet; letters are presented in a linear fashion.
         b. Procedure
            1) Position child 20 feet from the chart.
            2) Test one eye at a time.
            3) Determine the smallest line in which the child can read all the letters for each eye (must read all letters correctly above 20/40; may miss two letters on lines 20/20 and 20/30 and still receive a pass for the line).
         c. Interpretation
            1) Determine visual acuity.
            2) Numerator indicates the distance of the child from the chart.
            3) Denominator indicates the distance at which a normal eye can read the line.
            4) Passing is 20/30 or better before the age of 6, 20/20 after the age of 6 years.
      2. HOTV CHART
         a. Description: substitute for the Snellen alphabet chart if the child does not know the alphabet.

Table 30-1 Milestones of Normal Hearing Development

Age	Hearing
Birth to 3 months	Soothed by parent's voice Gives a startled response to loud sudden noises
3 to 6 months	Looks to see where sounds come from Becomes frightened by an angry voice Smiles when spoken to Wakes up when spoken to or when a loud noise is made nearby
6 to 12 months	Stops for a minute when someone says "no-no," "bye-bye," and own name Looks at objects or pictures when someone talks about them Enjoys rattle and similar toys for their sounds
12 to 18 months	Sings and hums spontaneously Discriminates between sounds such as doorbell, telephone, barking dog, and so forth "Dances" and makes sounds to music
18 to 24 months	Brings objects to others when asked Hears and identifies sounds coming from another room

    b. Procedure
        1) Position the child 10 feet from the chart.
        2) Place a matching card on the child's lap.
        3) Screen one eye at a time.
        4) Ask the child to point to the matching symbol on the lap chart as the examiner points to the symbol on the wall chart.
        5) Determine the smallest line in which the child can match the four symbols for each eye.
    c. Interpretation
        1) Kindergarten: pass is 10/15 or better in each eye without a two-line difference.
        2) Preschool: pass is 10/20 or better for each eye without a two-line difference.

3. COLOR VISION
    a. Description
        1) Ishihara-Pseudo-Isochromatic book of color plates is used to check for color vision deficiency.
        2) Usually test 4th-grade boys
    b. Procedure
        1) Position the book at a normal reading distance from the eyes away from glare.
        2) Instruct the child to read the numbers on each page carefully.
    c. Interpretation
        1) Pass: able to read all the numbers correctly on the numbered plates; unable to read a number on the last of these plates

4. HIRSCHBERG TEST (CORNEAL LIGHT REFLEX)
    a. Description: tests for alignment, may be done at any age
    b. Procedure
        1) Shine a light into the child's eyes from a distance of 12–16 inches.
        2) Observe the position of the light reflection on each cornea.
        3) It is helpful to perform this test in a darkened room when evaluating a very young infant.
    c. Interpretation
        1) Light should fall symmetrically on each pupil; asymmetric light reflexes indicate malalignment.
        2) Twin red reflexes should be observed.
        3) Consistent eye alignment should be observed between 4 and 6 months of age.

5. COVER TEST
    a. Description: a test for malalignment of the eyes
    b. Procedure
        1) Position the child 12–14 inches from an object held in front of her eyes by the examiner.
        2) Request the child to focus on the object with both eyes.
        3) Cover the right eye.
        4) Observe for movement in the uncovered (left) eye.
        5) Repeat the procedure, covering the left eye and observing for movement in right eye.
        6) Repeat the procedure for each eye at a distance of 20 inches.
    c. Interpretation
        1) Movement in the uncovered eye indicates malalignment.
        2) No movement in the uncovered eye indicates the eyes are aligned.

6. UNCOVER OR CROSS-COVER TEST
    a. Description: a test for malalignment of the eyes
    b. Procedure
        1) Position the child 12–14 inches from an object held by the examiner at eye level.
        2) Request that the child focus on the object with both eyes.
        3) Cover the right eye for a count of ≈ 3, then quickly cross over the bridge of the nose to the left eye and cover.
        4) Observe for movement in the right eye as it is uncovered.
        5) Repeat the procedure covering first the left eye and observing for movement as it is uncovered.
        6) Repeat the procedure two to three times on each side.
    c. Interpretation
        1) Movement in the eye that is covered as it is uncovered indicates malalignment.
        2) No movement in the covered eye as it is uncovered indicates the eyes are aligned.

B. AUDITORY TESTING
  1. EVOKED OTOACOUSTIC EMISSIONS (OAES)
    a. Description
        1) OAE analyzer delivers a quick series of clicks to the ear through a probe on the end of which is a tympanometry tip that is inserted into the external auditory canal of the neonate.
        2) Preferred method of screening newborn infants for sensorineural hearing loss

3) Requires specialized equipment and some training

4) A follow-up brainstem auditory evoked response (BAER) test is recommended because results do not indicate the severity of cochlear damage.

b. Preprocedure

1) Infants must be in a quiet sleep for testing.

2. BAER TEST

a. Description

1) Electrode wires attached to the infant's scalp transmit brain wave potentials from the auditory system to a computer for analysis.

2) Requires expensive equipment and specialized training of personnel

3) Normal results show a specific pattern of peaks and troughs that is reflective of the activation of cerebral neural structures.

b. Preprocedure

1) Infant must be sleeping or quiet.

3. AUDIOMETRY

a. Description

1) Measures the threshold of hearing for pure tone frequencies and loudness

2) Provides information regarding the severity of the hearing loss, the sound cycles involved, and the possible location of the defect

3) Air conduction audiogram: sound is transmitted through earphones.

4) Bone conduction audiogram: sound is transmitted through a plaque positioned over the mastoid bone.

5) Pure tone screening: child listens to a series of pure tones and the examiner notes whether there was a response to each one and identifies children with suspected hearing loss.

b. Preprocedure for pure tone screening

1) Requires cooperation from the child

2) Seat the child so the front of the audiometer cannot be seen.

3) Remove glasses, large earrings, or hair bands and put on earphones.

4) Instruct the child to raise either hand when a tone is heard.

c. Procedure

1) A sound is transmitted to the child's ear and reduced until the child indicates that the sound is no longer heard.

2) The procedure is repeated for several sounds, covering the range found in conversation.

3) Set the selector switch to the right to test the right ear.

4) Present 1000-Hz tone at 40 db (decibels) first to establish procedure then decrease to 20 db for tones 1000 Hz, 2000 Hz, and 4000 Hz on the right ear.

5) Turn the selector switch to the left to test the left ear.

6) Present tones of 4000 Hz, 2000 Hz, and 1000 Hz at 20 db on the left ear.

7) Turn frequency tone to 500 Hz at 25 db and present tone to the left ear.

8) Repeat on the right ear.

9) Recheck immediately if the child does not hear one or more tones. Increase by increments of 5 db until tone is heard to establish threshold.

10) Record on the screening form. Child should be able to hear pure tones of 1000–4000 Hz at 20 db and 500 Hz at 25 db.

11) Play audiometry can be used for children from 24 months to 5 years of age.

12) Requires specialized training and equipment

d. Postprocedure

1) Notify the physician if the child fails the screen.

4. TYMPANOMETRY

a. Description

1) Measures the mobility of the tympanic membrane and estimates middle ear air pressure

2) Can detect middle ear disease and abnormalities

3) Does not measure the degree of hearing loss or the interpretation of sound

b. Preprocedure

1) Requires cooperation of the child

2) Not useful in children less than 7 months because their ear canals are hypercompliant

c. Procedure

1) A soft rubber tip is placed over the external canal to produce an airtight seal.

    2) An automatic reading of air pressure registers on the machine.

5. PNEUMATIC OTOSCOPY

  a. Description: visual assessment of tympanic membrane mobility

  b. Preprocedure

    1) Requires stabilization of the child by a parent or the examiner to ensure an airtight seal with the speculum and otoscope

    2) Useful at all ages

    3) To best visualize the ear in a child under age 3 years, pull the earlobe down and back to straighten the ear canal; for a child older than age 3 years pull it up and back.

  c. Procedure

    1) Using an insufflator attached to the otoscope, a small tuft of air is blown into the ear canal toward the tympanic membrane while maintaining an airtight seal at the auditory meatus.

  d. Interpretation

    1) Brisk movement of the tympanic membrane indicates normal mobility.

    2) Altered movement of the tympanic membrane indicates impaired mobility resulting from middle ear pathology such as otitis media with effusion or tympanic membrane perforation.

C. LABORATORY TESTING

  1. THROAT CULTURE

    a. Description

      1) Rapid identification of group A beta hemolytic streptococcus (GABHS)

        a) Rapid immunologic test with antiserum against group A streptococcus antigen

      2) Standard culture (24 hour)

        a) May be used as backup culture for rapid strep test

    b. Preprocedure

      1) Explain the procedure to the client.

    c. Procedure

      1) Collect all cultures before antibiotic administration.

      2) Depress the tongue with a wooden tongue blade.

      3) Swab the posterior wall of the throat and areas of inflammation, exudation, or ulceration with a sterile cotton swab (two swabs if doing a rapid strep test and a backup throat culture).

    4) Avoid touching any part of the mouth.

    5) Place swabs in a sterile container.

  d. Postprocedure

    1) Label all specimens with the name, date, and source, and send to the lab.

    2) Notify the physician of positive results.

2. NASAL AND NASOPHARYNGEAL CULTURE

  a. Description

    1) Done to screen for infections and carrier states caused by various other organisms (*Staphylococcus aureus, Haemophilus influenzae, Neisseria meningitides,* respiratory syncytial virus)

    2) Done to detect infection in debilitated clients

  b. Preprocedure

    1) Explain the procedure to the client.

  c. Procedure

    1) Gently raise the tip of the nose and insert a flexible swab into the nares.

    2) Rotate the swab against the side of the nares.

    3) Remove the swab and place in an appropriate culture tube.

  d. Postprocedure

    1) Label all specimens and send to the lab.

    2) Notify the physician of positive results.

3. EYE CULTURE (CONJUNCTIVITIS)

  a. Description

    1) Conjunctival swab or smear of eye lesion or discharge, or both

    2) *Chlamydia* cultures in the neonate may require special handling and collection dependent on the lab.

  b. Preprocedure

    1) Explain the procedure.

    2) Requires the child's cooperation or immobilization, or both

  c. Procedure

    1) Swab the eye lesion with a sterile cotton-tipped swab or scrape with a sterile ophthalmic spatula.

    2) Smear on a clean glass slide or place in an appropriate culture tube.

  d. Postprocedure

    1) Label all specimens and send to the lab.

    2) Notify the physician of positive results.

4. ALLERGY TESTING
   a. Description
      1) Blood
         a) IgE antibody test: serum IgE increases in response to exposure to allergen.
         b) Radioallergosorbent test (RAST): a method of measuring IgE in which serum from the client is mixed with a specific allergen
         c) Presents less risk to the client more expensive
      2) Skin
         a) Prick-puncture test: allergen is injected into the epidermis.
         b) Intradermal test: allergen is injected into dermis; risk of local reaction or anaphylaxis.
   b. Preprocedure
      1) Blood
         a) Explain the procedure to the client and family.
         b) Remind the client that she will not experience any allergic reaction by this method of testing.
         c) Determine if the client has recently been treated with corticosteroid for allergy (increase levels of IgE).
      2) Skin
         a) Explain the procedure to the client and family.
         b) Observe skin testing precautions: emergency drugs and equipment available, physician on site, avoid spreading the allergen solutions during testing, record the skin reaction at the proper time, avoid bleeding due to injection, use caution if the client currently has allergic manifestations.
         c) Obtain a history to evaluate the risk of anaphylaxis (previous reactions and severity of response).
         d) Evaluate the client for dermographism (rub the skin with a pencil eraser and look for wheal development at the site). Positive response may predispose the client to false-positive results on the allergy skin test.
         e) Draw up aqueous epinephrine (0.05 ml of 1:1000) into a syringe to have

on hand in case of a pronounced allergic reaction.
         f) A negative prick-puncture test should be performed prior to an intradermal test.
   c. Procedure
      1) Cutaneous scratch or prick
      2) Intracutaneous infection
   d. Postprocedure
      1) Blood
         a) Apply pressure to the venipuncture site.
      2) Skin
         a) Assess the client for exaggerated allergic reaction.
         b) In the event of a systemic reaction, notify the physician immediately, place a tourniquet above the testing site, and administer epinephrine subcutaneously as prescribed by the physician.
         c) Circle the area of testing and note the allergen used.
         d) Read the skin test at the appropriate time (usually 15–20 minutes), measuring both the smallest and largest wheals as well as the flares in millimeters; average the measurements.
         e) Observe the client for 20–30 minutes before discharge.

D. RADIOGRAPHIC STUDIES
   1. SINUS STUDIES
      a. X-rays
         1) Description
            a) Water's view: x-ray done with the head tipped back; used to evaluate the maxillary sinuses
            b) Frontal view: frontal skull x-ray used to evaluate the frontal and ethmoid sinuses
            c) Useful if there is no response to antibiotic therapy
            d) Sinuses are not well developed or air filled until ages 4–6 years.
         2) Preprocedure
            a) Explain the procedure to the parent and child.
            b) Protect the child (reproductive organs) with a lead shield.
            c) NPO is not required.
         3) Procedure
            a) Requires child cooperation
         4) Postprocedure
            a) Notify the physician of findings.

2. COMPUTERIZED TOMOGRAPHY (CT) SCAN
   a. Description
      1) Series of rotational x-rays, each representing a cross section of facial bones and sinuses
      2) Useful in evaluation of complicated acute sinusitis, recurrent acute sinusitis, chronic sinusitis, and suspicion of sinus malignancy
      3) Superior to plain radiography and magnetic resonance imaging (MRI) in evaluating the paranasal sinuses, the mastoid sinuses, and the adjacent bones
   b. Preprocedure
      1) Administer drugs for relaxation and sedation as prescribed.
      2) Instruct the parent and child on the test.
      3) NPO for 4 hours before the procedure (in case contrast media used).
      4) Requires immobilization
   c. Postprocedure
      1) Encourage fluids if contrast is used.
E. THERAPEUTIC PROCEDURES
   1. MYRINGOTOMY WITH INSERTION OF PRESSURE-EQUALIZING (PE) TUBES
      a. Description
         1) Opening is made into the tympanic membrane and a small plastic spool-shaped tube is placed in the anteroinferior quadrant of the tympanic membrane.
         2) Relieves pressure and drains accumulated fluid in the middle ear
         3) Recommended after 4–6 months of bilateral otitis media with effusion, bilateral hearing loss, speech delay, recurrent otitis (OM) or severe eustachian tube dysfunction
         4) Also referred to as tympanostomy
      b. Preprocedure
         1) NPO is required after midnight.
         2) Instruct the parent and child on the procedure and need for anesthesia.
         3) Administer medications for relaxation and sedation as prescribed.
         4) Initiate intravenous access.
      c. Postprocedure
         1) Monitor vital signs.
         2) Monitor respiratory and cardiovascular status.
         3) Monitor level of consciousness and activity.
         4) Assess the surgical site for drainage.
      d. Nursing interventions
         1) Inform the parent and child that most tubes will fall out within 1 year and tubes should be removed at 2 years.
         2) Instruct the parent and child that diving, jumping, and submerging should be avoided and that bathwater and shampoo should be kept out of the ears; earplugs are recommended for these activities.
         3) Inform the parent that a sign of bacterial ear infection in child with PE tubes is otorrhea.
         4) Instruct the parent that the child should obtain follow-up every 6–12 months following the insertion of the tubes.

IV. **NURSING DIAGNOSIS**
   A. ACUTE OR CHRONIC PAIN
   B. INEFFECTIVE HEALTH MAINTENANCE
   C. RISK FOR INJURY
   D. DISTURBED SENSORY PERCEPTION
   E. ANXIETY
   Nursing Diagnoses: Definitions and Classification 2012–2014. Copyright © 2012, 1994–2012 by NANDA International. Used by arrangement with John Wiley & Sons Limited.

V. **DISORDERS OF THE EYE**
   A. STRABISMUS
      1. DESCRIPTION
         a. Malalignment of the eyes; may be referred to as "squint or cross-eyes"
            1) Types
               a) Esotropia is an inward deviation of the eye.
               b) Exotropia is an outward deviation of the eye.
            2) Etiology
               a) Muscle paralysis or imbalance
               b) Poor vision
               c) Congenital defect
            3) Complications
               a) Amblyopia (permanent vision loss) can result if not treated before the age of 6 years.
      2. ASSESSMENT
         a. Frowns or squints
         b. Difficulty accommodating (switching focus from one distance to another)
         c. Impaired judgment in picking up objects
         d. Fails to see print or moving objects clearly
         e. Closes one eye to see or tilts head to one side to see

      f. Diplopia (double vision)
      g. Photophobia (light sensitivity)
      h. Headache and fatigue
      i. Dizziness
      j. Cross-eye
      k. Unequal corneal light reflexes
      l. Positive cover test or uncover test

3. DIAGNOSTIC TESTING
      a. Hirschberg test (corneal light reflex)
      b. Cover test
      c. Uncover or cross-cover test

4. NURSING INTERVENTIONS
      a. Depends on the cause of the strabismus
      b. Perform occlusion therapy by patching the stronger eye.
      c. Surgery to increase visual stimulation to the weaker eye.
      d. Encourage early diagnosis to prevent vision loss.

B. REFRACTIVE ERRORS

    1. MYOPIA (NEARSIGHTEDNESS)
      a. Description
        1) Able to see clearly objects that are near but not objects that are at a distance
        2) Caused by elongated eyeball, which results in the image falling in front of the retina
      b. Assessment
        1) Difficulty reading or doing other close work
        2) May rub eyes excessively
        3) Reading materials held close to the eyes
        4) Positions head close to the table when writing or coloring
        5) Unsteady, may walk into objects
        6) May blink more than usual
        7) Fails to see objects clearly
        8) Dizziness, headache
        9) May experience nausea or irritability when doing close work
        10) May experience difficulty in school
      c. Diagnostic testing
        1) Snellen eye chart visual acuity testing
          a) Test with corrective lenses if history of refractive errors
        2) Assist with referral to an ophthalmologist or optometrist as ordered
      d. Nursing interventions
        1) Fit with biconcave lenses that focus rays on the retina to correct vision.

    2. HYPEROPIA (FARSIGHTEDNESS)
      a. Description
        1) The ability to see objects at a distance better than those that are close

        2) Caused by shortened eyeball, which results in the image falling beyond the retina
        3) Hyperopia is normal until age 7 years.
      b. Assessment
        1) A child may be able to see objects at all distances due to accommodative ability.
      c. Nursing interventions
        1) Fit with convex lens to focus rays on the retina if correction is required (correction is usually not required under the age of 7 years).
        2) Assist with referral to an ophthalmologist or optometrist as ordered.

    3. ASTIGMATISM
      a. Description
        1) Unequal curvatures in refraction
        2) Caused by unequal curvatures in the cornea or lens, resulting in light rays bending in different directions
      b. Assessment
        1) May show clinical manifestations similar to myopia, extent of which is dependent on the degree of refractive error
      c. Diagnostic testing
        1) Snellen eye chart visual acuity testing
      d. Nursing interventions
        1) Fit with lenses that compensate for refractive errors.
        2) Assist with referral to an ophthalmologist or optometrist as ordered.

    4. ANISOMETROPIA
      a. Description
        1) Refractive strength unequal in each eye
        2) Potential to develop amblyopia because the weaker eye is used less
      b. Assessment
        1) May show signs and symptoms similar to myopia, extent of which is dependent on the degree of refractive error
      c. Diagnostic testing
        1) Snellen eye chart visual acuity testing
      d. Nursing interventions
        1) Fit with corrective lenses or contact lenses (preferred).
        2) Assist with referral to an ophthalmologist or optometrist as ordered.

5. AMBLYOPIA
   a. Description
      1) May be referred to as "lazy eye"
      2) Decreased vision in one eye
      3) Etiology
         a) Insufficient stimulation to one eye
         b) Brain receives two images of one object and suppresses the less-clear image.
         c) Visual cortex eventually ceases to respond to visual stimulation of the weaker eye and vision is reduced in that eye.
   b. Assessment
      1) Poor vision in the "lazy" eye
      2) Strabismus or anisometropia often evident
   c. Diagnostic testing
      1) Snellen eye chart visual acuity testing
      2) Corneal light reflex
      3) Cover-uncover test
      4) Alternating cover test
   d. Nursing interventions
      1) Encourage early diagnosis because amblyopia is preventable if the primary visual defect is diagnosed and treated before age 6 years.
      2) Assist with referral to an ophthalmologist as ordered.
C. NASOLACRIMAL DUCT STENOSIS, OBSTRUCTION, AND INFLAMMATION
   1. DESCRIPTION
      a. Narrowing or complete obstruction of the nasolacrimal duct or tear sac
      b. Most common on the nasal side
      c. May be congenital or acquired (following infection or trauma)
      d. *Staphylococcus aureus* is the most common pathogen causing the inflammation.
      e. Spontaneous resolution common by 9–12 months of age
      f. Clinical signs appear 3–12 weeks after birth.
   2. ASSESSMENT
      a. Mucoid or mucopurulent discharge from the lacrimal duct
      b. Tearing from the affected eye(s)
      c. Area over the lacrimal duct may be tender or swollen.
      d. May be excoriation around the surrounding skin from continuous drainage
      e. May be concurrent blepharitis in the lids and lashes
      f. May be accompanied by nasal obstruction and drainage
      g. Fever possible in severe inflammation

3. DIAGNOSTIC TESTING
   a. Duct probing by an ophthalmologist
   b. White blood cell (WBC) count and eye culture if inflammation is severe
4. NURSING INTERVENTIONS
   a. Apply warm compresses to the affected area three to four times per day.
   b. Massage the lacrimal ducts from the mid eyelid downward toward the nose (make sure hands are clean).
   c. Instill antibiotic eyedrops or ointment as prescribed for inflammation.
   d. Assist with referral to an ophthalmologist if the condition persists after 6–12 months.

VI. **CRANIOFACIAL ABNORMALITIES**
   A. CLEFT LIP
      1. DESCRIPTION
         a. Embryonic structures around the oral cavity do not fuse completely
         b. Varying degrees of cleft, may be unilateral or bilateral
         c. Most common craniofacial malformation
         d. Genetic and sporadic etiology
         e. Associated abnormalities include cleft palate and nasal malformations.
      2. ASSESSMENT
         a. Varying cleft: slight notch to full separation of the lip extending to the nostril
         b. Depending on the severity of the cleft, may involve deformities of the nose
         c. Unilateral or bilateral presentation
         d. Dental abnormalities are common on the cleft side.
         e. May have feeding difficulties
      3. NURSING INTERVENTIONS
         a. Support the client and family with social and emotional adjustment.
         b. Assist with referral to a multidisciplinary team as needed.
         c. Promote maximal nutrition and hydration.
   B. CLEFT LIP AND CLEFT PALATE
      1. DESCRIPTION
         a. Cleft lip
            1) One of the most common congenital anomalies that results in a fissure of the upper lip up to the nasal septum
            2) Can be either unilateral or bilateral and may involve the separation of the nasal floor
            3) Surgical repair, cheiloplasty, is done either soon after birth or in early infancy.

b. Cleft palate
1) One of the most common congenital anomalies that may be seen with or without cleft lip
2) The condition results in a separation of the soft or hard palate that can be midline, unilateral, or bilateral.
3) Surgical repair, staphylorhaphy, is done usually during the toddler period (1–2 years of age) to allow for palate growth.

2. ASSESSMENT
   a. Cleft lip visible at birth
   b. Cleft palate is not usually obvious at birth unless accompanied by cleft lip. The condition can be detected by visual inspection or palpation, or both. Formula coming from the nose may be the first indication of the condition.

3. DIAGNOSTIC TESTS
   a. Physical examination of face and mouth
   b. If severe, may be detected by prenatal ultrasound

4. NURSING INTERVENTIONS
   a. Assess the infant's ability to suck, swallow, and feed.
   b. To improve quality of suck, use a soft nipple, special elongated nipple, or Brecht feeder (asepto syringe with a rubber tubing tip).
   c. Assess for respiratory problems related to aspiration.
   d. Assess the parents' reaction to the diagnosis, and provide information and emotional support.

5. SURGICAL MANAGEMENT
   a. Preoperative care
      1) Feed the infant in an upright position.
      2) Burp frequently.
      3) Use gavage feeding if the infant is unable to tolerate oral feedings.
      4) Encourage sucking between feedings to facilitate speech development.
      5) Instruct the parents on the anatomy of the anomaly and feeding techniques to maintain adequate nutrition.
      6) Instruct the parents on the surgery and anticipated care of the infant.
   b. Postoperative care
      1) Protect the suture line either by a Logan Bar for cleft lip and a cup for cleft palate.
      2) Rinse the suture line with water after feeding.
      3) Position the infant side lying after surgery to prevent damage to the suture line.
      4) Clean the lip after feeding with saline or half-strength peroxide to prevent crusting and scarring.
      5) Use elbow restraint to prevent touching or pulling the suture line.
      6) Monitor for respiratory distress and infection.
      7) Maintain a patent airway.
      8) Anticipate the infant's needs to prevent crying that could result in separation of the suture line.
      9) Administer pain medication as ordered.
      10) Instruct the parents on the care of the incision, feeding technique, and prevention of infection.
      11) Avoid straws or utensils that could damage the suture line.
      12) Start with a liquid diet initially post-op then progress to a soft diet.
      13) Have suction equipment at the bedside for an emergency.

VII. **INFECTIONS OF THE HEAD, EYES, EARS, NOSE, AND THROAT (HEENT) SYSTEM**
A. CONJUNCTIVITIS
   1. DESCRIPTION
      a. May be referred to as "pinkeye"
      b. Inflammation of the conjunctiva caused by allergy, bacterial or viral infection, or trauma
      c. Typically age related
      d. Chlamydial conjunctivitis is rare in older children and may indicate sexual abuse in the child who is not sexually active.
   2. ASSESSMENT
      a. Bacterial
         1) Typically bilateral but may begin unilaterally
         2) Crusting of eyelids
         3) Inflamed conjunctiva: itching, burning, or scratchy lids with redness
         4) Eyelids may be edematous.
         5) Photophobia (light sensitivity)
         6) Purulent or mucopurulent drainage
         7) Contagious
         8) May have concomitant otitis media or upper respiratory infection
      b. Viral
         1) Typically bilateral
         2) Serous (watery) drainage
         3) Inflamed conjunctiva: itchy, red
         4) Eyelids often edematous

      5) Contagious
      6) Usually occurs with an upper respiratory tract infection
   c. Allergic
      1) Typically bilateral
      2) Discharge is watery, may be stringy.
      3) Inflamed conjunctiva: redness, itchiness
      4) Eyelids may be edematous.
   d. Foreign body and corneal abrasion
      1) Typically unilateral
      2) Pain, scratchy sensation
      3) Inflamed conjunctiva
      4) Tearing
  3. DIAGNOSTIC TESTING
   a. Gram stain and bacterial culture
   b. Viral culture
   c. Chlamydial culture (special collection kit)
  4. NURSING INTERVENTIONS
   a. General
      1) Instruct the parent and child in infection control measures such as good hand washing, not sharing towels or washcloths.
      2) Remove accumulated secretions using a warm moist compress three to four times per day and cleansing from the inner canthus outward.
      3) Instruct the child to avoid rubbing the eye.
      4) Instruct the adolescent that existing eye makeup should be discarded and replaced.
      5) Instruct the child wearing contact lenses to discontinue wearing them and obtain new lenses to avoid reinfection.
      6) Avoid corticosteroid eyedrops, because they may make the eye more susceptible to infection.
      7) Administer antibiotic eyedrops or ointment as prescribed.
   b. Bacterial or foreign body
      1) Administer antibacterial eyedrops or ointment as prescribed.
      2) Instruct the child and parent on the administration of the prescribed drugs.
      3) Instruct the child and the parent that the child should not return to day care or school until the antibiotic eye preparation has been administered for 24 hours.
      4) Administer prophylactic eye treatment (silver nitrate 1% ophthalmic solution or 0.5% erythromycin ointment) in the eyes of the newborn after delivery.

      5) Encourage a referral if a foreign body is imbedded in the eye.
      6) Stabilize the client and provide support to the client and family.
   c. Viral
      1) Usually self-limiting, does not require treatment other than general management
   d. Allergic
      1) Administer antihistamines as prescribed and instruct the parent and child on use.
      2) Avoid allergy trigger.
B. ACUTE OTITIS MEDIA
  1. DESCRIPTION
   a. Infection of the middle ear
   b. Often follows eustachian tube dysfunction
   c. Risk factors: male gender in infancy, day care attendance, smoke exposure, family history, allergic rhinitis, hypertrophic adenoids, formula fed
   d. Peak incidence: 6 months to 2 years and during the winter months
   e. Common pathogens: *Streptococcus pneumoniae*, *Haemophilus influenzae*, and *Moraxella catarrhalis*
  2. ASSESSMENT
   a. Otalgia (ear pain) that may be exacerbated by sucking and chewing
   b. Tugging at the ears and irritability
   c. Fever
   d. Postauricular or cervical lymph node enlargement
   e. Concurrent respiratory or pharyngeal infection
   f. Vomiting and diarrhea and loss of appetite
   g. Disrupted sleep
   h. Hearing loss with persistent or recurrent otitis media
   i. Purulent drainage possible with perforation
   j. Tympanic membrane appears red, yellow, opaque, bulging, or retracted; landmarks are absent or obscured and there is increased vascularity.
  3. DIAGNOSTIC TESTING
   a. Tympanometry
   b. Pneumatic insufflation
   c. Tympanocentesis with culture of the middle ear fluid
  4. NURSING INTERVENTIONS
   a. Encourage fluids and maintain hydration.
   b. Instruct the parent to feed the infant upright and not to prop the bottle.
   c. Instruct the parent to avoid exposing the child to smoke.

d. Instruct the parent on the administration of analgesics and antipyretics.

e. Instruct the parent on the administration of the antibiotic as prescribed, stressing compliance.

f. If eardrops are prescribed, instruct the parent to pull the earlobe down and back in children younger than age 3 years to instill the drops and to pull the pinna up and back for a child older than 3 years.

g. Instruct the parents on the appropriate procedure for cleaning the ear canal, avoiding the use of cotton-tipped swabs or undiluted hydrogen peroxide.

h. Encourage the parent to keep the child up to date on immunizations.

i. When recurrent otitis media is present:

  1) Instruct the parent on the administration of prophylactic antibiotics as prescribed.

  2) Instruct the parent that screening for hearing loss may be necessary.

  3) Provide education on myringotomy or tympanostomy (pressure equalization tubes), or both, if prescribed.

C. OTITIS MEDIA WITH EFFUSION

1. DESCRIPTION

  a. Middle ear effusion

  b. Accumulation of fluid (secretory, nonsuppurative, or serous) in the middle ear and reduced mobility of the tympanic membrane with pneumatic otoscopy

  c. Consequence of acute otitis media and eustachian tube dysfunction

  d. May result in mild to moderate hearing impairment

2. ASSESSMENT

  a. Often asymptomatic without fever or pain

  b. May complain of a feeling of fullness in the ear

  c. Older children may complain of hearing loss.

  d. May demonstrate impaired balance (toddler age group) or dizziness

  e. Dull tympanic membrane, varying in appearance:

    1) Bulging and opaque with no visible landmarks

    2) Retracted and translucent with visible landmarks; air fluid levels may be seen

3. DIAGNOSTIC TESTING

  a. Pneumatic otoscopy reveals decreased tympanic membrane mobility.

  b. Tympanometry: tympanogram is flat.

  c. Audiogram is done to determine if the child has hearing loss of 15–30 db.

4. NURSING INTERVENTIONS

  a. Perform a hearing evaluation on a child who has fluid in both middle ears for 3 months.

  b. Instruct the parent on the administration of antibiotics if prescribed for a child who has had persistent effusion for more than 3 months.

  c. Provide information to the parent and child on tympanostomy tubes if prescribed for a child who has had persistent effusion for 4–6 months.

  d. Provide emotional support to the client and family.

D. OTITIS EXTERNA

1. DESCRIPTION

  a. Inflammation of the external auditory canal

  b. Results from infection by normal ear flora that become pathogenic under conditions of excessive wetness or dryness

  c. Can also result from fungus

2. ASSESSMENT

  a. Severe ear pain that may be aggravated by jaw movement or touching the ear, often preceded by an itching sensation

  b. Furuncles or small abscesses in hair follicles

  c. Impetigo or infection of the superficial layer

  d. Edema, redness, discharge that may be green, blue, yellow, gray in color

  e. Conductive hearing loss

  f. Fever

3. DIAGNOSTIC TESTING

  a. Culture of ear discharge in persistent or chronic otitis externa

4. NURSING INTERVENTIONS

  a. Remove the foreign body or debris from the ear canal if easily visualized.

  b. Administer an analgesic and an antipyretic.

  c. Administer antibiotic eardrops with steroid, as prescribed, using a wick to reach inflamed areas.

  d. Instruct the parent on administration of drugs, review use of the wick, warm eardrops prior to administration, and method of instilling.

e. Instruct the parent and child on the need to limit their stay in the water to less than 1 hour and to allow at least 2 hours before reexposure.

f. Instruct the parent and child to remove water from the ear after exposure using a cotton wick rather than a cotton-tipped swab.

g. Instruct the parent and child to instill 3–5 drops of a dilute solution (50/50) white vinegar and water or rubbing alcohol and water in the ears on rising, after swimming, and at bedtime to help decrease the recurrence of infection.

E. SINUSITIS
1. DESCRIPTION
   a. Inflammation and infection of the paranasal sinuses
   b. Risk factors: allergic rhinitis, nasal deformities, cystic fibrosis, nasal polyps, human immunodeficiency virus, day care attendance with recurrent viral URI, smoke exposure, older siblings
   c. Acute sinusitis: clinical manifestations last 10–30 days.
   d. Subacute sinusitis: clinical manifestations last more than 30 days.
   e. Chronic sinusitis: clinical manifestations last more than 120 days.
2. ASSESSMENT
   a. Upper respiratory manifestations lasting greater than 10 days
   b. Fever
   c. Tenderness over the involved sinuses
   d. Inflammation and edema of mucous membranes of the nose
   e. Postnasal discharge
   f. Clear or mucopurulent rhinorrhea
   g. Headache
   h. Facial pain or swelling, including periorbital edema
   i. Sore throat
   j. Bad breath
   k. Decreased appetite, especially in chronic sinusitis
   l. Cough
3. DIAGNOSTIC TESTING
   a. Not necessary if clinical picture is consistent with sinusitis
   b. Sinus radiograph (Waters view), ultrasound, or CT scan if the child has facial swelling, appears toxic, has chronic or recurrent sinusitis, or has asthma
4. NURSING INTERVENTIONS
   a. Instruct the parent and child on the administration of the antibiotic as prescribed; review adverse reactions.
   b. Instruct the parent on the administration of over-the-counter (OTC) antipyretic and analgesic.
   c. Instruct the parent and child on the clinical manifestations of complications or invasive infection (high fever, orbital cellulitis, brain abscess).
   d. Instruct the parent on the use of a humidifier to help relieve drying of mucous membranes.
   e. Encourage fluids and maintain hydration.
   f. Instruct the parent on the administration of antihistamines and decongestants, as prescribed, in a child with underlying allergies or chronic clinical manifestations, reviewing adverse reactions. Antihistamines and decongestants have not been found to be effective in the treatment of acute sinusitis in children less than age 6 years.
   g. Assist with referral to an otolaryngologist if needed.

F. ACUTE PHARYNGITIS AND TONSILLITIS
1. DESCRIPTION
   a. Inflammation and infection of the tonsils and adenoids caused by bacteria (group A beta-hemolytic streptococcus, *Neisseria gonorrheae,* or *Cornybacterium diphtheriae*) or virus (adenovirus common)
   b. Less commonly seen in children under age 2 years; most commonly found in children 5–11 years of age
2. ASSESSMENT
   a. Abrupt onset of clinical manifestations: fever, sore throat, malaise, dysphagia
   b. Mouth breathing and unpleasant mouth odor
   c. Abdominal pain and nausea and vomiting (especially in younger children)
   d. Headache
   e. Petechiae on the palate, beefy red uvula, red edematous tonsillopharyngeal tissue
   f. Tonsillopharyngeal exudate
   g. Tender anterior cervical lymph nodes
      1) Scarlatiform (sandpaper) rash (characteristic of group A beta-hemolytic streptococcus)
   h. Enlarged adenoids may cause nasal quality of speech, mouth breathing, hearing difficulty, snoring, and obstructive sleep apnea.
   i. Bacterial is usually not accompanied by URI symptoms, viral can be.

3. DIAGNOSTIC TESTING
   a. Rapid streptococcal test
   b. Throat culture
4. NURSING INTERVENTIONS
   a. Encourage fluids and rest.
   b. Instruct the parent and child on process of collecting throat culture, and collect the specimen.
   c. Notify the physician of positive results.
   d. Instruct the parent on the administration of the antibiotic as prescribed; review adverse reactions and need for compliance.
   e. Instruct the parent on the administration of antipyretics and analgesics to reduce fever and pain.
   f. Instruct the parent and child on the clinical manifestations of complications (acute glomerulonephritis, rheumatic fever).
   g. Instruct the parent that the child may return to school when afebrile and have been taking the antibiotic for 24 hours.
   h. Instruct the parent to discard the child's toothbrush after the antibiotics have been taken for 24 hours.
5. SURGICAL MANAGEMENT
   a. Tonsillectomy and adenoidectomy
      1) Removal of palatine tonsillar tissue or adenoids, or both, after persistent or recurrent sore throat, dysphagia, obstructed nasal breathing, development of peritonsillar abscess, significant hypertrophy, or malignancy
      2) Tonsillectomy is generally not performed under the age of 3 years, because of increased risk for blood loss and regrowth of tissue.
      3) Adenoidectomy without tonsillectomy is performed more commonly in children who have obstructed breathing due to enlarged adenoids and may be performed under the age of 3 years.
      4) Preprocedure
         a) NPO is required after midnight.
         b) Assess for signs of active infection (including upper respiratory infection).
         c) Assess bleeding and clotting studies because involved tissues are very vascular.
         d) Notify the physician of laboratory results.
         e) Provide education to the child and family regarding the surgery and recovery period such as anesthesia, sore throat, need to maintain hydration, signs of bleeding, avoidance of stress to affected tissues, and analgesics.
         f) Assess for any loose teeth to decrease the risk of aspiration during surgery.
      5) Postprocedure
         a) Monitor the vital signs.
         b) Monitor the respiratory and cardiovascular status.
         c) Monitor the level of consciousness and activity.
         d) Suction to prevent oropharynx trauma and irritation of the operative site.
         e) Apply an ice collar.
         f) Assess for signs of bleeding such as increased heart rate, vomiting of bright red blood or blood trickling down the throat, pallor, frequent clearing of the throat and notify the physician immediately if there are signs of hemorrhage.
         g) Maintain a side-lying or prone position to facilitate drainage.
         h) Place the child in a Fowler's position when alert.
         i) Administer analgesics rectally or intravenously in the initial postoperative period, then orally and topically as prescribed.
         j) Maintain hydration with clear liquids; avoid milk products because they may cause excessive clearing of the throat; carbonated, red-colored, and citrus beverages should also be avoided.
         k) Offer a diet of cold or frozen clear liquids; advance as tolerated to a soft diet.
         l) Monitor intake and output.
         m) Discourage coughing, clearing of the throat, or blowing of the nose to prevent stress to the operative site.
         n) Instruct the parent and child that the presence of dark brown blood in the oral

cavity and in emesis may be present and is normal.

o) Administer antibiotics and antiemetics as prescribed.

p) Provide discharge instruction: instruct the parents to notify the physician if bleeding, persistent earache, or fever occurs.

q) Instruct the parent to keep the child away from crowds for the first 1–2 weeks until healing has occurred.

G. STOMATITIS

1. DESCRIPTION
   a. May be referred to as "canker sores"
   b. Inflammation of the oral mucosa, including the cheek, lip, tongue, gingiva, palate, and floor of the mouth
   c. Infectious or noninfectious and caused by local or systemic factors
   d. Aphthous ulcer (canker sore): benign, painful, recurrent ulcers associated with mild trauma, allergy, and emotional stress
   e. Herpetic gingivostomatitis: caused by herpes simplex virus, usually type I associated with emotional stress, trauma, exposure to excessive sunlight

2. ASSESSMENT
   a. Aphthous ulcers
      1) Shallow pale white to yellow ulcers surrounded by a red border
      2) Can have concomitant fever, pharyngitis
      3) May be recurrent at 4–6-week intervals
      4) Ulcers persist for 4–12 days and heal uneventfully.
      5) Painful
      6) Decreased appetite and irritability
      7) May be associated with underlying inflammatory bowel disease or celiac disease
   b. Herpetic gingivostomatitis
      1) Primary infection: fever, edematous and erythematous pharynx, fluid-filled vesicles on the oral mucosa that eventually rupture and form ulcers, pain, cervical lymphadenitis, foul odor to breath, friable gums, headache, irritability, anorexia, weight loss and dehydration possible, duration 5–14 days
      2) Recurrent: vesicles appear on the lips singly or in groups

3) Immunosuppressed children at greater risk for developing it

3. DIAGNOSTIC TESTING
   a. Viral or bacterial culture of ulcers not usually necessary

4. NURSING INTERVENTIONS
   a. Administer oral OTC analgesics, topical anesthetics (may use those with lidocaine in older children), topical steroid rinses, or triamcinolone acetonide dental paste, as prescribed, for relief of pain and before meals.
   b. Administer antiviral medications such as acyclovir (Zovirax), as prescribed, for herpetic lesions.
   c. Administer antibacterial rinses, as prescribed, to reduce likelihood of secondary bacterial infections.
   d. Instruct the child not to swallow oral rinses and topical preparations.
   e. Encourage fluids and a soft diet; drinking fluids through a straw may be helpful.
   f. Recommend the use of a soft-bristled toothbrush or a disposable foam-tipped toothbrush.
   g. Instruct the child and parent on good hand washing to reduce the spread of infection or autoinoculation.
   h. Discourage placing fingers or objects in the mouth and recommend that any objects placed in the mouth be cleaned thoroughly.
   i. Instruct the parent that newborns and immunosuppressed clients should not be exposed to infected children until lesions are healed.

H. ORAL THRUSH

1. DESCRIPTION
   a. Infection of the mouth, mucous membranes, or corner of the mouth caused by *Candida albicans*
   b. May be concomitant candidal diaper rash

2. ASSESSMENT
   a. Furry white plaques on an erythematous base that adhere to the mucous membranes of the mouth including the tongue; may bleed when scraped; outer lips appear cracked
   b. Decreased appetite
   c. Irritability in infants
   d. If breastfeeding, mother's nipples may be sore and red appearing
   e. Often associated with bright red diaper rash with sharp borders and satellite lesions

3. NURSING INTERVENTIONS
   a. Administer the topical antifungal, as prescribed, for diaper rash and instruct the parent on usage.
   b. Instruct the mother on the treatment of nipples if breastfeeding to eliminate reinfection.
   c. Administer an oral antifungal, generally nystatin oral solution, (Mycostatin) after feedings, as prescribed, and instruct the parent and child on usage. (Administer other antifungal preparations orally, topically, or intravenously, as prescribed, for recalcitrant infections.)
   d. Apply gentian violet to the mouth, as prescribed, for unresponsive infections.
      1) Inform the parent that it is likely to stain clothing, teeth, and surrounding skin.
      2) Apply after eating or allow at least 20 minutes after application before feeding.
   e. Instruct the parent to thoroughly wash bottles and nipples, and to avoid use of the pacifier to reduce chance of reinfection.

VIII. LONG-TERM UPPER RESPIRATORY DYSFUNCTION
A. ALLERGIC RHINITIS
   1. DESCRIPTION
      a. A disorder that results in nasal edema caused by the release of chemical mediators from the antigen-antibody reaction
      b. Second most common atopic disorder (after asthma)
      c. Familial predisposition
      d. May occur seasonally or perennially depending on exposure and subsequent sensitization to the allergen; perennial allergic rhinitis is more common.
      e. Allergens include trees, grasses, weeds, foods, outdoor molds, dust mites, cockroaches, danders of household pets, feathers, indoor mold spores.
      f. Peak incidence occurs in the adolescent and postadolescent population.
   2. ASSESSMENT
      a. Watery or seromucoid rhinorrhea
      b. Nasal obstruction resulting in mouth breathing, snoring, nasal speech
      c. Nasal stuffiness, postnasal drip, sneezing, cough
      d. Nasal mucosa may appear hyperemic to purplish pallor with edema.
      e. Nasal turbinates may appear pale blue and swollen.
      f. Horizontal crease across the lower third of the nose
      g. Itching and rubbing of the nose; "allergic salute" may occur.
      h. Itching and rubbing of the eyes, palate, pharynx, or conjunctiva
      i. "Allergic shiners" (dark circles under the eyes) are common.
      j. Dennie lines (wrinkles below lower eyelids) are present.
      k. Fatigue and malaise
      l. Poor school performance may be a consequence.
      m. May have concomitant asthma or eczema
   3. DIAGNOSTIC TESTING
      a. Nasal smear for eosinophils is nonspecific, nonuniversal finding
      b. RAST test
      c. Skin or serological testing for IgE antibodies to specific allergens in severe cases
   4. NURSING INTERVENTIONS
      a. Encourage the child to avoid identified allergens.
      b. Administer immunotherapy (titrated allergen injections), as prescribed, to hyposensitize or desensitize the child to the allergen and observe for 20–30 minutes following injection.
      c. Instruct the parent and child on antihistamine use, as prescribed, reviewing adverse reactions such as drowsiness.
      d. Instruct the parent on use of nasal or oral decongestants, as prescribed; caution the parent and child on "rebound effects" of OTC nasal agents if used for more than 3–5 days.
      e. Instruct the parent and child on use of anti-inflammatory nasal inhalant medication, as prescribed, such as cromolyn sodium (Intal), or corticosteroid.
      f. Assist the parent and child to distinguish allergy manifestations from cold clinical manifestations.

PRACTICE QUESTIONS

1. A mother brings her infant to the clinic for a 9-month well-baby exam. She expresses concern to the nurse that her infant's "soft spot" in the front is still palpable. The nurse's response would be based on the understanding that the anterior fontanel closes
   1. by 6 months of age.
   2. before 18 months of age.
   3. shortly after birth.
   4. before 12 months of age.

2. A 5-year-old girl presents for a vision screen. A screening using an HOTV chart is completed with the following results: 10/15 right eye, 10/12.5 left eye. Which of the following interpretations by the nurse is correct?
   1. The results indicate that this is a failing response and the child requires immediate referral to an ophthalmologist
   2. The eyes should be retested at 20 feet for more accurate results
   3. These results are considered passing and no referral is required
   4. These results are inconclusive and the child should be rescreened using the Snellen alphabet chart

3. At a well-child exam, a 3-year-old boy is diagnosed with strabismus. Which of the following clinical manifestations does the nurse interpret as indicative of this disorder? Select all that apply:
   [ ] 1. Excessive eye rubbing
   [ ] 2. Squinting
   [ ] 3. Difficulty doing close work
   [ ] 4. Positioning self close to TV
   [ ] 5. Closing one eye to see
   [ ] 6. Tilting head to one side to see

4. On testing, a 3-year-old boy is found to have left esotropia. The physician directs the nurse to instruct the parent on "patching" to treat the strabismus. The nurse should instruct the parent to place
   1. the patch on the right eye.
   2. the patch on the left eye.
   3. patches on both eyes for a short time each day.
   4. the patch on the right and left alternately throughout the day.

5. In addition to instructing the mother on patching, the nurse informs her that it is important that the strabismus was recognized before the age of 6 years. This reflects the nurse's understanding that untreated strabismus may result in
   1. myopia.
   2. stigmatism.
   3. amblyopia.
   4. hyperopia.

6. To pass pure tone audiometry testing, the nurse understands that a child should be able to hear a frequency of 500 Hz at how many decibels (db)?
   1. 30 db
   2. 25 db
   3. 20 db
   4. 15 db

7. An 18-month-old child is to have a tympanogram. The mother asks what that is. Which of the following statements by the nurse best describes the purpose of tympanometry?
   1. "It is a diagnostic test that measures tympanic membrane compliance (mobility)."
   2. "It is a diagnostic test that is used most effectively in infants under age 6 months."
   3. "It is a diagnostic test that indicates the degree of hearing loss in a child."
   4. "It is a diagnostic test that measures external auditory canal air pressure."

8. A 2-year-old boy is sent home from day care because of red, itchy eyes. The nurse notes mucopurulent discharge from both eyes, and the physician treats the boy with antibiotic eyedrops. The nurse providing discharge education recognizes a need to repeat instruction when the mother states
   1. "He cannot return to day care for 24 hours after starting the eyedrops."
   2. "He needs to have the eyedrops regularly, so I will have to bring them to day care."
   3. "We should wash our hands frequently."
   4. "I need to clean his eyes from the outer corner inward."

9. The nurse evaluates which of the following laboratory tests and pathogens to cause acute otitis media in children?
   1. Group A beta-hemolytic *streptococcus*
   2. *Escherichia coli*
   3. *Haemophilus influenzae* and *Streptococcus pneumoniae*
   4. *Staphylococcus aureus* and *Pasteurella*

10. The mother of a 9-month-old infant calls the triage nurse with a concern that her child, who has a bad cold, might have an ear infection. The triage nurse elicits additional history. Which of the following can be identified from the health

history as a risk factor for the development of otitis media in children?

1. Day care attendance
2. Breastfeeding
3. Female gender in infants
4. Introduction of a new solid food

11. A 3-year-old boy is accompanied by his mother for follow-up of fluid in his middle ears. He had a bilateral ear infection 3 months ago and the fluid in his middle ears has persisted at all of his subsequent appointments. The nurse, based on an understanding of bilateral middle ear effusion, recognizes that this child should be
    1. reassured that this is a normal complication of otitis media.
    2. screened for hearing loss.
    3. rescheduled for follow-up at 6 months because not enough time has elapsed to reevaluate the ears.
    4. avoiding milk products because they thicken upper respiratory tract secretions.

12. A 5-year-old female has received tympanostomy tubes. The discharge nurse instructs the parent and child regarding tympanostomy tubes and their care. Which of the following would be included in the education plan?
    1. The child should never be allowed to go swimming
    2. The tympanostomy (PE) tubes will remain in place for 5 years
    3. The child with tympanostomy tubes in place will not experience any further episodes of otitis media
    4. Earplugs are recommended for activities such as diving, submerging, bathing, and shampooing

13. A 12-year-old child has experienced repeated otitis externa. The child swims daily on a swim team and is unwilling to give that up. The nurse instructs the child and parents on methods to prevent further episodes. Which of the following is included in the plan?
    1. Instruct parent and child to remove water from within the ear with a cotton-tipped swab
    2. Instruct the parent and child to instill rubbing alcohol into the ears after swimming
    3. Instruct the parent and child to instill a 50% solution of vinegar and water into the ears after swimming
    4. Instruct the parent and child to stay in the water for no more than 2 hours at a time

14. A 6-year-old child is scheduled for a tonsillectomy. The nurse is obtaining the preoperative history. Because of risks associated with this surgery, the nurse should report which of the following to the surgeon?
    1. There is a family history of bleeding tendencies
    2. Current upper respiratory infection is denied
    3. The child recently visited the dentist
    4. The child does not have cleft palate

15. The nurse is caring for a child following tonsillectomy. Which of the following observations should the nurse immediately report?
    1. The presence of dark brown blood on the teeth
    2. The presence of blood trickling down the throat
    3. An episode of vomiting
    4. A complaint of a sore throat

16. A 7-year-old child who has undergone tonsillectomy is alert, and the nurse is reviewing postoperative instructions. Which of the following should be included in the instructions?
    1. A soft diet will be ordered once the child is alert
    2. Coughing, clearing of throat, and blowing of the nose is discouraged
    3. The client should continue to be positioned prone or in a side-lying position for 24 hours
    4. Milk is the choice of fluid following the tonsillectomy to provide nutrients

17. The mother of a child asks the nurse when the frontal sinuses in children develop. Which of the following is the appropriate response by the nurse? "The frontal sinuses are fully developed
    1. at birth."
    2. by age 3 months."
    3. by age 7 years."
    4. in puberty."

18. A 9-year-old girl was diagnosed with strep throat and an antibiotic was prescribed. The mother asks the nurse when the child can return to school. Which of the following is the priority response by the nurse?
    1. "She may return immediately if she is afebrile."
    2. "She may return after 1 week if she is feeling better."
    3. "She may return after the 10-day course of antibiotic."
    4. "She may return after taking the antibiotic for a 24-hour period."

19. An adolescent experiences recurrent aphthous stomatitis. Which of the following should the nurse include in the instructions for a client with aphthous ulcers?

1. Encourage fluids through a straw and soft diet while the ulcers are present
2. Recommend the use of a hard-bristle toothbrush to remove affected tissue
3. Administer antiviral drugs such as acyclovir (Zovirax) to shorten course
4. Inform the client that the ulcers will last 1 to 2 days

20. The nurse understands that viscous lidocaine is sometimes prescribed for clients with aphthous ulcers. The nurse should question a physician's prescription for viscous lidocaine in which of the following clients?
1. An adolescent male with stomatitis
2. An adult female with stomatitis
3. A toddler male with stomatitis
4. An alert 60-year-old female with stomatitis

21. The nurse should assess for what related condition in a 4-month-old infant who has oral candidiasis?
1. Eczema
2. Diaper rash
3. Herpes simplex infection
4. Aphthous ulcers

22. A 2-month-old breast-fed infant has oral thrush. Which of the following is the most appropriate intervention to be included in the nurse's plan of care?
1. The oral lesions should be treated with an over-the-counter topical anesthetic such as Anbesol
2. Administer oral nystatin before feedings as prescribed
3. Instruct the mother on treatment of her nipples if she continues breastfeeding
4. Add cereal to the diet to decrease the need for sucking

23. The nurse is teaching a class on allergic rhinitis. The nurse should include which of the following in the class?
1. Unlike asthma, there is no familial predisposition to allergic rhinitis

2. Allergic rhinitis is a disorder that occurs seasonally
3. A nasal smear for eosinophils is the hallmark diagnostic test of allergic rhinitis
4. Peak incidence of allergic rhinitis occurs in the adolescent and postadolescent population

24. An 8-year-old boy will be undergoing skin allergy testing. The nurse should include which of the following precautions in the preparations?
1. Evaluate for dermographism before beginning the testing
2. Notify the physician if not on site that testing has begun
3. Reassure the parent and child that no allergic reactions generally occur with this method
4. Inject the allergen solution to a depth to elicit bleeding

25. A 13-year-old female has been prescribed allergy injections every 3 to 4 weeks. The nurse instructs the child that following the injection, she
1. must remain for observation for at least 5 minutes.
2. must remain for observation for at least 20 minutes.
3. must remain for observation for at least 1 hour.
4. does not need to remain for observation.

26. The registered nurse is preparing the nursing tasks for a pediatric eye, ear, nose, and throat disorder unit. Which of the following nursing tasks may be delegated to a licensed practical nurse?
1. Perform a nasopharyngeal culture
2. Refer the parent of a child with strabismus to an ophthalmologist
3. Instruct a client scheduled for a myringotomy on the procedure
4. Monitor the neurological status on a child with craniosynostosis

ANSWERS AND RATIONALES

1. 2. The anterior fontanel closes between 12 and 18 months of age, with average closure at 14 months. The parent of a 9-month-old should be reassured that the anterior fontanel is still palpable. The nurse should measure its size and plot it on the occipital frontal circumference chart.

2. 3. A 5-year-old child screened using the HOTV chart should achieve at least a 10/15 in both eyes without a two-line difference,

so this is considered a passing test. An HOTV test is the preferred test for children ages 3 to 5, because most children at these ages are unable to read the letters on a Snellen chart. The recommended testing distance is 10 feet.

3. 2. 5. 6. The child tilts the head to one side in an effort to improve visual alignment. In strabismus, the eyes are misaligned, so the child makes efforts to improve focus. Other clinical manifestations include squinting,

appearing cross-eyed, or closing one eye to see. Excessive eye rubbing, difficulty doing close work, and sitting close to the television are all manifestations of myopia.

4. 1.   For a client with esotropia, the stronger eye should be patched to increase visual stimulation in the weaker eye, thus strengthening the eye muscles. Patching the weaker eye would worsen the problem. Patching both eyes is impractical, unnecessary, and counter to the goals of treatment. Esotropia (convergent) occurs when the eye turns toward the midline.

5. 3.   Strabismus is a condition where the visual lines of the two eyes do not focus simultaneously on the same object in space because of a lack of muscle coordination, resulting in a cross-eyed appearance. If left untreated, it leads to eventual loss of vision in the weaker eye and may lead to blindness. Astigmatism, myopia, and hyperopia are disorders that, while significant, are refractory errors and can be corrected with special lenses.

6. 2.   Inability to hear any frequency at 25 db is considered a failure. Most children are able to hear frequencies higher than 500 Hz at 20 db.

7. 1.   Tympanometry is used to measure tympanic membrane compliance. It also estimates middle ear pressure. It does not indicate the degree of hearing loss. It is not useful in infants under age 6 months, because of hypercompliance of the tympanic membrane. It does not measure external auditory canal air pressure.

8. 4.   The eye should be cleaned from the inner canthus of the eye downward and outward. This will lessen the potential of infecting the other eye. It would be appropriate to prevent the child from returning to day care for 24 hours after starting antibiotics to prevent spreading the infection. It is also necessary to administer the antibiotic on a regular basis and to wash the hands frequently.

9. 3.   *H. influenzae* and *S. pneumoniae* are upper respiratory pathogens. These most often cause otitis media. Group A beta-hemolytic *streptococcus* is also an upper respiratory pathogen, but is not implicated in acute otitis media. *S. aureus* is commonly found on skin and *E. coli* is a bowel organism. *Pasteurella* is an infection associated with animal bites.

10. 1.   Day care attendance is recognized as a risk factor in otitis media because of increased exposure to bacterial pathogens and the likelihood that some of these pathogens may have developed resistance to antimicrobial therapy. Breastfeeding has been shown to decrease the incidence of otitis media in infants compared to bottle-feeding. Males less than school age are more at risk than females for the development of otitis media. There is currently no substantial evidence to support the link between the introduction of new foods and the development of otitis media, although some theories propose that allergies may play a role in the development of otitis media.

11. 2.   A child who has had fluid in both middle ears for 3 months should have a hearing screen because there is increased potential for conductive hearing loss. Over time, conductive hearing loss could negatively affect the development of speech, language, and cognition. Otitis media with effusion can be a normal consequence of otitis media but should resolve by 3 months. There is no evidence to support limiting milk products to treat otitis media effusion.

12. 4.   Although swimming does not increase the risk of infection, diving, jumping, and submerging may. Bath water carries a higher risk of infection because it is contaminated, as is lake water. The use of earplugs is recommended for these activities. Soap reduces the surface tension of water, facilitating its entry into the tube, so earplugs are also recommended when shampooing. Most tympanostomy (PE) tubes fall out by 12 months and should be removed after 2 years. Children with tympanostomy tubes in place most often experience otitis when there is otorrhea from the PE tube.

13. 3.   Instilling dilute vinegar and water into the ear of a child with otitis externa establishes an acidic environment, which is less conducive to bacterial growth. A cotton-tipped swab is not recommended for removal of water, because it may further damage the sensitive ear canal. Similarly, undiluted rubbing alcohol would be too harsh for the sensitive ear canal and may further damage tissue. The usual recommendation for water exposure is less than 1 hour at a time with a 1- to 2-hour interval between repeated exposures.

14. 1.   The operative site in a tonsillectomy is highly vascular, so family bleeding tendencies would require additional alertness for this potential problem in this client. It is ideal that the child does not have a concurrent upper respiratory infection, but this would not require notification of the surgeon. The child's mouth should be assessed for loose teeth prior to surgery, so this notation is of little significance. Cleft palate is a contraindication to tonsillectomy.

15. 2.   The presence of blood trickling down the throat following a tonsillectomy is a sign of bleeding and should be communicated to the surgeon immediately. The dark brown blood is old and is commonly found on the teeth, in the nose, and in the emesis following tonsillectomy. It does not signify hemorrhage. Vomiting may be a normal sequela following surgery and does

not need to be communicated to the surgeon. If, however, the vomitus contains bright red blood, then the surgeon should be notified immediately, as this is an indication of bleeding. A client complaint of a sore throat is an anticipated finding posttonsillectomy.

16. 2. Coughing, clearing of the throat, and blowing the nose should be discouraged following a tonsillectomy. A soft diet, an oral intake of milk, and positioning the client prone or side-lying once alert may all stress the operative site and cause bleeding or hemorrhage. Typically, a cold, clear liquid diet is begun and advanced slowly as tolerated. The client may prefer an upright position once alert. The prone and side-lying positions are recommended until the client is alert. Milk products can be given later in the course, but should be avoided if they cause excessive clearing of the throat.

17. 3. The frontal sinuses develop by age 7 years. The maxillary and ethmoid sinuses are present at birth, but they are very small. The sphenoid sinus does not develop fully until puberty.

18. 4. Twenty-four hours of antibiotic therapy decreases the number of colonies in respiratory secretions, thus lessening the infectious nature of strep throat. The child can return to school after 24 hours of antibiotic therapy when she is feeling better and is afebrile. This will likely be sooner than 1 week. The antibiotic is typically prescribed for 10 days, but this does not necessitate missing school for that period of time.

19. 1. Aphthous stomatitis is canker sores. Eating a soft diet and using a straw will help avoid additional trauma and contact with painful lesions, allowing the child to eat. A soft-bristle toothbrush is recommended to avoid further trauma and irritation of the ulcers. Antiviral drugs such as acyclovir (Zovirax) are helpful to treat herpetic lesions but are not used in the treatment of aphthous ulcers. Aphthous ulcers typically last 4 to 12 days.

20. 3. Viscous lidocaine can be prescribed for a client with aphthous ulcers. The client must be able to keep 1 teaspoon of the solution in the mouth for 2 to 3 minutes and then expectorate. The toddler patient would be unlikely to be able to do this. Adolescents and adults would likely be able to do this.

21. 2. Oral candidial lesions can spread to other body systems, including the gastrointestinal tract, and via poor hand washing by the caregiver. Concomitant monilial diaper rash is common. Although eczema, *herpes simplex* infection, and aphthous ulcers may be present, they are not directly related to the oral candidiasis.

22. 3. The nipples of a mother who is breastfeeding an infant with oral thrush should be treated with a topical antifungal to avoid reinfection of the infant. Anbesol is not recommended in the treatment of oral candidiasis. Oral nystatin is the treatment of choice, but should be administered after feeding. Current guidelines recommend introduction of cereal at 6 months; adding cereal to the diet of a 2-month-old is inappropriate.

23. 4. Allergic rhinitis can occur in any age group, but the peak incidence occurs in the adolescent and postadolescent population. Allergic rhinitis does have a familial component. It may occur seasonally or perennially. Perennial allergic rhinitis to common household allergens is more common. A nasal smear for eosinophils is a nonspecific, nonuniversal finding and is not considered a hallmark diagnostic test.

24. 1. The client should be tested for dermographism before beginning skin allergy testing because dermographism may result in false-positive test results. Clients undergoing skin testing for allergy are at risk for an allergic reaction; those undergoing blood testing are unlikely to suffer allergic reactions. The physician should be on site for testing as there is potential for anaphylactic response and certainly for allergic reaction. Bleeding should be avoided during injection because this would create the potential for systemic allergen exposure and resultant anaphylaxis.

25. 2. It is recommended that the client receiving allergy injections should remain for observation for 20 to 30 minutes following the injection to ensure that no delayed reaction occurs.

26. 1. A licensed practical nurse may perform a nasopharyngeal culture. Referring a child with strabismus to an ophthalmologist, instructing the parents of a child scheduled for a myringotomy, and monitoring the neurological status on a child with craniosynostosis are all nursing skills reserved for the registered nurse.

REFERENCES

Potts, N., & Mandleco, B. (2012). *Pediatric nursing: Caring for children and their families* (3rd ed). Clifton Park, NY: Delmar Cengage Learning.

Spratto, G. R., & Woods, A. L. (2012). *PDR nurse's drug handbook 2012.* Clifton Park, NY: Delmar Cengage Learning.

CHAPTER 31

RESPIRATORY DISORDERS

I. ANATOMY AND PHYSIOLOGY

A. DIFFERENCES IN THE RESPIRATORY SYSTEM BETWEEN THE CHILD AND THE ADULT

1. THE CHEST CIRCUMFERENCE OF THE NEWBORN'S CHEST IS CIRCULAR BECAUSE THE ANTEROPOSTERIOR AND TRANSVERSE DIAMETERS ARE EQUAL. (THE RATIO OF THE ANTEROPOSTERIOR TO LATERAL DIAMETERS REACH ADULT PROPORTION BY 6 YEARS OF AGE.)

2. THE INFANT'S CHEST WALL IS THIN BECAUSE OF THE DECREASED MUSCULARITY.

3. THE NEWBORN'S TRACHEA IS SHORT AT 2 INCHES (5 CM), 3 INCHES (7.6 CM) AT 18 MONTH'S OF AGE, AND 4–5 INCHES (10.2 TO 12.7 CM) BY ADOLESCENCE, WHICH IS EQUIVALENT TO THE ADULT SIZE.

4. THE RIBS IN THE INFANT ARE HORIZONTAL.

5. INFANTS BREATHE THROUGH THEIR NOSES UNTIL 3–4 MONTHS OF AGE.

6. INFANTS AND TODDLERS ARE ABDOMINAL BREATHERS.

7. CHILDREN UP TO 5 YEARS OF AGE ARE MORE SUSCEPTIBLE TO RESPIRATORY DISTRESS AND OBSTRUCTION BECAUSE THEIR RESPIRATORY TRACTS HAVE A NARROW LUMEN.

8. ACUTE RESPIRATORY ILLNESSES IN CHILDREN IS THE RESULT OF FREQUENT EXPOSURE TO INFECTION AND A LACK OF A DEVELOPED IMMUNE SYSTEM.

II. ASSESSMENT

A. HEALTH HISTORY

1. PAST HEALTH HISTORY

2. MEDICATIONS (PAST, PRESENT, OVER-THE-COUNTER [OTC], HERBAL)

3. SURGERIES

4. SOCIAL (ENVIRONMENTAL EXPOSURES)

5. ASSOCIATED CLINICAL MANIFESTATIONS (CHEST PAIN, DYSPNEA, WHEEZING, COUGH)

B. PHYSICAL EXAM

1. INSPECTION

a. Shape of the thorax
   1) Anterior-posterior dimensions
   2) Congenital anomaly
      a) Pectus carinatum (protrusion of the sternum)
      b) Pectus excavatum (funnel chest, depression in the lower body of the sternum)
      c) Kyphosis (humpback, excessive concavity of the thoracic vertebrae)
   3) Idiopathic
      a) Scoliosis (lateral curvature of the lumbar or thoracic vertebrae)
      b) Neuromuscular diseases, connective tissue diseases, rickets

b. Symmetry of the chest wall: shoulder height, presence of masses, anterior and posterior views, position of the scapula, scoliosis

c. Respirations: rate, pattern, depth, symmetry, preferred client position, mode of breathing, audibility (see Table 31-1)

d. Signs of respiratory distress
   1) Nasal flaring (significant in the infant)
   2) Head bobbing with each respiration in a sleeping infant
   3) Use of accessory muscles
   4) Intercostal spaces—retractions
   5) Grunting
   6) Cough and sputum production (color, odor, amount)

Table 31-1 Normal Respiratory Rates of Pediatric Clients by Age

Age	Rate (Breaths per Minute)
Birth–6 months	30–50
6 months–2 years	20–30
3–10 years	20–28
10–14 years	16–20
16–18 years	12–20

© Cengage Learning 2015

7) Clubbing (chronic hypoxia)
8) Color changes in the skin such as pallor, mottling, or cyanosis

2. AUSCULTATION
   a. General: anterior, posterior, lateral; compare contralateral sides; note quality and location
   b. Breath sounds
      1) Normal breath sounds
         a) Bronchial (expiration longer than inspiration, tubular over the trachea)
         b) Bronchovesicular (loud, high-pitched inspiration over the bronchial bifurcation)
         c) Vesicular (inspiration longer, louder than expiration, over the lungs)
      2) Adventitious breath sounds
         a) Fine crackle (strand of hair rolled between fingers)
         b) Coarse crackle (louder, lower in pitch than fine crackles)
         c) Wheeze (continuous high-pitched whistling or musical sound)
         d) Rhonchi (low-pitched snoring sounds)
         e) Pleural friction rub (grating sound)
         f) Stridor (crowing noise)

3. PERCUSSION
   a. General: anterior, posterior, and lateral
   b. Diaphragmatic excursion (percusses the position of the diaphragm)

4. PALPATION
   a. General: cephalocaudal direction, side to side, anterior, posterior, and lateral
   b. Pulsations
   c. Masses
   d. Thoracic tenderness
   e. Crepitus: crackling sound on palpation caused by air escaped from the lungs and trapped in the subcutaneous tissue

   f. Thoracic expansion (assesses bilateral chest wall movement)
   g. Tactile or vocal fremitus (palpable chest wall vibration produced by voice sounds)
   h. Tracheal position (midline)

III. **DIAGNOSTIC STUDIES**
   A. PULMONARY FUNCTION TESTS (SEE CHAPTER 3, DIAGNOSTIC TESTS RESPIRATORY DISORDERS, SECTION XI.)
   B. PEAK FLOWMETER
      1. DESCRIPTION
         a. Measures peak expiratory flow rate (PEFR)
         b. Used to assess how severe the airflow obstruction is
         c. Initially done one to two times daily to establish personal best then on a periodic and as-needed basis
         d. Used to evaluate the effectiveness of bronchodilator therapy (B_2-agonist)
         e. Cannot be used in children under 4 or 5 years old
      2. PREPROCEDURE
         a. Instruct the child and family on the purpose and method of use
      3. PROCEDURE
         a. Position the child in a standing position.
         b. Instruct the child to exhale sharply into the peak flowmeter, recording the volume of the breath.
         c. Reset after each breath and repeat three times.
      4. POSTPROCEDURE
         a. Establish personal best (highest volume of air exhaled in a single breath with maximal effort) and record on peak flowchart.
      5. INTERPRETATION OF RESULTS
         a. Green zone: highest volume achieved out of three breaths is 80–100% of the personal best volume.
         b. Yellow zone: highest volume achieved out of three breaths is 50–80% of the personal best volume.
         c. Red zone: highest volume achieved out of three breaths is below 50% of the personal best volume.
            1) Signifies serious airflow obstruction
            2) Requires medical intervention
   C. RADIOGRAPHY
      1. DESCRIPTION: X-RAY STUDY OF THE INTERNAL STRUCTURES OF THE CHEST, INCLUDING LUNGS, AIRWAYS, VASCULAR MARKINGS, HEART, AND GREAT VESSELS
      2. PREPROCEDURE
         a. Make certain that the infant or child receives protection from possible

hazards (protection of immature gonads, thyroid gland, ocular lens, and bone marrow). Lead shields may be used.

    b. Remove metal objects from the infant or child that could interfere with the x-ray.

  3. PROCEDURE

    a. Use play and technology modification to decrease potential trauma associated with the procedure and to gain the child's cooperation.

    b. Immobilize the child.

    c. The child is requested to take a deep breath and hold it while the x-ray is taken.

    d. Younger infants and children are placed upright when possible.

D. FLUOROSCOPY

  1. DESCRIPTION

    a. Electronically intensified images are projected on a viewing screen.

    b. Usually used to study respiratory motion of the lungs and the downward movement of the diaphragm

    c. Used also for examination of the barium-filled esophagus to outline mediastinal abnormalities

  2. PREPROCEDURE

    a. NPO for 8–12 hours

    b. No smoking in the adolescent client

    c. Requires immobilization of the child

  3. POSTPROCEDURE

    a. If used in conjunction with barium swallow:

      1) Increase fluids.

      2) Offer a laxative—stools may be white for 72 hours.

E. BRONCHOGRAPHY

  1. DESCRIPTION

    a. Instillation of contrast media directly into the brachial tree through an opaque catheter that is inserted through an orotracheal tube

    b. Used to demonstrate and inspect bronchiectasis, identify distal bronchial obstruction or detect malformations

    c. Used less frequently than other procedures

  2. PREPROCEDURE

    a. NPO for 8–10 hours to prepare for general anesthesia or conscious sedation

    b. No smoking in the adolescent client

    c. Immobilize the child.

    d. Establish IV access.

  3. POSTPROCEDURE

    a. Monitor vital signs.

    b. Assess pain level.

    c. Assess level of consciousness, activity.

F. BARIUM SWALLOW

  1. DESCRIPTION

    a. X-ray study with fluoroscopy and contrast medium such as barium

    b. Displacement of esophagus aids in defining mediastinal masses

    c. Aids in detecting swallowing disorders and malformations such as tracheoesophageal fistula

    d. Performed under fluoroscopy

  2. PREPROCEDURE

    a. NPO for 8–12 hours

    b. No smoking for the adolescent client

  3. POSTPROCEDURE

    a. Encourage 6–8 glasses of water daily.

    b. Offer a laxative—stool may appear white for 72 hours

G. ANGIOGRAPHY

  1. DESCRIPTION

    a. Image of pulmonary vasculature highlighted by injection of the dye

    b. Used for investigation of pulmonary hypertension and pulmonary vascular anomalies

  2. PREPROCEDURE

    a. Assess for allergy to iodinated dyes or shellfish.

    b. Determine if the child has ventricular arrhythmias.

    c. Child must be NPO for 8–12 hours.

    d. Administer preprocedural medications as ordered for sedation and relaxation.

  3. POSTPROCEDURE

    a. Monitor vital signs, level of consciousness, and activity.

    b. Observe the catheter insertion site for inflammation, hemorrhage, or hematoma, applying cold compresses as needed.

    c. Bed rest for 12–24 hours is required after the test.

    d. Inform the child that coughing may occur after the study.

H. COMPUTERIZED TOMOGRAPHY (CT) (SEE CHAPTER 3, RESPIRATORY DISORDERS, COMPUTED TOMOGRAPHY, SECTION III.)

I. MAGNETIC RESONANCE IMAGING (MRI)

  1. DESCRIPTION: NONINVASIVE DIAGNOSTIC SCANNING TECHNIQUE THAT USES A LARGE MAGNET AND RADIO WAVES TO PRODUCE TWO OR THREE-DIMENSIONAL IMAGES OF SOFT TISSUE, THE CENTRAL NERVOUS SYSTEM, AND BLOOD VESSELS

  2. PREPROCEDURE

    a. Assess the child for contraindications to test (internal or external metal objects).

b. You must have the child's cooperation or use sedation.

c. Immobilize the child (may require general anesthesia).

d. Prepare for anesthesia if ordered.

e. NPO for 8–12 hours is required if anesthesia is ordered.

3. POSTPROCEDURE

a. Monitor vital signs, level of consciousness, and activity if the child received sedation or anesthesia.

J. RADIOISOTOPE SCANNING

1. DESCRIPTION: INTRAVENOUS INJECTION OF RADIOISOTOPES OR INHALATION OF RADIOACTIVE AEROSOLS FOLLOWED BY RADIATION SCANNING TO IDENTIFY DISEASED AREAS IN THE LUNG, DEFECTS IN PULMONARY PERFUSION, OR THE LOCATION OF ASPIRATED FOREIGN BODIES

2. PREPROCEDURE

a. Must have cooperation of the child or use sedation

b. Adequate hydration, administer 2–3 glasses of water before test if alert

3. POSTPROCEDURE

a. No precautions need to be taken against radioactive exposure.

b. Encourage 6–8 glasses of water per day.

IV. **LABORATORY TESTING**

A. BLOOD OXYGENATION

1. TRANSCUTANEOUS O_2/CO_2 MONITORING (TCM)

a. Description: provides continuous and reliable trends of arterial O_2 and CO_2 via heated skin surface electrodes applied to a well-perfused area of the trunk; measured in mm Hg

2. OXIMETRY

a. Description: provides noninvasive, continuous photometric measurements of hemoglobin oxygen saturation (SaO_2)

3. CAPNOGRAPHY

a. Description: provides end-tidal CO_2 levels to identify trends and shunts by measuring CO_2 during inhalation and exhalation and producing a graph of CO_2 concentration over time

4. ARTERIAL PUNCTURE

a. Description: obtains arterial blood for gas analysis (PO_2, PCO_2, pH)

B. SPUTUM CULTURE AND SENSITIVITY

1. DESCRIPTION

a. Sputum sample is collected to determine the presence of pathogenic bacteria in clients with respiratory infections.

b. Gram stain is applied first to classify bacteria as gram positive or gram negative.

c. The sputum sample is subsequently applied to various bacterial culture plates.

d. Appropriate antimicrobial drug therapy is determined by identifying bacterial sensitivity to various antibiotics.

e. Tuberculosis sputum cultures: sputum smear for acid-fast bacillus from early morning specimen

2. PREPROCEDURE

a. Sputum specimens are best if collected when the child first awakens, before eating or drinking, and before antibiotic therapy is begun.

b. Coughing may be stimulated by lowering the head of the child's bed or by giving the child an aerosol administration of a warm hypertonic solution.

C. SPUTUM CYTOLOGY

1. DESCRIPTION

a. A collection of sputum examined to determine the presence of malignant cells. A positive test affirms the presence of malignant cells. A negative test is inconclusive.

b. Bronchoscopy and lung biopsy have largely supplanted the need for sputum cytology.

D. NASAL WASHING FOR RESPIRATORY SYNCYTIAL VIRUS

1. DESCRIPTION

a. Method of collecting a nasal specimen for culture

b. Especially useful in young infants

2. PROCEDURE

a. Place the child in a supine position and stabilize the head.

b. Instill 1–3 ml of sterile normal saline into one of the infant's nostrils using a sterile needleless syringe.

c. Use a sterile bulb syringe inserted immediately into the nare to gently aspirate the contents.

d. Send the contents to the lab in a sterile container.

e. Alternative is to use a sterile syringe attached to a short length of 18–20 gauge plastic tubing (piece of butterfly tubing works well) to quickly instill and aspirate the sterile normal saline.

3. POSTPROCEDURE

a. Comfort the infant and assess for respiratory distress.

b. Notify the physician of the results.

    c. Follow hospital infection control guidelines for RSV if results are positive.

E. MANTOUX TEST (PURIFIED PROTEIN DERIVATIVE [PPD]) (SEE CHAPTER 3, RESPIRATORY DISORDERS, SECTION VIII.)

   1. INTERPRETATION OF RESULTS

    a. An area of induration 15 mm or greater is considered to be a positive finding in children older than 4 years with risk factors.

    b. An area of induration 10 mm or greater is considered to be a positive finding in children less than age 4 years, in those with other medical risk factors such as chronic disease, and in those at increased risk for environmental exposure.

    c. An area of 5 mm or greater induration is considered to be a positive finding in children having close contact with persons who have known or suspected infectious cases of tuberculosis.

    d. Skin test results may not be valid in immunocompromised children, infants less than 6 months of age, children who have had bacilli Calmette-Guérin (BCG) vaccine, and those with early infection.

F. SWEAT CHLORIDE TEST

   1. DESCRIPTION

    a. Sodium and chloride content is analyzed from sweat induced by electrical current (pilocarpine iontophoresis).

    b. The degree of abnormality is no indication of the severity of the disease; it simply indicates that the child has cystic fibrosis.

   2. PREPROCEDURE

    a. Explain the test and procedure and reassure the child and family that the electrical current is small and there is usually no discomfort.

    b. Duration of test is about 90 minutes.

   3. PROCEDURE

    a. Positive and negative electrodes are placed over the test area.

    b. Positive electrode is covered with pilocarpine saturated gauze to induce sweating and the negative electrode is covered with bicarbonate solution.

    c. Electrical current is applied for 5–12 minutes.

    d. Electrodes are removed and the test area is rinsed with distilled water.

    e. Paper discs sealed with paraffin are placed over the test sites and left for 1 hour.

    f. Paper discs are removed and analyzed for sodium and chloride content.

   4. POSTPROCEDURE

    a. Educate the child and family and assist with referring to counseling for the child and parents if the test is positive (indicative of cystic fibrosis).

   5. INTERPRETATION OF RESULTS

    a. Sodium content less than 70 mEq/L is normal.

    b. Sodium content greater than 90 mEq/L is abnormal (positive).

    c. Sodium content between 70 and 90 mEq/L is inconclusive.

    d. Chloride content less than 50 mEq/L is normal.

    e. Chloride content greater than 60 mEq/L is abnormal (positive).

    f. Chloride content between 50 and 60 mEq/L is inconclusive.

V. DIAGNOSTIC PROCEDURES

  A. TRACHEAL ASPIRATION

   1. DESCRIPTION: SPUTUM IS DIRECTLY ASPIRATED FROM THE TRACHEA.

   2. PREPROCEDURE

    a. Performed in intubated children or during bronchoscopy

    b. Preparation dependent on circumstances

   3. POSTPROCEDURE

    a. Monitor vital signs.

  B. BRONCHOSCOPY (SEE CHAPTER 3, RESPIRATORY DISORDERS, SECTION IV.)

  C. THORACENTESIS

   1. DESCRIPTION

    a. Needle aspiration of lung fluid via a needle and syringe through the pleural space

    b. Obtains lung aspirate to relieve pain and dyspnea, for histologic study or culture, or for instillation of antibiotics directly into the pleural cavity

   2. PREPROCEDURE

    a. Provide explanation to the child and family.

    b. Sitting position with the arms and trunk bent forward is required in a child, semirecumbent position on the unaffected side for an infant.

   3. DURING THE PROCEDURE

    a. Monitor vital signs.

    b. Assess for changes in color, respirations, or pulse, and for alterations in behavior or level of consciousness.

    c. Provide emotional support.

   4. POSTPROCEDURE

    a. Record the amount and description of the fluid obtained.

    b. Send the specimen to the lab for culture.

c. Dress the wound and place the child on the unaffected side for at least 1 hour to permit the puncture site to heal.

d. Record any medications administered.

e. Monitor vital signs and respiratory status, assessing for signs of pneumothorax or infection.

f. Monitor level of consciousness and activity.

g. Assist with chest x-ray as prescribed to check for pneumothorax.

h. Watch for excessive coughing or hemoptysis (coughing of blood).

i. Manage closed chest drainage system if instituted.

D. LUNG BIOPSY (SEE CHAPTER 3, RESPIRATORY DISORDERS, SECTION V.)

E. BRUSH BIOPSY

  1. DESCRIPTION

    a. Lung tissue for culture and histologic examination is obtained with a nylon brush on the end of a wire that is passed through a tube placed via the nose, pharynx, trachea, and airways to the affected area of the lungs.

    b. Procedure is performed using fluoroscopy.

  2. PREPROCEDURE

    a. NPO is required for 8–12 hours.

    b. Administer drugs as ordered 30–60 minutes prior to the procedure.

    c. Immobilization of the child is required.

    d. Establish IV access.

  3. POSTPROCEDURE

    a. Monitor vital signs.

    b. Monitor level of consciousness (LOC).

VI. NURSING DIAGNOSES

A. INEFFECTIVE AIRWAY CLEARANCE

B. ANXIETY

C. INEFFECTIVE BREATHING PATTERN

D. FATIGUE

E. DISTURBED SLEEP PATTERN

F. RISK FOR INFECTION

Nursing Diagnoses: Definitions and Classification 2012–2014.
Copyright © 2012, 1994–2012 by NANDA International.
Used by arrangement with John Wiley & Sons Limited.

VII. RESPIRATORY DISEASES: INFECTIONS OF THE UPPER AIRWAYS

A. ACUTE VIRAL NASOPHARYNGITIS

  1. DESCRIPTION

    a. May be referred to as "the common cold"

    b. Caused by viruses such as rhinosinovirus, respiratory syncytial virus, adenovirus, influenza virus, or parainfluenza virus

    c. Higher incidence in children under 3 years of age (average six to eight colds per year) and in those attending large day care centers

    d. Self-limiting: resolves in 4–10 days

  2. ASSESSMENT

    a. Clinical manifestations are more serious in infants and children than in adults.

    b. Fever is common early in the illness.

    c. May be concomitant otitis media, especially in young children

    d. Infants and young children display irritability, restlessness, decreased appetite and activity, vomiting, and diarrhea.

    e. Open mouth breathing is common.

    f. Older children display dryness and irritation of the nasal passages and pharynx, sneezing, chilling, muscular aches, nasal discharge.

  3. NURSING INTERVENTIONS

    a. Instruct the parents on the administration of analgesics and antipyretics.

    b. Encourage fluids and maintain hydration.

    c. Instruct the parents on the administration of decongestants in children over age 6 months as prescribed.

    d. Instruct the parents on the administration of cough suppressants as prescribed; caution that they may contain alcohol and should not be used continuously.

    e. Inform the parents that antihistamines, antibiotics, and expectorants are not generally recommended for treatment of acute viral nasopharyngitis in children.

    f. Encourage good hand washing to prevent the spread of colds.

    g. Place the infant and young children in a comfortable position to maximize ventilation.

    h. Instill saline nose drops and gently suction the infant's nose with a bulb syringe to maintain patency of nares in obligatory nose breathers.

    i. Increased humidity may be helpful.

VIII. RESPIRATORY DISEASES: CROUP SYNDROMES

A. EPIGLOTTITIS

  1. DESCRIPTION

    a. Serious inflammation of the epiglottis that results in supraglottic obstruction; bacterial in origin

    b. Occurs primarily in children between 2 and 7 years, but it can occur from infancy to adulthood.

c. The onset is abrupt and usually preceded by a sore throat, but not by cold clinical manifestations.

d. Considered an emergency situation

e. Epiglottic swelling is diminished after 24 hours of antibiotic therapy and intubated children can usually be extubated by day 3.

f. Bacterial causative agent is usually *Haemophilus influenzae.*

2. ASSESSMENT

a. High fever

b. Irritability and restlessness

c. Red and inflamed throat with cherry edematous epiglottis (Note: Attempt throat inspection ONLY when immediate intubation can be performed if needed.)

d. Difficulty swallowing and drooling

e. Muffled voice

f. Inspiratory and sometimes expiratory stridor

g. Suprasternal and substernal retractions may be visible.

h. Tripod positioning: while supporting the body with the hands, the child thrusts the chin forward and opens the mouth in an attempt to widen the airway.

i. Sallow color of mild hypoxia, possibly progressing to cyanosis

3. DIAGNOSTIC TESTING

a. Blood cultures usually are ordered; restrain the child as needed.

b. Lateral neck radiograph may be obtained before the physical exam is taken (thumb sign is a classic finding).

4. NURSING INTERVENTIONS

a. Arrange for transport of the child to an emergency facility.

b. Monitor airway status and breath sounds. Assess for signs of respiratory distress: nasal flaring, the use of accessory muscles, stridor, and retractions.

c. Monitor vital signs; take axillary temperature, not oral temperature.

d. Maintain the child in a position that provides the most comfort and security.

e. Do not leave the child unattended and do not allow the child to lie down.

f. Do not restrain the child.

g. Do not attempt to visualize the posterior pharynx using a tongue depressor because this could result in spasm of the epiglottis and airway occlusion.

h. Prepare the child for lateral neck films to confirm the diagnosis.

i. Prepare the child with severe respiratory distress for possible endotracheal intubation or tracheostomy.

j. Establish IV access (any invasive procedure should be done in a setting in which intubation is available if needed).

k. Maintain NPO status.

l. Administer IV fluids and antibiotics as prescribed.

m. Monitor hydration status and record intake and output.

n. Administer corticosteroids, as prescribed, to reduce edema during the early hours of treatment and for 24 hours after extubation.

5. PREVENTION

a. *Haemophilus influenzae* type B conjugate vaccine beginning at age 2 months

B. LARYNGOTRACHEOBRONCHITIS (INFECTIOUS CROUP)

1. DESCRIPTION

a. Caused by inflammation of the mucosa lining the larynx and trachea, which results in airway narrowing

b. Narrowed airways impede inspiration, resulting in stridor.

c. Viral etiology is most common but may have viral or bacterial etiology.

d. Most common type of croup

e. Primarily affects children less than age 5 years

f. Gradual onset, often preceded by an upper respiratory infection

2. ASSESSMENT

a. Stage I

1) Anxiousness or fear

2) Hoarseness (primary complaint)

3) Croupy cough (like a seal barking)

4) May demonstrate inspiratory stridor when disturbed

b. Stage II

1) Respiratory stridor becomes continuous.

2) Soft tissue of the neck may retract.

3) Intercostal retractions of the lower ribs.

4) Accessory muscles of respiration are used.

5) Labored respiration, mild wheezing may be present.

c. Stage III

1) Signs of anoxia and carbon dioxide retention develop such as tachypnea, restlessness, anxiety.

2) Sweating

3) Pallor

d. Stage IV
   1) Intermittent cyanosis progressing to permanent cyanosis
   2) Respiratory failure (cessation of breathing)

3. DIAGNOSTIC TESTING
   a. Usually diagnosis is clinically evident.
   b. Radiography of the soft tissue of the chest and neck may be done

4. NURSING INTERVENTIONS
   a. Maintain a patent airway and provide for adequate respiratory exchange.
   b. Children with mild croup (defined as no stridor at rest) may be managed at home.
   c. Provide parent education on the clinical manifestations of respiratory distress such as tachypnea, use of accessory muscles, retractions, or restlessness.
   d. Children who progress to Stage II require medical attention.
   e. Administer cool temperature therapy, including cool mist humidifier, or night air.
   f. Monitor vital signs.
   g. Assess respiratory status: Look for nasal flaring, sternal retractions, inspiratory stridor.
   h. Monitor for cyanosis.
   i. Elevate the head at rest.
   j. Provide humidified oxygen as needed and as ordered.
   k. Provide fluids, begin intravenous if the child is unable to take oral fluids.
   l. Administer antipyretics such as acetaminophen to reduce fever.
   m. Avoid cough syrups and cold medicines.
   n. Administer nebulized epinephrine (racemic epinephrine) in children with severe disease.
   o. Administer corticosteroids as prescribed, because the anti-inflammatory effects decrease subglottic edema.
   p. Have resuscitation equipment available.

C. ACUTE SPASMODIC LARYNGITIS
   1. DESCRIPTION
      a. Brief attacks of laryngeal obstruction that occur suddenly, chiefly at night
      b. Absent to mild signs of inflammation
      c. Usually affects children ages 1 to 3 years and may be recurrent
      d. There is no associated fever.
      e. Duration of the attack is a few hours and the child feels well the next morning.

2. ASSESSMENT
   a. Child retires well and awakens suddenly with characteristic barking, metallic cough, noisy inspirations, hoarseness, and restlessness.
   b. Child may appear anxious and frightened.
   c. Excitement aggravates dyspnea.

3. NURSING INTERVENTIONS
   a. Administer steam from a hot bath or shower or cold steam from a humidifier in the bedroom to relieve mild clinical manifestations.
   b. Attempt exposure to night air to terminate laryngeal spasm.
   c. Administer cough and cold medicines as prescribed if the child has accompanying upper respiratory infection manifestations.
   d. Administer a bronchodilator such as albuterol, as prescribed, if bronchospasm is suspected.
   e. If moderately severe clinical manifestations, child may need to be hospitalized for observation and administration of cool mist and racemic epinephrine therapy.

D. BACTERIAL TRACHEITIS
   1. DESCRIPTION
      a. Bacterial infection involving the mucosa of the upper trachea
      b. Common pathogens include *Staphylococcus aureus,* group A beta-hemolytic streptococcus, and *Haemophilus influenzae*
      c. Exhibits features of both croup and epiglottitis
      d. Affects children ages 1 month to 6 years
      e. Usually preceded by upper respiratory infection with croupy cough
      f. May be a complication of laryngotracheobronchitis
      g. Early identification is essential to prevent airway obstruction.
      h. Usually follows a slower course than epiglottitis

   2. ASSESSMENT
      a. Fever
      b. Brassy cough
      c. Inspiratory stridor
      d. Hallmark: production of thick purulent tracheal secretions which can result in airway obstruction and even respiratory arrest

   3. DIAGNOSTIC TESTING
      a. Complete blood count (white blood cell count elevated)
      b. Lateral neck radiography as per epiglottitis (thumb sign absent)

4. NURSING INTERVENTIONS
   a. Inform the parent of the need for vigorous management and hospitalization.
   b. Administer humidified oxygen and airway support.
   c. Administer antipyretics as prescribed.
   d. Administer antibiotics as prescribed.
   e. Be prepared for endotracheal intubation and frequent suctioning to prevent airway obstruction.

IX. **RESPIRATORY DISEASES: INFECTIONS OF THE LOWER AIRWAYS**
  A. BRONCHIOLITIS
   1. DESCRIPTION
      a. An acute viral infection causing inflammation of the bronchioles and production of thick mucus that occludes the bronchiole tubes and small airways, impeding expiration
      b. Air becomes trapped behind the obstruction and leads to progressive overinflation of the lungs called emphysema.
      c. Usually occurs in children under the age of 2 years with peak incidence at ages 2–5 months during the winter months
      d. Most common causative agent is respiratory syncytial virus (RSV)
      e. Other causative agents include adenoviruses and parainfluenzae viruses.
      f. Transmission is through direct contact with respiratory secretions.
      g. Usually begins with an upper respiratory infection and has an incubation of 5–8 days
   2. ASSESSMENT
      a. Initial upper respiratory infection clinical manifestations include rhinorrhea, pharyngitis, coughing, sneezing, wheezing, possible ear or eye infection.
      b. Fever
      c. Signs of altered air exchange develop with progression of the disease: wheezing, retractions, crackles, dyspnea, tachypnea, nasal flaring, and diminished breath sounds.
      d. Cyanosis and apneic spells indicating severe disease
      e. Infants may exhibit irritability, poor feeding, or listlessness.
      f. Liver and spleen may be palpable due to hyperinflated lungs.
   3. DIAGNOSTIC TESTING
      a. Chest radiograph (anterior-posterior [AP] and lateral) shows hyperinflation of the lungs and increased AP diameter.
      b. RSV detection by nasal washing
         1) Viral culture: slower, may be less sensitive
         2) Direct fluorescent antibody (DFA) staining: rapid, sensitive
         3) Enzyme linked immunoabsorbent assay (ELISA): rapid, sensitive
   4. NURSING INTERVENTIONS
      a. Collect nasal or nasopharyngeal secretions for rapid immunofluorescent antibody (IFA) or ELISA testing for antigen detection.
      b. Elevate the head and maintain a patent airway.
      c. Monitor vital signs.
      d. Provide cool humidified oxygen.
      e. Assess for signs of dehydration such as sunken fontanel, decreased skin turgor, listlessness, decreased and concentrated urinary output.
      f. Assess for altered air exchange and respiratory distress.
      g. Maintain adequate fluid intake.
      h. Provide adequate rest.
      i. Inform the parents that hospitalization may be necessary for those who become dehydrated, have tachypnea greater than 70 breaths per minute, apneic spells, diminished breath sounds, and poor gas exchange.
      j. Inform the parents that the use of bronchodilators, corticosteroids, cough suppressants, and antibiotics is controversial and that they are not recommended routinely.
      k. Administer ribavirin (Copegus), an antiviral agent, in high-risk individuals.
   5. THE CHILD WITH RSV
      a. Isolate in a single room or group with other RSV-infected children.
      b. Maintain good hand washing.
      c. Limit the number of hospital personnel and visitors coming in contact with the child.
      d. Wear a protective gown if there is a likelihood of contamination of clothing.
      e. Avoid assigning nurses to care for other high-risk individuals when caring for the RSV-positive child.
      f. Administer ribavirin (Copegus) as prescribed.
      g. Avoid contact with ribavirin. Wear goggles, if soft contact lens wearer, and exposure to ribavirin is likely.

6. PREVENTION
   a. Administer RespiGam or respiratory syncytial virus immune globulin (RSV-IGIV) to high-risk infants as ordered; monitor for fluid overload during administration if there are underlying pulmonary problems. RespiGam is not approved by the Food and Drug Administration (FDA) for use in children with congenital heart disease and should not be used in clients with cyanotic congenital heart disease.

B. BRONCHITIS
   1. DESCRIPTION
      a. Inflammation of the large airways (trachea and bronchi) usually in combination with an upper or lower tract respiratory infection
      b. Viral agents are the primary cause in children under age 6 years, but it may have bacterial or asthmatic origin.
      c. *Mycoplasma pneumoniae* is a common cause in children older than age 6 years.
      d. Usual duration is 5–10 days.
   2. ASSESSMENT
      a. Dry, hacking, and initially nonproductive cough that is worse at night and becomes productive in 2–3 days
      b. May have fever
      c. Coarse breath sounds with rhonchi and crackles
      d. Evidence of nasopharyngitis common
   3. NURSING INTERVENTIONS
      a. Monitor for respiratory distress.
      b. Monitor vital signs.
      c. Administer antipyretics.
      d. Administer analgesics.
      e. Provide humidified air.
      f. Administer cough suppressants to promote rest but may impede clearance of secretions.
      g. Monitor weight and fluid status.
      h. Assess for signs of dehydration.
      i. Administer respiratory treatments such as postural drainage as prescribed.

C. PNEUMONIA
   1. DESCRIPTION
      a. Inflammation of the parenchyma of the lung caused by bacteria bacilli (*Streptococcus pneumoniae, Staphylococcus aureus, Haemophilus influenzae,* enteric chlamydia), virus, mycoplasma, or aspiration of foreign substance
      b. Subclassifications can be made by morphology, etiologic agent, or clinical form.

   c. It can occur at any age, but young infants have a higher risk.
   d. Primary atypical pneumonia (most common etiologic agent is mycoplasma) occurs during ages 5–12 years.
   2. ASSESSMENT
      a. Clinical manifestations vary depending on the etiologic agent, age of the child, the child's systemic reaction to the infection, the extent of the lesions, and the degree of bronchial and bronchiolar obstruction
   3. TYPES
      a. Viral pneumonia
         1) Varying degree of fever
         2) Increased pulse and respiratory rate
         3) Cough ranging from mild to severe
         4) Wheezes, fine crackles, or diminished breath sounds on auscultation
         5) Radiographic findings: patchy infiltration with a peribronchial distribution
      b. Bacterial pneumonia
         1) Often follows viral upper respiratory infection or is secondary to viral pneumonia in children
         2) Most common pathogen is *Streptococcus pneumoniae,* with the highest incidence in late winter and early spring, but pathogen varies with age.
         3) Fever, usually quite high
         4) Respiratory clinical manifestations include cough, tachypnea, rhonchi or fine crackles, dullness with percussion, diminished breath sounds, chest pain, retractions, nasal flaring, or circumoral pallor to cyanosis depending on severity.
         5) Behavior manifestations include irritability, restlessness, lethargy, poor feeding in infants.
         6) Gastrointestinal: anorexia, vomiting, diarrhea, abdominal pain
         7) Radiographic findings: diffuse or patchy infiltration with peribronchial distribution
      c. Primary atypical pneumonia (mycoplasma)
         1) Onset is variable: fever, chills, headache, malaise, anorexia, and muscle pain
         2) Followed by rhinitis, sore throat, and a dry, hacking cough

3) Fine crackles or rhonchi on auscultation

4) Radiographic findings of emphysema and consolidation may be evident before physical signs are apparent.

4. DIAGNOSTIC TESTS

   a. Chest x-ray (PA and lateral): lobar or segmental consolidation, possible pleural effusion

   b. Complete blood count (white blood cell count elevated)

   c. Arterial blood gases (ABGs) consistent with hypoxia

   d. Culture: nasopharyngeal scrapings, tracheal aspiration, blood, lung tap fluid

5. NURSING INTERVENTIONS

   a. Monitor vital signs, activity, and level of consciousness.

   b. Assess breath sounds and respiratory pattern.

   c. Instruct the parents to elevate the head of the bed to ease respirations, but avoid the use of infant seats because pressure may be placed on the diaphragm, which inhibits lung expansion.

   d. Monitor cardiac, respiratory, and pulse oximetry per monitors as needed.

   e. Administer oxygen therapy with cool mist as ordered.

   f. Schedule chest physiotherapy and postural drainage before meals and at bedtime as ordered.

   g. Administer antipyretics for fever management.

   h. Maintain hydration and monitor fluid intake and urine output.

   i. Monitor weight.

   j. Assess for signs of dehydration.

   k. Administer antibiotics as prescribed.

   l. Monitor for tension pneumothorax or empyema in staphylococcal pneumonia.

   m. Maintain continuous closed chest drainage, if required, in staphylococcal pneumonia with purulent effusions.

   n. Reduce anxiety and apprehension to promote relaxation and ease respiratory effort.

6. PREVENTION

   a. Immunization with the pneumococcal polysaccharide polyvalent vaccine is recommended for children under age 2 years and those over age 2 years who are immunocompromised.

X. **OTHER INFECTIONS OF THE RESPIRATORY TRACT**

A. TUBERCULOSIS

   1. DESCRIPTION

      a. A reportable contagious disease caused by the acid-fast bacillus, *Mycobacterium tuberculosis,* spread by a person with active tuberculosis who coughs or sneezes

      b. Transmission via inhalation of microdroplets into the respiratory tract

      c. Children most commonly infected by a member of the household or frequent visitor to the household

      d. Higher incidence of disease in infancy and again in puberty and adolescence versus middle childhood

   2. ASSESSMENT

      a. May be asymptomatic but can produce a wide variety of clinical manifestations

      b. General clinical manifestations: fever, weight loss, malaise, anorexia, lymphadenopathy

      c. Lung disease: may include cough, chest pain and tightness, hemoptysis

      d. Children ages 3–15 years are usually asymptomatic and often have normal chest x-ray results despite a positive skin test.

      e. Tachypnea, diminished breath sounds and crackles to auscultation, dullness to percussion over the affected area in more advanced disease

      f. Children (especially infants) may develop pallor and anemia in advanced disease.

      g. Positive Mantoux test (will produce positive result 3–6 weeks after initial exposure, occasionally as long as 3 months after infection)

      h. Positive risk factor screen (known exposure, children with immunosuppressive condition, frequent exposure to individual at risk for tuberculosis [TB])

      i. Radiographic findings: hilar adenopathy, tuberculous granulomatous polyp; other chronic intrathoracic diseases may simulate tuberculosis lesions

   3. DIAGNOSTIC TESTS

      a. Mantoux skin test

      b. Early morning gastric washings are the preferred method to obtain specimen for culture and smear. (Collecting sputum specimen in the usual manner is difficult because children are likely to swallow any mucus from the lower respiratory tract that is produced with cough.)

    c. Chest x-ray (PA and lateral): hilar adenopathy is suggestive of TB.

4. NURSING INTERVENTIONS

    a. Hospitalization is rare.

    b. Inform the parents that asymptomatic children may attend day care or school but should refrain from participating in vigorous activity or contact sports.

    c. Instruct the parents on the importance of adequate rest and diet.

    d. Instruct the parents to minimize exposure to other infections that further compromise the body's defenses.

    e. Administer isoniazid (INH), rifampin (Rifadin), and pyrazinamide (PZA) as prescribed.

        1) Recommended drug regimen to prevent latent infection from progressing to active TB is INH for 9 months or for 12 months in a child infected with the human immunodeficiency virus (HIV).

        2) Recommended drug regimen in active TB is a 2-month regimen of INH, rifampin, and PZA followed by a 4-month regimen of INH and rifampin.

        3) If drug resistance is present, ethambutol or streptomycin may be prescribed.

    f. Assist with filing the necessary paperwork for reporting tuberculosis to the state department of health as appropriate.

    g. Instruct the parents in measures to prevent transmission of TB to others.

    h. Instruct the parents to continue with regular immunization schedule.

B. PERTUSSIS (WHOOPING COUGH)

    1. DESCRIPTION

    a. An acute communicable respiratory infection caused by the bacterium *Bordetella pertussis*

    b. Occurs chiefly in children younger than 4 years who have not been fully immunized

    c. Young infants under 6 months of age are most at risk

    d. Higher incidence in spring and summer months

    e. Transmission by direct contact or droplet spread from an infected person or by indirect contact with articles that have been freshly contaminated

    f. Incubation period is 6–20 days.

2. ASSESSMENT

    a. Catarrhal stage

        1) Clinical manifestations of upper respiratory infection, including cough, coryza, sneezing, tearing, or low-grade fever

        2) Dry, hacking cough becomes more severe.

        3) Lasts 1–3 weeks

    b. Paroxysmal stage

        1) Staccato cough, usually at night followed by high-pitched crowing sound or "whoop" on sudden inspiration (may be no whoop in children under 6 months of age)

        2) Cheeks may be flushed or cyanotic, eyes may bulge, and the tongue may protrude during paroxysms.

        3) Paroxysms often continue until a thick mucus plug is dislodged.

            a) Vomiting may follow paroxysm.

            b) Exhaustion follows coughing paroxysm.

        4) Lasts 4–6 weeks

    c. Convalescent stage

        1) Paroxysmal coughing episodes wane.

        2) Lasts 2–3 weeks

3. DIAGNOSTIC TESTS

    a. Culture for *Bordetella pertussis* from nasopharyngeal swab

    b. Complete blood count (CBC) if ordered

4. NURSING INTERVENTIONS

    a. Monitor vital signs.

    b. Assess for signs of respiratory distress and maintain a patent airway.

    c. Use a bulb syringe or gentle mechanical suctioning to clear secretions.

    d. Inform the parents that hospitalization may be required for infants and children who are dehydrated or who have complications.

    e. Maintain bed rest until the fever subsides.

    f. Increase oxygen intake and provide humidity.

    g. Maintain a restful, irritant-free environment.

    h. Maintain adequate hydration and monitor intake and output.

    i. Administer antipyretic, analgesic, and antimicrobial medications as prescribed.

j. Administer antibiotic treatment with erythromycin, not to alter the course of the illness but to limit the spread of the organism if given in the paroxysmal stage.

k. Be prepared for endotracheal intubation in severe cases.

l. Apply respiratory precautions if hospitalized and isolate during catarrhal phase.

XI. CHRONIC RESPIRATORY DISORDERS

A. ASTHMA

1. **DESCRIPTION**
   a. Chronic inflammatory disorder of the airways involving mast cells, T-lymphocytes, and eosinophils
   b. Inflammation causes recurrent episodes of wheezing, cough, breathlessness, and chest tightness, especially at night or in the early morning.
   c. Inflammation also causes bronchial hyperresponsiveness to a variety of stimuli such as foods, pollen, dust, smoke, animal dander, temperature changes, upper respiratory infection (URI), activity, and stress.
   d. Chronic inflammation can result in airway remodeling and irreversible changes.
   e. Asthma prevalence, morbidity, and mortality are increasing worldwide.

2. **ASSESSMENT**
   a. Breathlessness or dyspnea with eventual cyanosis if prolonged
   b. End expiratory wheezing (also inspiratory in severe exacerbations)
   c. Hacking, irritating, paroxysmal, nonproductive cough progressing to rattling productive cough of gelatinous mucus
   d. Coarse, loud breath sounds (with severe bronchospasm, breath sounds and crackles may become inaudible)
   e. Nighttime cough or exercise-induced cough in the absence of respiratory infection
   f. Tachypnea
   g. Orthopnea
   h. Apprehension, restlessness, and inability to be comforted
   i. Infants may display retractions, nasal flaring, and use of accessory muscles

3. **CLASSIFICATIONS**
   a. Mild intermittent
      1) Clinical manifestations less than two times per week
      2) Exacerbations are brief
      3) Nighttime clinical manifestations occur less than 2 times per month
      4) Asymptomatic and normal peak flow between exacerbations
      5) Forced expiratory volume (FEV) in 1 second or peak expiratory flow (PEF) > 80% of predicted volume
      6) PEF variability less than 20%
   b. Mild persistent
      1) Clinical manifestations occur more than two times per week but less than one time per day.
      2) Exacerbations may affect activity.
      3) Nighttime clinical manifestations occur more than two times per month.
         a) PEF/FEV greater than 80% of predicted volume
         b) PEF variability 20–30%
   c. Moderate persistent
      1) Clinical manifestations occur daily.
      2) Daily use of inhaled short-acting B-agonist
      3) Activity affects exacerbations.
      4) Exacerbations occur at least two times per week.
      5) Exacerbations may last several days.
      6) Nighttime clinical manifestations occur more than one time per week.
      7) PEF/FEV > 60% to < 80% of predicted value
      8) PEF variability > 30%
   d. Severe persistent asthma
      1) Continuous clinical manifestations
      2) Frequent exacerbations
      3) Limited physical activity
      4) PEF/FEV < 60% of predicted value
      5) PEF variability > 30%

4. **DIAGNOSTIC TESTS**
   a. Laboratory tests
      1) CBC
      2) Allergic workup: RAST, skin testing, immunoglobulins
      3) Sweat test (if cystic fibrosis is considered)
      4) Chest x-ray
      5) Sinus x-ray
      6) Pulmonary function tests (PFTs)
      7) Peak expiratory flow rate (PEFR)

5. **NURSING INTERVENTIONS**
   a. General outcome criteria are to prevent lung remodeling and long-term disability, minimize or alleviate physical and psychological effects of the disease, and assist the child and family to live as normal a life as possible.

1) Instruct the parents on health care follow-up at least every 6 months, which includes clinical manifestations and a pharmacological review.
2) Instruct the parents and child to avoid triggers and allergens and compliance with the medication regimen as prescribed (see Table 31-2).
3) Inform the parents on pharmacologic management and environmental control.
4) Therapy should include objective measures that periodically monitor the severity of the disease and the effectiveness of treatment.

Table 31-2 Reducing Allergen Exposure in the Home and Outdoors

In the bedroom: Encase mattress, box springs, and pillows in vinyl covering or other similar barrier. Tape over zippers of barriers of bedding covers. Launder curtains, blankets, mattress pads, and comforters every 2 weeks. Launder bed linens and favorite stuffed animals weekly. Maintain laundry water at 130°F. Avoid nonessential fabric items and those made with feathers. Wash down the bedroom and closet every couple of months.
Pets and pests: Keep animals outside the home. Clean the home thoroughly if animals have lived indoors. Keep the indoor pet in uncarpeted areas that are easily cleaned. Premedicate the child before visiting a home with an animal. Eradicate cockroach populations in the home. Clean the home thoroughly if cockroaches have been present.
Throughout the house: Clean moldy surfaces with 1:10 solution of bleach and water. Use a dehumidifier to reduce mold growth in damp houses; keep humidity < 45%. If humidifier is used, change water regularly and clean with bleach solution. Avoid house plants. Damp mop and damp dust at least once per week. Vacuum carpets and upholstery at least once per week. Dry clean drapes and carpets. Remove carpeting and replace if possible with wood or vinyl. Replace furnace filters or use an electrostatic filter. Filter furnace vents. Close windows and use air conditioners when outdoor air quality is poor. Keep home a smoke-free environment (tobacco or wood). Avoid use of strong odors or sprays.
Outdoors: Keep the child from compost or leaf piles, woods, and other high-mold areas. Keep the child indoors when air quality is poor and when the mold/pollen counts are high. Keep the child from wood smoke, animals, and agriculture chemicals. Avoid exercise in cold, dry air.

© Cengage Learning 2015

b. Acute episode
  1) Assess cardiac, respiratory status, and pulse oximetry.
  2) Administer rescue medication bronchodilator, such as albuterol (beta-2 agonist), via nebulizer as prescribed.
  3) Monitor vital signs and PEFR.
  4) In severe cases or if PEFR is < 50%, transport to an emergency facility (if not already there).
  5) Initiate intravenous access.
  6) Prepare the child for x-ray, if needed, as ordered.
  7) Administer humidified oxygen as prescribed and maintain SaO_2 (oxygen saturation) > 90%.
  8) Administer bronchodilators, anticholinergics, and corticosteroids by IV if prescribed.
  9) Obtain blood gases and serum electrolytes as ordered.
  10) Administer IV sodium bicarbonate, as prescribed, to correct acidosis.
c. Long-term management
  1) Instruct the child and family about the disease process and management approach, including pharmacotherapy, respiratory treatments, and exercises as prescribed.
  2) Instruct the parents and child on the regular use of anti-inflammatory medications such as cromolyn (Intal) or nedocromil sodium (Tilade) and corticosteroids for persistent asthma as prescribed.
  3) Instruct the parents on the use of a bronchodilator such as albuterol (Proventil) as rescue medication for acute exacerbations.
  4) Encourage adequate rest, sleep, and a well-balanced diet.
  5) Instruct the parents in the importance of adequate fluid intake to assist in liquefying secretions.
  6) Allow the child to take control of daily self-care measures based on age appropriateness.
  7) Avoid exposure to allergens, triggers, and individuals with viral respiratory infections.
  8) Assist in developing an exercise program.
  9) Instruct the child on how to recognize early clinical

manifestations of an asthma attack: itchy chest or chin, cough, irritability, tired feeling, increased respiratory rate, dry mouth, or unusual dark circles under the eyes.

  10) Encourage the parents to keep immunizations up to date and to obtain an annual influenza vaccine.

  11) Instruct the child and parents on the use of the peak flowmeter, nebulizer, inhaler, and spacer as prescribed.

B. CYSTIC FIBROSIS

  1. DESCRIPTION

    a. Chronic congenital condition characterized by exocrine (mucous gland) dysfunction that results in multisystem involvement; pulmonary system is affected to some degree in most children with cystic fibrosis

    b. Inherited as autosomal recessive trait

    c. Mucus produced by the exocrine glands is abnormally thick, causing obstruction of the small passageways of organs such as the pancreas and bronchioles.

    d. Stagnant mucus provides an optimal medium for bacterial growth.

    e. Chloride channel defect in the sweat glands prevents reabsorption of sodium and chloride.

    f. Most common in Caucasians, extremely rare in other races

  2. ASSESSMENT

    a. Respiratory system

      1) Wheezing and nonproductive, dry cough initially

      2) Dyspnea with mucoid impactions, crackles, and diminished breath sounds on auscultation

      3) Repeated episodes of bronchitis and bronchopneumonia

      4) Purulent and copious sputum with infections

      5) Increased incidence of chronic sinusitis and nasal polyps

      6) Evidence of chronic obstructive pulmonary disease such as clubbing of fingers, barrel chest, emphysema, and atelectasis

      7) Signs of respiratory distress, including retractions, hypoxia, accessory muscle use, and cyanosis

      8) Cor pulmonale, heart failure (HF), spontaneous pneumothorax, or hemoptysis as the disease progresses

    b. Gastrointestinal system

      1) Meconium ileus in the neonate

      2) Steatorrhea; large, foul-smelling stools

      3) Abdominal distention or bowel obstruction, or both

      4) Malnutrition and growth failure despite a healthy appetite

      5) Rectal prolapse, impacted feces, and bowel obstruction

      6) Malabsorption of fat-soluble vitamins, resulting in anemia and bruising

      7) Biliary cirrhosis, portal hypertension, and esophageal varices as a result of obstruction of the bile ducts

      8) Pancreatic insufficiency due to obstructed pancreatic ducts

    c. Integumentary system

      1) Consistent abnormally high concentrations of sodium and chloride in the sweat because of a defect in the chloride channel in the sweat glands

      2) Prone to electrolyte imbalance and dehydration, especially during hot weather

      3) Dry mouth

      4) Increased susceptibility to infection

    d. Reproductive system

      1) Delayed puberty in females

      2) Sterility in males

      3) Difficulty becoming pregnant due to highly viscous cervical mucus

      4) Increased incidence of fetal loss and preterm birth

    e. Endocrine system

      1) Diabetes mellitus more common than in the general population

  3. DIAGNOSTIC TESTS

    a. Sweat chloride test

    b. Pancreatic function tests

    c. Pulmonary function tests

    d. Newborn screening for immunoreactive trypsinogen

  4. NURSING INTERVENTIONS

    a. General

      1) Provide information on adequate nutrition to promote growth.

      2) Assist the child and family in accessing resources to facilitate adaptation to a chronic disorder.

      3) Maintain pulmonary hygiene to prevent or minimize pulmonary complications, including chest physiotherapy.

      4) Regularly assess the child for pulmonary or gastrointestinal complications.

5) Administer antibiotic therapy as prescribed for infections.
6) Administer pharmacotherapy as prescribed, including medications for the blockade of the sodium pump, alteration of abnormal mucus in the airways, inhibition of neutrophil elastase (enzyme that causes inflammation), promotion of chloride secretion, and replacement gene therapy.
7) Encourage the parents to maintain up-to-date immunizations.
8) Administer pancreatic enzymes, as prescribed, within 30 minutes of eating meals and snacks.
9) Do not mix pancreatic enzymes with hot or starchy foods but with a small amount of nonfat, nonprotein food.
10) Avoid crushing or instruct the client to avoid chewing; enteric-coated pancreatic enzymes should not be crushed or chewed.
11) Administer multivitamins and iron supplements as prescribed.
12) Instruct the parents in the use of mucolytics, bronchodilators, hydrating agents, and steroids.
13) Instruct the parents not to give cough suppressants because they will inhibit expectoration of secretions and promote infection.
14) Protect the child from exposure to infections.
15) Supplement the child's diet with salt during extremely hot weather or if the child has a fever.
16) Provide emotional support to the child and family.

b. Acute
1) Assess respiratory status.
2) Elevate the head of the bed or support the child in an upright position if he is having difficulty breathing.
3) Administer low-flow oxygen.
4) Monitor vital signs.
5) Assess weight.
6) Maintain hydration and nutrition. Include the use of supplemental therapies as prescribed.
7) Encourage coughing and deep breathing.
8) Instruct the child on the forced expiratory technique to mobilize secretions.
9) Perform respiratory treatments as prescribed.

10) Administer chest physiotherapy before meals as prescribed (usually at least twice daily).
11) Administer bronchodilator therapy before chest physiotherapy as prescribed.
12) Administer pharmacotherapy such as a bronchodilator, a mucolytic, an antibiotic, or oxygen as prescribed.
13) Provide emotional support to the child and family.

XII. OTHER RESPIRATORY DISORDERS
A. SUDDEN INFANT DEATH SYNDROME
1. DESCRIPTION
   a. Unexpected death of an apparently healthy infant under the age of 1 year for which an autopsy, examination of the death scene, and review of clinical history fail to reveal an adequate cause of death
   b. Peak incidence is between 2–4 months of age, especially during the winter months.
   c. Risk factors include male gender, African American and Native American ethnicity, low socioeconomic status, prematurity, low birth weight, multiple births, prone sleeping position, overheating, central nervous system disturbances and respiratory disorders, history of an apparent life-threatening event (combination of apnea, color change, and decrease in muscle tone that could have led to death if intervention had not taken place), maternal factors such as smoking, young age, high-risk pregnancy.
   d. Breast-fed infants have a lower risk.
2. ASSESSMENT
   a. Death typically occurs during sleep.
   b. Appearance when found:
      1) Apneic
      2) Blue
      3) Lifeless
      4) Frothy blood-tinged fluid in the nose and mouth
      5) May be found in any position
      6) May be clutching bedding
3. DIAGNOSTIC TESTS
   a. No test can predict risk.
   b. Cardiopneumogram or pneumocardiogram are most widely used to provide accurate cardiorespiratory pattern.
4. NURSING INTERVENTIONS
   a. Apparent life-threatening event

     1) Home cardiorespiratory event monitor as prescribed
      a) Criterion for discontinuing monitor is 2–3 months without episodes.
     2) Administer respiratory stimulant medications such as theophylline or caffeine as prescribed.
   b. Emergency department
     1) Review scenario of events with the parents on arrival to the emergency department; determine if resuscitation was attempted.
     2) Allow the parents and family to say good-bye to their infant.
     3) Clean the infant before allowing the family to see him.
     4) Make appropriate referral for follow-up with the family.

   c. Public health nursing
     1) Encourage the expression of emotions.
     2) Explore coping mechanisms and evaluate effectiveness.
     3) Assess parental intellectual knowledge and understanding of the event.
     4) Provide written information about sudden infant death syndrome (SIDS).
     5) Discuss parental and sibling response to the infant's death.
     6) Refer to a support group or other parents who have lost a child to SIDS.
     7) Discuss fears related to subsequent pregnancies and births.

PRACTICE QUESTIONS

1. The nurse informs the parents of an infant that the primary difference between the chest of an infant and that of an adult is that the chest of an infant
   1. has a more flattened front-to-back diameter.
   2. is a cone-shaped structure.
   3. is rounded in shape.
   4. consists of cartilage, bone, and muscle.

2. A mother accompanies her 6-month-old male infant to the emergency room. She is concerned because the infant has not been feeding well. The infant has had a bad cold and cough, although the cough has subsided today. The nurse assessing the infant notes that the infant is very irritable and displays nasal flaring and intercostal retractions. Which of the following is the priority intervention for the nurse to take?
   1. Offer formula because the infant appears hungry
   2. Suction the infant's nose
   3. Acknowledge the mother's concern regarding the infant's diminished feeding
   4. Notify the physician that the infant needs to be seen quickly

3. Which of the following should the nurse include in a class on sudden infant death syndrome? Select all that apply:
   [ ] 1. Peak incidence is between 6 and 8 months
   [ ] 2. Being of female gender
   [ ] 3. Being African American
   [ ] 4. Being breast-fed infant
   [ ] 5. Being of low socioeconomic status
   [ ] 6. Have a respiratory disorder

4. While assessing a 13-year-old male following a motor vehicle accident, the nurse notes crepitus over the left lateral rib cage. Based on an understanding of crepitus, the nurse evaluates which of the following to cause the crepitus?
   1. Palpable vibrations over the chest wall that are produced by voice sounds
   2. The transmission of a pleural friction rub through the chest wall
   3. Remodeling of lung tissue secondary to asthma
   4. Air escaped from the lungs and trapped in the subcutaneous tissue

5. The parents of a 10-year-old child ask the nurse what pulmonary function testing is. Which of the following is the most appropriate response by the nurse? "Pulmonary function testing
   1. is an invasive test of pulmonary mechanics."
   2. is used to evaluate the severity of a respiratory disease."
   3. is used to diagnose specific respiratory diseases."

4. does not differentiate between restrictive and obstructive pulmonary disease."

6. A 15-month-old infant is seen in a well-child exam. Because the infant's family has recently emigrated from East Africa where tuberculosis (TB) is endemic, a Mantoux test is performed. No one in the infant's family has currently or has in the past had tuberculosis. The mother brings the infant back to the clinic in 48 hours to have the Mantoux test read. According to this infant's risk status and age, which is the smallest amount of induration that the nurse should consider a positive finding? An area of
   1. 5 mm induration.
   2. 10 mm induration.
   3. 15 mm induration.
   4. 20 mm induration.

7. The nurse is caring for a 5-year-old child suspected of having tuberculosis. Which of the following is the preferred method of obtaining a sputum specimen for culture and smear from this child?
   1. Endotracheal suctioning
   2. Sputum collected by elicited cough
   3. Sputum collected by early morning gastric washings
   4. Thoracentesis

8. A mother reports that her 15-month-old child has had three colds in three months during the winter while attending day care. The mother inquires whether she should use an over-the-counter antihistamine for this child, because she suspects allergies must be the cause of the frequent colds. Which of the following is the nurse's most appropriate intervention?
   1. Reassure the parent that frequent episodes of nasopharyngitis are common given the child's risk factors
   2. Notify the physician immediately because this information may be indicative of an immunodeficiency
   3. Inform the parent that the child might have asthma because of the frequency of upper respiratory infections
   4. Instruct the parent to use an over-the-counter antihistamine

9. A mother reports that her 4-month-old has a cold, but no fever. She reports noisy breathing at night and that the child's nose is very congested. The nurse advises the mother to promote maximum ventilation during sleep. Which of the following instructions about positioning would be appropriate for the nurse to include in the instructions?
   1. Elevate the infant's head on a pillow to open the airway
   2. Place infant in an upright (90 degrees) position
   3. Elevate the head of the crib 30 degrees
   4. Place the infant prone to promote drainage of secretions

10. A 3-year-old child is brought to the emergency room at night with a harsh cough, hoarseness, and noisy breathing. Although the nurse's initial assessment reveals a child who appears comfortable and whose respiratory status is within normal limits, a diagnosis of acute spasmodic laryngitis is made. Which of these instructions should the nurse include in the teaching plan?
    1. This is an isolated episode and will not recur
    2. This illness is usually accompanied by fever
    3. Stimulating the child may help terminate the episode
    4. Clinical manifestations may resolve on exposure to cool night air

11. Which of the following should the nurse include in a plan of care for a 5-year-old child admitted to the hospital with the diagnosis of epiglottitis?
    1. Perform a throat culture to identify the pathogen
    2. Administer cough syrup to the child
    3. Encourage the child to assume a tripod position
    4. Restrict fluids

12. A mother calls the medical information line and reports that her 6-year-old child has awakened with a complaint of sore throat and pain on swallowing. She reports that the child was fine when going to bed. The child has a fever of 39.2°C, or 102.5°F, orally and is restless and appears quite sick. Which of the following questions is a priority for the nurse to ask to triage this client?
    1. "Has the child been drooling?"
    2. "Has the child been exposed to strep throat?"
    3. "Did you give the child an antipyretic?"
    4. "Is the child up to date on immunizations?"

13. A child in the emergency room is suspected of having epiglottitis. Which of the following is the priority to include in this client's plan of care?
    1. Explain the course of the disease to the parents
    2. Ensure that the child has a patent airway
    3. Establish IV access
    4. Accompany the child to radiology for lateral neck x-ray

14. A 4-year-old child with epiglottitis is being transferred via ambulance to the hospital. The parents and child are very fearful. The mother

asks if her child can sit in her lap for transport. What is the nurse's best response?
1. "Your anxiousness is making your child upset. It is best to leave the child."
2. "Riding on your lap would be a dangerous practice and is not recommended."
3. "Letting your child ride on your lap may reduce your child's stress."
4. "Your child is very anxious so a sedative will be given so your child can sleep."

15. The father of a child with laryngotracheobronchitis asks the nurse what it is. Which of the following statements by the nurse best describes laryngotracheobronchitis?
1. "It is a reactive airway disease characterized by wheezing and cough."
2. "It is a viral illness that results in inflammation of the small airways and production of thick mucus."
3. "It is a bacterial illness that results in serious supraglottic inflammation."
4. "It is a viral illness that results in swelling around the level of the larynx characterized by a barking cough and hoarseness."

16. A child with a brassy cough, mild fever, and hoarseness is seen in the emergency department and diagnosed with croup. The physician orders discharge to home with management to include cool-temperature therapy. The nurse preparing discharge teaching notices that the child has developed continuous respiratory stridor. Which of the following is the priority nursing intervention?
1. Complete discharge instructions, including a review of the clinical manifestations of respiratory distress
2. Instruct the parent on how to perform cool-temperature therapy
3. Notify the physician of the child's status immediately
4. Request that the child follow up with the primary care provider in one week

17. The nurse administers which of the following vaccines to help prevent the development of epiglottitis?
1. Diphtheria/tetanus/acellular pertussis (DTaP) combination vaccine
2. Varicella vaccine (Varivax)
3. Haemophilus influenzae vaccine (HIB)
4. Pneumococcal polysaccharide vaccine (Prevnar)

18. The nurse is caring for a 5-year-old child diagnosed with bronchitis who is otherwise in good health. The child's mother verbalizes to the nurse that she is very upset that the physician did not prescribe antibiotics. The nurse's response would be based on the understanding that bronchitis is
1. treated by antihistamines, not antibiotics.
2. usually viral in a child under 5 years and not affected by antibiotic therapy.
3. a minor bacterial illness and antibiotics are not recommended because of the risk of developing bacterial resistance.
4. most appropriately controlled by cough syrup administered every 4 hours.

19. Which of the following infection control measures is the priority for the nurse to implement in the care provided to a 5-month-old infant admitted to the hospital with respiratory syncytial virus (RSV) bronchiolitis?
1. Hand washing is required by all personnel and visitors having contact with the infant
2. Gowns and masks must be worn by all personnel in the infant's room
3. Place the infant in a private room
4. Visitors are restricted to only the parents of the infant

20. The parents of a 5-month-old infant who has bronchiolitis ask the nurse what changes occur to the lung during the illness. The nurse informs these parents that which of the following lung changes occur?
1. Asthma
2. Emphysema
3. Atelectasis
4. Crepitus

21. The mother of a 4-month-old diagnosed with respiratory syncytial virus and bronchiolitis tells the nurse the infant has not been feeding well. Which of the following physical clinical manifestations indicates to the nurse that the client's condition is deteriorating and the client has become dehydrated?
Select all that apply:
[ ] 1. Bradycardia
[ ] 2. Oliguria
[ ] 3. Decreased respirations
[ ] 4. Decreased skin turgor
[ ] 5. Sunken anterior fontanel
[ ] 6. Dry mucous membranes

22. Which of the following methods should the nurse use to collect a respiratory syncytial virus (RSV) culture that has been ordered on a 6-month-old infant?
1. Use a nasopharyngeal swab
2. Perform a nasal washing
3. Venipuncture
4. Gastric lavage

23. The nurse screens which of the following pediatric age groups for atypical pneumonia caused by mycoplasma?
    1. Infancy
    2. Toddlerhood
    3. School age
    4. Adolescence

24. The nurse is teaching a class on sudden infant death syndrome to parents. Which of the following should the nurse include in the class?
    1. The peak incidence is between 6 and 8 months of age
    2. Occurrence is most frequent during the summer months
    3. Being a low-birth-weight male infant increases the risk
    4. Every infant under 1 year of age should be tested

25. Which of the following clinical manifestations does the nurse evaluate to be present in a child in the paroxysmal stage of pertussis?
    Select all that apply:
    [ ] 1. Sneezing
    [ ] 2. Low-grade fever
    [ ] 3. Flushed cheeks
    [ ] 4. Waning of paroxysmal coughing
    [ ] 5. High-pitched crowing
    [ ] 6. Protruding tongue

26. The clinical assignments on a pediatric respiratory unit have been made for the day. Which of the following assignments should be questioned?
    1. Unlicensed assistive personnel are assigned to walk children with croup
    2. A licensed practical nurse is assigned to teach a class to parents on sudden infant death syndrome
    3. Unlicensed assistive personnel are assigned to help children who have cystic fibrosis to eat
    4. A licensed practical nurse is assigned to administer a prescribed bronchodilator to a child with asthma

27. The nurse took respiratory rates on the following four pediatric clients. Which of the following clients should the nurse report as having an abnormal respiratory rate?
    1. A 6-month-old infant who has respirations of 45 breaths per minute
    2. A 2-year-old child who has respirations of 30 breaths per minute
    3. A 10-year-old who has respirations of 28 breaths per minute
    4. An 18-year-old who has respirations of 25 breaths per minute

28. Which of the following should the nurse include in the instructions given to parents of a child with an allergy on methods to reduce allergen exposure?
    Select all that apply:
    [ ] 1. Trim household plants of dead leaves daily
    [ ] 2. Exercise in cool, dry areas
    [ ] 3. Clean moldy areas with 1:10 bleach solution
    [ ] 4. Keep pets in uncarpeted areas
    [ ] 5. Avoid strong odors
    [ ] 6. Maintain laundry water at 37.8°C, or 100°F

29. Which of the following nursing interventions should the nurse include in the plan of care for a child with acute spasmodic laryngitis?
    1. Administer antipyretic
    2. Provide cold steam in the bedroom from a humidifier
    3. Avoid exposure to the night air
    4. Administer corticosteroids

30. The nurse is caring for a child suspected of having bacterial tracheitis. Which of the following is the primary clinical manifestation that the nurse assesses supporting this diagnosis?
    1. Fever
    2. Brassy cough
    3. Thick purulent tracheal secretions
    4. Inspiratory stridor

ANSWERS AND RATIONALES

1. 3. An infant's chest is almost circular in shape; in adults, the anterior-posterior diameter is less than the lateral diameter. The thoracic cavity for both infants and adults is cone-shaped and consists of bone, cartilage, and muscle.

2. 4. Poor feeding, irritability, nasal flaring, and intercostal retractions are signs of altered respiratory function and respiratory distress in infants. It is important for the nurse to recognize these clinical manifestations in order

to triage the infant, so that the physician sees this child before less ill clients. Infant feeding is likely decreased because the infant has air hunger and does not have the energy to feed. Suctioning the infant's nose would likely increase hypoxia. Although it is important to acknowledge the mother's concern regarding infant feeding, a more appropriate response is to have the physician see the infant as soon as possible.

3. 3. 5. 6. Male African-American infants who are formula fed have a higher incidence of sudden infant death syndrome. Other characteristics include being of low socioeconomic status or having a respiratory disorder. The peak incidence is between 2 and 4 months.

4. 4. Tactile fremitus is a palpable vibration over the chest wall that is produced by voice sounds. A pleural friction rub is auscultated as a grating sound. Remodeling in asthma does not cause crepitus.

5. 2. Pulmonary function testing (PFT) is used to evaluate the severity of the disease. It is a noninvasive test. PFT cannot diagnose specific diseases because different diseases may have the same functional abnormalities. It is used to differentiate between restrictive and obstructive disease.

6. 2. For a child under the age of 4 years and born in an area of the world where tuberculosis is prevalent, a reading of 10 mm induration would be the lowest value that would be considered a positive finding in accordance with current clinical standards. Although a 15-mm and 20-mm induration would also be considered positive findings, given the younger age of 15 months, a positive reading would occur at 10 mm.

7. 3. Because young children are likely to swallow any sputum that is produced by cough, gastric lavage is a more effective method of collecting a sputum sample. It is the preferred method of collecting sputum for culture and smear from a child who is suspected of having tuberculosis. Endotracheal suctioning, unless intubated, would not be well tolerated, and thoracentesis is both invasive and impractical on a routine basis.

8. 1. Nasopharyngitis occurs more frequently in infants and young children, especially in settings such as a day care center where many children interact in a small space. The most frequent transmission is by human hands, so good hand washing is essential to help prevent continuous colds. The fall and winter months are also prime times for colds. It is unlikely the child is immunosuppressed based on the circumstances and clinical manifestations. The nurse should not suggest that the child has asthma, because it is not in the scope of practice and the diagnosis is not supported by the data collected. It would not be appropriate to make a recommendation concerning over-the-counter antihistamine therapy for a child this young. Antihistamines have also been found to be ineffective in treating nasopharyngitis.

9. 3. Appropriate positioning is a significant means of easing respiratory efforts in infants and small children. Elevation of the head of the crib or maintaining the infant's head at 30 degrees will promote maximum lung expansion. Resting an infant's head on a pillow is not recommended, because of the risk of sudden infant death syndrome. Positioning an infant at 90 degrees would actually compress the diaphragm and diminish respiratory function. Prone positioning of infants is generally not recommended, because of its correlation with sudden infant death syndrome. It should be noted that in the rare case that the infant is experiencing gastroesophageal reflux, positioning the infant prone may be permitted.

10. 4. Exposure to cool night air or humidity may help relieve the spasm in acute spasmodic laryngitis. The parent should be advised that these attacks may be recurrent. The illness is usually not accompanied by fever. Stimulation may aggravate the dyspnea.

11. 3. Epiglottitis, also referred to as croup syndrome, is a life-threatening bacterial infection that can lead to a complete airway obstruction. Because of difficulty breathing and swallowing, the child is likely to assume a tripod position. This is characterized by the child sitting upright and leaning forward with chin thrust out, tongue protruding, and mouth open to facilitate breathing and swallowing. A throat culture should not be done, as this could cause additional or complete obstruction. Examination of the throat should only occur when emergency tracheostomy or intubation is possible. The onset of epiglottitis is usually abrupt and is more likely preceded by a sore throat than by cold manifestations. It is most common in children between the ages of 2 and 7 years. Fluids, antibiotics, and supportive care are included in the treatment plan.

12. 1. Clinical manifestations of a sore throat, difficulty swallowing, restlessness, and temperature of 39.2°C, or 102.5°F, orally is suggestive of epiglottitis, which is a medical emergency. Confirming that the child is drooling would be additional data to support the nurse's suspicions and assist to direct the parent and child to an emergency department for evaluation and treatment. Although asking about strep throat, administration of an antipyretic, and immunizations may be appropriate questions for any parent of a child, the priority question would be to inquire about drooling.

13. 2. Epiglottitis, or croup syndrome, is a bacterial infection that may lead to a complete airway obstruction. It should be managed in the same way as acute respiratory distress, with maintenance of the airway being the priority. Establishing IV access and assisting with x-ray will also be done, but only after the airway has been ensured and trained personnel are available. The nurse should not perform any procedures without additional medical team support. Communicating to the parents is important, but only after the client is stabilized.

14. 3. Being allowed to sit on a parent's lap may actually decrease the child's (and parent's) stress and facilitate easier breathing. Such a request would need to be approved by the physician and the ambulance personnel. Isolating the child from the parents would very likely increase the child's stress and consequently the respiratory dysfunction. This would be counterproductive. Sedation would be inappropriate in this situation, as it would further compromise respiratory effort.

15. 4. Laryngotracheobronchitis (croup) is a viral illness that results in swelling around the level of the larynx characterized by a barking cough and hoarseness. A reactive airway disease characterized by wheezing and cough is a description of asthma. A viral illness that results in inflammation of the small airways and production of thick mucus is a description of bronchiolitis. A bacterial illness that results in serious supraglottic inflammation is a description of epiglottitis.

16. 3. Stridor is a high-pitched sound produced by an obstruction of the trachea or larynx that can be heard during inspiration or expiration. Stridor even at rest signifies progression of the croup and requires medical management. The physician should be notified immediately. It would be inappropriate to discharge the client in view of the change in status without notifying the physician. Instructing the parents on cool-temperature therapy is an appropriate intervention but not the priority.

17. 3. *Haemophilus influenzae* is the most common causative organism of epiglottitis. The *H. influenzae* vaccine may help prevent it. Diphtheria/tetanus/acellular pertussis (DTaP) immunizes against diphtheria, tetanus, and pertussis. Varivax immunizes against varicella (chickenpox), and Prevnar immunizes against streptococcal pneumonia and to a lesser degree ear infections caused by *Streptococcus pneumoniae*.

18. 2. Laryngotracheobronchitis (croup) is usually caused by a virus, especially in young children. Antibiotics are ineffective against viral illnesses. It would be appropriate for the nurse to explain this rationale to the parent as part of client and family education. Bronchitis is not treated with antihistamines. Cough suppressants should be used with caution as they may make the child drowsy and may also impede the clearance of secretions. The issue in antibiotic resistance is to treat with an adequate dose of an antibiotic that is active against the offending pathogen, not whether or not to treat.

19. 1. Bronchiolitis is a viral infection causing inflammation of the bronchioles and production of thick mucus that occludes the bronchiole tubes and small airways, impeding expiration. Of the infection control measures implemented, consistent hand washing and not touching the nasal mucosa or conjunctivae have been shown to be most important. Wearing masks and gowns has not been shown to be of added benefit, although the gowns may help reduce the risk of fomite spread. Infants with RSV may be in rooms with children with similar diagnosis or isolated in private rooms, dependent on hospital policy. The advisability of limiting of visitors and staff in an effort to lessen the spread of infection is being studied.

20. 2. In bronchiolitis, the bronchioles and small airways become occluded due to inflammation and thick mucus. Air becomes trapped behind the occlusions, where it leads to progressive overinflation of the lungs called emphysema. While some infants may manifest asthmalike manifestations, this does not reflect the usual progression of bronchiolitis. Atelectasis is a collapse of the lung and is not a normal development in bronchiolitis. Crepitus is a crackling sound on palpation caused by the escape of air into the subcutaneous tissue and is also not common in bronchiolitis.

21. 2. 4. 5. 6. The sunken fontanel is the most specific clinical manifestation indicating that the infant is dehydrated. Other clinical manifestations include decreased skin turgor, oliguria, dry mucous membranes, and skin color changes. The infant may also become tachypneic and tachycardic.

22. 2. The nasal washing is identified as the method of choice for collecting the nasal specimen for respiratory syncytial virus (RSV). Although sometimes used, a nasopharyngeal swab is not as effective a collection technique. Venipuncture and gastric lavage are not used to obtain specimens for RSV determination.

23. 3. *Mycoplasma pneumoniae* is the most common causative agent of pneumonia in school-age children between the ages of 5 and 12 years.

Viral pneumonia is the most common pneumonia overall and is seen in all age groups. Bacterial pneumonias are more prevalent in children under age 5 years.

24. 3. Sudden infant death syndrome is the unexpected death of an apparently healthy infant under the age of 1 year. Peak incidence is between 2 and 4 months. It occurs more frequently between the ages of 2 and 4 months and in the winter months. Low-birth-weight male infants are at a greater risk than are females. There is no diagnostic test for sudden infant death syndrome.

25. 3. 5. 6. The classic clinical manifestation of pertussis (whooping cough) is the "whoop" or high-pitched crowing sound that is heard at the end of the cough during the paroxysmal stage of the disease. Other clinical manifestations found in the paroxysmal stage include flushed cheeks, bulging eyes, and a protruding tongue. Sneezing and a low-grade fever are found during the catarrhal stage, when manifestations of an upper respiratory infection occur. A waning of the paroxysmal coughing is characteristic during the convalescent stage.

26. 2. Unlicensed assistive personnel may help a child walk and eat. A licensed practical nurse may administer a bronchodilator to a child with asthma. It is inappropriate to assign a licensed practical nurse to teach a class on sudden infant death syndrome. A registered nurse should be given responsibility for teaching such a class.

27. 4. The respiratory rate of an infant from birth to 6 months is 30 to 50 breaths per minute. Children between 6 months and 2 years of age would have respirations from 20 to 30 breaths per minute. Children between 3 and 10 years of age have respirations between 20 and 28 breaths per minute. The respiratory rate of children between 10 and 14 years of age is between 16 and 20 breaths per minute. The respiratory rate of children between16 and 18 years of age would be between 12 and 20 breaths per minute. An 18-year-old who has respirations of 25 breaths per minute is experiencing some degree of respiratory distress and that finding should be reported.

28. 3. 4. 5. Household plants, strong odors, and exercising in cool, dry areas should be avoided in the plan of care for a child with an allergy. Moldy surfaces should be cleaned with a 1:10 bleach solution. Pets should be kept in uncarpeted areas that are easy to clean. Laundry water should be maintained at 54.4°C, or 130°F.

29. 2. Acute spasmodic laryngitis is characterized by sudden, brief laryngeal obstructions that occur primarily at night. There is no fever, so antipyretics are not administered. Corticosteroids are also not administered. Exposure to the night air may terminate the laryngeal spasm. It is appropriate to provide steam from a hot bath or shower or cold steam from a humidifier to relieve mild clinical manifestations.

30. 3. Bacterial tracheitis is a bacterial infection involving the mucosa of the upper trachea. Although fever, brassy cough, and inspiratory stridor are all clinical manifestations of bacterial tracheitis, the hallmark manifestation diagnostic of the condition is thick, purulent tracheal secretions. If left untreated, these secretions may result in airway obstruction or even respiratory arrest.

REFERENCES

Potts, N., & Mandleco, B. (2012). *Pediatric nursing: Caring for children and their families* (3rd ed.). Clifton Park, NY: Thomson Delmar Learning.

Spratto, G. R., & Woods, A. L. (2012). *PDR nurse's drug handbook 2012*. Clifton Park, NY: Delmar Cengage Learning.

CHAPTER 32

CARDIOVASCULAR DISORDERS

I. **ANATOMY AND PHYSIOLOGY**
   A. DEVELOPMENT OF THE PRENATAL AND POSTNATAL CIRCULATION
      1. PRENATAL AND TRANSITIONAL CIRCULATION
         a. Fetal circulation differs from postnatal circulation due to the oxygenation of blood via the placenta and the presence of shunts, the foramen ovale, the ductus arteriosus, and the ductus venosus, which direct a significant portion of blood flow to the brain and heart for most favorable perfusion and development.
         b. The ductus venosus carries oxygenated blood from the umbilical vein, bypassing the liver. When the umbilical cord is clamped, the ductus venosus closes.
         c. The foramen ovale allows oxygenated blood from the right atria to shunt from right to left, bypassing the lungs, which are nonfunctional in the fetus.
         d. The ductus arteriosus allows blood from the pulmonary artery to enter the aorta. This causes oxygenated blood coming from the umbilical cord to mix with the systemic circulation and bypass much of the pulmonary circulation.
         e. Circulatory transition begins at birth when gas exchange begins to occur in the lungs rather than the placenta. This causes the pressures to change in the heart, functionally closing the foramen ovale and the ductus arteriosus. Permanent closure of these shunts occurs within the first month of life.
         f. Systemic vascular resistance increases and pulmonary vascular resistance decreases as circulatory patterns change.
         g. Fetal circulation patterns may persist after birth if there is failure of any of the shunts to close.
      2. POSTNATAL HEMODYNAMICS
         a. Clinical pathologies are often the cause of alterations in hemodynamics.
         b. Blood takes the path of least resistance and will flow from higher pressure to lower pressure.
         c. Heart rate is largely affected by oxygenation of the blood.
         d. Cardiac output is a function of the heart rate until the child is near 5 years of age.
         e. Systolic pressure increases gradually with the age of the child corresponding to increased systemic vascular resistance and ventricular development. Pressures approach that of the adult near or during adolescence.
         f. Children have an increased risk for heart failure because the musculature of the heart is not as developed and the volume and pressure overloads are more difficult for the heart to compensate for.

II. **ASSESSMENT**
   A. HEALTH HISTORY
      1. PRENATAL AND BIRTH HISTORY INCLUDING MATERNAL INFECTIONS, DRUG AND ALCOHOL EXPOSURE, COMPLICATIONS OF PREGNANCY AND THE PERINATAL PERIOD, AS WELL AS GESTATIONAL AGE
      2. FAMILY HISTORY, ESPECIALLY CONGENITAL DEFECTS, SUDDEN INFANT DEATH SYNDROME (SIDS), AND FETAL LOSS
      3. FEEDING PATTERNS AND WEIGHT CHANGES
      4. EXERCISE TOLERANCE, CHEST PAIN, AND CYANOSIS

5. MEDICATIONS INCLUDING PAST, CURRENT, OR OVER THE COUNTER (OTC)
B. PHYSICAL EXAMINATION
  1. INSPECTION
    a. Nutritional status
    b. Skin color
    c. Position of comfort
    d. Clubbing of fingers
    e. Edema
    f. Respiratory effort
    g. Distended neck veins
  2. AUSCULTATION
    a. Heart sounds: rate, rhythm, presence of murmurs, S_1, S_2, also S_3 and S_4. S_4 is pathologic in children.
    b. Lung sounds: respiratory rate, presence of crackles, wheezing, grunting or decreased breath sounds
    c. Frequency of respiratory infections
    d. Reports of palpitations
    e. Blood pressure: monitor for hypertension or hypotension and syncope.
  3. PALPATION
    a. Capillary refill time
    b. Thrills
    c. Pulses of extremities
  4. OBSERVATION
    a. Infants with cardiac disease will exhibit restlessness, irritability, and inconsolability.
    b. Observe infants and older children for trends in height and weight monitoring for delays in physical development.

III. **DIAGNOSTIC STUDIES**
  A. CHEST X-RAY (SEE CHAPTER 4, CARDIOVASCULAR DISORDERS, SECTION III.)
  B. ELECTROCARDIOGRAPHY (SEE CHAPTER 4, CARDIOVASCULAR DISORDERS, SECTION III.)
  C. ECHOCARDIOGRAPHY (SEE CHAPTER 4, CARDIOVASCULAR DISORDERS, SECTION III.)
  D. CARDIAC CATHETERIZATION
    1. DESCRIPTION: THIS IS AN INVASIVE TECHNIQUE IN WHICH A RADIOPAQUE CATHETER IS INSERTED INTO THE HEART VIA A PERIPHERAL VENOUS OR ARTERIAL BLOOD VESSEL FOR THE PURPOSE OF OBTAINING DIRECT MEASUREMENTS OF PRESSURE CHANGES AND OXYGEN SATURATION LEVELS IN THE HEART CHAMBERS AND THE GREAT VESSELS, AS WELL AS A MEASUREMENT OF CARDIAC OUTPUT. CONTRAST MATERIAL INJECTED THROUGH THE CATHETER PROVIDES VISUALIZATION OF HEARD DEFECTS OR OBSTRUCTIONS TO BLOOD FLOW.
    2. PREPROCEDURE
      a. Use sensory and procedural preparation appropriate for developmental level.
      b. Minimize the child's fears.
      c. Assess allergies to iodine.
      d. Mark and document pedal pulses.
      e. Obtain accurate height, weight, and vital signs. Fever or infection may delay the procedure.
      f. Obtain baseline oxygen saturation and hemoglobin levels.
      g. Inform the parents of the need for the child to be NPO after midnight.
      h. Inform the parents and child that the child will be sedated during the procedure.
    3. POSTPROCEDURE:
      a. Observe closely for complications.
      b. Provide direct pressure to the catheterization site for a full 15 minutes.
      c. Monitor heart rate for 1 full minute during vital signs.
      d. Monitor for arrhythmias.
      e. Check pulses, color and temperature of the affected extremity.
      f. Monitor blood pressure. Hypotension may indicate hemorrhage.
      g. Monitor the occlusive pressure dressing. There is risk for hematoma formation or bleeding at the puncture site.
      h. Monitor for diuresis related to the contrast medium.
      i. Monitor IV and p.o. fluids, maintain hydration.
      j. Check blood glucose in infants.
      k. Keep the child quiet and positioned flat or according to institutional policy, 6 hours minimum.
  E. HYPEROXIA TEST
    1. DESCRIPTION
      a. The hyperoxia test is a method to discriminate between two potential causes of cyanosis in infants.
      b. Cardiac disease and pulmonary disease are the most common causes of cyanosis in infants, and this test assists to determine which is contributing to cyanosis in the client.
      c. The infant is supplied 100% oxygen via mask or tent, and blood gases are checked.
      d. A PaO_2 less than 100 mm Hg is an indication of inadequate pulmonary perfusion and thus cardiac in nature.

e. A PaO₂ at 150 mm Hg or higher is an indication of lung disease, which makes it difficult for the oxygen to move from the alveoli into the pulmonary capillaries.

IV. NURSING DIAGNOSES

A. DECREASED CARDIAC OUTPUT
B. EXCESS FLUID VOLUME
C. IMBALANCED NUTRITION: LESS THAN BODY REQUIREMENTS
D. ACTIVITY INTOLERANCE
E. DELAYED GROWTH AND DEVELOPMENT

Nursing Diagnoses: Definitions and Classification 2012–2014. Copyright © 2012, 1994–2012 by NANDA International. Used by arrangement with John Wiley & Sons Limited.

V. PATHOPHYSIOLOGY OF TWO COMMON COMPLICATIONS OF CONGENITAL HEART DISEASE

A. CONGESTIVE HEART FAILURE (CHF)
  1. DESCRIPTION: CHF IS UNUSUAL IN CHILDREN BUT MORE COMMON IN CHILDREN WITH CONGENITAL HEART CONDITIONS. VOLUME OVERLOAD AND PRESSURE OVERLOAD ARE THE MOST COMMON CAUSES OF CHF IN CHILDREN, BUT IT MAY ALSO BE ASSOCIATED WITH DEMAND FOR HIGH CARDIAC OUTPUT AND DECREASED CONTRACTILITY OF THE MYOCARDIUM.
    a. Left-sided heart failure: increased pressure in the pulmonary veins, causing pulmonary congestion and edema
    b. Right-sided heart failure: increased systemic venous pressure, causing peripheral edema and hepatomegaly
    c. In children, it is rare to see one side fail without the other.
    d. Compensatory mechanisms
      1) Hypertrophy and dilation of heart muscle increase ventricular pressure and force of contraction.
      2) Stimulation of the sympathetic nervous system: catecholamines increase the rate and force of contraction and also cause peripheral vasoconstriction.
  2. ASSESSMENT (SEE TABLE 32-1)
    a. Pulmonary congestion
      1) Tachypnea, retractions, nasal flaring
      2) Mild cyanosis
      3) Dyspnea, orthopnea
      4) Pulmonary edema: wheezing, cough, later gasping, grunting
      5) Developmental delays such as gross motor
    b. Systemic venous congestion
      1) Weight gain related to sodium and water retention

Table 32-1 Clinical Manifestations of Congestive Heart Failure in Newborns, Infants, Children, and Adolescents

Newborns/Infants	
Tachycardia	Tachypnea
Gallop rhythm	Retractions
Diminished pulses	Wheezing
Diaphoresis	Rales/rhonchi
Cool, mottled extremities	Hepatomegaly
Pallor	Low urine output
Edema	
Failure to thrive/poor weight gain	
Restlessness	

Children/Adolescents	
Jugular venous distention	Tachycardia
Wheezing	Gallop rhythm
Rales/rhonchi	Diminished pulses
Dyspnea	Pallor
Orthopnea	Edema
Hepatomegaly	Low urine output
Ascites	Exercise intolerance
Poor weight gain	

© Cengage Learning 2015

      2) Peripheral edema, ascites
      3) Distended neck veins and peripheral veins
    c. Altered myocardial function
      1) Tachycardia
      2) Diaphoresis—especially around the child's head
      3) Extra heart sounds, S₃, S₄
      4) Weak pulses, slowed capillary refill
      5) Hypotension
      6) Irritability, fussiness
      7) Decreased activity tolerance, poor feeding
      8) Cool extremities
      9) Pallor
  3. DIAGNOSTIC TESTS
    a. Clinical evaluation
    b. Chest x-ray: cardiomegaly, pulmonary vascular marking
    c. Electrocardiogram: hypertrophy
    d. Echocardiogram: pinpoint cause(s) of CHF, specific size and nature of defect
  4. NURSING INTERVENTIONS
    a. Administer drugs, as ordered, such as digoxin, diuretics, oxygen.
    b. Monitor vital signs and oxygen saturation closely.
    c. Monitor intake and output, daily weight, and restrict fluid as ordered.
    d. Monitor potassium intake and serum levels.
    e. Position the child in semi-Fowler's position to ease respiratory effort.

   f. Perform cardiac monitoring as ordered.
   g. Utilize developmentally appropriate techniques to instruct the child and family about procedures, equipment, and unit routines.
   h. Offer small frequent feedings or meals to the child.
   i. Gavage feed as necessary for poor oral intake.
   j. Maintain a quiet, nonstimulating environment of moderate temperature.
   k. Provide emotional support to the child and family.
   l. Prepare the family for home-going needs including:
      1) Instruct the family on the clinical manifestations of CHF.
      2) Instruct the parents about which clinical manifestations require immediate medical attention.
      3) Instruct the parents on medication administration, adverse reactions, and toxicity manifestations.
      4) Instruct the family on measures to prevent increased cardiac demand such as rest, quiet environment, and quiet play activities.
      5) Inform the family on the effects of CHF on growth and development.
      6) Provide phone support to the family and make referrals to home care as necessary.

5. MEDICAL MANAGEMENT
   a. Eliminate surplus sodium and fluid.
      1) Diuretics
      2) Fluid restriction
      3) Sodium restriction possible but not likely—children need Na for growth and development
   b. Improve myocardial function.
      1) Digitalis glycosides
      2) Angiotensin-converting enzymes
   c. Decrease cardiac demands.
      1) Quiet environment
      2) Rest, minimize activity
      3) Possible sedation
      4) Semi-Fowler's position
      5) Moderate room temperature: infants susceptible to cold stress
   d. Increase oxygenation of tissues.
      1) Conserve activity to decrease oxygen demand.
      2) Provide cool humidified oxygen.
      3) Prevent chilling.

B. HYPOXEMIA
   1. DESCRIPTION: HYPOXEMIA IS A LOW OXYGEN PRESSURE (PAO$_2$) OR, SIMILARLY, A LOW OXYGEN SATURATION (SAO$_2$). HYPOXEMIA OCCURS IN CHILDREN WITH CONGENITAL HEART DEFECTS WHEN VENOUS BLOOD MIXES WITH ARTERIAL BLOOD IN THE HEART DUE TO RIGHT-TO-LEFT SHUNTING OR THE ANATOMY OF THE DEFECT AND IS SENT BACK TO THE SYSTEMIC CIRCULATION BEFORE RETURNING TO THE PULMONARY VASCULAR BED.
   2. ASSESSMENT
      a. Cyanosis
      b. SaO$_2$ intermittent or continuous oximetry monitoring
      c. Increased respirations
      d. Difficult or labored respirations
      e. Polycythemia with chronic hypoxia—increases risk of clots and cerebrovascular accident (CVA)
      f. Clubbing with chronic hypoxia
      g. Hypercyanotic spells
   3. DIAGNOSTIC TESTS
      a. Clinical evaluation
      b. Family and medical history
      c. Chest x-ray: showing less than normal pulmonary blood flow
      d. Echocardiogram: cardiac defects and anomalies
      e. Hyperoxia test: discriminates between lung disease and cardiac disease
   4. NURSING INTERVENTIONS
      a. Monitor fluid status carefully: intake and output and daily weights
      b. Instruct the parents on the importance of avoiding dehydration and to notify the physician of any problems such as vomiting and diarrhea that may cause dehydration.
      c. Administer oxygen as ordered.
      d. Instruct the parents on the clinical manifestations of respiratory distress and respiratory infection.
      e. Prevent infection with good hand washing and careful pulmonary hygiene.
      f. Instruct the parents on hypercyanotic spells and their treatment.
      g. Assess for consequences of long-term hypoxemia such as clubbing or small stature.
      h. Provide emotional support and teaching regarding possible body image concerns.
   5. MEDICAL MANAGEMENT
      a. Newborns: prostaglandin E: enhances the patency of the ductus arteriosus after birth to increase oxygenation in cardiac defects
      b. During a hypercyanotic spell:
         1) Remain calm to decrease the client's anxiety.

2) Place the infant or child in a knee-chest position.

3) 100% oxygen administration

4) Morphine IV

5) IV fluids as needed

c. Improve O_2 saturation and prevent lung infections by:

1) Chest physiotherapy

2) Antibiotics as necessary

3) Oxygen administration

d. In the case of polycythemia, prevent CVA by:

1) Adequate hydration

2) Multiple phlebotomies to decrease hematocrit

3) Possible transfusions

VI. CONGENITAL HEART DEFECTS: OBSTRUCTIVE DEFECTS

A. DESCRIPTION: OBSTRUCTIVE DEFECTS ARE THOSE IN WHICH BLOOD LEAVING THE VENTRICULAR CHAMBERS MEETS WITH A RESISTANCE TO FLOW. THIS IS GENERALLY CAUSED BY A NARROWING OR STENOSIS OF A VALVE OR VESSEL.

B. COARCTATION OF THE AORTA (COA)

1. DESCRIPTION: A NARROWING OF THE AORTIC ARCH OR DESCENDING AORTA THAT CAUSES INCREASED RESISTANCE TO FLOW FROM THE LEFT VENTRICLE AND INCREASED BLOOD PRESSURE TO THE NECK, HEAD AND UPPER EXTREMITIES WHICH ARE PROXIMAL TO THE DEFECT, AND DECREASED BLOOD PRESSURE TO THE LOWER EXTREMITIES. UNTREATED, THE CHILD HAS AN INCREASED RISK FOR HEART FAILURE (HF) AND CVA.

2. ASSESSMENT

a. Bounding pulses and high blood pressure in the upper extremities

b. Hypertensive clinical manifestations such as headache, dizziness, and epistaxis may be seen.

c. Weak or absent pulses in the lower extremities, also cool to touch

d. Dyspnea and exercise intolerance

e. Rapid progression to HF and acidosis is a risk once the ductus arteriosus has closed.

3. DIAGNOSTIC TESTS

a. Echocardiogram

b. Chest x-ray

c. Electrocardiogram

4. NURSING INTERVENTIONS

a. Monitor blood pressure of upper and lower extremities.

b. Observe for signs of HF in the child such as fluid retention, dyspnea, activity intolerance, tachycardia, and increased respiratory effort.

c. Provide emotional support to the family.

d. Inform the family on the clinical manifestations of HF.

e. Prepare the family for the likelihood of cardiac surgery for their child.

f. Administer digoxin and angiotensin-converting-enzyme (ACE) inhibitors, as ordered, to improve cardiac function.

g. Administer oxygen, as ordered, to improve oxygenation.

h. Provide a restful, quiet environment to decrease cardiac demand.

i. Restrict fluids and administer diuretics, as ordered, to decrease cardiac demand.

j. Instruct the parents on the proper drug administration techniques and drug adverse reactions.

k. Inform the parents on the need for antibiotic prophylaxis during invasive procedures to prevent subacute endocarditis.

5. SURGICAL MANAGEMENT

a. Surgery may involve resection of the coarctation or a graft placement to the affected region of the aorta for the purposes of enlargement of the aortic lumen.

b. Balloon angioplasty may also be used to enlarge the aorta and treat residual coarctation postoperatively.

c. Treatment is very effective and mortality rates are less than 5%.

C. AORTIC STENOSIS

1. DESCRIPTION

a. This obstructive defect is a constriction at the aortic valve.

b. The resistance to blood flow caused by this constriction increases workload of the left ventricle.

2. ASSESSMENT

a. Most children with mild to moderate stenosis are asymptomatic.

b. Decreased cardiac output: tachycardia, hypotension, poor pulses, poor feeding in infants; older undiagnosed children may complain of chest pain, dizziness, or activity intolerance.

c. Hypertrophy of the left ventricle

d. Distinctive systolic ejection murmur

e. Pulmonary edema in the case of left-sided HF

3. DIAGNOSTIC TESTS

a. Echocardiogram: exact nature of the constriction, left ventricular hypertrophy

    b. Chest x-ray: cardiomegaly, left ventricular enlargement, possible dilation of the ascending aorta

    c. Electrocardiogram: generally normal

  4. NURSING INTERVENTIONS

    a. Monitor vital signs, pulses, continuous heart monitor if ordered.

    b. Assess feeding patterns and fatigue in infants.

    c. Assess regularly for signs of activity intolerance and chest pain.

    d. Instruct the family to monitor for clinical manifestations of HF.

    e. Inform the family on the proper medication administration and potential adverse reactions.

  5. NONSURGICAL MANAGEMENT

    a. Balloon angioplasty to dilate the aortic valve

    b. Complications may include valvular regurgitation, tearing of the valve.

  6. SURGICAL MANAGEMENT

    a. Aortic valvotomy is palliative; many will have need of further surgery for recurring stenosis.

    b. Valve replacement may be done as a second or third procedure.

    c. Complications include possible valve incompetence, dysrhythmias, aortic insufficiency.

D. PULMONARY STENOSIS

  1. DESCRIPTION: THIS OBSTRUCTIVE DEFECT IS A CONSTRICTION AT THE PULMONARY VALVE. THIS CONSTRICTION CAUSES INCREASED PRESSURE IN THE RIGHT VENTRICLE AND DECREASED PULMONARY BLOOD FLOW.

  2. ASSESSMENT

    a. Some children may be asymptomatic.

    b. Mild to severe cyanosis

    c. Right ventricular hypertrophy and eventual right ventricular failure leading to HF

    d. In severe cases, blood backs up into the right atrium, increasing atrial pressure and causing an increased likelihood of blood shunting right to left through an opened or reopened foramen ovale, which leads to systemic cyanosis.

    e. Distinctive murmur

  3. DIAGNOSTIC TESTS

    a. Chest x-ray: visualization of an enlarged pulmonary artery confirms the diagnosis.

    b. Echocardiogram: right ventricular hypertrophy

    c. Electrocardiogram: right axis deviation may indicate right ventricular hypertrophy.

    d. Cardiac catheterization: increased pressures on the right side of the heart, left-sided oxygen desaturation if right-to-left shunting is present

  4. NURSING INTERVENTIONS

    a. Monitor vital signs for indications of HF in severe stenosis.

    b. Assess the extremities for venous engorgement in severe stenosis.

    c. Inform the parents and child about the defect, clinical manifestations, and management in developmentally appropriate ways.

    d. Administer procedural and sensory preparation for surgery or intervention for the child.

    e. Instruct the family on proper drug administration techniques and potential adverse reactions of the drugs.

  5. NONSURGICAL MANAGEMENT

    a. Balloon angioplasty for dilation of the pulmonic valve

    b. Treatment of choice; low mortality and rare complications, which could include tearing of the valve and valve regurgitation

  6. SURGICAL MANAGEMENT

    a. Infants: Brock procedure (closed, transventricular valvotomy)

    b. Children: pulmonary valvotomy

    c. Complications are rare.

VII. CONGENITAL HEART DEFECTS: DEFECTS WITH INCREASED PULMONARY BLOOD FLOW

A. DESCRIPTION: INCREASED PULMONARY BLOOD FLOW IS CAUSED BY DEFECTS THAT ALLOW BLOOD TO MOVE FROM THE LEFT SIDE OF THE HEART TO THE RIGHT SIDE (HIGHER PRESSURE TO LOWER PRESSURE), INCREASING PULMONARY BLOOD FLOW AND DIMINISHING SYSTEMIC BLOOD FLOW.

B. ATRIAL SEPTAL DEFECT (ASD)

  1. DESCRIPTION

    a. In ASD there is a septal wall opening between the right atrium and left atrium. This is caused by the absence of part of the septal wall or nonclosure of the foramen ovale.

    b. Mixing of blood flowing is allowed from the slightly higher pressure left atrium to the lower pressure right atrium. This causes a left-to-right shunting of blood.

  2. ASSESSMENT

    a. May be asymptomatic

    b. Right atrium and right ventricular enlargement

    c. Pulmonary vascular changes may occur in middle age if ASD has remained undiagnosed.

    d. Dyspnea and pulmonary edema related to increased pulmonary blood flow; HF is rare.

    e. Distinctive systolic murmur, splitting S_2

    f. Risk for atrial dysrhythmias, obstructive pulmonary disease, emboli formation later in life

3. DIAGNOSTIC TESTS

    a. Electrocardiogram: possible dysrhythmias if unrepaired, right axis deviation

    b. Echocardiogram: exact nature and placement of the defect, confirms diagnosis

    c. Chest x-ray: cardiomegaly, pulmonary status

4. NURSING INTERVENTIONS

    a. Perform procedural and sensory preparation for surgery for the child at the appropriate developmental level.

    b. Monitor oxygen saturations.

    c. Provide family support.

    d. Instruct the parents to monitor the child's growth and development.

    e. Instruct the parents to monitor the nutritional status.

    f. Instruct the parents regarding the necessity for prophylactic antibiotics to prevent endocarditis.

5. SURGICAL MANAGEMENT

    a. Surgical management is best done by age 5 or 6 to prevent pulmonary complications.

    b. Method of choice is patch closure (Dacron patch or similar patch) via cardiac catheterization for defects large enough to be symptomatic. Suture closure may also be used.

    c. Open repair on bypass may be done for more severe defects or those with comorbid defects.

C. VENTRICULAR SEPTAL DEFECT (VSD)

1. DESCRIPTION

    a. In VSD there is an opening in the septum between the right and left ventricles. This is the most common of all heart defects.

    b. Mixing of blood occurs when blood shunts from the high pressure left ventricle to the lower pressure right ventricle. This causes increased load on the right ventricle and potential right ventricular hypertrophy.

    c. The size of the opening varies considerably from tiny to near absence or absence of the septum.

Up to 60% of VSDs may close spontaneously, most of these within the first year.

2. ASSESSMENT

    a. Distinctive loud systolic murmur and palpable systolic thrill, no murmur in neonates due to higher pulmonary vascular resistance

    b. Increased pressure in right ventricle and increased pulmonary resistance results in right ventricular hypertrophy.

    c. Tachypnea, dyspnea

    d. Poor growth

    e. Right-sided HF results when the right ventricle and right atrium can no longer absorb the increased workload. Left-sided failure quickly follows. HF is common with this type of defect.

3. DIAGNOSTIC TESTS

    a. Chest x-ray: cardiomegaly, pulmonary vascular changes

    b. Electrocardiogram: may be normal with small VSDs or may show ventricular hypertrophy and left atrial enlargement with larger lesions

    c. Echocardiogram: dimensions and position of the VSD, size of the heart chambers, estimate of internal pressures

    d. Cardiac catheterization: hemodynamics

4. NURSING INTERVENTIONS

    a. Provide support to the parents and family.

    b. Promote growth and development.

    c. Instruct the family regarding the clinical manifestations of HF.

    d. Instruct the family in measures to decrease cardiac workload of the child.

    e. Instruct the family on the administration of drugs such as digoxin, diuretics, ACE inhibitors, and oxygen.

    f. If surgery is to be performed, prepare the child and family using developmentally appropriate procedural and sensory techniques.

    g. Instruct the parents about the necessity of prophylactic antibiotics for the prevention of endocarditis.

5. NONSURGICAL MANAGEMENT

    a. Closure during cardiac catheterization, either patch closure or suture closure

6. SURGICAL MANAGEMENT

    a. Palliative care is sometimes undertaken by banding the pulmonary artery to decrease pulmonary blood flow. This is done in infants with complex defects or a number of VSDs.

b. The preferred approach is complete repair in infancy or early childhood—Dacron patch closure or possibly suture closure with cardiopulmonary bypass.

c. Complications include residual VSD, possible alterations in conduction.

D. PATENT DUCTUS ARTERIOSUS
   1. DESCRIPTION
      a. This defect is caused by the fetal ductus arteriosus failing to close soon after birth.
      b. At birth, the pressures of the systemic vasculature and the pulmonary vasculature are nearly equal; however, within a few weeks, the systemic pressures increase and shunting of the blood from the aorta to the pulmonary artery begins to occur. This is considered a left-to-right shunt.
      c. Oxygenated blood is sent back through the pulmonary circulation, increasing pulmonary vascular congestion and increasing workload on the left side of the heart due to the increase in volume returning from the lungs. Increased pulmonary pressures also may cause right ventricular hypertrophy.
   2. ASSESSMENT
      a. May be asymptomatic
      b. Characteristic murmur
      c. Widened pulse pressure
      d. Clinical manifestations of CHF, particularly left-sided failure
      e. Frequent respiratory infections are a risk.
      f. Poor weight gain
   3. DIAGNOSTIC TESTS
      a. Chest x-ray: left atrial and ventricular enlargement
      b. Electrocardiogram: usually normal, may show left-sided enlargement
      c. Echocardiogram: confirms diagnosis with visualization of the anatomy
   4. NURSING INTERVENTIONS
      a. Provide support to the parents and family.
      b. Promote growth and development.
      c. Instruct the family on the clinical manifestations of HF.
      d. Instruct the family in measures to decrease cardiac workload of the child.
      e. Instruct the family in administration of medications such as digoxin, diuretics, ACE inhibitors, and oxygen.

f. If surgery is to be performed, prepare the child and family using developmentally appropriate procedural and sensory techniques.

g. Instruct the parents about the necessity of prophylactic antibiotics for the prevention of endocarditis.

   5. MEDICAL MANAGEMENT
      a. Indomethacin (prostaglandin inhibitor) is given to premature infants and newborns to close the ductus arteriosus.
      b. If indomethacin is not successful, surgical closure is recommended before age 2 to decrease the risk of bacterial endocarditis.
   6. SURGICAL MANAGEMENT
      a. Coil embolization during cardiac catheterization results in a shorter hospital stay, minimal discomfort, and preclusion of surgery.
      b. Clip placement during video-assisted thorascopic surgery results in lower morbidity related to lack of the thoracotomy incision, less respiratory distress, less distress, and smaller incisions.
      c. Ligation and division of the ductus during left thoracotomy is very successful; however, a small morbidity rate is associated with the thoracotomy.

E. ATRIOVENTRICULAR CANAL (AVC)
   1. DESCRIPTION
      a. This defect allows blood to flow among all four heart chambers.
      b. An atrial septal defect is continuous with a ventricular septal defect along the septum, also affecting both atrioventricular (AV) valves (mitral and tricuspid) and creating essentially one large chamber.
      c. Blood flow direction depends on the client's peripheral resistance and pulmonary resistance as well as ventricular pressures. This is a defect seen in children with Down syndrome.
   2. ASSESSMENT
      a. May be asymptomatic
      b. Systolic murmur
      c. Mild cyanosis
      d. Signs of left HF, frequent respiratory infections, mild to moderate HF—clinical manifestations begin at 4 to 6 weeks when the pulmonary vascular resistance is less relative to systemic resistance
      e. Poor weight gain in infants
   3. DIAGNOSTIC TESTS
      a. Electrocardiogram: left axis deviation, right ventricular hypertrophy,

abnormal conduction such as first-degree AV block or bundle branch block

b. Chest x-ray: cardiomegaly—all four chambers, pulmonary vascular changes, enlarged pulmonary artery

c. Echocardiogram: exact nature of the defect, visualization of the chambers and the involvement of the valves

d. Cardiac catheterization: confirms septal defects, pulmonary hypertension, as well as degree and direction of shunting

4. NURSING INTERVENTIONS
a. Instruct the parents to recognize clinical manifestations of HF.
b. Inform the parents how to recognize and treat hypoxemia.
c. Instruct the parents and family in proper administration of cardiac drugs.
d. Instruct the parents in measures to decrease cardiac workload.
e. If surgery is to be performed, instruct the parents and child regarding surgical routines and post-op care, utilizing appropriate procedural and sensory techniques.

5. SURGICAL MANAGEMENT
a. Artery banding in infants for palliative care may be done in the case of severe symptoms.
b. Complete repair is recommended before 1 year of age to prevent the development of changes in pulmonary vasculature.
c. Repair is accomplished by the use of patch repair to close septal defects. This may require two patches. Repair will also most likely include repair of AV valves—possibly eventual valve replacement.
d. Complications include possible heart block, valvular incompetence, and dysrhythmias.

VIII. CONGENITAL HEART DEFECTS: DEFECTS WITH DECREASED PULMONARY BLOOD FLOW

A. TETRALOGY OF FALLOT (TOF)
1. DESCRIPTION
a. Four defects make up TOF. These are ventricular septal defect, right ventricular hypertrophy, overriding aorta, and pulmonic stenosis.
b. The size of the ventricular septal defect and the degree of pulmonic stenosis affect the hemodynamics widely. Systemic and pulmonary resistance also affect these hemodynamics.

c. Shunt direction may vary with changes in resistance.
d. Two factors contribute to cyanosis and hypoxemia. These are the decreased pulmonary blood flow related to pulmonic stenosis, and unoxygenated blood mixing with oxygenated in a right-to-left shunt.
e. A compensatory result is polycythemia.

2. ASSESSMENT
a. Mild to acute cyanosis
b. Clubbing of fingers and toes with chronic hypoxia
c. Pulmonic systolic ejection murmur
d. Activity intolerance
e. "Blue spells" or "tet spells" of acute hypoxia usually occurring during crying or exertion such as defecation or feeding, when oxygen demand is greater than supply
f. Difficulty feeding and failure to thrive
g. Squatting in ambulatory children as a compensatory mechanism—increases systemic resistance and decreased venous return, briefly decreasing hypoxia

3. DIAGNOSTIC TESTS
a. Electrocardiogram (EEG): right ventricular hypertrophy
b. Echocardiogram: nature and position of all defects
c. Chest x-ray: possible cardiomegaly, visualization of the shape of the heart
d. Cardiac catheterization: diminished pressure beyond the pulmonic valve, low oxygen saturation systemically (aorta)
e. Laboratory values: acidosis, polycythemia, poor PO_2

4. NURSING INTERVENTIONS
a. Instruct the parents on the clinical manifestations of congestive heart failure.
b. Instruct the family to promote nutrition, giving small frequent feedings.
c. Instruct the family to monitor for clinical manifestations of respiratory infections.
d. Instruct the parents and family to provide measures to decrease cardiac workload.
e. Assist the child into the knee-chest position during acute hypoxic spells.
f. Administer morphine or propranolol (Inderal) and oxygen during acute hypoxic episodes.
g. If surgery is scheduled, instruct the parents and child on the pre- and postoperative surgical routines and

nursing care. Utilize appropriate procedural and sensory teaching techniques.

h. Instruct the parents in the necessity of prophylactic antibiotics to prevent endocarditis.

5. SURGICAL MANAGEMENT

a. Prostaglandin E_1 is administered to maintain an open ductus arteriosus.

b. Palliative care, if necessary, involves a shunt from one of the subclavian arteries to the pulmonary arteries. This increases pulmonary blood flow and, consequently, oxygen saturation.

c. Elective complete repair is recommended in the first year of life; however, repair may be triggered by an increase in t spells and increasing cyanosis.

d. Corrective repair involves a patch for the VSD, enlargement of the pulmonary stenosis, and repair of the overriding aorta.

e. Complications include possible dysrhythmias and heart block.

B. TRICUSPID ATRESIA

1. DESCRIPTION

a. In tricuspid atresia, the tricuspid valve does not develop and thus there is no communication between the right atria and the right ventricle.

b. Associated defects include pulmonic stenosis, septal defects, very small or absent right ventricle, and enlarged left ventricle. Tricuspid atresia is also less commonly associated with transposition of the great arteries.

2. ASSESSMENT

a. Decreased pulmonary blood flow

b. Cyanosis, tachycardia, dyspnea

c. Chronic hypoxia leads to clubbing and polycythemia

d. Failure to thrive, growth retardation

e. Murmurs depend on the size and figuration of defects

3. DIAGNOSTIC TESTS

a. Chest x-ray: normal or minimally enlarged heart

b. Electrocardiogram: hypertrophy of both atria and the left ventricle

c. Echocardiogram: location of associated defects, left-to-right shunting

d. Cardiac catheterization: pressures and direction of blood flow, oxygen saturations, and specific locations of defects

4. NURSING INTERVENTIONS

a. Instruct the parents and family in nutrition support, providing small frequent meals.

b. Instruct the parents on mechanisms to reduce cardiac workload.

c. Instruct the family in proper administration of the drugs and monitoring the child for adverse reactions.

d. Administer pre-op and post-op teaching for the parents and child.

5. SURGICAL MANAGEMENT

a. Palliative surgery involves the positioning of a shunt from a systemic artery to a pulmonary artery for the purpose of increasing pulmonary blood flow. For clients who have increased pulmonary flow, a pulmonary artery banding may be necessary.

b. Corrective repair involves separating the systemic circulation from the pulmonary circulation. This is usually done by connecting the inferior and superior vena cava directly to the pulmonary artery. Closure of the septal defects is also done at this time.

c. Cardiac complications include dysrhythmias, dysfunction of the left ventricle, pleural effusions, and possible increases in pulmonary vascular resistance.

IX. **CONGENITAL HEART DEFECTS: MIXED DEFECTS**

A. TRANSPOSITION OF THE GREAT ARTERIES

1. DESCRIPTION

a. The pulmonary artery and the aorta have switched positions in this defect. The pulmonary artery rises from the left ventricle and the aorta from the right ventricle. This results in two entirely separate and closed circulatory systems—pulmonary and systemic.

b. There must be some other anomalies that provide communication and mixing of blood between the two systems for an infant to survive. This may be realized by an open foramen ovale or ductus arteriosus or by an associated septal defect.

2. ASSESSMENT

a. Defects with lesser communication cause severe cyanosis.

b. Larger septal defects result in less cyanosis but a higher risk of HF.

c. Heart sounds are variable with the associated defects—no murmur.

d. Hypoxia leads to tachycardia, tachypnea, and acidosis.

e. Poor feeding and failure to thrive

3. DIAGNOSTIC TESTS
   a. Chest x-ray: usually shows heart egg shaped, cardiomegaly several weeks postnatally
   b. ECG: right axis deviation
   c. Echocardiogram: to corroborate the diagnosis
   d. Cardiac catheterization: measures ventricular pressures, oxygen saturation; assesses anatomical landmarks
4. NURSING INTERVENTIONS
   a. Instruct the parents and family in provision of mechanisms to reduce cardiac workload.
   b. Instruct the family in pulmonary hygiene measures to reduce respiratory congestion.
   c. Instruct the family on safe drug administration.
   d. Instruct the parents to provide small, frequent nutritive meals.
   e. Provide procedural and sensory teaching for the parents and child regarding unit routines and nursing care.
5. SURGICAL MANAGEMENT
   a. Prostaglandin E_1 is administered to maintain open ductus arteriosus.
   b. Arterial switch procedure is the preferred method of treatment. This should occur as early as possible in the first few weeks of life. Coronary arteries must be carefully moved from the aorta and reimplanted after the switch. This procedure allows normal circulation, as the left ventricle pumps oxygenated blood to the systemic circulation.
   c. Cardiac complications include dysrhythmias, ventricular failure, coronary artery insufficiency, contraction or narrowing at the anastomosis sites.
   d. Palliative surgical procedures are performed if unable to do the arterial switch.

B. HYPOPLASTIC LEFT HEART SYNDROME
   1. DESCRIPTION
      a. The left side of the heart is underdeveloped in this defect. The left ventricle is hypoplastic—as is the ascending aorta.
      b. There is aortic atresia such that there is no blood flow from the left atrium to the left ventricle and aorta.
      c. Mitral valve and aortic valve are absent or stenosed.
      d. Oxygenated blood from the left atrium flows through the foramen ovale to the right atrium and into the

right ventricle, which becomes hypertrophied.
      e. Systemic circulation is supplied by blood flow through the patent ductus arteriosus from the pulmonary artery to the aorta.
   2. ASSESSMENT
      a. Ductus arteriosus open: mild cyanosis and HF, labored respirations, tachypnea, dyspnea, decreased peripheral pulses
      b. Ductus arteriosus closed: severe cyanosis, decreased cardiac output, and quick cardiac decompensation and arrest
      c. Mechanical ventilation is necessary to stabilize the infant.
      d. Prostaglandin E_1 administered for ductal patency.
      e. Fatal without surgical intervention
   3. DIAGNOSTIC TESTS
      a. Chest x-ray: absence of normal left ventricle, pulmonary vascular changes
      b. ECG: left axis alterations
      c. Echocardiogram: dimensions of the left ventricle, associated defects in anatomy
      d. Cardiac catheterization: assess ventricular pressure, measure oxygen saturation, anatomical landmarks
   4. NURSING INTERVENTIONS
      a. Administer prostaglandin E_1 as ordered.
      b. Prepare the parents and child for surgery when indicated.
      c. Instruct the parents on safe medication administration procedures.
      d. Instruct the family to provide care that minimizes cardiac workload.
   5. SURGICAL TREATMENT
      a. Survival rates are low.
      b. Prostaglandin E_1 is administered for patency of the ductus arteriosus.
      c. Palliative surgery may lengthen life expectancy.
      d. Heart transplant is a possible option.

C. TRUNCUS ARTERIOSUS
   1. DESCRIPTION
      a. This defect results from a failure of the aorta and pulmonary artery to divide embryonically. One vessel with one valve then empties both ventricles and blood flows to both pulmonary and systemic circulations.
      b. Direction of blood flow is determined by the vascular resistance of each circulation. Generally, the pulmonary resistance is lower, eventually resulting in HF.

   c. A ventricular septal defect is always associated with this defect.

   d. If pulmonary stenosis is present, the hemodynamics change due to increased pulmonary resistance.

2. ASSESSMENT
   a. Distinctive systolic murmur
   b. Cyanosis and HF vary with changes in pressure and blood flow
   c. Growth retardation
   d. Poor feeding and activity intolerance

3. DIAGNOSTIC TESTS
   a. Chest x-ray: cardiomegaly, hypertrophy of both ventricles, normal heart size if pulmonary stenosis is present
   b. ECG: biventricular hypertrophy
   c. Echocardiogram: position of defects, direction of blood flow, valvular incompetence
   d. Cardiac catheterization: saturation levels and pressures in addition to visualization of the defects

4. NURSING INTERVENTIONS
   a. Instruct the parents and family to recognize clinical manifestations of HF.
   b. Instruct the family to provide safe medication administration.
   c. Provide education for the family regarding measures to decrease cardiac workload.
   d. Instruct the parents on preoperative and postoperative routines and nursing care.
   e. Monitor for arrhythmias.

5. SURGICAL MANAGEMENT
   a. Repair is recommended early in the first months. This involves closure of the VSD and grafting the pulmonary arteries to the right ventricle using a homograft as conduit. Homograft is preferred over synthetic as it is less vulnerable to obstruction. Early repair prevents complications such as HF and pulmonary disease.
   b. The homograft conduit will require replacement as the child grows.
   c. Cardiac complications include HF, dysrythmias, residual septal defect, bleeding, pulmonary artery hypertension.

X. **ACQUIRED PEDIATRIC CARDIOVASCULAR DISORDERS**
  A. KAWASAKI DISEASE
    1. DESCRIPTION
     a. Kawasaki disease (KD) is an inflammation of primarily small- and medium-size vessels throughout the body, including a risk to coronary vessels. It most frequently affects young children.
     b. KD is a systemic vasculitis, which, in 20% to 25% of the cases, causes cardiac complications.
     c. Complications include aneurysms, thrombosis, and myocardial infarction.
     d. In the acute phase, the diagnostic clinical manifestations are noted and myocarditis may also develop during this phase of the disease.
     e. The subacute phase involves a continuation of clinical manifestations and a resolving fever. The risk of coronary aneurysm and thrombus formation is greatest during this phase. Palm and sole desquamation will likely occur during this period, causing irritability.
     f. All clinical signs and arthritis will resolve before the convalescent phase. Lab values will remain abnormal for up to 8 weeks.
     g. Most children recover completely from KD.

    2. ASSESSMENT
     a. Diagnosis is made if five of the first six clinical manifestations are noted.
      1) Fever for more than 5 days (first clinical manifestation), unresponsive to antipyretics
      2) Polymorphous rash, notable in the perineum
      3) Cervical lymphadenopathy
      4) Changes in the extremities such as edema, desquamation, and erythema of the soles and palms
      5) Bilateral conjunctival inflammation, absent exudates
      6) Strawberry tongue or other oral mucous membrane alterations
      7) Arthritis clinical manifestations may also be present after fever resolves.

    3. DIAGNOSTIC TESTS
     a. Complete blood cell count (CBC): leukocytosis (left shift) and deficiency of suppressor T cells are seen in the acute phase. In the subacute phase, significant thrombocytosis is observed.
     b. Echocardiograms: baseline and are necessary at intervals to monitor for cardiac changes such as arrhythmias, myocardial infarction, and HF.

    4. NURSING INTERVENTIONS
     a. Monitor fever.
     b. Assess for clinical manifestations of HF and aneurysms.

c. Monitor intake and output and vital signs closely.

d. Administer IV gamma globulin to decrease risk of coronary lesions and scarring.

e. Administer high-dose aspirin, as prescribed, to decrease inflammation.

f. Provide cardiac monitoring during gamma globulin infusion.

g. Provide symptomatic relief such as cool baths and oral care for fever and skin discomfort.

h. Provide a quiet environment and rest times to minimize irritability.

i. Provide therapeutic management of arthritis symptoms with pain relievers and passive range of motion.

j. Provide nutritional support and encourage oral fluids as needed.

k. Instruct the parents regarding the administration and adverse reactions of pertinent medications such as IVIG and aspirin.

B. RHEUMATIC FEVER AND RHEUMATIC HEART DISEASE

1. DESCRIPTION

a. Rheumatic fever is an inflammatory disease and is self-limiting. It occurs primarily in children between ages 5 and 15 years.

b. Inflammation primarily involves the joints, heart, central nervous system, skin, and other connective tissues.

c. Rheumatic fever occurs 2–6 weeks postpharyngeal infection with group A beta-hemolytic streptococcus.

d. Cardiac complications in 10% of clients occur when the streptococcal infection is untreated and scarring of cardiac anatomy transpires, leading to valve damage and regurgitation, which is known as rheumatic heart disease.

e. Antibiotic administration within the first 9–10 days of infection will typically prevent the onset of rheumatic fever.

2. ASSESSMENT

a. Jones criteria are used for diagnosis. Diagnosis is made in the presence of two major criteria or one major and two minor criteria.

b. Major criteria are:

1) Carditis, often with mitral regurgitation, tachycardia, and pericardial effusion. Murmurs, ECG changes, and friction rubs may be present, and HF occurs in some clients.

2) Polyarthritis: migrates from joint to joint and is reversible

3) Subcutaneous nodules over joints

4) Erythema marginatum: transitory rash largely located on the trunk

5) Chorea: sudden involuntary movements, possible speech involvement, and muscle weakness

c. Minor criteria:

1) Fever

2) Arthralgia

3) Elevated sedimentation rate, elevated C-reactive protein

4) Low red blood cell count

5) Prolonged P-R or Q-T intervals

d. Supporting evidence:

1) Throat culture positive for strep infection

2) Antibody titer for strep: increased

3) History of scarlet fever

4) Antistreptolysin-O (ASLO) titer elevated

3. NURSING INTERVENTIONS

a. Administer penicillin and salicylates as prescribed.

b. Administer prednisone for the treatment of inflammation.

c. Maintain bed rest or restricted activity during the acute phase, until the erythrocyte sedimentation rate is normal.

d. Monitor cardiac function.

e. Instruct the client and family on the importance of adherence to drug regimens and bed rest.

f. Provide quiet diversional activities.

g. Instruct the client and family on secondary prevention of recurrence of rheumatic fever with antibiotic prophylaxis.

h. Provide emotional support; encourage the client and family to verbalize feelings.

i. Instruct the client and family that chorea movements will eventually disappear.

C. HYPERTENSION

1. DESCRIPTION

a. Elevation of blood pressure is noted consistently above the levels of normal for age

b. Primary hypertension has no known cause and secondary hypertension is related to an underlying cause.

c. Secondary hypertension is the form of hypertension primarily seen in children often related to causes such as renal disease and cardiovascular disorders.

2. ASSESSMENT

a. Infants: irritability, head banging, screaming

b. Older children and adolescents: headaches, dizziness, vision changes

c. Measured on at least three separate occasions, blood pressure consistently between the 95th and 99th percentiles for age, sex, and height is "significant hypertension."

d. Blood pressure consistently above the 99th percentile for age, sex, and height is "severe hypertension."

3. DIAGNOSTIC TESTS

a. Blood pressure monitoring on at least three separate occasions for diagnosis, and frequent blood (BP) monitoring after beginning therapy

b. Laboratory data such as urinalysis, blood urea nitrogen (BUN), creatinine, lipid profile, complete blood count (CBC), electrolyte panel

for the purpose of searching out secondary causes

4. NURSING INTERVENTIONS

a. Administer drugs, as prescribed, in children resistant to non-pharmacologic approaches.

b. Instruct the child and parents on dietary changes such as sodium reduction.

c. Instruct the child and parents on the necessity of regular exercise.

d. Instruct the child and parents on stress reduction approaches.

e. Encourage the adolescents with hypertension to consider alternatives to oral contraceptives.

f. Instruct the adolescent and parents on the risks of smoking with the hypertension diagnosis.

PRACTICE QUESTIONS

1. When caring for a child with a ventricular septal defect (VSD), the nurse should monitor for which clinical manifestations of hemodynamic alterations?
Select all that apply:
[ ] 1. Pulmonic murmur
[ ] 2. Bradycardia
[ ] 3. Tachypnea
[ ] 4. Fatigue
[ ] 5. Dyspnea
[ ] 6. Anxiety

2. The nurse is reviewing the chart of a child with coarctation of the aorta. Which of the following findings would the nurse anticipate?
1. Congestive heart failure
2. Cerebral hypertension
3. Hypoxemia
4. Femoral artery hypertension

3. The nurse is planning care for a 2-year-old child immediately following cardiac catheterization. Which of these activities should have the highest priority?
1. Change the dressing at the puncture site
2. Apply direct pressure to the catheterization site for at least 15 minutes
3. Monitor the heart rate for at least 1 minute during vital signs
4. Start oral fluids

4. The nurse includes which of the following in a discharge teaching plan for parents of a child who has just undergone a cardiac catheterization for a cardiac defect?
1. Monitor the dressing and stitches until the return appointment
2. Maintain the postsurgical clear liquid diet for 48 hours
3. Use a home cardiac monitoring system
4. Administer antibiotics for two weeks

5. The nurse asks the mother of a child suspected of having a congenital heart defect about eating patterns and activities. Based on an understanding of this child's condition, which of the following should the nurse consider before recommending a plan of care?
1. Poor feeding and activity intolerance are common in children with congenital heart disease
2. The child's favorite foods and playtime activities are essential to compliance with therapy
3. The parenting techniques should be assessed
4. Mealtimes should be coordinated to the child's activity schedule

6. The nurse is evaluating heart sounds in four children. Which of the following heart sounds found in a 4-year-old child does the nurse report as pathologic?
1. S_1
2. S_2
3. S_3
4. S_4

7. A 5-year-old child is scheduled for an echocardiogram. She asks the nurse if the test will hurt. Which of the following is the nurse's best response?
   1. "It is different for everyone."
   2. "I'm not sure. You should ask your physician."
   3. "There will be a jelly that will feel cool, but it won't hurt."
   4. "The various positions you will have to assume may cause a little discomfort."

8. The nurse is caring for a child with tetralogy of Fallot who experiences an episode of acute cyanosis. Which of the following is the primary clinical manifestation the nurse will assess?
   1. Decreased respiratory rate
   2. Decreased pulse rate and blood pressure
   3. Loss of consciousness
   4. Anxiousness and irritability

9. Which of the following should be included in the discharge teaching the nurse is preparing for the parents of a child with tetralogy of Fallot?
   1. A demonstration of suctioning procedures
   2. The signs of infection
   3. Use of the knee-chest position for cyanotic spells
   4. Complete bed rest

10. The nurse is caring for a child with Kawasaki disease. Which of the following would indicate to the nurse that the client's condition is deteriorating?
    1. Bradycardia
    2. Strep throat
    3. Arrhythmias
    4. Hypotension

11. The nurse would expect which of the following clinical manifestations to be present in a 9-month-old infant with hypoplastic left heart? Select all that apply:
    [ ] 1. Heart murmur
    [ ] 2. Cyanosis
    [ ] 3. Hypertension
    [ ] 4. Heart rate of 130 beats per minute
    [ ] 5. Tachypnea
    [ ] 6. Syncope

12. The nurse is administering digoxin (Lanoxin) to a child with cardiac disease. The nurse should report which of the following manifestations indicative of digoxin toxicity? Select all that apply:
    [ ] 1. Hypertension
    [ ] 2. Cyanosis
    [ ] 3. Visual disturbances
    [ ] 4. Inconsolability
    [ ] 5. Weakness
    [ ] 6. Headache

13. The nurse is caring for a child with a possible diagnosis of rheumatic fever. Which of the following assessment findings does the nurse evaluate as a diagnostic criterion?
    1. Decreased erythrocyte sedimentation rate
    2. Bradycardia
    3. Elevation of antistreptolysin (ASO) levels
    4. Desquamation of the fingertips

14. When preparing discharge teaching for a family of a child recovering from rheumatic fever, the nurse's priority instruction is
    1. the child needs to take prophylactic antibiotics to prevent endocarditis.
    2. the child should resume school activities as soon as tolerated.
    3. parents should inform the school nurse of the child's illness.
    4. parents should monitor the child for poor appetite and growth.

15. Which of the following should the nurse include in the discharge instructions for an infant with an atrial septal defect?
    1. A discussion of speech development
    2. Cardiopulmonary resuscitation
    3. The necessity of monitoring for obesity
    4. Home oxygen saturation monitoring

16. A child's mother asks the nurse how her child got hypertension and what it means. In explaining hypertension in children, the nurse would most appropriately respond that in children, hypertension "is
    1. generally related to another disease process."
    2. generally not treated."
    3. usually nothing to worry about."
    4. related to cholesterol levels."

17. Which of the following should the nurse include in the preoperative teaching for the parents of a child scheduled for cardiac surgery?
    1. A warning to avoid bringing toys from home to the hospital
    2. A warning that siblings should not visit
    3. Concepts of pain management
    4. A tour of the general pediatric care unit

18. A nurse caring for a young child with a newly diagnosed atrial septal defect would
    1. prepare the child for echocardiogram.
    2. discuss life expectancy with the parents.
    3. assess for signs of liver damage.
    4. monitor the child for cyanotic spells.

19. To reduce cardiac workload, the nurse should implement which of the following nursing interventions for a child in heart failure?
    1. Place the child in Trendelenburg position
    2. Encourage fluids

3. Schedule regular meals three times a day
4. Provide a quiet environment

20. The parents of a 3-year-old child with tetralogy of Fallot tell the nurse that their child frequently squats during play. Based on an understanding of tetralogy of Fallot, the nurse recognizes that this is
    1. normal for the child's developmental age.
    2. a sign of constipation.
    3. a compensatory mechanism.
    4. a disinterest in engaging in play.

21. Which of the following should the nurse include in the plan of care for a child diagnosed with secondary hypertension?
    1. Weight control
    2. Managing cholesterol levels
    3. Use of diuretics
    4. Treatment of the underlying condition

22. The nurse caring for an infant with patent ductus arteriosus informs the parents that corrective surgery will prevent
    1. pulmonary vascular congestion.
    2. increased systemic venous pressure.
    3. cerebral vascular hemorrhage.
    4. hepatomegaly.

23. Which of the following is the nurse's priority intervention in a child with pulmonary stenosis?
    1. Monitor for indications of congestive heart failure
    2. Educate the parents regarding home medications
    3. Provide sensory preparation for a chest x-ray
    4. Discuss the child's nutritional and developmental needs

24. A child with an atrioventricular canal has been experiencing difficulty breathing and productive cough for 3 days. On admission, the nurse notes nasal flaring and retractions. At this point the nurse's priority action is to
    1. inform the physician of the client's worsening condition.
    2. administer oxygen via mask.
    3. reassure the parents.
    4. obtain the child's weight.

25. The nurse is assessing an infant who has been transferred from another facility for examination of possible cardiac anomalies. The child has congestive heart failure, is severely cyanotic, and is on mechanical ventilation. The chest x-ray shows an abnormally large right ventricle and a very small left ventricle. The nurse recognizes that this is most likely
    1. coarctation of the aorta.
    2. an atrioventricular canal defect.
    3. truncus arteriosus.
    4. hypoplastic left heart syndrome.

26. The registered nurse is preparing clinical assignments for a pediatric unit. Which of the following nursing assignments may be delegated to a licensed practical nurse?
    1. Instruct the parents of a child with septal defect in cardiopulmonary resuscitation
    2. Inform the parents of a child with an atrioventricular canal of the clinical manifestations of congestive heart failure
    3. Assist a child with tetralogy of Fallot to a knee-chest position during an acute hypoxic spell
    4. Assess a child with tricuspid atresia for growth retardation and failure to thrive

ANSWERS AND RATIONALES

1. 3. 4. 5. Ventricular septal defect is an abnormal connection between the right and left ventricles. Tachypnea, dyspnea, and fatigue are clinical manifestations that may indicate worsening hemodynamics and possible congestive heart failure. Pulmonic murmur, bradycardia, and anxiety are not manifestations of hemodynamic changes in ventricular septal defects.

2. 2. Coarctation of the aorta is a stenosis most commonly located within the thoracic aorta that increases systemic resistance at the site of the coarctation. This causes an increase in pressure proximal to the coarctation, causing hypertension in the cerebral arteries. Arteries distal to the coarctation have reduced pressure, causing lower extremity hypotension.

3. 2. Direct pressure on the site for 15 minutes and frequent monitoring of the occlusive pressure dressing will decrease the risk of complications from hematoma or hemorrhage following cardiac catheterization. The dressing should not be changed immediately postprocedure, as disruption of the clot may cause life-threatening hemorrhage. Monitoring the heart rate for 1 minute during vital signs and starting oral fluids are appropriate actions in postoperative care, but are of lower priority in the assessment and care of the child immediately post-op.

4. 4. After a cardiac catheterization, the dressing will be removed before discharge and stitches are not necessary for this procedure. The postprocedure diet is the child's usual diet, and home cardiac monitors are not used after cardiac catheterization. Antibiotics are used for children with heart defects prophylactically to minimize the risk of infection.

5. 1. Poor appetite and feeding patterns and activity intolerance are common to many congenital heart diseases. This is the primary consideration for the nurse before recommending the child's plan of care.

6. 4. The S_1 and S_2 are normal heart sounds at the beginning (closure of AV valves) and end (closure of semilunar valves) of ventricular systole. The S_3 sound occurs early in diastole and is considered normal in children and young adults, but is a sound of cardiac disease in older adults. S_4 is a rare sound and not heard in a normal heart.

7. 3. An echocardiogram is noninvasive and painless. The child needs to be reassured.

8. 4. Tetralogy of Fallot is comprised of a ventral septal defect, pulmonary stenosis, right ventricular hypertrophy, and an overriding aorta. During a cyanotic spell, pulse and respiratory rates increase to compensate for decreased oxygen levels. Anxiety and irritability are the most common manifestation in children with hypoxic spells. Loss of consciousness is more likely to be seen in states of severe heart failure.

9. 3. Tetralogy of Fallot is comprised of a ventral septal defect, pulmonary stenosis, right ventricular hypertrophy, and an overriding aorta. The use of the knee-chest position is effective in decreasing cardiac workload. Complete bed rest is inappropriate; as much normal activity as can be tolerated is encouraged. Signs of infection and suctioning are not a part of the care for a child with tetralogy of Fallot.

10. 3. Kawasaki disease is a multisystem vasculitis that affects the coronary arteries. Hypotension and strep throat are not manifestations seen in Kawasaki disease. Cardiac complications are the most serious and contribute to morbidity and mortality. Tachycardia, a gallop rhythm, and congestive heart failure may occur.

11. 1. 2. 5. Heart murmur and cyanosis would be characteristic of hypoplastic left heart. Heart rate of 130 at rest is within normal range for an infant. Increasing respiratory crackles could indicate an increased load on the right ventricle and increased potential for heart failure. Hypotension is also a manifestation.

12. 3. 5. 6. Clinical manifestations of digoxin toxicity are visual disturbances, weakness, headache, apathy, and psychosis.

13. 3. Streptococcal infection precedes the development of rheumatic fever by approximately 2 weeks. Elevation of antistreptolysin (ASO) levels indicates a recent strep infection.

14. 1. Rheumatic fever is thought to be an autoimmune disorder related to group A streptococcal infection. Future streptococcal infection and the risk for endocarditis can be prevented with prophylactic antibiotic administration. Resuming school activities and informing the school nurse about the illness may be appropriate interventions, but they are of lower priority. Poor appetite and growth do not generally occur with rheumatic fever unless the child already has experienced significant heart damage.

15. 2. An atrial septal defect is an abnormal connection between the right and left atria. Children with any heart defect are at a higher risk for heart failure. Instruction in cardiopulmonary resuscitation (CPR) increases parental confidence and prepares them to handle an emergency.

16. 1. Secondary hypertension is much more common in children than primary hypertension. It is usually a manifestation of another disease process. Hypertension in children is of concern and treatable. The association with cholesterol is not applicable.

17. 3. It is appropriate to instruct the parents of a child scheduled for cardiac surgery in the concepts of pain management. Toys from home can be comforting to a hospitalized child as can sibling visits. Siblings are also comforted by seeing the child in person. Although a tour of the intensive care unit is appropriate, the tour of general pediatrics can come later as necessary.

18. 1. An atrial septal defect is an abnormality between the left and right atria. A chest x-ray and an echocardiogram are generally performed to demonstrate the increase in the heart size and location and size of the defect. Cyanotic spells are generally not seen in atrial septal defects. Cyanosis itself is rare unless the defect in the septum is large enough to allow significant mixing of oxygenated and unoxygenated blood.

19. 4. Placing a child with a cardiac condition in a Trendelenburg position and encouraging fluids would actually increase cardiac workload. The preferred method of feeding to reduce cardiac workload is to feed five to six small meals a day. A quiet environment reduces stress and anxiety, resulting in a reduced cardiac workload.

20. 3. Tetralogy of Fallot is comprised of a ventral septal defect, pulmonary stenosis, right ventricular hypertrophy, and an overriding aorta. Squatting helps the child's circulatory system compensate for episodes of hypoxemia, especially during active periods.

21. 4. Secondary hypertension in a child is related to an underlying disease process. Treatment of that condition will most commonly significantly improve the hypertension. Weight control, use of diuretics, and managing the cholesterol level are common treatments for primary hypertension, which is rare in children.

22. 1. The ductus arteriosus is a direct connection between the main pulmonary artery and the aorta. When the connection remains open several weeks after birth in a full-term infant, it is a patent ductus arteriosus. Patent ductus arteriosus causes an increase in blood flow in the reverse of what it was in fetal life as systemic pressure increases relative to pulmonary pressures. This causes an increase in pulmonary flow through the pulmonary artery. Pulmonary vascular congestion is the risk in this case.

23. 1. Pulmonary stenosis is a narrowing of the pulmonary valve and obstruction of the blood flow from the right ventricle to the lungs. Monitoring the child for congestive heart failure is the priority as it is potentially life threatening. Provision of sensory preparation for the x-ray is also important but not as significant as monitoring for congestive heart failure (CHF). Educating the parents about

home medications and discussing the child's nutritional and developmental needs are appropriate interventions later in the hospitalization.

24. 2. An atrioventricular canal is a defect that allows blood to flow among all four chambers. An atrial septal defect is continuous with a ventricular septal defect along the septum, also affecting both AV valves (mitral and tricuspid), creating essentially one large chamber. Blood flow direction depends on the child's peripheral resistance and pulmonary resistance as well as ventricular pressures. This defect is seen in Down syndrome. This client is experiencing labored breathing and requires oxygen immediately. This can be applied quickly before calling the physician. Reassuring the parents and obtaining a weight are also important interventions, but immediate oxygen could reduce the difficulty of breathing for this child and help stabilize the condition.

25. 4. Hypoplastic left heart syndrome is characterized by a lack of development of the left ventricle secondary to mitral valve atresia or aortic atresia. The result is a small hypoplastic left ventricle not capable of cardiac function.

26. 3. Nursing assignments involving skills such as instructing, informing, or assessing should be performed only by a registered nurse. A licensed practical nurse may assist a child with tetralogy of Fallot to a knee-chest position during an acute hypoxic spell because the initial instruction has taken place.

REFERENCES

Potts, N., & Mandleco, B. (2012). *Pediatric nursing: Caring for children and their families* (3rd ed.) Clifton Park, NY: Delmar Cengage Learning.

Spratto, G. R., & Woods, A. L. (2012). *PDR nurse's drug handbook 2012*. Clifton Park, NY: Delmar Cengage Learning.

CHAPTER 33

GASTROINTESTINAL DISORDERS

I. **ANATOMY AND PHYSIOLOGY (SEE CHAPTER 5 GASTROINTESTINAL DISORDERS, SECTION I.)**
   A. DIFFERENCES IN THE GASTROINTESTINAL SYSTEM BETWEEN CHILDREN AND ADULTS
      1. SUCKING AND SWALLOWING ARE PRIMITIVE REFLEXES THAT BECOMES A VOLUNTARY ACTION BY APPROXIMATELY 6 WEEKS OF AGE.
      2. UNTIL APPROXIMATELY 2 YEARS OF AGE, THE STOMACH IS ROUND AND LIES HORIZONTALLY. AT THIS TIME, AN ELONGATION PROCESS BEGINS AND IS COMPLETED AT AROUND 7 YEARS OF AGE, WHEN IT TAKES THE SHAPE AND POSITION OF AN ADULT'S STOMACH.
      3. THE NEONATE'S STOMACH CAPACITY IS SMALL BUT EXPANDS RAPIDLY TO OVER 200 ML BY 1 MONTH OF AGE AND TO AN ADULT CAPACITY BY LATE ADOLESCENCE.
      4. DUE TO THE DECREASED OR RELAXED TONE OF THE LOWER ESOPHAGEAL SPHINCTER, REGURGITATION IS COMMON IN INFANCY.
      5. PERISTALSIS IS GREATER IN THE NEONATAL PERIOD, WITH EMPTYING TIME BEING APPROXIMATELY 2–3 HOURS AND GRADUALLY INCREASING TO 3–6 HOURS BY 1–2 MONTHS OF AGE. THE FREQUENCY AND CHARACTER OF THE STOOL ARE INFLUENCED BY THE PERISTALTIC RATE.
      6. THE SMALL INTESTINE OF AN INFANT IS SIX TIMES THE INFANT'S HEIGHT AS COMPARED TO AN ADULT'S BEING FOUR TIMES THE ADULT'S HEIGHT. EVEN THOUGH THE INFANT HAS THE SAME DIGESTIVE CAPACITY AS THE ADULT, MORE FLUID AND ELECTROLYTES ARE SECRETED DUE TO THE LENGTH OF THE INTESTINES, LEADING TO A HIGHER POTENTIAL FOR FLUID AND ELECTROLYTE IMBALANCE.
      7. THE LARGE INTESTINES ARE SHORTER, RESULTING IN A DECREASED ABILITY TO ABSORB WATER FROM THE GUT, WHICH CAUSES SOFTER AND MORE FREQUENT STOOLS.
      8. STARCH INTOLERANCE IS PRESENT DURING EARLY INFANCY DUE TO THE INSUFFICIENT PRODUCTION OF AMYLASE, A PANCREATIC ENZYME.
      9. LOW LEVELS OF LIPASE RESULTS IN IMPAIRED DIGESTION AND ABSORPTION OF FATS DURING INFANCY, THUS THE NEED TO SUPPLEMENT THE FAT-SOLUBLE VITAMINS A, D, E, AND K.

II. **ASSESSMENT**
   A. HEALTH HISTORY
      1. PRENATAL HISTORY
      2. DEVELOPMENTAL PROBLEMS
      3. MEDICATIONS
      4. HOSPITALIZATIONS
      5. SURGERIES
      6. HISTORY OF VOMITING, INCLUDING RELATIONSHIP TO FOOD, AMOUNT, COLOR, TYPE
      7. WEIGHT LOSS, WEIGHT GAIN, FOOD INTOLERANCE
      8. HISTORY OF BOWEL PATTERNS SUCH AS CONSTIPATION OR DIARRHEA
      9. NUTRITION PATTERN
   B. PHYSICAL EXAMINATION
      1. INSPECTION
         a. Measure the height and weight.
         b. Inspect the color.
         c. Measure the midarm circumference and tricep skinfold thickness.

d. Inspect the mouth for color and fissures.

e. Inspect skin integrity.

f. Observe for abdominal distention or peristaltic waves.

2. PALPATION

a. Palpate the abdomen for tenderness.

b. Palpate the liver.

c. Palpate the spleen.

3. PERCUSSION

a. Detects pain and tenderness

4. AUSCULTATION

a. Auscultate bowel sounds.

III. **DIAGNOSTIC STUDIES (SEE CHAPTER 5, GASTROINTESTINAL DISORDERS, SECTION III.)**

IV. **NURSING DIAGNOSES**

A. ACUTE PAIN

B. IMBALANCED NUTRITION: LESS THAN BODY REQUIREMENTS

C. CONSTIPATION OR DIARRHEA

D. IMPAIRED ORAL MUCOUS MEMBRANES

E. DEFICIENT FLUID VOLUME

F. NAUSEA

G. IMPAIRED SWALLOWING

Nursing Diagnoses: Definitions and Classification 2012–2014. Copyright © 2012, 1994–2012 by NANDA International. Used by arrangement with John Wiley & Sons Limited.

V. **UPPER GASTROINTESTINAL DISORDERS**

A. ESOPHAGEAL ATRESIA AND TRACHEOESOPHAGEAL FISTULA

1. DESCRIPTION

a. Esophageal atresia (EA)

1) The proximal end of the esophagus ends in a blind pouch.

2) A congenital anomaly usually associated with tracheoesophageal fistula

3) Surgical repair to reconnect the proximal and distal ends of the esophagus

b. Tracheoesophageal fistula (TEF)

1) An abnormal opening between the trachea and esophagus

2) Gastric content can enter and irritate the trachea.

3) Surgical repair to separate the trachea and esophagus is usually done in stages.

2. ASSESSMENT

a. Newborn presents with drooling and copious oral secretions.

b. Respiratory distress may be evident with pulmonary congestion, coughing, choking, and intermittent cyanosis.

c. Inability to pass a nasogastric (NG) tube

d. Stomach distention (TEF)

3. DIAGNOSTIC TESTS

a. History of polyhydramnios

b. Presence of respiratory distress during feeding

c. Inability to identify a stomach bubble in a prenatal ultrasound (EA)

d. Chest and abdominal x-rays to identify air in the stomach

4. NURSING INTERVENTIONS

a. Assess for respiratory distress.

b. Maintain a patent airway.

c. Elevate the head of the bed (HOB) at least 30 degrees to reduce reflux.

d. Feed the infant by intravenous fluids or by placement of a gastrostomy tube (GT) for enteral feedings.

e. Provide emotional support for the parent(s) and infant.

5. SURGICAL MANAGEMENT

a. Preoperative care

1) Maintain hydration and nutritional status.

2) Keep the head of the bed elevated, generally 30 degrees, and maintain a patent airway.

3) Maintain nothing by mouth, not even a pacifier.

4) Monitor for respiratory distress and nasopharyngeal suctioning as necessary.

5) Instruct the parents on the surgery and anticipated care of the infant.

b. Postoperative care

1) Maintain a patent airway and chest tube.

2) Monitor for adequate oxygenation.

3) Administer antibiotics, as ordered, to prevent infection.

4) Provide adequate nutrition via total parenteral nutrition (TPN) until GT or oral feedings are tolerated, starting with glucose water and progressing to small formula feedings.

5) Instruct the parents on the home care of the infant that includes feeding and clinical manifestations of problems, especially esophageal stricture (difficulty swallowing, increased drooling, and frequent coughing or choking).

B. PYLORIC STENOSIS

1. DESCRIPTION

a. A thickening of the muscular ring known as the pyloric sphincter that prevents the passage of food from the stomach to the duodenum

b. Surgical repair, a pyloromyotomy, to release the muscular fibers of the pyloric sphincter

2. ASSESSMENT
   a. Nonbilious projectile vomiting during or after feeding
   b. Palpable olive-shaped mass in the epigastric area
   c. Infant is hungry and will feed again in spite of vomiting.
   d. Infant does not appear ill.
   e. Weight loss and dehydration as condition worsens
3. DIAGNOSTIC TESTS
   a. Barium swallow (upper gastrointestinal [UGI] series)
   b. Abdominal ultrasound to evaluate for anomalies
   c. Blood chemistry to evaluate fluid balance (sodium, chloride, potassium, creatinine, and glucose)
   d. Blood gas to evaluate metabolic status, specifically alkalosis
4. NURSING INTERVENTIONS
   a. Maintain reflux precautions:
      1) Provide small, frequent thickened feedings.
      2) Burp frequently and position upright on the right side after feeding.
5. SURGICAL MANAGEMENT
   a. Preoperative care
      1) Assess vital signs for dehydration and to detect cardiac-pulmonary compromise.
      2) Maintain a strict intake and output and specific gravity to evaluate renal function.
      3) Weigh daily to evaluate growth.
      4) Maintain reflux precautions such as placing the child on the right side after feedings.
      5) NPO if feedings are not tolerated
      6) Insert the NG tube to decompress the stomach prior to surgery.
      7) Hydrate with intravenous fluids and correct electrolyte imbalance prior to surgery.
      8) Provide emotional support for the parents and infant.
      9) Instruct the parents on the surgery and anticipated care of the infant.
      10) Maintain a high-Fowler's position.
   b. Postoperative care
      1) Monitor vital signs.
      2) Maintain a strict intake and output.
      3) Assess the child's daily weights.
      4) Maintain intravenous fluids until the infant is able to tolerate feedings.
      5) Begin feedings slowly, gradually increase as tolerated, and monitor for "dumping syndrome."

      6) Keep the incision clean.
      7) Burp frequently and position the infant on the right side after feeding.
      8) Administer thickened formula or feedings for approximately 2 weeks to allow for muscle healing.
      9) Instruct the parents on the home care of the infant that includes feeding, positioning, and prevention of infection.

VI. **LOWER INTESTINAL DISORDERS**
   A. HIRSCHSPRUNG'S DISEASE
      1. DESCRIPTION
         a. A congenital aganglionic megacolon
         b. Motility slowed due to absence of parasympathetic ganglion cells in the large intestine needed for peristalsis
         c. Males affected three to four times more than females
         d. Most common cause of distal bowel obstruction in the newborn
         e. Surgical repair occurs in two stages of a colostomy for bowel rest then a resection of aganglionic segment and pull-through of normal colon to be connected to the rectum.
      2. ASSESSMENT
         a. Abdominal distention and no passage of meconium in the newborn
         b. History of constipation in the infant or child
         c. Episodes of vomiting
         d. Ribbonlike or pellet-shaped, foul-smelling stools
         e. Inadequate weight gain
         f. Easily palpable fecal mass
         g. Signs of enterocolitis with fever, foul-smelling diarrhea, and abdominal distention that can lead to bowel perforation
      3. DIAGNOSTIC TESTS
         a. Absence of stool on rectal exam
         b. Barium enema shows dilated bowel segments.
         c. Rectal biopsy to identify aganglionic cells
      4. NURSING INTERVENTIONS
         a. Prepare the parents and child for the anticipated surgery.
         b. Instruct the parents on the administration of enema (use only mineral oil or isotonic saline).
         c. Avoid treating the child for diarrhea because the child is actually constipated.
      5. SURGICAL MANAGEMENT
         a. Preoperative care
            1) Administer intravenous fluids to maintain fluid and electrolyte balance.

2) NPO
3) Assess for clinical manifestations of condition worsening or peritonitis.
4) Administer oral antibiotics and antibiotic enemas to reduce intestinal flora.
5) Provide emotional support for the parents and child.
6) Instruct the parents on the disease, surgery, and the anticipated care of the child.

b. Postoperative care
1) Monitor vital signs.
2) Maintain a strict intake and output.
3) Assess the daily weights to evaluate hydration status.
4) Administer analgesics for pain as needed.
5) Administer IV antibiotics to prevent infection.
6) Assess GI status by monitoring NG output, bowel sounds, and abdominal distention.
7) Provide ostomy care and change the diaper when soiled to prevent wound contamination.
8) Instruct and involve the parents in the immediate ostomy care of the child.
9) Instruct the parents on a low-residue diet.

B. IMPERFORATE ANUS
1. DESCRIPTION
a. An anorectal malformation that results in absence of a rectal opening
b. More common in males and associated with congenital anomalies of the urinary tract, esophagus, and intestines
c. Anoplasty surgery required to create an anal opening then anal dilation to prevent stenosis or temporary colostomy followed by pull-through connection of the blind pouch of the rectum to the anus

2. ASSESSMENT
a. Obvious absence of an anal opening on physical examination at birth
b. Presence of meconium in urine indicating a fistula between the bowel and urinary tract
c. A flat perineum and absence of an anal dimple noted on physical examination

3. DIAGNOSTIC TESTS
a. Physical examination of the perineum
b. Abdominal x-ray for presence of air in the blind pouch

c. Presence of gas in the urinary bladder or urethra on x-ray indicates presence of a fistula.

4. NURSING INTERVENTIONS
a. Prepare the parents and the child for the anticipated surgery.
b. Avoid taking a rectal temperature.

5. SURGICAL MANAGEMENT
a. Preoperative care
1) Administer intravenous fluids to maintain fluid and electrolyte balance.
2) NPO
3) Insert an NG tube to decompress the stomach.
4) Administer prophylactic antibiotics.
5) Maintain nutritional status with intravenous fluids.
6) Provide emotional support for the parents and child.
7) Instruct the parents on the surgery and the anticipated care of the child.

b. Postoperative care
1) Monitor vital signs.
2) Maintain a strict intake and output.
3) Assess daily weights to evaluate hydration status.
4) Administer analgesics for pain as needed.
5) Assess GI status by monitoring NG output and bowel sounds.
6) Change the diaper when soiled to prevent wound contamination.
7) Maintain meticulous wound care to prevent infection.
8) Provide ostomy care if a colostomy is present.
9) Instruct and involve the parents in the immediate ostomy care of the child.
10) Assist the child to the side-lying position or have the child lie prone with the hips elevated.

C. INTUSSUSCEPTION
1. DESCRIPTION
a. One segment of the bowel telescopes or invaginates into another.
b. Most frequent cause of intestinal obstruction in infants to toddlers
c. Potentially life-threatening if left untreated and usually requires hydrostatic reduction using water-soluble contrast and air pressure

2. ASSESSMENT
a. Abrupt onset of acute colicky episode
b. Intermittent abdominal pain
c. Vomiting and currant jellylike stool (bloody-mucoid stool)

d. Abdominal tenderness
e. As the severity of the condition occurs, signs of peritonitis will be present.

3. DIAGNOSTIC TESTS
a. Barium or air contrast enema to identify the telescoped area
b. Abdominal ultrasound to locate the obstruction

4. NURSING INTERVENTIONS
a. Administer intravenous fluids to maintain fluid and electrolyte balance.
b. NPO
c. Insert an NG tube to decompress the stomach.
d. Maintain nutritional status with intravenous fluids.
e. Provide emotional support for the parent(s) and child.
f. Instruct the parents on the hydrostatic reduction procedure and the anticipated care of the child.
g. Monitor the child for 12–24 hours after reduction for passage of barium or water-soluble contrast and stool.

D. MALROTATION AND VOLVULUS
1. DESCRIPTION
a. Congenital incomplete rotation of the midgut with the bowel twisted on itself
b. Results in arterial obstruction, ischemia, and necrosis of the intestine
c. Surgery done to rotate the intestine into the correct location and removal of any necrotic areas

2. ASSESSMENT
a. Diarrhea usually seen in infants
b. Abdominal distention
c. Bilious vomiting
d. Abdominal cramping and pain
e. Bowel obstruction
f. Perforation and peritonitis may occur.

3. DIAGNOSTIC TESTS
a. Abdominal x-ray to rule out free air
b. Abdominal ultrasound to locate the affected area
c. Barium swallow (UGI) to identify the area of obstruction

4. NURSING INTERVENTION
a. Prepare the parents and child for the anticipated surgery.

5. SURGICAL MANAGEMENT
a. Preoperative care
1) Administer intravenous fluids to maintain fluid and electrolyte balance.
2) NPO
3) Insert an NG tube to decompress the stomach.
4) Administer analgesics for pain and cramping.
5) Provide emotional support for the parents and child.
6) Instruct the parents on the surgery and the anticipated care of the child.
b. Postoperative care
1) Monitor vital signs.
2) Maintain a strict intake and output.
3) Monitor the daily weights to evaluate hydration status.
4) Administer analgesics for pain as needed.
5) Assess the GI status by monitoring NG output, bowel sounds, and abdominal distention.
6) Provide ostomy care if ostomy is required.
7) Instruct and involve the parents in the immediate ostomy care of the child.

VII. MOTILITY DISORDERS
A. GASTROESOPHAGEAL REFLUX (GER)
1. DESCRIPTION
a. Most commonly seen during infancy
b. The return of gastric contents into the lower esophagus through the lower esophagus sphincter (LES)
c. Condition usually improves around 6–12 months of age when the esophagus elongates and LES moves below the diaphragm.
d. Nissen fundoplication surgical procedure is performed if the condition is not controlled by medical regime.

2. ASSESSMENT
a. Vomiting
b. Nonbilious regurgitation consisting of undigested formula and mucus
c. Poor weight gain and malnutrition
d. Can develop into esophagitis
e. A more severe condition leads to apnea, repeated aspiration pneumonia, and respiratory infections.

3. DIAGNOSTIC TESTS
a. Physical examination and history of feeding habits
b. UGI to identify any anomalies
c. Barium swallow fluoroscopy to identify the degree of reflux and any inflammation or ulceration
d. Esophageal pH probe study to identify acidity of the distal esophagus, to determine the number of reflux episodes and the length of time it takes the acid to clear

4. NURSING INTERVENTIONS
a. Maintain reflux precautions.
1) Small, frequent thickened feedings
2) Burp frequently and position upright on the right side after feeding.

3) Elevate the head of the bed 30 degrees.
b. Administer prokinetic agents such as metaclopramide (Reglan), an H_2 blocker such as cimetadine (Tagamet), or ranitidine (Zantac).
c. If Nissen fundoplication becomes necessary, instruct the parents on the surgery and the anticipated care of the child.
d. Provide emotional support for parents and infant.

B. FAILURE TO THRIVE (FTT)
1. DESCRIPTION
a. A term used to describe a child with inadequate weight or height gain for age
b. Weight is below the third to fifth percentiles on standardized growth charts.
c. Usually diagnosed by the age of 2 years and classified as organic, nonorganic, or mixed (a combination of organic and nonorganic)
d. Organic failure to thrive (OFTT) is related to a physical condition such as GER, celiac disease, cystic fibrosis, and pyloric stenosis.
e. Nonorganic failure to thrive (NOFTT) is related to stress, poverty, anxiety, and failure to bond with the caregiver.
2. ASSESSMENT
a. Growth failure: less than third to fifth percentile in weight and height
b. Loss of subcutaneous fat
c. Reduced muscle mass
d. Developmental delays
e. Signs of neglect
f. Expressionless face, apathetic, and listless
g. Inadequate urination and stools
3. DIAGNOSTIC TESTS
a. History of previous illnesses and eating patterns
b. Review of family and social history
c. Diagnostic test related to specific physical conditions should be conducted once NOFTT is ruled out.
4. NURSING INTERVENTIONS
a. Maintain a supportive, nonblaming approach with caregivers.
b. Maintain the same caregiver with the child and provide consistency in care.
c. Maintain a feeding schedule.
d. Monitor the child's growth patterns.
e. Provide developmentally appropriate stimulation that is moderate and purposeful.
f. Observe family interaction with the child.

g. Educate the parents regarding the condition, normal growth and development, and appropriate parenting skills.
h. Praise positive parenting skills demonstrated by the family.
i. Provide emotional support for the parents and child.

C. NECROTIZING ENTEROCOLITIS (NEC)
1. DESCRIPTION
a. "Necrotizing" means causing death to tissue, "entero" refers to the small intestine, "colo" refers to the large intestine, and "itis" is inflammation.
b. An inflammation causing injury to the bowel.
c. NEC may involve only the innermost lining or the entire thickness of the bowel and variable amounts of the bowel.
d. Life threatening to the premature, low birth weight infant
e. Risk factors include intestinal ischemia, bacterial colonization of the bowel, and presence of hypertonic solutions (formula) in the intestinal lumen.
f. May require bowel resection and ostomy placement
g. Complications of NEC may be:
1) Malabsorption or inability of the bowel to absorb nutrients normally
2) Short bowel or too little bowel to absorb all the nutrients needed by the body
3) Scarring and narrowing of the bowel, resulting in its "obstruction" or blockage
4) Scarring within the abdomen, causing adhesions and pain
2. ASSESSMENT
a. General signs of acute illness: less active, more apnea, increased respiratory problems, difficulty maintaining normal body temperature
b. Poor tolerance to feedings
c. Vomiting or residuals that are greenish in color
d. Abdominal distention with increasing abdominal girth
e. Redness or abnormal abdominal skin color that may even appear shiny as distention worsens
f. Grossly positive blood in stool
g. Heme positive blood in the stool if blood is not visible in stool
3. DIAGNOSTIC TESTS
a. Abdominal x-ray to detect free air
b. Blood culture to check for bacteria

c. Serum electrolytes for fluid balance status
d. Stool for occult blood

4. NURSING INTERVENTIONS
   a. Administer intravenous fluids to maintain fluid and electrolyte balance.
   b. Administer packed red blood cells to improve oxygenation demands.
   c. NPO
   d. Insert an NG tube to decompress the stomach.
   e. Monitor abdominal girth.
   f. Administer IV antibiotics such as ampillicin and gentamicin.
   g. Maintain nutritional status with intravenous fluids.
   h. Provide emotional support for the parents and child.
   i. Instruct the parents on the condition, possible surgery, and the anticipated care of the child.

5. SURGICAL MANAGEMENT
   a. Preoperative care
      1) Inform the parents on the procedure.
   b. Postoperative care
      1) Monitor vital signs.
      2) Maintain a strict intake and output
      3) Assess the daily weights to evaluate hydration status.
      4) Administer analgesics for pain as needed.
      5) Assess the GI status by monitoring NG output and bowel sounds.
      6) Maintain meticulous wound care to prevent infection.
      7) Provide ostomy care if a colostomy is necessary.
      8) Instruct and involve the parents in the immediate ostomy care of the child.

VIII. OTHER GASTROINTESTINAL DISORDERS
A. BILIARY ATRESIA
1. DESCRIPTION
   a. The congenital absence or obstruction of the ducts that drain bile from the liver
   b. A progressive inflammatory process that begins very soon after birth
   c. The most common form, called extrahepatic biliary atresia
   d. Hepatic portenterostomy, Kasai procedure, is done to slow the pathologic process.
   e. The single most frequent indication for a liver transplant in children

2. ASSESSMENT
   a. Asymptomatic at birth but develops jaundice at approximately 2–3 weeks of age

b. Yellow eyes and skin
c. Light-colored stools
d. Dark tea-colored urine
e. Hepatomegaly present
f. Weight loss, irritability, severe pruritus, and FTT develop as the level of jaundice increases.

3. DIAGNOSTIC TESTS
   a. Serum fractionated bilirubin to identify liver dysfunction with increased bilirubin
   b. An ultrasound test may detect an absent or tiny gallbladder.
   c. Hydroxyiminodiacetic acid (HIDA) or gallbladder scan to identify the inability of the dye to flow from the liver through the damaged biliary system to the small intestine
   d. Liver biopsy to identify features typical of an obstruction to the biliary system
   e. Surgical exploration of the infant's abdomen is necessary in most cases to make a definitive diagnosis.

4. NURSING INTERVENTION
   a. Prepare the parents and child for surgery.

5. SURGICAL MANAGEMENT
   a. Preoperative care
      1) Administer intravenous fluids to maintain fluid and electrolyte balance.
      2) NPO
      3) Insert an NG tube to decompress the stomach.
      4) Administer analgesics for pain and cramping.
      5) Administer bile-binding drugs cholestyramine (Questran) and phenobarbital to reduce reabsorption of bile from the intestines and to improve the bile flow.
      6) Monitor the child for adverse reactions of cholestyramine (Questran) such as abdominal distention, steatorrhea, and abdominal cramping.
      7) Monitor the child for adverse reactions of phenobarbital such as sedation.
      8) Place mittens on the hands to prevent scratching the skin secondary to intense itching.
      9) Provide emotional support for the parents and child.
      10) Instruct the parents on the surgery and the anticipated care of the child.
   b. Postoperative care
      1) Monitor vital signs.
      2) Maintain a strict intake and output.

3) Assess daily weights to evaluate hydration status.
4) Administer analgesics for pain as needed.
5) Administer IV antibiotics and cholestyramine (Questran) or phenobarbital, or both.
6) Assess the GI status by monitoring NG output, bowel sounds, and abdominal distention. Report any changes immediately.
7) Assess for ascending cholangitis, a bacterial infection of the biliary tree. Signs include unexplained fever, increased jaundice, or lighter stools.
8) Give special formulas containing medium-chain triglycerides and water-soluble vitamin supplements to maximize the child's growth and development.
9) Monitor for complications of bleeding and clotting, esophageal varices, and ascites.
10) Instruct the parents regarding the long-term care of the child and the eventual need for a liver transplant.

B. CELIAC DISEASE
1. DESCRIPTION
a. A genetic digestive disease that damages the small intestine and interferes with absorption of a protein called gluten, which is found in wheat, rye, barley, and possibly oats
b. The immune system responds by damaging the small intestine, specifically, tiny fingerlike protrusions, called villi, that absorb food into the bloodstream.
c. Considered an autoimmune disorder; however, it is also classified as a disease of malabsorption.
d. Also known as celiac sprue, nontropical sprue, and gluten-sensitive enteropathy
e. An acute episode of watery diarrhea and vomiting leading to severe dehydration is called a celiac crisis and is life threatening.
f. The most common genetic disease in Europe

2. ASSESSMENT
a. Irritability (most common in children)
b. Depression
c. Recurring abdominal bloating and pain
d. Chronic diarrhea
e. Weight loss
f. Pale, foul-smelling, fatty stools called steatorrhea
g. Unexplained anemia
h. Flatus
i. Bone and joint pain
j. Behavior changes
k. Muscle cramps
l. Fatigue
m. FTT
n. Seizures
o. Tingling numbness in the legs (from nerve damage)
p. Pale sores inside the mouth, called aphthus ulcers
q. Painful skin rash, called dermatitis herpetiformis
r. Tooth discoloration or loss of enamel
s. Missed menstrual periods (related to excessive weight loss)

3. DIAGNOSTIC TESTS
a. Antigliadin, antiendomysium, and antireticulin antibodies are checked to measure levels of antibodies to gluten.
b. Biopsy of the small intestine to check for damage to the villi

4. NURSING INTERVENTIONS
a. Instruct the parents on the disease, including the need for strict adherence to a gluten-free diet (no wheat, barley, oats, or rye) for the rest of the child's life.
b. Administer dietary supplements of iron, foliate, calcium, and fat-soluble vitamins.
c. Provide emotional support for the parents and child.

C. GASTROSCHISIS/OMPHALOCELE
1. DESCRIPTION
a. Gastroschisis is a herniation (displacement) of the intestines through a defect on one side of the umbilical cord.
b. An omphalocele is a herniation of the abdominal contents through the umbilical cord and is covered with a sac.
c. A congenital defect of the abdominal wall
d. Surgical closure of the defect is required.
e. A mesh sack called a "silo" is inserted under the abdominal wall margins and the edges of the defect are pulled up. Gravity draws the herniated intestine back into the abdominal cavity, slowly stretching it to the point where the defect can be closed.
f. The abdominal contents should be pink to dark pink with serous or yellow-serous fluid covering the

majority of the contents. Fluid may also be above the abdominal contents.

2. ASSESSMENT
   a. Intestine is protruding through the abdominal wall near the umbilical cord (navel).
   b. The unprotected intestine is exposed to irritating amniotic fluid, and, as a result, gut motility and absorption may be affected.

3. DIAGNOSTIC TESTS
   a. Physical examination
   b. Perinatal history of polyhydramnios
   c. Prenatal ultrasonography often identifies the defect.

4. NURSING INTERVENTIONS
   a. Maintain temperature regulation due to the large surface area exposed.
   b. Monitor for complications of infection, respiratory distress, and bowel necrosis.

5. SURGICAL MANAGEMENT
   a. Preoperative care
      1) Administer intravenous fluids to maintain fluid and electrolyte balance.
      2) NPO
      3) Insert an NG tube to decompress the stomach.
      4) Administer IV antibiotics for bowel contamination and analgesics for pain.
      5) Provide emotional support for the parents and infant.
      6) Instruct the parents on the condition, surgery, and the anticipated care of the child.
   b. Postoperative care
      1) Monitor vital signs.
      2) Maintain a strict intake and output.
      3) Assess daily weights to evaluate hydration status.
      4) Administer analgesics for pain as needed.
      5) Administer IV antibiotics.
      6) Assess GI status by monitoring NG output, bowel sounds, and abdominal distention.

D. HYPERBILIRUBINEMIA
   1. DESCRIPTION
      a. Hyperbilirubinemia is a high level of bilirubin in the blood.
      b. Normal increase is < 5 mg/dl/day.
      c. Be alert for bilirubin increases of > 5 mg/dl/day.
      d. Jaundice is the yellow color to the skin that is often seen in the first few days after birth. The yellow color is due to bilirubin.
      e. Types (see Table 33-1)
         1) Physiologic jaundice: gradual rise in bilirubin of 8 mg/dl at 3–5 days after birth
         2) Pathologic jaundice: an extreme elevation in bilirubin within the first 24 hours
         3) Breast-fed jaundice: an increase in bilirubin due to substances in maternal milk, such as ß-glucuronidases, and nonesterified fatty acids, which may inhibit normal bilirubin metabolism
      f. Common risk factors are fetal-maternal blood group incompatibility, prematurity, cephalohematoma, bruising, birth trauma, and delayed meconium passage.
      g. Kernicterus, bilirubin toxicity, refers to the neurologic consequences of the deposition of unconjugated bilirubin

Table 33-1 Types of Hyperbilirubinemia

Type of Jaundice	Physiological	Pathological	Breast-Fed Infant
Onset	Appears after 24 hours of age and disappears by the end of day 5–7 of life	Appears before 24 hours of age	Early onset: appears by day 4 of life Late onset: appears between days 6 and 14 of life and may persist 2–3 months
Incidence	50% full-term infant; 80% premature infant	Approximately 0.3% of bottle-fed and 2% of breast-fed infants	Approximately 2% of breast-fed infants develop jaundice.
Bilirubin level	Usually does not exceed 12 mg/100 dl in full-term infant and 15 mg/100 dl in premature infant	Increases by more than 5 mg/dl in 24 hours	Early onset: Bilirubin peaks < 17 mg/dl Late onset: Bilirubin often 12–20 mg/dl
Etiology	Liver immaturity leading to the inability to convert fat-soluble unconjugated bilirubin to water-soluble conjugated bilirubin	The most common causes are Rh and ABO blood incompatibilities, liver disease, or infection.	Exact etiology unknown but suspected to be substances in maternal milk, such as glucuronidases and nonesterified fatty acids, which may inhibit normal bilirubin metabolism

in brain tissue leading to subsequent damage and scarring of the basal ganglia and brainstem nuclei.

2. ASSESSMENT
   a. Jaundiced discoloration primarily of the skin and sclera

3. DIAGNOSTIC TESTS
   a. Physical examination to check for cephalocaudal progression of dermal icterus
   b. Serum fractionated bilirubin to detect the conjugated and unconjugated bilirubin levels in the blood

4. NURSING INTERVENTIONS
   a. Phototherapy (bilirubin lights) is used to help convert unconjugated bilirubin to conjugated and move from the skin to the blood plasma and then excreted.
   b. Place under phototherapy lights. Completely undress the infant except for the diaper area and place under phototherapy with eye patches to protect the eyes from the high-intensity fluorescent lights.
   c. A fiberoptic blanket that is placed around the infant or the panel that is placed under the infant may be used and does not require eye patches.
   d. Remove eye patches during assessment and feedings to allow for eye rest.
   e. Maintain temperature regulation due to the large surface area being exposed to environmental temperatures.
   f. Maintain adequate hydration due to increased excretion of conjugated bilirubin through the bowel and urinary system.
   g. Monitor serial fractionated bilirubin levels to evaluate the infant's condition.
   h. Instruct the parents on the disease and the expected care of the infant.

IX. **PRIORITY CARE IN PEDIATRIC CLIENTS WITH GI DISORDERS (SEE TABLE 33-2.)**

Table 33-2 Priority of Care in Pediatric Clients with Gastrointestinal Disorders

Priority in Care	Nursing Interventions
Oxygenation	Keep oxygen saturation at 90%. Keep airway open. Monitor vital signs. Insert an orogastric or a nasogastric tube to decompress the stomach. Measure abdominal girth. Assess for clinical manifestations of respiratory distress.
Hydration	Monitor vital signs. Assess daily weights. Maintain a strict intake and output. Maintain hydration through intravenous fluids or total parenteral nutrition (TPN). Assess for clinical manifestations of obstruction.
Comfort	Monitor vital signs. Assess pain through a standardized pain scale appropriate for age. Assess for clinical manifestations of pain. Provide comfort measures—turning, positioning, egg-crate type mattress pad, dim lights, minimal stimulation, quiet environment. Administer analgesics.
Elimination	Monitor vital signs. Monitor intake and output. Assess for clinical manifestations of GI obstruction. Document GI output.
Psychosocial needs	Assess child and family interaction. Keep the family informed of the child's status. Include the family in care of the child. Educate the child and family on the disease and expected care. Encourage expression of feelings and concerns. Answer questions.

PRACTICE QUESTIONS

1. A mother brings an 8-month-old infant into the health clinic. An examination reveals that the infant's height and weight are below the fifth percentile, skin is dry and wrinkled, the abdomen protrudes, and muscle wasting is evident. The most appropriate nursing diagnosis for this child at this time would be
   1. risk for injury related to parental abuse.
   2. failure to thrive related to unknown causes.
   3. diarrhea related to deficiency in essential nutrients.
   4. social isolation related to lack of maternal-infant bonding.

2. Which assessment provides the nurse with the most accurate information regarding a 6-month-old child admitted with a tentative diagnosis of nonorganic failure to thrive (NFTT)? Select all that apply:
   [ ] 1. Irritable
   [ ] 2. Periorbital edema
   [ ] 3. Taut skin
   [ ] 4. Muscle wasting
   [ ] 5. Uninterested in the environment
   [ ] 6. Responds to stimulation

3. An infant, who has had a cleft palate repair, is positioned side-lying or on the back. The rationale for this positioning is that it
   1. allows observation of the suture line.
   2. decreases anxiety.
   3. promotes drainage.
   4. facilitates oral intake.

4. The mother of an infant who has had a cleft lip repair tells the nurse that the physician said it was very important not to let the baby cry and wants to know why. Which of the following is the appropriate response by the nurse? "Crying
   1. impairs breathing."
   2. stresses the sutures."
   3. may result in gagging."
   4. leads to crusting."

5. Which of the following interventions is a priority for the nurse to implement in the postoperative care of a child with a cleft lip repair?
   1. Assess for edema of the tongue, lips, and mucous membranes
   2. Place the child prone to facilitate drainage
   3. Encourage the parents to limit their visits to allow the child to rest
   4. Restrain the child's arms with blankets to prevent the rubbing the suture line

6. Which of the following is the first intervention to include in the initial postoperative care of an infant following a bilateral cleft lip and palate repair?
   1. Clean the suture line to prevent formation of crusts
   2. Maintain nothing by mouth until the incision is sealed
   3. Restrain all extremities to prevent rubbing of the face and lip
   4. Administer sedation to prevent picking at the incision site

7. Ongoing nursing measures for the infant with a tracheoesophageal fistula (TEF) include
   1. observing respiratory status.
   2. isolating for respiratory precautions.
   3. keeping the room lights dimmed.
   4. giving slow oral feedings.

8. When planning the care of an infant suspected of having a tracheoesophageal fistula (TEF), it is critical for the nurse to
   1. hold the infant in an upright position after feeding.
   2. feed the infant by enteral feedings.
   3. feed the infant slowly.
   4. hold all feedings.

9. When evaluating the assessment data of a preterm infant who has bloody stools, apnea, and bradycardia, the nurse should suspect
   1. intraventricular hemorrhage (IVH).
   2. necrotizing enterocolitis (NEC).
   3. meconium aspiration syndrome.
   4. esophageal atresia.

10. An infant with short bowel syndrome will be discharged home on total parenteral nutrition (TPN) and gastrostomy feedings. The nurse should include which of the following in the discharge instructions?
    1. Maintain a strict NPO status
    2. Provide a pacifier for nonnutritive sucking
    3. Calculate the caloric needs of the infant
    4. Secure TPN and gastrostomy tubing under diaper

11. A mother who brings a 6-week-old infant into the clinic reports that the baby has been spitting up for about 3 weeks. The vomitus has become more frequent and projectile since yesterday. In reviewing the child's record, the nurse notes that the child has gained only 1 pound since birth and suspects that the child may have pyloric stenosis. Which of the following

assessment findings would confirm a diagnosis of pyloric stenosis?
1. Immediate postfeeding vomiting
2. Bile-stained vomitus
3. An axillary temperature of 38°C, or 101°F
4. A refusal to eat

12. Which of the following is the nurse's priority in the plan of care for a child admitted with pyloric stenosis?
1. Assess the respiratory status
2. Maintain thermoregulation
3. Evaluate fluid status
4. Assess perfusion

13. A priority nursing diagnosis in the care of a child with pyloromyotomy is
1. trauma related to break in skin integrity.
2. fluid deficit related to loss of gastric secretions.
3. imbalanced nutrition: less than body requirements related to NPO status.
4. ineffective breathing related to tissue trauma from vomiting.

14. In which of the following positions should the nurse place an infant following a pyloromyotomy?
1. On the right side in a low-Fowler's position at all times
2. In a prone position while sleeping
3. On the right side with the head elevated after feeding
4. On the left side in a semi-Fowler's position after feeding

15. The parents of a child with Hirschsprung's disease ask the nurse what the expected treatment is. Which of the following is the most appropriate response by the nurse?
1. "You will be taught how to do daily neomycin enemas at home."
2. "The nutritionist will discuss a gluten-free diet with you."
3. "Surgery will be scheduled for a permanent colostomy."
4. "The affected bowel segment will be surgically removed."

16. When planning the postoperative care of a child with Hirschsprung's disease, which of the following interventions should the nurse include?
Select all that apply:
[ ] 1. Monitor vital signs
[ ] 2. Assess gastric pH
[ ] 3. NPO
[ ] 4. Strict intake and output
[ ] 5. Administer daily enemas
[ ] 6. Colostomy care

17. The nurse caring for a child with Hirschsprung's disease documents the stools to have what characteristic appearance?
1. Tarry and tenacious
2. Currant jellylike
3. Frothy and foul smelling
4. Ribbonlike

18. When preparing a child with probable intussusception for a hydrostatic reduction procedure, the nurse should explain which of the following aspects of the procedure? The procedure will
1. blow air into a cavity of the bowel.
2. empty the bowel of all stool.
3. relax the bowel.
4. facilitate mixing the currant jellylike stool with normal stool.

19. The nurse assists a child with celiac disease to make which of the following menu selections?
Select all that apply:
[ ] 1. Whole-wheat toast
[ ] 2. Cornbread
[ ] 3. Oatmeal
[ ] 4. Green beans
[ ] 5. Reuben sandwich with rye bread
[ ] 6. Canned tomato soup

20. Which of the following should the nurse perform to minimize reflux in a 4-month-old infant who has gastroesophageal reflux without other complications?
1. Place the infant in a Trendelenburg position after eating
2. Thicken formula with rice cereal
3. Administer continuous nasogastric tube feedings
4. Offer three meals

21. While assisting another nurse with the postoperative care of neonate with an omphalocele repair, the nurse explains that it is a priority to monitor which of the following?
1. Blood pressure
2. Pulse
3. Respiration
4. Skin

22. The triage nurse in the emergency department is evaluating the following four clients. Which client is the priority and a surgical emergency?
1. A child with gastroschisis
2. A child with hypertrophic pyloric stenosis
3. A child with celiac disease
4. A child with malrotation/volvulus

23. Which of the following serum bilirubin levels supports a diagnosis of pathologic jaundice?
1. Concentrations greater than 2 mg/dl in cord blood
2. An increase of more than 1 mg/dl in 24 hours

3. Levels greater than 10 mg/dl in a full-term newborn

4. An increase of 5 mg/dl or greater in 24 hours

24. Which of the following nursing actions takes priority in the plan of care for an infant receiving phototherapy?
   1. Provide opportunities for parent–infant interaction
   2. Avoid bathing the infant who is receiving treatment
   3. Remove eye patches to allow assessment
   4. Interrupt treatment for 60 minutes per shift for tactile stimulation

25. Which of the following in a newborn's assessment should be reported as a critical sign of an imperforate anus?
   1. The first rectal temperature of 36.8°C, or 98.3°F
   2. The infant has not passed a meconium stool in the first 48 hours
   3. The infant has not voided six times in 24 hours
   4. There is a family history of congenital defects

26. The registered nurse is making the day's clinical assignments for a pediatric unit. Which of the following clinical assignments would be most appropriate to delegate to a licensed practical nurse?
   1. An infant with volvulus
   2. A child with short bowel syndrome
   3. An infant with esophageal atresia and tracheoesophageal fistula
   4. A child with celiac disease

27. The nurse is caring for a preterm neonate who has necrotizing enterocolitis. Which of the following is a clinical manifestation that this infant's condition is deteriorating?
   1. Cyanosis
   2. Bloody stools
   3. Decreased bowel sounds
   4. Hypotension

28. Which of the following clinical manifestations should the nurse assess in a child suspected of having extrahepatic biliary atresia? Select all that apply:
   [ ] 1. Jaundice
   [ ] 2. Regurgitation
   [ ] 3. Light tan stools
   [ ] 4. Nocturnal asthma
   [ ] 5. Dark urine
   [ ] 6. Failure to thrive

29. The nurse is reviewing the diagnostic criteria in a child with necrotizing enterocolitis. Which of the following findings is indicative of severe disease and perforation of the bowel?
   1. Dilated bowel loops
   2. Pneumatosis intestinalis
   3. Pneumoperitoneum
   4. Deep crypts on the intestinal mucosa

30. The nurse is caring for a child with inflammatory bowel disease. Which of the following should the nurse include in the plan of care?
   1. Place the child on a gluten-free diet
   2. Administer omeprazole (Prilosec)
   3. Provide the child with increased calories
   4. Monitor the child for melena

ANSWERS AND RATIONALES

1. 2. A diagnosis of failure to thrive is an appropriate nursing diagnosis for an 8-month-old infant who falls below the fifth percentile, and has dry and wrinkled skin, a protruding abdomen, and muscle wasting. Although a child with diarrhea may have the clinical manifestations of failure to thrive, diarrhea is not a presenting manifestation. Diarrhea is a diagnosis in itself, but may be a defining characteristic of imbalanced nutrition.

2. 4. 5. In cases of nonorganic failure to thrive, the cause may be a variety of psychosocial factors such as lack of interest in the environment. Muscle wasting results from the disinterest in food. These children may be below normal in intellectual development, language skills, and social interactions, and their weight falls below the third to fifth percentiles. Irritability is found in a variety of gastrointestinal disorders such as colic. Periorbital edema and taunt skin are typical manifestations of dehydration.

3. 3. After surgery for a cleft lip and palate repair, increased salivation is expected and aspiration is a potential complication. Positioning the child in a side-lying position maintains an open airway and facilitates drainage. The suture line is usually not observed unless bleeding is suspected. The rationale for the side-lying is to maintain a patent airway and promote drainage, which in turn will relieve

anxiety. Prone position is not suggested as a means to facilitate feeding unless the medical condition prevents any other positioning.

4. 2. Crying stretches the facial muscles, especially those around the lips, which stresses the suture line and leads to potential separation of the incision site following a cleft lip and repair. Impairment of breathing and gagging are more of an issue with cleft palate. Scarring occurs as a result of suture line crusting and tissue trauma from rubbing.

5. 1. Trauma to the mucous membranes of the mouth that occurs with a cleft lip repair causes edema, leading to the respiratory distress and potential closing of the airway. Trauma to the suture line would occur in the prone position. Family-centered care is very important; because the parents can help calm the child, their visits are not limited. Elbow restraints, not blankets, are used to keep the child's hands away from the suture line.

6. 1. Crusting of the suture line following a bilateral cleft lip and palate repair can lead to scarring and uneven closure of the incision. The child is not kept NPO and can take oral feedings when fully awake from anesthesia. Only the elbows are restrained to protect the suture line and only analgesics are used to control the pain.

7. 1. Because the fistula links the trachea and esophagus, acidic substances from the gastrointestinal tract can irritate the pulmonary system. Aspiration can occur from any secretions in the oropharyngeal cavity. There is no evidence of infection. Close observation of respiratory status is critical. The child is NPO until after surgical repair, because of the risk for aspiration.

8. 4. In a tracheoesophageal fistula, the fistula forms an open connection between the trachea and esophagus. Because the client can aspirate anything entering the oral cavity, the goal of treatment is to prevent aspiration.

9. 2. In necrotizing enterocolitis (NEC), the bowel is perforated as a result of necrosis, causing blood loss. Apnea and bradycardia are secondary to the hemorrhaging. The clinical manifestations are not always specific. Apnea and a low hematocrit are consistent with bleeding in the ventricles of the brain. Central apnea without hemorrhaging is expected with meconium aspiration. Evidence is not present for esophageal atresia.

10. 2. To ensure adequate growth and development in the infant, it is important to maintain developmentally appropriate behaviors even though the infant is not allowed anything by mouth. Since the child will be given enteral feeds through a gastrostomy tube, the child is not considered NPO. Calculating the caloric

needs of the infant and securing the TPN and gastrostomy tube under the diaper do not promote developmentally appropriate behaviors.

11. 1. In pyloric stenosis, the circular muscle of the pylorus thickens, causing constriction and obstruction of the gastric outlet. Projectile vomiting immediately after feeding is a cardinal indicator of pyloric stenosis. Bile-stained vomitus is not expected since bile is passed through the pyloric valve. Fever is an indication of an infection and is not usually seen with pyloric stenosis. With pyloric stenosis, a child will usually eat immediately after vomiting if a feeding is offered.

12. 3. Fluid and electrolyte imbalance is a problem because of the loss of gastric secretions and poor nutrition secondary to projectile vomiting in pyloric stenosis. Respiratory status and perfusion may be affected by severe imbalance, making it a priority to evaluate fluid status. Thermoregulation is not an issue with pyloric stenosis. Altered perfusion is a result of altered fluid balance.

13. 2. The priority nursing diagnosis following a pyloromyotomy is fluid status, because the loss of gastric secretions can lead to more serious dysfunction of the respiratory and cardiac systems. Tissue trauma is important but is not a priority at this time. The child is not placed NPO without maintaining nutritional status by parenteral fluids until the child is able to take nutrition by mouth. Mucous membrane irritation secondary to vomiting usually does not lead to ineffective breathing.

14. 3. Placing an infant on the right side with the head elevated after feeding facilitates gastric emptying and decreases the possibility of "dumping syndrome" following a pyloromyotomy. Prior to surgery, placing the infant on the left side with the head elevated reduces the risk of severe pyloric spasm. To reduce the risk of sudden infant death syndrome (SIDS), the infant is placed supine for sleep.

15. 4. Hirschsprung's disease, a congenital aganglionic megacolon, is a motility disorder of the bowel caused by the absence of parasympathetic ganglion cells in the large intestine. Feces accumulate proximal to the defect. The aganglionic segment must be removed to enable peristalsis to return, producing normal evacuation of fecal material. Antibiotic enemas are only given prior to surgery to reduce the intestinal flora. The colostomy is temporary, to allow the colon to rest before resection.

16. 1. 3. 4. 6. After the aganglionic segment has been removed in a child with Hirschsprung's disease, the child must be NPO until peristalsis returns. Monitoring vital signs and maintaining a strict intake and output are important to evaluate the fluid and nutritional status of the child. The child will have a temporary colostomy for several months to allow the colon to rest secondary to the tissue trauma. Gastric pH checks are performed with enteral tube placement, and the child would not have an ileostomy. Enemas are done prior to surgery and not after surgery.

17. 4. Ribbonlike stool is characteristically seen with Hirschsprung's disease. Tarry and tenacious stools would be related to high gastrointestinal bleeding. Currant jellylike stools are related to the presence of blood and mucus seen with intussusception. Frothy and foul-smelling stool would indicate cystic fibrosis.

18. 1. Intussusception occurs when one segment of the bowel telescopes into the lumen of an adjacent segment of intestine. The purpose of the hydrostatic reduction procedure is to pull the invaginated bowel out from another section of bowel, allowing normal fecal material to pass. The procedure uses barium or air insufflation; air insufflation is considered to be safer than barium insufflation. The procedure will not empty the bowel completely nor relax it. The currant jelly stools will stop when the bowel is no longer irritated.

19. 2. 4. Celiac disease is called a gluten-sensitive enteropathy and is caused by an intolerance to gluten, the protein component of wheat, rye, barley, and oats. Beans and corn do not contain the protein gluten. It is important to read labels of all prepared foods because many of these products contain flour made from wheat, barley, rye, or oats, all of which contain gluten.

20. 2. Gastroesophageal reflux is the reflux of the gastric contents into the lower portion of the esophagus through the lower esophageal sphincter. Thickened formula decreases acid reflux and increases the emptying time of the stomach. Reflux precautions include positioning the child supine or on the right side with head elevated. Continuous NG feedings are not necessary because the child can tolerate bolus feedings. To reduce the reflux process, small, frequent feedings are more appropriate than three large meals.

21. 3. An omphalocele is a congenital malformation that results from a failure of the intestines to reenter the abdominal cavity at approximately 7 weeks of gestation. The defect, which permits the abdominal contents to herniate through the abdominal cavity, is located centrally and includes the umbilical cord. Surgical intervention is the treatment of choice. Once the abdominal contents have been replaced into the peritoneal cavity, the organs place pressure on the diaphragm, which can lead to respiratory compromise. Decreased cardiac output, altered hemodynamics, and congestive heart failure occur secondary to a respiratory compromise.

22. 4. Malrotation is an incomplete rotation of the midgut during the period of fetal development when the gut returns from the umbilical pouch to the abdominal cavity. With this condition, the bowel fails to rotate normally as it returns to the abdominal cavity and obstructs blood flow to the mesentery organs. This leads to bowel death and necrosis, which is not compatible with life. Malrotation is considered a surgical emergency. Gastroschisis is a congenital malformation where a defect in the abdominal wall allows a segment of the abdominal contents to herniate outside the abdominal cavity. Although surgery is the recommended treatment, it is not a priority. Hypertrophic pyloric stenosis involves a hypertrophic pyloric sphincter generally with a width four times normal that results in a narrow opening and gastric outlet obstruction. A pyloromyotomy is the surgical repair but not an emergency. Celiac disease is a gluten-sensitive enteropathy in which there is a permanent intolerance to gluten. Treatment involves providing a gluten-free diet.

23. 4. Pathologic jaundice is present when serum bilirubin exceeds 15 mg/dl at any time. Jaundice appears within the first 24 hours and is diagnosed when the serum bilirubin concentration in cord blood is greater than 4 mg/dl and there is an increase of 5 mg/dl or greater in 24 hours.

24. 1. Phototherapy is the use of high-intensity fluorescent lights as a way of reducing serum bilirubin levels to prevent kernicterus. Although the infant needs to stay under phototherapy, the infant can be removed for brief periods that should not last longer than 30 minutes. Because phototherapy interrupts parent–infant attachment during the first few days of life, it is considered very stressful for the child and family. Encouraging all opportunities for parent–infant interaction is the priority.

25. 2. An imperforate anus is an anorectal condition in which there is no obvious anal opening. A meconium stool is expected to pass within 48 hours after the neonate's birth. A rectal temperature would be indicative of a patent anus. Urine output is not indicative of an imperforate anus. A family history of congenital defects is not usually associated with an imperforate anus.

26. 4. A volvulus is a complication of malrotation. It occurs when an incompletely rotated bowel twists on itself. This leads to arterial obstruction, ischemia, and necrosis and is a surgical emergency. Short bowel syndrome is a condition that results from surgical resection of the intestine in cases of volvulus, Crohn's disease, or necrotizing enterocolitis. There is an inadequate surface area of the small intestine. Treatment focuses on maintaining optimal nutrition. This usually involves administration of total parenteral nutrition by a central line and enteral feeding by a nasogastric or gastrostomy tube, which require the skills of a registered nurse. Esophageal atresia and tracheoesophageal fistula generally occur together when the esophagus is incomplete and terminates before it reaches the stomach. After preventing aspiration pneumonia, treatment generally requires surgery and neonatal intensive care, which require the skills of a registered nurse. Celiac disease is a gluten-sensitive enteropathy caused by a permanent intolerance to gluten. Control involves medical management and control through a gluten-free diet. The licensed practical nurse can assist a child and parents of a child with celiac disease to select foods free of gluten.

27. 4. Necrotizing enterocolitis is a necrosis of the mucosa of the small and large intestine generally in preterm neonates. Classical features include abdominal tenderness and distention, bloody stools, decreased bowel sounds, increased gastric residuals, erythema of the abdominal wall, and bilious vomiting after feeding. Clinical manifestations of deterioration include bradycardia, apnea, lethargy, temperature instability, decreased urine output, and evidence of shock. A late deteriorating sign is hypotension.

28. 1. 3. 5. 6. Extrahepatic biliary atresia is a progressive inflammatory process causing intrahepatic and extrahepatic bile duct fibrosis. Regurgitation and nocturnal asthma are clinical manifestations of gastroesophageal reflux. Jaundice, light tan stools, dark urine, and failure to thrive are clinical manifestations of extrahepatic biliary atresia.

29. 3. Necrotizing enterocolitis is a necrosis of the mucosa of the small and large intestine. Radiographic findings found in necrotizing enterocolitis include dilated bowel loops and pneumatosis intestinalis. Pneumoperitoneum or free air in the peritoneal cavity or portal circulation indicates severe disease and perforation of the bowel. Deep crypts on the intestinal mucosa are found in celiac disease.

30. 3. Inflammatory bowel disease (IBD) consists of ulcerative colitis and Crohn's disease because of an inflammation or ulceration of the small and large intestine. A gluten-free diet is the diet of choice with celiac disease. Although some children with inflammatory bowel disease poorly tolerate lactose, there is no special diet for IBD. Omeprazole (Prilosec) is a proton pump inhibitor used in the treatment of peptic ulcers. The goal of nutritional therapy is to replace nutrients and increase calories in the diet to maintain normal metabolic functions. Melena or black tarry stools occur in peptic ulcer disease.

REFERENCES

Potts, N., & Mandleco, B. (2012). *Pediatric nursing: Caring for children and their families* (3rd ed). Clifton Park, NY: Delmar Cengage Learning.

Spratto, G. R., & Woods, A. L. (2012). *PDR nurse's drug handbook 2012.* Clifton Park, NY: Delmar Cengage Learning.

CHAPTER 34

METABOLIC AND ENDOCRINE DISORDERS

I. **ANATOMY AND PHYSIOLOGY (SEE CHAPTER 6, ENDOCRINE DISORDERS, SECTION I.)**
   A. DIFFERENCES IN THE ENDOCRINE SYSTEM BETWEEN THE CHILD AND ADULT
      1. GROWTH HORMONE IS NOT AFFECTED BY PRENATAL GROWTH.
      2. IMMEDIATELY AFTER BIRTH, THE NEWBORN'S LEVEL OF THYROID-STIMULATING HORMONE (TSH) RAPIDLY RISES TO AS MUCH AS 10 TIMES HIGHER THAN SEEN IN OLDER CHILDREN, FOLLOWED BY A PERIOD OF DECLINE OVER THE NEXT SEVERAL DAYS TO A NORMAL LEVEL.
      3. THE LEVELS OF TRIIODOTHYRONINE (T_3) AND THYROXINE (T_4) SIMILARLY RISE IN THE FIRST 24 HOURS OF LIFE.
      4. TSH SECRETION DECREASES THROUGHOUT CHILDHOOD THEN INCREASES AT PUBERTY.
      5. A SMALL AMOUNT OF ADRENOCORTICOTROPIC HORMONE (ACTH) IS PRODUCED THROUGHOUT CHILDHOOD.
      6. ACTH BECOMES ACTIVE IN ADOLESCENCE.

II. **ASSESSMENT**
   A. HEALTH HISTORY
      1. PAST HEALTH HISTORY
      2. MEDICATIONS (PAST, PRESENT, OVER THE COUNTER [OTC], HERBALS)
      3. FAMILY HISTORY
   B. PHYSICAL EXAMINATION
      1. INSPECTION
         a. General appearance
            1) Appears stated age; within growth (height and weight) parameters for age; accurate measurement is important.
            2) Appropriate sexual development for age and gender
            3) Alert, oriented, attentive, appropriately responsive

      2. AUSCULTATION
         a. Cardiac: tachycardia or bradycardia
      3. PALPATION
         a. Neck: for enlarged thyroid gland

III. **DIAGNOSTIC STUDIES**
   A. PROVOCATIVE GROWTH HORMONE TESTING (GROWTH HORMONE STIMULATION TEST)
      1. DESCRIPTION: GROWTH HORMONE (GH) IS A HORMONE SECRETED BY THE ANTERIOR PITUITARY GLAND. IT IS USEFUL IN CLINICAL EVALUATION OF SHORT STATURE IN CHILDHOOD AND HELPS TO DIFFERENTIATE BETWEEN ABNORMAL GH PRODUCTION AND OTHER CAUSES OF GROWTH FAILURE. GH IS RELEASED IN AN INTERMITTENT MANNER; THEREFORE, RANDOM TESTING IS NOT USUALLY HELPFUL AND PROVOCATIVE TESTING IS USUALLY RECOMMENDED. MEASUREMENT OF GH IS DONE AFTER STIMULATION BY GROWTH STIMULANT, USUALLY CLONIDINE, INSULIN, GLUCAGON, ARGININE, OR L-DOPA. USUALLY TWO OR MORE TESTS ARE NEEDED WITH PEAK GH LEVELS BELOW 7–10 NG/L.
      2. PREPROCEDURE
         a. Instruct the child and parents on NPO the night before the test.
         b. Inform the parents of the need for multiple blood samples at specific intervals after stimulating substance is given—heparin lock or other line is left in place to minimize need for painful needle sticks.
         c. The test may take several hours.
         d. Inform the parents and child of potential temporary adverse reactions of the test, such as sleepiness, nausea, and weakness.
      3. POSTPROCEDURE
         a. Resume normal diet and activity.

B. X-RAY FOR BONE AGE
1. DESCRIPTION: X-RAY OF THE HAND AND WRIST COMPARING BONE MINERALIZATION WITH NORMS FOR AGE; CHILDREN WITH GH DEFICIENCY MAY HAVE A BONE AGE MUCH LESS THAN THEIR CHRONOLOGICAL AGE.
2. PREPROCEDURE
   a. Instruct the child and parents that the x-ray is painless.
   b. Instruct the child to hold still during the procedure.
3. POSTPROCEDURE
   a. Resume normal activity.
C. LUTEINIZING HORMONE (LH)/FOLLICLE-STIMULATING HORMONE (FSH)
1. DESCRIPTION: LH IS A HORMONE PRODUCED BY THE ANTERIOR PITUITARY GLAND. IT STIMULATES OVULATION AND PRODUCTION OF ESTROGEN AND PROGESTERONE IN FEMALES AND TESTOSTERONE IN MALES. FSH IS ALSO PRODUCED BY THE ANTERIOR PITUITARY GLAND. IT STIMULATES FOLLICULAR GROWTH IN FEMALES. IN MALES, FSH STIMULATES TESTICULAR GROWTH. THESE TESTS MAY BE ELEVATED IN PRECOCIOUS PUBERTY.
D. ESTRADIOL
1. DESCRIPTION: BLOOD TEST TO MEASURE THE LEVEL OF ESTRADIOL, WHICH IS THE MAJOR BIOACTIVE ESTROGEN PRODUCED BY THE OVARY; LEVELS CAN BE USED TO MONITOR FOLLICULAR DEVELOPMENT.
E. TESTOSTERONE
1. DESCRIPTION: BLOOD TEST TO MEASURE LEVELS OF TESTOSTERONE, WHICH IS SECRETED BY THE TESTES OF MALES AND INDIRECTLY BY BOTH ADRENALS AND OVARIES IN FEMALES
F. URINE SODIUM AND OSMOLALITY
1. DESCRIPTION: MEASUREMENT OF SODIUM LEVEL AND CONCENTRATION OF OSMOTICALLY ACTIVE PARTICLES IN THE URINE; DECREASED IN DIABETES INSIPIDUS
G. URINE SPECIFIC GRAVITY
1. DESCRIPTION: URINE SAMPLE TO DETERMINE URINE CONCENTRATION; DECREASED IN DIABETES INSIPIDUS
H. SERUM SODIUM AND OSMOLALITY
1. DESCRIPTION: MEASUREMENT OF SODIUM LEVEL AND CONCENTRATION OF OSMOTICALLY ACTIVE PARTICLES IN THE SERUM; ELEVATED IN DIABETES INSIPIDUS
I. THYROID FUNCTION TESTS
1. TYPES
   a. Triiodothyronine (T_3): used to diagnose and monitor treatment of hyperthyroidism
   b. Thyroxine (T_4): also known as thyroid hormone; released by the thyroid gland; used to diagnose and monitor treatment of hypothyroidism
   c. Thyroid-stimulating hormone (TSH): made in the pituitary gland and sends message to the thyroid gland to make T_4; used to diagnose and monitor treatment of hypothyroidism (see Chapter 6, Endocrine Disorders, Section IV.)
J. THYROID SCAN (SEE CHAPTER 6, ENDOCRINE DISORDERS, SECTION III.)
K. THYROID ANTIBODIES
1. DESCRIPTION: BLOOD TEST TO MEASURE ANTIBODIES AGAINST THE THYROID GLAND
L. SERUM 17-HYDROXYPROGESTERONE
1. DESCRIPTION: 17-HYDROXYPROGESTERONE IS AN ADRENAL STEROID INTERMEDIATE IN THE SYNTHESIS OF CORTISOL. IT IS USED TO CONFIRM THE DIAGNOSIS OF ADRENAL INSUFFICIENCY IN INFANTS WITH SIGNS OF AMBIGUOUS GENITALIA, HYPOTENSION, VOMITING, FEVER, HYPOGLYCEMIA, AND HYPERKALEMIA.
M. PLASMA PHENYLALANINE
1. DESCRIPTION: PHENYLALANINE IS AN ESSENTIAL AMINO ACID; LEVELS ARE ELEVATED IN THE DISORDER PHENYLKETONURIA (PKU).
N. FASTING BLOOD SUGAR
1. DESCRIPTION: BLOOD TEST TO MEASURE FASTING GLUCOSE LEVEL
O. ISLET CELL ANTIBODY
1. DESCRIPTION: BLOOD TEST TO MEASURE ANTIBODIES AGAINST ISLET CELLS
P. URINE KETONES
1. DESCRIPTION: URINE KETONES REFLECT THE BREAKDOWN OF FAT BY THE BODY.
Q. GLUCOSE TOLERANCE TEST (SEE CHAPTER 6 ENDOCRINE DISORDERS, SECTION III.)
R. PARATHYROID HORMONE (PTH)
1. DESCRIPTION: PTH IS A HORMONE RELEASED BY THE PARATHYROID GLAND; IT IS INSTRUMENTAL IN CALCIUM METABOLISM. A FASTING SPECIMEN MAY BE REQUESTED.
S. CALCIUM METABOLISM TESTS
1. DESCRIPTION: TESTS TO MEASURE THE LEVELS OF CALCIUM; OVERNIGHT FASTING MAY BE REQUESTED.
T. SERUM CORTISOL
1. DESCRIPTION: CORTISOL IS THE MAJOR GLUCOCORTICOID SECRETED BY THE ADRENAL GLAND. IT IS REGULATED BY ACTH IN A DIURNAL

FASHION, PEAKING IN EARLY MORNING HOURS. AN EARLY MORNING SPECIMEN IS BEST MEASURED BEFORE 8:00 A.M. TO EVALUATE FOR ADRENAL INSUFFICIENCY, AND AFTERNOON OR EVENING (4:00–11:00 P.M.) FOR CUSHING'S SYNDROME.

U. 17-HYDROXYPROGESTERONE
  1. DESCRIPTION: 17-HYDROXYPROGESTERONE IS A MARKER FOR ADRENAL DEFICIENCY.

V. ADRENOCORTICOTROPIC HORMONE (ACTH) STIMULATION TEST
  1. DESCRIPTION: THIS TEST USES ACTH TO STIMULATE THE ADRENAL GLAND TO MAKE CORTISOL. ADRENAL INSUFFICIENCY IS DIAGNOSED IF THE CORTISOL LEVEL DOES NOT RISE AFTER ACTH IS GIVEN BY IM INJECTION OR BY IV. A NORMAL RESPONSE RULES OUT ADRENAL INSUFFICIENCY.
  2. PREPROCEDURE
    a. Instruct the child and parents that a baseline blood sample will be drawn, then an injection or IV dose will be given.
    b. Blood will be drawn 60 minutes later.
  3. POSTPROCEDURE
    a. Instruct the child and parents on the importance of observing the blood draw site for bleeding and infection.

W. DEXAMETHASONE SUPPRESSION TEST
  1. DESCRIPTION: THIS TEST IS USED TO DIAGNOSE CUSHING'S SYNDROME, AND IS USEFUL IN DISTINGUISHING CUSHING'S DISEASE FROM OTHER CAUSES OF CUSHING'S SYNDROME, SUCH AS EXOGENOUS STEROIDS. BASELINE BLOOD IS DRAWN, AND DEXAMETHASONE IS ADMINISTERED AS A SINGLE DOSE OR FOR MULTIPLE DAYS AND BLOOD IS MEASURED AT DESIGNATED TIME PERIODS. THOSE WITH CUSHING'S SYNDROME DO NOT HAVE SUPPRESSED LEVELS OF CORTISOL.

IV. **NURSING DIAGNOSES**
  A. INEFFECTIVE HEALTH MAINTENANCE
  B. DISTURBED BODY IMAGE
  C. CHRONIC LOW SELF-ESTEEM
  D. NONCOMPLIANCE

Nursing Diagnoses: Definitions and Classification 2012–2014. Copyright © 2012, 1994–2012 by NANDA International. Used by arrangement with John Wiley & Sons Limited.

V. **ENDOCRINE DISORDERS**
  A. DISORDERS OF THE ANTERIOR PITUITARY
    1. GROWTH HORMONE DEFICIENCY/ SHORT STATURE
      a. Description
        1) Short stature caused by decreased production of GH by the pituitary gland
        2) Occurs equally in boys and girls, but more psychologically devastating for boys
        3) Causes include injury and destruction of the anterior pituitary gland by a tumor, an infection, or radiation, but most commonly idiopathic.
      b. Assessment
        1) Decreased velocity of height and weight on growth charts (height and weight usually proportional, or weight somewhat above height); height is 2–3 standard deviations below mean for age.
      c. Diagnostic tests
        1) Blood tests: measurement of GH—random testing is not useful because growth hormone is released in intermittent spurts.
        2) Provocative GH testing: given medication (arginine, clonidine, glucagons, insulin, or L-dopa) to stimulate release of GH, which is then measured.
        3) Bone age x-ray: determines bone age and potential for growth; once the epiphyses are closed, growth potential is minimal; bone growth is often delayed when compared to age-related norms.
        4) Need to rule out familial short stature (short parents), constitutional growth delay (nutritional), or skeletal dysplasia.
      d. Nursing interventions
        1) Instruct the parents on subcutaneous injections of GH—given 6–7 days weekly or as intramuscular depot shot (slowly absorbed) every 2–4 weeks.
        2) Accurately monitor growth over time and plot on growth curves at least every 6 months.
        3) Instruct the family about the disorder and treatment and instruct the parents to give shots if appropriate.
        4) Evaluate the need for help with financial coverage for treatment— not covered by many insurance plans.
        5) Offer support to the child because short stature may be emotionally difficult, especially for boys, who are expected to be tall.
    2. PRECOCIOUS PUBERTY
      a. Description
        1) Secretion of hypothalamic releasing factors, stimulating release of gonadotropic hormones, which

trigger development of secondary sexual characteristics, increased growth, and reproductive capacity

    2) Central (true) precocious puberty: premature activation of hypothalamic-pituitary-gonadal axis; its causes are idiopathic (most common), brain tumors, and postinflammatory.

      a) Girls: Caucasian—breast development before age 7; African American—breast development before age 6

      b) Boys: secondary sex characteristics before age 9

  b. Assessment

    1) Evaluate sexual development.

    2) Evaluate linear growth.

  c. Diagnostic tests

    1) Lab tests: LH, FSH, estradiol, testosterone

    2) Bone age x-ray: look for premature skeletal maturation. Children with precocious puberty may have advanced bone age relative to their chronological age.

  d. Nursing interventions

    1) Instruct the family on the administration of leuprolide (Lupron), as appropriate, to slow puberty by shutting down the puberty hormones in the brain until the child reaches the appropriate age for puberty. It is important that the child receives injections as scheduled. Missing doses or giving a dose late may cause puberty to advance.

    2) Provide emotional support.

    3) Evaluate the need for financial help—often not covered by insurance.

B. DISORDERS OF THE POSTERIOR PITUITARY

  1. DIABETES INSIPIDUS (DI)

    a. Description

      1) Disorder of water regulation

      2) The usual function of antidiuretic hormone (ADH) is to concentrate urine.

      3) In DI, a deficiency in ADH causes excretion of large amounts of dilute urine.

      4) Causes include head trauma, complication after cranial surgery (especially in the hypothalamus/ pituitary area), vascular anomalies, infection, and genetic defect in ADH synthesis.

    b. Assessment

      1) Polyuria (including nocturnal enuresis)

      2) Polydipsia

  c. Diagnostic tests

    1) Urine (first morning specimen): for osmolality, specific gravity, and sodium

    2) Serum sodium, osmolality

  d. Nursing interventions

    1) Instruct the family on the administration of desmopressin acetate (DDAVP)—a long-acting form of ADH—intranasally or orally.

      a) Take regularly as directed.

      b) Rhinorrhea may affect absorption.

    2) Instruct the family to monitor fluid intake and hydration status of the child.

      a) Increased or decreased urine output

      b) Thirst

      c) Headache

      d) Rapid weight gain

      e) Confusion or lethargy

      f) Dehydration

      g) Sunken fontanel on infants

    3) Monitor the child if NPO because dehydration can easily occur.

C. DISORDERS OF THE THYROID

  1. CONGENITAL HYPOTHYROIDISM

    a. Description

      1) Decrease or lack of production of thyroid hormones (T_3 and T_4) at birth

      2) Results from congenital lack of thyroid gland, or thyroid gland is present but unable to produce the hormones

    b. Assessment

      1) Screening thyroid function is test done on all newborns by law (T_4—if abnormal TSH is done).

      2) Clinical manifestations are often absent or minimal and may include a large fontanel, low temperature, breathing or feeding difficulty, constipation, jaundice, or low activity.

      3) If untreated, brain damage or mental retardation will occur.

    c. Diagnostic tests

      1) T_4

      2) T_3

      3) Thyroid scan

    d. Nursing Interventions

      1) Instruct the parents about safe administration of thyroid replacement—take at the same time daily.

      2) Instruct the client on the clinical manifestations of decreased thyroid hormone function.

      3) Evaluate growth and perform thyroid function tests

periodically—medication must be increased to maintain therapeutic range as the child grows.

4) Instruct the family on the importance of planning ahead so they do not run out of medication.

5) Instruct the family that although a lifelong condition, prognosis is excellent with replacement therapy.

2. ACQUIRED HYPOTHYROIDISM

a. Description

1) Decreased ability of the body to produce thyroid hormone (T_4 or T_3) or TSH

2) Caused by an abnormality of the immune system resulting in damage/destruction of the thyroid gland (T_4 and T_3) or cyst, disease, tumor, radiation, or trauma to the pituitary gland (decreased TSH production) or thyroid gland

b. Assessment

1) Decreased linear growth rate

2) Weight gain

3) Cool, coarse, dry skin

4) Cold intolerance

5) Fatigue, decreased activity

6) Constipation

7) Coarse or thinning hair

8) Facial edema

9) Mild anemia

10) Slow speech

11) Delayed sexual maturation, delayed dentition

c. Diagnostic tests

1) T_4

2) Free T_4

3) TSH

4) Thyroid antibodies

d. Nursing interventions

1) Same as for acquired hypothyroidism

3. HYPERTHYROIDISM (GRAVES' DISEASE)

a. Description

1) Excessive production of thyroid hormones (T_4, T_3), which increase the metabolic rate

2) The most common cause is autoimmune—thyroid antibodies cause an increase in hormone production.

3) Other causes: toxic nodules, goiter, or thyroiditis

4) Too much thyroid replacement

b. Assessment

1) Tachycardia, palpitations

2) Elevated blood pressure

3) Weight loss despite excellent appetite

4) Difficulty sleeping

5) Tremors

6) Heat intolerance

7) Exophthalmos

c. Diagnosis

1) Thyroid function tests

2) Thyroid antibody

d. Nursing interventions

1) Administer antithyroid medication as ordered—propylthiouracil (PTU) or methimazole (MTZ, Tapazole)—to block the ability of the thyroid gland to use iodine and make thyroid hormone.

2) Support the family if radioactive iodine is used—absorbed by the thyroid gland, damages the thyroid cells and decreases the ability to make thyroid hormone, and eliminated in urine. Takes 3–6 months, and may require a second or third dose. If too much is given, the child can become hypothyroid and require replacement therapy.

3) Inform the parents that if most of thyroid gland is removed it will require replacement therapy for life.

D. DISORDERS OF THE ADRENAL GLAND

1. CONGENITAL ADRENAL HYPERPLASIA

a. Description

1) Autosomal recessive disorder

2) Deficiency of the enzyme needed for synthesis of cortisol, leading to increased ACTH and excessive production of androgens

3) Two forms: salt losing (aldosterone also affected), and nonsalt losing (simple virilization)

b. Assessment

1) Pseudohermaphrodism (ambiguous genitalia due to virilizing effect of excessive androgens on female genitalia); there are no physical changes to male genitalia.

2) Dehydration, electrolyte imbalance (salt wasting)

3) Shock

c. Diagnostic tests

1) Serum 17-hydroxyprogesterone (required newborn screening in some states)

2) Chromosome studies (karyotype)

d. Nursing interventions

1) Administer replacement hormones, as ordered, to suppress adrenal secretion of androgens.

2) Administer replacement glucocorticoids, which then suppress secretion of ACTH, resulting in decrease in androgen production.

3) In salt-wasting type, salt may need to be added to food and

fludrocortisone (Florinef, a mineralocorticoid medication) taken to replace aldosterone.

    4) Monitor for signs of fluid and electrolyte imbalance/shock.

    5) Increase hormone dosage during the stress of illness, injury, or surgery.

    6) Offer emotional support—it can be very difficult at initial diagnosis and as the child is raised due to sexual ambiguity.

E. DISORDERS OF THE PANCREAS

    1. DIABETES MELLITUS—TYPE 1 (PREVIOUSLY KNOWN AS JUVENILE OR INSULIN-DEPENDENT DIABETES)

      a. Description

        1) Autoimmune—antibodies attack and destroy insulin-producing islet cells

        2) Genetic predisposition, environmental trigger, such as virus or bacteria

        3) Impaired carbohydrate and lipid metabolism

      b. Assessment

        1) Polyuria—enuresis in previously toilet-trained child

        2) Polydipsia

        3) Polyphagia

        4) Weight loss

        5) Fatigue

        6) Stomachaches

        7) Frequent infections, such as vaginal infections in adolescent girls

        8) Clinical manifestations develop gradually, may present in ketoacidosis

      c. Diagnostic tests

        1) Blood glucose: results may be over 200

        2) Islet cell antibodies: positive

        3) Blood and urine ketones: often positive

        4) Glucose tolerance test: not required with classic symptoms

      d. Nursing interventions

        1) Instruct the child and parents on the technical and self-management skills at their learning level, including:

          a) Home testing—blood glucose and urine ketones

          b) Subcutaneous injections—rotate arms, legs, stomach, buttocks to prevent lipodystrophy. Insulin injections timed and frequent enough to cover needs over a full 24-hour period; intense management is necessary.

          c) Insulin types and actions (see Table 34-1)

          d) Safe treatment of blood sugar extremes (fast-acting glucose for hypoglycemia; extra insulin may be necessary for hyperglycemia or during illness to prevent ketoacidosis)

          e) Ongoing changes in management plan, stressing the importance of dietary choices—current recommendation is for carbohydrate counting

          f) Impact of physical activity—helps body to use insulin, can cause hypoglycemia

        2) Communication with the school personnel for daily support

        3) Support the family because they are adjusting to a chronic, lifelong condition—often express disbelief at diagnosis.

    2. TYPE 2 DIABETES

      a. Description

        1) Decreased insulin production or insulin resistance

        2) Becoming more common in youth—possibly due to diets of high-carbohydrate/high-calorie junk food and decreasing physical activity in children

Table 34-1 Insulin Types and Actions

Name	Type	Onset	Peak	Duration
Lispro (Humalog)	Rapid-acting	5–12 min	30–90 min	5 hrs
Regular	Short-acting	20–60 min	2–3 hrs	6–8 hrs
NPH	Intermediate-acting	2-4 hrs	4-10 hrs	10–16 hrs
Detemir (Levernir)	Long-acting	1–2 hrs	Minimal	22–24 hrs
Glargine (Lantus)	Long-acting	1–2 hrs	None	20–24 hrs
Premixed 70/30	70% NPH with 30% regular or Novolog	20 min–4 hrs	4–10 hrs	10–16 hrs
Premixed 75/25	75% NPH with 25% Humalog	5 in–4hrs	4–10 hrs	10–16 hrs

b. Assessment
1) Most often overweight
2) Acanthosis—darkened "dirty" appearance of skin, especially of the neck, axilla, antecubital areas

c. Diagnostic tests
1) Glucose tolerance test

d. Nursing interventions
1) Instruct the parents about medications, including oral hypoglycemics such as metformin (Glucophage), which is the only currently approved oral hypoglycemic for children.
2) Instruct the parents about the importance of exercise.
3) Instruct the parents and child on the importance of diet.

F. OTHER ENDOCRINE DISORDERS (GENERALLY RARE IN CHILDREN)

1. HYPOPARATHYROIDISM

a. Description
1) Deficiency in secretion of parathyroid hormone (PTH)
2) Involved in calcium metabolism
3) Congenital or acquired
4) Most common cause: removal or manipulation during thyroid or neck surgery, but can be idiopathic

b. Assessment
1) Signs of hypocalcemia
   a) Neonate: jitteriness, convulsions, apnea, poor feeding
   b) Older child: tetany, stridor, Chvostek's sign (muscle spasm tapped), Trousseau's sign (carpopedal spasm), paresthesia, irritability, seizure

c. Diagnostic tests
1) PTH levels: decreased or absent
2) Calcium: decreased
3) Phosphorus: elevated
4) Alkaline phosphatase: normal or decreased

d. Nursing interventions
1) Administer oral replacement of calcium (calcium gluconate) as ordered.
2) Administer vitamin D metabolite (calcitriol) as ordered.
3) Administer IV calcium gluconate, as ordered, for seizures or tetany.
4) Monitor serum and urinary calcium levels.
5) Closely monitor the IV insertion site; calcium gluconate is caustic and causes severe tissue burns with extravasation.
6) Monitor the child for kidney stones that may occur as a result of treatment.

7) Instruct the parents about medication and signs of hypocalcemia and hypercalcemia.
   a) Hypocalcemia: in neonate, jittery movements, seizures, apnea, lethargy, poor feeding, vomiting; in older children, tetany, stridor, Chvostek's sign facial muscle spasm elicited by tapping the facial nerve, tingling of the hands or around mouth, diarrhea, seizures, papilledema, changes in dental enamel
   b) Hypercalcemia: vomiting, bradycardia (acute)—frequently iatrogenic from medication

2. ADDISON'S DISEASE

a. Description
1) Chronic adrenal insufficiency of glucocorticoids (cortisol) and mineralocorticoids (aldosterone)
2) Causes: trauma, infection, or autoimmune process that damages the adrenal glands

b. Assessment
1) Clinical manifestations may be acute or chronic.
   a) Acute: hypotension, shock, acute electrolyte imbalance, dehydration, weakness, cardiovascular changes, fever, mental changes, hypoglycemia
   b) Chronic: fatigue, anorexia, salt-craving, hyperpigmentation of the skin, abdominal pain, nausea, vomiting, diarrhea
2) Stress (surgery, injury, illness) can cause adrenal crisis and will require stress doses of medication.

c. Diagnostic tests
1) Serum cortisol (early morning): decreased
2) Urinary 17-hydroxycorticoid levels (early morning): decreased
3) ACTH levels: increased with ACTH stimulation testing

d. Nursing interventions
1) Inform the parents on the recognition and prevention of acute episodes (signs of hypotension, shock, electrolyte imbalance, dehydration, weakness, cardiovascular changes, fever, changes in mental status, and hypoglycemia).
2) Instruct the parents on the administration of oral hydrocortisone to replace cortisol.
   a) Give regularly; do not stop administration abruptly.

b) Child should wear identification stating corticosteroid use.

c) Dose may need to be increased during stressful times such as illness.

d) Alert all care providers to steroid use; care when receiving live immunizations.

e) Watch for adverse reactions— weight gain, growth failure, mood swings, acne, abnormal hair growth.

3) Instruct the parents on the administration of fludrocortisone (Florinef) to replace aldosterone.

3. CUSHING'S SYNDROME
   a. Description
      1) Increased free cortisol levels
      2) Cause: most common in childhood from excessive or prolonged corticosteroid therapy for other disorders
      3) Other causes: rare in childhood— adrenal tumor or pituitary tumor
   b. Assessment
      1) Rapid weight gain, especially the abdomen and face (moon face)
      2) "Buffalo hump" (fat pad over the shoulders and upper back)
      3) Slowed linear growth, delayed bone age
      4) Hypertension
      5) Striae
      6) Hirsutism (abnormal hair growth)
      7) Osteoporosis
      8) Acne
      9) Delayed puberty
      10) Infections and poor wound healing
   c. Diagnostic tests
      1) Cortisol and 17-hydroxycorticosteroid levels: increased
      2) Fasting blood sugar (FBS): elevated blood glucose
      3) Dexamethasone (cortisone) suppression test: cortisol levels remain elevated in those with Cushing's syndrome.
   d. Nursing interventions
      1) Inform the parents on the disorder.
      2) Give steroid on every-other-day or early-morning schedule to minimize adverse reactions, but avoid sudden discontinuation of the drug.
      3) Support the child and parents on body image changes, especially weight gain, short stature, striae, and acne.
      4) Instruct the parents on how to protect the child from infection because increased cortisol is immune suppressive.

4. SYNDROME OF INAPPROPRIATE ANTIDIURETIC HORMONE (SIADH)
   a. Description
      1) Hypersecretion of antidiuretic hormone (ADH) vasopressin by the posterior pituitary
      2) Causes: infections, tumors, trauma, intracranial surgery, some medications (analgesics, barbiturates, chemotherapy)
   b. Assessment
      1) Fluid retention
      2) Decreased urine output
      3) Weight gain (fluid)
      4) Hypotonicity
      5) Anorexia, nausea, vomiting
      6) Lethargy, decreased level of consciousness, seizures
   c. Diagnostic tests
      1) Serum osmolality: low; urine osmolality: high
      2) Serum sodium: decreased
   d. Nursing interventions
      1) Monitor fluid and electrolyte balance and weight.
      2) Instruct the child about necessary fluid restrictions.
      3) Monitor for possible SIADH in susceptible children (postcranial surgery, etc.).
      4) Administer antibiotics as ordered.

VI. **METABOLIC DISORDER**
   A. PHENYLKETONURIA (PKU)
      1. DESCRIPTION
         a. Genetic, autosomal-recessive disorder of amino acid metabolism
         b. Absence of enzyme phenylalanine hydroxylase, necessary to convert phenylalanine to tyrosine
         c. Results in increase in phenyl acids
         d. Tyrosine is needed to form the pigment melanin and hormones epinephrine and thyroxine; without it, characteristic coloration is blond or light hair color, blue eyes, fair skin.
         e. Increased levels of phenylalanine affect normal brain and central nervous system development, causing mental retardation.
      2. ASSESSMENT
         a. Failure to thrive, vomiting
         b. Vomiting
         c. Irritability, hyperactivity, seizures
         d. Musty body odor, musty urine odor
         e. Eczemalike rash
      3. DIAGNOSTIC TESTS
         a. Screening mandatory in all 50 states
         b. No later than 7 days of age; should have ingested protein in formula or breast milk before being tested
         c. If elevated plasma levels of phenylalanine, repeat test

4. NURSING INTERVENTIONS
  a. Instruct the parents on the importance of sticking to prescribed low-protein formula (Lofenolac, Pro-Phree, Phenex-1) or breast milk for the infant.
  b. Instruct the parents that as the child grows, high-protein foods should be avoided; specially calculated diet to

keep serum phenylalanine levels no higher than 2–6 mg/dl.
  c. Instruct the parents on the importance of maintaining a low-phenylalanine diet until late school age or adolescence to prevent decrease in IQ.
  d. Instruct affected women to resume low-phenylalanine diet before conception to prevent congenital defects in the infant.

PRACTICE QUESTIONS

1. Which of the following should the nurse include in the nursing assessment of the endocrine system in a child?
   1. The number and type of pets in the home
   2. Family health history
   3. Dietary intake of calcium
   4. History of streptococcus infection

2. A nurse is caring for a client with short stature from a growth hormone (GH) deficiency. Which of the following measures would be essential to include in the child's plan of care?
   1. Monitor linear growth
   2. Encourage at least two glasses of milk per day
   3. Assess the skin for bruising
   4. Instruct the child on weight-control issues

3. Which of the following children being cared for by the nurse is in need of treatment for precocious puberty?
   1. A 10-year-old Caucasian girl with beginning breast development
   2. An 8-year-old African-American girl with breast development
   3. An 8-year-old boy with secondary sex characteristics
   4. A 10-year-old boy with beginning pubic hair

4. Which of the following instructions is most appropriate for the nurse to give the parents of a child with diabetes insipidus?
   1. Technique for administering desmopressin acetate (DDAVP)
   2. Directions for performing a urine dipstick
   3. Procedure for giving an insulin injection
   4. Provisions necessary for providing a safe home environment

5. The nurse is caring for a 10-year-old child who has been diagnosed with acquired hypothyroidism. The parents ask the nurse for information on the disorder. Which of the following should the nurse include in the information given to the parents?
   1. Infection is the most likely cause

   2. Weight loss is a common clinical manifestation
   3. A thyroid replacement drug will be given
   4. Fevers and diarrhea are common

6. The nurse should include which of the following in the preprocedure instructions given to the parents of a child scheduled for a thyroid function test?
   1. NPO after midnight
   2. A high-carbohydrate meal should be eaten the day before the test
   3. A concentrated glucose will be given just prior to the test
   4. It is important that the child remain still during the procedure

7. The nurse is assessing a child's thyroid status. Which of the following assessment findings should the nurse document as a subjective finding?
   1. Fatigue
   2. Weight loss
   3. Hypertension
   4. Tachycardia

8. The nurse is caring for a child with Cushing's syndrome. Which of the following should the nurse include in the plan of care?
   1. Encourage a diet high in carbohydrates
   2. Administer medication to slow growth
   3. Offer emotional support for premature puberty
   4. Encourage a diet low in sodium

9. The nurse is working with the parents of a newborn with ambiguous genitalia due to congenital adrenal hyperplasia (CAH). Which of the following instructions should the nurse provide the parents?
   1. Glucose monitoring should be performed
   2. Salt should be restricted in the daily formula
   3. Extra blankets will be used because of heat intolerance
   4. An assignment of sex may be delayed

10. When planning the education for the parents of a child with type 1 diabetes mellitus, which of the following should the nurse include?
    1. Restrict the activity of the child
    2. Rotate insulin injection sites
    3. Avoid letting the child perform the home testing of blood sugar
    4. Encourage a high-carbohydrate diet

11. The nurse is admitting a child with suspected type 1 diabetes mellitus. Which of the following questions should the nurse ask the parents?
    1. "Has the child's number and type of bowel movements changed?"
    2. "Has the child experienced nocturia or bedwetting?"
    3. "How much exercise does the child get?"
    4. "Does the child complain of headaches?"

12. Which of the following is a priority for the nurse to include in the discharge instructions for the family of a child with type 2 diabetes?
    1. How to recognize complex blood sugar patterns
    2. Changes the family will need to make
    3. Daily blood sugar and ketone testing
    4. Accurate carbohydrate counting

13. Which of the following statements by a child with type 2 diabetes mellitus indicates a lack of understanding about the disease and a need for further instructions?
    1. "I will exercise regularly."
    2. "I will count the carbohydrates I eat."
    3. "I will avoid junk food high in calories."
    4. "I will take my injections of insulin on time."

14. The parents of a child with newly diagnosed type 2 diabetes mellitus want to know more about the condition. The nurse should include which of the following?
    1. Activity is not important with type 2 diabetes
    2. Daily insulin injections are required
    3. Type 2 diabetes does not require intervention
    4. Type 2 diabetes is increasing in frequency in children

15. The nurse should implement which intervention when caring for a child with hypoparathyroidism?
    1. Instruct the parents about the signs of hypocalcemia
    2. Administer a daily thyroid hormone replacement drug
    3. Instruct the parents that the child should wear a medical alert bracelet
    4. Weigh the child daily

16. Leuprolide acetate (Lupron) is prescribed for a child with precocious puberty. Based on an understanding of this drug, the nurse caring for this child should
    1. inform the parents that shakiness and a general malaise are common adverse reactions.
    2. administer the drug intramuscularly once every 4 weeks.
    3. encourage the child to increase fluids.
    4. assess blood pressure and respiration prior to giving the drug.

17. Which of the following tasks may the registered nurse delegate to unlicensed assistive personnel?
    1. Documentation of the urinary output after toileting of a child with diabetes mellitus
    2. Informing a child with growth hormone deficiency that a growth hormone injection will be given
    3. Monitoring a neonate suspected of having hypoparathyroidism for jittery movements during the bath
    4. Assessing the presence of arthralgia, fatigue, and tachycardia when ambulating a child with hyperthyroidism

18. The nurse receives a report on a newborn who is lethargic and exhibiting jittery movements during morning care. Which of the following is the priority nursing intervention?
    1. Administer oral calcium gluconate
    2. Evaluate the response to feeding
    3. Administer intravenous calcium
    4. Assess for the presence of bone deformities

19. The nurse should monitor a child receiving propylthiouracil (PTU) for which of the following adverse reactions indicating toxicity?
    Select all that apply:
    [ ] 1. Tachycardia
    [ ] 2. Headaches
    [ ] 3. Sore throat
    [ ] 4. Loss of taste
    [ ] 5. Nausea
    [ ] 6. Fever

20. The nurse is admitting a child suspected of having hyperglycemia. Which of the following assessment findings would support a diagnosis of hyperglycemia?
    Select all that apply:
    [ ] 1. Hunger
    [ ] 2. Pallor
    [ ] 3. Tachycardia
    [ ] 4. Blurred vision
    [ ] 5. Polydipsia
    [ ] 6. Headaches

21. The nurse is preparing discharge for a child with type 1 diabetes. Which of the following should the nurse include in the discharge instructions?
    1. A physical examination should be performed every other year
    2. Sugar-free products are not always carbohydrate-free
    3. Conserve energy by restricting activity
    4. Test the blood glucose once daily

22. A school nurse should include which of the following in the assessment of a child who has type 1 diabetes mellitus for adherence to the treatment plan?
    Select all that apply:
    [ ] 1. Assess the finger pads for small marks
    [ ] 2. Ask the child if high-sugar foods are avoided
    [ ] 3. Evaluate the injection sites for bruising
    [ ] 4. Ask the child to describe the symptoms of hypoglycemia
    [ ] 5. Ask the child how long it takes to use a bottle of insulin
    [ ] 6. Obtain a blood glucose level

23. The nurse identifies which of the following adolescents with type 1 diabetes mellitus as being at greatest risk for complications? An adolescent
    1. with frequent *Candida albicans* urinary infections.
    2. who has an eating disorder.
    3. who has a fever and a sore throat.
    4. who is sexually active and taking birth control.

24. Which of the following is a priority for the nurse to include in the assessment of a child admitted with dehydration who is to begin on intravenous potassium?
    1. Obtain a weight
    2. Assess the child for edema
    3. Evaluate the output
    4. Monitor blood pressure

25. The nurse is admitting a child suspected of having acquired hypothyroidism. Which of the following assessments should the nurse evaluate as confirming the diagnosis?
    1. Goiter
    2. Exophthalmos
    3. Proptosis
    4. Hirsutism

ANSWERS AND RATIONALES

1. 2. The family health history is important, as many endocrine disorders run in families. The number of pets, calcium intake, and history of streptococcus infection are not specifically relevant to the endocrine system.

2. 1. Growth hormone deficiency is an endocrine disorder in which there is a poor growth in stature as a result of a failure of the pituitary to produce sufficient growth hormone. Linear growth is monitored to evaluate the need for medication prior to treatment and the effectiveness of medication during treatment. Bruising and weight control are not part of growth hormone deficiency. Monitoring milk intake is part of a normal healthy diet in children and not just in growth hormone deficiency.

3. 3. The development of secondary sex characteristics in boys before age 9 years is abnormal and in need of treatment for precocious puberty. A 10-year-old Caucasian girl with beginning breast development, an 8-year-old African-American girl with breast development, and a 10-year-old boy with beginning pubic hair are considered within the normal range. Precocious puberty is defined as breast development occurring in Caucasian girls before 7 years of age and before 6 years of age in African-American girls. Children with precocious puberty have accelerated growth rates, develop secondary sex characteristics earlier than normal, and exhibit advanced bone age, acne, body odor, and some behavioral changes. Psychosocial development is generally age appropriate.

4. 1. Desmopressin acetate (DDAVP) is the drug of choice for the child with diabetes insipidus. It is a synthetic antidiuretic hormone that acts to increase the absorption of water in the kidney. It is important that the parents learn how to administer the drug intranasally or orally. Diabetes insipidus is a disorder of water regulation in which there is a deficiency of the antidiuretic hormone. Urine dipstick and insulin administration would be used by parents of a child with diabetes mellitus. Home safety is important for all children.

5. 3. Acquired hypothyroidism is an endocrine disorder that generally has an autoimmune cause. It is associated with weight gain, hypothyroidism, and constipation. Thyroid replacement medication must be taken daily.

6. 4. There is no special preparation for thyroid function tests except for the child to hold still during the procedure. There is no need for a child to be NPO or eat a high-carbohydrate diet or concentrated glucose before the test.

7. 1. A subjective finding is something the client tells the nurse. An objective finding is one the nurse detects through evaluative procedures. Fatigue, something felt and described by the child, is a subjective finding. Weight loss, hypertension, and tachycardia are all objective findings.

8. 4. Hypertension is common in a child with Cushing's syndrome due to sodium retention, so limiting the salt intake will help control blood pressure. Weight gain is common, and a high-carbohydrate intake would contribute to weight gain. Premature puberty is not part of Cushing's syndrome because growth is slowed.

9. 4. Congenital adrenal hyperplasia is a group of inherited disorders characterized by a deficiency of an enzyme essential for the synthesis of cortisol and occasionally aldosterone. Ambiguous genitalia are difficult for parents to adjust to and accept. The process of gender selection is controversial, which is stressful for the family, and an assignment of sex may be delayed. There is no heat intolerance with congenital adrenal hyperplasia; heat intolerance occurs with hyperthyroidism.

10. 2. Rotation of injection sites is one of the most important things to teach a child with type 1 diabetes mellitus. Rotating the site allows for the best absorption and most accurate dosing of insulin. Blood sugar testing is often one of the earliest skills a child with type 1 diabetes mellitus acquires. A high-carbohydrate diet would contribute to an elevated blood sugar level. Activity is important in the treatment and management of diabetes.

11. 2. Frequent urination (polyuria) is one of the classic clinical manifestations of diabetes mellitus, along with increased appetite (polyphagia) and increased thirst (polydipsia). Weight loss is also common in children.

12. 3. In type 2 diabetes mellitus, the pancreas still produces some insulin. However, the body is unable to use the insulin effectively and is unable to produce enough insulin to lower the glucose. Type 2 diabetes can usually be managed with an oral hypoglycemic agent, exercise, diet, and home glucose monitoring. Testing of blood sugar and ketone levels is the priority and basis for all care for children with diabetes. Recognition of complex blood sugar patterns, carbohydrate counting, and changes the family needs to make are important but not the priority.

13. 4. Because the pancreas still produces some insulin in type 2 diabetes mellitus, it is generally managed with oral hypoglycemic drugs and lifestyle changes such as a healthy diet, regular exercise, carbohydrate counting, and avoidance of high-calorie junk food.

14. 4. Type 2 diabetes is increasing in frequency, even in youth. Type 2 diabetes mellitus generally can be controlled with oral hypoglycemic drugs, diet, exercise, and home glucose monitoring.

15. 1. Hypoparathyroidism is a disorder of the parathyroid hormone. The primary function of the parathyroid hormone is to maintain the serum calcium. Thyroid replacement is used with hypothyroidism. Weight is not directly affected by the parathyroid glands and daily weighing is not necessary. A medical alert bracelet is also unnecessary. A medical alert bracelet should be worn for disorders such as Addison's disease.

16. 2. Leuprolide acetate (Lupron) depot injection is a GnRH analog administered once every 3 to 4 weeks by subcutaneous or intramuscular injection or intranasally two to three times a day for precocious puberty. Shakiness and a general malaise are not common adverse reactions, and assessing blood pressure or respiration prior to administration is not necessary. Fluids need not be increased with Lupron.

17. 1. Although unlicensed assistive personnel may ambulate and bathe a child, assessing and monitoring for the presence of an abnormality are not tasks that can be delegated to them. Unlicensed assistive personnel can never inform or instruct new information. Unlicensed assistive personnel may document the urinary output after toileting a child.

18. 3. Jittery movements in a lethargic newborn indicate the presence of hypoparathyroidism and of tetany. This poses an emergency situation, and intravenous calcium is the treatment of choice and the priority. Poor feeding behavior would be assessed in any newborn but is not the priority. Oral gluconate is reserved for the nonacute treatment of transient hypocalcemia. Assessing for the presence of bone deformities would be done on a growing child and is not a priority in a newborn.

19. 3. 6. Propylthiouracil (PTU) is an antithyroid drug used to treat hyperthyroidism. It relieves the clinical manifestations of tachycardia, restlessness, and tremors associated with hyperthyroidism. Nausea, headaches, and loss of taste are mild adverse reactions. A sore throat and high fever are adverse reactions indicating agranulocytosis, which is serious and potentially fatal.

20. 1. 4. 5. Hunger, polydipsia, and blurred vision are clinical manifestations of hyperglycemia. Tachycardia, pallor, and headaches are clinical manifestations of hypoglycemia.

21. 2. In type 1 diabetes mellitus, glucose accumulates in the blood, and the body cannot make efficient use of the glucose. Daily insulin doses are required. Sugar-free products are not necessarily carbohydrate-free. A physical examination should be performed annually. Activity is not restricted, but insulin should be adjusted according to exercise level. Increased insulin is necessary with increased activity. A blood glucose test should be performed before every insulin dose.

22. 1. 3. 5. To evaluate a child's compliance to the type 1 diabetes mellitus treatment plan, the nurse should assess the finger pads for small stick marks and the injection sites for bruising. Asking the child how long it takes to use a bottle of insulin can serve as a way to determine whether all of the insulin was administered over the prescribed time frame. Obtaining a blood glucose level would not be an accurate evaluation of adherence to the treatment plan; it would only indicate the glucose level at the time of the test and not long-term compliance. Asking a child if high-sugar foods are avoided and what the clinical manifestations of hypoglycemia are merely evaluate the child's knowledge but not necessarily compliance.

23. 2. An eating disorder poses a serious health hazard in the management of diabetes. Not only do bulimic behaviors such as binging and vomiting pose serious complications, but starvation that occurs with anorexia nervosa also raises the potential for serious complications. The omission of insulin can lead to serious complications too. A urinary infection with *Candida albicans* is often an early sign in adolescents that type 2 diabetes may be present. Sore throat and fever do not necessarily pose serious health risks but simply may indicate that an insulin adjustment may be necessary during the illness. Sexual activity and birth control do not directly alter an adolescent's risk for complications.

24. 3. The priority assessment in a child admitted with dehydration who is to begin on intravenous potassium is to evaluate the child's output. The child must have functioning kidneys necessary for excretion. Intravenous potassium should never be given to a child with an impaired renal output. Obtaining a blood pressure and a weight and evaluating for edema may be appropriate interventions, but not the priority.

25. 1. Acquired hypothyroidism generally results from an autoimmune cause. The thyroid gland becomes inflamed, is infiltrated by the antibodies, and is progressively destroyed. Goiter is an indication found in acquired hypothyroidism. Exophthalmos and proptosis are present in hyperthyroidism. Hirsutism is a clinical manifestation in congenital adrenal hyperplasia.

REFERENCES

Potts, N., & Mandleco, B. (2012). *Pediatric nursing: Caring for children and their families* (3rd ed.). Clifton Park, NY: Delmar Cengage Learning.

Spratto, G. R., & Woods, A. L. (2012). *PDR nurse's drug handbook 2012*. Clifton Park, NY: Delmar Cengage Learning.

CHAPTER 35

NEUROLOGICAL DISORDERS

I. **ANATOMY AND PHYSIOLOGY (SEE CHAPTER 7, NEUROLOGICAL DISORDERS, SECTION I.)**

A. DIFFERENCES IN THE NEUROLOGICAL SYSTEM BETWEEN THE CHILD AND THE ADULT

1. THE INFANT PRIMARILY FUNCTIONS AT THE SUBCORTICAL LEVEL BECAUSE THE CORTICAL FUNCTIONS RESPONSIBLE FOR FINE MOTOR COORDINATION ARE NOT FULLY DEVELOPED.

2. MEMORY AND MOTOR COORDINATION ARE APPROXIMATELY THREE-FOURTHS DEVELOPED BY 2 YEARS OF AGE.

3. AS A RESULT OF THE INFANT BEING UNABLE TO VERBALLY EXPRESS HIS LEVEL OF CONSCIOUSNESS, ASSESS HIS LEVEL OF ACTIVITY, POSITIONING, ABILITY TO CRY, AND OVERALL APPEARANCE.

4. CRANIAL NERVE ASSESSMENT IS DIFFICULT TO PERFORM ON AN INFANT LESS THAN 1 YEAR OF AGE AND IN TODDLERS BECAUSE THEY CANNOT FOLLOW DIRECTIONS OR COOPERATE.

5. RAPID HEAD GROWTH OCCURS DURING CHILDHOOD, WITH THE BRAIN BEING 25% OF ADULT WEIGHT AT BIRTH, 75% AT 2½ YEARS, AND REACHING 90% BY AGE 6 YEARS.

6. THE BONES OF THE INFANT'S SKULL DO NOT FUSE UNTIL 18 MONTHS OF AGE.

7. THE ANTERIOR AND POSTERIOR FONTANELS ARE NOT COVERED BY THE SKULL AND SHOULD FEEL FLAT AND FIRM BUT MAY BECOME SUNKEN WITH DEHYDRATION OR BULGE WITH INCREASED INTRACRANIAL PRESSURE.

   a. The anterior fontanel closes between 9 and 18 months.
   b. The posterior fontanel closes by 2 months of age.

8. THE AUTONOMIC NERVOUS SYSTEM, ALTHOUGH INTACT AT BIRTH, IS IMMATURE.

9. THE INFANT'S NEUROLOGICAL EXAM IS PRIMARILY REFLEXIVE, SUCH AS THE BABINSKI'S REFLEX BEING NORMAL AT BIRTH BUT DISAPPEARING WHEN THE CHILD BEGINS TO WALK.

10. BECAUSE MYELINATION DOES NOT OCCUR UNTIL LATE INFANCY AND THE PERIPHERAL NEURONS ARE NOT MYELINATED, MOTOR DEVELOPMENT IS CRUDE AND NOT DEVELOPED.

11. THE INFANT'S FLEXOR MUSCLES ARE DOMINANT AND PRESENT A GOOD PORTION OF THE TIME, SUCH AS WHEN HE IS SLEEPING.

12. THE INFANT MAY EXHIBIT MINUTE TREMORS DURING THE FIRST SEVERAL MONTHS OF LIFE.

13. THE CEREBROSPINAL FLUID IS MANUFACTURED AT A RATE OF 100 ML PER DAY AS COMPARED TO 500 ML IN THE ADULT CLIENT.

14. THE CEREBRAL BLOOD FLOW IS LESS THAN 45–50 ML/G OF BRAIN TISSUE PER MINUTE IN THE YOUNG CHILD (45–50 ML IS CONSIDERED NORMAL IN THE OLDER CHILD AND ADULTS).

15. HEAD CIRCUMFERENCE IS 34–35 CM IN THE INFANT AND APPROXIMATELY 47 CM BY 1 YEAR OF AGE.

II.   ASSESSMENT

A. HEALTH HISTORY
  1. FAMILY HISTORY
      a. Seizure disorders
      b. Neurological disorders
      c. Mental retardation
  2. MOTHER'S PREGNANCY HISTORY
      a. Infant Apgar scores
      b. Maternal illness
      c. Intrapartal fetal distress
  3. CHILD'S DEVELOPMENTAL HISTORY

B. PHYSICAL EXAMINATION
  1. INSPECT THE SIZE AND SHAPE OF THE HEAD, MEASURING THE HEAD CIRCUMFERENCE.
  2. INSPECT THE FONTANELS.
  3. EVALUATE THE DEVELOPMENTAL LEVEL.
  4. INSPECT THE POSTURE AND ACTIVITY.
      a. Decorticate: flexor posturing; associated with bilateral cerebral hemisphere injury
      b. Decerebrate: rigid extensor posturing; secondary to midbrain or pons trauma
      c. Flaccid areflexia: absence of response; indicative of severe brainstem injury
  5. PERFORM THE GLASGOW COMA SCALE (GCS).
  6. ASSESS AVPU.
      A = ALERT AND AWAKE
      V = RESPONSIVENESS TO VERBAL STIMULI
      P = RESPONSIVENESS TO PAINFUL STIMULI
      U = UNRESPONSIVENESS
  7. ASSESS THE MOTOR RESPONSE: CHECK STRENGTH, SYMMETRY, SPONTANEITY; PRESENCE OF POSTURING.
  8. ASSESS THE SENSORY RESPONSE: CHECK TEMPERATURE (HOT OR COLD), RESPONSE TO PRESSURE (MILD, MODERATE, SEVERE) AND PAIN (SHARP OR DULL), AND PROPRIOCEPTION.
  9. ASSESS THE REFLEXES: NOTE PRESENCE, ABSENCE, SYMMETRY, AND STRENGTH OF CRANIAL NERVES AND BABINSKI, BICEPS, TRICEPS, PATELLAR, AND ANKLE REFLEXES.
  10. ASSESS THE CHILD'S PHYSICAL ABILITIES.
  11. INSPECT THE CHILD FOR CONTRACTURES AND SKIN BREAKDOWN.

III.   DIAGNOSTIC STUDIES (SEE CHAPTER 7, NEUROLOGICAL DISORDERS, SECTION III.)

IV.   NURSING DIAGNOSES

A. IMPAIRED PHYSICAL MOBILITY
B. INEFFECTIVE HEALTH MAINTENANCE
C. INEFFECTIVE BREATHING PATTERN
D. HIGH RISK FOR INJURY
E. IMBALANCED NUTRITION: LESS THAN BODY REQUIREMENTS
F. RISK FOR IMPAIRED SKIN INTEGRITY
G. PAIN

Nursing Diagnoses: Definitions and Classification 2012–2014. Copyright © 2012, 1994–2012 by NANDA International. Used by arrangement with John Wiley & Sons Limited.

V.   NEUROLOGICAL DISORDERS

A. SEIZURES
  1. DESCRIPTION
      a. Spontaneous electrical discharge of hyperexcited brain cells in an epileptogenic focus
          1) Triggered by environmental or physiologic stimuli
          2) The exact location and number of discharges determine the nature of the seizure.
              a) If small area: focal (localized) seizure
              b) If electrical discharge continues, or the focal area is located in the brainstem, midbrain, or reticular formation: generalized seizure
      b. Causes include birth injury, anoxic episodes, infection, intraventricular hemorrhage, or congenital brain anomaly in infants and trauma, infection, changes in diet or hydration status, fatigue, or not taking prescribed medications in older children
  2. TYPES (SEE TABLE 35-1)
      a. Febrile seizures: these are tonic or clonic seizures that are usually associated with rapid rise in temperature (a minimum of 39°C [102.2°F], usually occurring in children between 6 months and 5 years of age with a positive family history). They frequently accompany infectious processes (e.g., upper respiratory infection [URI], pneumonia, pharyngitis, shigella, urinary tract infection [UTI], otitis media [OM], roseola, meningitis) and are often self-limiting, with a postictal period lasting less than 15 minutes.
      b. Infantile spasms: also known as salaam seizures, these are spasms that begin at 3 months of age with a history of gestational difficulties, developmental delay, or other neurological abnormalities; twice as common in males. During seizure, the infant's head may suddenly drop forward while both arms and legs are flexed, the eyes may roll upward or downward, and the infant may cry out and turn pale, cyanotic, or flushed. There may be a loss of consciousness or awareness.

Table 35-1 Types and Clinical Manifestations of Seizures

Seizure	Manifestations
Partial simple (focal)	Due to abnormal activity in a small area of the brain. Symptoms are associated with the area affected. No aura; consciousness generally is not lost. Motor: may involve one extremity, a part of that extremity, or ipsilateral extremities, with the head and eyes twisting in the opposite direction (the arm toward which the head is turned is abducted and extended with the fingers clenched). Numbness, tingling, or painful sensations beginning in one body area and spreading out to other areas may be seen. Sensory: visual hallucinations, buzzing sounds, unusual odors, odd tastes. Emotional: anxious feelings.
Jacksonian	Motor episodes begin with tonic contractions of the fingers of one hand, the toes of one foot, or one side of the face. Spasms progress into tonic-clonic movements that "march" up the adjacent muscles of the affected extremity or side of the body.
Rolandic	Tonic-clonic movements of the face with increased salivation and arrested speech, commonly occurring during sleep.
Complex	Generally seen in age 3 through adolescence; aura is present (feelings of anxiety, fear, déjà vu; abdominal pain, unusual taste; smelling odd odor; visual or auditory hallucinations). Consciousness is not completely lost; presence of confusion or being dazed. During seizure: activity is stopped and purposeless behaviors (staring into space, assuming usual posture, automatisms [repeated nonpurposeful actions—lip smacking, chewing, sucking,] uttering the same word over and over, wandering aimlessly, removing clothing) are started; rare violent acts or rage. Postictal period: drowsiness, confusion, aphasia, sensory or motor impairments displayed; no memory of the event.
General	Secondary to diffuse electrical activity throughout the cortex and into the brainstem; loss of consciousness with bilateral and symmetrical uncontrolled motor involvement and spasms; arises from both cerebral hemispheres; can occur at any time; lasts from several seconds to hours; no aura; loss of consciousness is always seen; if in children under 4 years of age, frequently associated with developmental delays, learning disabilities, and behavior disorders.
Tonic-clonic (grand mal)	Occurs at any age; abrupt onset; begins with loss of consciousness and fall to the ground. Initial phase is tonic (intense muscle contractions); jaw clenches shut; abdomen and chest become rigid; a cry or grunt is emitted as exhaled air is forced through the taut diaphragm; pallor or cyanosis may occur (oxygenation and ventilation impaired); airway is compromised due to increased salivation not being managed because of muscular contractions and diminished mental status; neck and legs extended; arms flexed or contracted; eyes roll upward or deviate to one side; pupils dilate; bladder or bowel incontinence may occur; persists 10–30 seconds. During the clonic phase: jerking movements are produced due to muscle contraction and relaxation; spasms dissipate as the seizure ends; lasts from 30 seconds to 30 minutes. Postictal or postconvulsive state follows somnolence, or if awake, confusion or combativeness; no memory of the event. Hypertension, diaphoresis, headache, nausea, vomiting, poor coordination, slurred speech, or visual disturbances may occur as well.
Absence (formerly called petit mal)	Seizures generally begin to occur around the fourth birthday, disappearing near adolescence; characterized by transient loss of consciousness (may appear as cessation of current activity); seem to stare into space or eyes roll upward with ptosis or fluttering lids; lip smacking or loss of muscle tone causes head to droop or objects in hands to be dropped; lasts from 5 to 10 seconds; can occur as often as 20 or more times per day. Children with this type of seizure are often accused of daydreaming and being inattentive in school.
Myoclonic	Usually seen during school age or adolescence; sudden repeated muscle contractures of head, extremities, or torso; quickly recover; occurs when the child is drowsy and just falling asleep or just waking up; usually no loss of consciousness and no postictal period.
Atonic or astatic-akinetic	Seen between 2 and 5 years of age; manifested by sudden loss of muscle tone, with the head dropping forward for a few seconds; more significant events occur when consciousness lost with fall to the ground (often face down); amnesia seen; may cause repetitive head injuries if not protected by wearing a football or hockey helmet. Many have underlying brain abnormalities and are mentally challenged.
Akinetic seizures	Manifested by total lack of movement; child appears frozen in a position; mental status is diminished during the event.

© Cengage Learning 2015

c. Status epilepticus: generally refers to generalized prolonged tonic-clonic seizure without regaining consciousness; it is unresponsive to treatment and may result in a decrease in oxygen supply and possible cardiac arrest.

3. ASSESSMENT (SEE TABLE 35-1 CLINICAL MANIFESTATIONS FOR THE SPECIFIC TYPE OF SEIZURE.)
4. DIAGNOSTIC TESTS
   a. Comprehensive history
   b. Computerized tomography (CT) scan
   c. Magnetic resonance imaging (MRI) scan
   d. Electroencephalogram (EEG)
   e. Laboratory tests such as complete blood count (CBC), serum chemistry, and urinalysis (UA)
   f. Lumbar puncture
   g. Cerebral angiography
   h. Positron emission tomography (PET) scan
5. NURSING INTERVENTIONS
   a. Provide patent airway.
   b. Administer prescribed medications and monitor for adverse reactions.
   c. Administer ketogenic diet generally in absence, akinetic, or myoclonic seizures by limiting the intake of protein and carbohydrate, forcing the body to use ketones. The mechanism of action is not very well understood.

(Protein is regulated, so 90% of calories are derived from fat; fat-to-carbohydrate ratio is 4:1.)

    d. Observe and record the seizure.

    e. Pad bed side rails.

    f. Have suction and oxygen equipment available.

    g. Gently help the child to the ground and place him on the side if the event occurs when he is in a chair or standing.

    h. Encourage the child to wear a protective helmet if he suffers from recurrent seizures.

    i. Provide emotional support to the child and family.

    j. Encourage responsibility for self-care.

    k. Instruct the child to avoid contact sports and swimming.

    l. Instruct the child's teachers and associated personnel on what to do during a seizure at school.

    m. Refer the child and family to seizure support groups.

    n. Instruct the child to wear a Medic Alert bracelet.

VI. CRANIAL DEFORMITIES

  A. MICROCEPHALY

    1. DESCRIPTION

      a. Refers to a small brain

        1) Primarily is due to a congenital abnormality, or toxic exposure during the critical phase of development in the first trimester of pregnancy.

        2) Secondarily is due to an insult in the third trimester.

    2. ASSESSMENT

      a. Occipital-frontal circumference (OFC) > .3 standard deviations below the mean

      b. A correlation between microcephaly and some degree of mental retardation exists.

    3. DIAGNOSTIC TESTS

      a. Skull x-rays

      b. CT scan

      c. Laboratory testing

      d. Genetic counseling

    4. NURSING INTERVENTIONS

      a. Monitor OFC, measuring around the fullest part of the head just above the eyebrows.

      b. Provide supportive care.

  B. CRANIOSYNOSTOSIS

    1. DESCRIPTION: EARLY CLOSURE OF THE CRANIAL SUTURES, RESULTING IN EARLY FUSION OF THE SKULL BONES AND DEFORMITY OF THE SKULL

    2. ASSESSMENT

      a. Fontanels close earlier than normal.

      b. Deformity of the skull is dependent on which sutures close early, how quickly they close, and whether or not the other sutures accommodate for the early closure (may be frontal bossing, ridging of suture lines).

      c. Sagittal suture is most commonly involved; ridging is palpable.

      d. Mental retardation is possible.

    3. DIAGNOSTIC TESTS

      a. Skull x-ray

      b. CT scan

    4. NURSING INTERVENTIONS

      a. Measure OFC and look for prolonged molding.

      b. Postoperative management of children who have had surgery before 6 months of age to correct deformity:

        1) Monitor neurological status.

        2) Observe for hemorrhage or infection.

        3) Apply pressure bandages to reduce swelling.

        4) Administer analgesics as prescribed.

        5) Maintain hydration and nutritional status.

        6) Provide support to the parents and family.

  C. PLAGIOCEPHALY

    1. DESCRIPTION

      a. Molding of the skull due to pressure continually applied to it

        1) Positional (back-lying infants): occiput is flattened.

          a) Does not involve stenosis of cranial sutures

    2. ASSESSMENT

      a. Measure OFC.

      b. Observe for flattened surfaces; palpate the fontanels and sutures.

    3. DIAGNOSTIC TESTS

      a. Skull x-ray

      b. CT scan

    4. NURSING INTERVENTIONS

      a. Instruct the parents on infant positioning and recommend varied positioning.

      b. Apply a helmet, as prescribed, between 4 and 10 months.

        1) Monitor postoperatively if surgery was performed (usually between 3 and 6 months).

  D. CAPUT SUCCEDANEUM

    1. DESCRIPTION

      a. Soft tissue of the scalp is swollen and possibly bruised.

      b. Result of trauma to the baby while passing through the birth canal

2. ASSESSMENT
   a. Swelling usually crosses the suture lines.
   b. Usually involves the parietal areas
   c. Often associated with pronounced molding
3. DIAGNOSTIC TESTS
   a. Skull x-ray
   b. CT scan
4. NURSING INTERVENTIONS
   a. Provide reassurance to the parents because the condition usually resolves within 3–4 days.

E. CEPHALHEMATOMA
1. DESCRIPTION
   a. Swelling caused by collection of blood in the scalp between the bone and the periosteum
   b. Results from trauma secondary to a difficult delivery
   c. Rare possibility of concurrent skull fracture, intracranial hemorrhage, or coagulopathy
2. ASSESSMENT
   a. Parietal area involved
   b. Swelling does not cross the suture lines.
   c. Swelling may occur within hours to days after delivery.
3. DIAGNOSTIC TESTS
   a. Skull x-ray
   b. CT scan
4. NURSING INTERVENTIONS
   a. Provide reassurance because hematoma reabsorbs within weeks to months.
   b. Monitor neurological status and vital signs.
   c. Assess for blood loss, hypovolemia, and infection.
   d. Observe for evidence of hyperbilirubinemia (jaundice, lethargy).
   e. Instruct the parents that as calcification of the hematoma occurs, there may be a palpable bony prominence on the scalp.

F. HYDROCEPHALUS
1. DESCRIPTION
   a. Communicating: 1%; obstruction outside the ventricular system; causes decreased absorption of cerebrospinal fluid (CSF) in the subarachnoid space
   b. Noncommunicating (obstructive): 99%; impediment of CSF flow within the ventricular system; often secondary to congenital malformation (aqueductal stenosis, meningomyelocele [MMC], Dandy-Walker syndrome, Arnold-Chiari deformity), intraventricular hemorrhage, infection, tumors, head injury
   c. Causes include increased production, impaired absorption, or block in the flow of CSF, acquired or congenital cause, and excessive amount of CSF within the ventricles.
2. ASSESSMENT
   a. Infant
      1) Increased OFC
      2) Disproportionately large head
      3) Bossing of the forehead
      4) Translucent skin covering the forehead
      5) Prominent scalp veins
      6) Wide palpable sutures
      7) Wide bridge between the eyes
      8) Sunsetting sign
      9) Bulging anterior fontanel
      10) Positive Macewen's sign
      11) Fussy
      12) Restless
      13) Irritable
      14) Apathetic
      15) Altered or diminished level of consciousness
      16) Sluggish pupillary response
      17) Posturing
      18) Atypical reflex reaction
      19) Lower extremity spasticity
      20) Poor feeding
      21) High-pitched cry
      22) Cardiopulmonary depression
   b. Child and adolescent
      1) Headache on awakening
      2) Nausea
      3) Vomiting
      4) Irritability
      5) Lethargy
      6) Apathy
      7) Confusion
      8) Impaired judgment and reasoning skills
      9) Incoherence
      10) Ataxia, spasticity
      11) Papilledema
      12) Strabismus
      13) Decrease in visual acuity
3. DIAGNOSTIC TESTS
   a. CT scans
   b. MRIs
   c. Ultrasound
   d. EEG
   e. Plain skull x-rays
4. NURSING INTERVENTIONS
   a. Prepare the child for shunt insertion.
      1) Ventriculoperitoneal shunt: most common shunt in infants and children from the ventricle to the peritoneum, or ventriculoatrial

Figure 35-1 Ventriculoperitoneal shunt

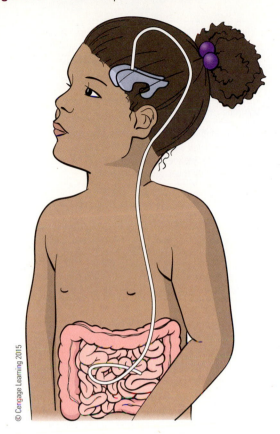

© Cengage Learning 2015

from the ventricle to the left
atrium (see Figure 35-1)
2) Monitor the child for infection.
3) Administer prescribed
antibiotics.
b. Preoperative management
1) Measure the head circumference
daily.
2) Monitor the child for increased
intracranial pressure.
3) Assess respiratory status.
4) Measure intake and output.
5) Offer small, frequent feedings
with intermittent burping.
6) Position the child carefully,
supporting the neck muscles.
7) Place a sheepskin under the
child's head.
c. Postoperative management
1) Assess vital signs.
2) Perform neurological checks
every 2 hours.
3) Monitor intake and output.
4) Assess skin integrity.
5) Monitor for manifestations of
infection such as fever, increased
heart and respiratory rate, poor
feeding, vomiting, altered mental
status, seizures, and focal

manifestations such as redness or
CSF leakage at the surgical site.
6) Place the child in a flat position
on the unoperative side to
prevent rapid CSF drainage and
pressure on the valves.
7) Gradually elevate the head of the
bed to avoid a too-rapid drainage
of the CSF, which places the child
at risk for subdural hematoma.
d. Offer support to the parents of the
child.
e. Inform the parents that
hydrocephalus is a lifelong condition
requiring follow-up.
f. Instruct the parents on the
manifestations of infection and failure.
G. NEURAL TUBE DEFECTS (SPINA BIFIDA)
1. DESCRIPTION
a. Failure of the neural tube to close
completely during the fourth week
of gestation
b. Development of fissure because of
increased CSF pressure
c. Unknown cause, but environmental
factors have been implicated
(exposure to chemicals, medications,
poor maternal nutrition, or decreased
folic acid intake)
d. Prognosis related to type and level of
defect, presence of other congenital
anomalies, or complicating factors
2. TYPES (SEE TABLE 35-2)
3. ASSESSMENT
a. Neurological deficits
1) Lower extremities are partially
or completely paralyzed.
2) Bowel and bladder may or may
not be affected.
3) Hydrocephalus
b. Orthopedic deficits
1) Flexion or extension contractures
2) Talipes valgus
3) Varus contractures
4. DIAGNOSTIC TESTS
a. Prenatally
1) Amniocentesis
2) Ultrasound
b. Natally
1) Transillumination
2) Radiologic studies (CT scans,
MRIs, flat-plate films of the
spinal column)
3) Neuroimaging
4) Neurological examination
5. NURSING INTERVENTIONS
a. Preoperative management
1) Place the child in a prone
position to prevent urine and
feces from coming in contact
with the defect.

Table 35-2 Types of Neural Tube Defects

Types of Spina Bifida	Description
Anencephaly	Absence of the cranial vault, with cerebral hemispheres either completely missing or greatly reduced in size; brainstem may be intact; vital functions maintained for weeks or months; death usually due to respiratory failure
Cranioschisis	Defect in the skull through which neural tissue protrudes
Exencephaly	Brain totally exposed/herniated through a skull defect
Encephalocele	Protrusion of the brain and meninges into fluid-filled sac through a skull defect
Spina bifida occulta	Failure of the posterior vertebral arches to fuse, most often at the fifth lumbar or first sacral vertebrae; no herniation of the spinal cord or meninges; not usually visible externally, although a dimple or small depression may be noted; can be seen on x-ray. During toddlerhood, abnormal gait with foot weakness or deformity may be apparent; may have disturbances in controlling the bladder or bowel, or both, when toilet training attempted.
Rachischisis	Fissure in the vertebral column; meninges and spinal cord exposed
Spina bifida cystica	Defect in closure of the posterior vertebral arch
Meningocele	Saclike herniation through a bony malformation containing the meninges and CSF; sac covering may be thin and translucent or membranous
Meningomyelocele	Saclike herniation through a bony defect containing the meninges, CSF, and portion of the spinal cord or nerve roots; poorly covered; may be CSF leakage at the site; occurs most often at the lumbar or lumbosacral area

© Cengage Learning 2015

2) Place the child in an isolette to maintain temperature.
3) Cover the sac with sterile dressing moistened with normal saline.
4) Place a towel roll between the knees with the hips flexed slightly and the legs abducted.
5) Provide meticulous skin care.
6) Place sheepskin, lamb's wool sheet, or an egg-crate mattress pad under the infant.
7) Monitor the child for manifestations of infection.
8) Measure OFC as ordered.
9) Perform frequent neurological exam.
10) Monitor for presence or absence of extremity movement as well as evidence of flaccidity or spasticity.
11) Monitor for the presence of dribbling urine or continuous stooling.
12) Place the child in a prone position on a pillow for feeding, with the head turned to one side (breastfeeding is generally contraindicated pre-op).
b. Postoperative management
1) Place the child in a prone position until the incision is healed.
2) Administer prescribed antibiotics.
3) Monitor for signs of infection and hydrocephalus.
4) Assess bowel and bladder dysfunction, administering stool softeners and a diet high in fiber.
5) Perform a neurological assessment of the extremities.
6) Monitor vital signs frequently.
7) Assess the child for signs of local or systemic infection, meningitis, hydrocephalus, and increased intracranial pressure (ICP).
8) Instruct the parents on the importance of positioning, casting, splinting, bracing, traction, or surgeries to enhance ambulation and decrease the risk of complications (walkers, crutches, canes, and lightweight braces are used with L2 to L5 lesion, whereas a customized wheelchair may be used at an L2 or above).
9) Assess for urinary retention or infection (perform intermittent catheterization with medications to enhance bladder storage and continence).
10) Hold the child prone, side-lying, or upright while leaning against the caretaker's chest.
11) Maintain skin integrity (protect bony prominences, massage the area, and change linen frequently).
c. General interventions
1) Offer the growing child and parents support.
2) Inform the parents that this is a lifelong condition with physical challenges.
3) Encourage independence in the older child or adolescent.

H. ARTERIOVENOUS MALFORMATION (AVM)
  1. DESCRIPTION
     a. A weblike tangle of vessels between the arteries and veins due to failure of the cerebral capillaries to form during fetal development
     b. Vessels in malformation dilated and thin-walled, causing increased blood volume at high pressure
     c. Most common cause of intracranial hemorrhage in children under 10 years of age
     d. Etiology is unknown.
     e. May result in ischemia to the area near the malformation, congestive heart failure (CHF), cardiomegaly, intracranial hemorrhage, or aneurysm
  2. ASSESSMENT
     a. Neonates
        1) Heart failure (HF)
        2) Cardiomegaly
        3) Cerebral bruit
        4) Hydrocephalus
     b. Children
        1) Seizure
        2) Headache (migrainelike)
        3) Clinical manifestations of increased ICP
  3. DIAGNOSTIC TESTS
     a. Cerebral angiography
     b. CT with contrast
     c. MRI
     d. Skull films
     e. EEG
     f. Lumbar puncture (LP)
     g. Cerebral blood flow studies
     h. Chest x-ray
  4. NURSING INTERVENTIONS
     a. Monitor airway, breathing, and circulation (ABCs) and the vital signs.
     b. Assess for increased ICP.
     c. Check the pupils.
     d. Calculate the GCS score.
     e. Adhere to AVM precautions.
     f. Watch for sequelae of treatment such as surgery or radiology.
     g. Educate the family about the deformity and treatment options.

VII. **INFECTIONS OR POSTINFECTION CONDITIONS**
  A. BACTERIAL MENINGITIS
     1. DESCRIPTION
        a. Inflammation of the meninges due to trauma, neurosurgery, infection, dental caries
        b. Bacteria enter the blood supply into the CSF and spread throughout the subarachnoid space.
        c. Inflammatory response occurs with thick, purulent exudate (*Neisseria meningitides* over the parietal, occipital, and cerebellar regions; *Streptococcus pneumoniae* over the anterior lobes).
        d. Brain becomes hyperemic and edematous, resulting in increased ICP.
        e. Prognosis depends on the age of the child, organism, treatment efficacy, and whether complications occur.
        f. Sequelae (hearing loss, blindness, paresis of facial muscles, intellectual impairments) are common.
        g. Children under 5 years of age account for 90% of cases.
        h. Males are affected more often than females.
        i. Causative organisms:
           1) In neonates include *Escherichia coli*, *Haemophilus influenzae* type B, group B *Streptococcus*, *N. meningitides*, *S. pneumoniae*, herpes
           2) In infants and children include *H. influenzae* type B, *N. meningitides*, *S. pneumoniae*, enterovirus, adenovirus, mumps virus
           3) In adolescents include *N. meningitides*, *S. pneumonia*, herpes, adenovirus, arbovirus
        j. Complications include sepsis, seizures, subdural effusions, brain abscess, hydrocephalus, disseminated intravascular coagulation (DIC), and syndrome of inappropriate antidiuretic hormone (SIADH).
     2. ASSESSMENT
        a. Infant less than 3 months of age
           1) Lethargy
           2) Fussiness
           3) Irritability
           4) Fever may or may not be present.
           5) Hypothermia may be seen.
           6) Alterations in feeding or sleeping patterns
           7) Vomiting or diarrhea with or without weight loss
           8) Bulging anterior fontanel
           9) Seizures
           10) Diminished level of consciousness (LOC)
           11) Depressed respiratory state

    b. Infants over 3 months of age and toddlers
      1) Same as for infant less than 3 months of age
      2) Change in activity level
      3) Fever
    c. Child over 2 years
      1) Gastrointestinal (GI) upset
      2) Coldlike prodromal signs
      3) Chills
      4) Fever
      5) Cortical involvement, manifested by:
        a) Irritability
        b) Agitation
        c) Confusion
        d) Delirium
        e) Lethargy
        f) Somnolence
        g) Nausea
        h) Projectile vomiting
      6) If cranial nerves are involved:
        a) Photophobia
        b) Diplopia
        c) Tinnitus
      7) If cervical nerves are irritated:
        a) Nuchal rigidity with or without opisthotonic position (see Figure 35-2)
        b) Headache
        c) Myalgias
        d) Joint pain
        e) Malaise
      8) If seriously compromised:
        a) Shock
        b) Increased ICP
        c) Hyperreactive reflexes
        d) Positive Kernig and Brudzinski's responses
      9) Petechial, purpuralike, or ecchymotic rash suggests meningococcemia.
  3. DIAGNOSTIC TESTS
    a. Microscopic examination of urine
    b. CSF culture and Gram stain
    c. CBC

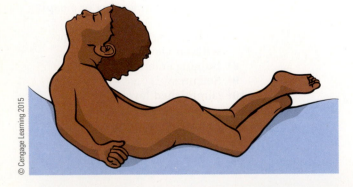

Figure 35-2 Nuchal rigidity with or without opisthotonic position

    d. Serum electrolytes and osmolarity
    e. Clotting studies
    f. LP, except in the presence of increased ICP
    g. Chest x-ray
    h. CT or MRI
  4. NURSING INTERVENTIONS
    a. Wear appropriate protective attire (gown, gloves, mask) before giving care if the cause is bacterial.
    b. Instruct the family on the precautions that must be adhered to.
    c. Assess the need for prophylactic antibiotics.
    d. Assess vital signs frequently, including blood pressure (BP) and capillary refill time.
    e. Assess the skin for petechiae or purpura.
    f. Assess the child for irritability, fussiness, and LOC.
    g. Palpate the anterior fontanel (in infants) for bulging or depression.
    h. Measure OFC daily (infants).
    i. Monitor for seizure activity and notify the physician if seizures occur.
    j. Administer prescribed antibiotics.
    k. Maintain normothermia.
    l. Administer acetaminophen or ibuprofen for fever.
    m. Monitor intake, output, and urine specific gravity.
    n. Provide comfort measures (quiet, dark environment).
    o. Manage pain with acetaminophen or nonsteroidal anti-inflammatory.
    p. Assess developmental and social needs.
    q. Instruct the family about the Hib vaccine.
  B. VIRAL (ASEPTIC) MENINGITIS
    1. DESCRIPTION
      a. Inflammatory response of the leptomeninges
      b. More common in adolescents
      c. More common in summer or fall
      d. May follow inappropriately or partially treated bacterial disease
      e. May be caused by herpes, adenovirus, arbovirus, mycoplasma, *Chlamydia trachomatis,* fungi, enterovirus, or various protozoa
    2. ASSESSMENT
      a. Clinical manifestations usually subside within 3–10 days.
      b. Irritability
      c. Lethargy
      d. Malaise
      e. Myalgia
      f. Headache

  g. Photophobia

  h. Anorexia

  i. Nausea or vomiting, or both

  j. Upper respiratory manifestations

  k. Maculopapular rash

  l. Nuchal rigidity

  m. Back pain

  n. Positive Kernig and Brudzinski's signs

  o. Fever rarely over 40°C (104°F)

  p. Seizures

3. DIAGNOSTIC TESTS

  a. LP

  b. CSF analysis and culture

4. NURSING INTERVENTIONS

  a. Assist the child to be comfortable.

  b. Provide a quiet and dark room.

  c. Provide IV or oral fluids.

  d. Administer prescribed drugs.

  e. Instruct the parents and child on follow-up care.

C. REYE'S SYNDROME

1. DESCRIPTION

  a. An acute life-threatening encephalopathy with accompanying microvascular fatty deposits in the liver and kidney

  b. Generally follows a mild viral illness (e.g., varicella, influenza B, influenza A, Epstein-Barr, adenovirus, coxsackievirus)

  c. Suspected link with aspirin

2. ASSESSMENT

  a. Initially, mild viral infection with apparent recovery generally within 24 to 48 hours

    1) Vomiting

    2) Presence or absence of fever

    3) Behavior changes (confusion, fear, irritability, anxiety, flat affect, speech patterns)

    4) Deterioration of level of consciousness with periods of screaming, ranting, and raving

      a) Dilated and light-sensitive pupils

  b. Deep coma within 24 hours, with:

    1) Decorticate or decerebrate posturing

    2) Loss of cranial nerve reflexes

  c. Death can occur within 2–3 days of onset.

3. DIAGNOSTIC TESTS

  a. CBC

  b. Blood chemistries

  c. Blood urea nitrogen (BUN)

  d. Amylase

  e. Liver biopsy

  f. Liver function tests

  g. Clotting times

  h. Urinalysis

  i. pH of arterial blood

  j. LP (avoided if symptoms of increased ICP)

  k. CT scan

4. NURSING INTERVENTIONS

  a. Intensive care unit (ICU)

  b. Frequent monitoring of vital signs, respiratory effort, neurologic status, laboratory values

  c. Select appropriate play activities and interactions with others after recovery from acute clinical manifestations.

  d. Instruct the parents about using salicylates in children with viral illness such as medications containing aspirin: Alka-Seltzer, Anacin, Aspergum, Bufferin, Coricidin, Dristan, Excedrin, Pepto-Bismol, and Triaminicin.

D. ENCEPHALITIS

1. DESCRIPTION: DIFFUSE OR LOCALIZED INFLAMMATION OF THE BRAIN DUE TO INVASION BY A PATHOGEN THROUGH THE CNS

2. ASSESSMENT

  a. Intense headache

  b. Signs of respiratory infection

  c. Nausea or vomiting

  d. Meningeal irritation

  e. Disorientation

  f. Confusion

  g. Personality and behavior changes

  h. Hemiplegia

  i. Ataxia

  j. Weakness

  k. Slurred speech

  l. Alterations in the cranial nerve and other reflex responses

  m. Generalized or focal seizure activity with intermittent periods of screaming, hallucinating, or moving in bizarre fashions

  n. Deteriorating level of consciousness

3. DIAGNOSTIC TESTS

  a. CSF analysis

  b. CT

  c. MRI

  d. EEG

4. NURSING INTERVENTIONS

  a. Close monitoring in ICU if acutely ill with intubation, mechanical ventilation, oxygenation, treatment of cerebral edema

  b. Administer intravenous (IV) or nasogastric (NG) nutrition.

  c. Perform frequent vital signs, with special attention to airway and respiratory function.

  d. Perform a complete neurological assessment, including pupil checks and GCS.
  e. Monitor for seizure activity.
  f. Perform range-of-motion (ROM) activities.
  g. Provide meticulous skin care.
  h. Offer good adequate nutrition.

VIII. TRAUMA AND INJURY
  A. HEAD TRAUMA
   1. DESCRIPTION
    a. Primary injury
     1) Direct blow to the head produces coup injury
     2) Acceleration or deceleration movement of the brain within the skull causes coup-contrecoup injury
     3) Shearing of small veins and arteries
    b. Secondary injury (involves the brain and body's response immediately or several minutes, hours, days, weeks, or months later)
     1) Increased ICP due to brain tissue destruction
     2) If left unresolved will lead to irreversible brain damage and death
    c. Examples of head trauma include scalp injury, concussive injuries, skull fractures, cerebral contusion or laceration, intracranial hematomas and hemorrhage such as epidural, subdural, subarachnoid, or intracerebral, and penetrating injuries.
    d. More frequent in males
    e. Causative factors include mechanical force such as falls, abuse, competitive sports, and motor vehicle accidents.
   2. ASSESSMENT
    a. Mild (concussion)
     1) No loss of consciousness or very short episode (less than 2 minutes)
     2) Amnesia may or may not be present.
     3) Headache, nausea, vomiting
     4) Initially, behavior within normal limits
    b. Moderate
     1) Loss of consciousness
     2) By the time the emergency room is reached, LOC may improve.
      a) Infant: lethargic; history of vomiting, seizures
      b) Child: headache, nausea, vertigo, fatigue, vomiting, seizures, irritability, amnesic of event, aggressiveness, combativeness
    c. Severe
     1) Clinical manifestations of increased ICP

     2) Long period of seriously diminished mental status or unconsciousness
     3) Coma for up to 2 weeks
     4) After 2 weeks, either subtle signs of improvement or further deterioration and may be declared brain dead
   3. DIAGNOSTIC TESTS
    a. Head x-rays
    b. EEG
    c. CT scan
    d. Laboratory tests such as CBC, chemistries, urine assays, and clotting time
   4. NURSING INTERVENTIONS
    a. Maintain ventilation, oxygenation, and perfusion.
    b. Monitor LOC.
    c. Monitor intake and output.
    d. Monitor vital signs and ICP.
    e. Monitor oxygen and carbon dioxide levels.
    f. Assess for changes in respiratory status.
    g. Restrict fluids.
    h. Maintain the bed in a flat position.
    i. Keep the room quiet and dark, with the head in midline of the body.
    j. Avoid hyperflexing the hips and knees.
    k. Manage pain with acetaminophen or narcotics.
    l. Maintain comfortable room temperature.
    m. Monitor arterial blood gases (ABGs) and pulse oximetry.
    n. If intubated:
     1) Position the child comfortably and assess for signs of pain or need for sedation.
     2) Evaluate respiratory status and perfusion frequently.
    o. Work with the child and family to accept the disability (if present) and with the rehabilitation team to evaluate and improve physical, developmental, and social needs.
    p. Inform the parents about the recovery process of the brain injury.
  B. SPINAL CORD INJURY
   1. DESCRIPTION
    a. Loss of movement or sensation below the site of the injury is due to transection, contusion, compression, vascular damage, or hemorrhage.
    b. Number of young adults (20 to 24 years) injured is four times greater than children and adolescents together.
    c. Causes in young children include pedestrian-vehicle, bike-vehicle, passenger-vehicle injuries, balls (thrown or hit), or abuse.

d. Causes in older children and adolescence include passenger- and driver-related injuries, gymnastics, or contact sports such as football.

e. In children under age 8 years, 75% of injuries are in the cervical area, especially at C3.

f. The second most common site of injury is the thoracolumbar region, probably due to improperly placed seat belts.

2. ASSESSMENT

a. Deficits displayed secondary to level of lesion (see Table 35-3)

b. Neurogenic and spinal shock (see Table 35-4)

Table 35-3 Deficits Displayed Secondary to Level of Lesion

Level	Deficits
C1 to C2	Quadriplegia with total loss of respiratory function Flaccid paralysis
C2 to C4	Quadriplegia with loss of phrenic innervation to diaphragm
C4 to C5	Quadriplegia with possible phrenic nerve involvement caused by edema resulting in loss of respiratory function
C5 to C6	Quadriplegia but with gross arm movements Diaphragmatic breathing No intercostal respirations
C6 to C7	Quadriplegia but with biceps intact Diaphragmatic breathing Complete loss of shoulder movement
C7 to C8	Quadriplegia with biceps and triceps intact Diaphragmatic breathing No function of intrinsic hand muscles
T1 to T2	Paraplegia with loss of leg, bowel, bladder, and sexual function Some loss of intercostal muscles Arm function intact
T2 to L2	Paraplegia with loss of varying degrees of intercostal and abdominal muscles
Below L2	Varying amounts of motor and sensory loss
Cauda equina	Bowel and bladder dysfunction

© Cengage Learning 2015

Table 35-4 Comparison of Neurogenic and Spinal Shock

Neurogenic Shock	Spinal Shock
Neurogenic shock is a form of distributive shock that accompanies complete high spinal cord injury. It is caused by interruption of sympathetic impulses from the spinal cord in the cervical/thoracic region. The hallmark signs include: • Vasodilation • Hypotension • Bradycardia • Warm flushed skin • Inability to perspire • Hypothermia	Spinal shock is the complete loss of all reflex activity after spinal cord injury. This is a transient event that often occurs shortly after the trauma and can persist for as long as 7 to 10 days. Signs include: Below the level of the lesion Flaccid, areflexic extremities Loss of deep tendon reflexes No sensory response Autonomic dysfunction Hypotension Bradycardia Decreased peripheral vascular resistance Impaired temperature control Warm, flushed, dry skin Loss of sphincter control with urinary retention Priapism

© Cengage Learning 2015

3. DIAGNOSIS
   a. Based on clinical manifestation
   b. Radiologic findings
4. NURSING INTERVENTIONS
   a. Immediately following injury:
      1) Ensure airway patency.
      2) If high injury, the client may need intubation or a tracheostomy.
      3) Ensure proper perfusion and hydration.
      4) Monitor vital signs.
      5) Immobilize.
   b. Later:
      1) Monitor vital signs.
      2) Monitor intake and output.
      3) Protect bony prominences.
      4) Maintain skin integrity.
      5) Monitor surgical sites.
      6) Maintain immobility.
      7) Provide pin or screw care (if appropriate).
      8) Provide adequate nutrition.
      9) Provide catheter care if an indwelling urinary catheter is present.
      10) Provide bowel training when appropriate.
      11) Avoid being solicitous or overprotective.
      12) Encourage independence and normal activities.
      13) Assist the child and family with grief and loss.

C. SUBMERSION
   1. DESCRIPTION
      a. Drowning is death from a submersion incident in a liquid medium within the first 24 hours postinjury.
      b. Wet drowning results from aspiration of fluid into the lungs and is most common in infants and toddlers.
      c. Dry drowning secondary to hypoxemia is due to laryngospasm in which fluid has not entered the lungs.
      d. Near drowning is survival for more than 24 hours regardless of outcome.
      e. Secondary drowning is the rapid deterioration of respiratory function from several hours to several days after successful resuscitation.
      f. Drowning claims around 2000 per year, second only to transportation injuries as the most common cause of unintentional injury in children.
      g. Approximately one-half of victims are under 4 years of age (peak incidence between 1 and 2 years of age, and then again during adolescence).
      h. Drowning is 10 times more common in males.
      i. Over 90% occur in fresh water (50% in swimming pools).
      j. Most occur between 4:00 p.m. and 6:00 p.m.
   2. ASSESSMENT
      a. Child is trapped, panics and struggles if in a body of water.
      b. Child holds his breath before swallowing some water.
      c. Child vomits then aspirates; laryngospasms, lasting less than 2 minutes, follow.
      d. Child panics again.
      e. Hypoxia occurs.
      f. Child swallows more fluid.
      g. If dry drowning, profound laryngospasms occur, with the child becoming severely hypoxic; the child seizes and dies.
      h. If wet drowning, child goes unconscious, laryngospasms lessen as reflexes are lost and large amounts of fluid passively enter the airway and stomach.
      i. Initially the body tries to compensate by shunting blood to the lungs to increase circulating oxygen, resulting in pulmonary edema.
      j. When combined with aspirated liquid, decreased lung compliance occurs, which may be further complicated by inactivation of pulmonary surfactant.
      k. Hypoxia and resulting acidosis lead to physiologic complications.
      l. Cardiac dysrhythmias (asystole, bradycardia, ventricular fibrillation) frequently are manifested.
      m. Neurological dysfunctions
      n. Renal failure
      o. Hypothermia
   3. DIAGNOSTIC TESTS
      a. History from witnesses at the scene and prehospital providers, including length of submersion; fluid temperature; salt or freshwater and source (e.g., hot tub, spa, cleaning solution in a bucket, creek); presence of other injuries (head trauma, cord trauma); initial response after rescue; presence or absence of spontaneous respirations or heartbeats; neurological status (awake, semiconsciousness, or totally unresponsive); actions taken by bystanders, including cardiopulmonary resuscitation (CPR), and the child's response; and the time prehospital providers arrived and the interventions taken.

b. Upon arrival at the acute care center, physical assessment with evaluation of airway, ventilatory status, circulation, LOC, and pupil checks

c. ABGs

d. Serum chemistries

e. BUN

f. Creatinine

g. Clotting factors

h. Blood, urine, and tracheal aspirate cultures

i. Chest x-ray

j. Head CT

k. If concurrent injury is suspected, lateral cervical spine and pelvis x-ray

4. NURSING INTERVENTIONS

a. Monitor the minimally impaired child.

b. For the child who is more impaired:

1) ICU care for continual monitoring of respiratory, cardiac, and neurologic status

2) Monitor for condition changes in laboratory values as well as head CT.

3) Make arrangements for occupational therapy (OT) and physical therapy (PT) as appropriate.

D. CEREBRAL PALSY

1. DESCRIPTION: DAMAGE TO THE CEREBRUM OR CEREBELLUM RESULTING IN ABNORMAL MUSCLE TONE AND MOVEMENT WITH MILD TO SEVERE DEVELOPMENTAL DELAYS

2. ASSESSMENT (SEE TABLE 35-5)

Table 35-5 Early Warning Signs for Cerebral Palsy

Age	Warning Signs
Neonate	• Weak or absent sucking or swallowing difficulties • Periods of apnea or bradycardia • Encephalopathic (high-pitched) cry • Extreme fussiness and irritability • Poor tone • Twitching of an arm or leg • Not moving extremities normally • Absent or weak primitive reflex responses
3 months	• Feeding difficulties, may be caused by tongue thrust or poor swallowing, or both • Irritability or listlessness, or both • Hypotonia, but may have head control in prone position • One or both hands in fisted position • Strabismus • Presence of primitive reflexes • Brisk tendon reflex response
6 months	• Delay in reaching developmental milestones (motor, speech) • Continued primitive reflexes • Hands remain clenched; one hand becomes dominant • Hypertonia • Arching or tendency to stand when held up • Lack of interest in people or toys • Unaware of or indifferent to stimuli in environment • Little if any spontaneous actions
9 months	• Persistent delay in motor milestones • Reach may be atypical as fingers are extended and arms tremble with purposeful movement • Arms flexed
12 months	• Inability to sit alone • Scissoring of lower extremities • Toe walking while held, but unable to stand alone • Crawl, if present, may be abnormal as only arms may be used • Athetoid (irregular, twisting) movement • Poor articulation or lack of speech

3. DIAGNOSTIC TESTS
   a. Based on clinical manifestations
4. NURSING INTERVENTIONS
   a. Provide the child with technical aids such as braces, walkers, customized wheelchairs, and computers or voice synthesizers.
   b. Coordinate speech therapy, PT, or OT.
   c. Inform the parents on surgical interventions such as tendon lengthening, hamstring release, hip or foot surgery, and rhizotomy.
   d. Administer prescribed muscle relaxants and antianxiety drugs generally reserved for the older child and adolescent.
   e. Ensure that the body is in best alignment, using pillows or bolsters.
   f. Protect bony prominences.
   g. Instruct the parents on home care.
   h. Provide the family with referral services.

PRACTICE QUESTIONS

1. During hospitalization, a child experiences a tonic-clonic seizure. To provide for the client's safety, which of the following actions should the nurse take?
   1. Put a padded tongue blade between the child's teeth
   2. Perform a jaw thrust and administer oxygen
   3. Securely restrain the child in the bed
   4. Administer a benzodiazepine intramuscularly

2. Postoperatively, for placement of a shunt for hydrocephalus, the nurse should place a child in which of the following positions?
   1. Elevated 45 degrees in a supine position
   2. Flat and lying on the unoperated side
   3. Flat and lying on the operated side
   4. Elevated 30 degrees and prone

3. The parents of a 2-year-old toddler who has cerebral palsy notice the child does not sit up alone. They ask the nurse whether the child will be able to learn to walk alone or with crutches. Which of the following is the appropriate response by the nurse?
   1. "Your child will most likely not be able to walk alone or with crutches."
   2. "The chances of your child walking without crutches is good, but it is unlikely that your child will walk alone."
   3. "It is very difficult to say because every child is different."
   4. "Your child will most probably be able to walk alone and without the use of crutches."

4. The parents of a child with cerebral palsy ask the nurse what the most common cause of cerebral palsy is. The most appropriate response by the nurse is which of the following?
   1. "It results when the cord gets wrapped around the neck in the birth canal."
   2. "It is the result of a forceps delivery."
   3. "It is the result of a premature birth or very low birth weight."
   4. "It is the result of preeclampsia in the mother."

5. When caring for a child with meningitis, it is essential that the nurse evaluate for a positive Brudzinski's sign, which would indicate
   1. increased intracranial pressure.
   2. meningeal irritation.
   3. encephalitis.
   4. intraventricular hemorrhage.

6. A nurse is providing discharge instructions to the parents of a child who suffered a head injury 6 hours ago. Which statement by the parents indicates additional teaching is needed?
   1. "We will call the doctor immediately if vomiting occurs."
   2. "We won't give anything stronger than Tylenol for headache."
   3. "We will provide for uninterrupted sleep when we get home."
   4. "We know continued amnesia regarding the events of the injury is expected."

7. The nurse is assigned to administer bismuth subsalicylate (Pepto-Bismol) to a 10-year-old child who has Reye's syndrome and is experiencing gastrointestinal clinical manifestations. Which of the following is the priority action for the nurse to take?
   1. Administer the prescribed dose of 1 tablet
   2. Inform the child and parents that stools will be dark in appearance
   3. Instruct the child to chew the tablet thoroughly
   4. Question the physician's order

8. The nurse identifies which of the following as warning signs in a 12-month-old with cerebral palsy?
   Select all that apply:
   [ ] 1. Weak or absent sucking
   [ ] 2. Hypotonia

[ ] 3. Toe walking but unable to stand alone
[ ] 4. Absent or weak primitive reflex responses
[ ] 5. Toe walking while held, but unable to stand alone
[ ] 6. Athetoid (irregular, twisting) movement

9. The nurse assesses cranial nerve VII in a pediatric client by which of the following techniques?
   1. Gently swab the cornea with a sterile cotton-tipped applicator
   2. Hold the eyes open and turn the head from side to side
   3. Place the child's head in the midline position with the head elevated and inject ice water into the ear canal
   4. Irritate the pharynx with a tongue depressor or cotton swab

10. The nurse should monitor a child for which of the following clinical manifestations of meningeal irritation?
    Select all that apply:
    [ ] 1. Nuchal rigidity
    [ ] 2. Nausea and vomiting
    [ ] 3. Anxiousness
    [ ] 4. Heightened sense of environment
    [ ] 5. Headache
    [ ] 6. Decreased resistance to pain and extension of the leg

11. With an infant who has anencephaly, the most appropriate nursing intervention is to
    1. inform the parents that an abnormal gait with foot weakness or deformity will appear by toddlerhood.
    2. assess the infant for cerebrospinal fluid leak at the site of the defect.
    3. instruct the parents to notify the physician if difficulties in controlling bowel and bladder functions develop when toilet training is attempted.
    4. monitor the infant for respiratory failure and prepare the parents that death is imminent.

12. When planning client assignments for the day, which of the following nursing tasks would be appropriate for the registered nurse to assign to unlicensed assistive personnel?
    1. Assess a child for signs of increased intracranial pressure
    2. Explain the procedure for a skull x-ray to the parents and child
    3. Document the temperature of a child with bacterial meningitis
    4. Monitor a child for urinary retention following surgery for spina bifida

13. The nurse is caring for a child who had a seizure 15 minutes after sustaining a head injury. After assuring a patent airway, which of the following is the priority intervention?
    1. Assess fluid and electrolyte status
    2. Administer prescribed benzodiazepine
    3. Monitor for postconcussive syndrome
    4. Observe for signs of increased intracranial pressure

14. A child has received an external ventricular drainage (EVD) for treatment of an infection following shunt insertion. For which of the following clinical manifestations of overdraining ventricles should the nurse monitor the child? Select all that apply:
    [ ] 1. Tachycardia
    [ ] 2. Nausea and vomiting
    [ ] 3. Ataxia
    [ ] 4. Polydipsia
    [ ] 5. Headache
    [ ] 6. Apnea

15. The nurse receives report from an emergency room nurse that a child is being admitted with a C7 spinal cord injury. Based on this information, the nurse prepares to care for a child with which of the following deficits?
    1. Quadriplegia with total loss of respiratory function and flaccid paralysis
    2. Paraplegia with loss of leg, bowel, and bladder function
    3. Quadriplegia but with gross arm movements and diaphragmatic breathing
    4. Paraplegia, arm function intact, loss of some degree of intercostal and abdominal muscle use

16. The nurse should monitor a child who has survived a submersion injury in a hot tub for pneumonia caused by which of the following organisms?
    1. *Escherichia coli*
    2. *Pseudomonas aeruginosa*
    3. *Staphylococcus aureus*
    4. *Streptococcus*

17. The nurse is preparing to teach a class to educate parents about common neurological injuries in children. Which of the following should the nurse include in the class? Select all that apply:
    [ ] 1. Most drownings occur between 12 p.m. and 2 p.m.
    [ ] 2. Improperly placed seat belts are the second most common cause of spinal injuries
    [ ] 3. Fifty percent of drownings occur in lakes and oceans
    [ ] 4. A lap belt in an automobile is the best way to prevent spinal cord trauma in children under the age of 13 years

[ ] 5. Seventy-five percent of spinal injuries in children under the age of 8 years occur at the C3 level

[ ] 6. Most spinal cord injuries in young children are the result of pedestrian-vehicle, bike-vehicle, or passenger-vehicle injuries

18. The nurse assesses a child who cries, withdraws from painful stimuli, and opens the eyes to pain to have a Glasgow Coma Scale score of
1. 3.
2. 6.
3. 9.
4. 12.

19. The nurse observes a child having a seizure that begins with tonic contractions of the fingers in the left hand and progresses into tonic-clonic movements that proceed up the muscles of the left side of the body. The nurse should report these seizures as
1. Jacksonian.
2. Rolandic.
3. general.
4. complex.

20. Which of the following statements indicates the family of a child with a seizure disorder has followed the nurse's discharge instructions?
1. "Our child has had a growth spurt, so we made an appointment to review the medication to prevent seizures."
2. "We remind our child every day of what activities should be restricted."
3. "Most of our time is spent with our child who has seizures, so we have little time for the other children."
4. "Our child knows to take a dose of seizure medicine after remembering a dose that was accidentally forgotten."

21. The parents of a child suspected of having a shunt malfunction ask the nurse what caused it. The appropriate response by the nurse is which of the following?
1. Increased flow of cerebrospinal fluid
2. Increased reabsorption of cerebrospinal fluid
3. Obstructed flow of cerebrospinal fluid
4. Decreased production of cerebrospinal fluid

22. The nurse assists the parents of a child with myoclonic seizures to make which of the following menu selections?
1. Baked potato
2. Creamed corn
3. Roast beef
4. Pecan pie with ice cream

23. The nurse is planning the care for a child who has an elevated blood pressure and slow pulse, is flushed, has profuse facial perspiration, and is experiencing urinary retention and constipation 4 days after sustaining a C3 injury. Which of the following is the priority nursing intervention?
1. Administer the prescribed antihypertensive
2. Insert a prescribed Foley catheter
3. Remove the blankets on the bed
4. Encourage fluids

24. The nurse should monitor a client for which of the following signs of neurogenic shock after a C5 injury?
Select all that apply:
[ ] 1. Hypotension
[ ] 2. Tachycardia
[ ] 3. Hypothermia
[ ] 4. Cool and pale skin
[ ] 5. Vasoconstriction
[ ] 6. Inability to perspire

ANSWERS AND RATIONALES

1. 2. To provide for the safety of the child during a tonic-clonic seizure, the nurse should perform a jaw thrust and administer oxygen. Holding the child down, restraining the child, or putting a padded tongue blade between the child's teeth may cause injury to the child. Benzodiazepine is not used to treat a tonic-clonic seizure but is used in status epilepticus.

2. 2. A child who has had a shunt revision for hydrocephalus should be placed flat in bed, lying on the unoperated side. The head-elevated position may cause the cerebrospinal fluid to drain too quickly from the ventricles. Lying on the operated side can cause injury to the shunt, and the prone position may cause interference with respiration.

3. 1. If a child cannot sit up by the age of 2, there is every indication that the child has cerebral palsy affecting voluntary motor control. As a result, the child will not be able to walk with or without crutches.

4. 3. Although the cord getting wrapped around the neck in the birth canal, a forceps delivery, and preeclampsia in the mother all place a child at

risk for cerebral palsy, children born prematurely or those who have very low birth weights are the most at risk.

5. 2. Brudzinski's sign, when the legs flex at both hips and knees in response to flexing the head and neck, indicates meningeal irritation.

6. 3. Waking children to check neurological status following a head injury is important, no matter the time of day. Vomiting could indicate increased intracranial pressure requiring further evaluation. Narcotics should be avoided after a head injury. Amnesia following a head injury is not uncommon.

7. 4. Bismuth subsalicylate (Pepto-Bismol) contains aspirin, and there is a suspected link between aspirin and the etiology of Reye's syndrome. It is a priority to question the order for Pepto-Bismol to be given to this child. One tablet is appropriate for a child 10 years of age. Chewing the tablet and informing the child and parents that the stool will be dark in appearance are all appropriate interventions in the plan of care for a child taking Pepto-Bismol, but not for a child with Reye's syndrome.

8. 3. 5. 6. Warning signs for cerebral palsy in a 12-month-old include toe walking while being held because the child is unable to stand alone. When crawling occurs, it is abnormal because only the arms may be used and it may be athetoid, which refers to irregular, twisting movements. Weak or absent sucking reflex and absent or weak primitive reflex responses are present in the neonate. Hypertonia is present in a 6-month-old.

9. 1. Gently swabbing the cornea with a sterile cotton-tipped applicator assesses cranial nerve VII, which evaluates the corneal reflex. Holding the eyes open and turning the head from side to side evaluates cranial nerves II, IV, and VI and the oculocephalic reflex. Placing the child's head in a midline position with the head elevated prior to injecting ice water into the ear canal evaluates cranial nerves III and VIII, or the oculovestibular reflex. Irritating the pharynx with a tongue depressor or cotton swab evaluates cranial nerves IX and X, or the gag reflex.

10. 1. 2. 5. Clinical manifestations of meningeal irritation are nuchal rigidity, positive Kernig's sign (resistance to pain and extension of the leg), positive Brudzinski's sign, severe headache, loss of consciousness, photophobia, nausea, vomiting, fever, and convulsions.

11. 4. Anencephaly is the absence of the cranial vault, with the cerebral hemisphere missing or reduced in size. Although the brainstem may be intact, respiratory failure and death are imminent. The abnormal gait with foot

weakness or deformity appears in toddlerhood with spina bifida. Leakage of cerebrospinal fluid occurs with meningomyelocele. Difficulties in bowel and bladder functions occur at the time of toilet training with spina bifida occulta.

12. 3. It is appropriate for a registered nurse to assign only those activities that are basic cares and do not involve assessing, explaining or teaching, or monitoring for change. Unlicensed assistive personnel are trained only to take a temperature.

13. 2. If a seizure occurs within 30 minutes of a head injury, benzodiazepine is administered intravenously to stop the seizure. If the seizure continues, phenytoin may be administered. Although the remaining interventions of assessing fluid and electrolyte status, monitoring for postconcussive syndrome, and observing for increased intracranial pressure are appropriate, the priority intervention is to stop the seizure.

14. 2. 5. 6. The clinical manifestations of overdraining ventricles following placement of an external ventricular drainage include bradycardia, apnea, severe headache, nausea, vomiting, lethargy, drowsiness, and irritability, and there is a possibility that seizures will occur.

15. 3. C1 to C2 spinal cord lesions result in quadriplegia with total loss of respiratory function and flaccid paralysis. Spinal cord lesions at C7 to C8 would result in quadriplegia with biceps intact and diaphragmatic breathing. Spinal cord lesions at T1 to T2 would result in paraplegia with loss of leg, bowel, bladder, and sexual function. Spinal cord lesions at C5 to C6 would result in paraplegia with loss of varying degrees of intercostals and abdominal muscle use, but gross arm movements would be present.

16. 2. Because *Pseudomonas aeruginosa* is an organism commonly found in hot tubs, a child who suffers a submersion injury in a hot tub is at risk for pneumonia caused by this organism.

17. 2. 5. 6. Most drownings occur between 4 p.m. and 6 p.m. when the caregiver is busy preparing dinner and not closely supervising the child. Over 90% of drownings occur in fresh water, with 50% of those in swimming pools. Lap belts are dangerous because when a crash occurs, the lap belt is positioned on the abdomen of a child of this age. In a crash, the child is hyperflexed over the belt, which snaps back upright. The force of the lap belt continues posteriorly to the spinal column and cord, causing trauma.

18. 3. Crying to painful stimuli is a 3, withdrawing from pain is a 4, and opening the eyes to painful stimuli is a 2 on the Glasgow Coma Scale. This gives a total score of 9. A score of 3 means there is neither a verbal nor a motor response to painful stimuli. A score of 12 indicates the child opens the eyes on command, withdraws at simple touch, and has an irritable cry to painful stimuli. A score of 6 is a minimal response to all of the categories, but still a response.

19. 1. Jacksonian seizures begin with tonic contractions of the fingers in the left hand and progress into tonic-clonic movements that proceed up the muscles of the left side of the body. Rolandic seizures include tonic-clonic movements of the face, with increased salivation and arrested speech; they commonly occur during sleep. Complex seizures have an aura, and consciousness may not be completely lost. Children are rarely violent, but may demonstrate confusion or purposeless behaviors. General seizures are secondary to diffuse electrical activity throughout the cortex and into the brain.

20. 1. As children gain weight, the dose of the seizure medication may need to be altered. Dosages of medications should not be missed at all. Children with seizure disorders should be allowed to participate in most activities and should not be overprotected by parents, and parents should divide their time equally among all their children. Reminders of what an affected child can and cannot do should not be necessary.

21. 1. Decreased reabsorption is a common cause of hydrocephalus. Increased flow of and decreased production of cerebrospinal fluid (CSF) do not relate to hydrocephalus, intracranial pressure (ICP), or shunt malfunction.

22. 4. A ketogenic diet, in which 90% of calories come from fat, and protein and carbohydrates are limited, is used in the treatment of myoclonic seizures. Roast beef is high in protein. Baked potato and creamed corn are high in carbohydrates. Pecans and ice cream are high in fat, so that menu selection is appropriate to a ketogenic diet. Why ketones affect seizures is not understood, but researchers theorize that ketones change lipid concentrations, reduce fluid and electrolyte imbalances, modify the seizure threshold, and stabilize the central nervous system.

23. 2. Spinal shock occurs shortly after the injury and may persist for up to 10 days with a high cervical or thoracic injury. After the spinal shock has resolved and reflex activity has returned, high cervical or thoracic lesions may react with a potential life-threatening sympathetic nervous system response to stimuli such as a distended bladder, constipation, or fecal impaction. Spasms of the pelvic viscera and arterioles produce vasoconstriction below the lesion, resulting in hypertension, superficial vasodilatation, flushing, piloerection, and profuse perspiration above the injury. To compensate for the increased blood pressure, the heart rate is slowed via vagal stimulation. Without prompt reversal of the clinical manifestations, which is usually just removal of the stimulant, the client may stroke, have a seizure, or die.

24. 1. 3. 6. Neurogenic shock is a form of distributive shock that accompanies complete high spinal cord injury. It is caused by an interruption of sympathetic impulses from the spinal cord in the cervical-thoracic region. Clinical manifestations include vasodilatation, hypotension, bradycardia, warm, flushed skin, inability to perspire, and hypothermia.

REFERENCE

Potts, N., & Mandleco, B. (2012). *Pediatric nursing: Caring for children and their families* (3rd ed.). Clifton Park, NY: Delmar Cengage Learning.

CHAPTER 36

INTEGUMENTARY DISORDERS

I. ANATOMY AND PHYSIOLOGY (SEE CHAPTER 8, INTEGUMENTARY DISORDERS, SECTION I.)

A. DIFFERENCES IN THE INTEGUMENTARY SYSTEM BETWEEN THE CHILD AND THE ADULT

1. THE INTEGUMENTARY SYSTEM AT BIRTH IS IMMATURE.
2. THE SKIN IS VERY THIN IN THE NEWBORN AND THE EPIDERMIS IS LOOSELY BOUND TO THE DERMIS.
3. THE SKIN OF A PREMATURE INFANT IS SUSCEPTIBLE TO DAMAGE CAUSED BY FRICTION EVEN WITH MINOR CONTACT.
4. BECAUSE THE NEWBORN'S SKIN IS VERY THIN, THERE IS AN INCREASED ABSORPTION OF SUBSTANCES AND DRUGS.
5. THE NEWBORN IS UNABLE TO ADAPT TO ENVIRONMENTAL TEMPERATURE CHANGES BECAUSE OF LIMITED SUBCUTANEOUS FAT.
6. THE NEWBORN IS MORE SUSCEPTIBLE TO INFECTION DURING THE FIRST WEEK OF LIFE BECAUSE THE PH OF THE SKIN IS ALKALINE (WITH AGE, THE SKIN BECOMES MORE ACIDIC).
7. THE SEBACEOUS GLANDS OF THE NEWBORN ARE ACTIVE AT BIRTH BECAUSE OF THE INFLUENCE OF THE MOTHER'S HORMONES.
8. THE INFANT'S SEBACEOUS GLANDS SECRETE SEBUM, WHICH LUBRICATES THE SKIN AND MAY RESULT IN THE APPEARANCE OF NEONATAL ACNE.
9. THE PROTECTIVE FUNCTIONS OF THE SKIN MATURE AS THE CHILD REACHES THE PRESCHOOL YEARS.
10. SECRETORY IGA DECREASES UNTIL THE CHILD IS BETWEEN 2 AND 5 YEARS OF AGE.
11. UP UNTIL 5 YEARS OF AGE, THE CHILD HAS A DECREASED MUCOSAL RESISTANCE TO ORGANISMS.
12. ECCRINE GLANDS ARE DISTRIBUTED OVER THE BODY, PERMITTING PERSPIRATION, AND DO NOT REACH MATURITY UNTIL THE CHILD IS 2–3 YEARS OF AGE, WHICH WILL PERMIT ADEQUATE THERMOREGULATION.
13. APOCRINE GLANDS ARE SWEAT GLANDS THAT ARE CONCENTRATED IN THE AXILLAE, SCALP, FACE, ABDOMEN, AND GENITAL AREA THAT DO NOT FUNCTION UNTIL BETWEEN 8 AND 10 YEARS OF AGE.
14. PERSPIRATION BEGINS A FEW YEARS BEFORE PUBERTY.
15. SEBUM SECRETION OCCURS DURING THE SCHOOL-AGE YEARS WITH AN INCREASED SEBACEOUS ACTIVITY UNDER THE INFLUENCE OF STIMULATION FROM NORMAL ANDROGEN SECRETION IN ADOLESCENCE, LEADING TO THE DEVELOPMENT OF ACNE.
16. AXILLARY AND PUBIC HAIR DEVELOPMENT OCCURS IN ADOLESCENCE.
17. WATER LOSS IS GREATER IN INFANTS AND SMALL CHILDREN.

II. ASSESSMENT

A. HEALTH HISTORY
1. PAST MEDICAL HISTORY (ALLERGIES)
2. MEDICATIONS (ORAL AND TOPICAL)
3. HISTORY OF CURRENT CONDITION (DURATION, SITE, PRESENTATION, SYMPTOMS)
4. FAMILY HISTORY

B. PHYSICAL EXAMINATION
1. DISTRIBUTION OF LESIONS
2. TYPE OF LESION
   a. Primary lesion
      1) Papule: superficial raised solid lesion up to 1 cm

2) Plaque: a well-defined raised lesion greater than 1 cm

3) Macule: flat circumscribed area with change in color, up to 1 cm, not palpable

4) Patch: flat, nonpalpable area with color change greater than 1 cm

5) Pustule: well-defined, superficial lesion that contains purulent fluid, less than 1 cm in size

6) Abscess: well-defined, superficial lesion, pus-filled, greater than 1 cm in size

7) Vesicle: well-defined, elevated lesion containing fluid, up to 1 cm in size (blister)

8) Bulla: well-defined, elevated lesion containing fluid, greater than 1 cm (large blister)

9) Nodule: solid, elevated lesion with palpable deeper portion, up to 2 cm

10) Tumor: solid, elevated lesion with palpable deeper portion greater than 2 cm

11) Wheal: edematous round or flat-topped papule or plaque, usually disappears within hours

12) Cyst: raised lesion with sac containing solid material

b. Secondary lesions

1) Crust: dried exudates (serum, blood, pus), scabs

2) Scale: flakes of dead skin. Various types (whitish, silvery, platelike), result of abnormal keratinization

3) Erosion: superficial break in the skin, does not penetrate the dermis, heals without scarring (base of blister)

4) Ulcer: clearly defined, deep break in the skin, involving both the epidermis and the dermis, heals with scarring

5) Fissure: deep linear break in the skin

6) Atrophy: skin surface is depressed

7) Scar: abnormal formation of connective tissue, present at the site of the injury, surgery

8) Lichenification: thickening of the skin caused by chronic scratching, rubbing

III. DIAGNOSTIC STUDIES (SEE CHAPTER 8, INTEGUMENTARY DISORDERS, SECTION III.)

A. CULTURES

1. BACTERIAL: EXUDATE FROM LESION IS COLLECTED AND PLACED IN CULTURE MEDIUM AND SENT TO THE LAB FOR PROCESSING.

2. VIRAL: LESION IS UNROOFED, EXCESS FLUID IS REMOVED, AND THE FLOOR OF THE LESION IS GENTLY SCRAPED; THE SPECIMEN IS PLACED IN VIRAL CULTURE MEDIUM AND SENT TO THE LAB.

3. FUNGAL: AREA IS BRUSHED VIGOROUSLY WITH A CYTOLOGY BRUSH, IMPLANTED IN DTM OR MYCOSEL TEST MEDIUM, AND SENT TO THE LAB FOR PROCESSING.

B. SCRAPINGS

1. FUNGAL: SCRAPING FROM THE EDGE OF THE LESION IS PLACED ON A SLIDE. KERATIN IS DISSOLVED WITH KOH 10% AND LOW HEAT AND EXAMINED UNDER A MICROSCOPE FOR HYPHAE.

2. INFESTATIONS—MINERAL OIL SCRAPING (SCABIES PREP): MINERAL OIL IS APPLIED TO THE LESION, WHICH IS THEN SCRAPED WITH A #15 BLADE OR FOMAN BLADE; THE DEBRIS IS PLACED ON A SLIDE AND VIEWED UNDER THE MICROSCOPE FOR MITES, EGGS, AND FECAL MATERIAL.

C. WOOD'S LAMP

1. WOOD'S LAMP (A HIGH-PRESSURE MERCURY LAMP THAT EMITS A BLACK LIGHT) IS USED TO EXAMINE THE SKIN FOR CHANGES IN PIGMENTATION OR TO IDENTIFY VARIOUS INFECTIONS THAT FLUORESCE (MOSTLY FUNGAL INFECTIONS SUCH AS *MICROSPORUM CANIS* AND ERYTHRASMA).

D. SKIN BIOPSY

1. PUNCH BIOPSY: SKIN IS ANESTHETIZED AND A BIOPSY PUNCH IS USED TO REMOVE A PLUG OF SKIN THAT CONTAINS EPIDERMIS, DERMIS, AND SUBCUTANEOUS TISSUE FOR MICROSCOPIC EXAMINATION.

2. SHAVE BIOPSY: A MORE SUPERFICIAL SKIN SAMPLE IS OBTAINED FROM A RAISED LESION.

a. Postprocedure for punch and shave biopsies

1) Instruct the child or parent to keep the area dry for 24 hours and covered with a Band-aid.

2) If a small amount of bleeding is seen, instruct the parent to apply firm pressure for 10 minutes. If the bleeding becomes heavier or does not stop, instruct the parent to continue to apply pressure and to call the dermatology office.

3) Instruct the parent that the area may get wet after 24 hours, but direct pressure from the shower should be avoided.

4) Instruct the parent to apply antibiotic ointment twice daily.

5) Instruct the parent to take acetaminophen (Tylenol, Tempra) for any discomfort.

6) Instruct the parent to make an appointment to have sutures removed in 10–14 days (unnecessary for a shave biopsy because sutures are not used).

3. EXCISIONAL BIOPSY: LESION IS REMOVED WITH AN ELLIPTICAL EXCISION TO OBTAIN A FULL-THICKNESS SPECIMEN. IT IS USED TO REMOVE VARIOUS LESIONS, INCLUDING ATYPICAL NEVI, RECURRENT LESIONS, OR AGGRESSIVE FORMS OF SKIN CANCER.

a. Postprocedure instructions

1) Provide written instructions for the child or parent.

2) Instruct the parent to leave the pressure dressing in place for 24–48 hours.

3) Instruct the parent to keep the site as dry as possible until the sutures are removed. This helps to optimize healing and prevent infection.

4) Instruct the parent to give acetaminophen (Tylenol, Tempra) for any discomfort.

5) Instruct the parent that the child should avoid vigorous physical activity for 2–4 weeks. Each case is different, and the physician will specify the appropriate activity level for each client based on the size and location of the wound. Provide a written excuse for physical education at school, if necessary.

6) Instruct the parent that if bleeding should occur, apply gentle pressure with a clean gauze or washcloth for 15 minutes. If bleeding continues, maintain pressure and call the dermatology office immediately.

7) Instruct the parent to watch for clinical manifestations of infection (redness, soreness, drainage, or fever). If any of these occur, call the dermatology office immediately.

4. CURETTAGE: A ROUND SCALPEL IS USED TO SCRAPE A LESION; IT CAN BE SENT TO PATHOLOGY.

IV. NURSING DIAGNOSES
A. RISK FOR INFECTION
B. IMPAIRED SKIN INTEGRITY
C. ACUTE PAIN
D. LOW SELF-ESTEEM
E. DISTURBED SENSORY PERCEPTION
F. DISTURBED BODY IMAGE
G. INEFFECTIVE HEALTH MAINTENANCE
Nursing Diagnoses: Definitions and Classification 2012–2014. Copyright © 2012, 1994–2012 by NANDA International. Used by arrangement with John Wiley & Sons Limited.

V. SKIN DISEASES
A. ACNE VULGARIS
1. DESCRIPTION
a. Inflammation of the pilosebaceous follicles
1) Hair follicle may get plugged with dead skin cells.
2) Sebum and bacteria may accumulate at the site, resulting in pimples and comedones.
b. More common in males than females
c. Peak prevalence in teen years
d. Can severely affect the self-image of the teenager
e. Left untreated, can cause scarring
f. Contributing factors include familial tendency, hormones, and bacteria *(Propionibacterium acnes)*.
2. ASSESSMENT
a. Closed (whiteheads) and open (blackheads) comedones
b. Inflammatory lesions
1) Papules
2) Pustules
3) Nodules
4) Cysts
5) Scars
3. DIAGNOSTIC TESTS
a. None
4. MEDICAL MANAGEMENT
a. Topical antibiotics (clindamycin, erythromycin, sodium sulfacetamide): destroy skin bacteria
b. Benzoyl peroxide: decreases inflammation and bacteria
c. Oral antibiotics (tetracycline, doxycycline, minocycline, erythromycin, azithromycin, cephalexin): decrease inflammation and bacteria
d. Topical retinoid (Retin-A, Differin, Avita, Tazorac): peeling agent that loosens the plugs of skin cells; used to treat comedones (blackheads and whiteheads)
e. Isotretinoin (Accutane, Amnesteem): for treatment of severe or recalcitrant acne only; many side effects
1) Strict pregnancy prevention program—must use two forms of birth control
2) Monthly labs to monitor liver function, lipid levels, complete blood count (CBC), and serum pregnancy test

        3) Smart Program or Amnesteem Information Guide (booklet provided by the drug company) must be used. Includes education, consent form, discussion of adverse reactions, guide to contraception

        4) Monitor closely for clinical manifestations of depression.

        5) Adverse reactions include chelitis, dryness, epistaxis, sun sensitivity, musculoskeletal discomfort, triglyceride elevation, and severe teratogenicity.

    f. Oral contraceptives: used to treat adolescents over the age of 16 who have not responded to oral antibiotics, when the acne flares coincide with menses; must have baseline gynecological exam

5. NURSING INTERVENTIONS

    a. Instruct the adolescent that it may take 6–8 weeks before improvement is seen.

    b. Instruct the adolescent on the use and significant adverse reactions for the medication prescribed.

    c. Instruct the adolescent to gently cleanse the skin and to avoid use of harsh soaps.

    d. Inform the adolescent that acne treatments may cause dryness of the skin.

    e. Instruct the adolescent that if cosmetics are used, the products should be water based and oil-free. Skin creams that do not cause acne (noncomedogenic) may be used if necessary.

    f. Inform the adolescent that foods do not cause acne, but eating sensibly and in moderation is always advisable.

    g. Instruct the adolescent to use sun protection because the medications cause photosensitivity.

    h. Inform the adolescent that antibiotics can decrease the effectiveness of oral contraceptives.

    i. Instruct the adolescent on isotretinoin (Accutane, Amnesteem) therapy.

        1) Strict contraception must be followed. Pregnancy tests should be done prior to starting isotretinoin (Accutane, Amnesteem) and monthly during therapy.

        2) Blood levels must be monitored monthly.

        3) Family should be instructed to monitor the adolescent for any changes in personality and notify the physician immediately.

B. **ATOPIC DERMATITIS**

1. DESCRIPTION

    a. A chronic relapsing inflammation of the dermis and epidermis

    b. Cause is unknown

    c. Can occur at any age; most common in infants and young children

    d. Affects 10% of American children

2. ASSESSMENT

    a. Major criteria include:

        1) Pruritus

        2) Characteristic distribution and morphology of the rash

            a) During infancy, more generalized: lesions occur primarily on the face, scalp, and extensor surfaces of the extremities. Diaper area is usually spared.

            b) Older children, adults: lesions are more common on flexural surfaces—antecubital, popliteal fossae, wrists, ankles, and neck.

        3) Chronic relapsing course

        4) Atopic history (hereditary predisposition to develop allergies) in clients or family members (e.g., hay fever, asthma, or atopic dermatitis)

    b. Minor criteria include:

        1) Elevated serum IgE levels

        2) Xerosis

        3) Early age of onset

        4) Hand or foot dermatitis

        5) Cheilitis

        6) Keratosis pilaris

        7) Hyperlinear palms

        8) Susceptibility to cutaneous infection

        9) Midfacial pallor

       10) Infraorbital fold

       11) Food intolerances

3. DIAGNOSTIC TESTS

    a. Criteria for diagnosis: need three major and three minor criteria

4. MEDICAL MANAGEMENT

    a. Daily baths or shower

    b. Topical steroids as prescribed; use the least potent steroid necessary to relieve clinical manifestation, taper as clinical manifestations improve.

    c. Nonsteroidal ointments (topical immunomodulators): tacrolimus (Protopic) and pimecrolimus (Elidel) as prescribed

    d. Emollients (see Table 36-1)

    e. Oral antibiotics (cephalexin, dicloxicillin) if secondary infection is present

Table 36-1 Use of Emollients

In order to promote hydration of the skin, moisturizing creams and ointments must be applied within 3 minutes of the bath or shower. Agents should be applied thinly in smooth downward strokes in the direction of hair growth to minimize trapping heat and increasing the potential for pruritus.

Emollients are substances containing varying amounts of lipids and water and are used to promote hydration and softening of the skin. Application of emollients provides a thin film over the surface of the skin, trapping water and preventing further water loss.

Numerous preparations of emollients are available for use. Selection of an emollient product should be individualized based on the child's condition. An appropriate understanding of available products and indications for use can assist you in providing education to children and their caregivers.

Lotions contain the greatest proportion of water. Their consistency is lighter and less greasy. Their high water content may promote evaporative water loss. Lotions often contain fragrances that can be irritating to the skin. Caregivers should be instructed to select products that do not contain added fragrances.

Creams are heavier products than lotions and have a greater capacity to trap water under the skin. Creams are more readily absorbed than ointments.

Ointments are thicker, greasier, and contain the least water. Ointments have the greatest capacity to trap moisture but may not be practical because of their greasy consistency.

Bath oils provide benefit by allowing an emollient film to form on the skin during bathing.

  f. Systemic corticosteroids (Orapred, Pediapred, Prelone) as prescribed, in severe cases only
  g. Cyclosporin as prescribed (used in very severe, recalcitrant cases)
  h. Antihistamines (Atarax, Benadryl, Zyrtec) to help control itching, primarily by causing drowsiness
5. NURSING INTERVENTIONS
  a. Instruct the parents to give the client short baths (no longer than 10 minutes). Avoid very hot or very cold water and bubble baths. Pat the skin dry. Apply emollients immediately after bathing.
  b. Instruct the parents to apply moisturizers frequently during the day. Use creams rather than lotions. Creams are heavier products and have a greater capacity to trap moisture under the skin.
  c. Instruct the parents to apply a thin layer of the prescribed topical steroid twice a day. Rub in thoroughly. It must be applied before the emollient. If the emollient is applied first, the steroid will not be able to penetrate it.
  d. Instruct the parents to avoid substances that cause itching such as wool, soaps, detergents, and grass.
  e. Instruct the parents to avoid using fabric softeners.
  f. Instruct the parents to keep the temperature and humidity in the home fairly constant.
  g. Instruct the parents to keep the nails short and well filed and avoid scratching.
  h. Instruct the parents to make sure the child wears loose-fitting, cotton clothing.
  i. Address psychological factors. Promote self-esteem, encourage participation in normal activities. Avoid being overprotective. Counseling may be necessary for the child and parents.
  j. Stress the importance of follow-up visits to evaluate the treatment plan.
C. SCABIES
  1. DESCRIPTION
    a. Caused by *Sarcoptes scabiei*
    b. Affects humans only, all ages, all races
    c. Rash is the result of infestation and immune response.
    d. Transmission is via skin-to-skin contact.
    e. Fomite transmission is less likely but possible.
  2. ASSESSMENT
    a. History
    b. Papules, vesicles, nodules, and burrows (linear lesions, home of the female mite)
    c. Severe itching, especially intense at night
    d. Distribution and grouping of lesions
      1) Infants: more generalized; includes the face, neck, scalp, palms, and soles
      2) Children and adolescents: intertriginous sites, interdigital spaces, flexural regions, intertriginous zones, wrists, waistline, genitals, and buttocks
  3. DIAGNOSTIC TESTS
    a. Mineral oil scraping (scabies prep)
  4. MEDICAL MANAGEMENT
    a. Permethrin 5% cream (Elimite, Acticin)
    b. Lindane (Kwell): reports of neurotoxicity
    c. 5% sulfur in petrolatum: irritating, unpleasant odor
    d. Crotamiton (Eurax): high failure rate
    e. Oral ivermectin
  5. NURSING INTERVENTIONS
    a. Instruct the parents to treat all household members and close contacts prophylactically.

b. Instruct the parents to avoid warm shower or bath prior to application—may increase absorption and possibility of toxicity.

c. Instruct the parents to apply the cream from the neck down in a thin layer. The cream should be left on for 8–14 hours and then washed off.

d. Instruct the parents to treat the entire body, especially the skin folds, under the nails, postauricular areas, and the scalp (in infants).

e. Instruct the parents to wash all clothing, linens, and bedding in hot water and dry in a hot dryer.

f. Inform the parents that itching may persist for a few weeks after treatment. Use of moisturizers may help alleviate the itch.

D. PEDICULOSIS CAPITIS

1. DESCRIPTION
   a. Most common in school-age children
   b. Lice are not responsible for the spread of human disease.
   c. Affects all socioeconomic classes
   d. Less common in African Americans—most likely related to the shape of the hair shaft
   e. Lice are not a sign of uncleanliness.
   f. Transmission in most cases is via head-to-head contact. Indirect spread, although less likely, may occur by contact with personal belongings of an infested individual.
   g. Eggs (nits) are firmly attached to the hair shaft close to the scalp.
   h. Eggs hatch in 10–14 days.

2. ASSESSMENT
   a. Pruritus
   b. Live lice on the head—grayish-white wingless insect
   c. Nits—oval in shape, whitish, firmly attached to one side of the hair close to the scalp; most often found in the hairs above the ears and in the occipital region
   d. Papules, excoriations

3. DIAGNOSTIC TESTS
   a. Inspection of the hair close to the scalp

4. MEDICAL MANAGEMENT
   a. Permethrin 1% (Nix) as prescribed
   b. Pyrethrin (RID) as prescribed
   c. Lindane (Kwell) as prescribed—reports of neurotoxicity
   d. Malathion (Ovide) as prescribed
   e. Oral ivermectin
   f. Nit removal: use of a 50% distilled white vinegar solution or formic acid solution may help loosen the nits from the hair shaft.

5. NURSING INTERVENTIONS
   a. Give the parents specific instructions for the use of the prescribed treatment.
   b. Instruct the parents to apply permethrin 1% (Nix) to clean, slightly damp hair. Leave on for 10 minutes. Rinse thoroughly.
   c. Instruct the parents that after application of the product, hair should be combed using the fine-toothed comb (included with the pediculosis product) to remove all nits and lice.
   d. Instruct the parents to wash all clothing, linens, and bedding in hot water and dry in a hot dryer.
   e. Inform the parents that nonwashable articles can be dry-cleaned or stored in plastic bags for 2 weeks.
   f. Instruct the parents to clean hairbrushes and combs with boiling water.

E. TINEA CAPITIS

1. DESCRIPTION
   a. Most common fungal infection in children
   b. Causes include dermatophytes—*Trichophyton tonsurans* (90%) or *Microsporum canis.*
   c. Occurs most frequently between ages 2 and 10
   d. More common in African American children
   e. Transmission occurs by direct contact with an infected person, a fomite, or an animal.

2. ASSESSMENT
   a. Scaling with or without hair loss
   b. Pustules
   c. Black dots—site of broken hairs
   d. Kerion: hypersensitive reaction to the fungus; boggy, moist nodules, may leave scar
   e. Lymphadenopathy
   f. Tinea corporis

3. DIAGNOSTIC TESTS
   a. Potassium hydroxide (KOH)
   b. Fungal culture
   c. Wood's lamp exam (*M. canis* fluoresces)

4. MEDICAL MANAGEMENT
   a. Topical treatments alone are ineffective—they are unable to penetrate the hair follicle.
   b. Griseofulvin: 6- to 8-week course as prescribed
   c. Terbinafine (Lamisil), itraconazole (Sporanox), or fluconazole (Diflucan) for 4 weeks as prescribed
   d. Seborrheic shampoo used daily (ketaconazole, selenium sulfide 2.5%) as prescribed
   e. Treat kerions with corticosteroids (Orapred, Pediapred, Prelone) as prescribed.

5. NURSING INTERVENTIONS
   a. Instruct the child or parents to take griseofulvin with a fatty meal; it is better absorbed.
   b. Instruct the parents to wash and disinfect linens, combs, brushes, barrettes.
   c. Reinforce need for long-term therapy as ordered.
   d. Instruct the child to continue to attend school. Provide written explanation for school.

F. TINEA CORPORIS
   1. DESCRIPTION
      a. Superficial fungal infection of the skin
      b. Asymmetrical distribution
      c. Affects all ages
      d. Causes include *Trichophyton rubrum*, *Epidermophyton floccosum*, *M. canis*, and *T. tonsurans*.
      e. Transmission is via direct contact with an infected person, soil, or animal (kittens or puppies).
   2. ASSESSMENT
      a. Annular well-circumscribed scaly patch; may have central clearing and scaly vesicular, papular, or pustular border
      b. Asymmetrical distribution of lesions
      c. Occur on nonterminal hair-bearing areas of the body
   3. DIAGNOSTIC TESTS
      a. KOH
      b. Fungal culture
   4. MEDICAL MANAGEMENT
      a. Topical medications (terbinafine cream, econazole cream, ketoconazole cream) applied twice daily for 2–3 weeks
      b. Avoid combination products (steroid and antifungal).
      c. If lesions are widespread or the client is immunocompromised and not improving with topical treatment, systemic antifungal treatment may be necessary.
   5. NURSING INTERVENTIONS
      a. Reinforce the need to continue topical medication for 5–7 days after clinical manifestations resolve.
      b. Instruct the child or parents that careful hand washing is important in preventing the spread of the infection.

G. TINEA PEDIS
   1. DESCRIPTION
      a. Dermatophyte infection of the feet
      b. More common in adolescents and adults
      c. Causes include *T. rubrum*, *Trichophyton mentagrophytes*, and *E. floccosum*.
      d. Transmission is via contact with a contaminated surface.
      e. Commonly called "athlete's foot"
   2. ASSESSMENT
      a. Scaly, erythematous, pruritic lesions between the toes
      b. Usually seen between the fourth and fifth toes
      c. May have fissuring, maceration, vesicles, and papules
      d. Erythema, scaling on the plantar surface of the foot, called "moccasin distribution"
   3. DIAGNOSTIC TESTS
      a. KOH
      b. Fungal culture
   4. MEDICAL MANAGEMENT
      a. Topical antifungal agents for 4–6 weeks
      b. If no improvement, systemic antifungal for 3–4 weeks
   5. NURSING INTERVENTIONS
      a. Instruct the adolescent to avoid tight-fitting shoes.
      b. Instruct the adolescent to keep the feet dry.
      c. Instruct the adolescent to wear cotton socks.
      d. Reinforce the need to continue medication 5–7 days after clinical manifestations resolve.

H. TINEA VERSICOLOR
   1. DESCRIPTION
      a. Most common in adolescents
      b. Cause includes *Pityrosporum ovale*.
   2. ASSESSMENT
      a. Hyper- or hypopigmented scaly reddish brown plaques
      b. Occur on face, trunk, and arms
      c. May be itchy
      d. Pigment changes persist for months.
      e. High incidence of recurrence
   3. DIAGNOSTIC TESTS
      a. KOH
      b. Fungal culture
      c. Wood's lamp examination
   4. MEDICAL MANAGEMENT
      a. Topical treatment with selenium sulfide 2.5% or ketoconazole (Nizoral) shampoo as body wash
      b. Oral ketoconazole (Nizoral) as prescribed
      c. Use topical treatment (selenium sulfide or ketaconazole shampoo) weekly after clinical manifestations resolve as prophylaxis.

5. NURSING INTERVENTIONS
   a. Instruct the adolescent that if ketoconazole (Nizoral) is prescribed, take the medicine and exercise to work up a sweat. Do not shower until the next morning.
   b. Instruct the adolescent to use topical treatment weekly to help prevent recurrence.

I. ONYCHOMYCOSIS
   1. DESCRIPTION
      a. Fungal infection of the nails
      b. Transmitted via contact with a contaminated surface or tinea pedis
      c. Affects toenails more often than fingernails
      d. Causes include *T. rubrum* and *T. mentagrophytes*.
   2. ASSESSMENT
      a. Yellowing of the nail
      b. Thickening of the nail
      c. Subungual debris
      d. Superficial opaque white scale
      e. Loss of the nail
      f. Presence of tinea pedis
   3. DIAGNOSTIC TESTS
      a. KOH
      b. Fungal culture
   4. MEDICAL MANAGEMENT
      a. Topical therapy: ciclopirox solution 8% (Loprox) as prescribed
      b. Oral antifungal therapy: itraconazole (Sporanox), terbinafine (Lamisil) as prescribed
      c. CBC and liver function tests (LFTs) should be monitored before, during, and after systemic therapy.
   5. NURSING INTERVENTIONS
      a. Instruct the child to avoid wearing tight-fitting shoes.
      b. Instruct the child to keep the feet clean and dry.
      c. Instruct the child to wear absorbent cotton socks and change frequently.
      d. Instruct the child to avoid going barefoot in public places.

J. MOLLUSCUM CONTAGIOSUM
   1. DESCRIPTION
      a. Viral infection of the skin
      b. Cause includes DNA pox virus.
      c. Most common in children less than 6 years of age
      d. No association with immunodeficiency in childhood
      e. Transmission is via person-to-person contact; autoinoculation.
      f. May resolve without treatment
   2. ASSESSMENT
      a. Flesh-colored, dome-shaped papules with central umbilication
      b. Eczema is common, called "molluscum dermatitis"

3. DIAGNOSTIC TESTS
   a. Inspection
4. MEDICAL MANAGEMENT
   a. Cantharidin: applied with a wooden applicator directly to the lesion
   b. Liquid nitrogen
   c. Tretinoin cream (Retin-A): used to treat molluscum on the face
   d. Curettage: area is numbed with a topical anesthetic and the lesions are scraped off.
   e. Imiquimod (Aldara): applied three times a week, increasing as tolerated to every day
   f. Cimetidine (Tagamet): believed to stimulate the immune system
5. NURSING INTERVENTION
   a. If lesions are treated with cantharidin, instruct the parents to wash off the medicine in 4–6 hours.
   b. Instruct the parents that a small blister usually occurs after treatment with cantharidin. When the scab falls off the lesion will be gone.
   c. Because all of the treatments may cause some discomfort, acetaminophen (Tylenol) or ibuprofen (Motrin, Advil) may be given.
   d. Instruct the parents that although molluscum is contagious, the child may attend school.

K. VERRUCA
   1. DESCRIPTION
      a. Most common in childhood
      b. Cause includes the human papilloma virus.
      c. Transmission is via direct contact, autoinoculation, or via the birth canal.
   2. ASSESSMENT
      a. Verruca vulgaris: flesh-colored verrucous papules; can occur anywhere on the body. Most common on the knees, elbows, hands, and feet
      b. Subungual/periungual: around and beneath the nail beds
      c. Filiform: on a stalk
      d. Verrucae plantaris: occur on the plantar surface of the feet. Walking may be painful.
      e. Flat warts: occur primarily on the face, neck, arms, and legs. Usually small, flat-topped, pink to brownish colored papules
      f. Condyloma: genital warts. A thorough history must be obtained from the client and the family. If there is any suspicion of sexual abuse, it must be reported to the child protection team immediately for further investigation.

3. DIAGNOSTIC TESTS
   a. Based on clinical presentation
4. MEDICAL MANAGEMENT
   a. Chemical: works by peeling away the virus from the underlying skin that is needed for growth
      1) Salicylic acid preparations: available over the counter
      2) Tretinoin cream (Retin-A): acts as a keratolytic for flat warts
      3) Podophyllin and trichlororcetic acid: used to treat condyloma; applied in the physician's office
      4) Cryotherapy: liquid nitrogen is very painful and is best used on children over 8 years of age. The wart is pared prior to application. It is applied with a cotton-tipped applicator directly to the wart. A blister may form at the site.
   b. Immunotherapy
      1) Cimetidine (Tagamet): stimulates the immune system; often used in conjunction with other therapies
      2) Squaric acid: topical immunomodulator
         a) Client is sensitized with a 2% solution that is applied with a cotton-tipped applicator to an area about the size of a quarter on the arm.
         b) One to 2 weeks after sensitization, the client begins to apply squaric acid 0.2% to the warts three times weekly, gradually increasing to nightly applications. If there is no improvement, the strength of the squaric acid may be increased up to 0.8%.
         c) This treatment is painless, the recurrence rate is low, and there are no systemic side effects.
      3) Imiquimod (Aldara): used in treatment of condyloma; applied three times weekly, gradually increasing to daily applications
   c. Laser surgery: pulsed dye laser is used to destroy the wart tissue.
      1) This treatment is painful. It requires local or general anesthesia.
      2) It usually requires multiple treatments and is very expensive.
      3) It is reserved for multiple, recalcitrant warts that have failed all other treatments.

5. NURSING INTERVENTIONS
   a. Instruct the parents that warts can be stubborn and treatment can be frustrating. Encourage patience and persistence.
   b. If podophyllin is used, instruct the parents to wash the medication off in 4–6 hours.
   c. If squaric acid is the prescribed treatment, instruct the parents to have the child wear gloves to avoid sensitization, and to apply the squaric acid with a cotton-tipped applicator directly to the warts.

L. HEMANGIOMAS
   1. DESCRIPTION
      a. Benign proliferation of blood vessels in the skin
      b. Rarely present at birth, although congenital hemangiomas can occur
      c. Most appear 1–4 weeks after birth.
      d. Grow rapidly during the first year of life, with most rapid growth between 1 and 4 months. Maximum growth is usually reached by 1 year of age.
      e. Spontaneous involution begins after 6–10 months. Area becomes gray in color and begins to soften; 50% are gone by age 5, and 90% are gone by age 12.
      f. Lesions do not always leave normal skin; atrophy, wrinkling, redundant tissue, telangiectasias, and pallor are common.
      g. More common in females than males
      h. Can occur anywhere on the body, most common sites being the head and neck
   2. ASSESSMENT
      a. Superficial hemangiomas tend to be bright red and elevated with an uneven surface. They may fluctuate in size and volume with crying or activity.
      b. Deeper hemangiomas tend to be smooth on the surface and blue in color.
      c. By history, usually not present at birth
      d. Rapid growth
      e. Involution may begin to occur within the first year of life—color changes to violaceous gray; lesion flattens, feels softer, and may fluctuate less during crying or activity.
   3. DIAGNOSTIC TESTS
      a. Inspection
   4. MEDICAL MANAGEMENT
      a. No therapy required except when certain complications occur.
         1) Life threatening or causing alteration in function
            a) Laryngeal, beard distribution: may cause respiratory distress or stridor

    b) Eyelid: may obstruct vision, cause pressure on the globe, strabismus, myopia

    c) Nasal tip: distorts underlying cartilage

  2) Ulceration: occurs in less than 5% of clients

    a) Bleeds and may leave scars

    b) May get infected; painful

b. Treatment includes the following:

  1) Topical antibiotics—ulcerated lesions

  2) Barriers and occlusive dressings

  3) Oral antibiotics—infected lesions

  4) Pulsed dye laser—ulcerated lesions

  5) Intralesional steroids—ulcerated lesions

  6) Analgesics

  7) Oral corticosteroids (Orapred, Pediapred, Prelone) slow the growth of blood vessels in hemangiomas.

    a) Used to treat ulcerated lesions as well as eyelid, nasal tip, and laryngeal hemangiomas

  8) Magnetic resonance imaging (MRI) to assess if pushing on structures, causing obstruction

  9) Direct laryngoscopy for stridor

  10) Interferon alfa or vincristine for life-threatening hemangiomas

    a) Interferon alfa causes spastic diplegia in 10–20% of clients. Close neurologic follow-up is essential.

5. NURSING INTERVENTIONS

a. Instruct the parents to give oral corticosteroid (Orapred, Prelone, Pediapred) with food.

b. Instruct the parents to measure medication carefully with a medicine cup or syringe.

c. Instruct the parents that medication should not be stopped without notifying the physician.

d. Instruct the parents to avoid exposure to people who are sick.

e. Instruct the parents that live attenuated vaccines (MMR and varicella) should not be given while the client is on oral corticosteroids and for at least 2–3 months afterward.

f. Inform the parents that blood pressure and weight will be checked at each visit, along with a physical exam by the physician.

g. Instruct the parents with a child with hemangiomas in beard distribution to watch for clinical manifestations of respiratory distress. Go to the emergency room immediately if the child develops stridor or difficulty breathing.

M. PORT-WINE STAINS

1. DESCRIPTION

a. Capillary malformation present at birth

b. Grows with the child, does not become raised

c. Composed of dilated capillary vessels

d. Darken and thicken with age (color changes to dark crimson or deep purple), may develop angiomatous papules

e. Most port-wine stains are not associated with any other problems.

f. Some facial port-wine stains may be associated with Sturge-Weber syndrome (eye and neurologic problems).

g. Some port-wine stains of the arms and legs may be associated with Klippel-Trénaunay syndrome (overgrowth of the extremity underlying the stain).

2. ASSESSMENT

a. Irregularly shaped, reddish purple macular, vascular lesion

3. DIAGNOSTIC TESTS

a. Clinical observation

4. MEDICAL MANAGEMENT

a. Treatment with pulsed dye laser

b. Treat early to prevent thickening and darkening of the stain and the development of angiomas.

5. NURSING INTERVENTIONS

a. After laser treatment, instruct the parents to keep the area moist with bacitracin.

b. Instruct the parents to prevent sun exposure to the treated area.

c. Instruct the parents to administer analgesics for pain.

N. PYOGENIC GRANULOMA

1. DESCRIPTION

a. Benign growth of blood vessels on the surface of the skin

b. Bleed profusely with trauma

c. May occur at any age

d. Cause is unknown; may occur at sites of trauma

e. Grows rapidly

2. ASSESSMENT

a. Single dull red raised nodule

b. Smooth surface; may be crusted if it has been bleeding

3. DIAGNOSTIC TESTS

a. Clinical observation

4. MEDICAL MANAGEMENT

a. Lesion is shaved off and the base is cauterized under local anesthesia.

5. NURSING INTERVENTIONS

a. Instruct the parents to keep the area dry for 24 hours.

b. Instruct the parents to apply antibiotic ointment (bacitracin, Polysporin) daily.

O. IMPETIGO
1. DESCRIPTION
   a. Highly contagious superficial skin infection
   b. Causes are group A beta-hemolytic streptococci and *Staphylococcus aureus*.
   c. Most common in infants and children
   d. Common complication following bites, varicella, eczema, and scabies
2. ASSESSMENT
   a. Bullous impetigo: begins as small red macules; may be clustered or single lesions, rapidly progressing to distinct vesicles, which may enlarge to fragile bullae. The bullae contain clear yellow to slightly cloudy fluid. Ruptured bullae may result in shiny erosions or may form a honey-colored crust.
   b. Nonbullous impetigo: small vesicles that rupture easily to expose denuded erythematous skin. A honey-colored crust forms on the surface. Superficial localized infection; may be more generalized when presents as secondary infection on diseased skin (impetiginized atopic dermatitis).
3. DIAGNOSTIC TESTS
   a. Clinical observation
4. MEDICAL MANAGEMENT
   a. Topical antibiotic therapy such as mupirocin (Bactroban)
   b. If lesions are extensive or do not respond to topical therapy, systemic antibiotics such as cephalexin (Keflex) or dicloxacillin (Dynapen)
5. NURSING INTERVENTIONS
   a. Instruct the parents to use the medication as prescribed even if the infection appears to have cleared.
   b. Inform the parents that impetigo is highly contagious and good hand washing is essential to prevent the spread of infection.

P. PSORIASIS
1. DESCRIPTION
   a. One of the most common skin problems
   b. Occurs in 1–3% of the population
   c. Affects all ages, races, genders
   d. Chronic, no cure
   e. Complex physical and emotional factors
   f. Totally unpredictable
   g. Controllable with various treatments
   h. Cause is unknown
   i. Hereditary
2. ASSESSMENT
   a. Plaque psoriasis (nummular, discoid)
      1) Single and multiple lesions
      2) Macular—papular
      3) Covered with silvery white scales
      4) Sharply delineated lesions
      5) Lesions occur at sites of trauma (Koebner phenomenon); the most common sites are the knees, elbows, and scalp.
      6) Nail pitting
   b. Guttate psoriasis
      1) Usually follows a strep infection
      2) Very small scaly plaques over the entire body
   c. Pustular psoriasis
      1) Sudden onset
      2) May be life threatening
      3) Burning erythema with pinpoint pustules
      4) Fever, generalized weakness, severe malaise
3. DIAGNOSTIC TESTS
   a. Clinical observation
4. MEDICAL MANAGEMENT
   a. Steroid ointments
   b. Tars
   c. Vitamin D ointments (Dovonex)
   d. Anthralin
   e. Topical retinoid
   f. Topical immunomodulators: tacrolimus (Protopic) and pimecrolimus (Elidel)
   g. Ultraviolet (UV) light therapy
   h. Systemic retinoids, methotrexate, and antibiotics for severe cases
5. NURSING INTERVENTIONS
   a. Instruct the parents that the child should wear protective guards when participating in sports to avoid trauma to the skin.
   b. Instruct the parents that the child should avoid wearing tight-fitting clothing and shoes.

Q. CONGENITAL NEVI
1. DESCRIPTION
   a. Tan or brown macules or plaques; may have hair growth
   b. The risk of melanoma with small to medium congenital nevi is slightly increased.
   c. Giant nevi measuring greater than 20 cm have a 2–10% risk of melanoma developing, most often between the ages of 3 and 15 years.
2. ASSESSMENT
   a. Asymmetry: if a mole is divided in half, it should be the same on both sides. Asymmetry can include color, size, shape, or surface texture.
   b. Border: not sharply delineated; blends into the area of normal skin
   c. Color: variable and includes multiple colors such as red, dark black, or blue
   d. Diameter: larger than the size of a pencil eraser (greater than 0.6 cm)

3. DIAGNOSTIC TESTS
  a. Clinical manifestations
4. MEDICAL MANAGEMENT
  a. Evaluation of changing nevi
  b. Excision
5. NURSING INTERVENTIONS
  a. Instruct the parents that the child should avoid sun exposure.
  b. Instruct the parents that the child should use sunscreen daily, including during the winter months.
  c. Encourage the parents to do frequent self-examinations and to notify the dermatologist of any changes.
  d. Instruct the parents that the child should have yearly examinations by the dermatologist.

R. SUNBURN
  1. DESCRIPTION
    a. Damage to the skin as a result of penetration of the skin by UVA and UVB rays
    b. The majority of sun damage occurs before the age of 18.
    c. Skin cancer accounts for one-half of all cancers diagnosed in the United States each year.
    d. Factors affecting sun exposure include:
      1) Time of day: sun is strongest between 11 a.m. and 3 p.m.
      2) Location: sun is most intense near the equator and at high altitudes.
      3) Weather: UV rays are strongest on clear sunny days, but clouds and fog do not totally block UVA and UVB rays.
      4) Reflectivity: sand, water, cement, roads and snow reflect the sun's rays.
      5) Skin type: people with darker skin have more natural protection from the sun.
  2. ASSESSMENT
    a. Pink to bright red areas of skin; may include vesicles
    b. Current medications: certain medications cause photosensitivity.
  3. DIAGNOSTIC TESTS
    a. Clinical observation
  4. MEDICAL MANAGEMENT
    a. Cool compresses
    b. Topical corticosteroids
    c. Ibuprofen for pain
  5. NURSING INTERVENTIONS
    a. Instruct the parents that the child should avoid sun exposure.
    b. Instruct the parents to apply sunscreen or sunblock with a sun protection factor (SPF) of 15 or greater.
    c. Instruct the parents to apply sunscreen 20–30 minutes prior to sun exposure.
    d. Instruct the parents to apply an adequate amount of sunscreen on the child. One ounce covers the average body.
    e. Instruct the parents to reapply the child's sunscreen at least every 2 hours, more often if perspiring excessively, swimming, or frequent towel drying.
    f. Instruct the parents to use waterproof sunscreen in water.
    g. Instruct the parents that infants under 6 months of age should avoid sun exposure. Sun protective clothing and a hat should be worn.

S. BURNS
  1. DESCRIPTION
    a. Fires and burns are major causes of death in children under age 18, second only to deaths from motor vehicle accidents.
    b. Burns cover a wide spectrum range, from minor local injury to a major burn with multisystem involvement.
  2. ASSESSMENT
    a. Systemic evaluation
    b. Evaluation of airway is most important. Screen for presence/possibility of airway edema.
    c. Assess level of consciousness (LOC).
    d. Immediate evaluation of eye and ear—edema may hamper evaluation later.
    e. Type of burn—classified by depth of tissue destroyed
      1) Superficial thickness (first-degree) burn: involves only the epidermis (minor sunburn)
        a) Skin is red, dry, and very painful—often deeper than appears.
        b) Heals spontaneously in about 5–10 days without scarring
        c) Rarely systemic effects
      2) Partial-thickness (second-degree) burn: epidermis and upper layers of dermis are destroyed.
        a) Skin is moist, bright red, extremely painful, and sensitive to cold air.
        b) Wide variations in depth, healing, and scar formation
        c) Commonly caused by exposure to hot liquids. Scald burns most common in children under 4 years of age
      3) Full-thickness (third-degree) burn: involves the dermis, epidermis, and subcutaneous tissue
        a) Dry, waxy, with decreased pain sensation
        b) Presence of eschar—thick leathery dead skin
        c) Most commonly caused by flame

4) Full-thickness (fourth-degree) burns: extend into the underlying subcutaneous tissues, tendons, muscles, and bone

    a) Usually caused by electrical burns or prolonged exposure to flame

    b) Result in scarring and contractures; complicated healing issues

f. Extent of burn: expressed as percentage of the total body surface area affected

  1) Mapped on body chart: the Lund and Browder chart is preferred because it accounts for changes of body proportion with growth. If unavailable, use the palm of the child's hand (represents 0.5% of body surface) to estimate the extent of the burn.

  2) Careful evaluation of the size of the burn is important in determining resuscitation, transfer decisions, and prognosis.

g. Presence of other injuries

h. Age of the client

i. Chronic health problems or social problems that may affect treatment/outcome

j. Obtain detailed history of burn—16% of burns in children are the result of child abuse.

  1) Red flags include inconsistency in history and clinical findings, unclear history of the injury, a delay in seeking treatment, and conflicting stories about how the burn occurred.

  2) Immersion burns (stocking and glove burns with a clearly demarcated line at the wrist or ankle), doughnut-shaped burns on the buttocks, and burns from a cigarette or iron are classic signs of child abuse.

  3) If child abuse is suspected, documentation must be complete and accurate and the child protection team must be notified immediately to further investigate the case.

k. If the client has major burns or those involving the hands, feet, face, eyes, ears, and genitalia, she should be stabilized and transferred to a pediatric burn unit or pediatric intensive care unit.

l. Minor burns can be treated on an outpatient basis.

3. DIAGNOSTIC TESTS

  a. Clinical observation

4. MEDICAL MANAGEMENT

  a. Respiratory management

    1) Pulmonary complications are the leading cause of death in thermal burns.

    2) Assess for patency of the airway; establish or maintain it.

    3) Airway obstruction from edema may result from burns to the client's upper body and face or smoke inhalation.

    4) Intubation may be performed for clients with face and neck edema, soot in the nose or mouth, or singed nose hairs due to increased risk of airway edema.

    5) Arterial blood gases (ABGs) to evaluate for smoke inhalation and adequacy of gas exchange

    6) Oxygen should be administered if hypoxia is present.

    7) Assess the client's ability to expand the chest. Full-thickness burns around the trunk may interfere with breathing.

    8) An escharotomy incision may be necessary to release the chest constriction and restore peripheral circulation.

  b. Fluid resuscitation

    1) Severe burns alter capillary permeability, causing fluid and electrolyte loss; requires fluid replacement to prevent hypovolemic shock.

    2) Goal: infuse intravenous fluids at a rate and volume to compensate for loss of intravascular fluids.

    3) Central venous catheter is used to deliver massive amounts of fluid (usually lactated Ringer's solution).

    4) Volume and rate of fluid administration is based on the body weight and the total body surface area burned.

    5) Fluid formula requirements: usually 2–4 ml/kg of body weight times the total body surface affected (TBSA); administration rate should be regulated by the client's response and based on various factors, including electrolyte results, level of consciousness, urine output.

    6) Success of fluid resuscitation based on:

      a) Urine output of 1–2 mL/kg/hr, measured via a foley catheter; if urine output is below this amount, fluids must be increased. If not corrected quickly, renal tubular obstruction may develop.

  b) A sudden increase in urine output indicates a capillary leak has been sealed. Intravenous fluids should be reduced to maintenance rate to prevent pulmonary edema and fluid overload.

  c) Results of electrolyte tests will determine type of fluid and rate of administration.

  d) Stable vital signs

  e) Alert and oriented mental status

c. Pain management
  1) Pain can be very severe and prolonged, compounded by procedures such as dressing changes.
  2) Fear and anxiety contribute to the child's perception of pain.
  3) Morphine sulfate is indicated for major burns.
  4) Acetaminophen with codeine is given for minor burns.
  5) Pain medication should be given prior to all procedures.
  6) Children also respond well to distraction, imagery, relaxation therapies, and hypnosis.

d. Wound care: excision and closure of full-thickness wounds to prevent wound sepsis and systemic inflammation
  1) Medicate for pain prior to any procedure.
  2) Debridement: removal of the dead tissue
    a) Soak the wound for about 10 minutes to soften the tissue.
    b) Using aseptic technique, wound is then washed with a firm circular motion from inner to outer edge.
    c) Remove loose or dead tissue by gently lifting and cutting it away.
    d) Topical antimicrobial is applied to minimize bacterial proliferation and prevent infection.
    e) Dressings are then applied.
  3) Hydrotherapy: used to soften dead tissue and improve circulation
    a) Painful and frightening— requires premedication for pain
    b) Helpful if caregivers are present to comfort and distract the client
  4) Dressings are changed once or twice a day.

e. Skin grafting: used after the wound is debrided and begins to heal
  1) Temporary grafts: homografts (cadaver skin) and heterografts (pig skin) speed wound healing by promoting growth of granulation tissue; helpful in maintaining pain control.
  2) Permanent grafts: required for extensive full-thickness burns
    a) Adequate granulation tissue must be present before permanent grafting can be done.
    b) Autograft: skin is taken from an unburned area of the client's own skin. After application, the client must be immobilized.
    c) Cultured epithelial autograft: sheets of skin are grown in the lab from a skin biopsy of the client.
  3) After the grafts heal, pressure dressings are applied to prevent formation of contractures and to minimize scarring.

f. Prevention of contractures
  1) Increased risk for developing contractures due to prolonged bed rest, muscular atrophy, and shortening and stiffening of burned tissues
  2) Range of motion should be performed three times a day.
  3) Splint application to maximize extension of joints

g. Nutritional support
  1) Child with burns: greater nutritional needs, requires two to three times the normal amount of calories to promote healing
  2) Require vitamin supplements

h. Psychological support
  1) Develop network of support that includes counselors, social workers, teachers, and community outreach groups.
  2) Caregivers need support in dealing with long-term care and family and financial issues.

5. NURSING INTERVENTIONS
  a. Develop a discharge teaching book, so that the parents will have a reference at home.
  b. Instruct the parents on nutrition and diet requirements.
  c. Instruct the parents on daily dressing changes and skin care.

d. Have the parents demonstrate the dressing changes before discharge.

e. Instruct the parents on a pain control program.

f. Set up support services and supplies for home care.

g. Arrange for nursing visits to help with dressing changes and wound evaluation.

h. Instruct the parents to watch for clinical manifestations of infection, increasing pain or anxiety associated with the wound cleansing and dressing changes, inability to carry out treatments, delayed healing, or a change in wound appearance. If any of these changes are noted, call the physician's office.

i. Stress the importance of keeping follow-up appointments to the client.

j. Instruct the parents on range-of-motion exercises. Involve physical and occupational therapy.

k. Arrange for home tutors to help the client keep current in school.

l. Encourage the child to do as many independent tasks as possible.

m. Discuss burn prevention.
  1) Working smoke detectors in the home and a planned escape route
  2) Turn pot handles inward on the stove; keep young children away from containers of hot liquids.
  3) Keep electrical cords out of reach of young children.
  4) Insert plastic plugs in electrical sockets.
  5) Cleaning solutions and caustic products should be kept out of reach of children and stored in locked cabinets.
  6) Use sunscreen and wear protective clothing to avoid excessive exposure to UV light.

PRACTICE QUESTIONS

1. Which of the following instructions should the nurse include in the teaching plan for a 16-year-old client with comedonal acne being treated with topical Retin-A?
   1. Avoid sun exposure
   2. Severe headaches may be experienced
   3. Improvement will be seen in 24 hours
   4. Scrub the skin prior to application

2. Which of the following should the nurse include in the discharge instructions for a child who had a punch biopsy done on the back?
   1. Leave the site open to air
   2. Make an appointment to have the sutures removed in 5 days
   3. Keep the site clean, dry, and covered for 24 hours
   4. Avoid physical activity

3. Which of the following should the nurse include when preparing a teaching plan for a child with atopic dermatitis regarding application of steroid ointments?
   1. Apply the steroid ointment over the emollient
   2. Apply the ointment sparingly and rub into the skin
   3. Use a large amount of the ointment
   4. Apply the steroid frequently

4. The nurse should prepare an 18-year-old adolescent with acne who has not responded to antibiotic therapy for which of the following tests prior to starting treatment with isotretinoin (Accutane)?
   1. Skin biopsy
   2. Hearing test
   3. Pregnancy test
   4. Urinalysis

5. A mother calls the pediatric office and states that her 8-year-old child is complaining of intense itching around the nape of her neck. Which of the following is the priority intervention?
   1. Inspect the child for lice or nits
   2. Cut the child's nails shorter
   3. Wash the hair with a mild shampoo
   4. Administer a topical steroid ointment

6. Which of the following should the nurse include when instructing the mother of a child with pediculosis capitis on the use of permethrin 1% (Nix)?
   1. Apply the Nix and cover the hair with a shower cap
   2. After rinsing the hair, comb to remove the nits
   3. Apply the Nix at bedtime
   4. Leave the Nix on for 8 to 14 hours

7. Following application of permethrin 5% (Elimite) for scabies, the nurse should anticipate that the pruritus will
   1. subside within 24 hours.
   2. be relieved immediately.
   3. continue for 12 hours.
   4. subside within 14 to 21 days.

8. Which of the following is a priority for the nurse to include in the plan of care for a child using a pediculocide?
   1. Apply a cream rinse following the application of the pediculocide
   2. Avoid washing the hair for two days following treatment with the pediculocide
   3. Shampoo the hair with a mild shampoo before using the pediculocide
   4. Wash the hair with a combination shampoo and conditioner before the use of a pediculocide

9. Following excision of a nevus on the arm, which of the following should the nurse include in this child's discharge instructions?
   1. Shower after 24 hours
   2. Remove the dressing after 24 hours, leaving the wound open to the air
   3. All activities may be resumed
   4. Take acetaminophen (Tylenol) for discomfort

10. The nurse should inform a child with atopic dermatitis that which of the following may cause a flare?
    1. Bathing with mild soap
    2. Moisturizing the skin
    3. Wearing cotton clothing
    4. Sudden changes in temperature

11. The parent of a child infested with scabies asks the nurse how the child got scabies. Based on the nurse's knowledge of scabies, the most likely method of contracting scabies is
    1. swimming in a pool.
    2. being in close contact with an infested individual.
    3. having contact with an infected pet.
    4. airborne.

12. Which of the following assessments does the nurse conclude supports a diagnosis of a second-degree burn?
    Select all that apply:
    [ ] 1. Skin is red and dry
    [ ] 2. Skin is moist, bright red, and extremely painful
    [ ] 3. Wide variations in depth, healing, and scar formation
    [ ] 4. Commonly caused by exposure to hot liquids
    [ ] 5. Results in scarring and contacturess
    [ ] 6. Heaaling spontaneously in about 5–10 days without scarring

13. The nurse should assess a child suspected of having tinea capitis for which of the following? Select all that apply:
    [ ] 1. Scalp scaling with alopecia
    [ ] 2. Warts on the periungual regions
    [ ] 3. Orolabial lesions
    [ ] 4. Presence of kerions
    [ ] 5. Scale and black dots
    [ ] 6. Creamy-white plaques on the buccal mucosa

14. The client with tinea capitis asks the nurse what the treatment for a kerion is. Based on the treatment of tinea capitis, the nurse replies
    1. "apply warm, moist soaks."
    2. "apply permethrin 1% (Nix)."
    3. "shave the hair."
    4. "oral corticosteroids (Orapred, Prelone, Pediapred)."

15. Which of the following should the nurse include in the medication instructions for a child with tinea capitis for whom griseofulvin (Grifulvin V, Fulvicin P/G, Grisactin) has been prescribed?
    1. Stop taking the drug when the scalp improves
    2. Take the drug on an empty stomach
    3. Take the drug with a fatty meal
    4. Take the drug at bedtime only

16. The mother of a 4-week-old infant with a small hemangioma asks the nurse if the hemangioma will get any bigger. Which of the following is the most appropriate response by the nurse?
    1. "Hemangiomas generally grow rapidly during the first year of life, followed by a gradual spontaneous involution."
    2. "The hemangioma will not grow and get any bigger."
    3. "The hemangioma will fade over time, leaving just a pink scar."
    4. "Hemangiomas gradually get smaller with each passing month of life, until there is normal skin where the hemangioma was."

17. Which of the following nursing interventions should the nurse include in the plan of care for a child with tinea pedis?
    1. Apply warm soaks to the feet
    2. Keep the feet dry
    3. Wear wool socks
    4. Administer oral steroids

18. Which of the following should the nurse include in the information given to the parents of an infant born with a port-wine stain?
    1. The port-wine stain does not grow bigger with age
    2. Most port-wine stains are the result of a medical condition
    3. Port-wine stains generally become darker and thicker with age
    4. The port-wine stain becomes raised over time

19. The nurse prepares to include which of the following in the plan of care of a child with molluscum contagiosum?
    1. Instruct the child to scratch with the knuckles instead of the fingers
    2. Instruct the parents to keep the child out of school as long as the child is contagious
    3. Administer cantharidin directly to the lesion
    4. Administer oral Prelone

20. A client with molluscum contagiosum has read on the Internet that no treatment is required and asks why the molluscum should be treated. The nurse's most appropriate response is which of the following?
    1. "It will not clear spontaneously."
    2. "It is contagious, and your child cannot attend school until the molluscum is treated."
    3. "The lesions may resolve spontaneously, but they may continue to spread."
    4. "If the lesions are not treated, they grow larger."

21. The child with molluscum contagiosum is going to be treated with cantharidin. The parents of the child ask the nurse how the cantharidin is given. The nurse's response would be which of the following?
    1. "It is injected into each lesion."
    2. "An oral tablet is given twice a day."
    3. "A wooden applicator is used to apply the cantharidin directly to each lesion."
    4. "You will receive a prescription for the topical ointment to rub on twice a day."

22. The nurse prepares a 10-year-old child who presents with a single wart on the hand for which of the following treatments?
    1. Liquid nitrogen
    2. Tagamet
    3. Aldara
    4. Retin-A

23. The parents of a 3-month-old infant who has a hemangioma on the nasal tip asks the nurse what the treatment is. Based on an understanding of hemangiomas, which of the following is the nurse's response?
    1. "Hemangiomas are generally not treated because they are never life threatening."
    2. "Liquid nitrogen is usually applied to nasal tip hemangiomas."
    3. "Surgical excision is generally performed within the first year of life."
    4. "Nasal tip hemangiomas are treated with oral corticosteroids."

24. The nurse is admitting a 4-month-old infant with an irregularly shaped reddish-purple macular vascular lesion on the face. The mother states it was present at birth. The nurse documents this as which of the following?
    1. Hemangioma
    2. Port-wine stain
    3. Congenital melanocytic nevus
    4. Pyogenic granuloma

25. The nurse should prepare a child with a pyogenic granuloma on the chin that has been bleeding for which of the following treatments?
    1. Elliptical excision
    2. Punch biopsy
    3. Shave excision and electrodessication
    4. Pulsed dye laser

26. The registered nurse is delegating nursing tasks for the day. Which of the following tasks should the nurse delegate to a licensed practical nurse?
    1. Instruct the parents of a child with a wart to wash off the podophyllin used in the treatment in 4 to 6 hours
    2. Inform the parents of a child with a hemangioma that generally no treatment is required
    3. Administer Prelone to a child with tinea capitis who has a kerion
    4. Assess and report the characteristics of a child's port-wine stain

ANSWERS AND RATIONALES

1. 1. Tretinoin (Retin-A) is a retinoid used in the treatment of acne vulgaris. An adverse reaction of topical tretinoin (Retin-A) is photosensitivity. It is important to avoid excessive sun exposure. Retin-A does not cause headaches. Improvement with use of any acne treatment usually takes 6 to 8 weeks. Scrubbing the skin prior to application irritates and inflames the skin.

2. 3. Following a punch biopsy, the area should be kept clean, dry, and covered for 24 hours to protect the wound and promote healing. No physical restrictions are necessary following a skin biopsy. Sutures should be removed in 10 to 14 days.

3. 2. Atopic dermatitis is a chronic relapsing inflammation of the dermis and epidermis. It may be referred to as "eczema" but is only one

disorder in a group of eczematous disorders. Topical corticosteroids are the most often prescribed. Steroid ointments should be applied in a thin layer and rubbed into the skin twice a day. Because the steroid cannot penetrate the emollient, it must be applied before the emollient.

4. 3. Isotretinoin (Accutane) is a retinoid used in the treatment of severe recalcitrant nodular acne that does not respond to standard therapies. It has severe teratogenic effects. Two negative pregnancy tests are required prior to starting Accutane therapy.

5. 1. The main clinical manifestation of pediculosis capitis, or head lice, is intense pruritus. Nits are commonly found on the hairs of the occipital area of the scalp.

6. 2. Permethrin 1% (Nix) is both pediculocidal and ovicidal and generally considered the treatment of choice. Nix should be applied to clean, damp hair. It should be left on for 10 minutes followed by rinsing and combing with fine-toothed comb to remove nits.

7. 4. Permethrin 5% is considered the treatment of choice for scabies. The pruritus is a hypersensitivity response to the nit and its ova and feces. Following application of Elimite, the pruritus may continue for 14 to 21 days. Emollients may help to relieve the discomfort.

8. 2. Following the use of a pediculocide for pediculosis capitis, or head lice, the hair should not be washed for 1 to 2 days. A combination shampoo and conditioner or a cream rinse should not be used before using a pediculocide.

9. 4. Following excision of a nevus, the wound should be kept dry until sutures are removed to avoid infection. Physical activity should be avoided for 2 to 4 weeks to prevent wound dehiscence.

10. 4. Atopic dermatitis is a chronic inflammation of the dermis and epidermis resulting in pruritus, erythema, edema, papules, serous discharge, and crusting. Cotton clothing, daily baths, and moisturizing are all part of the plan of care for atopic dermatitis. Sudden temperature changes can cause dryness or sweating, which may contribute to a flare.

11. 2. Scabies is an infestation of the scabies mite with *Sarcoptes scabiei* and is dependent on a human host for survival. It is transmitted by skin-to-skin contact with an infested individual. It is less likely to contract through fomites. Animals do not carry scabies. The mite can survive for 24 to 36 hours away from the host.

12. 2. 3. 4. Characteristics of second-degree burns include moist skin, bright red, and extremely painful. There are wide variations in depth, healing, and scar formation. The most common cause is exposure to hot liquids. The skin of a first-degree burn is red, dry, and heals in 5–10 days spontaneously. Third-degree burns appear waxy and dry and have a decreased pain sensation.

13. 1. 4. 5. Scalp scaling with alopecia is a clinical manifestation of tinea capitis. Kerions are moist, boggy scalp nodules. Scale and black dots may also be present. Warts on the periungual region around the nail are seen in verrucae. Orolabial lesions occur in the herpes simplex virus type 1. Creamy-white plaques on the buccal mucosa are characteristic of candidiasis.

14. 4. Oral corticosteroids (Orapred, Prelone, Pediapred) are used to treat a kerion. It is not necessary to shave the hair or apply soaks. Topical treatment is ineffective.

15. 3. Griseofulvin (Grifulvin V, Fulvicin P/G, Grisactin) is the standard treatment for tinea capitis. It is best absorbed when taken with fatty foods. Treatment generally lasts for a minimum of 8 weeks.

16. 1. Hemangiomas are benign proliferations of the blood vessels of the skin. Although rarely present at birth, most appear by 1 to 4 weeks of life. They grow rapidly during the first year of life and then have a spontaneous involution that may begin as early as 6 to 10 months. They become soft and gray. About 50% of hemangiomas are gone by age 5 years and 90% are gone by age 12 years.

17. 2. Tinea pedis is a dermatophyte infection of the feet. Because it is generally acquired from shower room floors, the feet should be kept dry. It must be treated for 4 to 6 weeks with topical antifungals. Clients should avoid tight-fitting shoes and wear cotton socks.

18. 3. A port-wine stain is a capillary malformation present at birth. It generally is not associated with any medical condition. Port-wine stains usually grow with the child, but do not become raised.

19. 3. Molluscum contagiosum is a viral infection of the skin caused by a DNA pox virus. The main feature is a flesh-colored, dome-shaped papule with central umbilication. Cantharidin is applied with a wooden applicator directly to the lesion. Although contagious, the child does not have to be kept out of school. Corticosteroids, such as Prelone, are used in the treatment of tinea capitis.

20. 3.   Molluscum contagiosum is a viral infection of the skin characterized by flesh-colored, dome-shaped papules with central umbilication. Although molluscum will eventually resolve, lesions spread easily, may become infected, may be itchy or irritated, and are sometimes cosmetically objectionable. For these reasons, they are usually treated with cantharidin applied directly to the lesion.

21. 3.   Molluscum contagiosum is a viral infection of the skin that causes flesh-colored, dome-shaped papules with central umbilication. Cantharidin is very potent and can cause significant burns if not used properly. It must be applied carefully to each lesion with a wooden applicator. This treatment is only done in the doctor's office. A prescription is never given and the drug is never administered in the home by the client.

22. 1.   Verrucae, or cutaneous warts, are benign tumors of the epidermis caused by a human papillomavirus. For a 10-year-old child with a single wart, the most likely treatment would be liquid nitrogen. Cryotherapy with liquid nitrogen is reserved for children over the age of 8 years. Tagamet is given for multiple warts and is often used in younger children who cannot tolerate liquid nitrogen. Aldara and Retin-A are used to treat flat warts on the face. In addition, Aldara is used to treat genital warts.

23. 4.   Hemangiomas are benign proliferations of the blood vessels in the skin. They are rarely present at birth. Most of them develop within 1 to 4 weeks after birth. To prevent excessive tissue growth on the nasal tip (Cyrano nose deformity) in a nasal tip hemangioma, oral corticosteroids (Prelone, Pediapred, Orapred) are given. Surgical intervention is recommended only after the hemangioma has involuted. It will continue to grow for up to 1 year of age. Some hemangiomas can be life threatening.

24. 2.   Port-wine stains are capillary malformations present at birth. They are generally irregularly shaped reddish-purple macular vascular lesions. Hemangiomas are not usually present at birth and grow rapidly during the first year of life. Congenital nevi are brown. Pyogenic granulomas are raised reddish-purple papules that bleed profusely with trauma.

25. 3.   Pyogenic granulomas are benign growths of blood vessels that can bleed profusely with trauma. Treatment is to shave the lesion and cauterize the base to prevent recurrence. A pulsed dye laser is used to destroy wart tissue.

26. 3.   Instructing, informing, and assessing are all nursing skills that are most appropriately performed by the registered nurse. A licensed practical nurse may administer a prescribed drug.

REFERENCES

Potts, N., & Mandleco, B. (2012). *Pediatric nursing: Caring for children and their families* (3rd ed.). Clifton Park, NY: Delmar Cengage Learning.

Spratto, G. R., & Woods, A. L. (2012). *PDR nurse's drug handbook 2012.* Clifton Park, NY: Delmar Cengage Learning.

CHAPTER 37

MUSCULOSKELETAL DISORDERS

I. **ANATOMY AND PHYSIOLOGY (SEE CHAPTER 9, MUSCULOSKELETAL DISORDERS, SECTION I.)**
   A. DIFFERENCE IN THE MUSCULOSKELETAL SYSTEM BETWEEN A CHILD AND AN ADULT
   1. THE CHILD'S BONES CONTAIN LARGER AMOUNTS OF CARTILAGE, MAKING THEM MORE FLEXIBLE AND MORE POROUS WHILE ALSO CAUSING THEM TO FRACTURE MORE EASILY.
   2. THE PERIOSTEUM, WHICH IS THE THIN TOUGH MEMBRANE THAT COVERS ALL BONES AND CONTAINS BLOOD VESSELS TO NOURISH THE BONES, IS STRONGER AND TOUGHER IN CHILDREN THAN IN ADULTS.
   3. THE BONES OF CHILDREN ARE ABLE TO ABSORB MORE ENERGY BEFORE BREAKING AND HEAL MORE QUICKLY.
   4. THE EPIPHYSEAL GROWTH PLATE, WHICH PLAYS AN IMPORTANT ROLE IN LONGITUDINAL BONE GROWTH, IS ONE OF THE WEAKEST POINTS OF LONG BONES, CAUSING THIS TO BE THE LOCATION OF MANY FRACTURES IN CHILDREN.
   5. TENDONS AND LIGAMENTS IN CHILDREN ARE STRONGER THAN BONE UNTIL CHILDREN REACH PUBERTY.
   6. SKULL BONES ARE NOT RIGID AT BIRTH.
      a. Sutures between the skull bones fuse during the early months.
      b. The posterior fontanel closes at 2–3 months and the anterior fontanel closes at 16–18 months.
      c. Increased intracranial pressure before fontanel closure leads to separation of the sutures, resulting in the enlargement of the infant's head.
   7. ALL MUSCLES ARE PRESENT AT BIRTH AND AS THE CHILD GROWS, THE LENGTH AND CIRCUMFERENCE INCREASE.
   8. BONE FORMATION BEGINS IN THE SECOND MONTH OF LIFE AND OSSIFICATION IS NEARLY COMPLETE AT BIRTH.
   9. THE GROWING CELLS OF THE EPIPHYSIS ARE SENSITIVE TO HORMONAL CHANGES AND NUTRITION.
   10. MATURATION AND SHAPING OF BONE IS A CONTINUOUS PROCESS THAT OCCURS UNTIL APPROXIMATELY 21 YEARS OF AGE.

II. **ASSESSMENT OF MUSCULOSKELETAL SYSTEM**
   A. HEALTH HISTORY
   1. PAST HEALTH HISTORY
   2. MEDICATIONS (PAST, PRESENT, OVER THE COUNTER [OTC], INCLUDING HERBS/LOTIONS/ OINTMENTS)
   3. ILLNESSES, INJURIES, AND SURGERIES
   4. GAIT AND POSTURE
   5. JOINT MOVEMENTS
   6. MUSCLE STRENGTH
   7. ACTIVITY LEVEL
   B. PHYSICAL EXAMINATION
   1. INSPECTION
      a. Bones and muscles: differences in alignment, contour, skin folds, length, and deformities
      b. Joints: compare bilaterally for size, discoloration, and ease of voluntary movement
      c. Head and spine: shape and symmetry of the head, muscle strength of the head and neck, alignment and symmetry of the spinal column
      d. Upper extremities
         1) Arms: alignment, muscle strength
         2) Hands: count digits, palmar creases

e. Lower extremities
   1) Hips: dislocation, subluxation, skin folds
   2) Legs: alignment, length
   3) Feet: alignment, number of toes, deformities

2. PALPATION
   a. Bones and muscles: muscle tone, muscle strength, masses, tenderness
   b. Joints: range of motion, swelling, masses, heat, or tenderness

3. AGE-APPROPRIATE MOTOR DEVELOPMENT
   a. Gross motor: muscle development continues throughout childhood (see Table 37-1).
   b. Fine motor: muscle development increased by 36 months and refined throughout school age (see Table 37-2)

III. DIAGNOSTIC STUDIES

A. RADIOGRAPHY (SEE CHAPTER 9, MUSCULOSKELETAL DISORDERS, SECTION III.)

B. COMPUTERIZED TOMOGRAPHY (CT)
   1. DESCRIPTION
      a. Sequence of x-ray films that represent a cross section of tissue at different levels
      b. Tomography allows the examination of a single layer of tissue that may be obscured by other surrounding tissue.

c. May be done with or without administration of contrasting material

2. PREPROCEDURE
   a. Explain the procedure to the child and family.
   b. Obtain written consent if required.
   c. Administer sedation if ordered.
   d. If iodine contrast dye is to be used, assess the child for allergy to iodine or shellfish.

3. POSTPROCEDURE
   a. Continue to monitor the child's condition.
   b. If contrast material was used, offer the child fluids to assist in dye excretion.
   c. Monitor the child for delayed allergic reaction to contrast material, which may occur within 2–6 hours after the test.

C. MAGNETIC RESONANCE IMAGING (MRI) (SEE CHAPTER 9 MUSCULOSKELETAL DISORDERS, SECTION III.)

D. BONE SCAN (SEE CHAPTER 9, MUSCULOSKELETAL DISORDERS, SECTION III.)

Table 37-1 Summary of Gross Motor Development

Age	Motor Skill
2–3 months	Some head lag when pulled to sitting position
	Holds head up and supports weight on forearms when prone
	Some head bobbing while supported in sitting position
	Rolls from abdomen to back
	Tonic neck and Moro reflexes disappearing
4–6 months	Good head control with no head lag, holds chest and abdomen up with weight supported by hands while prone
	Sits with support
	Rolls from back to abdomen
	Bears weight in standing position with support
7–8 months	Sits alone without support
	Bears weight with some support
9–12 months	Moves from prone to sitting to standing position without assistance
	Stands alone without support
	Goes from crawling to creeping to cruising
	Attempts to walk alone

© Cengage Learning 2015

Table 37-2 Summary of Fine Motor Development

Age	Motor Skill
2–3 months	Follows object past midline
	Holds hands open
	Regards own hands and fingers when held in front of face
	Places hand in mouth
	Briefly reaches at a dangling object
4–5 months	Reaches for object beyond grasp
	Looks from object to hand and back again
	Places object in mouth
	Uses whole hand to grasp object
	Plays actively with hands and feet
6–7 months	Holds objects securely and bangs them together
	Actively drops objects
	Transfers object between hands
8–9 months	Pincer grasp beginning
	Releases object at will
	Dominant hand preference emerging
10–12 months	True pincer grasp present
	Can self-feed finger foods
	Can place small objects into a container
	Can remove small objects from a container
	Can hold and mark with a crayon
	Can turn multiple pages in a book

© Cengage Learning 2015

E. ELECTROMYOGRAPHY
1. DESCRIPTION
   a. The placement of a recording electrode into skeletal muscle for the purpose of monitoring electrical activity in skeletal muscle
   b. Used to assess muscle weakness and spontaneous muscle movement
2. PREPROCEDURE
   a. Explain the procedure to the child and family.
   b. Obtain written consent if required.
   c. Administer sedation if ordered.
3. POSTPROCEDURE
   a. Observe the intravenous injection site for redness or swelling.
   b. Provide pain medication if needed.
F. ELECTRONEUROGRAPHY (NERVE CONDUCTION STUDIES)
1. DESCRIPTION
   a. Initiation of an electrical impulse at the proximal end of the nerve and the recording of time required for that impulse to travel to the distal end of the same nerve
   b. Used to identify peripheral nerve injury in clients with noted weakness and to differentiate peripheral nerve disease from muscular injury
2. PREPROCEDURE
   a. Explain the procedure to the child and family.
   b. Obtain written consent if required.
   c. Administer sedation if ordered.
3. POSTPROCEDURE
   a. Provide skin care at the site of electrode placement.
   b. Provide pain medication if indicated.

IV. NURSING DIAGNOSES
A. RISK FOR PERIPHERAL NEUROVASCULAR DYSFUNCTION (FRACTURES)
B. ACUTE PAIN
C. RISK FOR IMPAIRED SKIN INTEGRITY
D. IMPAIRED PHYSICAL MOBILITY
E. DISTURBED BODY IMAGE
F. INEFFECTIVE HEALTH MAINTENANCE

Nursing Diagnoses: Definitions and Classification 2012–2014. Copyright © 2012, 1994–2012 by NANDA International. Used by arrangement with John Wiley & Sons Limited.

V. IMMOBILITY DEVICES
A. CASTS AND BRACES
1. PURPOSE
   a. Hold bones immobile during healing
   b. Protect from injury after injury or surgery
2. PLASTER CASTS
   a. Most commonly used because they are less expensive
   b. Mold well to body parts and have a smooth exterior
   c. Heavy and bulky; must be kept dry and have a long drying time
3. SYNTHETIC (FIBERGLASS) CASTS
   a. Lightweight, less bulky, fast drying, and may tolerate immersion
   b. More expensive than plaster, less able to mold easily (especially on small body parts), and have a rough exterior
4. TYPES OF CASTS
   a. Long and short leg casts
   b. Long and short arm casts
   c. Hip spica casts and shoulder spica casts (See Chapter 9, Musculoskeletal Disorders, Section V.)
5. NURSING CARE
   a. Nursing care of clients with casts or splints should include regular neurovascular checks (see Table 37-3).
   b. Educate families on how to care for the child with a cast at home before discharge (see Table 37-4).
B. TRACTION
1. PURPOSE OF TRACTION
   a. Realign bone fragments
   b. Provide rest for an extremity
   c. Prevent or improve contracture deformity
   d. Correct a deformity
   e. Treat a dislocation
   f. Allow preoperative and postoperative positioning and alignment
   g. Provide for immobilization of a body part
   h. Reduce muscle spasms
2. TYPES OF TRACTION
   a. Manual: applied to a body part by the hand placed distal to the injury
   b. Skin traction: pull is applied with adhesive material or elastic to the skin surface and indirectly to the skeletal structures.
   c. Skeletal traction: pull is applied directly to the skeletal structure by a pin, wire, or tongs inserted into or through the diameter of the bone distal to the fracture.
3. SITES OF TRACTION USE
   a. Skin traction: Buck extension (lower extremity), Bryant's traction (lower extremity), Russell traction (lower extremity), and cervical traction (head and neck)
   b. Skeletal traction: Crutchfield tongs (head), balanced suspension (lower extremity), 90/90 femoral traction (lower extremity), Dunlop or sidearm traction (upper extremity) (See Chapter 9, Musculoskeletal Disorders, Section V.)

Table 37-3 Assessment of Neurovascular Status

Technique	Normal	Abnormal
Pain Assess using behavioral and physiological cues and age-appropriate rating scales.	Some pain is normal after an injury or surgery.	Excessive or increasing pain, especially with passive motion or unrelieved with analgesia may indicate neurovascular compromise.
Skin Color Inspect area distal to the injury.	No change in color compared with unaffected extremity	Pallor, cyanotic, or dusky
Pulses Palpate pulses distal to the injury or immobilizing device if possible.	Pulses are strong; no different in affected and unaffected extremity.	Weak or absent pulse (pulselessness)
Sensation Ask the child if numbness or tingling is present. Touch the fingers or toes of the affected and unaffected extremity, especially the web space between the thumb and index finger and between the first and second toes.	No difference in sensation in both extremities	Numbness or tingling (paresthesia); decreased sensation
Motion Ask the child to move the fingers or toes of the affected extremity.	Able to move fingers or toes of affected extremity	Unable to move fingers or toes of the affected extremity; paralysis
Skin Temperature Palpate the extremity (the back of the hand is most sensitive to temperature).	Skin is warm or comparable to unaffected extremity.	Cool or cold (may be caused by cool environment; if so, apply a blanket to the extremity, then reassess)
Capillary Refill Press each nail bed and note the time until color returns.	Returns to usual color in less than 3 seconds	Returns to usual color in more than 3 seconds

© Cengage Learning 2015

Table 37-4 Home Care for the Child with a Cast

1. After application of a plaster cast, let it dry thoroughly. This will take from 24 to 48 hours. Handle the cast gently. Use the palms of the hands to pick up the cast to prevent dents. Use of a fan or cool-air hair dryer will facilitate drying.
2. Elevate the cast on a pillow above the level of the heart to reduce swelling and improve circulation.
3. Do not hit or bang the cast, as this may damage the cast or cause reinjury.
4. Avoid getting plaster casts wet. Plastic wrap or a plastic bag can be used to protect the cast from moisture during bathing.
5. "Petal" the edges with moleskin or adhesive tape to protect the child's skin from rough and irritating edges. The edges are rounded with scissors, and each of these "petals" is placed over the edge of the cast, with each slightly overlapping the previous one to form a smooth, finished edge. "Petaling" the cast around the edges, especially the groin and perineum, will protect it from urine and stool.
6. Do not allow the child to push small or sharp objects under the cast, such as a pencil, pen, or small game piece, as these may injure the skin.
7. Assess neurovascular status frequently on the extremity distal to the cast.
8. For itching, a hair dryer set on a cool setting can be used to blow air into the cast. An antihistamine can be used if the itching is bothersome.
9. Report any foul-smelling odors, excessive swelling, bleeding, or excessive pain to the health care provider. The odor may indicate infection or skin breakdown. Bleeding, excessive pain, or swelling indicate problems and are not to be ignored.
10. Report any slippage, cracking, softness, or looseness of cast to the health care provider.

© Cengage Learning 2015

VI. MUSCULOSKELETAL DYSFUNCTION

A. CLUBFOOT

1. DESCRIPTION
   a. Congenital anomaly of the foot and lower leg with rotation at the ankle caused by abnormal bone and soft tissue structure
   b. Incidence is 1.5 per 1000 live births.
   c. Can be unilateral (most common) or bilateral
   d. Males are affected twice as often as females.
   e. Caused by arrested fetal development in utero
   f. Genetic predisposition

2. ASSESSMENT
   a. Affected foot is rotated, rigid, fixed, and difficult to move.
   b. Types of clubfoot:
      1) Varus (inward rotation) or valgus (outward rotation)
      2) Calcaneous (upward rotation) or equinus (downward rotation)
      3) Most common (95%) is talipes equinovarus, with inward and downward rotation

3. DIAGNOSTIC TESTS
   a. Diagnosis is made by visual inspection and confirmed by radiographs.
   b. Magnetic resonance imaging (MRI) may be used in further diagnosis.

4. MEDICAL MANAGEMENT
   a. Exercises
   b. Serial cast changes to change the angle of the foot
   c. Splint (with shoes attached to metal bar) to hold correct angle of the foot
   d. Surgery with casting

5. NURSING INTERVENTIONS
   a. Support and educate the family about the condition.
   b. Provide or teach the family passive exercises on the affected foot.
   c. Provide or teach the family about a cast or brace for the affected foot.

B. DEVELOPMENTAL DYSPLASIA OF THE HIP (DDH)

1. DESCRIPTION
   a. Femoral head is not properly placed in the acetabulum at birth.
   b. Congenital disorder, although it is not always diagnosed at birth
   c. Occurs in 1 to 1.5 live births per 1000 and affects females more than males (6:1 ratio)
   d. Cause is unknown; however, it may be associated with family history, breech or knee prenatal position, ligament laxity, small uterine size, postnatal positioning (swaddling).

2. ASSESSMENT
   a. May be unilateral or bilateral, partial or complete
   b. Asymmetry of thigh and gluteal folds
   c. Limited abduction of the hip
   d. Barlow's sign (apparent shortening of femur): with the infant on his back, bend the knees and the affected knee will be lower because the head of the femur dislocates and lowers in this position.
   e. Positive Ortolani's sign: with the infant supine, flex the knees and hips to 90 degrees; while placing the middle finger over the greater trochanter, abduct the hips, and listen for a clicking sound.
   f. Trendelenburg test (for walking child): when standing on the affected leg, the pelvis will dip on the normal side.

3. DIAGNOSTIC TESTS
   a. Positive Barlow or Ortolani test
   b. Confirmation is made by radiographs.

4. MEDICAL MANAGEMENT
   a. Goal is to deepen the hip socket in order to stabilize the joint.
   b. Surgery (open reduction) is followed by a hip spica cast.

5. NURSING INTERVENTIONS
   a. Maintain or provide teaching for parents to maintain the hip in the proper flexed abducted position by triple diapering, splints, harness, casts, or braces for 24 hours each day by using the Pavlik harness.
   b. Adapt feeding and care to the immobilized child.
   c. Provide developmental stimulation in all ways except in hip and leg mobility.
   d. Assess neurovascular status.

C. OSTEOGENESIS IMPERFECTA (OI)

1. DESCRIPTION
   a. Inherited disease (autosomal dominant) of connective tissue
   b. Characterized by fragile bones that break easily caused by poor collagen formation
   c. Fractures may result from trauma or normal daily activities.
   d. Other manifestations may include deafness, dental deformities, blue sclera, hyperlaxity of ligaments, and short stature.
   e. Types of OI:
      1) OI congenital, which is autosomal recessive (poor prognosis)
      2) OI retarda, which is autosomal dominant and is less severe in form

2. ASSESSMENT
   a. OI congenital may have multiple fractures at birth, skeletal deformity, soft skull bones, and possible intracranial hemorrhage.
   b. OI retarda may have delayed walking, fractures, scoliosis, hypermobility of joints, and dental caries.
3. MEDICAL MANAGEMENT
   a. Early intervention of fractures and prevention of deformities using splints, braces, casts, or surgery
   b. Surgery may include insertion of rods into long bones to prevent fractures.
   c. Allow for long healing time to promote remineralization of bones.
4. NURSING INTERVENTIONS
   a. Educate the caregivers about care of splints, braces, or casts at home.
   b. Perform and teach the caregivers to do neurovascular checks.
   c. Provide and teach the caregivers about a diet high in vitamins and minerals.
   d. Educate the caregivers about promoting growth and development within the child's limitations.
   e. Educate the parents about injury prevention.
D. FRACTURES
   1. DESCRIPTION
      a. Most common musculoskeletal injury in childhood
      b. Incidence peaks between ages 6 and 16 years for both sexes.
      c. A break or interruption in bone structure is caused by placing more stress on a bone than it can absorb.
      d. Early diagnosis and treatment are necessary to avoid complications.
   2. TYPES OF FRACTURES
      a. Closed or simple
      b. Open or compound
      c. Transverse
      d. Oblique
      e. Spiral
      f. Greenstick
   3. ASSESSMENT
      a. Pain
      b. Tenderness
      c. Edema
      d. Decreased range of motion
      e. Deformity
      f. Bruising
      g. Muscle spasms
      h. Crepitus
   4. DIAGNOSTIC TESTS
      a. Radiography

   b. Be alert to signs of child abuse:
      1) History inconsistent with injury or developmental stage
      2) Multiple fractures in various stages of healing
      3) Spiral fractures of the leg when the child is not yet walking
      4) Multiple or depressed skull fractures
5. MEDICAL MANAGEMENT
   a. Realign bone fragments:
      1) Closed reduction occurs when the alignment is done by manual manipulation or traction.
      2) Open reduction occurs when the alignment is done surgically with wires, pins, screws, or plates.
   b. Immobilize realigned fracture for duration of healing with casts, traction, or splints.
6. NURSING INTERVENTIONS
   a. Perform neurovascular checks.
   b. Provide cast, traction, or splint care or teach caregivers to do care.
   c. Provide necessary interventions for any physiological effects of immobilization that are evident (see Table 37-5).
   d. Observe the child for complications of the fracture such as nerve or vascular injury, infection, malunion, or nonunion.
   e. For fracture involving the growth plate of long bones, observe for or teach caregivers to observe for limb length discrepancy.
   f. Observe for compartment syndrome:
      1) Deep pain that is unrelieved by analgesics
      2) Caused by swelling or bleeding, or both, within a fibrous covering that surrounds groups of muscles and nerves
   g. Observe for signs of pulmonary embolism.
E. SPORTS INJURIES
   1. DESCRIPTION
      a. Injuries sustained in recreational and sporting events that involve any part of the body, ranging from minor injury such as cuts, bruises, and abrasions to serious central nervous system injury or death
      b. Acute trauma is a sudden, acute injury from a major force and includes fractures to the long bones and the axial skeleton, sprains of joint ligaments, strains of muscle tendons, and contusions.

Table 37-5 Physiological Effects of Immobilization and Nursing Interventions

Body System	Clinical Manifestations	Nursing Interventions
Respiratory	Decreased lung expansion Weakness of respiratory muscles Stasis of secretions Increased potential for pneumonia and atelectasis	Frequent repositioning Turn, cough, and deep breathing Incentive spirometer
Cardiovascular	Increased venous stasis Decreased cardiac output and circulatory fluid volume Formation of thrombus Potential for pulmonary emboli	Passive and active range-of-motion (ROM) exercises Antiembolism stockings Mobilize child as soon as possible.
Musculoskeletal	Decreased muscle strength and mass Atrophy of muscle Decreased bone density Joint contractures Footdrop	Passive and active ROM exercises Foot support
Gastrointestinal	Constipation Anorexia	Increased intake of fiber and fluids Stool softeners and rectal suppositories as ordered Small frequent meals Encourage family to bring child's favorite foods.
Urinary	Decreased urine output Increased urine concentration Retention of urine Renal calculi Urinary tract infection	Increased fluid intake Maintain acidic urine with cranberry juice. Monitor intake and output. Monitor urine concentration.
Integumentary	Skin breakdown Pressure ulcers	Frequent repositioning Keep skin clean and dry. Use pressure-reducing devices, such as sheepskin.

© Cengage Learning 2015

c. Microtrauma is repetitive injury to tissue over a long period of time and includes stress fractures, bursitis, tendonitis, and trauma to joint surfaces.

d. Of sports injuries, 95% occur in soft tissues.

e. Types of injuries:

  1) Contusions are damage to the soft tissues, subcutaneous structures, and muscles.

  2) Dislocations occur when the force of stress on a ligament causes displacement of the bone ends or the bone end into a socket.

  3) Sprains occur when trauma to a joint causes a ligament to stretch or become partially or completely torn by the force created on the joint itself.

  4) Strains are caused by microscopic tears to the musculotendinous space.

  5) Overuse syndrome occurs with repetitive microtrauma to a particular anatomic structure, including structures such as the bursae, tendons, muscles, ligaments, joints, and bones.

2. ASSESSMENT

  a. Swelling, redness, bruising, bulges, and soft tissue damage

  b. Pain, change in range of motion and mobility, and asymmetry of all joints and extremities

  c. Popping, burning, tearing, looseness of any joint, bone, or soft tissue

3. DIAGNOSTIC TESTS

  a. Radiography

  b. MRI

  c. Bone scan

4. MEDICAL MANAGEMENT

  a. Diagnosis is critical in the early stages of the injury.

b. Immobility devices such as harnesses, braces, splints, and casts may be used to stabilize the affected area.

c. Fractures and some dislocations may require surgical procedures.

5. NURSING INTERVENTIONS
   a. Apply ice for the first 6–12 hours.
   b. Maintain compression, elevation, and support.
   c. Maintain ice, compression, elevation, and support (ICES) and rest, ice, compression, and elevation (RICE).
   d. Educate the parents on the correct procedures for cast and immobility devices care, including neurovascular checks.
   e. Support and assist with age-appropriate diversional activities that promote bed rest and the healing process.
   f. Encourage follow-up visits to monitor the healing process.

F. LEGG-CALVE-PERTHES (LCP) DISEASE
   1. DESCRIPTION
      a. Disturbance of circulation to the femoral capital epiphysis that causes an ischemic, aseptic necrosis of the femoral head
      b. Incidence is predominant in Caucasian males 4–8 years of age (range is 2–12 years): 1 in 12,000 children.
      c. The cause is unknown but may be familial predisposition, trauma, inflammation, or coagulation defects.
   2. ASSESSMENT
      a. Mild pain in the hip and anterior thigh
      b. Limp aggravated by increased activity and relieved by rest
      c. Stiffness in the morning or after rest
      d. Progressive stages may have limited ROM, weakness, muscle wasting, shortening of affected limb, and positive Trendelenburg sign.
   3. DIAGNOSTIC EVALUATION
      a. Radiographs
      b. Bone scan
   4. MEDICAL MANAGEMENT
      a. Goal of treatment is to keep the femoral head in the acetabulum.
      b. Bed rest and use of abduction traction to reduce pain and improve range of motion
      c. Immobility devices such as a brace, harness, traction, casting, or surgery may be used during the healing process.
   5. NURSING INTERVENTIONS
      a. Promote rest to decrease inflammation.

b. Avoid weight bearing on the lower extremities.

c. Assist in selecting age-appropriate developmental activities.

d. Provide appropriate preoperative and postoperative care, if needed, including neurovascular checks, pain management, and appropriate activity.

G. SLIPPED CAPITAL FEMORAL EPIPHYSIS (SCFE)
   1. DESCRIPTION
      a. The upper femoral epiphysis gradually slips from its functional position.
      b. Incidence is greatest during growth spurt of adolescence (11–14 years for females and 13–16 years for males).
      c. Prevalence is most common in African Americans and obese males.
   2. ASSESSMENT
      a. Persistent aching to mild pain in the hip that may be referred to the thigh and knee
      b. Decreased ROM and internal rotation of the hip
      c. Gait may show an external rotation of the hip and leg to relieve stress and pain in the hip joint.
   3. DIAGNOSTIC TESTS
      a. Radiographs
   4. MEDICAL MANAGEMENT
      a. Stabilization of the femoral head via pinning or open reduction surgical correction, or both
   5. NURSING INTERVENTIONS
      a. Prepare the child and family for the surgical procedure, including the possibility of pinning and external fixation of the femoral head.
      b. Maintain strict bed rest with non-weight-bearing activity.
      c. Assist with selection of age-appropriate diversional activities.
      d. Provide postoperative care for immobilized extremity, neurovascular checks, and pain management.
      e. Provide postoperative education, including nutrition for healing, ambulation and weight-bearing activities, restricted contact sports, and follow-up visits for close monitoring of closure of the epiphyseal plates.

H. SPINAL DEFORMATION
   1. DESCRIPTION
      a. Curvature of the spine with vertebral body malalignment
      b. Types of spinal curvature:
         1) Kyphosis is an increased posterior convex angle in the curvature of the thoracic spine.

2) Lordosis is an increased anterior curvature of the lumbar spine.

3) Scoliosis is an increased lateral curvature of the spine with vertebral body rotation.

  c. Incidence of scoliosis is 100 out of 1000 children and is greater in males than females; however, more females progress to need for treatment.

  d. Scoliosis occurs most often during the growth spurt of adolescence (11–14 years for females; 13–16 years for males).

2. ASSESSMENT

  a. Painless, slower progression in the early stages

  b. Unequal shoulder and hip level with prominence of one scapula or a curved spinal column and asymmetry of the trunk are visible on inspection.

  c. Begin screening in the late school-age years (4th or 5th grade).

3. DIAGNOSTIC TESTS

  a. Routine physical examination

  b. Radiographs

4. MEDICAL MANAGEMENT

  a. Treatment involves observation, bracing, or surgery.

  b. Periodic evaluation, including radiographs, is suggested for children with an immature skeletal system.

  c. For therapy that includes bracing, the most common used are the Boston brace, TLSO custom-molded jacket, and the Milwaukee brace.

5. SURGICAL MANAGEMENT

  a. For curvatures greater than 40 degrees, surgery for placement of rods, screws, and wires next to the spinal curvature; spinal fusion; or both may be necessary.

  b. In some cases, halo traction may be used postoperatively to stabilize the spine.

6. NURSING INTERVENTIONS

  a. Educate the child and family about the importance of periodic evaluation (every 3–6 months) during the rapid growth period.

  b. Educate the child and family about the use of immobility devices such as braces and harnesses.

  c. Preoperatively, educate the child about deep breathing, coughing, and turning and use of the incentive spirometry.

  d. Educate the child and family about postoperative pain management, use of special nutritional intake such as a nasogastric (NG) tube, ROM exercises, and possible stay in an intensive care unit (ICU).

  e. Assist with postoperative care activities, including ROM exercises, log rolling, neurovascular checks, pain management, pulmonary hygiene (pulmonary toilet), antibiotic administration, and antiembolism stockings.

  f. Prepare the child and family for discharge by teaching appropriate posture, mobility, and activity restrictions.

  g. Encourage the child and family to comply with periodic follow-up visits.

  h. Assist and promote age-appropriate diversional activities.

I. OSTEOMYELITIS

1. DESCRIPTION

  a. Infection of the bone caused by bacteria, virus, or fungus and includes the entire bone

  b. Incidence is most common in children 3–12 years of age and males are affected two to four times more often than females.

2. ASSESSMENT

  a. Check for history of trauma to the bone as well as past infections in any area of the body.

  b. Malaise, fever, irritability, rapid pulse, and possible dehydration

  c. Pain, tenderness, swelling, and redness at the bone site

  d. Decreased mobility of the affected extremity

3. DIAGNOSTIC TESTS

  a. White blood cell (WBC) count, C-reactive protein, sedimentation rate, and positive blood cultures

  b. Radiographs may reveal bone changes 5–10 days after the beginning of the infection.

  c. Computed tomography (CT) scan

4. MEDICAL MANAGEMENT

  a. Limitation of weight bearing on the affected extremity.

  b. Intravenous antibiotics for 3 to 6 weeks followed by 2 weeks of oral antibiotic therapy

  c. Surgery is indicated if the infection site needs an incision and drainage.

5. NURSING INTERVENTIONS

  a. Provide age-appropriate diversional activities to maintain activity restrictions.

  b. Provide routine intravenous and wound site care.

c. Administer antibiotic therapy as indicated by the physician.

d. Promote healing through education on food sources high in calcium and protein.

e. Prepare the child and family for discharge by teaching appropriate antibiotic administration, activity, and diversional activities at home.

J. JUVENILE RHEUMATOID ARTHRITIS (JRA)

1. DESCRIPTION

a. Chronic autoimmune inflammatory disease of the connective tissue

b. Incidence is 1 in 1000 children, with Native Americans being the population most affected.

c. Of children affected by JRA, 10% become adults with moderate to significant functional impairments.

d. The peak age of onset is 2–4 years (most common in girls) and 10–12 years (most common in boys). Overall, females are affected 2:1 over males.

2. ASSESSMENT

a. Morning immobility

b. Stiffness

c. Joint pain

3. DIAGNOSTIC TESTS

a. No specific tests are done; however, blood work is monitored for elevated erythrocyte sedimentation rate (ESR), elevated C-reactive protein (CRP), elevated WBC count, decreased hemoglobin, and increased platelet count.

b. Antinuclear antibody (ANA) and rheumatoid factor (RF) are monitored.

c. Radiographs may be used to monitor changes in soft tissues and joints.

4. MEDICAL MANAGEMENT

a. Goal is to decrease inflammation, maintain joint function, and promote normal physiological and psychosocial development.

b. Treatment may include medications, physical and occupational therapy, as well as health teaching.

c. Common medication therapy includes nonsteroidal anti-inflammatories, slow-acting anti-rheumatic drugs, corticosteriods, or small doses of chemotherapy drugs such as methotrexate.

5. NURSING INTERVENTIONS

a. Support the medical regimen, including medication administration and teaching.

b. Assist the child with appropriate level of mobility and activity.

c. Promote developmental health with age-appropriate diversional activities.

K. MUSCULAR DYSTROPHY

1. DESCRIPTION

a. Group of progressive degenerative inherited disorders that cause muscle wasting

b. Composed of disorders of various types, ages of onset, and inheritance patterns

c. Duchenne muscular dystrophy (DMD) is the most common, with an onset at 3–6 years and an X-linked recessive inheritance pattern.

d. DMD occurs in 0.3 in 1000 live male births (females may be carriers only).

e. Pathophysiology includes an absence of the muscle protein dysprophin, which leads to degeneration of the skeletal or voluntary muscles that control movement.

2. ASSESSMENT

a. Normal early motor development with clinical manifestations becoming apparent or acute at 2–4 years of age

b. Initial clinical manifestations (due to weakening of pelvic muscles) include waddling gait and difficulty climbing stairs, running, or riding a bicycle.

c. At 5–6 years, the seated child with DMD must use his hands to walk up the legs to achieve the standing position (Gowers' sign).

d. As the disease progresses, the shoulder, arm, and leg muscles become more involved so that by 9–12 years, most boys are confined to a wheelchair.

e. Muscles may appear enlarged and feel woody on palpation (pseudohypertrophy).

f. Atrophy of muscles may lead to scoliosis or fractures, or both.

g. Later stages include respiratory muscle involvement and cardiomyopathy, which may lead to death in the late teens or early 20s.

3. DIAGNOSTIC TESTS

a. Observation of clinical manifestations

b. Muscle biopsy reveals replacement of normal muscle with connective and fatty tissue.

c. Electromyogram (EMG) reveals decreased electrical impulses on placement of an electrode in the muscle.

d. Nerve conduction velocity (NCV)

e. Blood enzymes are usually elevated because enzymes leak from the muscles.

4. MEDICAL MANAGEMENT
   a. Use supportive treatment to prevent complications because there is no cure.
   b. Use a team approach to incorporate caregivers, physician, nurse, physical therapist, occupational therapist, and social worker.
   c. Assist the child to achieve maximum level of functioning within the confines of the degenerative process.
   d. Splinting and bracing may be used to assist in lower extremity stability and to avoid contractures.
   e. Surgery may be performed to treat contractures.
5. NURSING INTERVENTIONS
   a. Organize or work with the health care team.

   b. Monitor respiratory or cardiac status frequently.
   c. Promote mobility without increasing muscular stress with water exercises.
   d. Diversional activities such as books, tapes, and computers may be used to promote development as much as possible.
   e. In later stages, administer good skin care, ensure adequate hydration and nutrition, prevent constipation, and assess and prevent heart and lung complications as much as possible.
   f. Families should be referred for genetic counseling or support, or both, from local agencies or support groups.

PRACTICE QUESTIONS

1. The parents of a 4-year-old child whose femur is fractured at the growth plate ask the nurse what type of fracture this is. Based on an understanding of the growth plate, the nurse should respond, "The growth plates
   1. serve no function after birth."
   2. are found in every bone in the body."
   3. serve to produce red blood cells."
   4. control the growth of long bones."

2. The nurse completes an orthopedic assessment of a 6-year-old child who has a new cast applied for a fractured radius. Which of the following clinical manifestations is a priority for the nurse to report immediately to the physician?
   1. Skin around the cast is warm
   2. The child states that hand feels "asleep"
   3. Edema in fingers that lessens with elevation
   4. Capillary refill of 3 seconds in affected hand

3. The nurse is told in a report that an infant has talipes equinovarus. In doing the physical assessment of this infant, the nurse would expect to find which of the following?
   1. Asymmetry of gluteal and thigh skin folds
   2. One foot is rotated upward slightly, but the foot is easily moved to a normal position
   3. One foot is rotated in and down and is fixed and difficult to move
   4. One knee is lower when flexing both legs

4. While assessing a newborn infant for developmental hip dysplasia (DDH), the nurse evaluates which of the following signs as indicating the presence of DDH?
   1. One knee is lower when both legs are flexed
   2. Thigh and gluteal skin folds are symmetrical
   3. Hip adduction of affected side is limited
   4. Negative Ortolani sign when hips are abducted

5. The nurse evaluates the musculoskeletal systems of children to be different from adults in which of the following ways?
   1. Tendons and ligaments are weaker in children until puberty
   2. The periosteum is not as strong in children
   3. The bones of children are less porous and dense than adult bones
   4. The skull bones are not rigid or fused at birth

6. While caring for a 4-year-old child with a fractured femur in skeletal traction, the nurse notes that the child is crying with pain and the foot of the affected leg is pale and pulseless. Which of the following nursing actions is a priority?
   1. Remove the weight from the traction
   2. Notify the physician of the changes noted
   3. Give the child a prescribed analgesic
   4. Document the observations and check the extremity in 15 minutes

7. The nurse is caring for a child with a new full-leg cast. Which of the following is an appropriate nursing intervention for this client?
   1. Avoid changing the child's position for 24 hours after application of the cast
   2. Handle the cast with the tips of the fingers
   3. Avoid elevating the casted extremity until the cast is completely dry
   4. Make sure that all cast edges are smooth and free of irritating projections

8. When providing information about osteogenesis imperfecta (OI) to the parents of a newly diagnosed child, the nurse should include which of the following information about the disorder?
   1. It is an inherited disease of the connective tissue
   2. When treated early, it is easily controlled
   3. With later onset, the disease usually runs a more difficult course than with early onset
   4. Braces and splints are not of therapeutic value for this condition

9. While teaching 9- and 10-year-old children about safety measures to prevent injuries, the school nurse considers which of the following as the priority influence in the risk-taking behavior in this age group?
   1. Concrete thinking patterns
   2. The lack of a well-developed identity
   3. Inadequate rule enforcement
   4. Pressure from peers

10. When caring for a 4-year-old child whose left leg is in traction, the nurse notices that the traction weights are resting on the floor at the foot of the bed. What is the best action that the nurse should take in this situation?
    1. Elevate the foot of the bed
    2. Lower the head of the bed
    3. Cut the ropes to make them shorter
    4. Pull the child up in the bed

11. A mother of an infant asks the nurse when the anterior fontanel usually closes. The most appropriate response by the nurse is
    1. 6 months.
    2. 12 months.
    3. 18 months.
    4. 24 months.

12. The nurse assesses which of the following to be gross motor developments of a 4- to 6-month-old?
    [ ] 1. Holds chest and abdomen up with weight supported by hands while prone
    [ ] 2. Sits alone without support
    [ ] 3. Goes from crawling to creeping to cruising
    [ ] 4. Rolls from back to abdomen
    [ ] 5. Good head control with no head lag
    [ ] 6. Holds head up and supports weight on forearms when prone

13. The nurse should assess a child admitted with a diagnosis of slipped capital femoral epiphysis for which of the following additional health problems?
    1. Emaciated appearance
    2. Nutritional anemia
    3. Developmental delays
    4. Obesity

14. The nurse should assess a teenage child suspected of having early stage scoliosis for which of the following clinical manifestations?
    Select all that apply:
    [ ] 1. Unequal shoulder level
    [ ] 2. Curved spinal column
    [ ] 3. Altered gait with a limp
    [ ] 4. Truncal asymmetry
    [ ] 5. Prominence of one scapula
    [ ] 6. Limited use of one arm

15. Based on an understanding of the treatment for moderate scoliosis, which of the following is a priority?
    1. Assess for more severe clinical manifestations
    2. The use of a Boston or TLSO brace
    3. Stretching and exercising
    4. Surgery to place rods or wires

16. A school nurse is conducting a screening program for scoliosis. At which grade level should the school nurse begin testing for scoliosis?
    1. 3rd grade
    2. 5th grade
    3. 7th grade
    4. 9th grade

17. A 3-year-old child is admitted with a fractured femur and a diagnosis of osteogenesis imperfecta. On physical examination of this child, the nurse also assesses this child to have which of the following clinical manifestations?
    Select all that apply:
    [ ] 1. Blue sclera
    [ ] 2. Chronic anemia
    [ ] 3. Dental deformities
    [ ] 4. Open posterior fontanel
    [ ] 5. Hyperlaxity of ligaments
    [ ] 6. Bowed legs

18. The mother of an 8-year-old with osteogenesis imperfecta asks the nurse if there is a sport in which her child could safely participate. Which of the following sports should the nurse suggest?
    1. Soccer
    2. Track
    3. Baseball
    4. Swimming

19. The nurse correctly assesses which of the following children for the onset of Duchenne's muscular dystrophy?
    1. An infant at birth
    2. A preschool child
    3. A school-age child
    4. An adolescent

20. The nurse caring for a child with muscular dystrophy observes the child use the Gower maneuver while trying to
    1. sit.
    2. walk.
    3. stand.
    4. bend over.

21. A nurse is teaching a class to parents of children with spinal deformities. Which of the following should the nurse include in the class?
    1. Lordosis is an increased posterior convex angle in the curvature of the thoracic spine
    2. The child should be evaluated annually for progress during growth spurts
    3. Scoliosis occurs most often during infancy and childhood
    4. Spinal deformities may be painless and have a slow progression in the early stages

22. The nurse is assessing four infants for fine and gross motor development. The nurse should report which of the following infants as having a problem with motor development?
    1. A 7-month-old infant who cannot sit without support
    2. A 3-month-old infant whose tonic neck and Moro reflexes are disappearing
    3. A 5-month-old infant who uses the whole hand to grasp an object
    4. A 6-month-old infant who does not have a pincer grasp

23. Which of the following should the nurse include in the home care instructions given to the parents of a child with a cast?
    Select all that apply:
    [ ] 1. With time, the cast may give off a foul-smelling odor
    [ ] 2. Instruct the child to use a small object such as a pencil to scratch under the top of the cast
    [ ] 3. Elevate the cast on a pillow above the level of the heart
    [ ] 4. Avoid "petaling" the edges of the cast around the groin or perineum
    [ ] 5. For itching, blow air into the cast with a hair dryer set on the cool setting
    [ ] 6. Cover the cast with plastic wrap before bathing

24. The nurse evaluates a child who can self-feed finger foods to have the fine motor development of what age group? _____

25. Which of the following pictures of traction should the nurse include in the preparation given to the parents of a child to be placed in Bryant's traction? _____

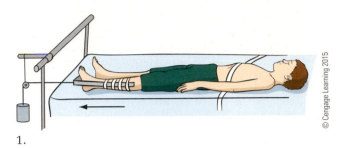

1.

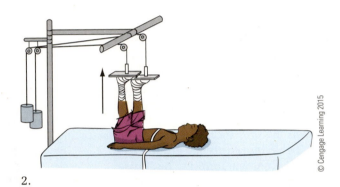

2.

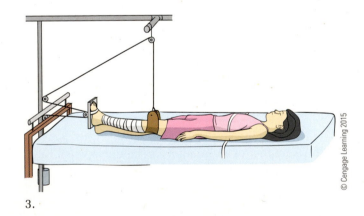

3.

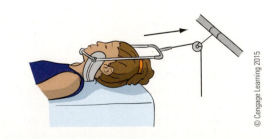

4.

26. The registered nurse is preparing the clinical assignments for a pediatric musculoskeletal unit. Which of the following nursing tasks should the nurse delegate?

1. Assess a child for juvenile rheumatoid arthritis
2. Bathe a client with a hip spica cast
3. Prepare a child with slipped femoral capital epiphysis for surgery, including a pinning and external fixation of the femoral head
4. Monitor a child with Bryant's traction following a fracture of the femur for compartment syndrome

27. The nurse should report which of the following pediatric musculoskeletal assessment findings as abnormal?
    1. An increased muscle tone in a 2-year-old child
    2. An 18-month-old infant who is bowlegged
    3. A 1-year-old toddler who has a wide-based gait
    4. An infant with a lumbar curvature of the spine and protuberant abdomen

ANSWERS AND RATIONALES

1. 4. Growth plates are located in the metaphysis of long bones. They control bone growth until about 21 years of age. Fractures of the growth plate retard the growth of the affected long bone. Red blood cells are produced in the marrow of the bone, not the growth plate.

2. 2. The sensation of numbness or tingling indicates neurovascular impairment. If not reported immediately, the impairment can lead to permanent tissue or nerve damage. The skin around the cast often feels warm. Capillary refill of 3 seconds is acceptable. As long as edema is decreasing, this is not an adverse sign.

3. 3. Talipes equinovarus, referred to as clubfoot, is a congenital abnormality characterized by the affected foot being rotated in and down while in a fixed position. Clinical manifestations of developmental hip dysplasia include asymmetry of gluteal and thigh skin folds and one knee being lower when both legs are flexed. An upward rotation of the foot is known as talipes calcaneus.

4. 1. Developmental hip dysplasia (DDH) is characterized by one knee being lower when both knees are flexed, asymmetrical gluteal and thigh skin folds, limited abduction of hip on affected side, and a positive Ortolani sign when the hips are abducted.

5. 4. In the musculoskeletal systems of children, the tendons, ligaments, and periosteum are stronger that those of adults. The bones of children are more porous and less dense than the bones of adults. The skull bones of children are not rigid or fused at birth to allow for ease of delivery and growth of the brain.

6. 2. It is a priority to notify the physician when a child with a fractured femur in skeletal traction complains of pain in the affected foot and the foot is pale and pulseless. This may be an indication of neurovascular damage. Traction weights are not removed unless there is a doctor's order to do so. The nurse should administer an analgesic and chart the observations after notifying the physician.

7. 4. The child's position can be changed carefully using the palms of hands to allow the cast to dry on all sides. The casted extremity should be elevated above the level of the heart to encourage venous return while the cast is drying. To prevent skin irritation and breakdown, the cast edges should always be smooth and free of projections.

8. 1. Osteogenesis imperfecta (OI) is an inherited disease of the connective tissue that is very difficult to treat and control. Earlier onset usually means a more difficult course of the disease. Braces and splints may be of therapeutic value to treat fractures and prevent deformity.

9. 4. Although 9- and 10-year-olds have concrete thinking patterns and lack well-developed identities, peer pressure is the most likely cause of risk-taking behavior in this age group. Inadequate rule enforcement is less likely to cause risk-taking behavior.

10. 4. When the traction weights are resting on the floor, the child needs to be pulled up in bed so that the weights can hang freely and the proper traction can be applied to the leg. Elevating the foot of the bed or lowering the head of the bed would not allow the proper traction to be applied to the child's leg. Cutting the ropes would not improve the traction if the child remains down at the foot of the bed.

11. 3. An infant's anterior fontanel normally closes at 18 months.

12. 1. 4. 5. Gross motor developments of a 4- to 6-month-old include being able to hold the chest and abdomen up with weight supported by the hands while prone, rolling over from back to abdomen, and good head control with no head lag. Holding the head up and supporting weight on forearms when prone is a gross motor development of a 2- to 3-month old. Sitting alone without support is characteristic of a 7- to 8-month-old. Going from crawling to creeping to cruising is a gross motor development of a 9- to 12-month-old.

13. 4. The upper femoral epiphysis slips from its functional position in slipped capital femoral epiphysis. The incidence of slipped capital femoral epiphysis is greatest in African-American obese males. An emaciated appearance, anemia, and developmental delays are not usually associated with this diagnosis.

14. 1. 2. 4. 5. Scoliosis is a lateral curvature of the spine with vertebral body rotation. Clinical manifestations in the early stages include an unequal shoulder level, curved spinal column, truncal asymmetry, and prominence of one scapula. Severe back pain does not usually occur in the early stages. Neither a limp nor limited use of an arm is usually apparent at this time.

15. 2. When moderate scoliosis is found, the priority treatment is usually to fit the child with a brace to limit progression of the disease. The Boston brace is a prefabricated plastic shell that fits under the arm and is used for curves of the low thoracolumbar and lumbar spine. The TLSO brace is a molded custom jacket used for thoracolumbar curves. Stretching and exercising may be done in mild forms of the disease, and surgery may be performed for more severe forms of scoliosis.

16. 2. In order to detect scoliosis in the early stage, the school nurse should begin testing for scoliosis in the 5th grade and continue testing until mid-adolescence. The 3rd grade is too early to begin testing.

17. 1. 3. 5. Osteogenesis imperfecta, also called brittle bone disease, is a connective tissue disease characterized by a disturbance of the formation of the periosteal bone. Along with fragile bones and frequent fractures, an affected child may also have blue sclerae, dental deformities, and hyperlaxity of the ligaments.

18. 4. Participating in sports is a problem for children with osteogenesis imperfecta, or brittle bone disease. Swimming is a sport that would not place stress on the child's bones. Soccer, track, and baseball are all sports that would be too dangerous for a child with osteogenesis imperfecta.

19. 2. Duchenne's muscular dystrophy is a group of progressive degenerative inherited diseases that cause muscle wasting. It has an onset between the ages of 3 and 6 years.

20. 3. At about 5 or 6 years of age, children with muscular dystrophy must use their hands to walk up their legs to achieve the standing position. This is called the Gower maneuver.

21. 4. Spinal deformities are generally painless and have a slow progression in the early stages. Lordosis is an increased anterior curvature of the lumbar spine. The child and family should be taught that periodic evaluation (every 3 to 6 months) during rapid growth spurts is indicated. Scoliosis most often occurs during the growth spurt of adolescence.

22. 1. A 6-month-old infant should be able to sit without support. The tonic neck and Moro reflexes begin to disappear between 2 and 3 months. Using the whole hand to grasp an object occurs between 4 and 5 months. The pincer grasp begins to develop between 8 and 9 months.

23. 3. 5. 6. At no time should a foul-smelling odor from the cast be ignored; an odor indicates the presence of infection. Using objects to scratch under the cast can cause injuries to the skin. "Petaling"—covering the edges of the cast with moleskin or adhesive tape to protect the child's skin from rough, irritating edges—should be done in the groin and perineum to protect the cast from urine and stool.

24. 10–12. The fine motor development of self-feeding of finger foods is characteristic of a 10- to 12-month-old child.

25. 2. Choice 1 is Buck's extension. Choice 3 is Russell's traction. Both of these are types of skin traction, as is Bryant's traction. Choice 4 is balanced suspension and a form of skeletal traction.

26. 2. Assessing, monitoring, and preparing a child for surgery are nursing tasks that require the skills of a registered nurse. A licensed practical nurse may bathe a client with a cast.

27. 1. An increased muscle tone in a 2-year-old child is abnormal. It may indicate cerebral palsy. It is normal for an 18-month-old child to be bowlegged. A wide-based gait is normal in a 1-year-old toddler. Infants normally have lumbar curvatures of the spine and protuberant abdomens.

REFERENCES

Daniels, R. (2012). *Delmar's manual of laboratory tests* (2nd ed.). Clifton Park, NY: Delmar Cengage Learning.

Potts, N., & Mandleco, B. (2012). *Pediatric nursing: Caring for children and their families* (3rd ed.). Clifton Park, NY: Delmar Cengage Learning.

Spratto, G. R., & Woods, A. L. (2012). *PDR nurse's drug reference 2012*. Clifton Park, NY: Delmar Cengage Learning.

CHAPTER 38

GENITOURINARY DISORDERS

I. **ANATOMY AND PHYSIOLOGY (SEE CHAPTER 10, GENITOURINARY DISORDERS, SECTION I.)**
   A. DIFFERENCES IN THE RENAL SYSTEM BETWEEN THE CHILD AND THE ADULT (SEE TABLE 38-1)
      1. THE FUNCTIONAL DEVELOPMENT OF THE KIDNEY IS NOT COMPLETE UNTIL AFTER THE FIRST YEAR OF LIFE.
      2. THE STRUCTURAL DEVELOPMENT OF THE KIDNEY CONTINUES DURING CHILDHOOD AND IS NOT COMPLETE UNTIL ADOLESCENCE.
      3. GLOMERULAR FILTRATION AND ABSORPTION ARE INSUFFICIENT AT BIRTH AND DO NOT REACH ADULT VALUES UNTIL 2 YEARS OF AGE.
      4. THE LOOP OF HENLE IS SHORT AT BIRTH, ACCOUNTING FOR A DECREASED REABSORPTION OF SODIUM AND WATER, RESULTING IN DILUTE URINE.
      5. SHORTER TUBULES UNTIL THE THIRD MONTH OF LIFE RESULT IN THE RETENTION OF ESSENTIAL ELECTROLYTES AND NITROGEN.
      6. REDUCED HYDROGEN ION EXCRETION, ACID SECRETION, AND PLASMA BICARBONATE LEVELS AT BIRTH MAKE NEWBORNS MORE SUSCEPTIBLE TO METABOLIC ACIDOSIS.
      7. REDUCED SODIUM EXCRETION AT BIRTH RESULTS IN SODIUM DEFICIENCIES OR EXCESSES.
      8. INSUFFICIENT REABSORPTION OF GLUCOSE AND INABILITY TO PRODUCE AMMONIUM ION DURING THE FIRST SEVERAL DAYS OF LIFE
      9. FIRST VOIDING OCCURS WITHIN THE FIRST 48 HOURS OF LIFE.
      10. THE RATIO OF FLUID TO BODY SURFACE IS GREATER IN NEWBORNS AND SMALL CHILDREN.
      11. AS A RESULT OF THE DEFICIENCY IN ACID-BASE BALANCE AND ELECTROLYTE REGULATION AT BIRTH, THE RISK OF VOLUME EXCESS AND DEHYDRATION IS GREATER WITHIN THE FIRST 2 YEARS OF LIFE.

Table 38-1 Characteristics of the Urinary System in Infants and Children

Infants	Preschoolers and School Age
Decreased ability to concentrate urine	Immature kidneys during the first 2 years
Involuntary control of urine	Recognition of a full bladder does not come until 18–24 months of life
	Full urine control at 4–5 years of age
	Daytime control of urine at 3 years of age
	Kidneys are growing in proportion to the body
Urine output	**Urine output**
10 days to 2 months: 250–400 ml	1 to 3 years of age: 500–600 ml
2 months to 1 year: 400–500 ml	3 to 5 years of age: 600–700 ml
	5 to 8 years of age: 700–1000 ml
	8 to 14 years of age: 800–1400 ml

12. INCREASED INCIDENCE OF URINARY TRACT INFECTIONS OCCURS IN CHILDREN BECAUSE OF THE SHORTER URETHRA.
13. LESS ADIPOSE TISSUE IN CHILDREN PREDISPOSE THEM TO A GREATER INCIDENCE OF KIDNEY TRAUMA.

II. ASSESSMENT

A. HEALTH HISTORY
  1. PRENATAL HISTORY
  2. DEVELOPMENTAL PROBLEMS
  3. MEDICATIONS (NEPHROTOXIC PROBLEMS)
  4. HOSPITALIZATIONS
  5. SURGERIES
  6. VOIDING HISTORY

B. PHYSICAL EXAMINATION
  1. INSPECTION
     a. Inspect the area of the kidneys and bladder for texture, turgor, bruises, and edema.
     b. Inspect the urinary meatus, penis, and vagina for visible abnormalities.
     c. Failure to gain weight
     d. Crying or pain on urination
     e. Presence of diaper rash
     f. Color and odor of urine
  2. PALPATION
     a. Palpate the kidneys for enlargement.
     b. Palpate the bladder for distention.
  3. PERCUSSION
     a. Detects pain and tenderness
  4. AUSCULTATION
     a. Assess for hypertension.

III. DIAGNOSTIC STUDIES

A. URINALYSIS
  1. DESCRIPTION: EXAMINATION OF URINE FOR COLOR, ODOR, PH, SPECIFIC GRAVITY, PROTEIN, GLUCOSE, KETONES, BILIRUBIN, RED AND WHITE BLOOD CELLS, AND BACTERIA

B. URINE CULTURE AND SENSITIVITY (MIDSTREAM)
  1. DESCRIPTION: COLLECTION OF URINE SPECIMEN FOLLOWING CLEANING OF THE URINARY MEATUS IN CHILDREN AND ADOLESCENTS OR AFTER THE APPLICATION OF A URINE COLLECTION BAG IN INFANTS
  2. PREPROCEDURE AND POSTPROCEDURE FOR CHILDREN AND ADOLESCENTS (SEE CHAPTER 10, GENITOURINARY DISORDERS, SECTION III.)
  3. APPLICATION OF URINE COLLECTION BAG IN INFANTS
     a. Don gloves, remove the diaper, remove gloves, wash hands, don gloves, and cleanse the genital area with three soapy cotton balls. Then rinse with sterile water-soaked cotton balls and dry the area.
     b. For the female infant, cleanse the genital area with one warm soapy cotton ball at a time from front to back and rinse with sterile water-soaked cotton balls.
     c. For the male infant, cleanse the penis toward the penis with one warm soapy cotton ball at a time and rinse with sterile water-soaked cotton balls.
     d. After drying the skin around the genital area, remove the adhesive on the back of the urine collection bag, place the bag around the urinary meatus on the female and around the scrotum on the male, and firmly secure the bag to prevent leakage.
     e. Diaper the infant and obtain a minimum of 20 ml for the specimen. Gently remove the adhesive from the skin, close the bag, place the bag in a specimen container, and send to the lab.

C. BLOOD CHEMISTRIES
  1. COMPLETE BLOOD COUNT (CBC)
     a. Hemoglobin, hematocrit decreased in anemia
     b. Presence of white blood cells (WBCs) and bacteria indicates infection.
  2. BLOOD UREA NITROGEN (BUN)
     a. Reflects urea nitrogen in the blood (end product of protein metabolism) used to diagnose renal impairment
     b. Normal level is 3–12 mg/dl for a newborn and 5–18 mg/dl for a child.
     c. Elevated levels indicate renal disease, dehydration, increased catabolism of protein, hemorrhage, or corticosteroid therapy.
  3. CREATININE
     a. Measures creatinine, a by-product of protein metabolism
     b. Normal level is 0.2–0.4 mg/dl for an infant, 0.3–0.7 mg/dl for a child, and 0.5–1 mg/dl for an adolescent.
     c. Elevated levels indicate severe renal disease.
  4. URIC ACID
     a. Product of purine metabolism
     b. Normal level is 2–5.5 mg/dl.
     c. Elevated levels indicate severe renal disease.
  5. SERUM ELECTROLYTES: CHILDREN LESS THAN 2 YEARS OF AGE HAVE A GREATER PERCENT OF WATER IN THE URINE AS A RESULT OF

IMMATURE GLOMERULI, TUBULES, AND NEPHRONS, INCREASING THE INCIDENCE OF ELECTROLYTE IMBALANCES AND DEHYDRATION.

   a. Sodium: normal level is 136–146 mEq/L for a newborn, 139–146 mEq/L for an infant, and 138–145 mEq/L for a child.

   b. Potassium: normal level is 3.9–5.9 mEq/L for a newborn, 4.1–5.3 mEq/L for an infant, and 3.4–4.7 mEq/L for a child.

   c. Calcium: normal level is 9–10.6 mg/dl for a newborn and 8.8–10.8 mg/dl for a child.

   d. Chloride: normal level is 96–106 mEq/L for a newborn and 90–110 mEq/L for a child.

   e. Magnesium: normal level is 1.4–2 mEq/L for a newborn and 1.4–1.7 mEq/L for a child.

IV. RADIOLOGICAL STUDIES

  A. DEVIATIONS FROM ADULT INTRAVENOUS PYELOGRAPHY (IVP) OR EXCRETORY UROGRAM

    1. FOR INFANTS UNDER 2 YEARS OF AGE, PERFORM THE TEST EARLY IN THE DAY AFTER WITHHOLDING THE MORNING BOTTLE AND SOLID FOOD TO PREVENT FLUID RESTRICTION.

    2. FOR CHILDREN OVER 2 YEARS OF AGE, ORAL RESTRICTION MAY RANGE FROM 2 TO 8 HOURS AND A CATHARTIC MAY BE ADMINISTERED THE EVENING BEFORE THE PROCEDURE (FLEET ENEMA IS CONTRAINDICATED IN CHILDREN WITH CHRONIC RENAL FAILURE BECAUSE OF HYPERPHOSPHATEMIA).

V. URINARY AND RENAL TUBES

  A. URINARY CATHETERIZATION

    1. DESCRIPTION: INSERTION OF A CATHETER INTO THE BLADDER THROUGH THE URINARY MEATUS INTO THE URETHRA WHEN THE CHILD HAS AN ABILITY TO VOID OR TO PROVIDE A STERILE URINE SPECIMEN

    2. PREPROCEDURE

     a. Instruct the child how to blow a pinwheel while pressing the hips against the bed to relax the pelvic and perineal muscles.

     b. Select an appropriate size of catheter to prevent kinking of the catheter in the bladder (see Table 38-2).

     c. Avoid using a feeding tube for indwelling catheterization because of

Table 38-2 Size of Foley Catheter for Age-Related Catheterizations

	Female	Male
Newborn	5–6	5–6
Infants to 3 years	5–8	5–8
4–8 years	8	8
8–13 years	10–12	8–10
14–17 years	12–14	12–14

© Cengage Learning 2015

the high incidence of kinking, which may necessitate surgical removal (feeding tube may be used for intermittent catheterization).

     d. Assess the child for an allergy to povidone-iodine or latex.

     e. Instruct the child and parent that a 2% lidocaine lubricant is used to decrease discomfort associated with catheterization.

     f. Explain the procedure to the child and parent.

     g. Reassure the parent of varying cultures that catheterization does not affect the child's virginity.

    3. PROCEDURE

     a. Use distractions such as singing to music or playing with small toys during the procedure.

     b. Encourage the parent to hold the small child's hand during the procedure to offer support.

     c. Ask the older child if the parent should stay during the procedure.

     d. For female children:

      1) Separate the labia with the nondominant gloved hand.

      2) Cleanse the urinary meatus with three povidone-iodine swabs (one at a time from front to back).

      3) Apply 1–2 ml of lidocaine lubricant to both the periurethral and urethral meatus.

      4) Add additional lubricant to the catheter.

      5) Wait 2–3 minutes before inserting the catheter to increase the effects of the anesthesia.

      6) Advance the catheter 1–2 inches.

      7) Inflate the balloon if a closed drainage system is to be used.

     e. For male children:

      1) Retract the foreskin with the nondominant gloved hand.

    2) Cleanse the penis with three povidone-iodine swabs.

    3) Hold the penile shaft under the glans to prevent contaminating the area with the foreskin.

    4) Lift the penis to a 90-degree angle to the body.

    5) With the lidocaine applicator inserted 1–2 cm into the urethra, apply 5–10 ml of lubricant followed by holding the end of the penis closed for 2–3 minutes.

    6) Add additional lubricant to the catheter.

    7) Insert the catheter until there is a return of urine.

    8) Inflate the balloon if a closed drainage system is to be used.

  4. POSTPROCEDURE

    a. Praise the child after the procedure.

    b. Remove supplies and tidy the room.

    c. Ensure the child is covered up.

    d. Send a urine specimen to the lab if ordered.

B. SUPRAPUBIC CATHETER

  1. DESCRIPTION

    a. Aspiration of urine from the bladder when the child cannot void, a catheter cannot be passed through the urethra because of a congenital abnormality, or the risk of infection associated with passing a catheter is increased

    b. May be used to obtain a sterile specimen in newborns and very young infants who have not voided for over 1 hour because the bladder is easily accessed through the abdomen

    c. Less-desirable procedure than bladder catheterization because the procedure is painful and the child is restrained

    d. Performed less frequently because smaller-size catheters such as a French 5 or 6 available for catheterization

  2. PREPROCEDURE

    a. Prepare the skin approximately 1 cm above the symphysis pubis for insertion of the needle.

  3. PROCEDURE

    a. Insert a 20- to 21-gauge needle for aspiration 1 cm above the symphysis pubis.

    b. Comfort the child as much as possible and implement pain management techniques.

    c. Obtain urine as ordered.

VI. NURSING DIAGNOSES

  A. ACUTE PAIN

  B. RISK FOR IMBALANCED FLUID VOLUME

  C. INEFFECTIVE HEALTH MAINTENANCE

  D. IMPAIRED URINARY ELIMINATION

  E. RISK FOR INFECTION

Nursing Diagnoses: Definitions and Classification 2012–2014. Copyright © 2012, 1994–2012 by NANDA International. Used by arrangement with John Wiley & Sons Limited.

VII. URINARY DISORDERS

  A. URINARY TRACT DISORDERS

    1. DESCRIPTION

      a. Classified as lower urinary tract infections (urethritis, cystitis) or upper urinary tract infections (pyelonephritis)

      b. Clinical manifestations may or may not be present (worse with pyelonephritis).

      c. With the exception of the newborn period, which has a higher incidence in males, the incidence is higher in females.

      d. Most common causative organism is *Escherichia coli* (common to the perineal and anal areas).

      e. Other organisms include *Klebsiella pneumoniae*, *Enterobacter*, *Proteus* species, *Pseudomonas*, and *Candida*.

      f. The shorter urethra in females accounts for their higher incidence of urinary tract infections.

      g. The longer urethra in males and antibacterial properties of prostatic fluid account for the decreased incidence in uncircumcised males.

      h. Urinary stasis caused by incomplete bladder emptying, dysfunctional voiding, or anatomical abnormalities is the most common condition influencing the onset of urinary tract infections.

      i. Extrinsic causative factors causing urinary tract infections include catheters, tight diapers, poor hygiene, bubble baths, sexual intercourse, local inflammation, and antimicrobial agents.

      j. Controversial research on the benefits of cranberry juice in the prevention of urinary tract infections dispute the increased acidity theory and suggest that antiadherence properties exist most frequently in urinary tract infections caused by *E. coli*.

      k. *E. coli* urinary tract infections most often occur in healthy children with a urinary tract infection and less frequently in children with abnormalities of the urinary tract or chronic health problems.

Table 38-3 Age-Related Clinical Manifestations of Urinary Tract Infections in Children

Infants and Children Under the Age of 2 Years	Children 2 Years and Older	Adolescence
Nonspecific	Enuresis	Frequency
Failure to thrive	Incontinence	Dysuria
Abdominal distention	Dysuria	Hematuria
Nausea	Urgency	Fever
Vomiting	Frequency	Chills
Feeding problems	Fever	Abdominal pain
Diarrhea	Dribbling	Flank pain
Jaundice	Strong, foul-smelling urine	Strong, foul-smelling urine
	Flank pain	
	Straining at urination	

© Cengage Learning 2015

2. ASSESSMENT
   a. Characteristics of clinical manifestations are age related (see Table 38-3).
3. DIAGNOSTIC TESTS
   a. History and physical
   b. Urinalysis
   c. Urine culture and sensitivity
   d. Suprapubic aspiration
   e. WBC count
   f. Erythrocyte sedimentation rate (ESR)
   g. C-reactive protein
   h. Renal scanning
   i. Renal ultrasound
   j. Voiding cystourethrogram
4. NURSING INTERVENTIONS
   a. Assess for clinical indications of dehydration.
   b. Instruct the child and parent on the prevention of urinary tract infections.
   c. Assess the diaper of an infant frequently straining, showing hesitancy before voiding, dribbling, and dysuria.
   d. Encourage increased fluids (100 ml/kg or 50 ml/lb of body weight).
   e. Instruct the child and parent to avoid bubble baths and perfumed soaps.
   f. Instruct a sexually active adolescent to void as soon as possible after intercourse.
   g. Instruct the child and parent to take the prescribed antibiotics until completed.
   h. Instruct the female child and parent on appropriate perineal hygiene such as wiping from front and back.
   i. Instruct the child and parent to wear cotton underwear.
   j. Instruct the child on the importance of completely emptying the bladder.

B. VESICOURETERAL REFLUX
   1. DESCRIPTION
      a. Retrograde flow of urine into the bladder, resulting in increased incidence of infection
      b. May be primary (congenital abnormality of the ureterovesical junction) or secondary (acquired)
      c. Most common cause of pyelonephritis in children
      d. Most commonly occurs in children under the age of 3 years
      e. Often results in renal scarring
      f. Tends to run in families
      g. Staged in grades I to V
   2. ASSESSMENT
      a. Chronic urinary tract infections
      b. Enuresis
      c. Flank pain
      d. Abdominal pain
   3. DIAGNOSTIC TESTS
      a. Evaluation of a child with frequent urinary tract infections
      b. Cystogram
      c. Voiding cystourethrogram
   4. NURSING INTERVENTIONS
      a. Administer prescribed antibiotics (generally for grades I, II, and III).
      b. Instruct the child and parent on the prevention of urinary tract infections.
      c. Administer prescribed anticholinergics such as oxybutynin chloride (Ditropan) to decrease bladder pressure.
      d. Implement postoperative nursing measures in children who have ureterovesical junction abnormality, chronic urinary tract infections, unsuccessful antibiotic therapy, or vesicoureteral reflux after puberty in females.

e. Inform the child and parent on appropriate surgical follow-up, including renal ultrasonography 1 month post-op, to assess for ureteral obstruction, voiding cystourethrogram, and renal ultrasound at 6 months and 1 year to evaluate renal growth.

f. Instruct the child and parent on the importance of taking medications as scheduled.

g. Encourage the parents to have other children screened for vesicoureteral reflux.

C. GLOMERULONEPHRITIS

1. **DESCRIPTION**
   a. Considered to be a classification indicating a primary disorder or a manifestation of a systemic disorder
   b. Ranges in severity from mild to severe
   c. The classic form is a postinfectious inflammation of the glomeruli within the kidney caused by a streptococcal, pneumococcal, or viral infection.
   d. Acute poststreptococcal is the most common form, frequently affecting school-age children.
   e. May have acute glomerulonephritis that successfully responds to treatment or chronic glomerulonephritis that leads to renal failure
   f. Hypertensive encephalopathy, acute cardiac decompensation, and acute renal failure are complications that may occur.

2. **ASSESSMENT**
   a. Periorbital edema (worse in the morning)
   b. Dark, smoke-colored urine (hematuria)
   c. Pale
   d. Irritability
   e. Anorexia
   f. Decreased urine output
   g. Hypertension
   h. Proteinuria

3. **DIAGNOSTIC TESTS**
   a. History and physical
   b. Urinalysis
   c. Urine culture and sensitivity
   d. Streptococcal antibody titers
   e. Serum complement level
   f. Chest x-ray
   g. Renal biopsy

4. **NURSING INTERVENTIONS**
   a. Monitor vital signs.
   b. Assess the body weight.
   c. Maintain an accurate intake and output (I & O).

d. Administer prescribed diuretics if renal failure is not severe.
e. Administer prescribed antihypertensives.
f. Encourage a regular diet with no added salt.
g. Avoid high-potassium foods during the oliguria phase.
h. Avoid protein foods with azotemia.
i. Assess characteristics of the urinary output.
j. Restrict and distribute fluid intake evenly during the day.
k. Encourage frequent rest periods but bed rest is not required.

D. NEPHROTIC SYNDROME

1. **DESCRIPTION**
   a. Results from a glomerular injury
   b. Primarily occurs in children between the ages of 2 and 6 years
   c. May be primary (confined to the glomerular injury) or secondary (result of systemic disease)

2. **ASSESSMENT**
   a. Weight gain
   b. Edema (generally periorbital and worse in the morning)
   c. Abdominal swelling and lower extremity edema develops during the day.
   d. Slow development of generalized edema initially confused with normal growth (may lead to anasarca, severe generalized edema)
   e. Diarrhea
   f. Anorexia
   g. Decreased dark frothy urine with a pale scent
   h. Pallor
   i. Irritability
   j. Fatigue
   k. Muercke (white) line on nail beds
   l. Decreased or normal blood pressure

3. **DIAGNOSTIC TESTS**
   a. History and physical
   b. Serum albumin level (hypoalbuminemia)
   c. Urinalysis (hyperalbuminuria, small amount of red blood cells, and high specific gravity)
   d. Serum cholesterol (elevated)
   e. Hemoglobin and hematocrit (decreased)
   f. Platelet count (elevated)
   g. Renal biopsy

4. **NURSING INTERVENTIONS**
   a. Encourage bed rest during the edematous phase.
   b. Administer prescribed prednisone until the proteinuria subsides for a

period of 10–14 days and then gradually discontinue.

c. Administer prescribed oral alkylating drug, generally cyclophosphamide (Cytoxan), for 2–3 months.

d. Inform the parents of possible adverse reactions to Cytoxan (leukopenia, azoospermia).

e. Administer prescribed furosemide (Lasix) with metolazone (Zaroxolyn) for situations in which edema interferes with respiration or hypotension, hyponatremia, and normal skin integrity.

f. Maintain strict I & O.

g. Assess the urinalysis for albumin.

h. Monitor the vital signs.

i. Assess the presence and location of edema.

j. Monitor for infection.

k. Restrict salt and fluids when edema is present.

l. Promote attractive and tasteful meals.

m. Instruct the parents on the signs of relapse.

n. Instruct the parents how to test the urine for albumin.

o. Instruct the parents to ensure the child does not have contact with sick children.

p. Monitor the child for adverse reactions of corticosteroid therapy.

E. HEMOLYTIC UREMIC SYNDROME (HUS)

1. DESCRIPTION

a. Uncommon acute renal disease responsible for one of the most common causes of acute renal disease in children

b. Occurs primarily in infants and children between the ages of 6 months and 3 years in developing countries

c. No etiologic agent identified but theories suggest endotoxins (especially *Shigella*), deficiencies of antioxidants, antithrombin III, prostacyclin, neuraminidase, agglutination, and platelet aggregation

d. Most commonly occurs after an acute gastrointestinal (GI) infection such as from contaminated beef

e. Results less often from a respiratory infection

f. Characterized by a triad of clinical manifestations (acute renal failure, thrombocytopenia, and anemia)

2. ASSESSMENT

a. Diarrhea and vomiting are prodromal clinical manifestations associated with a GI infection.

b. Anorexia, irritability, and lethargy make up the hemolytic phase lasting several days to 2 weeks.

c. Pallor

d. Bruising

e. Purpura

f. Rectal bleeding

g. Anuria

h. Hypertension

i. Seizures

3. DIAGNOSTIC TESTS

a. History and physical

b. Urinalysis

c. Complete blood count

d. Serum electrolytes

4. NURSING INTERVENTIONS

a. Administer carefully calculated fluid replacement or restrict fluids as prescribed.

b. Maintain accurate I & O.

c. Assist with peritoneal or hemodialysis if prescribed (anuria or oliguria has been present for 24 hours, hypertension, or seizures).

d. Administer prescribed Kayexalate enema for an elevated serum potassium.

e. Administer prescribed glucose or parenteral nutrition if hypoglycemia is present.

f. Administer prescribed calcium gluconate or calcium chloride if prescribed.

g. Administer prescribed aluminum hydroxide gel to bind with rising phosphorus.

h. Monitor serum electrolytes, hemoglobin, and hematocrit.

i. Assess for indications of dehydration.

j. Assess daily weight.

k. Auscultate the lungs.

l. Implement safety measures to protect the child from bruising and bleeding.

m. Administer prescribed antihypertensive drugs such as hydralazine (Apresoline) and captopril (Capoten).

n. Monitor the vital signs.

o. Monitor for seizure activity.

p. Instruct the parents on the proper cooking of meat such as ensuring the internal temperature is 165°, the color inside the meat is not pink, and to use a meat thermometer.

q. Instruct the parents to avoid giving the child unpasteurized apple juice or raw vegetables that have not been washed.

r. Avoid the use of antimotility drugs.

F. RENAL FAILURE

1. DESCRIPTION
   a. Failure of the kidneys to excrete waste, concentrate urine, and conserve electrolytes
   b. Generally considered an uncommon disorder in children, in whom the renal failure is transient and most frequently caused by dehydration that responds to the administration of fluids
   c. May be the result of prerenal, intrarenal, or postrenal causes (see Table 38-4)

2. ASSESSMENT
   a. Oliguria
   b. Edema
   c. Fluid and electrolyte imbalances such as hyperkalemia, hyponatremia, and hypocalcemia
   d. Metabolic acidosis
   e. Pallor
   f. Listlessness
   g. Anorexia
   h. Vomiting
   i. Tachypnea
   j. Seizures
   k. Arrhythmia
   l. Azotemia (nitrogen wastes in the blood)
   m. Uremia (toxic manifestations caused by retention of nitrogen products)

3. DIAGNOSTIC TESTS
   a. History and physical
   b. 24-hour urine collection
   c. BUN (elevated)
   d. Creatinine (elevated)
   e. Blood pressure readings (elevated)
   f. Complete blood count (anemia)

4. NURSING INTERVENTIONS
   a. Assess vital signs.
   b. Monitor fluids and electrolytes.
   c. Limit fluid intake as prescribed.
   d. Provide nutritious foods that are high in carbohydrates and fat, but low in potassium and protein, in an attractive manner.
   e. Assess for indications of irritability, restlessness, and anxiousness, and be supportive.
   f. Provide a supportive environment for the parents.
   g. Monitor the child closely who is taking a nephrotoxic drug.
   h. Administer prescribed IV fluids for dehydration.
   i. Monitor central venous pressure.
   j. Maintain an accurate urinary output.
   k. Administer prescribed mannitol or furosemide (Lasix) to induce urination (output may be generated to 6–10 ml/kg in 1 to 3 hours).
   l. Maintain a strict I & O.
   m. Monitor the child for cardiac arrhythmias (electrocardiogram [ECG] abnormalities and serum potassium over 7 mEq/L).
   n. Administer prescribed calcium gluconate to ensure cardiac conduction.
   o. Administer prescribed sodium bicarbonate to transport potassium from the extracellular to intracellular fluid and elevate the pH.
   p. Administer prescribed glucose and insulin to transport glucose into the cells.

Table 38-4 Prerenal, Intrarenal, and Postrenal Causes of Acute Renal Failure

Prerenal	Intrarenal	Postrenal
Most common etiology in acute renal failure in children	Damage to the tissues of the kidneys is sustained.	Renal function may be restored after relieving the obstruction.
Dehydration	Nephrotoxic drugs such as antibiotics, including aminoglycosides, methicillin, neomycin, polymyxin, kanamycin, and sulfonamides	Ureterovesical or ureteropelvic obstruction, neurogenic bladder, Wilms' tumor, or renal calculi
Shock	Contrast dyes	
Burns	Glomerulonephritis	
Hypovolemia	Pyelonephritis	
Renal artery stenosis	Hemolytic uremic syndrome	
Sepsis	Ingestion of heavy metals	
Perirenal asphyxia	Inhalation of carbon tetrachloride	

    q. Administer prescribed Kayexalate to remove excess potassium from the body.

    r. Administer prescribed antihypertensives.

    s. Administer blood transfusions if anemia is present.

    t. Monitor the child for seizure activity.

G. CHRONIC RENAL FAILURE

  1. DESCRIPTION

    a. Progressive disease with the destruction of over 50% of kidney function occurring over the years

    b. End-stage renal disease is permanent, irreversible, and results from uremia that does not resolve.

    c. Causes include indiscriminate use of nephrotoxic drugs, prematurity, congenital renal or urinary obstruction, hemolytic uremic syndrome, glomerulonephritis, pyelonephritis, and immunologic disorders.

  2. ASSESSMENT

    a. Lack of energy

    b. Fatigue on exertion

    c. Hypertension

    d. Pallor

    e. Retarded growth for age

    f. Enuresis

    g. Lack of interest in normal play activities

    h. Anorexia

    i. Anemia

    j. Nausea

    k. Vomiting

    l. Muscles cramps

    m. Headache

    n. Joint and bone pain

    o. Ecchymosis

    p. Amenorrhea

    q. Dry and itchy skin

  3. DIAGNOSTIC TESTS

    a. History and physical (reveals previous renal disease)

    b. Serum electrolytes

    c. BUN

    d. Creatinine

    e. Complete blood count (CBC)

    f. Long bone x-rays

  4. NURSING INTERVENTIONS

    a. Provide a supportive environment for the parents and child for a chronic irreversible condition for which there is no known cure.

    b. Administer prescribed diuretic, immunosuppressive, and antihypertensive drugs.

    c. Encourage a diet low in protein, potassium, and phosphorus.

    d. Maintain a strict I & O.

    e. Administer prescribed aluminum hydroxyl gel or calcium carbonate to bind phosphorus.

    f. Administer prescribed vitamin D to raise calcium level.

    g. Administer prescribed erythropoietin or blood transfusion.

    h. Monitor blood pressure.

    i. Avoid supplementation with vitamins A, E, and K (fat-soluble vitamins and may accumulate).

    j. Encourage frequent dental care and monitor the child for dental complications (teeth abnormalities, malocclusion, and hypermineralization).

  5. RENAL REPLACEMENT THERAPY

    a. Movement of fluid and waste products in the blood across a semipermeable membrane into a dialysis solution that restores chemical and electrolyte balance

    b. Types of dialysis include hemodialysis, peritoneal dialysis, or hemofiltration.

    c. Generally reserved for end-stage renal disease

  6. HEMODIALYSIS

    a. Requires the use of a machine with an artificial semipermeable membrane referred to as an artificial kidney

    b. Graft or fistula surgically created, facilitating access to the circulatory system

    c. Generally the preferred dialysis method for life-threatening conditions such as hyperkalemia or when family situations do not permit dialysis at home

    d. Results in less protein loss than peritoneal dialysis

    e. Not a good option for infants and small children because of their small size, difficulty in accessing vascular capabilities, and a cardiovascular system easily upset by blood pressure and blood volume changes

  7. PERITONEAL DIALYSIS

    a. Involves the process of inserting a catheter into the anterior abdominal wall, which serves as a semipermeable membrane

    b. Generally an ideal method for parents and children to perform and prefer this method of dialysis at home if live a distance from a medical facility where hemodialysis is available

c. Contraindicated in children who have had recent abdominal surgery, have peritoneal adhesions, or have significant abdominal scarring

d. Prevention of infection (peritonitis) is a major risk with peritoneal dialysis.

8. HEMOFILTRATION

a. A simultaneous process where a filtrate of blood is circulated outside the body and across a semipermeable membrane

b. A good option for infants, small children, children experiencing fluid volume overload from surgery such as cardiovascular surgery, or need volume-expanding fluids such as packed red blood cells, albumin, or parenteral nutrition

c. Has become a viable option for children who may not otherwise survive hemodialysis or peritoneal dialysis

9. PROCEDURE AND NURSING INTERVENTIONS FOR HEMODIALYSIS AND PERITONEAL DIALYSIS (SEE CHAPTER 10, GENITOURINARY DISORDERS, SECTION VII.)

10. RENAL TRANSPLANTATION

a. The most desirable method of renal replacement therapy for children because it is the only method that offers a choice for a normal life

b. Children with end-stage renal disease must be cancer-free for a period of no less than 2 years or have no indications of an infection.

c. The greatest risk for noncompliance with the postoperative course includes adverse reactions to drugs and discontinuing those drugs or a lack of family support.

d. Higher risk of complication in children who have abnormal urinary tracts

e. Nursing interventions for renal transplantation (See Chapter 10, Genitourinary Disorders, Section VII.)

H. ENURESIS

1. DESCRIPTION

a. Involuntary voiding of urine beyond the expected age at which continence is generally established (5 years), occurs at least twice a week for a period of 3 months, or is not the result of a structural abnormality

b. Generally daytime and nocturnal bowel is first to be achieved by age 2½ to 3½ years

c. Commonly referred to as bedwetting

d. Classified as primary (never been dry during a 3-month period), secondary (period of enuresis after continence has been established for at least 3–6 months), diurnal (enuresis occurring only during the day), or nocturnal (enuresis occurring only at night)

e. More common in boys and usually is primary nocturnal enuresis

f. No single etiology but organic (delayed neurological development, urinary tract infections, renal failure, diabetes mellitus, constipation, and structural disorder of urinary tract) and nonorganic (sleep disorders such as sleep apnea, enlarged tonsils, or sound sleep; psychological stress; attempts to toilet train at too early an age; or punishment for failure to toilet train)

2. ASSESSMENT

a. Urinary urgency manifested by leg-crossing, holding genitals, or inability to stand still

b. Dysuria

c. Restlessness

d. Urinary frequency

e. Difficulty in awakening to urinate

f. Spontaneous voiding during sleep

g. Dribbling after voiding

h. Incontinence with laughing

3. DIAGNOSTIC TESTS

a. History and physical

b. Urinalysis

c. Urine culture

d. Renal ultrasound

4. NURSING INTERVENTIONS

a. Obtain an accurate voiding history.

b. Implement the use of a bedwetting alarm, such as placing the alarm under the bottom sheet or attaching the alarm to the child's pajamas.

c. Instruct the child and parents on the use of the bedwetting alarm, such as that the purpose of the alarm is to recognize a full bladder, to turn the alarm off when it goes off, and to go to the bathroom immediately to void after the alarm.

d. Use caution when implementing a behavior motivational star chart to reward the child when progress is made (discontinue the chart if the child consistently fails to achieve continence) (see Figure 38-1).

e. Instruct the parents to eliminate foods that may be irritants to the bladder such as carbonated beverages, beverages containing caffeine, and artificially sweetened

Figure 38-1 Behavior modification star chart is often used to reward desired behavior in children with enuresis

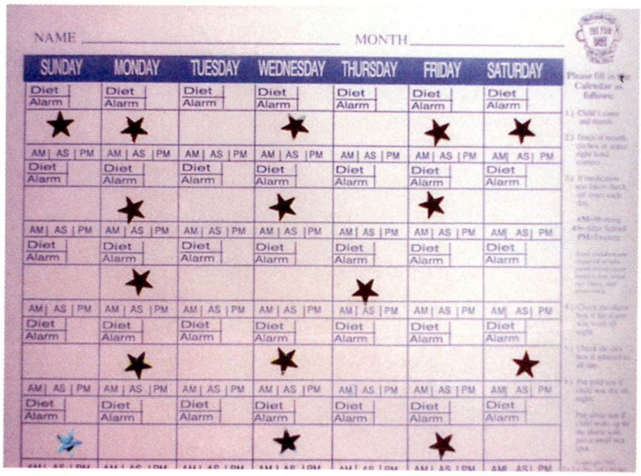

© Cengage Learning 2015

beverages; dairy products; citrus fruits; and heavily sugared foods.

f. Encourage foods high in fiber and fluids to prevent constipation.

g. Encourage the parents to be supportive and not punitive with both successes and failures.

h. Administer prescribed oxybutynin chloride (Ditropan), desmopressin (DDAVP), and imipramine hydrochloride (Tofranil) (see Table 38-5).

i. Avoid administration of DDAVP to a child with cystic fibrosis or renal disease because of fluid and electrolyte imbalances such as hyponatremia or water intoxication.

j. Instruct the parents to keep all medications out of reach of the child and administer them to the child (overdose of imipramine [Tofranil] may cause fatal arrhythmias).

I. CRYPTORCHIDISM

1. DESCRIPTION

a. Failure of one or both testes to normally descend into the scrotum through the inguinal canal

b. May be retractile (testes that have normally descended but may be retracted with exam or physical stimulation), ectopic (testes that are located outside the normal path of descent between the abdominal cavity and the scrotum), or anorchia (absence of testes)

c. More common in premature male infants

d. Generally, testes spontaneously descend during the first year but rarely descend after the first year.

2. ASSESSMENT

a. Unilateral or bilateral absence of testes in the scrotum

b. Intermittently palpable testes noted in the scrotum with retractile testes (testes generally appear in the scrotum when the child is in warm water such as bathing)

c. Smaller hemiscrotum on the side of the undescended testes

Table 38-5 Common Medications to Treat Enuresis

Name of Medication	Actions	Adverse Reactions
Oxybutynin chloride (Ditropan)	Anticholinergic used for children with small functional bladder capacity. Ditropan affects the bladder muscle by reducing uninhibited bladder contractions, inhibiting voiding, and increasing voluntary control of the urethral sphincter.	Facial flushing Dry mouth Constipation Heat intolerance Drowsiness Insomnia Blurred vision
Imipramine hydrochloride (Tofranil)	Tricyclic antidepressant. Decreases depth of sleep during latter part of night	Dry mouth Nervousness Insomnia Changes in personality
Desmopressin acetate (DDAVP)	A synthetic analog of vasopressin that works by increasing water retention and urine concentration. By concentrating urine and decreasing the amount of urine produced, the child may not reach bladder capacity and therefore stays dry.	Headaches Nausea Nasal congestion Nosebleeds

© Cengage Learning 2015

3. DIAGNOSTIC TESTS
   a. Physical examination (undescended testes cannot be "milked" in and out of the scrotum where retractile testes can be)
   b. Pelvic ultrasound
   c. Magnetic resonance imaging (MRI)
   d. Computerized tomography (CT) scan
   e. Abdominal laparoscopy
4. NURSING INTERVENTIONS
   a. Assess the cremasteric reflex in a squatting child by application of firm pressure by the finger on the external ring before palpating the abdomen or genitalia (the cremasteric reflex is active in an infant and up to age 5 years and results in withdrawal of the testes above the scrotum).
   b. Administer prescribed human chronic gonadotropin (HCG) injection or luteinizing-hormone-releasing nasal spray to induce the descent of the testes.
   c. Inform the parents that if the testes fail to spontaneously descend, orchiopexy surgery is generally performed between 1 and 2 years of age.
   d. Inform the parents why surgery is necessary (to avoid exposure of the undescended testis to body temperature, an increased risk of infertility, increased risk of tumors, physical or psychological trauma due to an empty scrotum, and closure of the processus vaginalis).
   e. Postoperatively, apply loose clothing, administer prescribed acetaminophen (Tylenol), and perform frequent diaper changes.
   f. Instruct the parents to prevent the child from engaging in strenuous activities or using riding toys.
   g. Instruct the parents on the importance of monthly testicular examinations to detect early tumor formation.
   h. Instruct the parents on information necessary to answer the child's questions as adolescence is reached.
J. HYPOSPADIAS
   1. DESCRIPTION
      a. Common congenital defect in which the urethral meatus appears on the ventral surface of the penis
      b. Exact etiology is unknown but some theories suggest a deficit in the testosterone metabolism that affects the development of the male genitalia.

c. Complications include urethral fistula.
2. ASSESSMENT
   a. Small ventral prepuce that is redundant dorsally
   b. May have a circumcised appearance
   c. May have chordee (curvature downward of the penis and incomplete foreskin, undescended testes, and inguinal hernia)
   d. Downward urinary stream
3. DIAGNOSTIC TESTS
   a. Physical examination
4. NURSING INTERVENTIONS
   a. Inform the parents that the treatment of choice is surgery, generally before the age of 18 months, to ensure correct placement of the urethral meatus and facilitate voiding in a standing position.
   b. Inform the parents that circumcision is avoided in these infants.
   c. Administer prescribed testosterone cream or injections to enhance tissue growth.
   d. Instruct the parents on the adverse reactions of the testosterone cream and that they will disappear when the cream is discontinued.
   e. Instruct the parents that a penile dressing or no dressing may be applied postoperatively.
   f. Monitor the infant for purulent drainage from the incision, foul-smelling urine, increased temperature, or erythema.
   g. Administer prescribed oxybutynin chloride (Ditropan) for bladder spasms.
   h. Encourage fluids.
   i. Maintain an accurate intake and output.
   j. Assess the penis for bruising, edema, and wrinkled appearance for several days to weeks.
   k. Instruct the parents on the care of the dressing and how to remove the dressing in 5 days.
   l. Instruct the parents to soak the child up to the waist in the tub for 20 minutes prior to removal of the layered dressing.
K. BLADDER EXSTROPHY/EPISPADIAS COMPLEX
   1. DESCRIPTION
      a. Rare, severe congenital anomaly characterized by an exposed urinary urethra and bladder, pelvic bone

separation, and genital and anal abnormalities

b. More common in males

2. ASSESSMENT

a. Difficulty walking and waddling gait from separation of the pelvic bone

b. Undescended testes

c. Short penis

d. Inguinal hernia

e. Absence of a vagina

f. Cleft or bifid clitoris

g. Completely separated labia

h. Exposed bladder mucosa

3. DIAGNOSTIC TESTS

a. Visible deformity

4. NURSING INTERVENTIONS

a. Initially cover the bladder with a thin dressing or clear plastic wrap.

b. Avoid adhesives or petroleum jelly, which may damage the bladder mucosa.

c. Inform the parents that the treatment of choice is surgery to close the bladder within 2 days of life, followed by additional surgeries to create a successful urethral sphincter mechanism and correct genital anomalies.

d. Provide the parents with psychological support.

e. Instruct the parents on how to recognize urinary infections.

L. INGUINAL HERNIA

1. DESCRIPTION

a. A swelling in the scrotum or inguinal area containing abdominal contents protruding into the processus vaginalis

b. Increased incidence in preterm births

c. Strangulation or cessation of the blood supply to the herniated area leads to ischemia, obstruction of the bowel, necrosis, and perforation.

2. ASSESSMENT

a. May be asymptomatic

b. Generally painless

c. Inguinal swelling (may be reducible with compression or rest)

d. Thickened cord in the groin

e. Strangulation (red scrotum, pain, irritability, abdominal distention, tachycardia, and vomiting)

3. DIAGNOSTIC TESTS

a. Physical examination of the scrotal area

b. Silk glove test (the sides of the empty hernial sac will be able to be rubbed together)

4. NURSING INTERVENTIONS

a. Assess the area for bagginess and reducibility (inguinal hernia) or firmness and irreducibility (hydrocele).

b. Inform the parents that the treatment of choice is surgery.

c. Postoperatively, keep the incision clean and dry.

d. Administer analgesics as ordered.

e. Instruct the parents to frequently change the diapers to prevent infection.

f. Instruct the parents that there are no activity restrictions.

g. Instruct the parents of older children that strenuous activities, riding bicycles, or contact sports should be avoided for 3 weeks.

h. Instruct the parents on the signs of strangulation if surgery is postponed.

M. HYDROCELE

1. DESCRIPTION

a. A collection of peritoneal fluid in the scrotum

b. May be communicating hydrocele (processus vaginalis remains continually open with peritoneal fluid that may enter after increased intra-abdominal pressure) or noncommunicating (common in newborns, subsides spontaneously, and the result of an obliterated processus vaginalis and tunica vaginalis filled with peritoneal fluid)

2. ASSESSMENT

a. May be asymptomatic

b. Firm palpable bulge in the inguinal area that is irreducible

3. DIAGNOSTIC TESTS

a. Physical examination

4. NURSING INTERVENTIONS (SEE NURSING INTERVENTIONS FOR INGUINAL HERNIA, SECTION VII.)

a. Inform the parents that the treatment of choice is surgery.

PRACTICE QUESTIONS

1. The parents of a newborn with bladder exstrophy ask the nurse why a suprapubic catheter is being inserted. Which of the following is the most appropriate response by the nurse? "Suprapubic catheterization
   1. is a less painful procedure on a newborn than bladder catheterization."
   2. does not require restraining the newborn like bladder catheterization."
   3. is performed to aspirate urine when the newborn has not voided for more than 1 hour."
   4. is the only procedure that allows a small catheter to be used on a newborn."

2. The nurse assesses a 6-year-old child suspected of a urinary tract infection for which of the following clinical manifestations?
   Select all that apply:
   [ ] 1. Enuresis
   [ ] 2. Straining at urination
   [ ] 3. Dribbling
   [ ] 4. Urinary retention
   [ ] 5. Jaundice
   [ ] 6. Dysuria

3. Which of the following should the nurse include in the postoperative management of a child who had surgery for vesicoureteral reflux?
   1. Cover the bladder with a thin, clear, nonadhesive dressing
   2. Encourage the parents to have the child wear loose clothing
   3. Inform the parents that a renal ultrasound should be done at 6 months and again at 1 year
   4. Administer prescribed oxybutynin chloride (Ditropan) and desmopressin acetate (DDAVP)

4. When working with a child with postinfectious glomerulonephritis, which of the following is most appropriate to consider when planning the goals of care?
   1. Most children fully recover from this illness
   2. Visible blood in the urine may persist for 1 to 2 years
   3. Blood pressure medications will need to be taken permanently
   4. There is a high incidence of recurrent urinary tract infections

5. When providing care for a child who is on oxybutynin chloride (Ditropan) for enuresis, the nurse should monitor the child for which of the following?
   Select all that apply:
   [ ] 1. Facial flushing
   [ ] 2. Nasal congestion
   [ ] 3. Diarrhea
   [ ] 4. Blurred vision
   [ ] 5. Dry mouth
   [ ] 6. Nosebleeds

6. The parents of a child in end-stage renal disease have received dietary instructions. Which of the following statements by the parents would indicate that they understood which foods to avoid in end-stage renal disease? "We will avoid foods high in
   Select all that apply:
   [ ] 1. calcium."
   [ ] 2. sodium."
   [ ] 3. phosphorus."
   [ ] 4. magnesium."
   [ ] 5. potassium."
   [ ] 6. cholesterol."

7. The nurse identifies which of the following three characteristics in a child suspected of nephrotic syndrome?
   Select all that apply:
   [ ] 1. Hypoalbuminemia
   [ ] 2. Hyperalbuminuria
   [ ] 3. Periorbital edema
   [ ] 4. Thrombocytopenia
   [ ] 5. Oliguria
   [ ] 6. Hypocalcemia

8. The post-op care for a child who has had surgery for cryptorchidism, the nurse should perform which of the following priority nursing interventions?
   1. Encourage protein in the diet
   2. Assess the cremasteric reflex
   3. Change the diapers frequently
   4. Encourage activity

9. Because a 3-year-old child has diurnal enuresis, plans for nursing interventions should include which of the following?
   Select all that apply:
   [ ] 1. Restrict citrus fruits and foods high in sugar
   [ ] 2. Implement a bedwetting alarm on the child's pajamas
   [ ] 3. Implement a behavior motivational star chart
   [ ] 4. Restrict fluids in the diet
   [ ] 5. Encourage a diet high in fiber
   [ ] 6. Administer prescribed luteinizing-hormone-releasing hormone nasal spray

10. A mother of a 4-year-old child asks the nurse whether control of urine or stool comes first. Which of the following responses is appropriate?
    1. "Control of urine at night occurs first."
    2. "Control of stool during the day occurs first."
    3. "Control of stool at night occurs first."
    4. "Control of urine during the day occurs first."

11. The nurse is admitting a client with glomerulonephritis and assesses for which of the following manifestations?
    Select all that apply:
    [ ] 1. Elevated serum cholesterol
    [ ] 2. Periorbital edema
    [ ] 3. Hematuria
    [ ] 4. Metabolic acidosis
    [ ] 5. Urinary urgency
    [ ] 6. Proteinuria

12. Which of the following nursing interventions is a priority for the nurse to implement in the plan of care for a child with hemolytic uremic syndrome?
    1. Administer prescribed sodium polystyrene sulfonate (Kayexalate) rectally
    2. Restrict glucose foods
    3. Administer prescribed trimethoprim-sulfamethoxazole (Bactrim)
    4. Encourage phosphorus-rich foods

13. The nurse evaluates which of the following children with end-stage renal failure to be the most appropriate candidate for a renal transplant?
    1. A 12-year-old child with osteosarcoma
    2. A 2-year-old child born with the HIV virus
    3. A 3-year-old child with hemolytic uremic syndrome
    4. An 18-year-old adolescent with Hodgkin's disease

14. Which of the following is the priority for the nurse to monitor in a child who has had hypospadias surgery?
    1. Urethral fistula
    2. Urinary tract infections
    3. Dysuria
    4. Bladder spasms

15. Which of the following changes in a child's assessment should the nurse report as a critical indication of a toxic reaction to oxybutynin chloride (Ditropan)?
    1. Constipation and urinary retention
    2. Dry mouth and blurred vision
    3. Tachycardia and hypertension
    4. Heat intolerance and insomnia

16. In planning the post-op care for a child following reimplantation of the ureters, the nurse should include which of the following in the plan of care to prevent urinary tract infections?
    1. Assess the tubing and ureteral stents for breaks in their integrity
    2. Monitor the intake and output
    3. Perform frequent bladder irrigations
    4. Maintain a diet high in protein and fiber

17. The nurse evaluates which of the following laboratory tests and assessment findings in a 6-month-old infant to support a diagnosis of hemolytic uremic syndrome?
    Select all that apply:
    [ ] 1. Blood pressure of 110/70 mm Hg
    [ ] 2. Blood urea nitrogen (BUN) of 20 mg/dl
    [ ] 3. A platelet count of 95,000/ml
    [ ] 4. Serum calcium of 11.0 mg/dl
    [ ] 5. Serum potassium of 6.1 mEq/L
    [ ] 6. Serum sodium of 131 mEq/L

18. The registered nurse in charge of a busy genitourinary unit should most appropriately delegate which of the following nursing tasks to the appropriate unit personnel considering budget, time, and qualifications of the employee?
    1. Assign unlicensed assistive personnel (UAP) to take the vital signs on a child suspected of being hypertensive and in renal failure
    2. Assign a registered nurse (RN) to assess an infant with hemolytic syndrome for signs of intracranial pressure
    3. Assign a licensed practical nurse (LPN) to teach the parents of a child with a urinary obstruction about an intravenous pyelography scheduled for their child and obtain an informed consent
    4. Assign unlicensed assistive personnel (UAP) to evaluate the laboratory tests of a child with acute glomerulonephritis for hematuria and elevated serum sodium and potassium levels

19. The nurse is preparing the client assignments for the day on a genitourinary unit. Which of the following assignments would be appropriate to delegate to a licensed practical nurse (LPN)?
    1. Develop the plan of care for a client with vesicoureteral reflux
    2. Instruct the parents about the surgery scheduled for an infant with hypospadias
    3. Administer the prescribed prednisolone (Prelone) to a child with nephrotic syndrome
    4. Monitor the central venous pressure of a child with hemolytic uremic syndrome

20. The nurse should assess a child suspected of being in acute renal failure for which of the following?

Select all that apply:
[ ] 1. Urine output of less than 1 ml/kg/hr
[ ] 2. Hematuria
[ ] 3. Listlessness
[ ] 4. Anorexia
[ ] 5. Pain
[ ] 6. White blood cell count of greater than 100,000 CFU/ml

21. The nurse is discharging a 2-month-old infant after a recurrent urinary tract infection. Which of the following are common signs of a urinary tract infection that the nurse should instruct the parents to monitor the infant for at home? Select all that apply:
[ ] 1. Urinary frequency
[ ] 2. Failure to thrive
[ ] 3. Nausea and vomiting
[ ] 4. Enuresis
[ ] 5. Chills
[ ] 6. Abdominal distention

22. The nurse should assist a 4-year-old child experiencing primary enuresis to make which of the following menu selections?

1. Hamburger, orange, and cola
2. Hot dog and a chocolate milk shake
3. Pizza, vanilla ice cream, and tea
4. Fried chicken and mashed potatoes

23. The nurse anticipates cyclophosphamide (Cytoxan) is prescribed for how many months in a client who has nephritic syndrome?

_____

24. The nurse is assessing the following four children for the risk of developing an inguinal hernia. The nurse should recognize that which of the following children has the highest risk of developing this condition?
1. A 3-week-old male who was premature and has a low birth weight
2. A 7-year-old male who has been exposed to an infectious agent
3. A 2-year-old female who has a history of urinary tract infections
4. A 1-year-old female who lives in an underdeveloped country and is known to have eaten beef contaminated with *Escherichia coli*

ANSWERS AND RATIONALES

1. 3. Suprapubic catheterization allows the aspiration of urine when a child cannot void because of a congenital abnormality such as bladder exstrophy. Generally, suprapubic catheterization is performed when a child hasn't voided for more than an hour. It is a less desirable procedure than bladder catheterization because it is painful and the child must be restrained. It is performed less frequently now than in the past because small catheters are now available for bladder catheterization.

2. 1. 2. 3. 6. Clinical manifestations of a urinary tract infection in a child 2 years of age or older include enuresis, dysuria, frequency, urgency, fever, dribbling, foul-smelling urine, flank pain, and straining at urine.

3. 3. Postoperative care of a child who has had surgery for a vesicoureteral reflux should include a renal ultrasound at 6 months and again at 1 year to evaluate renal growth. Covering the bladder with a thin, nonadhesive dressing is an appropriate intervention before surgery for a bladder exstrophy. Encouraging the parents to have the child wear loose clothing is an appropriate intervention for cryptorchidism. Oxybutynin chloride (Ditropan) is an anticholinergic used in the treatment of enuresis. Desmopressin acetate

(DDAVP), a synthetic analog of vasopressin that acts by increasing water retention and urine concentration, is also used for enuresis.

4. 1. Glomerulonephritis is a primary disorder or a manifestation of a systemic disorder that may range from mild to severe. The most common form is a postinfectious inflammation of the glomeruli caused by a streptococcal, pneumococcal, or viral infection. A full recovery generally occurs. Although hypertension and hematuria are clinical manifestations, they generally resolve with recovery. Recurrent urinary infections do not occur in glomerulonephritis but in vesicoureteral reflux.

5. 1. 4. 5. Oxybutynin chloride (Ditropan) is an anticholinergic used in the treatment of enuresis by inhibiting voiding and enhancing voluntary urethral control. Common adverse reactions include facial flushing, dry mouth, constipation, heat intolerance, drowsiness, insomnia, and blurred vision. Nasal congestion and nosebleeds are adverse reactions to desmopressin acetate (DDAVP).

6. 2. 3. 5. Chronic renal failure is a progressive disease with the gradual destruction of over 50% of kidney function. Potassium, sodium, and phosphorus are to be avoided. Potassium and phosphorus are not well excreted, and

sodium is restricted because it is associated with edema and blood pressure.

7. 1. 2. 3. Hypoalbuminemia, hyperalbuminuria, and periorbital edema are the correct choices. Nephrotic syndrome results from a glomerular injury and is manifested by periorbital edema that is generally worse in the morning. Significant laboratory data includes hypoalbuminemia and hyperalbuminuria. Thrombocytopenia is characteristic of hemolytic uremic syndrome. Oliguria and hypocalcemia are clinical manifestations of renal failure.

8. 3. Cryptorchidism is failure of one or both testes to descend normally into the scrotum. Surgery is necessary to avoid exposure of the undescended testis to the body temperature, increased incidence of infertility, tumors, and physical or psychological trauma as a result of an empty scrotum. The priority nursing intervention is frequent diaper changes to prevent infection. There are no dietary restrictions, although protein will promote wound healing. Assessing the cremasteric reflex is the application of firm pressure on the external ring before palpating the abdomen or genitalia. The reflex is active in an infant and child up to 5 years of age and may result in withdrawal of the testes above the scrotum. Activity is not encouraged, and engaging in strenuous activity and playing on riding toys are to be avoided.

9. 1. 3. 5. Diurnal enuresis is enuresis that occurs only during the day, so a bed-wetting alarm is not necessary. Citrus fruits and heavily sugared foods are to be avoided because they are irritants to the bladder mucosa. Fiber and fluids should be increased to avoid constipation. A behavior motivational star chart is implemented to reward the child when progress is made and serves as a visual chart of successes. Luteinizing-hormone-releasing hormone nasal spray is used in the treatment of cryptorchidism.

10. 3. Control of the bowel occurs first at night followed by control of the bowel during the day. Subsequently, urine is controlled during the day; control of urine at night occurs last.

11. 2. 3. 6. Assessment findings of glomerulonephritis include periorbital edema, hematuria, and proteinuria. Metabolic acidosis is found in renal failure. Urinary urgency manifested by leg-crossing, holding the genitals, or inability to stand is an assessment finding in enuresis. An elevated serum cholesterol is an assessment finding in nephritic syndrome.

12. 1. A priority nursing intervention for hemolytic uremic syndrome is the administration of rectal sodium polystyrene sulfonate (Kayexalate) to

bind potassium in the body and remove it through the rectum. Glucose may be administered if hypoglycemia is present. Trimethoprim-sulfamethoxazole (Bactrim) is a sulfonamide that is nephrotoxic. Aluminum hydroxide gel may be given to bind with phosphorus.

13. 3. Renal transplantation for children with end-stage renal disease is the only treatment that offers these children a chance at a normal life. The child must be free of cancer for a period of no less than 2 years and have no indications of an infection.

14. 1. Hypospadias is a congenital defect in which the urethral meatus appears on the ventral surface of the penis. A urethral fistula results in urine leaking from the urethra and may necessitate surgery if it does not spontaneously resolve. Although dysuria, bladder spasms, and urinary tract infections may occur following urinary surgery, the priority is the leakage of urine that may occur from the urethra with a urethral fistula.

15. 3. Oxybutynin chloride (Ditropan) is an anticholinergic used in the treatment of enuresis. Common adverse reactions include constipation, urinary retention, dry mouth, blurred vision, heat intolerance, and insomnia. Tachycardia and hypertension are serious adverse reactions that are indications of toxicity.

16. 1. Assessing the ureteral stents and tubing for breaks in their integrity is a priority nursing intervention to prevent urinary tract infections following implantation of the ureters.

17. 1. 2. 3. Hypertension, thrombocytopenia, and an elevated blood urea nitrogen are laboratory findings in hemolytic uremic syndrome. In a 6-month-old infant, normal blood pressure is approximately 90/61 mm Hg; normal blood urea nitrogen should be between 4 mg/dl and 16 mg/dl; a normal platelet count is between 84,000 and 478,000 (a platelet count less than 75,000 indicates thrombocytopenia); normal serum calcium is 9.0 mg/dl to 10.6 mg/dl; normal serum sodium is 136 mEq/l to 146 mEq/L; and a normal serum potassium is 3.9 mEq/L to 5.9 mEq/L.

18. 2. Only a registered nurse can perform assessments. Also, a child suspected of having signs of intracranial pressure may not be stable. It is not appropriate to delegate to unlicensed assistive personnel the task of taking the vital signs of a child suspected of being hypertensive and in renal failure. Taking the vital signs of this client would be an assessment and evaluation of the client's status, which can only be performed by a registered nurse. A licensed practical nurse cannot provide education or evaluate; such tasks must be performed by the registered nurse.

19. 3. Prednisolone (Prelone) may be administered by a licensed practical nurse (LPN). An LPN cannot plan nursing care, perform education, or perform a central venous pressure reading. These assignments may only be performed by a registered nurse.

20. 1. 3. 4. Clinical manifestations of acute renal failure include anuria or a urine output of less than 1 ml/kg/hr, listlessness, and anorexia. Other clinical manifestations associated with acute renal failure include pallor, vomiting, lethargy, and signs of dehydration. Hematuria is a clinical manifestation of acute glomerulonephritis, not renal failure. Pain and an elevated white blood cell count are not features associated with acute renal failure.

21. 1. 2. 3. 6. Clinical manifestations of a urinary tract infection in a 2-month-old infant include urinary frequency, failure to thrive, feeding problems, nausea, vomiting, abdominal distention, diarrhea, and jaundice.

22. 4. Foods such as dairy products, citrus fruits, heavily sugared foods, and beverages with artificial coloring, carbonation, and caffeine can be irritants to the bladder and increase the child's enuresis.

23. 2–3 months. Cyclophosphamide (Cytoxan) is an alkylating drug prescribed for nephritic syndrome for 2–3 months.

24. 1. Infantile inguinal hernias are more common within the first month of life in males. The incidence is greatly increased in males born prematurely and with a low birth weight. A 7-year-old male exposed to an infectious agent may have acute glomerulonephritis. A 2-year-old female with a history of urinary tract infections may have vesicoureteral reflux. A 2-year-old female living in an undeveloped country who ate *E. coli*–contaminated beef may have hemolytic uremic anemia, a disorder that is distributed equally between the sexes.

REFERENCES

Daniels, R. (2012). *Delmar's manual of laboratory tests* (2nd ed.). Clifton Park, NY: Delmar Cengage Learning.

Potts, N., & Mandleco, B. (2012). *Pediatric nursing: Caring for children and their families* (3rd ed.). Clifton Park, NY: Delmar Cengage Learning.

Spratto, G. R., & Woods, A. L. (2012). *PDR nurse's drug reference 2012*. Clifton Park, NY: Delmar Cengage Learning.

CHAPTER 39

ONCOLOGY DISORDERS

I. BIOLOGIC BASIS OF PEDIATRIC ONCOLOGY

A. OVERVIEW

1. FEW ENVIRONMENTAL FACTORS ARE ASSOCIATED WITH PEDIATRIC MALIGNANCIES, WHICH IS CONTRARY TO THE ADULT ONCOLOGY EXPERIENCE.

2. PEDIATRIC MALIGNANCIES USUALLY ORIGINATE FROM AN EMBRYONIC VERSUS THE EPITHELIAL ORIGIN OF ADULT MALIGNANCIES.

3. PEDIATRIC CANCER ETIOLOGY

   a. Ecogenetics: the interaction between environmental exposures and genetic variations

   b. Hereditary: refers to familial cancer syndromes such as the familial form of retinoblastoma

   c. Two-hit model: theorizes that two mutations are needed for cancer to develop. Mutations occur when errors are made during the process of cellular division. Normal cells can repair the damage; however, a faulty DNA repair gene cannot control the abnormal proliferation of mutated cells, which may lead to uncontrolled growth and proliferation, leading to a malignant condition.

4. CANCER IS THE LEADING CAUSE OF DEATH BY DISEASE IN CHILDREN.

5. LEUKEMIA IS THE MOST COMMON TYPE OF MALIGNANCY.

6. CENTRAL NERVOUS SYSTEM (CNS) TUMORS ARE THE MOST COMMON TYPE OF PEDIATRIC SOLID TUMOR.

B. DIFFERENCES BETWEEN CHILDHOOD AND ADULT CANCERS (SEE TABLE 39-1)

C. MULTIMODAL CANCER TREATMENT: COMBINATION OF INTERVENTIONS TO ERADICATE THE EXISTING MALIGNANCY

1. CHEMOTHERAPY

   a. Systemically prevents malignant cells from proliferating

   b. Agents can be cell-cycle specific (most effective when the cell is in a certain phase of replication) or cell-cycle nonspecific.

   c. Methods of delivery
      1) Oral
      2) Intramuscular
      3) Subcutaneous

Table 39-1 Differences Between Adult and Childhood Cancers

Adult	Childhood
Most tumors are carcinomas of epithelial origin.	Most common tumors are lymphoma and sarcoma which are of primitive embryonic origin.
Strong relationship to environmental factors.	Not a strong relation to environmental factors. Genetic factors may be involved.
Routine screening for certain malignancies, such as mammograms for breast cancer is recommended.	Routine screening is not recommended except in cases of known genetic abnormalities associated with a particular childhood malignancy.
Many adult cancers are preventable.	Few preventive strategies known.
Often present with localized disease.	Metastatic disease often present at diagnosis.
Less responsive to treatment.	More responsive to treatment.
Less than a 60% cure rate.	Greater than 70% cure rate.

4) Intravenous
5) Intrathecal
6) Intra-arterial
7) Intraventricular
d. Categories of agents
1) Alkylating agents interact with the DNA of the cell to create inaccuracy in cellular division or hinder DNA replication. Common agents include cisplantin (Platinol), ifosphamide (Ifex), and busulfan (Myleran).
2) Antibiotic agents bind to DNA in order to affect replication and transcription. Common agents include doxorubicin (Adriamycin), bleomycin (Blenoxane) and dactinomycin (Actinomycin-D).
3) Antimetabolite agents hinder essential enzymes or alter nucleic acid coding. Common agents include Methotrexate (Mexate), cytarabine (cytosine arabinoside) and 6-mercaptopurine (Purinethol).
4) Plant alkaloid agents are miotic inhibitors. Common agents include etoposide (VP-16), vincristine (Oncovin), and vinblastine (Velban).
5) Hormonal agents exhibit a lytic effect on lymphoid cells. Corticosteroids are commonly used.
6) Miscellaneous agents are a unique category in which the mechanism of action is not fully understood or cannot be categorized. The enzyme L-asparaginase (Elspar) is an example.
2. RADIATION THERAPY
a. High-energy particles aimed at a particular anatomic site to eradicate malignancy while sparing surrounding tissues
b. Types
1) External beam: well-defined beam aimed at a specific anatomic site
2) Brachytherapy: implantation of high-dose radionuclides directly into tissue or a body cavity
3. SURGICAL MANAGEMENT
a. Types
1) Biopsy: remove a portion of tissue for pathological examination to aid in diagnosis
2) Staging: visually examine anatomical sites infiltrated by malignancy

3) Resection: removal of malignancy
4) Debulking: removing a portion of the tumor when anatomically impossible to remove entire malignancy
5) Debridement: removing necrotic tissue
6) Clinical manifestation relief: decompress structures affected by the tumor or to relieve pain
4. STEM CELL TRANSPLANTATION (HISTORICALLY CALLED BONE MARROW TRANSPLANTATION—STEM CELLS ARE THE ACTUAL CELLS USED IN TRANSPLANTATION, BONE MARROW REFERS ONLY TO ONE SOURCE OF STEM CELLS COLLECTION): REPLACE DYSFUNCTIONAL HEMATOPOIETIC SYSTEM OR REPLENISH HEMATOPOIETIC SYSTEM AFTER HIGH-DOSE CHEMOTHERAPY
a. Types of transplants
1) Autologous: stem cells are collected from the child for infusion after high-dose chemotherapy.
2) Allogeneic: stem cells are collected from a source other than the child.
a) Donor types
1. Goal: human leukocyte antigen (HLA) typing as close to the recipient as possible to reduce risk of graft-versus-host disease or graft failure. HLA refers to the proteins that help the body identify foreign cells. Six antigens are typed for compatibility.
2. Matched related: usually a sibling, at least 6/6 antigens match
3. Mismatched related: usually a sibling or parent, 3/6–5/6 antigen match
4. Matched unrelated: unrelated source with a 5/6 or 6/6 match
5. Matched related cord: stem cells harvested from a sibling's umbilical cord, can range from 3/6 to 6/6
6. Matched unrelated cord: stem cells harvested from an unrelated umbilical cord, can range from 3/6 to 5/6
b. Collection of stem cells
1) Peripheral blood stem cell: pheresis machine separates stem cells from

circulating blood. Collection requires large-bore double-lumen catheter placement for pheresis procedure; may require more than one collection to procure an adequate cell count.

2) Bone marrow aspiration: numerous aspirations from punctures in the iliac crest of the donor under general anesthesia

3) Umbilical cord blood: collected immediately after birth

c. Preparatory regimens

1) Goal(s)

a) Eradicate malignancy

b) Immunosuppress the recipient to prevent graft rejection

c) Create space in the marrow for the new hematopoietic system

2) High-dose chemotherapy

a) Cyclophosphamide (Cytoxan)

b) Thiotepa (Thiotepa)

c) Busulfan (Myleran)

d) Melphalan (Alkeran)

e) Cytarabine (Cytosine Arabinoside)

f) Etoposide (VP-16)

3) Radiation therapy: eradicate malignancy in the sanctuary sites

a) Total body irradiation: given in fractionated doses for 4–5 days

b) Local control: radiation can be given before or after transplantation for those children with a solid tumor or central nervous system (CNS) disease.

5. BIOLOGICAL RESPONSE MODIFIERS: ACTIVATE IMMUNOLOGIC RESPONSE AGAINST MALIGNANCY

a. Types

1) Monoclonal antibodies: immunoglobulin molecules created to bind to a specific target site on a tumor-associated antigen; may have a toxin or radionuclide or drug attached

2) Cytokines: nonantibody antigens that regulate the immune response

a) Interferons: antiproliferative effect on tumor cells and activate natural killer cells

b) Interleukins: natural proteins that act as messengers between the immune system and cells

c) Hematopoietic growth factors: differentiate and maturate blood cells; commonly used to accelerate bone marrow recovery after chemotherapy

II. **DIAGNOSTIC TESTS**

A. BONE MARROW ASPIRATION AND BIOPSY

1. DESCRIPTION: INSERTION OF A BONE MARROW ASPIRATE/BIOPSY NEEDLE IN THE ANTERIOR OR POSTERIOR ILIAC CREST TO OBTAIN A SPECIMEN OF BONE AND BONE MARROW FOR MICROSCOPIC EXAMINATION OF THE HEMATOPOIETIC SYSTEM

2. PREPROCEDURE

a. Day before the test

1) Obtain informed consent.

2) NPO for 6 hours prior to the procedure if sedation is ordered

b. Day of the test

1) Obtain baseline vital signs.

2) Apply EMLA Cream (a eutectic mixture of lidocaine and prilocaine) to the site at least 1 hour, but no more than 4 hours, prior to the procedure.

3) Provide an age-appropriate description of the procedure.

4) Place the child prone with a folded sheet or blanket under the pelvis.

5) Assist with firm restraining during the procedure, if needed.

6) Monitor sedated child until alert and oriented.

3. POSTPROCEDURE

a. Monitor the pressure dressing for bleeding.

b. Monitor the client for sedation side effects such as respiratory depression and loss of protective reflexes.

c. Maintain the integrity of the pressure dressing for 24 hours.

B. LUMBAR PUNCTURE

1. DESCRIPTION: INSERTION OF A SPINAL NEEDLE BETWEEN THE THIRD AND FOURTH OR FOURTH AND FIFTH LUMBAR VERTEBRAE INTO THE INTERSPACE TO OBTAIN A CEREBROSPINAL FLUID (CSF) SAMPLE OR ADMINISTER MEDICATION

2. PREPROCEDURE

a. Day before the test

1) Obtain written consent.

2) NPO for 6 hours prior to the procedure if the client is to be sedated

b. Day of the test

1) Obtain baseline vital signs.

2) Apply EMLA Cream (a eutectic mixture of lidocaine and prilocaine) to the site at least 1 hour, but no more than 4 hours, prior to procedure.

3) Provide an age-appropriate description of the procedure.

4) Position the child on the side with the knees drawn up under the chin and head bent over the chest or seated on the exam table bent over in a curved position.

3. POSTPROCEDURE
   a. Monitor the dressing for bleeding and CSF leakage.
   b. Monitor the child for sedation adverse reactions such as respiratory depression and loss of protective reflexes.
   c. Instruct the child to lie flat for 30 minutes to prevent headache.
   d. Maintain the integrity of the pressure dressing for 24 hours.

C. SURGICAL BIOPSY
   1. DESCRIPTION: SURGICAL REMOVAL OF TUMOR TISSUE FOR DIRECT EXAMINATION FOR PATHOLOGICAL ANALYSIS
   2. PREPROCEDURE
      a. Day before the procedure
         1) Obtain informed consent.
         2) NPO after midnight
         3) Type and cross match
      b. Day of the procedure
         1) Obtain baseline vital signs.
         2) Provide an age-appropriate description of the procedure.
   3. POSTPROCEDURE
      a. Monitor the dressing for bleeding.
      b. Monitor vital signs.
      c. Monitor the child for anesthesia adverse reactions such as respiratory depression, loss of protective reflexes, nausea, and vomiting.
      d. Provide appropriate pain management.

D. PLAIN FILM RADIOGRAPHY
   1. DESCRIPTION: UTILIZING ELECTROMAGNETIC ENERGY TO VISUALIZE ORGANS AND STRUCTURES WITHIN THE BODY
   2. DAY OF THE TEST
      a. Provide an age-appropriate explanation of the test.
      b. Assist the child in positioning site for examination.

E. ULTRASOUND
   1. DESCRIPTION: UTILIZING SOUND WAVES TO VISUALIZE ORGANS AND STRUCTURES WITHIN THE BODY
   2. DAY OF THE TEST
      a. Provide an age-appropriate explanation of the test.
      b. Instruct the child to maintain a full bladder prior to and during the examination.
      c. Assist the child in positioning to maximize visualization.

F. COMPUTED TOMOGRAPHY WITHOUT CONTRAST
   1. DESCRIPTION: MULTIPLE X-RAY BEAM RECEPTORS TRANSMIT DATA TO A COMPUTER FOR DATA ANALYSIS AND CONVERSION TO AN IMAGE ON A VIDEO SCREEN, WHICH MAY BE PHOTOGRAPHED OR STORED IN THE COMPUTER OR ON VIDEOTAPE
   2. PREPROCEDURE
      a. Obtain informed consent.
      b. NPO if child is to be sedated
   3. DAY OF THE TEST
      a. Provide an age-appropriate explanation of the test.
      b. Instruct the child to maintain position once testing begins.
      c. NPO 6 hours before the test if sedation is ordered
      d. Administer contrast (IV or PO) as ordered.
   4. POSTPROCEDURE
      a. Monitor the child for sedation adverse reactions such as respiratory depression and loss of protective reflexes.

G. COMPUTED TOMOGRAPHY WITH CONTRAST
   1. DESCRIPTION: RADIOIODINATED CONTRAST MATERIAL (IV OR PO) IS ADMINISTERED TO ENHANCE THE IMAGE OF PARTICULAR ORGANS.
   2. PREPROCEDURE
      a. Obtain informed consent.
      b. NPO after midnight if the child is to be sedated
   3. DAY OF THE TEST
      a. Provide an age-appropriate explanation of the test.
      b. Instruct the child to maintain position once testing begins.
      c. NPO 6 hours before the test if sedation is ordered
      d. Administer contrast (IV or PO) as ordered.
   4. POSTPROCEDURE
      a. Monitor the child for sedation adverse reactions such as respiratory depression and loss of protective reflexes.

H. MAGNETIC RESONANCE IMAGING (MRI)
   1. DESCRIPTION: UTILIZING A LARGE, ROUND MAGNET, A RADIOFREQUENCY SIGNAL IS PERIODICALLY BEAMED INTO THE MAGNETIC FIELD, STIMULATING AND HALTING PROTON ACTIVITY. THIS ENERGY IS MEASURED AND TRANSMITTED TO A COMPUTER, WHICH INTERPRETS THE DATA AND CREATES AN IMAGE ON A TELEVISION MONITOR.

2. PREPROCEDURE
   a. Day of the test
      1) Provide an age-appropriate explanation of the test.
      2) Instruct the child to maintain position once testing begins.
      3) NPO 6 hours before the test if sedation is ordered
      4) Administer IV contrast if ordered.
3. POSTPROCEDURE
   a. Monitor the child for sedation adverse reactions such as respiratory depression and loss of protective reflexes.

I. NUCLEAR MEDICINE SCANS
   1. DESCRIPTION: INJECTED ISOTOPES (RADIOACTIVE MATERIAL) DEMONSTRATE PHYSIOLOGIC ACTIVITY IN TISSUES. THE CAMERA DETECTS GAMMA RAYS, WHICH PROJECT AN IMAGE ON THE SCREEN.
   2. PREPROCEDURE
      a. Day of the test
         1) Assess for allergy to the radiopharmaceutical.
         2) Provide an age-appropriate explanation of the test.
         3) Inject the isotope.
         4) Instruct the child to maintain position once testing begins.

J. ECHOCARDIOGRAM
   1. DESCRIPTION: HIGH-FREQUENCY SOUND WAVES DEFINE THE SIZE, MOTION, AND SHAPE OF CARDIAC STRUCTURES
   2. PREPROCEDURE
      a. Day of the test
         1) Provide an age-appropriate explanation of the test.
         2) Instruct the child to maintain position once testing begins.

III. **NURSING DIAGNOSES**
   A. ACUTE PAIN
   B. NAUSEA
   C. IMBALANCED NUTRITION: LESS THAN BODY REQUIREMENTS
   D. IMPAIRED ORAL MUCOUS MEMBRANES
   E. IMPAIRED URINARY ELIMINATION
   F. FATIGUE
   G. IMPAIRED SKIN INTEGRITY
   H. INEFFECTIVE COPING
   I. GRIEVING
   J. DISTURBED BODY IMAGE
   K. HOPELESSNESS

Nursing Diagnoses: Definitions and Classification 2012–2014. Copyright © 2012, 1994–2012 by NANDA International. Used by arrangement with John Wiley & Sons Limited.

IV. **NURSING CARE OF THE CHILD RECEIVING CHEMOTHERAPY OR RADIATION THERAPY**
   A. EDUCATE THE CHILD REGARDING SAFE ADMINISTRATION OF ANTIEMETICS.
   B. MAINTAIN ADEQUATE NUTRITION; ENCOURAGE SMALL, FREQUENT MEALS AND ORAL SUPPLEMENTS TO MEET CALORIC NEEDS.
      1. NASOGASTRIC (NG) FEEDINGS IF UNABLE TO TAKE IN ADEQUATE CALORIES
      2. TOTAL PARENTERAL NUTRITION (TPN) IF UNABLE TO TOLERATE ORAL INTAKE OR GASTRIC FEEDINGS
   C. PREVENT CONSTIPATION BY MAINTAINING ADEQUATE HYDRATION, ACTIVITY LEVEL, AND A WELL-BALANCED DIET.
   D. MANAGE FATIGUE BY PROMOTING REST PERIODS AND GROUPING CARE.
   E. MONITOR FOR CLINICAL MANIFESTATIONS OF NEUROPATHY (TINGLING IN THE HANDS AND FEET, ALTERED GAIT, CHRONIC CONSTIPATION, CHANGES IN GROSS OR FINE MOTOR SKILLS RELATED TO STRUCTURES IN THE RADIATION FIELD).
   F. MONITOR LABORATORY VALUES.
      1. COMPLETE BLOOD COUNT (CBC) FOR NEUTROPENIA (LOW WHITE BLOOD CELL [WBC] COUNT), ANEMIA (LOW RED BLOOD CELL [RBC] COUNT), AND THROMBOCYTOPENIA (LOW PLATELET COUNT)
      2. LIVER FUNCTION TESTS (LFTS) FOR ELEVATIONS CAUSED BY CHEMOTHERAPY OR MALIGNANCY
      3. SERUM CHEMISTRIES FOR ELECTROLYTE IMBALANCES CAUSED BY CHEMOTHERAPY OR MALIGNANCY
   G. EDUCATION
      1. IMMUNOSUPPRESSION
         a. Neutropenia
            1) Defined as an absolute neutrophil count (ANC) of less than 1000
            2) Severe neutropenia: defined as an ANC of less than 500
         b. Clinical manifestations of infection
            1) General: fever, chills, pain
            2) Respiratory: productive or nonproductive cough, chest pain, shortness of breath, fever
            3) Gastrointestinal (G1): retrosternal chest pain, dysphagia, anorexia, dehydration, right lower quadrant pain, diarrhea, perirectal tenderness, fever
            4) Skin: redness, swelling, pain, possible drainage around the central venous access device exit site, fever

c. Fever greater than or equal to 38.3°C (101°F)

d. Hand washing as primary preventive measure against infection

e. Avoid close contact with individuals who display clinical manifestations of infection.

2. BLEEDING

a. Instruct the child and parent to call the treatment team immediately if the child is bleeding (typical sites: skin, gums, nose, rectal).

b. Introduce the potential need for platelet infusion(s).

3. FATIGUE

a. Anemia: introduce the potential need for blood product support to maintain the hemoglobin between 8 g/dl and 9 g/dl

or asymptomatic.

b. Promote rest by grouping activities of daily living (ADLs).

4. NUTRITION

a. Promote a well-balanced diet.

b. Encourage small, frequent meals.

c. Support oral hygiene.

5. CENTRAL LINE CARE

a. Type of central line

1) Indwelling catheter: a catheter and reservoir are surgically placed under the skin—requires the skin to be punctured when accessing the catheter for use. The catheter tip dwells in the superior vena cava. The catheter requires occlusive dressing only when accessed (e.g., Port-A-Cath).

2) External catheter: a surgically placed catheter is inserted through the skin and tunneled into a main vein. The catheter tip dwells in the superior vena cava. The exit site is secured with an occlusive dressing (e.g., Broviac, Hickman).

3) Peripherally inserted central catheter (PICC): the PICC can be placed with or without sedation. The catheter is inserted through the skin and threaded into a main vein. The catheter tip dwells in the superior vena cava. The exit site is secured with an occlusive dressing.

b. Daily care

1) Flush the central line with heparin to maintain patency.

2) Inspect the line for holes, leaks, and breaks. Report any catheter damage to the treatment team immediately to initiate repair.

3) Inspect the insertion site for signs and symptoms of infection

Table 39-2 Holiday-Segar Method of Assessing Fluids

Body Weight	ml/kg/day
First 10 kg	100 ml/kg/day
Second 10 kg	50 ml/kg/day
Each additional kg	20 ml/kg/day

© Cengage Learning 2015

Table 39-3 Example: 9-Year-Old Weighing 23 kg

Body Weight	ml/day
100 (for first 10 kg) × 10	1000 ml/day
50 (for second 10 kg) × 10	500 ml/day
20 (for each additional kg) × 3	60 ml/day
Total	1560 ml/day

© Cengage Learning 2015

(redness, tenderness, drainage, edema, warmth).

c. Dressing changes

1) Instruct the parents on occlusive, sterile dressing changes.

2) Instruct the parents on sterile cap/extension tubing changes.

6. SKIN CARE

a. Instruct the parents about the application of approved topical skin creams, ointments, or lotions during radiation therapy to rehydrate irradiated skin and avoid further cellular damage.

b. Instruct the parents to maintain adequate hydration to sustain appropriate skin turgor: Holiday-Segar method for assessing fluid needs (not to be used for neonates less than 14 days old). (See Tables 39-2 and 39-3.)

c. Maintain diligent perirectal skin care to decrease incidence of skin tears or fissures, which may lead to infection.

V. **NURSING CARE OF THE CHILD RECEIVING ONCOLOGIC SURGICAL MANAGEMENT**

A. PREOPERATIVELY

1. PREVENT TRAUMA TO THE TUMOR.

2. MONITOR STRICT INTAKE AND OUTPUT.

3. MONITOR VITAL SIGNS.

4. MONITOR LABORATORY VALUES.

a. Correct electrolyte imbalances

b. Blood product support

5. MONITOR AND MANAGE PAIN.

6. MAINTAIN ADEQUATE NUTRITION.

a. TPN if unable to tolerate appropriate oral intake of nutritional needs

7. PREPARE THE CLIENT AND FAMILY FOR THE SURGICAL PROCEDURE AND CONCOMITANT CENTRAL LINE PLACEMENT.

B. POSTOPERATIVELY
1. MONITOR FOR CLINICAL MANIFESTATIONS OF INFECTION (FEVER, REDNESS, EDEMA, DRAINAGE, TENDERNESS AT THE OPERATIVE SITE).
2. MONITOR VITAL SIGNS, TEMPERATURE.
3. MONITOR FLUID BALANCE.
   a. Strict intake and output
   b. Daily weights
   c. Monitor edema
4. MANAGE NAUSEA AND VOMITING.
5. MANAGE PAIN.
6. PROVIDE NUTRITIONAL SUPPORT VIA TPN.

VI. **NURSING MANAGEMENT OF TREATMENT OF ADVERSE REACTIONS**
A. BONE MARROW SUPPRESSION
1. ANEMIA: DECREASED NUMBER OF CIRCULATING RED BLOOD CELLS
   a. Symptoms include fatigue, pallor, tachycardia, headache.
   b. Administer packed red blood cells (PRBCs) at 10–15 ml/kg if clinical symptoms are present.
2. NEUTROPENIA: DECREASED NUMBER OF CIRCULATING NEUTROPHILS
   a. Can be asymptomatic, determined by examining CBC and calculating the ANC
   b. Severe neutropenia: ANC less than 500. The child is a greater risk for developing infection during periods of severe neutropenia.
   c. Granulocyte colony-stimulating factor (Neupogen): cytokine administered to stimulate bone marrow to release neutrophils
3. THROMBOCYTOPENIA: DECREASED NUMBER OF CIRCULATING PLATELETS
   a. Symptoms include petechiae and gingival or nasal bleeding.
   b. Transfuse platelets with active bleeding or a platelet count less than 20,000/mm^3 or 50,000/mm^3 for children with CNS tumors.
   c. Oprelvekin (Neumega): cytokine administered to stimulate the bone marrow to release platelets
B. CENTRAL NERVOUS SYSTEM (CNS) COMPLICATIONS
1. DIABETES INSIPIDUS: DECREASED PRODUCTION OF THE ANTIDIURETIC HORMONE
   a. Risk factors: CNS tumors, CNS leukemia, radiation to the hypothalamic-pituitary axis

   b. Clinical manifestations include polyuria with a urine specific gravity less than 1.005, hypernatremia, and lethargy.
   c. Management includes vasopressin (Pitressin) replacement, strict intake and output, fluid replacement, urine specific gravity monitoring, serum electrolyte monitoring.
2. POSTERIOR FOSSA SYNDROME: TRANSIENT OR PERMANENT DEFICITS AFTER POSTERIOR FOSSA SURGERY
   a. Clinical manifestations include mutism or speech alterations, dysphasia, decreased gross motor function, emotional liableness, and cranial nerve palsies appearing 24–48 hours after surgery and may persist for 2–6 months postoperatively.
   b. Management includes instituting rehabilitative services after surgical recovery is complete.
C. ENDOCRINE ABNORMALITIES
1. HORMONE DEFICITS: LOW LEVELS OF HORMONES SECRETED BY THE BODY
   a. Neuroendocrine injury can occur from the disease or treatment.
   b. Hypothyroidism
   c. Gonadal dysfunction
   d. Growth hormone deficiency
   e. Clinical manifestations include abnormal hormone and thyroid levels, fatigue, delayed development of secondary sexual characteristics or precocious puberty, and a decrease in linear growth.
   f. Management includes hormone replacement and symptom management.
D. CARDIAC AND PULMONARY COMPLICATIONS
1. ACUTE CARDIOMYOPATHY: ALTERED CARDIAC FUNCTION RELATED TO DAMAGED MYOCYTES
   a. Clinical manifestations include hypertension or hypotension, fatigue, chest pain, activity intolerance, and shortness of breath.
   b. Management includes monitoring cardiac function throughout the course of therapy, administering antiarrhythmic drugs, and adjusting chemotherapy agents associated with cardiac damage.
2. PNEUMONITIS: INFLAMMATION OF THE LUNG
   a. Clinical manifestations include dyspnea, fatigue, fever, and nonproductive cough.

b. Management includes prophylactic treatment with TMP-SMZ (Bactrim) or pentamidine (Pentam 300) to prevent *Pneumocystis carinii,* oxygen therapy, and antibiotic therapy for bacterial infections.

E. GASTROINTESTINAL COMPLICATIONS

1. MUCOSITIS: AN INFLAMMATION OF THE MUCOUS MEMBRANES OF THE BUCCAL CAVITY AND MAY INCLUDE THE ESOPHAGUS

   a. Clinical manifestations include mucous membranes with whitish plaques and indurated borders caused by *Candida albicans,* herpetic ulcerations, pallor, or erythema. Drooling or difficulty speaking or swallowing may also be present.

   b. Management includes oral rinses to clean and moisturize the oral mucosa; antifungal, antiviral, or antibiotic therapy for confirmed secondary infections; pain management; and fluid management. Nutritional considerations include:

      1) A soft diet that maximizes nutritional content
      2) Avoiding mechanical injuries
      3) Limits to mastication for pain control; if unable to tolerate oral feedings, implement TPN.

2. DIARRHEA: INCREASE IN THE FREQUENCY OR QUANTITY OF STOOL OR A CHANGE IN THE CONSISTENCY OF THE STOOL

   a. Clinical manifestations include frequent loose stools, stool with mucus or blood, abdominal cramping, hyperactive bowel sounds, altered electrolytes, and fever.

   b. Management includes correcting electrolyte imbalances, intravenous therapy, and antibiotic therapy for identified infection.

3. CONSTIPATION: INFREQUENT STOOLING OR EXPULSION OF HARD AND DRY FECES

   a. Clinical manifestations include straining during defecation, abdominal cramping, bleeding, and rectal soreness.

   b. Management includes initiating the use of stool softeners or laxatives, increasing fluid intake, and increasing fiber intake. In severe cases, surgical intervention may be required for obstructions. Rectal manipulation or irrigation should not be implemented for the pediatric oncology client.

   c. Chemotherapy agents that decrease peristalsis include vincristine (Oncovin) and vinblastine (Velban).

4. NAUSEA AND VOMITING

   a. Nausea: wavelike feelings of gastrointestinal discomfort

   b. Vomiting: expulsion of gastric contents

   c. Types

      1) Acute: most severe within the first 24 hours after receiving chemotherapy
      2) Delayed: symptoms lasting up to 2 weeks after chemotherapy administration
      3) Anticipatory: preexisting anxiety stimulating a conditioned response to a trigger (sight of hospital, oncology clinic, nursing staff)
      4) Management includes minimizing and preventing nausea and vomiting.
         a) Nonpharmacologic: relaxation; distraction; guided imagery
         b) Pharmacologic: ondansetron (Zofran); prochlorperazine (Compazine); diphenhydramine (Benadryl); dexamethasone (Decadron); metoclopramide (Reglan)
         c) Antianxiety therapy: lorazepam (Ativan)

F. RENAL COMPLICATIONS

1. KIDNEY IMPAIRMENT: DECREASED ABILITY TO PERFORM NORMAL FUNCTIONS

   a. Clinical manifestations include elevated creatinine, blood urea nitrogen (BUN), proteinuria, hematuria, and altered fluids and electrolytes.

   b. Management includes renal function analysis prior to each renal-offensive chemotherapy course, urine alkalinization, hyperhydration, and careful monitoring during concomitant therapy with other nephrotoxic drugs.

2. HEMORRHAGIC CYSTITIS: CONDITION RANGING FROM MILD DYSURIA AND SLIGHT HEMATURIA TO SIGNIFICANT DAMAGE TO THE EPITHELIAL LINING OF THE BLADDER, LEADING TO HEMORRHAGE

   a. Clinical manifestations include dysuria (painful or difficulty urinating) and hematuria.

   b. Management includes maintenance of adequate hydration, concomitant use of mesna (a bladder protective agent) during the administration of cyclophosphamide (Cytoxan) and ifosfamide (Ifex), monitoring renal function via laboratory values (BUN, creatinine, electrolytes), and urinalysis (specific gravity, microscopic hematuria).

3. TUMOR LYSIS SYNDROME: RAPID RELEASE OF INTRACELLULAR METABOLITES IS GREATER THAN THE KIDNEY'S CAPACITY TO EXCRETE THEM. PROCESS POTENTIALLY OCCURS WHEN THE CHILD HAS A LARGE TUMOR BURDEN, SUCH AS IN LEUKEMIA OR LYMPHOMA.

   a. Clinical manifestations include cramping, vomiting, flank pain, and cardiac arrhythmias caused by severe electrolyte imbalances.

   b. Management

     1) Close monitoring of the child's vital signs

     2) Frequent laboratory assessment of electrolytes

     3) Hyperhydration with alkalinization

     4) Correct electrolyte imbalances

     5) Administer rasburicase (Elitek) to facilitate uric acid excretion

     6) Administer allopurinol (Aloprim [IV form] or Zyloprim [oral form]) to inhibit the formation of uric acid.

G. PAIN MANAGEMENT

1. RISK FACTORS

   a. Disease related: infiltration of malignant cells can lead to compression of normal structures and excite pain receptors.

   b. Treatment related: invasive procedures (e.g., lumbar punctures) and side effects of therapy (e.g., mucositis) may initiate painful processes.

2. CLASSIFICATIONS

   a. Acute: sudden onset or self-limiting

   b. Chronic: persistent pain usually lasting 6 months or greater

3. MANAGEMENT

   a. Pharmacologic

     1) Mild pain: nonopioid analgesics; consider adjuvant.

     2) Moderate pain: weak opioids; consider nonopioid and adjuvant analgesic.

     3) Severe pain: strong opioids; consider nonopioid and adjuvant analgesic.

     4) Nonopioid analgesics

       a) Acetaminophen (Tylenol)

       b) Nonsteroidal anti-inflammatory drugs ([NSAIDs] Advil)

     5) Weak opioids

       a) Codeine with acetaminophen (Tylenol with Codeine)

       b) Hydrocodone with acetaminophen (Vicodin, Lortab)

     6) Strong opioids

       a) Morphine (MS Contin)

       b) Hydromorphone (Dilaudid)

       c) Fentanyl (Sublimaze)

     7) Adjuvants

       a) Lorazepam (Ativan)

       b) Dexamethasone (Decadron)

       c) Clonazepam (Klonopin)

   b. Nonpharmacologic: to support successful teaching of nonpharmacological techniques, instruction must occur when the child is not experiencing pain.

     1) Guided imagery

     2) Distraction

     3) Relaxation techniques

   c. Assessment

     1) Based on the child's developmental age

     2) Utilize established pain assessment tools.

       a) Visual analogue scale (0–10): rate pain on a scale of 0 to 10, with 0 being no pain and 10 being the worst pain imaginable

     3) Use the same pain scale among caregivers for consistency.

H. GROWTH AND DEVELOPMENT

1. CANCER TREATMENT CAN INTERFERE WITH THE PHYSICAL AND PSYCHOLOGICAL GROWTH AND DEVELOPMENT OF THE CHILD.

2. RISK FACTORS

   a. Treatment less than 6 years old

   b. Treatment after onset of puberty

   c. Combination chemotherapy

   d. Radiation therapy

   e. Steroid therapy

   f. Chemotherapy combined with radiation therapy

3. CLINICAL MANIFESTATIONS

   a. Delay: developmental, social, motor, language

   b. Musculoskeletal abnormalities (e.g., asymmetrical features, poor linear growth, scoliosis)

   c. Neuroendocrine dysfunction (e.g., luteinizing hormone [LH] or follicle-stimulating hormone [FSH] deficiency, thyrotropin deficiency, adrenocorticotropic hormone deficiency)

   d. Management

     1) Monitoring velocity (cm/year) of physical growth

     2) Height and weight documentation

     3) Neuropsychological evaluations

     4) Educational intervention

5) Tanner stage evaluation
6) Laboratory analysis
   a) Thyroid function
   b) Growth hormone status

I. NUTRITIONAL COMPLICATIONS
1. DESCRIPTION: CHANGE IN NUTRITIONAL INTAKE THAT LEADS TO WEIGHT LOSS OR GAIN
2. RISK FACTORS
   a. Radiation to the head and neck (can lead to mucositis) or abdomen and pelvis (can lead to intestinal dysfunction)
   b. Chemotherapy
   c. Steroid therapy
   d. Disease state: metastatic or recurrent disease
3. MANAGEMENT
   a. Oral supplementation with commercial products such as Ensure and Pediasure
   b. Enteral feedings via nasogastric or gastrostomy tube
   c. TPN intravenously if the gastrointestinal tract is unable to tolerate intake required to meet the nutritional needs of the child

VII. **NURSING DISORDERS**
A. WILMS' TUMOR (NEPHROBLASTOMA)
1. DESCRIPTION
   a. Malignant tumor of the kidney(s)
   b. Peak age of onset is 2–3 years of age
   c. Rarely associated with anomalies such as aniridia (congenital absence of the iris), hemihypertrophy (a relative increase in size of one-half of the body as compared to the other side), and genitourinary anomalies
2. ASSESSMENT
   a. Asymptomatic mass in the abdomen
   b. Hypertension
   c. Microscopic or gross hematuria
   d. Malaise
   e. Fever
   f. Anemia
   g. Pain
3. DIAGNOSTIC TESTS
   a. History
      1) Incidence and duration of clinical manifestations
      2) Predisposing factors
      3) Family history
   b. Physical exam
      1) Presence of mass
      2) Hypertension
      3) Congenital anomalies
         a) Aniridia
         b) Hemihypertrophy
         c) Genital or renal malformations

4) Distended abdominal veins
5) Neurologic status, as initial diagnosis may include metastasis to the brain
c. Tumor evaluation
   1) Abdominal ultrasound
   2) Computed tomography (CT)
   3) Magnetic resonance imaging (MRI)
d. Metastatic search
   1) Chest x-ray
   2) Chest CT
   3) Bone scan
   4) Brain CT
e. Laboratory testing
   1) Complete blood count to monitor hematopoiesis
   2) LFTs for baseline evaluation
   3) Renal functions for baseline evaluation
   4) Urinalysis
4. STAGING
   a. Stage I: tumor is limited to the kidney and completely resected.
   b. Stage II: tumor extends beyond the kidney but is completely resected.
   c. Stage III: residual nonhematogenous tumor is localized to the abdomen.
   d. Stage IV: hematogenous metastases; deposits are beyond stage III to the lung, liver, bone, and brain.
   e. Stage V: both kidneys are affected at the time of diagnosis.
5. MULTIMODAL MANAGEMENT
   a. Surgical removal or resection of the affected kidney(s)
   b. Chemotherapy
      1) Vincristine (Oncovin)
      2) Dactinomycin (Actinomycin-D)
      3) Doxorubicin (Adriamycin)
      4) Cyclophosphamide (Cytoxan)
6. NURSING INTERVENTIONS
   a. Preoperatively
      1) Prevent trauma to the tumor, including avoiding palpating the abdomen.
      2) Obtain abdominal girth.
      3) Monitor vital signs and manage hypertension.
   b. Postoperatively
      1) Monitor vital signs, specifically blood pressure (BP) and temperature.
      2) Measure abdominal girth.
      3) Maintain gastric decompression.
   c. During chemotherapy and radiation
      1) Laboratory monitoring
         a) Urinalysis to monitor for hematuria
      2) Education
         a) Activity: eliminate contact sports to protect the remaining kidney.

B. NEUROBLASTOMA
1. DESCRIPTION
   a. Tumor derived of primordial neural crest cells that develop into the sympathetic nervous system (most common extracranial solid tumor)
   b. Etiology unknown
   c. Incidence truly unknown because of spontaneous tumor regression or maturation, most commonly seen in neonates or infants
   d. Average age of child at diagnosis is 2 years, with most being below 5 years of age.
   e. Most common sites
      1) Abdominal mass, often involving the adrenal gland
      2) Pelvic
      3) Thoracic
      4) Cervical
   f. Most common metastatic sites
      1) Lymph nodes
      2) Bone
      3) Bone marrow
      4) Liver
      5) Skin
2. ASSESSMENT
   a. Clinical manifestations may vary, depending on disease site and metastasis.
   b. Distended abdomen with a mass that is hard, fixed, and painful
   c. Bowel and bladder difficulties
   d. Edema
   e. Low-grade fever
   f. Weight loss
   g. Fatigue
   h. Proptosis: the forward displacement of one or both eyeballs
   i. Periorbital ecchymosis: raccoon eyes
   j. Lymphadenopathy
   k. Pallor
   l. Pain
3. DIAGNOSTIC TESTS
   a. History
      1) Presence and onset of clinical manifestations associated with catecholamines (hypertension, flushing, irritability)
      2) Weight loss
      3) Pain
      4) Refusal to walk
      5) Family history of cancer
   b. Physical exam
      1) Abdominal mass
      2) Baseline vital signs
      3) Lymphadenopathy
      4) Cutaneous masses
      5) Extremity weakness

      6) Periorbital ecchymosis (raccoon eyes)
      7) Proptosis (the forward displacement of the eyeball[s])
   c. Tumor evaluation and metastatic search
      1) Bone scan to assess for metastasis
      2) CT of the chest, abdomen, and pelvis
      3) MRI of the primary site
      4) Iodine-131-metaiodobenzylguanidine (MIBG) scan
      5) Bilateral bone marrow aspirate and biopsy
      6) Surgical tissue sample
   d. Laboratory testing
      1) Urine catecholamine metabolites (VMA, HVA, dopamine) are excessively produced in clients with neuroblastoma.
      2) Ferritin level is often elevated in clients with neuroblastoma.
      3) Lactate dehydrogenase (LDH) level is often elevated in clients with neuroblastoma.
      4) GD2 level (GD2 is present on the surface of neuroblastoma cells and is shed by tumor cells and easy to detect)
      5) CBC to monitor hematopoiesis
      6) Serum chemistries to monitor abnormalities
4. STAGING
   a. Stage I: localized tumor confined to the site of origin
   b. Stage IIA: identifiable ipsilateral and contralateral lymph nodes
   c. Stage IIB: positive ipsilateral and contralateral lymph nodes
   d. Stage III: tumor has infiltrated across the midline, with possible regional lymph node involvement
   e. Stage IV: tumor disseminates to the distant lymph nodes
   f. Stage IVS: tumor disseminates to the liver, skin, or bone
5. MULTIMODAL MANAGEMENT
   a. Based on staging
   b. Surgical removal or debulking of the tumor
   c. Chemotherapy
      1) Cyclophosphamide (Cytoxan)
      2) Ifosfamide (Ifex)
      3) Cisplatin (Platinol)
      4) Doxorubicin (Adriamycin)
      5) Etoposide (VP-16)
      6) Vincristine
   d. Tandem hematopoietic stem cell transplantation for high-risk clients

e. Radiation therapy for residual disease management

f. Biological modifiers to induce growth arrest and apoptosis (cell death)

   1) 13-*cis*-retinoic acid introduced after stem cell transplantation

6. NURSING INTERVENTIONS

  a. Preoperatively

    1) Obtain abdominal girth.

    2) Monitor vital signs and manage hypertension.

  b. Postoperatively

    1) Monitor vital signs, specifically temperature and BP.

    2) Monitor abdominal girth as ordered.

    3) Maintain gastric decompression as ordered.

    4) Manage pain.

  c. During chemotherapy and radiation

    1) Monitor laboratory values.

      a) Ferritin levels as a measure of tumor responsiveness (level should decrease)

      b) Urine catecholamine metabolites as a measure of tumor responsiveness (levels should decrease)

    2) Educate the client about radiation recall: inflammatory reaction of affected tissues.

      a) Associated with chemotherapy agents such as

        1. Cyclophosphamide (Cytoxan)

        2. Doxorubicin (Adriamycin)

        3. Etoposide (VP-16)

C. EWING'S SARCOMA, SOFT TISSUE AND PERIPHERAL PRIMITIVE NEUROECTODERMAL TUMORS

  1. DESCRIPTION

    a. Primitive, highly malignant, radiosensitive tumor of neural origin that arises from the bone or soft tissue (extraosseous Ewing's sarcoma)

    b. Peripheral primitive neuroectodermal tumors (PNET): similar pathology with the most cellular differentiation

    c. Peak age of onset in older children and young adults

    d. Most common sites

      1) Long bones

      2) Pelvis

      3) Rib cage

    e. Most common metastatic sites

      1) Lung

      2) Bone

      3) Bone marrow

  2. ASSESSMENT

    a. Palpable mass

    b. Pain

    c. Pathological fractures

    d. Fever

3. DIAGNOSTIC TESTS

  a. History

    1) Incidence and duration of clinical manifestations, specifically intermittent pain (usually present 3–9 months prior to diagnosis)

    2) Family history of cancer

  b. Physical exam

    1) Presence of mass; assess warmth, tenderness, and bilateral limb circumference, if applicable

    2) Range of motion, if applicable

    3) Pain

  c. Tumor evaluation

    1) MRI scan

    2) Bone scan

    3) Tumor biopsy

  d. Metastatic search

    1) Bone marrow biopsy

    2) Chest CT

  e. Laboratory testing

    1) CBC to monitor hematopoiesis

    2) LFTs for baseline evaluation; alkaline phosphatase is often elevated in bone tumors.

    3) Serum chemistries for baseline evaluation

4. MULTIMODAL MANAGEMENT

  a. Local tumor control

    1) Surgical resection

      a) Limb salvage: wide resection including biopsy site; ORIF: reconstruction with open reduction internal fixation; arthroplasty: surgical replacement with metallic implantation; arthrodesis: fuses a joint

      b) Rotationplasty: combines amputation and limb salvage by removing the tumor, amputating the lower portion of the leg, rotating it 180 degrees, and reattaching the leg in order to use the now reversed foot as a stable knee joint

      c) Amputation: complete surgical removal of the affected site

    2) Radiation therapy

      a) Local control if the tumor is surgically unresectable

      b) Adjuvant radiation therapy if surgical margins are close to eradicate the microscopic residual tumor

  b. Chemotherapy

    1) Vincristine (Oncovin)

    2) Dactinomycin (Actinomycin-D)

    3) Doxorubicin (Adriamycin)

    4) Cyclophosphamide (Cytoxan)

    5) Ifosfamide (Ifex)

c. Radiation
   1) Local tumor control based on location of the tumor (not surgically accessible) and response to systemic control (chemotherapy)
   2) Lung irradiation if lung metastases are present at the time of diagnosis
5. NURSING INTERVENTIONS
   a. Prelocal control
      1) Support pathological fractures with casting or bracing.
      2) Prepare the child and family for timing of local control (surgical procedure vs. radiation therapy after several predetermined courses of chemotherapy).
      3) Administer neoadjuvant chemotherapy (chemotherapy given before local control to shrink the tumor).
      4) Preoperative tumor evaluation: assess tumor response to neoadjuvant chemotherapy (chemotherapy given before local control to shrink the tumor).
         a) MRI of tumor site
         b) Chest CT
         c) Bone scan
   b. Postlocal control
      1) Monitor vital signs, specifically the temperature and respiratory status, if thoracic surgery was performed.
         a) O_2 saturation
         b) Respiratory rate and effort
         c) Quality of breath sounds bilaterally
      2) Monitor circulation, movement, sensation (CMS) distal to the operative site, if applicable.
      3) Perform chest tube management if thoracic surgery was performed.
      4) Initiate physical therapy and rehabilitation services.
   c. During chemotherapy and radiation
      1) Monitor for signs and symptoms of neuropathy.
      2) Education
         a) Promote child safety: physical therapy to promote safe locomotion; occupational therapy to promote safe performance of ADLs.
         b) Educate the child and parent about radiation recall: inflammatory reaction of affected tissues.
         c) Associated with chemotherapy agents such as
            1. Cyclophosphamide (Cytoxan)
            2. Dactinomycin (Actinomycin-D)
            3. Doxorubicin (Adriamycin)
            4. Etoposide (VP-16)
D. OSTEOGENIC SARCOMA (OSTEOSARCOMA)
   1. DESCRIPTION
      a. Malignant nonradiosensitive tumor of the bone arising from the bone-forming mesenchyme (most common bone cancer)
      b. Peak age of onset in adolescence and young adults
      c. Most common sites are long bones
      d. Most common metastatic sites
         1) Lung
         2) Bone
   2. ASSESSMENT
      a. Palpable mass
      b. Pain that increases with activity and may result in limping
      c. Pathological fractures that may be the first clinical manifestation
      d. Fever
   3. DIAGNOSTIC TESTS
      a. History
         1) Incidence and duration of clinical manifestations, specifically intermittent pain (usually present 3 months prior to the diagnosis)
         2) Associated with trauma
         3) Altered function of the affected body part (gait variances, limited range of motion)
         4) Prior irradiation therapy increases the risk of developing a secondary malignancy, often osteosarcoma in the radiation field.
         5) Hereditary retinoblastoma or Li-Fraumeni syndrome, which are genetic predispositions for osteosarcoma
         6) Family history of cancer
      b. Physical exam
         1) Presence of mass; assess warmth, tenderness, and bilateral limb circumference, if tumor site is located within an extremity
         2) Range of motion, if tumor site is located within an extremity
         3) Pain
      c. Tumor evaluation
         1) X-ray of primary tumor site
         2) MRI
         3) Bone scan
         4) Tumor biopsy required to confirm diagnosis
      d. Metastatic search
         1) Chest x-ray
         2) Chest CT

e. Laboratory testing
   1) Complete blood count to monitor hematopoiesis
   2) LFTs for baseline evaluation; alkaline phosphatase is often elevated in bone tumors
   3) Serum chemistries for baseline evaluation

4. MULTIMODAL MANAGEMENT
   a. Surgery
      1) Limb salvage: wide resection including the biopsy site
         a) ORIF: reconstruction with open reduction internal fixation
         b) Arthroplasty: surgical replacement with metallic implantation
         c) Arthrodesis: fuses a joint
      2) Rotationplasty: combines amputation and limb salvage by removing the tumor, amputating the lower portion of the leg, rotating it 180 degrees, and reattaching the leg in order to use the now reversed foot as a stable knee joint
      3) Amputation: complete surgical removal of the affected site
   b. Chemotherapy
      1) High-dose methotrexate
      2) Cisplatin (Platinol)
      3) Doxorubicin (Adriamycin)
      4) Etoposide (VP-16)
      5) Ifosfamide (Ifex)

5. NURSING INTERVENTIONS
   a. Preoperative
      1) Support pathological fractures with casting or bracing.
      2) Prepare the client and family for timing of surgical intervention after several predetermined courses of chemotherapy.
      3) Administer neoadjuvant chemotherapy (chemotherapy given before surgical resection to shrink the tumor).
      4) Preoperative tumor evaluation: assess tumor response to neoadjuvant chemotherapy.
         a) MRI of tumor site
         b) Chest CT
         c) Bone scan
   b. Postoperative
      1) Monitor vital signs, specifically temperature and respiratory status if thoracic surgery was performed to remove lung metastases.
         a) O₂ saturation
         b) Respiratory rate and effort
         c) Quality of breath sounds bilaterally

2) Monitor CMS distal to the operative site, if applicable.
3) Perform chest tube management if thoracic surgery was performed.
4) Initiate physical therapy and rehabilitation services.

c. During chemotherapy and radiation
   1) Monitor for clinical manifestations of neuropathy.
   2) Education
      a) Promote client safety.
         1. Physical therapy to promote safe locomotion
         2. Occupational therapy to promote safe performance of ADLs

E. CENTRAL NERVOUS SYSTEM (CNS) TUMORS
   1. DESCRIPTION
      a. Malignant or benign tumor occurring in the regions of the brain
      b. Most common types
         1) Astrocytoma
            a) Description
               1. Astrocyte: a star-shaped cell in the central nervous system's supportive tissue
               2. Classified according to loss of distinctive cell features
               3. Benign or malignant, depending on the level of cellular activity, vascularization, and necrosis
            b) Occurs at any age
            c) Most common type of brain tumor
            d) Most common sites
               1. Cerebellum
               2. Cerebral hemispheres
               3. Brainstem
               4. Optic chiasm or optic nerve
               5. Hypothalamus
         2) Medulloblastoma
            a) Description: small, round, blue cell tumor; fast growing; most common malignant primary CNS tumor
            b) Occurs at any age
            c) Most common sites: posterior fossa; cerebellar hemispheres; fourth ventricle
            d) Most common metastatic sites: spine; bone; bone marrow
         3) Brainstem tumors
            a) Description: fast growing; subcategorized into focal or diffuse; histology: low grade glioma (a tumor composed of connective tissue [neuroglial tissue] of the nervous system); anaplastic astrocytoma;

malignant glioblastoma multiforme; poorer prognosis due to inoperability
      b) Age of onset less than 10 years
    4) Ependymoma
      a) Description: ependymal cells line the central canal of the spinal cord and the ventricles; invasively spreads to contiguous brain tissue
      b) Age of onset less than 6 years
      c) Most common sites: infratentorial; supratentorial; spinal cord, particularly the lumbosacral area
  2. ASSESSMENT
    a. Neurological changes, depending on location of the tumor
      1) Increased intracranial pressure (ICP) caused by:
        a) Hydrocephalus
        b) Tumor pressure
      2) Seizures
      3) Visual changes
        a) Nystagmus
        b) Diplopia
      4) Irritability
      5) Ataxia
    b. Headache
    c. Vomiting
  3. DIAGNOSTIC TESTS
    a. History
      1) Incidence and duration of clinical manifestations
      2) Predisposing factors
        a) Prior radiation therapy
        b) Prior chemotherapy
        c) Genetic abnormalities
      3) Family history of cancer
    b. Physical exam
      1) Neurological examination
        a) Cranial nerve testing
        b) Mental status
        c) Gait analysis
        d) Sensory exam
        e) Strength testing
      2) Growth and development
      3) Pain assessment
    c. Tumor evaluation
      1) MRI scan of the brain—gold standard
      2) Tumor biopsy
    d. Metastatic search
      1) MRI scan of the spine
      2) Lumbar puncture, if indicated: timing is crucial to avoid herniation in the presence of increased ICP
      3) Bone marrow biopsy, if medulloblastoma is suspected
      4) Bone scan, if medulloblastoma is suspected

    e. Laboratory testing
      1) Complete blood count to monitor hematopoiesis
      2) Serum chemistries for baseline evaluation
  4. MULTIMODAL MANAGEMENT
    a. Local tumor control
      1) Surgery
        a) Surgical excision is the primary treatment.
        b) Immediate intervention to relieve symptoms and obtain tissue sample for diagnosis
        c) Client may need ventriculoperitioneal (VP) shunt placed to manage hydrocephalus.
      2) Radiation therapy if tumor is surgically unresectable
    b. Systemic chemotherapy
      1) Vincristine (Oncovin)
      2) Carmustine (BiCNU)
      3) Lomustine (CeeNU)
      4) Cyclophosphamide (Cytoxan)
      5) Ifosfamide (Ifex)
      6) Cisplatin (Platinol)
      7) Carboplatin (Paraplatin)
      8) Etoposide (VP-16)
    c. Sanctuary therapy: the CNS is protected by the blood-brain barrier, so chemotherapy is administered intraventricularly via Ommaya reservoir if cerebral spinal fluid examination reveals presence of tumor cells.
    d. Radiation
      1) Cranial irradiation of the tumor bed to eradicate microscopic residual
      2) Craniospinal radiation if metastasis to spine is present
  5. NURSING INTERVENTIONS
    a. Preoperative
      1) Prepare the child and family for neurosurgical intervention.
      2) Preoperative tumor evaluation
        a) MRI scan of the brain
        b) Brain CT scan if the child's condition cannot tolerate MRI
    b. Postoperative
      1) Monitor mental status.
      2) Monitor fluid balance.
        a) Strict intake and output: CNS tumors have a higher incidence of syndrome of inappropriate diuretic hormone (SIADH) or diabetes insipidus (DI).
        b) Monitor for cerebral edema (increased ICP, mental status changes).

    3) Monitor for posterior fossa syndrome (symptomatology includes mutism, ataxia, nerve palsies, and hemiparesis).

    4) Monitor laboratory values.

       a) Serum electrolytes, correct imbalances: CNS tumors have a higher incidence of SIADH or DI

       b) CBC; initiate blood product support if indicated: maintain platelet count greater than 50,000/mm^3 to decrease incidence of intracranial hemorrhage.

    5) Initiate physical therapy and rehabilitation services.

c. During chemotherapy and radiation

    1) Monitor for signs and symptoms of neuropathy.

    2) Monitor laboratory values.

       a) Serum chemistries to monitor for SIADH or DI

    3) Education

       a) Clinical manifestations of VP shunt malfunction (headache, vomiting, changes in neurological status)

       b) Promote client safety: physical therapy to promote safe locomotion; occupational therapy to promote safe performance of ADLs; eliminate contact sports.

       c) Bleeding: introduce potential need for platelet infusion(s) if count falls below 50,000/mm^3; Educate client about radiation recall: inflammatory reaction of affected tissues. Associated with chemotherapy agents: cyclophosphamide (Cytoxan); lomustine (CeeNU); etoposide (VP-16)

F. HODGKIN'S DISEASE

  1. DESCRIPTION

    a. Malignancy of the immune system

    b. Presence of Reed-Sternberg cells (large, multinucleated cells with copious cytoplasm)

    c. Peak age of onset is adolescent and young adult

    d. Varies in histology

       1) Nodular sclerosing (NS)

       2) Mixed cellularity (MC)

       3) Lymphocyte prominence (LP)

       4) Lymphocyte depletion (LD)

  2. ASSESSMENT

    a. Asymptomatic enlarged lymph node(s)

    b. Persistent, nonproductive cough

    c. Malaise

    d. Intermittent fever

    e. Anorexia

    f. Weight loss

    g. Night sweats

    h. Hepatosplenomegaly

  3. DIAGNOSTIC TESTS

    a. History

       1) Incidence and duration of clinical manifestations

       2) Predisposing factors

          a) Prior radiation therapy

          b) Prior chemotherapy

          c) Genetic abnormalities

       3) Family history

    b. Physical exam

       1) Presence of lymphadenopathy

       2) Hepatosplenomegaly

       3) Respiratory assessment

          a) Dyspnea caused by mediastinal mass

    c. Tumor evaluation

       1) Chest x-ray

       2) CT of the neck, chest, abdomen and pelvis

       3) Gallium scan

       4) Tumor biopsy

    d. Metastatic search

       1) Bilateral bone marrow biopsy

       2) Bone scan

    e. Laboratory testing

       1) CBC to monitor hematopoiesis

       2) LFTs for baseline evaluation, elevations indicative of liver involvement

       3) Serum electrolytes for baseline evaluation

       4) Erythrocyte sedimentation rate (ESR), usually elevated

       5) Serum copper level, often elevated at the time of diagnosis

       6) Serum ferritin level, often elevated at the time of diagnosis

  4. STAGING

    a. Stage I: single lymph node region or single extralymphatic site

    b. Stage II: two or more lymph node regions on the same side of the diaphragm or local involvement of an extralymphatic site and one or more lymph node regions on the same side of the diaphragm

    c. Stage III: lymph node regions on both sides of the diaphragm, may involve spleen or localized involvement of extralymphatic site or both

    d. Stage IV: disseminated involvement of one or more extralymphatic sites or tissues with or without related lymph node involvement

5. CLINICAL MANIFESTATION CLASSIFICATION
   a. B classification
      1) Profuse night sweats
      2) Unexplained weight loss
      3) Unexplained recurrent fevers
   b. A classification is the absence of B clinical manifestations.
6. MULTIMODAL MANAGEMENT
   a. Radiation therapy
      1) Low-dose involved field radiation
      2) Radiation dose dependent on tumor involvement and adjuvant chemotherapy
   b. Chemotherapy
      1) Vincristine (Oncovin)
      2) Doxorubicin (Adriamycin)
      3) Cyclophosphamide (Cytoxan)
      4) Prednisone (Deltasone)
      5) Procarbazine (Matulane)
      6) Vinbalstine (Velban)
      7) Bleomycin (Blenoxane)
      8) Dacarbazine (DTIC)
      9) Meethotrexate
7. NURSING INTERVENTIONS
   a. Preoperatively
      1) Prepare the child and family for biopsy and concomitant central line placement.
      2) Maintain a patent airway if a large chest mass is present.
   b. Postoperatively
      1) Monitor respiratory status if a large chest mass is present.
         a) Oxygen saturation
         b) Quality and effort of respirations (rate, stridor, retractions, child's position for ease of respirations)
   c. During chemotherapy and radiation
      1) Monitor for clinical manifestations of neuropathy.
      2) Monitor laboratory values.
         a) ESR, serum copper and serum ferritin levels to monitor tumor responsiveness (should decrease)

G. LEUKEMIA
   1. DESCRIPTION
      a. Malignancy that involves the blood-forming tissues of the bone marrow, spleen, and lymph nodes
      b. WBC precursors produced in an unregulated manner, manufacturing abnormal blast cells.
      c. Most common types of pediatric leukemia
         1) Acute lymphocytic leukemia (ALL): abnormal proliferation of immature lymphoblasts
         2) Acute myelogenous leukemia (AML):
            a) Abnormal proliferation of immature myeloblasts
            b) Predisposing factors: Down syndrome (trisomy 21); Fanconi's anemia; certain types of chemotherapy (e.g., alkylating agents, etoposide); ionizing radiation; myelodysplastic syndrome (monosomy 7); common secondary malignancy after certain types of cancer chemotherapy
      d. Etiology unknown, suggested links with viruses, genetic predisposition, or environmental conditions
      e. The peak age of onset is 2–5 years old.
   2. ASSESSMENT
      a. Symptomatic anemia
         1) Fatigue
         2) Pallor
      b. Thrombocytopenia (low platelet count)
         1) Petechiae, capillaries break and bleed into pores
         2) Bleeding, especially gingival or nasal
      c. Neutropenia (low WBC count)
         1) Fever
         2) Infection
      d. Enlarged lymph node(s)
      e. Hepatosplenomegaly
      f. Bone pain
      g. Neurological symptoms
         1) Less than 10% of clients present with metastatic CNS disease at the time of diagnosis
         2) Increased intracranial pressure
            a) Headache
            b) Vomiting
            c) Visual disturbances
   3. DIAGNOSTIC TESTS
      a. History
         1) Incidence and duration of clinical manifestations
         2) Predisposing factors
            a) Prior radiation exposure
            b) Prior chemotherapy
            c) Genetic abnormalities
         3) Family history
      b. Physical exam
         1) Presence of lymphadenopathy
         2) Hepatosplenomegaly
         3) Cranial nerve testing
         4) Gait and weight-bearing evaluation
      c. Tumor evaluation
         1) Bone marrow aspiration and biopsy
            a) Greater than 25% blasts indicate leukemia.

b) Cytogenetics, immunophenotyping, and special stains are performed to identify the type of leukemia.

d. Metastatic search
  1) Lumbar puncture to examine cerebrospinal fluid (CSF) for leukemia cells
  2) Chest x-ray to check for mediastinal mass

e. Laboratory testing
  1) Complete blood count to monitor hematopoiesis
  2) LFTs for baseline evaluation; may be elevated
  3) Serum electrolytes for baseline evaluation; may demonstrate hyperkalemia and hyperphosphatemia related to lysis of lymphoblasts
  4) Uric acid level, which may be elevated
    a) Elevated serum uric acid levels can lead to renal failure. Assess baseline prior to initiating chemotherapy, as levels typically increase once chemotherapy has started and leukemia cells die.

4. MANAGEMENT OF ACUTE LYMPHOCYTIC LEUKEMIA
  a. Chemotherapy
    1) Sanctuary chemotherapy
      a) Central nervous system prophylaxis or treatment
      b) Intrathecal methotrexate (Mexate): administered during all three phases of therapy; administered more frequently if there is evidence of CNS disease at the time of diagnosis
    2) Systemic chemotherapy
      a) Two phases
        1. Three-drug induction: vincristine (Oncovin); prednisone (Deltasone); L-Asparaginase (Elspar)
        2. Four drug induction: vincristine (Oncovin); prednisone (Deltasone); L-Asparaginase (Elspar); daunomycin (Daunorubicin)
  b. Consolidation
    1) Intravenous methotrexate (Mexate)
  c. Maintenance
    1) Oral or intramuscular methotrexate (Mexate)
    2) 6-Mercaptopurine (Purinethol)
    3) Prednisone (Deltasone) scheduled pulses
    4) Vincristine (Oncovin) scheduled with prednisone (Deltasone) pulses

5. MANAGEMENT OF ACUTE MYELOGENOUS LEUKEMIA
  a. Sanctuary chemotherapy
    1) CNS prophylaxis or treatment
      a) Intrathecal methotrexate (Mexate), administered throughout treatment
  b. Systemic chemotherapy
    1) Induction goal: bone marrow aplasia
    2) Chemotherapeutic agents
      a) Cytarabine (Cytosine)
      b) Daunomycin (Daunorubicin)
      c) Thioguanine (6-TG)
      d) Prednisone (Deltasone)
      e) Etoposide (VP-16)
  c. Stem cell transplantation
    1) Goal: to replace dysfunctional hematopoietic system
    2) Progress to transplantation
      a) Child is in remission (no evidence of disease).
      b) Matched related donor is identified.
      c) Chromosomal analysis reveals a positive Philadelphia chromosome (associated with a very poor prognosis).
  d. Continuation therapy (if the child is not a stem cell transplant candidate)
    1) High-dose cytarabine (Cytosine)
    2) L-Asparaginase (Elspar)
    3) Etoposide (VP-16)
    4) Thioguanine (6-TG)
    5) Daunomycin (Daunorubicin)
    6) 6-Mercaptopurine (Purinethol)

6. NURSING INTERVENTIONS
  a. Preprocedure
    1) Prepare the child and family for bone marrow aspirate and biopsy.
    2) Maintain a patent airway if a large chest mass is present.
  b. Postprocedure
    1) Monitor respiratory status if a large chest mass is present.
      a) Oxygen saturation
      b) Quality and effort of respirations (rate, stridor, retractions, child's position for ease of respirations)
    2) Monitor pressure dressing at the site of the bone marrow aspirate and biopsy for bleeding.
  c. During chemotherapy
    1) Monitor for clinical manifestations of neuropathy.
    2) Monitor laboratory values, specifically an elevated uric acid level during induction chemotherapy.

H. RETINOBLASTOMA
1. DESCRIPTION
   a. Tumor arising from the embryonic retinal cells of the eye(s)
   b. Two patterns
      1) Familial
         a) Initial mutation is in the germ cell.
         b) Increased incidence of bilateral disease
      2) Sporadic
         a) All mutation occurs in the retinal cells.
         b) Increased incidence of unilateral disease
   c. Average age of the child at diagnosis is less than 1 year for bilateral retinoblastoma; unilateral retinoblastoma typically diagnosed by age 5
2. ASSESSMENT
   a. Leukokoria (cat's eye reflex): white pupil
   b. Strabismus
      1) Esotropia: eye turning inward
      2) Exotropia: eye turning outward
   c. Erythematous conjunctiva (red eyes)
3. DIAGNOSTIC TESTS
   a. History
      1) Presence and onset of clinical manifestations
      2) Family history of retinoblastoma
   b. Physical exam
      1) Direct and indirect examination of the retina under anesthesia
   c. Tumor evaluation and metastatic search
      1) MRI of the orbits
      2) CT of the brain and orbits to establish the extent of the disease
      3) Bilateral bone marrow aspirate and biopsy
      4) Lumbar puncture for collection of CSF to examine for tumor cells
      5) Surgical tissue sampling is omitted due to a high incidence of tumor cell spillage, which will negatively affect the prognosis.
4. MULTIMODAL MANAGEMENT
   a. Enucleation of the affected eye
   b. Radiation therapy to the affected eye with useful vision in cases of bilateral disease
   c. Chemotherapy
      1) Vincristine (Oncovin)
      2) Carboplatin (Paraplatin)
      3) Cyclophosphamide (Cytoxan)
      4) Etoposide (VP-16)
5. NURSING INTERVENTIONS
   a. Preoperatively
      1) Educate the child and parent about enucleation and alterations in visual fields.
   b. Postoperatively
      1) Initiate referral for ophthalmic prosthetic device once enucleation has healed.
      2) Accommodate the child's visual field when providing care.
      3) Initiate rehabilitative services: occupational therapy
   c. During chemotherapy and radiation
      1) Provide frequent fundal examination.
      2) Educate the client about radiation recall: inflammatory reaction of affected tissues.
         a) Associated with chemotherapy agents
            1. Cyclophosphamide (Cytoxan)
            2. Etoposide (VP-16)

PRACTICE QUESTIONS

1. The nurse should include which of the following statements when providing education to the parents of a child who has had a bone marrow aspirate procedure?
   1. "Your child can take a shower, if desired."
   2. "You should not give your child a tub bath for 24 hours."
   3. "Your child should not sit for prolonged periods of time."
   4. "You should restrict your child's activity to quiet play for the next 12 hours."

2. The nurse is caring for a child who is experiencing severe mucositis. Which of the following measures would be essential to include in the child's plan of care?
   1. Offer oral liquid nutritional supplements
   2. Provide nasogastric feedings
   3. Maintain hydration with intravenous fluids
   4. Provide total parenteral nutrition (TPN)

3. A child is admitted to the day infusion area for two units of packed red blood cells. Which of the following clinical manifestations indicates to the nurse that the child is experiencing anemia? Select all that apply:
   [ ] 1. Gingival bleeding
   [ ] 2. Petechiae

[ ] 3. Tachycardia
[ ] 4. Pale mucous membranes
[ ] 5. Dry mucous membranes
[ ] 6. Headache

4. The father of a child newly diagnosed with acute lymphocytic leukemia (ALL) asks the nurse why trimethoprim-sulfamethoxazole (Bactrim) has been prescribed. The nurse would best describe the purpose of trimethoprim-sulfamethoxazole (Bactrim) therapy as a means to prevent which of the following?
   1. A certain type of pneumonia
   2. Diarrhea caused by a certain type of bacteria
   3. Upper respiratory infections caused by a certain type of virus
   4. A certain type of fungal infection in the mouth

5. An adolescent with newly diagnosed osteosarcoma of the femur asks the nurse why a computerized tomography (CT) scan of the chest was ordered. The nurse should give this client which explanation of what the CT scan will show?
   1. "The CT scan will show well your lungs are functioning."
   2. "The CT scan will show your oxygenation status."
   3. "The CT scan will reveal any metastatic lesions, if present."
   4. "The CT scan will show how well your heart is pumping."

6. Before setting out for an appointment at the hematology/oncology clinic, an adolescent begins experiencing anticipatory nausea and vomiting. When informed of this situation, the nurse should instruct the adolescent to follow which of the following medication regimens?
   1. Oral lorazepam (Ativan), 1 hour before arriving at the clinic
   2. Intravenous lorazepam (Ativan) upon arrival at the clinic
   3. Oral dexamethasone (Decadron) half an hour before arriving at the clinic
   4. Intravenous dexamethasone (Decadron), with ondansetron (Zofran) upon arrival at the clinic

7. Which of the following assessments should the nurse perform on a child with newly diagnosed Wilms' tumor?
   1. Urine dipstick for microscopic hematuria
   2. Deep abdominal palpation
   3. Cranial nerve testing
   4. Urine electrolyte analysis

8. The nurse is caring for a child diagnosed with stage IV neuroblastoma. The nurse recognizes that the child may require which of the following?
   1. Total parenteral nutrition (TPN) to maintain nutritional requirements

   2. Rehabilitative services after tumor resection
   3. Placement of a ventriculoperitoneal (VP) shunt
   4. Thyroid replacement therapy after completion of chemotherapy

9. The nurse is providing postoperative care for an adolescent immediately following a limb salvage procedure of the left femur. Which of the following assessments should the nurse perform during the immediate postoperative period?
   1. Abduction of the left lower extremity
   2. Adduction of the left lower extremity
   3. Weight-bearing capacity of operative leg
   4. Circulation, movement, sensation (CMS) checks distal to operative site

10. The nurse is caring for a child receiving radiation therapy to the scapula as part of the treatment for Ewing's sarcoma. Which of the following interventions should the nurse include when performing skin care?
   1. Perform deep tissue massage of the radiation site
   2. Apply baby oil to the skin prior to daily radiation treatment
   3. Apply ice to irritated skin three times a day
   4. Apply prescribed lotion to reddened skin daily after radiation treatment

11. The nurse is caring for a child with neutropenia secondary to chemotherapy. Which of the following measures would be essential to include in the child's discharge instructions?
   1. Call the doctor if the child has a fever greater than or equal to 38.3°C, or 101°F
   2. Do not send the child to school
   3. Discontinue granulocyte colony-stimulating factor (Neupogen)
   4. Administer acetaminophen (Tylenol) if the child complains of pain

12. The nurse is collecting a nursing history from a child with a pathological fracture of the right tibia. Which of the following questions should the nurse ask first to elicit the most accurate assessment?
   1. "Have you had any fevers recently?"
   2. "Did you experience any trauma to your right leg?"
   3. "Is there a family history of cancer?"
   4. "Are you having pain in any area other than your right leg?"

13. The nurse is collecting a nursing history from an adolescent diagnosed with Hodgkin's disease. Which of the following reported clinical manifestations are classified as B category manifestations?
   Select all that apply:
   [ ] 1. Anorexia
   [ ] 2. Productive cough

[ ] 3. Unilateral numbness in lower extremity
[ ] 4. Nausea and vomiting
[ ] 5. Night sweats
[ ] 6. Recurrent fevers

14. The nurse is caring for a child with a brain tumor. Which of the following observations should the nurse immediately report? Select all that apply:
[ ] 1. Headache
[ ] 2. Visual changes
[ ] 3. Abdominal discomfort
[ ] 4. Diarrhea
[ ] 5. Decreased urine output
[ ] 6. Vomiting

15. The child newly diagnosed with acute lymphocytic leukemia is scheduled to have a lumbar puncture. With which of the following statements can the nurse best describe the purpose of the lumbar puncture?
    1. "It will relieve the headaches you are having."
    2. "It will allow for collection of fluid to examine for metastasis."
    3. "It will allow for collection of fluid to examine for meningitis."
    4. "It will relieve the bone pain you are having."

16. Which of the following does the nurse assess as a major presenting clinical manifestation in the child with a retinoblastoma?
    1. Icteric sclera
    2. Cat's eye reflex
    3. Chronic conjunctivitis
    4. Aniridia

17. The nurse is caring for a child with left-sided hemiparesis after a brain tumor resection. Which of the following nursing interventions is appropriate?
    1. Place the call light near the child's left hand
    2. Secure a peripheral intravenous catheter in the child's left hand
    3. Support the child's right side during transfer to a bedside commode
    4. Instill natural tears in both eyes four times a day

18. In preparing a child for a magnetic resonance image (MRI) with sedation, the nurse should include which of the following preprocedure instructions?
    1. Nothing by mouth 6 hours prior to exam
    2. Clear liquids until time of the test
    3. The child will need to be admitted to the hospital after the exam
    4. The child can go home immediately after the scan

19. The nurse is discharging a child with Wilms' tumor after a resection. Which of the following measures would be a priority to include in the client's discharge instructions?
    1. Low-sodium diet
    2. Restrict fluid intake
    3. Avoid contact sports
    4. Limit protein intake

20. The nurse should monitor a child with a brain stem glioma receiving vincristine sulfate (Oncovin) for which of the following adverse reactions?
    1. Constipation
    2. Diarrhea
    3. Appendicitis
    4. Typhlitis

21. The parents of a child with acute lymphocytic leukemia, positive for Philadelphia chromosome, ask the nurse to describe the treatment plan. The priority response by the nurse is "Chemotherapy
    1. until the child achieves remission."
    2. and biologic modifiers until the child achieves remission."
    3. until the child achieves remission, then radiation therapy."
    4. until the child achieves remission, then stem cell transplantation."

22. The nurse caring for a child with neuroblastoma includes which of the following assessments as a measure of tumor responsiveness?
    1. Serum copper levels
    2. Erythrocyte sedimentation rate (ESR)
    3. Urine catecholamines
    4. Urinalysis with a culture and sensitivity

23. When planning the discharge of a child newly diagnosed with a malignancy, which of the following instructions should be included regarding infection prevention?
    1. Isolation is the most effective method of infection prevention
    2. Hand washing is the most effective method of infection prevention
    3. Restrict the intake of fresh fruits and vegetables
    4. Remove the carpet from the child's bedroom and play area

24. When caring for a child who has a ventriculoperitoneal (VP) shunt secondary to hydrocephalus from medulloblastoma, the nurse should include which of the following interventions?
    1. Darken the room to decrease photosensitivity
    2. Administer platelets when the platelet count drops below 50,000/mm^3
    3. Instruct the child to wear a hat instead of a wig for alopecia
    4. Restrict dietary sodium intake to 2 g/day

25. An adolescent with Ewing's sarcoma asks why radiation therapy will be needed because the entire tumor was surgically removed. In describing the purpose of multimodal therapy, the nurse should give this client which explanation of why radiation is needed?
    1. "It destroys remaining microscopic tumor cells."
    2. "It eliminates the cells damaged by chemotherapy."
    3. "It assists the injured tissue in the healing process."
    4. "It maintains function of the operative site."

26. The registered nurse is delegating the clinical assignments for a pediatric oncology unit. Which of the following clinical assignments is most appropriate for the nurse to delegate to unlicensed assistive personnel?
    1. Bathe and position a child with a Wilms' tumor
    2. Provide the care to a child who is neutropenic and has a temperature of 39°C, or 102.2°F
    3. Dispose of the bodily fluids from a child receiving radioactive fluids
    4. Bathe a child with acute lymphocytic leukemia

ANSWERS AND RATIONALES

1. 2. Tub bathing and showering will compromise the integrity of the pressure dressing applied to the bone marrow aspirate site; the dressing needs to be in place for 24 hours postprocedure. Sitting for prolonged periods of time has no ill effect on the site of injury or the iliac crest. Activity restriction is regulated by the child's comfort level, as there are no activity restrictions associated with a bone marrow aspiration procedure.

2. 4. The most appropriate intervention for a child with mucositis is to provide total parenteral nutrition. Because mucositis severely alters oral cavity mucosa, oral feeding would be painful. Nasogastric feedings would not be an option, because intubation could potentially cause mechanical damage to the already injured oral and esophageal mucosa. Maintaining hydration does not allow for nutrition needs, only fluid needs.

3. 3. 4. 6. Anemia, or a decrease in the number of red blood cells with oxygen-carrying hemoglobin that are circulating, produces clinical manifestations of rapid heart rate, headache, and paleness. Gingival bleeding and petechiae are manifestations of thrombocytopenia. Dry mucous membranes can indicate dehydration.

4. 1. Leukemia is a malignant disease in which normal marrow cells are replaced by abnormal, immature lymphocytes known as blast cells. It is the most common form of childhood leukemia. Trimethoprim and sulfamethoxazole (Bactrim) is prophylactic treatment for pneumonia caused by *Pneumocystis carinii*. Bactrim is ineffective against fungal and viral agents as well as ineffective in treating diarrhea.

5. 3. Osteosarcoma is a bone tumor that usually occurs in the growth metaphysis or the long ends of the bone. It is usually not diagnosed until there is a trauma to the bone. A chest computerized tomography (CT) scan is performed during the metastatic search. A test to determine how well the lungs are functioning would be a pulmonary function test. A test determining oxygenation would be arterial blood gas (ABG), or oxygen-saturation monitoring. A test to determine how well the heart is pumping would be an echocardiogram.

6. 1. Lorazepam (Ativan) is an antianxiety medication that is effective against anticipatory nausea and vomiting. Administration of IV lorazepam (Ativan) is the incorrect route. Oral dexamethasone (Decadron) is not an antianxiety medication. Dexamethasone (Decadron) with ondansetron (Zofran) upon arrival to the clinic is not effective against anticipatory nausea and vomiting.

7. 1. Wilms' tumor, or nephroblastoma, is the most common tumor of the kidney in children. Microscopic hematuria is often seen in clients diagnosed with Wilms' tumor. Deep palpation is avoided in order to keep the malignancy encapsulated. Cranial nerve testing is assessed in suspected central nervous system tumors. Urine electrolyte analysis is performed when syndrome of inappropriate antidiuretic hormone or diabetes insipidus is suspected.

8. 1. Neuroblastoma is a tumor that originates from cells that are precursors of the adrenal medulla and sympathetic nervous system. With stage IV neuroblastoma, the tumor has spread to the liver, skin, or bone marrow. Nutritional support is needed when a child is not capable of

maintaining requirements. Rehabilitation services after tumor resection is needed for children undergoing limb salvage procedures. Placement of a VP shunt is needed for children experiencing hydrocephalus from a brain tumor. Thyroid replacement therapy after completion of chemotherapy is needed if the thyroid was in the radiation field and can no longer function adequately.

9. 4. Circulation, movement, and sensation (CMS) checks distal to the operative site are imperative perfusion assessments following a limb salvage of the left femur. Abduction and adduction of the left lower extremity would not be assessed immediately after surgery, due to tissue trauma and the potential for tissue injury. Assessment of the weight-bearing capacity of the operative leg would occur only after 24 to 48 hours of strict bed rest.

10. 4. Ewing's sarcoma is a highly malignant bone tumor usually present in the pelvis, tibia, fibula, and femur. It would be appropriate to apply prescribed lotion to reddened skin after radiation treatment. Massage would increase pain and mechanical cellular damage to already irritated skin. Baby oil prior to therapy would affect the efficacy of the radiation beam during therapy. Ice application would decrease circulation to the site, which needs an adequate blood supply for tissue healing.

11. 1. Fever is often the first sign of infection in a child with neutropenia. Not sending the child to school does not prevent infection caused by intrinsic organisms. Neupogen should be discontinued only after the neutrophil count has recovered. Administering acetaminophen (Tylenol) can mask a fever.

12. 2. Bone tumors alter the integrity of the bone, which often leads to pathological fractures. A fracture can be correlated with the onset of clinical manifestations, an important component in obtaining a health history. Recent fevers do not always give the nurse information about onset of manifestations. Family history and pains in other areas do not give the nurse information about the timing of onset of clinical manifestations.

13. 1. 5. 6. Hodgkin's disease originates in the cervical lymph nodes and spreads to other lymph node regions. If treatment is not initiated, it may spread to the organs. Anorexia, night sweats, and recurrent fevers are B category clinical manifestations of Hodgkin's disease. Productive cough may be an indication of an upper respiratory infection. Altered gait and unilateral numbness in a lower extremity are clinical manifestations of a neurologic injury. Nausea, vomiting, and diarrhea are indications of a viral illness or adverse reactions to chemotherapy.

14. 1. 2. 6. Headache, visual changes, and vomiting are clinical manifestations of space-occupying intracranial lesions or ventriculoperitoneal (VP) shunt malfunction. Abdominal discomfort, diarrhea, and decreased urine output are all general clinical manifestations that a child may exhibit, but they do not necessarily require immediate attention.

15. 2. The purpose of a lumbar puncture is to obtain cerebral spinal fluid to be examined for leukemic cells. Telling the client that it will relieve headaches is not appropriate, because there is a high incidence of headaches after a lumbar puncture. Examination of collected fluid for meningitis is not part of a new diagnosis evaluation of acute lymphocytic leukemia. Relieving bone pain is not correlated with accessing the intrathecal space.

16. 2. Retinoblastoma tumors are tumors of the eye that create a cat's eye reflex when the light hits the eye at the right angle; the reflex is also identifiable in photographs. An icteric sclera would be associated with hepatic dysfunction. Chronic conjunctivitis is not identified as a precursor or a clinical manifestation of retinoblastoma. Aniridia is associated with Wilms' tumor.

17. 2. A peripheral intravenous catheter should be inserted in the child's left hand. The child's right hand should not be used because it would further limit the function of a compromised right side. Securing the call light near the child's left hand would not allow the child to independently call for the nurse. Supporting the child's right side does not consider safety during transfer. Instilling natural tears in both eyes four times a day suggests a bilateral intervention for a unilateral functional disability to keep the cornea protected.

18. 1. Children receiving sedation for a magnetic resonance image (MRI) need to be NPO in order to prevent aspiration. Clear liquids would not be permitted. Hospital admission is not required. Postsedation monitoring is all that is required until the child is awake and alert. Immediate discharge is not allowed because the child needs to recover from sedation.

19. 3. Wilms' tumor is the most common childhood tumor of the kidney. Avoiding contact sports is a priority to protect the remaining kidney. A low-sodium diet is part of hypertension management. Fluid restriction and limiting protein intake are part of renal failure management.

20. 1. Vincristine sulfate (Oncovin) is an antineoplastic drug that inhibits mitosis at metaphase. It can cause neuropathy, including the gut, leading to constipation. Appendicitis and typhlitis are infectious processes that may arise during neutropenic episodes.

21. 4. Acute lymphocytic leukemia accounts for 80% of childhood leukemias. Children positive for Philadelphia chromosome require related or unrelated stem cell transplantation in order to eradicate the chromosomal defect. Biologic modifiers and radiation therapy will not eradicate the chromosomal defect.

22. 3. Neuroblastoma is a tumor that originates from the adrenal medulla and sympathetic nervous system. Clients with neuroblastoma produce excessive amounts of urine catecholamine metabolites (VMA, HVA, dopamine). Serum copper levels and erythrocyte sedimentation rates are tumor markers for Hodgkin's disease. Urinalysis with culture and sensitivity is an assessment conducted when urinary tract infection is suspected.

23. 2. Hand washing has been identified as the most effective method for preventing infection. Isolation, restricting the intake of fresh fruits and vegetables, and removing the carpet from the child's bedroom are measures instituted when a child is discharged to home after a stem cell transplant.

24. 2. Platelets should be administered when the platelet count drops below 50,000/mm³ in children with brain tumors to decrease the incidence of intracranial hemorrhage. Darkening the room to decrease

photosensitivity is an intervention for migraine headaches or dilated eyes. A ventriculoperitoneal (VP) shunt has no impact on the type of head covering a child can wear. Restricting dietary sodium intake is an intervention for a child experiencing hypernatremia.

25. 1. Radiation therapy is often used with radiosensitive tumors to eradicate microscopic disease in the tumor beds if surgical margins are close in cancers such as Ewing's sarcoma, a highly malignant bone tumor.

26. 4. Great care is to be used in the bathing and handling of a child with a Wilms' tumor. It is essential to limit manipulation of the abdomen to prevent spread of the malignancy should the encapsulated mass rupture. It would not be appropriate to delegate bathing this child to unlicensed assistive personnel. A child who is neutropenic and has a fever of 39°C, or 102.2°F, would most appropriately be cared for by a nurse because of the risk of infection. Because precautions should be taken when handling the bodily fluids of a client receiving radioactive fluids, this would not be the most appropriate clinical assignment for unlicensed assistive personnel. It would be appropriate to permit unlicensed assistive personnel to bathe a child with acute lymphocytic leukemia.

REFERENCES

Potts, N., & Mandleco, B. (2012). *Pediatric nursing: Caring for children and their families* (3rd ed.). Clifton Park, NY: Delmar Cengage Learning.

Spratto, G. R., & Woods, A. L. (2012). *PDR nurse's drug handbook 2012*. Clifton Park, NY: Delmar Cengage Learning.

CHAPTER 40

HEMATOLOGICAL DISORDERS

I. **ANATOMY AND PHYSIOLOGY (SEE CHAPTER 11, HEMATOLOGY DISORDERS, SECTION I.)**

II. **ASSESSMENT**
   - A. HEALTH HISTORY
     1. PAST MEDICAL HISTORY (ILLNESSES, SURGERIES, TRAUMA)
     2. MEDICATIONS (PAST, PRESENT, OVER THE COUNTER [OTC], HERBAL REMEDIES)
     3. NUTRITIONAL HISTORY (FEEDING HABITS, DIET RECALL, PICA)
     4. ONSET AND DURATION OF SYMPTOMS
     5. BLOOD FLOW DURING MENSES
   - B. PHYSICAL ASSESSMENT
     1. INSPECTION
        - a. Growth parameters: height and weight (prolonged anemia may cause growth retardation)
        - b. Vital signs: heart rate (increased with anemia), blood pressure (decreased with anemia), respiratory rate (may be increased or decreased)
        - c. Skin: color (pallor or jaundice), bruising, rashes (petechiae)
        - d. Mouth and tongue: cheilosis and glossitis
        - e. Eyes: jaundice often seen in conjunctivae
     2. AUSCULTATION
        - a. Heart sounds: evaluate for murmur, gallop, tachycardia
     3. PALPATION
        - a. Lymph nodes: increase in size, tenderness, warmth; lymphadenopathy common with malignancies
        - b. Liver: may be palpable with a variety of hematological conditions
        - c. Spleen: commonly enlarged with many hematological conditions

III. **DIAGNOSTIC STUDIES**
   - A. COMPLETE BLOOD COUNT (CBC)
     1. DESCRIPTION
        - a. A basic diagnostic exam that measures the number, quality, variety, concentrations, and percentages of the blood cells
        - b. Includes a white blood cell (WBC) count (with or without differential [see later discussion]), a red blood cell (RBC) count, hematocrit, hemoglobin, mean corpuscular volume (MCV), mean corpuscular hemoglobin concentration (MCHC), mean corpuscular hemoglobin (MCH), platelet count, and may include a peripheral smear (see later discussion)
        - c. Normal values vary for sex and age.
        - d. Specimen is obtained via venipuncture.
     2. PREPROCEDURE
        - a. Explain the procedure to the child and parent, including the risk for discomfort with venipuncture.
        - b. Clean the skin covering the vessel well with alcohol or Betadine.
        - c. Instruct the child to be as still as possible during the procedure, or have a parent or other adult restrain the child during the procedure.
     3. POSTPROCEDURE
        - a. Apply pressure and a bandage to the site after removing the needle.
        - b. Instruct the child or parent to notify the physician if bleeding continues from the site or if the site becomes warm, erythematous, or tender to touch.
     4. THE PRECEDING PRE- AND POSTPROCEDURE INSTRUCTIONS WILL BE CONSISTENT FOR ALL TESTS REQUIRING VENIPUNCTURE TO OBTAIN A SPECIMEN.

B. DIFFERENTIAL
  1. DESCRIPTION
   a. Measures the percentage of each type of WBC present in circulation
   b. Has little value if not compared to the total number of circulating WBCs
   c. Increases or decreases in various types of WBCs may be clinically significant according to the type of WBC that is affected.
   d. Specimen is obtained via venipuncture, usually in conjunction with a WBC count.

C. PERIPHERAL SMEAR
  1. DESCRIPTION
   a. An opportunity for the clinician to view the various types of blood cells present in circulation under a microscope
   b. A drop of blood is applied in a thin layer to a glass slide for clinician review.
   c. Specimen is obtained via venipuncture.

D. RETICULOCYTE COUNT
  1. DESCRIPTION
   a. A measure of how rapidly the bone marrow is producing new red blood cells by counting the number of reticulocytes present in circulation
   b. Specimen is obtained via venipuncture.

E. SERUM IRON
  1. DESCRIPTION
   a. A measure of the amount of iron present in serum
   b. Important in the diagnosis of iron deficiency anemia, as well as in ruling out other hematological disorders
   c. Specimen is obtained via venipuncture.

F. SERUM FERRITIN
  1. DESCRIPTION
   a. A measure of the amount of iron stored by the body
   b. May be indicated in the evaluation of clients with various types of anemia
   c. Specimen is obtained via venipuncture.

G. TOTAL IRON-BINDING CAPACITY (TIBC)
  1. DESCRIPTION
   a. A representation of the body's capacity to bind iron with available globin chains in order to create a hemoglobin molecule
   b. If iron stores or circulating iron is low, the TIBC will be high.
   c. This is due to the fact that there is an inadequate supply of iron available to bind with globin chains.
   d. Specimen is obtained via venipuncture.

H. HEMOGLOBIN ELECTROPHORESIS
  1. DESCRIPTION
   a. A measure of normal and abnormal hemoglobins
   b. Used to detect the presence of hemoglobinopathies, such a sickle cell anemia or thalassemia
   c. Specimen is obtained via venipuncture.

I. BONE MARROW ASPIRATION
  1. DESCRIPTION
   a. The evaluation of the presence or absence of the various types of cells in the bone marrow
   b. May help to diagnose or rule out a variety of hematological or oncologic disorders
   c. Specimen is obtained through a large-bore needle inserted into the bone.
   d. The best sites for this procedure are the posterior iliac crest (preferred site in children) and the sternum.
  2. PREPROCEDURE
   a. Explain the procedure to the child and the parents and prepare them for the discomfort associated with both insertion of the needle and aspiration of the specimen.
   b. Position the child on the abdomen for the procedure.
   c. Parents or other adults may be needed to help restrain the child during the procedure.
   d. Cleanse the site with alcohol and Betadine and drape the area to maintain a sterile field.
   e. Local anesthetics, such as lidocaine, or conscious sedation with midazolam (Versed) may be used if ordered by a physician.
   f. The needle, with stylet, should be inserted through the iliac crest into the marrow cavity.
   g. After reaching the cavity, remove the stylet and aspirate marrow through the needle into a syringe, for a total volume of 1–3 ml, depending on the number and type of tests to be run on the specimen.
   h. Remove the needle carefully after aspiration.
  3. POSTPROCEDURE
   a. Apply pressure for at least 5 minutes after the procedure, then apply a pressure dressing to the site.
   b. Instruct the child or parents that the site will be sore for 1–2 days after the procedure.
   c. Site should be monitored for signs of bleeding or infection.

J. PLATELET COUNT
  1. DESCRIPTION
     a. A measure of the number of platelets in circulation
     b. Specimen is obtained via venipuncture.
K. BLEEDING TIME
  1. DESCRIPTION
     a. A measure of the length of time it takes the blood to form a platelet plug for the vessel wall
     b. Specimen is obtained by creating a small "stab" wound in the forearm.
  2. PREPROCEDURE
     a. Explain the procedure to the child and parents.
     b. Cleanse the selected area of the forearm.
     c. Stretch the skin between the fingers and puncture a 3 mm × 5 mm area.
     d. Begin the stopwatch as soon as bleeding commences.
     e. Stop the timer once a clot has formed.
  3. POSTPROCEDURE
     a. Apply a sterile dressing to the wound.
L. PROTHROMBIN TIME (PT)
  1. DESCRIPTION
     a. Utilized in the diagnosis of coagulation disorders
     b. One of the proteins necessary for clotting to occur
     c. Specimen is obtained via venipuncture.
M. PARTIAL THROMBOPLASTIN TIME (PTT)
  1. DESCRIPTION
     a. Can identify abnormalities in the intrinsic coagulation system of the body and measure the body's response to heparin therapy
     b. Utilized in the diagnosis of coagulation disorders
     c. Specimen is obtained via venipuncture.
N. VON WILLEBRAND'S PROFILE
  1. DESCRIPTION
     a. Utilized to identify children with von Willebrand's disease
     b. A series of tests, including von Willebrand's factor antibody, von Willebrand's factor antigen, platelet count, bleeding time, and ristocetin cofactor
     c. May include other tests at varying facilities
     d. Specimen is obtained via venipuncture.
O. SERUM FIBRINOGEN
  1. DESCRIPTION
     a. Fibrinogen is a protein that is converted to fibrin and is essential for clot formation.
     b. Utilized to establish a diagnosis of disseminated intravascular coagulation (DIC)
     c. Specimen is obtained via venipuncture.

P. FIBRIN DEGRADATION PRODUCTS
  1. DESCRIPTION
     a. Utilized to establish a diagnosis of DIC
     b. Measures by-products produced when fibrin is split by plasmin
     c. These by-products inhibit normal clotting.
     d. Specimen is obtained via venipuncture.

IV. NURSING DIAGNOSES
  A. INTERRUPTED FAMILY PROCESSES
  B. IMBALANCED NUTRITION: LESS THAN BODY REQUIREMENTS
  C. FATIGUE
  D. ACTIVITY INTOLERANCE
  E. RISK FOR INFECTION
  F. INEFFECTIVE THERAPEUTIC REGIMEN MANAGEMENT

Nursing Diagnoses: Definitions and Classification 2012–2014.
Copyright © 2012, 1994–2012 by NANDA International.
Used by arrangement with John Wiley & Sons Limited.

V. HEMATOLOGICAL DISORDERS
  A. ANEMIA
    1. DESCRIPTION
       a. A reduction in the total number of circulating RBCs or a decrease in the quality or quantity of hemoglobin, resulting from impaired RBC production, blood loss, RBC destruction, or a combination of the three
       b. Not a disease but the most common hematological disorder in children
       c. Defined as a hemoglobin of less than 11 g/dl or a hematocrit less than 33%
       d. Described by the cause of the anemia or the characteristics of the RBCs, including their size and color
    2. ASSESSMENT (SEE TABLE 40-1.)
    3. TYPES
       a. Iron deficiency anemia
       b. Sickle cell anemia
       c. Thalassemias
          1) Beta thalassemia major
          2) Beta thalassemia minor
       d. Aplastic anemia
    4. DIAGNOSTIC TESTS
       a. There is a wide variety of tests available to evaluate the cause or type of anemia (see Table 40-2 on page 779).
    5. NURSING INTERVENTIONS
       a. Will be specific to the type of anemia present
  B. IRON DEFICIENCY ANEMIA
    1. DESCRIPTION
       a. Anemia resulting from impaired RBC production due to inadequate iron intake, blood loss, impaired iron absorption, or periods of rapid growth, leading to depletion of iron stores in the body and a subsequent decrease in erythropoiesis

Table 40-1 Clinical Manifestations of Anemia

Level of Anemia	Associated Manifestations
Mild	Slightly lowered hematocrit and hemoglobin Most often asymptomatic Dyspnea and fatigue with exertion
Moderate	Moderately lowered hematocrit and hemoglobin Tachycardia Shortness of breath Lightheadedness, dizziness Pallor Easy fatigability Irritability
Severe	Severely lowered hematocrit and hemoglobin Headache, irritability Tachycardia Shortness of breath Lightheadedness, dizziness Pallor or jaundice, or both Moist, cool skin Easy fatigability Audible heart murmur Cheilosis, glossitis Low blood pressure, weak pulse

© Cengage Learning 2015

b. Present in as many as 25% of children 10–15 months of age
c. Groups at risk include infants, older children of lower-socioeconomic status, African-American children, and adolescent females.
d. Characterized by small (microcytic), pale (hypochromic) RBCs
e. Major complications include fatigue, apathy, impaired growth and development, and impaired intellectual capacity.

2. ASSESSMENT
   a. Clinical manifestations are directly related to the severity of the anemia.
   b. Clinical manifestations include:
      1) Dyspnea
      2) Fatigue with exertion
      3) Headache
      4) Poor concentration
      5) Heart palpitations
      6) Irritability
      7) Pallor
      8) Tachycardia
      9) Heart murmur
      10) Anorexia
      11) Glossitis
      12) Cheilosis
      13) Brittle concave nails

3. DIAGNOSTIC TESTS
   a. CBC
   b. Peripheral smear
   c. Serum iron
   d. Serum ferritin
   e. Reticulocyte count
   f. TIBC
   g. History should include:
      1) Onset and duration of clinical manifestations
      2) Nutritional evaluation
      3) Menstrual flow
      4) Presence of pica
      5) Current or recently ingested medications
   h. Physical exam should include:
      1) Growth parameters
      2) Vital signs
      3) Skin inspection
      4) Thorough oral, cardiovascular, and abdominal examination

4. MEDICAL MANAGEMENT
   a. Resolution of the cause of the anemia
   b. Replenishment of body iron stores
   c. Prescription of elemental iron 3–6 mg/kg/day divided t.i.d., for 2–4 months after anemia has resolved
   d. Ferrous sulfate (Feosol, Apo-Ferrous Sulfate, ED-IN-SOL, Fer-gen-sol, Fer-Iron Drops, Fero-Grad, Mol-Iron) is the drug of choice.

5. NURSING INTERVENTIONS
   a. Instruct the parents in the proper administration of iron supplements.
      1) Medication should be given on an empty stomach with a source of vitamin C to increase absorption.
      2) If stomach upset occurs, give medication between meals to decrease gastrointestinal (GI) adverse reactions.
      3) Because liquid iron stains teeth, it should be administered through a straw and the mouth should be rinsed after administration.
   b. Instruct the parents on the adverse reactions of the drug.
      1) Tarry black or green stools
      2) GI discomfort
      3) Vomiting
      4) Diarrhea or constipation
   c. Instruct the parents that iron is toxic if consumed in large doses.
   d. Do not make up missed doses.
   e. Keep medication in a child-safe container and out of the child's reach.
   f. Provide the child and parents diet education.

Table 40-2 Laboratory Tests Commonly Used to Evaluate Causes of Anemia

Lab Test	Increased in:	Decreased in:	Normal in:
Hemoglobin		Iron deficiency Sickle cell Beta thalassemia Aplastic anemia	
Hematocrit		Iron deficiency Sickle cell Beta thalassemia Aplastic anemia	
Reticulocyte count	Sickle cell	Aplastic anemia	Beta
Mean corpuscular volume (MCV)*	Hemolytic anemia	Iron deficiency	thalassemia
Serum iron		Iron deficiency	Sickle cell Aplastic anemia Beta thalassemia
Ferritin	Sickle cell	Iron deficiency	Aplastic anemia Beta thalassemia
Total iron-binding capacity (TIBC)	Iron deficiency	Sickle cell	Aplastic anemia
Other Lab Tests Associated with Evaluation of Anemia			

Hemoglobin electrophoresis: will be normal in iron deficiency and aplastic anemia. Sickle cell disease and beta thalassemia will show abnormal levels of certain hemoglobins, depending on disease type.

Peripheral smear: will reveal the character, quality, size, and color of the red blood cells.

Iron deficiency: microcytic, hypochromic cells

Sickle cell anemia: normocytic, normochromic with sickled cells and target cells

Beta thalassemia: microcytic, hypochromic cells

Aplastic anemia: normocytic, normochromic cells

© Cengage Learning 2015

*This value will fluctuate in sickle cell disease according to the disease type experienced by the child.

1) Encourage foods high in iron (iron-fortified formulas and cereals, red meat, organ meats, oysters, spinach, cooked legumes, oatmeal, soybean products, dried fruits, potatoes, and greens—both collard and turnip).

2) Refer to Women, Infants, and Children (WIC) program, if not already enrolled.

3) In infants less than 12 months of age, avoid introducing whole milk into the diet.

C. SICKLE CELL ANEMIA
   1. DESCRIPTION
      a. A group of autosomal recessive disorders that result from a mutation of a single amino acid in the beta globin chain
      b. Characterized by the presence of hemoglobin S (sickle hemoglobin)
      c. One of the most prevalent genetic disorders
      d. Most commonly affects African-American, Mediterranean, Middle Eastern or Indian populations
      e. Pathophysiology
         1) Hemoglobin S forms polymers when it becomes deoxygenated.
         2) Its tendency to polymerize is based on its concentration.
         3) When this occurs, the affected RBC becomes rigid, sticky, and crescent shaped.
         4) These changes cause membrane damage and a shorter life span for the RBC, and lead to vasoocclusion.
         5) Vasoocclusion occurs when sickled cells fail to move through blood vessels, creating a blockage.
         6) This prevents oxygen delivery to the tissues below the blockage.
         7) This process can occur anywhere in the body where blood flows.

Figure 40-1 Clinical manifestations of sickle cell anemia.

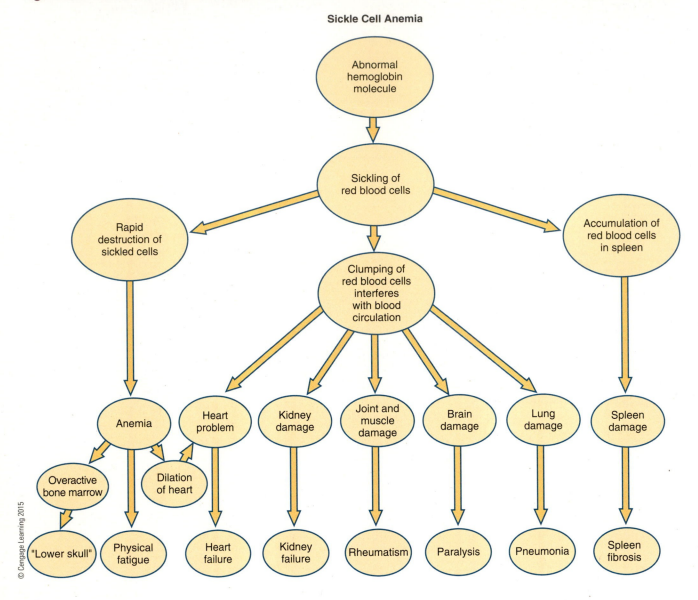

Sickle Cell Anemia

© Cengage Learning 2015

2. TYPES
   a. Hemoglobin SS disease
      1) True sickle cell anemia
      2) Most severe of the sickle disorders
      3) Level of severity 9–10 on a scale from 0 to 10
   b. Hemoglobin S beta zero thalassemia
      1) Similar to hemoglobin SS in types of complications experienced
      2) Characterized by smaller RBCs
      3) Level of severity 7–10 on a scale from 0 to 10
   c. Hemoglobin SC disease
      1) Combination of hemoglobin S and hemoglobin C
      2) Produces a milder sickle syndrome
      3) Level of severity 5–8 on a scale from 0 to 10
   d. Hemoglobin S beta plus thalassemia
      1) The mildest sickle disorder
      2) Like hemoglobin S beta zero thalassemia in that it is characterized by smaller RBCs
      3) Has some normal hemoglobin, so does not experience large number of clinical problems
      4) Level of severity 3–6 on a scale from 0 to 10
3. ASSESSMENT (SEE FIGURE 40-1.)
   a. Dependent of the type of sickle disorder

b. Most commonly experienced manifestations include:
  1) Varying levels of anemia
  2) Elevated reticulocyte count
  3) Recurrent episodes of vasoocclusion
  4) Increased susceptibility to pneumococcal infection (especially in children from 0 to 6 years of age)
  5) Pallor
  6) Jaundice
  7) Splenomegaly
  8) Respiratory disease
  9) Delayed growth and development

4. DIAGNOSTIC TESTS
  a. Based on the results of newborn screening for sickle cell disease, family history, and confirmatory hemoglobin electrophoresis
  b. Newborn screening results
    1) FS (hemoglobin SS or S beta zero thalassemia)
    2) FSA (hemoglobin S beta plus thalassemia)
    3) FSC (hemoglobin SC disease)
    4) FAS (sickle cell trait)

5. MAJOR COMPLICATIONS
  a. Pain
    1) Due to vasoocclusion
    2) Most common reason for emergency room (ER) visits and hospital admission
    3) Occurs in response to infection, decreased oxygenation, dehydration, fever, stress, and extremes of temperature
  b. Dactylitis
    1) Swelling of the hands or feet with or without tenderness and warmth at the site due to vasoocclusion
    2) The first painful episode occurs between 6 months and 3 years of age.
    3) If experienced prior to 1 year of age, it may indicate a more severe clinical course.
  c. Infection
    1) Most common cause of death in pediatric clients with sickle cell disease
    2) Children with sickle cell disease at risk due to impaired splenic function
    3) Greatest risk due to pneumococcal infection
    4) Any client with fever greater than 38.3°C (101°F) must seek medical treatment.

d. Anemia
  1) Due to rapid destruction and shorter life span of RBCs
  2) Signs and symptoms include pallor, jaundice, fatigue, and dark urine.
  3) May occur with aplastic crisis, the temporary cessation of RBC production in clients with chronic anemia, caused by infection with parvovirus B-19
e. Stroke
  1) Occurs in approximately 8% of clients with hemoglobin SS/hemoglobin S beta zero thalassemia disease
  2) Usually a result of infarction of one of the major vessels of the brain
  3) Most common presenting symptom is hemiparesis.
f. Acute chest syndrome (ACS)/pneumonia
  1) Due to vasoocclusion in the vessels of the lungs
  2) Will see infiltrate on chest x-ray
  3) Most commonly affects lower lobes
  4) Episodes tend to recur and have a high mortality rate.
  5) Signs and symptoms include fever, cough, dyspnea, and chest, rib, sternal, or back pain.
g. Splenic sequestration
  1) Sudden, unexplained change in spleen function
  2) Causes severe anemia and massive splenomegaly
h. Gallstones
  1) Common complication
  2) Due to buildup of by-products from RBC destruction
  3) Client will have complaints of abdominal pain, especially after eating high-fat meals.
  4) Diagnosis based on abdominal ultrasound results
i. Priapism
  1) Only affects males
  2) A prolonged, sustained, painful erection
  3) Recurrences are common.
j. Avascular necrosis
  1) Most common in clients with hemoglobin SC disease
  2) Occurs when RBCs sickle inside the bone, causing death to a portion of that bone
  3) Tends to affect the larger joints such as the hip, shoulder, and knee

k. Retinopathy
  1) Vision damage or loss that occurs when RBCs sickle inside the vessels in the eyes
  2) Most commonly affects clients with hemoglobin SC disease

6. NURSING INTERVENTIONS
  a. Pain
    1) Evaluate for precipitating factors or causes of pain other than vasoocclusion.
    3) Maintain adequate hydration through oral or intravenous fluids.
    4) Maintain adequate pain control with acetaminophen (Tylenol), nonsteroidal anti-inflammatory medications (NSAIDs), or narcotic pain medications.
    5) Promote rest and relaxation.
    6) Hydroxyurea is a chemotherapeutic drug used for prevention of painful crises prescribed for a child with greater than three painful episodes in a year due to the potential for serious adverse reactions.
    7) Apply warm compresses to the affected area.
  b. Dactylitis
    1) Increase oral fluid intake.
    2) Administer acetaminophen alternating with ibuprofen every 4 to 6 hours on a scheduled basis for the first 24–48 hours, then decrease to p.r.n.
    3) Administer a narcotic pain reliever if acetaminophen is not effective.
  c. Infection
    1) Instruct the parents that the most effective treatment is prevention, and that medical asepsis is crucial.
    2) Draw blood cultures.
    3) Administer prescribed antibiotics such as daily penicillin.
    4) Monitor the child's temperature and seek medical treatment for a fever greater than 38.3°C (101°F).
    5) Instruct the parents to keep the immunizations up to date.
  d. Anemia
    1) Instruct the parents that treatment is usually not indicated unless reticulocyte count is low.
    2) Avoid administering iron supplements.
    3) Administer blood transfusion for aplastic crisis.
  e. Stroke
    1) Immediate admission to the hospital for exchange transfusion is required.
  2) Instruct the client that posthospitalization, the child will require monthly blood transfusions and chelation therapy.
  f. Acute chest syndrome (ACS)/ pneumonia
    1) Instruct the parents that any child with hemoglobin SS/S beta zero thalassemia and respiratory clinical manifestations such as fever, and chest, back, sternal, or rib pain may need workup for ACS.
    2) Perform a chest x-ray.
    3) Monitor the pulse oximetry.
    4) Administer IV antibiotics.
    5) Maintain IV fluids.
    6) Encourage the child to use the incentive spirometry.
    7) Administer oxygen for sats < 92%, possible blood transfusion if not responsive to conservative measures.
  g. Splenic sequestration
    1) Administer blood transfusion to reverse anemia.
    2) Prepare for surgery to remove the spleen in children greater than 5 years of age.
    3) Administer penicillin prophylaxis after splenectomy.
  h. Gallstones
    1) Prepare the child for surgery to remove gallstones or the gallbladder.
  i. Priapism
    1) Increase fluids and provide symptomatic pain relief.
    2) Administer hydroxyurea (Hydrea).
  j. Avascular necrosis
    1) Perform symptomatic pain relief.
    2) Instruct the parents that the child may eventually require joint replacement surgery and rehabilitation.
  k. Retinopathy
    1) Instruct the parents that the best treatment is prevention.
    2) Instruct the parents that yearly eye exams are performed on all clients with Hgb SC disease after 12 years of age.

D. BETA THALASSEMIA MAJOR
  1. DESCRIPTION
    a. Also called Cooley's anemia
    b. An autosomal recessive disorder characterized by decreased synthesis of beta globin chains and subsequent decrease in hemoglobin content of the RBCs

c. Children with this disorder inherit the thalassemia gene from both parents.

d. Most children are of Mediterranean background.

e. Severe hemolytic anemia develops by 2–6 months of age.

f. Major complications include heart failure, pathologic fractures, and iron overload due to chronic blood transfusions.

2. ASSESSMENT
   a. Severe anemia
   b. Jaundice
   c. Bone marrow hyperplasia, which leads to frontal bossing, maxillary hypertrophy, and prominent cheekbones
   d. Hepatosplenomegaly
   e. Delayed growth and development

3. DIAGNOSTIC TESTS
   a. Family history
   b. Clinical manifestations
   c. Hemoglobin electrophoresis

4. MEDICAL MANAGEMENT
   a. Refer to a hematologist for management of this condition.
   b. Genetic counseling of family should be initiated.
   c. Chronic, monthly blood transfusions, chelation therapy with deferoxamine (Desferal), or bone marrow transplant are the only treatment options.
   d. Some clients may require a splenectomy.

5. NURSING INTERVENTIONS:
   a. Instruct families on the proper use and adverse reactions of Desferal.
   b. Offer family support to help parents cope with the diagnosis.
   c. Encourage social services to assist with financial needs.
   d. Follow hospital or agency protocols for administration of blood products.

E. BETA THALASSEMIA MINOR
   1. DESCRIPTION
      a. An autosomal recessive disorder characterized by decreased synthesis of beta globin chains
      b. Produces a mild, microcytic, hypochromic anemia
      c. Clients with this disorder inherit the thalassemia gene from one parent and do not display clinically significant clinical manifestations.
   2. ASSESSMENT
      a. Healthy child with occasional, mild anemia
      b. Mild jaundice
      c. Limited bone marrow hyperplasia

   3. DIAGNOSTIC TESTS
      a. Family history
      b. Hemoglobin electrophoresis
   4. NURSING INTERVENTIONS
      a. Inform the parents that treatment is generally not necessary.
      b. Encourage the family to seek counseling from a genetic counselor if additional pregnancies are planned.

F. APLASTIC ANEMIA
   1. DESCRIPTION
      a. Failure of the bone marrow which results in a dramatic decrease in production of RBCs, WBCs, and platelets
      b. Can be inherited (Fanconi's anemia) or acquired (autoimmune)
      c. Other causes include infections, toxic agents, medications, and radiation or chemotherapy.
   2. ASSESSMENT
      a. Marrow failure, resulting in decreased hemoglobin and hematocrit, decreased RBC count, decreased WBC count, and decreased platelet count
      b. Easy bruising
      c. Increased infections
      d. Pallor
      e. Fatigue
      f. Impaired growth and development
   3. DIAGNOSTIC TESTS
      a. History
      b. Clinical manifestations
      c. Complete blood count with differential
      d. Bone marrow aspiration, including chromosomal studies
   4. MEDICAL MANAGEMENT
      a. Alleviate the causative factor, if it can be identified.
      b. Symptomatic treatment of anemia, neutropenia, and thrombocytopenia
         1) Anemia: blood transfusions may be indicated.
         2) Neutropenia: extensive evaluation of fever and aggressive treatment of all infections
         3) Thrombocytopenia: platelet transfusions may be indicated.
      c. Treatment will also include immunosuppressive therapy with antithymocyte globulin (Atgam) and cyclosporine (Neoral, Sandimmune, SangCya).
      d. Bone marrow transplant is the only curative option available.
   5. NURSING INTERVENTIONS
      a. Assess the child for clinical manifestations of anemia, neutropenia, and thrombocytopenia.

b. Carefully monitor the client's temperature to evaluate for fever.

c. Educate the family on techniques to prevent infection, such as avoiding contacts with clients who are ill and proper hand washing.

d. Follow hospital or agency protocols for administration of blood products, including packed RBCs for anemia and platelets for thrombocytopenia.

e. Provide emotional support for family.

G. HEMOPHILIA
   1. DESCRIPTION
      a. An X-linked recessive genetic bleeding disorder that results in a defect or deficiency of factor VIII (hemophilia A) or IX (hemophilia B) and only affects males
      b. Hemophilia B is also known as Christmas disease and is not as common as hemophilia A.
      c. This disorder causes prolonged bleeding, either spontaneously or due to trauma.
      d. Incidence of hemophilia A is 1:5,000 male births.
   2. TYPES OF HEMOPHILIA A
      a. Mild
         1) Factor VIII level greater than 5%
         2) Clients bleed after surgery, dental procedures, or severe trauma.
      b. Moderate
         1) Factor VIII level 1–5%
         2) Clients bleed with trauma but not spontaneously.
      c. Severe:
         1) Factor VIII level < 1%
         2) Clients bleed longer and often spontaneously, even without trauma.
   3. ASSESSMENT
      a. Varies, depending on factor levels
      b. Excessive bruising
      c. Prolonged bleeding
      d. Bleeding into muscles or joints
      e. Prolonged PTT
   4. DIAGNOSTIC TESTS
      a. Based on family history, laboratory values, and clinical manifestations
      b. Family history is usually significant for mother being the carrier of the hemophilia gene.
      c. Prenatal amniocentesis at 12–15 weeks of gestation can detect hemophilia.
      d. Coagulation testing is used to confirm the diagnosis but should be delayed until 6 months of age due to the presence of lower factor levels at birth.

5. MAJOR COMPLICATIONS
   a. Intracranial hemorrhage
      1) Primary concern at birth
      2) Leading cause of death for clients with hemophilia
      3) Serious head trauma should always be treated even in the absence of neurological clinical manifestations.
   b. Circumcision
      1) Often the first episode of prolonged bleeding
      2) May be instrumental in making a diagnosis
   c. Hematomas
      1) Pockets of blood under the skin that occur after injections or injury to soft tissue
   d. Tooth eruption
      1) May see excessive bleeding with teething
   e. Hematuria
      1) Blood in the urine
   f. Hemarthrosis
      1) Bleeding into the joint that causes a hot, swollen joint and loss of joint stability
      2) May lead to severe, crippling arthritis if the client repeatedly bleeds into the same joint
   g. Inhibitors
      1) Antibodies to factor that develop in frequently treated clients and make hemostasis difficult to achieve
   h. Hepatitis/AIDS
      1) Due to contaminated clotting factor
      2) Has decreased in recent years due to use of recombinant factor and increased safety with blood products
6. MEDICAL MANAGEMENT
   a. Clients require comprehensive, multidisciplinary care.
   b. It must involve the primary care physician, hematologist, orthopedist, physical/occupational therapist, social worker, dentist, and case manager.
   c. Client will need a Medic Alert bracelet.
   d. Education
   e. Factor replacement
      1) Many types are available.
      2) Each client needs an individualized treatment plan with a prescription for factor replacement from a hematologist.
      3) The replacement dosage and schedule will depend on the client's level of severity and the type of complication experienced by the child.

4) Some clients will also receive prophylactic treatment, giving factor on a scheduled basis, rather than during bleeding episodes

5) Desmopressin (DDAVP, Stimate) may be utilized in clients with the mild type.

6) In addition, aminocaproic acid (Amicar) is frequently used in clients who experience mouth bleeds.

f. Exercise

1) Goals include building flexibility, strength, and cardiovascular endurance.

2) Exercise may help decrease the frequency and severity of bleeding episodes.

3) Exercise regimen should be prescribed and followed closely by a physical therapist.

g. Nutrition

1) May need iron supplements if anemia develops from frequent bleeding episodes

7. NURSING INTERVENTIONS

a. Instruct the child and family to recognize clinical manifestations of bleeding episodes such as visible bleeding, pain, swelling, limited motion in a joint, excessive bruising, history of trauma, headache or changes in level of consciousness (LOC), and black tarry stools.

b. Instruct the child and family to calculate factor dosages specific to the client.

c. Instruct the child and family to administer factor.

d. Instruct the child and family methods to prevent bleeding episodes such as avoiding trauma, providing close supervision of activities, using protective equipment, using soft-bristled toothbrushes, and avoiding contact sports.

e. Instruct the child and family on how to deal with acute bleeding episodes such as applying pressure to the site of bleeding for 10–15 minutes, immobilizing and elevating the area, and applying ice to decrease bleeding.

f. Encourage genetic counseling.

g. Refer families to hemophilia support groups or organizations.

h. Administer immunizations subcutaneously (s.q.).

H. VON WILLEBRAND'S DISEASE

1. DESCRIPTION

a. An autosomal-dominant mild bleeding disorder that affects both males and females

b. Causes a decrease in the amount of circulating von Willebrand's protein, which normally functions to facilitate platelet adhesion

c. Incidence is not known.

d. It is believed to be one of the most common bleeding disorders.

e. Present in up to 1% of the general population

2. ASSESSMENT

a. Prolonged oral bleeding with teething or dental procedures

b. Epistaxis

c. Excessive menstrual bleeding

d. GI bleeds

e. Excessive bruising

f. Prolonged postoperative bleeding

3. DIAGNOSTIC TESTS

a. Family history

b. Laboratory findings—diagnosis complex and may require repeated testing

c. Clinical manifestations

d. Commonly underdiagnosed due to mild symptoms

4. MEDICAL MANAGEMENT

a. Referral to a hematologist for diagnosis and management. Desmopressin (DDAVP, Stimate) is utilized for treatment of acute bleeding episodes as well as for prophylactic treatment, before dental procedures, surgery, and the like.

b. For clients who do not respond to desmopressin (DDAVP, Stimate), cryoprecipitate or antihemophilic factor (Humate-P) can be used.

c. Aminocaproic acid (Amicar) can also be used for oral bleeding in these clients.

d. Comprehensive care is essential.

5. NURSING INTERVENTIONS (SEE THE NURSING INTERVENTIONS FOR HEMOPHILIA, SECTION IV.)

I. IDEOPATHIC (IMMUNE) THROMBOCYTOPENIC PURPURA (ITP)

1. DESCRIPTION

a. Most common bleeding disorder of childhood

b. Characterized by acute development of thrombocytopenia (low platelet count) and purpura (petechiae beneath the skin)

c. Low platelet count results from premature destruction of platelets in the spleen.

d. Prevents the formation of platelet plugs when injury occurs to a vessel wall

e. Cause is unknown, but believed to be an autoimmune process

f. A self-limiting disorder, even if not treated

g. Frequently occurs in children 2–5 years of age but can occur at any age

2. ASSESSMENT

a. Physical exam is normal with the exception of petechiae or bruising, or both.

b. Decreased platelet count (usually less than 50,000), with an otherwise normal complete blood count (CBC)

3. DIAGNOSTIC TESTS

a. Client history (may be significant for preceding viral illness)

b. Laboratory values, including a CBC

c. Bone marrow aspiration, which will show large numbers of megakaryocytes (platelet precursors)

4. MEDICAL MANAGEMENT

a. Short course of corticosteroids is the treatment of choice.

b. Oral prednisolone (Pediapred) 2 mg/kg/day on a tapering schedule

c. Weekly platelet counts to monitor progress

d. If not responsive to prednisone, may use (intravenous immune globulin [IVIG]) or Rho (D) globulin (Win Rho D) intravenously

e. Splenectomy usually indicated for clients with chronic or recurrent episodes of ideopathic (immune) thrombocytopenic purpura (ITP)

5. NURSING INTERVENTIONS

a. Instruct the family on the measures to avoid trauma.

b. Avoid medications that enhance bleeding such as aspirin and nonsteroidal and anti-inflammatory drugs

c. Elevate the involved area, apply pressure, and apply ice during active bleeding episodes.

d. Instruct the family to recognize clinical manifestations of bleeding.

J. DISSEMINATED INTRAVASCULAR COAGULATION (DIC)

1. DESCRIPTION

a. A disorder of coagulation characterized by inappropriate and accelerated coagulation

b. May lead to hemorrhage or thrombosis, or both.

c. Occurs in response to a variety of precipitating events in the body

d. Begins during the first stage of coagulation that stimulates an overproduction of thrombin, resulting in fibrinogen being converted to fibrin more rapidly and causing clot formation to occur; this leads to obstruction of blood vessels and subsequent ischemia and tissue necrosis and may result in massive hemorrhage

2. ASSESSMENT

a. Acute DIC

1) Oozing from puncture sites

2) Bleeding from the nose, mouth, or eyes

3) Purpura and petechiae

4) GI bleeding

5) Hypotension

6) Organ dysfunction

b. Chronic DIC

1) Jaundice

2) Hypoxia

3) Oliguria

4) Changes in mental status

3. DIAGNOSTIC TESTS

a. PT: prolonged

b. PTT: prolonged

c. Platelet count: decreased

d. Fibrinogen: decreased

4. MEDICAL MANAGEMENT

a. Identify and treat the underlying cause.

b. Will usually spontaneously resolve the coagulation abnormalities

c. Replacement therapy

1) Administration of platelets and fresh frozen plasma

2) Possible blood transfusion

3) Cryoprecipitate administration to increase fibrinogen

d. Heparin administration

1) Utilized only in severe cases

5. NURSING INTERVENTIONS

a. Assess the child for clinical manifestations of bleeding such as pallor, hypotension, and changes in LOC.

b. Administer replacement products.

c. Provide supportive care for the child and family.

PRACTICE QUESTIONS

1. In examining a child with suspected anemia, the nurse would recognize which of the following as a significant objective finding?
   1. History of pica
   2. Daily aspirin therapy
   3. Cheilosis and glossitis
   4. Tonsillectomy three days ago

2. A child is being admitted to the hematology unit of the hospital with physician orders to obtain a complete blood count (CBC). The parent inquires about the purpose of this test. The nurse's best response would be which of the following?
   1. "It provides a basic description of the types of cells present and measures the quantity of all the cells in the blood."
   2. "It provides the physician with an opportunity to view the red blood cells under a microscope."
   3. "It measures the body's stores of iron and its ability to bind iron and create hemoglobin."
   4. "It allows for the evaluation of the presence of abnormal hemoglobins and can detect hemoglobinopathies."

3. In preparing the client and family for bone marrow aspiration, the nurse should explain the procedure thoroughly. Which of the following statements represents appropriate family preparation?
   1. "The child will be required to lie perfectly still while the physician obtains the specimen from the sternum."
   2. "This procedure is virtually painless and well tolerated by all children, so anesthesia is not necessary."
   3. "The test measures with a stopwatch the length of time it takes the child to stop bleeding once the procedure is completed."
   4. "The physician will use sterile technique while obtaining a small sample of bone marrow through a needle inserted into the child's hip bone."

4. Which of the following should be included in the discharge instructions for a child with iron deficiency anemia?
   1. Take two iron supplements after missing a dose
   2. Iron supplements should be taken between meals with orange juice and monitor for black, tarry stools
   3. Increase vitamin D milk consumption in infants less than 12 months of age to increase dietary iron
   4. Avoid foods high in vitamin C, because they decrease the absorption of iron supplements

5. After assessing four clients with sickle cell anemia, which of the following clients is the priority for the nurse to administer care to first?
   1. A client whose speech is slurred and has hemiparesis
   2. A client complaining of painful swelling of the hands or feet
   3. A client who is experiencing pallor, icteric sclera, and fatigue
   4. A client complaining of abdominal pain after eating a high-fat meal

6. A nurse is caring for a child with sickle cell anemia. Which of the following measures would be a priority to include in the plan of care to prevent infection?
   1. Increase oral fluid intake and administer prescribed analgesics
   2. Administer penicillin twice daily and immunize with Pneumovax
   3. Infuse packed red blood cells monthly as prescribed
   4. Administer prescribed antipyretics for temperatures greater than 38.3°C, or 101°F

7. The nurse is admitting a child suspected of having beta thalassemia major. Which of the following findings should be reported?
   Select all that apply:
   [ ] 1. Excessive bruising
   [ ] 2. Hematuria
   [ ] 3. Severe anemia
   [ ] 4. Pallor
   [ ] 5. Maxillary hyperplasia
   [ ] 6. Joint pain

8. In caring for a child with aplastic anemia, the nurse should immediately report which of the following assessment findings?
   1. Fever of 39°C, or 102°F
   2. Splenomegaly
   3. Pallor and fatigue
   4. Amenorrhea

9. The nurse should include which of the following instructions for the parents of a child with hemophilia A (factor XIII deficiency)?
   1. Participation in contact sports is permitted with supervision and protective equipment
   2. All forms of physical activity should be avoided in order to prevent bleeding episodes
   3. Apply warm packs to hemarthroses to decrease associated discomfort
   4. Encourage age-appropriate immunizations

10. The nurse is caring for a child suspected to have ideopathic thrombocytopenic purpura (ITP). Which of the following questions would be most important to ask while obtaining the history?
    1. "Has your child been sick recently?"
    2. "What blood type does your child have?"
    3. "What medications have you given your child?"
    4. "Are there any pets in the home?"

11. The nurse is caring for a child suspected of having von Willebrand's disease. The nurse should prepare the client for which of the following laboratory tests?
    Select all that apply:
    [ ] 1. Complete blood count (CBC) with differential
    [ ] 2. Platelet count
    [ ] 3. Bone marrow aspiration
    [ ] 4. Hemoglobin electrophoresis
    [ ] 5. Bleeding time
    [ ] 6. Ristocetin cofactor

12. Which of the following characteristics should the nurse include in a class on beta thalassemia major?
    Select all that apply:
    [ ] 1. Causes prolonged bleeding
    [ ] 2. Produces a mild, microcytic, hypochromic anemia
    [ ] 3. Severe hemolytic anemia develops by 2–6 months
    [ ] 4. Major complications include heart failure, pathologic fractures, and iron overload due to chronic blood transfusions
    [ ] 5. Most common hematological disorder in children
    [ ] 6. Also called Cooley's anemia

13. Which of the following should the nurse include in the plan of care for a child with disseminated intravascular coagulation (DIC)?
    1. Administer blood thinners
    2. Monitor the child for signs of bleeding
    3. Administer intravenous analgesics
    4. Monitor the child's respiratory status

14. Which of the following laboratory findings would the nurse expect to be ordered for a child with disseminated intravascular coagulation (DIC)?
    Select all that apply:
    [ ] 1. Prolonged partial thromboplastin time (PTT)
    [ ] 2. Decreased white blood cell count (WBC)
    [ ] 3. Increased red blood cell count (RBC)
    [ ] 4. Decreased platelet count
    [ ] 5. Increased reticulocyte count
    [ ] 6. Decreased fibrinogen

15. Which of the following drugs should the nurse administer to a child with sickle cell anemia to decrease painful episodes and prevent hospitalizations?
    1. Morphine sulfate (MS Contin)
    2. Meperidine (Demerol)
    3. Acetaminophen with codeine (Tylenol #3)
    4. Hydroxyurea (Hydrea)

16. The parent of a child with a hematological disorder inquires about the purpose of the red blood cells in the body. The nurse should respond, "Red blood cells
    1. serve as the body's defense against infection."
    2. assist in the formation of blood clots."
    3. carry oxygen to the tissues."
    4. are primarily responsible for removing debris from the bloodstream."

17. The nurse is caring for a child with anemia. Which of the following would indicate to the nurse that the client's condition is deteriorating?
    1. Circumoral pallor
    2. Fatigue with exertion
    3. Cardiac murmur
    4. Irritability

18. The nurse is instructing the family of a child with iron deficiency anemia about the importance of increasing iron in the diet. Which of the following foods should the nurse include?
    Select all that apply:
    [ ] 1. Fortified cereals
    [ ] 2. Green leafy vegetables
    [ ] 3. Vitamin D milk
    [ ] 4. Pasta
    [ ] 5. Dried fruits
    [ ] 6. Tea

19. The nurse is caring for a child with sickle cell disease who is experiencing hematuria. Which of the following actions is an appropriate intervention?
    1. Restrict activity
    2. Administer ibuprofen (Motrin)
    3. Push fluids
    4. Check the child's temperature

20. The nurse is discharging an infant who was recently diagnosed with sickle cell anemia, or hemoglobin SS disease. It is a priority to provide the infant's parents with information on which of the following complications?
    1. Avascular necrosis
    2. Retinopathy
    3. Gallstones
    4. Dactylitis

21. Which of the following drugs should the nurse administer to a child with beta thalassemia major who has been on chronic transfusion therapy for several years?
    1. Acetaminophen with codeine (Tylenol #3)
    2. Deferoxamine (Desferal)
    3. Hydroxyurea (Hydrea)
    4. Cyclosporine (Sandimmune, Neoral)

22. The nurse is caring for a child with aplastic anemia. Which of the following measures should be included in the child's plan of care?
    1. Recommendation of genetic counseling
    2. Education on the proper administration of iron supplements
    3. Administration of antithymocyte globulin (ATG)
    4. Encourage interaction with other children at day care

23. The nurse is caring for a child with severe hemophilia A (factor XIII deficiency). Which of the following measures is most appropriate for the nurse to implement in this child's plan of care?
    1. Pad the bed rails
    2. Force fluids
    3. Administer intravenous immune globulin (IVIG)
    4. Monitor temperature

24. After a health interview with an adolescent child, which of the following findings should the nurse report as significant?
    1. Heavy menstrual flow
    2. Accelerated growth curve
    3. Delayed puberty
    4. Spinal curvature

25. Parents who are both carriers of the beta thalassemia gene have one child with the disease and want to have another child. They ask the nurse what the chances are of having another child with this disorder. The appropriate response by the nurse is which of the following?
    1. "There is a 25% chance."
    2. "There is approximately a 50% chance."
    3. "There is no chance for the next child to be affected."
    4. "The second child will be born with the disorder."

26. The registered nurse is delegating the nursing tasks for a pediatric hematology unit. Which of the following tasks should the nurse delegate to a licensed practical nurse?
    1. Administer deferoxamine (Desferal) IV to a child with beta thalassemia major
    2. Monitor the platelet count in a child with aplastic anemia
    3. Assess a child with immune thrombocytopenia purpura for indications of bleeding
    4. Administer desmopressin (DDAVP) intranasally to a child with mild hemophilia A

ANSWERS AND RATIONALES

1. 3. Cheilosis (fissures in the angles of the lips) and glossitis (inflammation of the tongue) are observable physical abnormalities that tend to occur in clients experiencing significant anemia. A history of pica, daily aspirin therapy, and tonsillectomy 3 days ago are all examples of subjective findings that may be associated with anemia.

2. 1. The CBC (complete blood count) is a basic diagnostic exam that measures the number, quality, variety, concentrations, and percentages of the blood cells. A peripheral smear allows the clinician to view blood cells under a microscope. Serum iron and TIBC

(total iron-binding capacity) measure iron stores and the capacity of the body to bind with iron and form hemoglobin. Hemoglobin electrophoresis measures both normal and abnormal hemoglobins and is the diagnostic test required to identify hemoglobinopathies.

3. 4. Children will be positioned on the abdomen for the procedure because the posterior iliac crest is the preferred site for bone marrow aspiration in children. Sterile technique is used during the procedure to minimize the risk for infection. The sternum is an acceptable site for bone marrow aspiration

in adults, but not in children. Bone marrow aspiration is associated with discomfort during needle insertion and specimen aspiration. The length of time it takes a client to form a clot is a measure of bleeding time.

4. 2. Iron supplements should be given on an empty stomach with a source of vitamin C to increase absorption and may be given between meals to decrease stomach upset. Black, tarry stool is a common side effect of iron therapy. Making up for missed doses of iron supplements is never recommended. Whole milk consumption by young infants is responsible for a large number of cases of iron deficiency anemia. The immature gastrointestinal (GI) tract in infants cannot process whole milk, and this can lead to GI bleeding, blood loss, and anemia. Vitamin C increases the absorption of iron from the GI tract.

5. 1. Hemiparesis and slurred speech may be indicative of stroke. Stroke requires immediate admission to the hospital for an exchange transfusion to prevent permanent motor damage. Painful swelling of the hands or feet is called dactylitis and can be managed at home with fluids and analgesics, unless fever is present. Pallor, icteric sclera, and fatigue are continuously present in a large number of clients with sickle cell disease due to underlying anemia. Abdominal pain that occurs after eating greasy foods is associated with gallstones and is not a medical emergency.

6. 2. All children with sickle cell anemia who are less than 6 years of age should be on penicillin twice daily to prevent pneumococcal sepsis. In addition to regular immunizations, these children should receive Pneumovax, to further protect them from infection. Increasing fluids and administering analgesics are measures aimed at treating painful episodes. Monthly blood transfusions increase a client's hematocrit and decrease the risk for stroke, but do not prevent infection in sickle cell clients. Antipyretics are not effective in preventing infection.

7. 3. 4. 5. Maxillary hypertrophy results from bone marrow hyperplasia in response to the severe anemia that occurs in beta thalassemia major. Pallor is also a result of the severe anemia. Excessive bruising and hematuria are common manifestations of hemophilia, not beta thalassemia major. Joint pain is not a common manifestation of beta thalassemia major; however, it is experienced in clients with sickle cell anemia and hemophilia.

8. 1. Children with aplastic anemia are at increased risk for overwhelming sepsis due to neutropenia. Any fever greater than 38.3°C, or 101°F, is considered a medical emergency and requires immediate treatment. Splenomegaly is not commonly associated with aplastic anemia. Pallor and fatigue are common in clients with aplastic anemia, but do not usually require immediate evaluation. Amenorrhea is actually induced in many clients with aplastic anemia to prevent further blood loss and increasing anemia.

9. 4. Immunizations should be administered in children with hemophilia, but should be given s.q. In addition, pressure should be applied to the site of injection for 15 minutes. Children with hemophilia are allowed participation in noncontact sports only. Exercise is important for children with hemophilia to build flexibility, strength, and cardiovascular endurance. Ice should be applied to areas of bleeding to constrict blood vessels and decrease bleeding.

10. 3. Drugs such as aspirin products and nonsteroidal anti-inflammatory drugs (NSAIDs) can adversely affect children and cause bleeding. This needs to be ruled out before making a diagnosis of ideopathic thrombocytopenic purpura (ITP). Many children with ITP have a history of preceding viral illness, although it is not a definitive indication that the child will develop ITP. The child's blood type does not play a role in the diagnosis of ITP, although it might be necessary to know this if initial treatment options are unsuccessful. Pets in the home are insignificant for ITP.

11. 2. 5. 6. Platelet count, bleeding time, and ristocetin cofactor are all essential to confirm a diagnosis of von Willebrand's disease. A complete blood count (CBC) and hemoglobin electrophoresis are instrumental in the diagnosis of hemoglobinopathies. Bone marrow aspiration looks at the cellular components of the bone marrow and is utilized in the diagnosis of many hematological conditions, but not von Willebrand's disease.

12. 3. 4. 6. Another name for beta thalassemia major is Cooley's anemia. It is a severe hemolytic anemia that develops by age 2–6 months of age. Major complications include heart failure, pathologic fractures, and iron overload due to chronic blood transfusions. Hemophilia is a disorder that causes a prolonged bleeding. Beta thalassemia minor produces a mild, microcytic, hypochrimic anemia. Anemia is the most common hematological disorder in children.

13. 2. The nurse should be acutely aware of any bleeding that occurs, as hypovolemic shock can be a complication of disseminated intravascular coagulation (DIC). Blood thinners, such as heparin, are usually administered only in severe cases because they create a risk for bleeding. IV analgesics are not routinely utilized in clients with disseminated intravascular coagulation. The child's respiratory status is not usually compromised in DIC.

14. 1. 4. 6. Prolonged partial thromboplastin is common in clients with disseminated intravascular coagulation (DIC), due to the body's attempt to dissolve the clots formed as a result of the increased activity of coagulation factors. The platelet count and fibrinogen may drop, due to the fibrinolysis which may occur. The white blood cell count (WBC) does not play a role in the pathophysiology of DIC and is unrelated to this condition. The red blood cell count (RBC) is usually decreased from bleeding. An increased reticulocyte count is associated with certain types of anemia.

15. 4. Hydroxyurea (Hydrea) is a daily drug prescribed to decrease painful crises and prevent hospitalization of a child with sickle cell anemia. Morphine sulfate, meperidine (Demerol), and acetaminophen with codeine are all drugs utilized during acute pain episodes.

16. 3. Red blood cells are responsible for carrying oxygen to the tissues and removing carbon dioxide from them. White blood cells are the body's primary defense against infection. Platelets are the cellular components of blood that assist in the formation of blood clots. Phagocytosis is the process of removing debris from the bloodstream and is carried out by white blood cells.

17. 3. Cardiac murmurs are only present in children with significant anemia and indicate their condition is deteriorating. Pallor, fatigue with exertion, and irritability are findings that may be present with all levels of anemia.

18. 1. 2. 5. Fortified cereals, leafy green vegetables, and dried fruits are all excellent sources of iron and should be included in the child's diet. Vitamin D milk is high in calcium. Tea blocks the absorption of iron and should be excluded from the child's diet. Pasta is not a significant source of dietary iron.

19. 3. Increasing fluid intake will dilute the urine and reduce further kidney damage and may possibly correct the hematuria. Restricting activity is not specific to hematuria. Ibuprofen has no indication in the treatment of hematuria. Evaluation of temperature is not indicated in the treatment of sickle cell anemia and hematuria.

20. 4. Dactylitis is the first painful episode a sickle cell client may experience and usually occurs between 6 months and 3 years of age. This information would be most relevant for the parents of an infant who was just diagnosed. A vascular necrosis and retinopathy tend to be complications experienced in adolescence and adulthood. Gallstones are not common in infancy.

21. 2. Children who are receiving chronic transfusion therapy are at risk for iron overload and subsequent organ damage. Deferoxamine (Desferal) is a chelation agent that binds with iron and helps the body remove the excess. Tylenol with codeine and hydroxyurea (Hydrea) are drugs used in the treatment and prevention of sickle cell pain. Cyclosporine (Sandimmune, Neoral) is an immunosuppressive agent used in the treatment of aplastic anemia.

22. 3. Antithymocyte globulin (ATG) is routinely used to treat clients with aplastic anemia. Genetic counseling is not indicated for families experiencing aplastic anemia, as it is not a hereditary condition. Iron supplementation is not usually indicated for clients with aplastic anemia. Because children with this disease should avoid exposure to sources of infection, they should not be encouraged to interact in day care. Day care centers and schools are common sources of infection.

23. 1. Padding the bed rails may help to decrease the chances of injury in a child with hemophilia. Forcing fluids is not part of routine care for hemophilia clients. Intravenous immune globulin (IVIG) is utilized in clients with ideopathic thrombocytopenic purpura (ITP). Monitoring temperatures is necessary in all clients, but is not the most appropriate intervention for this child.

24. 3. Delayed puberty is common in adolescents with sickle cell disease. Heavy menstrual flow is more commonly associated with bleeding disorders, such as von Willebrand's disease. Children with sickle cell anemia have a strong tendency to be smaller and weigh less than their peers and often do

not follow a normal growth curve. Spinal curvature is not associated with having sickle cell disease.

25. 1. If both parents are carriers of the disease gene of beta thalassemia major, there will be a 25% chance of having a child with the condition with each pregnancy. The parents are both

carriers of a recessive gene that has a 25% chance of being expressed with each pregnancy.

26. 4. Administering a drug IV, monitoring a platelet count, and assessing a child for indications of bleeding are all tasks that require the skills of a registered nurse. A licensed practical nurse may administer a drug intranasally.

REFERENCES

Daniels, R. (2012). *Delmar's manual of laboratory and diagnostic tests* (2nd ed.). Clifton Park, NY: Delmar Cengage Learning.

Potts, N., & Mandleco, B. (2012). *Pediatric nursing: Caring for children and their families* (3rd ed.). Clifton Park, NY: Delmar Cengage Learning.

Spratto, G. R., & Woods, A. L. (2012). *PDR nurse's drug handbook 2012*. Clifton Park, NY: Delmar Cengage Learning.

CHAPTER 41

INFECTIOUS AND COMMUNICABLE DISORDERS

I. **INTRODUCTION TO INFECTIOUS AND COMMUNICABLE DISORDERS**
  A. HISTORY OF INFECTIOUS DISORDERS
   1. RESPONSIBLE FOR HIGH INFANT AND CHILDHOOD MORTALITY IN EARLY TWENTIETH CENTURY
   2. THE DISCOVERY AND USE OF ANTIBIOTICS HAS REDUCED MORBIDITY AND MORTALITY RATES.
   3. IMPROVED METHODS OF TREATMENT INCLUDE:
     a. Prevention of infection
     b. Potent antibiotics
     c. Stringent immunization
     d. Modern sanitation
   4. DESPITE IMPROVEMENTS, INFECTION STILL ACCOUNTS FOR MANY SERIOUS ILLNESSES.
   5. IN DEVELOPING COUNTRIES, INFECTION CONTINUES TO BE A PRESSING HEALTH CONCERN.
   6. PREVENTION OF INFECTION IS A MAJOR GOAL OF THE WORLD HEALTH ORGANIZATION.
     a. Prevention of disease
     b. Prevention of disability and death from infection
     c. Prevention through immunization
  B. DEFINITIONS
   1. INFECTIOUS DISEASE
     a. Any disease caused by invasion and multiplication of microorganisms
     b. May not be communicable
     c. Commonly occur in infancy, childhood, and adolescence
     d. Until 3 years of age, children typically experience 6–10 infectious illnesses per year.
   2. COMMUNICABLE DISEASE
     a. Disease caused by an infectious agent
     b. Transmitted to a person by direct or indirect contact, vehicle or vector, or airborne route
   3. PATHOGEN
     a. Disease-producing microorganism
     b. Infectious microorganisms can include bacteria, viruses, fungi, and parasites.
   4. VIRULENCE
     a. The degree or power of organisms to cause disease classifications
       1) Extent of involvement
         a) Local infection: limited to one locality of the body; may have systemic repercussions such as fever and malaise
         b) Focal infections: a local infection from which organisms spread to other body parts
         c) Systemic infections: the infectious agent is spread throughout the body
     b. Length of the infectious process
       1) Acute infection
         a) Develops rapidly
         b) Usually results in high fever and severe sickness
         c) Resolves in a short period of time
         d) Sometimes an acute infection becomes chronic.
       2) Chronic infection
         a) Develops slowly
         b) Milder but longer lasting clinical manifestation
         c) Sometimes a chronic infection becomes acute.

C. ANATOMY AND PHYSIOLOGY OF
   INFECTION
   1. MOST INFECTIOUS DISEASES ARE
      TRANSMITTED IN ONE OF FOUR WAYS,
      AND ISOLATION METHODS ARE
      ALIGNED ACCORDING TO METHOD
      OF TRANSMISSION.
      a. Contact: the susceptible host comes
         into direct contact, such as in sexually
         transmitted diseases, or in indirect
         contact, such as contaminated
         inanimate objects or spread of
         respiratory droplets, with the source.
   2. AIRBORNE TRANSMISSION: RESULTS
      FROM INHALATION OF
      CONTAMINATED EVAPORATED SALIVA
      DROPLETS, SUCH AS PULMONARY
      TUBERCULOSIS, WHICH MAY BE
      SUSPENDED IN AIRBORNE DUST
      PARTICLES OR VAPORS.
   3. ENTERIC (FECAL-ORAL)
      TRANSMISSION: THE ORGANISMS ARE
      FOUND IN FECES AND ARE INGESTED
      BY SUSCEPTIBLE CLIENTS MOST
      LIKELY THROUGH CONTAMINATED
      FOOD OR WATER.
   4. VECTOR-BORNE TRANSMISSION:
      OCCURS WHEN AN INTERMEDIATE
      CARRIER (VECTOR) SUCH AS A FLEA
      OR MOSQUITO TRANSFERS THE
      ORGANISM.
D. TRANSMISSION THAT THE DISEASE IS
   DEPENDENT ON
   1. INFECTIOUS AGENT
      a. Must be present in sufficient numbers
         to cause disease
      b. Some organisms have greater virulence
         than others.
      c. Human response is dependent on age
         and development of the immune system.
   2. RESERVOIR
      a. Where pathogens can survive without
         multiplication
      b. May be alive in humans, animals, or
         insects
      c. May be inanimate (not living) in soil,
         water, other environmental sources, or
         medical equipment
   3. PORTAL OF EXIT FROM RESERVOIR
      a. Pathogens leave through blood or body
         secretions such as saliva, urine, feces,
         respiratory secretions, and saliva.
   4. MODE OF TRANSMISSION
      a. Spread by direct contact from person to
         person through saliva, droplets from
         the respiratory tract, body contact, or
         blood and body fluids in urinary,
         gastrointestinal, and reproductive
         systems
      b. Transmitted on objects

      c. May be in contaminated food or water
      d. Spread by vectors, animals or insects
         that carry infectious organisms from
         one host to another
   5. PORTAL OF ENTRY TO THE HOST
      a. Pathogens enter the body through the
         respiratory tract, gastrointestinal tract,
         urinary tract, skin and mucous
         membranes, or across the placenta
   6. SUSCEPTIBLE HOST
      a. Lacks immunity to a specific
         organism
      b. Dysfunctional immune system
   7. OTHER FACTORS
      a. Pathogens may survive the
         environment because many organisms
         remain viable from hours to several
         weeks on the surfaces of toys or
         tabletops (rotavirus).
      b. Clients who are asymptomatic may be
         able to transmit pathogens before they
         become ill, as in varicella.
      c. Carriers can harbor and spread
         the organism to others without
         exhibiting clinical manifestations
         of illness.
      d. The concentration of a pathogen
         determines whether or not an infection
         occurs after a single exposure.
E. PREVENTION OF INFECTION
   1. DRUG PROPHYLAXIS
   2. STANDARD PRECAUTIONS
   3. HAND WASHING
   4. COMPREHENSIVE IMMUNIZATION
   5. IMPROVED NUTRITION, LIVING
      CONDITIONS, AND SANITATION
   6. CORRECTION OF ENVIRONMENTAL
      FACTORS

II. **RISK OF INFECTION BY DEVELOPMENTAL AGE**
A. EACH DEVELOPMENTAL STAGE BRINGS
   UNIQUE RISKS FOR INFECTION
   1. PRENATAL (FETUS)
      a. Susceptible to maternal infection
      b. Process is known as vertical
         transmission (mother to fetus)
      c. May occur through the placenta
      d. May occur during the birth process
      e. Examples include human immune
         deficiency virus (HIV), rubella,
         and herpes.
   2. INFANCY
      a. May be acquired infection through
         consumption of breast milk
      b. Infection by organisms that later in life
         are considered normal flora
         (*e.g., Escherichia coli*) may occur
      c. Exposed to objects and surfaces that are
         contaminated with pathogens such
         as toys, tabletops, or the hands
         of caregivers

   d. May occur as a result of hand-to-mouth behavior
   e. More susceptible to gastrointestinal and respiratory viruses
   f. At a greatest risk for metabolic problems resulting from fever, decreased appetite, fluid intake, diarrhea, and dehydration

3. TODDLERS AND PRESCHOOLERS
   a. Infections caused by fecal-oral routes
   b. May occur from encounters with other children wearing diapers, as in day care settings
   c. Continued hand-to-mouth exploration increase the risk
   d. Developing toileting and handwashing skills
   e. Increased exposure to pets and outside environments

4. SCHOOL AGE
   a. Substandard hygienic practices (hand washing)
   b. Strict school schedules
   c. Sharing of clothes, food, or toys
   d. Overnight stays with other children and sharing of grooming devices
   e. Exposure to contagious disease in school settings such as pneumonia or Fifth disease

5. ADOLESCENCE
   a. Generally do not seek care unless ill
   b. Fail to have continuity of care
   c. Requires booster immunizations to maintain immunity
   d. Generally lack immunity to hepatitis B
   e. Have an increased exposure to sexually transmitted diseases (STDs)
   f. Have difficulty assessing and utilizing confidential health care
   g. Fail to believe they are at risk of infection or pregnancy
   h. Increased frequency of sexual intercourse or multiple partners
   i. Increase in high-risk behaviors such as unprotected sex, drug and alcohol use

B. GENERAL INTERVENTIONS IN THE PREVENTION OF INFECTION
   1. PERFORM FAMILY EDUCATION ABOUT DISEASE TRANSMISSION.
   2. PROVIDE EDUCATION FOCUSED ON PERSONAL HYGIENE, WAYS OF STAYING HEALTHY, AND BASIC NUTRITION.
   3. REVIEW THE GERM THEORY AND ILLNESS PREVENTION WITH THE CHILD AND FAMILY.
   4. ENCOURAGE THE PARENTS TO OPENLY DISCUSS STDS WITH THE CHILD.

5. ASSESS ADOLESCENTS FOR AT-RISK BEHAVIORS SUCH AS UNPROTECTED SEX, DRUG USE, OR GANG RELATIONSHIPS.
6. ENCOURAGE THE FAMILY TO BE FAMILIAR WITH THE LAWS OF THEIR STATE REGARDING CONFIDENTIAL TREATMENT AND DIAGNOSIS.

III. IMMUNIZATIONS
   A. DESCRIPTION
      1. AN IMPORTANT PART OF HEALTH PROMOTION AND DISEASE PREVENTION
      2. INTRODUCED INTO THE BODY TO EVOKE AN IMMUNE RESPONSE
      3. THE TERMS *IMMUNIZATION* AND *VACCINE* ARE INTERCHANGEABLE.
      4. MOST VACCINES ARE GIVEN BY INJECTION, ALTHOUGH SOME ARE AVAILABLE IN ORAL OR AEROSOL ROUTES.
   B. IMMUNIZATION SCHEDULES
      1. REINFORCES AND ENSURES REGULAR HEALTH CARE SUPERVISION
      2. SCHEDULES CHANGE BASED ON INCREASED KNOWLEDGE OF EFFICACY.
      3. SCHEDULES CHANGE BASED ON NEW VACCINE DEVELOPMENT.
      4. RECOMMENDATIONS ARE BASED ON CONSENSUS OF FOUR REGULATORY GROUPS: ADVISORY COMMITTEE ON IMMUNIZATION PRACTICES (ACIP), CENTERS FOR DISEASE CONTROL AND PREVENTION (CDC), AMERICAN ACADEMY OF PEDIATRICS (AAP), AND AMERICAN ACADEMY OF FAMILY PHYSICIANS (AAFP).
      5. PROPOSED IMMUNIZATION SCHEDULE IS UPDATED ANNUALLY.
      6. MISSED VACCINE DOSES SHOULD BE RESCHEDULED, BUT IT IS NOT NECESSARY TO REPEAT THE ENTIRE VACCINE SERIES.
      7. ALL STATES REQUIRE CHILDREN TO BE IMMUNIZED PRIOR TO ENTRY INTO LICENSED DAY CARE SETTINGS OR SCHOOL.
   C. COMBINATION VACCINES
      1. COMBINATION VACCINES REDUCE THE NUMBER OF INJECTIONS AN INFANT MUST ENDURE; MANUFACTURERS HAVE RESEARCHED METHODS OF COMBINING VACCINES INTO A SINGLE DOSE.
      2. COMBINATION VACCINES ARE SUBJECT TO FEDERAL DRUG ADMINISTRATION (FDA) APPROVAL.

3. EXAMPLES OF CURRENT COMBINED VACCINES INCLUDE MEASLES, MUMPS, RUBELLA (MMR); INACTIVE POLIO VIRUS (IPV); AND DIPHTHERIA, TETANUS, AND PERTUSSIS (DTAP).

4. COMBINATION VACCINES MAY REQUIRE A DIFFERENT SCHEDULE.

D. NATIONAL CHILDHOOD VACCINE INJURY ACT

1. PASSED IN 1986

2. ESTABLISHED IN RESPONSE TO CONCERNS ABOUT SERIOUS VACCINE-RELATED INJURIES AND DEATHS

3. A PERSON INJURED OR KILLED BY VACCINES MAY SEEK COMPENSATION.

4. NO NEGLIGENCE MUST BE PROVEN.

5. PROVIDES AN ALTERNATIVE TO A CIVIL SUIT

6. REQUIRES EVERY PERSON TO HAVE A PERSONAL IMMUNIZATION RECORD MAINTAINED IN A PERMANENT MEDICAL RECORD

7. INFORMATION MUST BE RECORDED AT THE TIME OF EACH IMMUNIZATION.

   a. Month, day, and year of administration
   b. Vaccine administered
   c. Manufacturer
   d. Lot number and expiration date
   e. Site and route of administration
   f. Name, address, and title of health care provider administering the vaccine

8. PARENTS ARE ASKED TO READ INFORMATION AND SIGN A CONSENT FORM PRIOR TO ADMINISTRATION OF VACCINES.

E. INTERVENTIONS FOR IMMUNIZATION

1. PRIMARY SOURCE OF VACCINES

2. PROVIDE EDUCATION ON IMMUNIZATION REQUIREMENTS.

3. ADMINISTER INJECTABLE VACCINES IN THE APPROPRIATE SITES.

4. STORE VACCINES APPROPRIATELY ACCORDING TO MANUFACTURER INSTRUCTIONS.

5. PROVIDE EDUCATION ON THE NATIONAL CHILDHOOD SAFETY VACCINE INJURY ACT OF 1986.

6. INSTRUCT THE PARENTS ON THE EXPECTED REACTIONS AND REPORTABLE VACCINE-RELATED EVENTS.

7. ASSESS FOR CONTRAINDICATIONS TO SPECIFIC VACCINES.

8. UTILIZE CDC GUIDELINES FOR SCHEDULE ADJUSTMENT WHEN VACCINES ARE MISSED.

9. ENSURE THAT APPROPRIATE DOCUMENTATION FOR EACH IMMUNIZATION OCCURS.

10. OFFER TO SERVE AS A RESOURCE IN DAY CARE AND SCHOOL SETTINGS TO STAFF AND STUDENTS ABOUT PREVENTION OF COMMON ILLNESSES AND HOW TO MANAGE OUTBREAKS AS THEY OCCUR.

IV. **NURSING DIAGNOSES**

A. IMPAIRED SKIN INTEGRITY

B. DEFICIENT KNOWLEDGE

C. INEFFECTIVE HEALTH MAINTENANCE

D. RISK FOR INFECTION

Nursing Diagnoses: Definitions and Classification 2012–2014. Copyright © 2012, 1994–2012 by NANDA International. Used by arrangement with John Wiley & Sons Limited.

V. **INFECTIOUS DISEASES**

A. VARICELLA (CHICKENPOX)

1. DESCRIPTION

   a. Caused by varicella zoster virus
   b. Incubation 10–21 days, communicable from 48 hours before lesions appear until after all lesions are crusted over
   c. Highly contagious by direct contact and airborne spread from respiratory secretions
   d. Occurs most often in children under the age of 10 years
   e. Occurs most often in late winter and early spring months
   f. Vaccine available: varicella vaccine (Varivax)
   g. Complications include superinfection of lesions, thrombocytopenia, arthritis, hepatitis, encephalitis, meningitis, glomerulonephritis, and Reye's syndrome.

2. ASSESSMENT

   a. Mild fever
   b. Generalized pruritic rash
   c. Exposure within the past 2–3 weeks to someone with chickenpox

3. DIAGNOSIS STUDIES

   a. Clinical findings
   b. Although usually not necessary, the virus can be isolated from vesicular fluid within the first 3–4 days of the rash.

4. NURSING INTERVENTIONS

   a. Maintain strict isolation until all vesicles are crusted over.
   b. Instruct the parents that the child may return to school if only a few scabs remain.
   c. Apply local or systemic antipruritics such as calamine lotion or diphenhydramine to reduce discomfort and itching.

d. Administer cool sponge baths with baking soda or oatmeal to promote skin care comfort.

e. Dress the child in light clothing and maintain a cool environment to promote comfort.

f. Administer acetaminophen (Tylenol) as an analgesic and antipyretic. Salicylates are contraindicated because of their link with Reye's syndrome.

g. Administer IV acyclovir to reduce visceral complications such as pneumonitis and meningitis in clients with immune suppression or are immunocompromised.

h. Monitor the child for complications such as severe skin pain, burning, or purulent discharge, which may indicate secondary infection and require prompt medical attention.

i. Maintain hydration with cool nonacidic fluids such as gelatin and popsicles.

B. MUMPS

1. DESCRIPTION

a. Swelling of the salivary and parotid glands

b. Generally does not occur in children less than 1 year of age because of passive immunity from maternal antibodies

c. Approximately 50% of cases occur in young adults, with the remainder occurring in young children or immunocompromised adults.

d. Meningeal signs occur in about 30% of cases.

e. Peak incidence takes place during late winter and early spring months.

f. Prognosis for complete recovery is good, although postpubertal males may have serious complications.

g. One attack of mumps generally results in lifelong immunity.

h. Transmitted by droplet or direct contact with respiratory secretions

i. Incubation period is usually 16–18 days; may be as long as 25 days.

j. Vaccine available: MMR

2. ASSESSMENT

a. Inadequate immunization

b. Exposure to someone with mumps within the preceding 2–3 weeks

c. Clinical manifestations vary widely; up to 50% of susceptible persons have subclinical illness without clinical manifestations.

d. Myalgia, anorexia, malaise, headache, and earache aggravated by chewing and pain when drinking acidic fluids

e. Fever

f. Swelling of the parotid and salivary glands

g. Complications include CNS involvement such as altered level of consciousness (LOC) and nuchal rigidity.

3. DIAGNOSTIC TESTS

a. Glandular swelling confirms the diagnosis.

b. Serologic testing can detect mumps antibodies, even if the client's glands do not swell.

c. Serum amylase levels may be elevated.

4. NURSING INTERVENTIONS

a. Administer analgesics.

b. Apply warm or cool compresses to the neck area to relieve pain.

c. Administer antipyretics and tepid sponge baths for fever.

d. Increase fluids to prevent dehydration.

e. Provide a high-calorie diet, avoiding spicy, irritating foods that trigger salivation or require a lot of chewing.

f. Implement airborne and droplet precautions until all clinical manifestations subside. The mumps virus remains in the saliva throughout the disease course.

g. Instruct the parents that the child should stay home from school until 9 days after the onset of parotid swelling.

h. Provide comfort measures such as supporting the scrotum with a small pillow if the child has scrotal swelling.

i. Report all cases of mumps to local health authorities.

C. MEASLES (RUBEOLA)

1. DESCRIPTION

a. Rash begins light on the upper body and head on the first day.

b. By the third day the upper body rash has increased and progressed to the lower body.

c. Transmitted by direct contact with infected droplets and occasionally by airborne spread

d. Peak incidence in winter and spring, primarily in nonimmunized individuals

e. Incubation period is 8–12 days.

f. Vaccine available: MMR

g. Complications include otitis media, bronchopneumonia, croup, diarrhea, or encephalitis, resulting in permanent brain damage and death.

2. ASSESSMENT

a. Fever

b. Cough

c. Coryza

d. Conjunctivitis

e. Koplik spots

3. DIAGNOSTIC TESTS
   a. Viral tissue culture from nasopharyngeal secretions
   b. Acute and convalescent antibody titers
4. NURSING INTERVENTIONS
   a. Initiate respiratory isolation for 4 days after the onset of the rash.
   b. Administer vitamin A if a deficiency is suspected.
   c. Instruct the parents that hospitalization for infants and children with severe case or complications may be necessary.
   d. Implement fever control measures if fever is present.
   e. Offer comfort measures, including dimming the lights in the presence of photophobia.

D. RUBELLA (GERMAN MEASLES)
   1. DESCRIPTION
      a. Of all cases, 25–50% are asymptomatic.
      b. On the first day the rash appears heavily on the head and upper torso.
      c. By the third day the lower half of the body is heavily covered by the rash, with the upper body rash lessening in severity.
      d. Transmitted by direct or droplet contact with nasopharyngeal secretions
      e. Peak occurrence is late winter and early spring.
      f. Incubation period is 14–21 days.
      g. Universal immunization using the MMR vaccine and good hygiene practices, including hand washing and disposal of contaminated tissues, are helpful in controlling the spread of rubella.
      h. Complications include transient polyarthralgia and, rarely, encephalitis and thrombocytopenia.
   2. ASSESSMENT
      a. Slight fever
      b. Red maculopapular discrete rash
      c. Lymphadenopathy
   3. DIAGNOSTIC TESTS
      a. Nasal secretion cultures
      b. Acute and convalescent antibody titers
   4. NURSING INTERVENTIONS
      a. Initiate isolation.
      b. Instruct the parents that school should be avoided for 7 days after the onset of the rash.
      c. Provide supportive care and comfort measures.

E. ROSEOLA (HUMAN HERPES VIRUS 6)
   1. DESCRIPTION
      a. Transmitted by contact with respiratory secretions
      b. Highest incidence is in children between 6 and 24 months of age; rare in infants less than 3 months of age and in children over the age of 4 years.
      c. There is no seasonal pattern for roseola.
      d. Complications include seizures or encephalitis.
   2. ASSESSMENT
      a. High fever for 3–5 days
      b. A red maculopapular rash lasting up to several days
   3. DIAGNOSTIC TESTS
      a. Clinical presentation
   4. NURSING INTERVENTIONS
      a. Administer antipyretics for fever.
      b. Encourage fluids.
      c. Provide comfort measures.

F. CYTOMEGALOVIRUS (CMV)
   1. DESCRIPTION
      a. Generally asymptomatic
      b. CMV is a member of the herpes family of viruses.
      c. Transmitted by direct person-to-person contact with the virus containing secretions and from the mother to the infant before, during, or after childbirth
      d. CMV infection is distributed worldwide; most humans have become infected by the time they reach adulthood.
      e. CMV causes congenital infection in 1–2% of all live births.
      f. Incubation period is unknown.
      g. Susceptible pregnant women are at the greatest risk when exposed to the urine and saliva of CMV-infected children.
      h. Complications include psychomotor retardation, microcephaly, hearing loss, seizures, and learning disabilities.
   2. ASSESSMENT
      a. Generally asymptomatic
      b. Fetal damage such as intrauterine growth retardation
      c. Jaundice
      d. Hepatitis
      e. Hepatosplenomegaly
      f. Brain damage
      g. Petechial rash, retinitis
   3. DIAGNOSTIC TESTS
      a. Viral culture specimens from urine, pharynx, cervical secretions, human milk, semen, serum leukocytes, or presence of IgM CMV antibodies in cord blood identifies congenitally infected infants; polymerase chain reaction detects CMV DNA in tissues.
   4. NURSING INTERVENTIONS
      a. Administer ganciclovir (Cytovene), an antiviral drug, to treat life-threatening CMV infections in immunocompromised hosts and to treat retinitis.
      b. Hand washing and simple hygiene should be reinforced.

G. DIPHTHERIA
  1. DESCRIPTION
     a. Transmitted by intimate contact with discharges from the nose, throat, eye, or skin lesions
     b. Most frequently occurs in fall and winter
     c. Most common and most severe in nonimmunized or inadequately immunized individuals
     d. Incubation period is 2–5 days.
     e. Universal immunization with diptheria toxoid helps to control diptheria.
     f. Prophylactic treatment of frequent close contacts with erythromycin or penicillin Benzedrine
     g. Public health officials must be notified.
     h. Complications include thrombocytopenia, myocarditis, vocal cord paralysis, and ascending paralysis.
  2. ASSESSMENT
     a. Low-grade fever
     b. Gradual onset of membranous nasopharyngitis
     c. Obstructive laryngotrachitis
  3. DIAGNOSTIC TESTS
     a. Nose and throat cultures
  4. NURSING INTERVENTIONS
     a. Administer a single-dose equine antitoxin IV after sensitivity testing.
     b. Administer erythromycin or penicillin.
     c. Initiate strict isolation of the hospitalized child until two sequential nose and throat cultures are negative.
     d. Monitor respiratory status.
     e. Offer comfort measures such as rest, fluids, and fever management.

H. ERYTHEMA INFECTIOSUM (FIFTH DISEASE)
  1. DESCRIPTION
     a. Rash can recur for weeks with exposure to heat or sun.
     b. Transmitted by contact with respiratory secretions
     c. Contagious before onset of illness
     d. Often has outbreaks in elementary and junior high schools during the spring
     e. Incubation is 4–14 days and can be as long as 20 days.
     f. Good hygienic practices are effective measures of control.
     g. Caused by parvovirus B19
     h. Complications include arthralgia and arthritis.
  2. ASSESSMENT
     a. Mild systemic symptoms
     b. Occasional fever
     c. Red facial rash, giving a "slapped cheek" appearance
     d. Circumoral pallor
     e. Symmetric lacy rash on the trunk and limbs
     f. Rarely seen in dark-skinned individuals
  3. DIAGNOSTIC TESTS
     a. Clinical findings
  4. NURSING INTERVENTIONS
     a. Manage fever.
     b. Offer comfort measures.
     c. Instruct the parents that the child may attend school; no longer contagious after the appearance of the rash.

I. INFECTIOUS MONONUCLEOSIS
  1. DESCRIPTION
     a. Caused by the Epstein-Barr virus (EBV), a member of the herpes group
     b. EBV is spread by contact with oral secretions.
     c. Frequently transmitted from adults to infants and among young adults by kissing
     d. Has been transmitted during bone marrow transplantation and blood transfusion
     e. Primarily affects young adults and children, although in children, it is usually so mild that it is often overlooked
     f. Prognosis is excellent and complications are uncommon.
     g. Incubation period of 4–6 weeks
     h. May cause hepatic dysfunction, increased lymphocytes and monocytes
  2. ASSESSMENT
     a. Fever
     b. Sore throat
     c. Cervical lymphadenopathy
     d. May have had contact with a person who has infectious mononucleosis
     e. Headache
     f. Malaise
     g. Profound fatigue
     h. Possible abdominal discomfort
     i. After 3–5 days, the child may develop a sore throat and dysphagia related to adenopathy.
     j. Cervical adenopathy with slight tenderness
     k. Inguinal adenopathy
  3. DIAGNOSTIC TESTS
     a. White blood cell count: increased to 10,000–20,000/mm^3 during the second and third week of the illness
     b. Lymphocytes and monocytes: account for 50–70% of the total WBC count.
     c. Ten percent of the lymphocytes are atypical splenic rupture.
  4. NURSING INTERVENTIONS
     a. Administer prescribed steroids.
     b. Encourage rest.

c. Manage fever.

d. Promote fluid intake with cool, nonacidic fluids, jello, and popsicles.

e. Encourage saline gargles.

f. Avoid contact sports if splenomegaly present.

J. BORDATELLA PERTUSSIS (WHOOPING COUGH)

   1. DESCRIPTION

     a. Transmitted by close contact with respiratory secretions

     b. Most contagious during mild respiratory clinical manifestations

     c. Occurs in nonimmunized or partially immunized infants and children

     d. Adolescents and adults are a major source.

     e. There is no seasonal pattern.

     f. Incubation period is 6–20 days.

     g. Vaccine available: DPT

   2. ASSESSMENT

     a. Starts with mild upper respiratory clinical manifestations known as the catarrhal stage

     b. Progresses to severe paroxysms of cough; often with inspiratory whoop followed by vomiting

     c. Apnea is common in infants under 6 months of age.

   3. DIAGNOSTIC TESTS

     a. Nasopharyngeal cultures

   4. NURSING INTERVENTIONS

     a. Instruct the parents that infants under 6 months of age and other children with severe disease are usually hospitalized.

     b. Administer erythromycin orally for 14 days.

     c. Place the child in respiratory isolation for 5 days after initiation of antibiotic treatment.

     d. Maintain a patent airway.

     e. Maintain fluid intake.

     f. Provide a restful environment.

     g. Offer supportive care for respiratory distress and feeding difficulties.

     h. Support anxious parents by explaining about the illness and nature of the cough.

K. POLIOMYELITIS

   1. DESCRIPTION

     a. Nonspecific illness with low-grade fever and sore throat

     b. Fecal-oral and possibly respiratory transmission

     c. More common in infants and young children

     d. Most common in summer and fall

     e. All endemic cases since 1979 have been associated with oral poliovirus vaccine.

     f. Incubation period is 3–6 days.

     g. Complications include aseptic meningitis, rapid onset of asymmetric acute flaccid paralysis and residual paralytic disease involving the motor neurons, and paralysis of respiratory muscles.

   2. ASSESSMENT

     a. Nonspecific illness with low-grade fever and sore throat

   3. DIAGNOSTIC TESTS

     a. Stool culture

   4. NURSING INTERVENTIONS

     a. Offer comfort measures and supportive treatment depending on the extent of complications present.

     b. Refer to physical therapy if required.

L. ROCKY MOUNTAIN SPOTTED FEVER (*RICKETTSIA RICKETTSII*)

   1. DESCRIPTION

     a. Occurs in spring and summer

     b. Widespread in the United States

     c. Most cases are reported in South Atlantic, southeastern, and south-central states.

     d. Incubation period ranges from 2 to 14 days.

     e. Transmitted to humans through bites of infected ticks

     f. Dogs and wild rodents act as reservoir for infected ticks.

     g. Complications include CNS disease, multisystem organ failure, DIC, shock, and death.

   2. ASSESSMENT

     a. Fever

     b. Vomiting

     c. Anorexia

     d. Confusion

     e. Begins with erythematous and macular rash on the ankles and wrists, which may spread to the rest of the body.

   3. DIAGNOSTIC TESTS

     a. History

     b. Serologic tests

   4. NURSING INTERVENTIONS

     a. Administer chloramphenicol or doxycycline.

M. LYME DISEASE

   1. DESCRIPTION

     a. Caused by *Borrelia burgdorferi,* a spirochete

     b. Transmitted to humans through the bite of an infected tick, especially a deer tick

     c. Localized to three regions in the United States: Northeast, Midwest, and Northwest California

     d. Incidence is highest in children 5–10 years of age.

     e. Incubation is 7–14 days.

2. ASSESSMENT
   a. In the early stages, a rash begins as a small papule and spreads peripherally.
   b. Rash is characterized by a raised red margin and clearing in the center at the site of the tick bite.
   c. Fever
   d. Malaise
   e. Fatigue
   f. Headache
   g. Stiff neck
   h. Arthralgia
   i. In the late stages, arthritis of large joints, especially the knee, beginning months after the initial infection, may occur.
3. DIAGNOSTIC TESTS
   a. Client history
   b. Serologic testing
4. NURSING INTERVENTIONS
   a. Administer antibiotics doxycycline or amoxicillin.
   b. Instruct the parents to avoid tick-infested areas; use insect repellant with DEET, wear light-colored, long-sleeved tops and pants.
   c. Instruct the parents to inspect clothing and body daily after possible tick exposure.
   d. Remove ticks from the body immediately.
   e. Immunize persons over 15 years of age who reside or recreate in geographical areas of high risk.

N. SCARLET FEVER
   1. DESCRIPTION
      a. Caused by group A beta hemolytic streptococci (GAS)
      b. Transmitted through contact with respiratory secretions
      c. Incubation period is 2–5 days
      d. Most frequently occurs among school-age children in late fall, winter, and spring
      e. Complications include otitis media, sinusitis, peritonsillar and retropharyngeal abscesses, cervical adenitits, rheumatic fever, and acute glomerulonephritis.
   2. ASSESSMENT
      a. Acute fever
      b. Sore throat
      c. Rhinitis
      d. Headache
      e. Red, sandpaperlike rash, prominent in creases
      f. White strawberry tongue (day 1)
      g. Flushed cheeks, red strawberry tongue (day 2)

3. DIAGNOSTIC TESTS
   a. Throat culture
4. NURSING INTERVENTIONS
   a. Administer antibiotics for 10 days (penicillin, erythromycin, amoxicillin, or cephalosporins).
   b. Instruct the parents to have the child avoid school for at least 24 hours after the initiation of treatment and until afebrile.
   c. Perform measures to manage fever.
   d. Maintain fluid intake with cool, nonacidic fluids, gelatin, and popsicles.
   e. Encourage saline gargles for older children.
   f. Offer comfort measures.

O. TETANUS
   1. DESCRIPTION
      a. Caused by *Clostridium tetani,* a spore-forming bacillus that produces a neurotoxin
      b. Transmitted to humans through a wound in the skin from contact with soil contaminated with animal feces
      c. Incubation is 4–14 days.
      d. Occurs worldwide
      e. Prevalent in nonimmunized populations
      f. High mortality rate
      g. Complications include airway obstruction and asphyxiation due to laryngeal and respiratory muscle spasms and death.
      h. Tetanus vaccine available
   2. ASSESSMENT
      a. Headache
      b. Restlessness
      c. Spasms of chewing (masticatory) muscles follow
      d. Difficulty opening the mouth (trismus)
      e. Dysphagia
      f. Opisthotonos
      g. Seizures
      h. Dysuria and urinary retention
      i. Bowel incontinence
      j. Fever
   3. DIAGNOSTIC TESTS
      a. Clinical presentation
   4. NURSING INTERVENTIONS
      a. Administer human tetanus immune globulin (TIG) to neutralize neurotoxin and halt the spread of infection.
      b. Administer penicillin G IM initially for 10–14 days.
      c. Clean and debride the wound.
      d. Administer diazepam (Valium) to reduce muscle spasms and control seizures.
      e. Provide respiratory support as needed.
      f. Provide a quiet environment because muscle spasms are aggravated by external stimuli.

P. INTESTINAL PARASITES
  1. GIARDIA
    a. Description
      1) Giardia is caused by *Giardia lamblia,* a protozoan.
      2) Direct transmission is hand-to-mouth transfer of cysts from the feces of an infected person.
      3) Indirect transmission ingestion of a cyst through contaminated food or water
      4) More common in children than in adults
      5) Endemic in areas of the world with poor sanitation
      6) Associated with day care centers and residential institutions
      7) Incubation period is 1–4 weeks.
      8) Complications include lactose intolerance.
    b. Assessment
      1) May be asymptomatic
      2) Chronic or relapsing diarrhea
      3) Cramping abdominal pain
      4) Anorexia leading to weight loss and failure to thrive
      5) Flatulence
    c. Diagnostic tests
      1) Identification of cysts in fecal sample
      2) Enzyme immunoassay to detect *G. lamblia* antigens
    d. Nursing interventions
      1) Administer furazolidone.
      2) Giardia may also be treated with quinacrine hydrochloride and metronidazole.
  2. PINWORMS
    a. Description
      1) Caused by the parasite *Enterobius vermicularis*
      2) Most common helminth infection in the United States
      3) Occurs frequently in preschoolers and school-age children
      4) Occurs frequently in crowded conditions, institutions, and families
      5) Incubation period is 1–2 months.
      6) Transmitted by fecal-oral ingestion or inhalation of eggs of worms
      7) Eggs are transmitted by fingers and hands from scratching the anal area.
      8) Eggs remain infective in indoor environments for 2–3 weeks.
      9) Eggs contaminate anything they come in contact with such as bedding, toys, clothing, toilet seats, baths, and food.

      10) Complications include migration of the worm to the appendix, female genital tract, and peritoneal cavity.
    b. Assessment
      1) Nocturnal anal itching
      2) Sleeplessness
    c. Diagnostic tests
      1) Direct visualization of worms or microscopy
      2) Eggs detected on a transparent tape pressed against the perianal region in the morning, before the child has a bowel movement
    d. Nursing interventions
      1) Administer mebendazole or pyrantel pamoate.
      2) All household members should be treated simultaneously.
  3. ASCARIASIS
    a. Description
      1) Caused by the roundworm *Ascaris lumbricoides*
      2) Transmitted through ingestion of eggs via contact with contaminated soil, food, fingers, toys
      3) Food may be contaminated wherever human feces is used as fertilizer.
      4) Most common in warm climates
      5) Common in areas where sanitation is poor
      6) Occurs most often in children aged 1–4 years
      7) Prolonged incubation period of 4–8 weeks
      8) Complications include intestinal obstruction, pulmonary involvement with cough and blood-stained sputum; perforation of the intestines by migration of worms, resulting in peritonitis; and obstruction of the common bile duct by migration of worms.
    b. Assessment
      1) May be aymptomatic
      2) Abdominal pain
      3) Distention
      4) Anorexia
      5) Weight loss
      6) Fever
    c. Diagnostic tests
      1) Eggs can be detected by microscopic stool examination.
    d. Nursing interventions
      1) Administer mebendazole or pyrantel pamoate.
      2) Reexamine stool 3 weeks after therapy to determine if the worms have been eliminated.
      3) Assess for intestinal obstruction related to a large number of worms in the intestinal tract.

Q. SEXUALLY TRANSMITTED DISEASES (STDS)
  1. GONORRHEA
     a. Description
        1) Caused by infection with the bacterium *Neisseria gonorrhoeae,* a gram-negative diplococcus
        2) Occurs in 132/100,000 persons in the United States
        3) Most common among 15- to 19-year-olds
        4) Incubation period is 2–7 days.
        5) Transmitted through intimate contact via sexual intercourse
        6) When gonorrhea is diagnosed in a child who is not sexually active, a diagnosis of sexual abuse should be considered.
        7) Can be transmitted perinatally
     b. Assessment
        1) Purulent discharge
        2) Urethritis
        3) Endocervicitis
        4) Pelvic inflammatory disease (PID)
        5) Pharyngitis
        6) Conjunctivitis
        7) Proctitis
        8) Infection of the eyes in neonates
        9) Scalp abscesses related to fetal monitor probe
     c. Diagnostic test
        1) Gram stain
     d. Nursing interventions
        1) Administer ceftriaxone (Rocephin) IM, a single dose plus doxycycline (Vibramyacin) twice a day for 7 days or azithromycin PO in a single dose.
        2) Evaluate for other STDs, including syphilis, HIV, chlamydia, hepatitis B.
        3) Chlamydia occurs in 45% of cases of gonorrhea and should be treated.
        4) Encourage abstinence until treated and symptom-free.
        5) Offer education regarding medication administration and importance of adherence to the treatment regimen.
        6) Avoid all sexual contacts until cured.
        7) Instruct the parents about signs of complications, including acute epididymitis, acute PID, arthritis, dermatitis, meningitis, disseminated gonococcal infection, and infertility.
  2. SYPHILIS
     a. Description
        1) Caused by infection with the spirochete *Treponema pallidum*
        2) May be transmitted congenitally during pregnancy or at the time of delivery
        3) May be acquired by intimate contact, sexual intercourse, or sexual abuse
        4) Sexual abuse should be considered if a diagnosis of acquired syphilis is made in a child who is not sexually active.
        5) Occurs in 2.6/100,000 in the United States
        6) Incubation period is 3 weeks, with a range of 10–90 days.
     b. Assessment
        1) Congenital
           a) Stillbirth
           b) Prematurity
           c) Hydrops fetalis
           d) Multisystem sequelae including hepatosplenomegaly, mucocutaneous lesions, lymphadenopathy, and thrombocytopenia
        2) Acquired
           a) In the primary stage, the client will have one or more painless ulcers on the mucous membranes and skin, usually on the genitalia.
        3) Secondary syphilis
           a) Maculopapular rash on the palms and soles
           b) Fever
           c) Enlarged lymph glands
           d) Sore throat
           e) Headache
           f) Splenomegaly
           g) Arthralgia
        4) Tertiary stage
           a) Neurosyphilis
           b) Skin, bone, and visceral changes
           c) Aortitis
     c. Diagnostic tests
        1) Serologic VDRL
        2) Serologic RPR
     d. Nursing interventions
        1) Administer penicillin G IV every 12 hours for 7 days then every 8 hours for 3 additional days for a total of 10 days or a single dose of procaine penicillin G, IM for 10 days.
        2) In early-acquired syphilis a single dose of penicillin G benzathine IM is effective treatment.
        3) If the client is pregnant, administer penicillin G benzathine IM two doses, 1 week apart.

4) When the client has a penicillin allergy, administer tetracycline four times a day for 14 days or erythromycin twice a day for 14 days (except to a client who is pregnant).

5) Instruct the adolescent on the importance of adherence to medication administration.

6) Refer the adolescent to disclose any sexual contacts for evaluation and treatment.

7) Instruct the adolescent to avoid sexual activity until cured.

8) Encourage follow-up to monitor serology as recommended.

9) Instruct in use of latex condoms to prevent reinfection.

3. CHLAMYDIA
   a. Description
      1) Caused by the bacterium *Chlamydia trachomatis*
      2) Transmitted by sexual contact
      3) Neonates may be infected during contact with an infected genital tract during delivery.
      4) Most common STD in adults less than 25 years of age
      5) Occurs in 6–12% of pregnancies
      6) Rates during adolescence is as high as 37%
      7) Incubation period is about 1 week.
      8) Incidence is 236/100,000.
   b. Assessment
      1) May be symptomatic or asymptomatic
      2) Mucopurulent cervicitis
      3) Urethritis
      4) Salpingitis
      5) Proctitis
   c. Diagnostic tests
      1) Chlamydia culture
      2) Enzyme immunoassay
   d. Nursing interventions
      1) Administer doxycycline (Vibramycin) b.i.d. for 7 days or azithromycin (Zithromax) 1 gram in a single dose or erythromycin four times a day for 7 days.
      2) Encourage abstinence until treated and free of clinical manifestations.
      3) Provide education regarding medication administration and importance of adherence to the treatment regimen.
      4) Instruct the adolescent to avoid sexual contact until cured.
      5) Instruct the adolescent in the use of latex condoms to prevent reinfection.

4. HERPES GENITALIS (HSV-2)
   a. Description
      1) Characterized by periods of latency between the initial outbreak and recurrence
      2) Occurs in one out of five adults over the age of 12
      3) 30,000,000 new cases reported annually
      4) Incubation period is about 6 days.
      5) Caused by the herpes simplex type 2 virus
      6) Complications in neonates include generalized systemic infection including CNS and liver involvement, and infections of the skin, eyes, and mouth. There is a high mortality rate in neonatal herpes infection.
   b. Assessment
      1) Itching and intense burning at the site of outbreak
      2) May be accompanied by flulike clinical manifestations
      3) Inguinal lymphadenopathy
      4) Initial lesions are painful raised vesicles.
      5) Recurrent lesions are less painful and resolve more quickly.
      6) Virus can be shed when the client is asymptomatic and is contagious.
      7) Transmitted in neonates through the placenta or contact with an infected genital tract during delivery
      8) Transmitted through sexual intercourse
   c. Diagnostic test
      1) Viral culture
   d. Nursing interventions
      1) Administer oral acyclovir within 6 days of onset to shorten median duration of viral shedding from primary lesions by 3–5 days.
      2) Administer acyclovir (Zovirax) for recurrent infection, which decreases the frequency of recurrence.
      3) Instruct the adolescent about asymptomatic viral shedding and potential for recurrent outbreaks.
      4) Keep the lesions clean and dry.
      5) Encourage abstinence during the active stage when lesions are present.
      6) Instruct the adolescent on the use of latex condoms to prevent infection in sexual partners.

5. HUMAN PAPILLOMAVIRUS (HPV)
   a. Description
      1) Over 20 types of HPV; most common are types 6 and 11
      2) Transmitted by direct sexual contact
      3) Perinatal contact during delivery
      4) Occurs in 50/100,000 in the population
      5) 3,000,000 cases annually
      6) Incubation period is 3 months to several months.
      7) Complications include cervical, anal, or vaginal dysplasia. HPV can lead to cervical cancer, cancer reoccurrence, and laryngeal papilloma in newborns.
   b. Assessment
      1) Soft, flesh, single or multiple papules that occur in the anogenital area and are known as genital warts
      2) Pain
      3) Pruritus
      4) May be asymptomatic or subclinical
      5) In females, the warts are located on the perineum, vulva, cervix, vagina, urethra, anus, and oral cavity.
      6) Caused by the human papilloma virus
      7) In males, the warts are located on the penis, perineum, anus, and oral cavity.
   c. Diagnostic tests
      1) Clinical presentation
      2) Biopsy
   d. Nursing interventions
      1) Inform the adolescent that treatment depends on the location of the lesions.
      2) Instruct the adolescent in self-application of prescribed ointments or solutions.
      3) Support the adolescent through cryotherapy with liquid nitrogen every 1–2 weeks.
      4) Assist in surgical removal by excision or laser surgery.
      5) Instruct the adolescent about the need for periodic screening for cervical cancer as well as examination of sexual partners for presence of warts.
      6) Counsel sexual partners of the adolescent with HPV if appropriate.
      7) Perform cervical cancer screening on the adolescent with HPV.

R. HEPATITIS B
   1. DESCRIPTION
      a. Caused by hepadnavirus
      b. Transmitted by contact with infected blood or body fluids, sexual contact, or perinatal transmission
      c. 10,258 new cases annually
      d. Of case, 5–10% become chronic carriers.
      e. Incubation period averages 120 days with a range of 45–160 days.
      f. An infected person can infect others approximately 4–6 weeks before symptoms appear.
      g. Client may become a chronic carrier.
      h. Complications include progressive liver disease with cirrhosis or hepatocellular carcinoma.
   2. ASSESSMENT
      a. General fatigue
      b. Muscle and joint pain
      c. Loss of appetite
   3. DIAGNOSTIC TESTS
      a. History of illness including sexual history
      b. IV drug use
      c. Hepatitis panel
   4. NURSING INTERVENTIONS
      a. There is no specific treatment for hepatitis B.
      b. Provide symptomatic management.
      c. Administer interferon alfa 2b antiviral medication, which is 40% effective in eliminating chronic HBV infection.
      d. Administer hepatitis B immune globulin when exposed to HBV.
      e. Provide counseling to adolescents who are chronic carriers of hepatitis.
      f. Instruct the adolescent to use condoms for sexual activity.

S. HUMAN IMMUNODEFICIENCY VIRUS (HIV)
   1. DESCRIPTION
      a. Caused by retrovirus, RNA virus
      b. 40,000 to 80,000 new infections reported annually
      c. Clinical manifestations may appear 2–12 weeks after infection.
      d. Seroconversion (the ability of antibodies to HIV to be detected in the blood) may not occur until 4–12 weeks or longer after infection.
      e. The period when antibodies remain undetected is known as the window period.
      f. Transmitted by contact with infected blood or body fluids, sexual contact, perinatal transmission

g. Progression to AIDS as a late manifestation in 85% of all cases within 17 years of infection

h. Complications include opportunistic infections such as *Pneumocystis carinii* (PCP), Kaposi's sarcoma (KS), mycobacterium avium complex (MAC), and AIDS.

2. ASSESSMENT
   a. Fever
   b. Sore throat
   c. Skin rash
   d. Lymphadenopathy
   e. Malaise
   f. Arthralgia
   g. Myalgia
   h. Headache
   i. Nausea
   j. Vomiting

3. DIAGNOSTIC TESTS
   a. HIV RNA polymerase chain reaction (PCR) test in infants less than 18 months of age
   b. HIV antibody test in children greater than 18 months of age and Western Blot
   c. HIV culture

4. NURSING INTERVENTIONS
   a. Inform the client that there is no known cure.
   b. Obtain a written consent for HIV testing.
   c. Pre- and posttest counseling by trained professionals is essential.
   d. Inform the client that treatment assists to slow the decline of the immune system.
   e. Current treatment includes antiretroviral therapies.
   f. Treatment is individualized based on the client's immune status and sensitivity to the specific drug.
   g. Treatment goals include maintaining high CD4 counts and decreased viral loads.
   h. Refer the client for counseling, social support, behavioral change, and care.
   i. Encourage the client to avoid sex with an individual having multiple partners and consistent use of a latex condom.
   j. Instruct the adolescent to avoid needle sharing.
   k. Offer testing to HIV-positive women during pregnancy.

T. TUBERCULOSIS (SEE CHAPTER 3, RESPIRATORY DISORDERS TUBERCULOSIS, SECTION XI.)

U. ROTAVIRUS
1. DESCRIPTION
   a. Most common cause of severe diarrhea among children
   b. Results in approximately 55,000 hospitalizations in the United States annually

c. Annually over 600,000 deaths related to rotavirus occur worldwide
d. Incubation period is approximately 2 days.
e. Immunity after infection is incomplete, but reinfections are less severe than the original infection.
f. Primarily transmitted through fecal-oral route
g. Most often occurs in winter and spring
h. Most children in the United States have had rotavirus by 2 years of age.
i. About 1 out of 40 children with rotavirus will require hospitalization.
j. Vaccine available: RotaShield, pulled from use in 1998 because of association with intussusception

2. ASSESSMENT
   a. Vomiting and watery diarrhea lasting 3–8 days
   b. Fever
   c. Abdominal pain

3. DIAGNOSTIC TESTS
   a. Rapid antigen detection in stool specimen

4. NURSING INTERVENTION
   a. Provide rehydration.
   b. Maintain contact isolation and standard precautions.
   c. Instruct family members in hand hygiene and assessment of hydration.

V. RESPIRATORY SYNCYTIAL VIRUS (RSV)
1. DESCRIPTION
   a. Most common cause of bronchiolitis and pneumonia among infants and children under 1 year of age
   b. Most children recover from the illness in 8–15 days.
   c. The majority of children hospitalized for RSV are under 6 months.
   d. Infection occurs when infectious material comes in contact with mucous membranes and through inhalation of infectious droplets.
   e. Occurs in late fall, winter, and early spring months
   f. Most children have evidence of infection from RSV by 2 years of age.

2. ASSESSMENT
   a. Moderate-to-severe coldlike symptoms
   b. Lower respiratory tract disease may occur.

3. DIAGNOSTIC TESTS
   a. Virus isolation
   b. Viral antigen detection
   c. Rise in serum antibodies

4. NURSING INTERVENTIONS
   a. Inform the parents that symptomatic treatment may be sufficient.
   b. Administer acetaminophen (Tylenol) or ibuprofen (Motrin) for fever, discomfort.
   c. Oxygen therapy and mechanical ventilation may be necessary.

W. **MULTIPLE-RESISTANT ORGANISMS (MROS)**
  1. DESCRIPTION
     a. Methicillin-resistant *Staphylococcus aureus* (MRSA) and vancomycin-resistant enterococcus (VRE)
     b. Organisms are highly resistant to antibiotics and difficult to treat.
     c. Great potential for transmission between clients in acute health care settings
     d. Associated with outbreaks in client populations and can cause morbidity and mortality
     e. Once colonized, a client may harbor organisms for months to years.
     f. MRSA is emerging as a cause of skin infection in the community (community acquired MRSA, or CA-MRSA).
  2. ASSESSMENT
     a. Cuts or abrasions that do not heal normally
     b. Infections that are not responsive to usual antibiotic therapies
  3. DIAGNOSTIC TESTS
     a. MRSA cultures from anterior nares, and any body site that is open or draining
     b. VRE cultures are best obtained from a stool or rectal swab.
     c. Colonization and infection are confirmed through laboratory testing.
  4. NURSING INTERVENTIONS
     a. Meticulous hand hygiene before and after contact is essential.
     b. Place the child in a single-bed room.
     c. Place the child in contact isolation for MRO and droplet precautions for the child who has MRSA pneumonia.
     d. Instruct family members and visitors on use of protective barriers and good hygiene.
     e. Instruct the family not to visit other clients' rooms.
     f. Coordinate care activities in order to provide continuous isolation precautions.
     g. Avoid sharing equipment between children; if that is not possible, adequate cleaning of equipment is essential.
X. **SEVERE ACUTE RESPIRATORY SYNDROME (SARS)**
  1. DESCRIPTION
     a. One or more clinical findings of respiratory illness: cough, shortness of breath, difficulty breathing, or hypoxia
     b. Travel within 10 days of onset of symptoms to an area with current or previously documented or suspected community transmission of SARS

     c. Close contact within 10 days of onset of symptoms with a person known or suspected to have SARS
  2. ASSESSMENT
     a. Asymptomatic or mild respiratory illness
     b. Moderate respiratory illness
     c. Temperature greater than 40°C (100.4°F)
     d. One or more clinical findings of respiratory illness
  3. DIAGNOSTIC TESTS
     a. Radiographic evidence of pneumonia
     b. Respiratory distress syndrome
     c. Autopsy findings consistent with pneumonia or respiratory distress syndrome without identifiable cause
     d. Detection of SARS-associated coronavirus in a serum sample
     e. Detection of SARS-CoV RNA by RT-PCR confirmed by second PCR assay
  4. NURSING INTERVENTIONS
     a. Implement standard precautions together with airborne and contact precautions.
     b. Until the mode of transmission has been defined, eye protection should also be worn.
Y. **WEST NILE VIRUS**
  1. DESCRIPTION
     a. Most West Nile virus infections are mild.
     b. Approximately 20% of those infected develop a mild illness.
     c. Incubation period is 3–14 days.
     d. Symptoms last 3–6 days.
     e. Approximately 1 in 150 infections result in severe neurological disease.
     f. Encephalitis is more commonly reported than meningitis.
  2. ASSESSMENT
     a. Malaise
     b. Loss of appetite
     c. Nausea
     d. Vomiting
     e. Eye pain
     f. Headache
     g. Muscle pain (myalgia)
     h. Rash
     i. Lymphadenopathy
     j. Fever
     k. Changes in mental status
  3. DIAGNOSTIC TESTS
     a. Clinical presentation
     b. Detection of IgM antibody in cerebrospinal fluid (CSF) collected within 8 days of illness onset
     c. Elevated protein levels
  4. NURSING INTERVENTIONS
     a. Provide supportive treatment.
     b. Administer IV fluids for rehydration.
     c. Provide respiratory support.
     d. Prevention of secondary infections for children with severe disease is essential.

PRACTICE QUESTIONS

1. The nurse instructs a group of nurses about the impact of infectious diseases in the childhood population of the world. The nurse should include which of the following statements in the discussion?
   1. Since the development of vaccines, infectious diseases are no longer a worldwide concern
   2. Severe infectious diseases have been eliminated
   3. Most infectious diseases are minor childhood ailments
   4. Despite improved methods of treatment, infectious diseases continue to be a health concern

2. The nurse is educating a group of health care providers on the great strides toward eradicating infectious diseases in the world that were made during the twentieth century. Which of the following events should the nurse include as having played a major role?
   1. Decreased fertility and birth rates
   2. Steroid-enhanced dairy products
   3. Modern sanitation
   4. The Immunization Act of 1986

3. When instructing a client, which of the following statements should the nurse include in explaining communicable diseases?
   1. They commonly occur in infancy, childhood, and adolescence.
   2. They are transmitted by direct or indirect contact.
   3. They are limited in physiologic involvement.
   4. They are insidious and develop rapidly.

4. The parent of a child asks the nurse what the term "local infection" means. The nurse's appropriate response is, "A local infection
   1. occurs in many individuals in a common geographic area."
   2. is minor and easily treated."
   3. can be spread to others in close contact with the infected individual."
   4. is limited to one area of the body."

5. When considering the diagnosis of Lyme's disease in a child, the nurse evaluates the incubation period to be how many days?

_____

6. A child is hospitalized with an infection that develops rapidly and resolves in a short period of time. The nurse informs the parents that the diagnosis is which of the following?
   1. A local infection
   2. A childhood illness
   3. Varicella
   4. An acute infection

7. The nurse instructs the parents of a child that the greatest weapon and priority available to reduce the spread of disease is which of the following?
   1. Antibiotics
   2. Isolation techniques
   3. Ethyl alcohol wipes before injections
   4. Hand washing

8. The nurse instructs student nurses that the Centers for Disease Control (CDC) recommends that isolation be based on which of the following?
   1. Method of disease transmission
   2. Severity of client illness
   3. Availability of personal protective equipment
   4. The client's health care coverage and ability to pay for private room

9. The mother of a child whose chickenpox rash first appeared 8 days ago asks the nurse when her child may return to school without being contagious. Which of the following is the nurse's most appropriate response?
   1. "Your child cannot return to school until all the lesions disappear."
   2. "Your child is contagious as long as your child is itching."
   3. "The contagious state of chickenpox is generally 2 weeks."
   4. "Your child is not contagious and may return to school now."

10. When planning the care of a client diagnosed with asymptomatic herpes simplex virus type 2 (HSV-2), which of the following should the nurse consider?
    1. There is no risk of transmitting the condition to anyone else
    2. After prescribed treatment, herpes simplex virus type 2 is cured
    3. An antibiotic is used successfully in the treatment
    4. The client is a carrier, and still able to transmit the disease

11. Which of the following interventions should the nurse include in the plan of care of a child with mumps?
    1. Initiate respiratory isolation with the appearance of a rash
    2. Administer ganciclovir (Cytovene)
    3. Provide a high-calorie diet
    4. Monitor the white blood cell count

12. The nurse is teaching a class on how to prevent infectious diseases. Which of the following are priorities for the nurse to include in the class? Select all that apply:
    [ ] 1. Hand washing
    [ ] 2. Rest
    [ ] 3. Immunization
    [ ] 4. Nutrition
    [ ] 5. Drug prophylaxis
    [ ] 6. Herbal therapy

13. A mother asks the nurse how her child became infected with rotavirus. The most appropriate response by the nurse is, "Rotavirus is primarily spread by
    1. the fecal-oral route."
    2. inhalation of infected droplets."
    3. infected blood."
    4. sexual contact."

14. The nurse should consider which of the following when planning the care of a child infected with hepatitis B?
    1. Treatment is aimed at symptom management
    2. Administer oral acyclovir (Zovirax)
    3. Administer doxycycline (Vibramycin) and azithromycin (Zithromax)
    4. Treatment is directed by the results of the white blood cell test

15. The nurse assesses which of the following to be present in an infant born prematurely with congenital syphilis? Select all that apply:
    [ ] 1. Hepatosplenomegaly
    [ ] 2. Pain in the chest
    [ ] 3. Weight loss
    [ ] 4. Mucocutaneous lesions
    [ ] 5. Lymphadenopathy
    [ ] 6. Generalized pruritic rash

16. The nurse is caring for a child with varicella (chickenpox). Which of the following assessments are priorities to report and indicate a secondary infection requiring prompt medical attention?
    1. Generalized pruritic rash and mild fever
    2. Skin pain and purulent discharge
    3. Body rash and Koplik's spots
    4. Red facial (slapped cheek) rash and circumoral pallor

17. A mother of a child diagnosed with erythema infectiosum (Fifth's disease) asks the nurse when the child may return to school without being contagious. The nurse should tell the mother that her child may return to school after
    1. the appearance of the rash.
    2. the appearance of a generalized pruritic rash.
    3. being immunized.
    4. the diarrhea disappears.

18. The nurse is instructing the adolescent client about birth control and sexually transmitted diseases. Which of the following methods of birth control should the nurse include that is 100% effective in protecting against sexually transmitted disease?
    1. Birth control pills
    2. Abstinence from sexual behavior
    3. Withdrawal method
    4. Latex condoms and spermicidal foam

19. The nurse assesses what clinical manifestation to be the priority in a child with *Enterobius* (pinworm)?
    1. Nocturnal anal itching
    2. Weight loss
    3. Chronic or relapsing diarrhea
    4. Flatulence

20. Which of the following is a priority nursing intervention when caring for an adolescent client to lessen the client's risk of infection?
    1. Assess for high-risk behaviors, such as unprotected sex, drug use, and gang relationships
    2. Encourage continuity of health care providers
    3. Provide personal privacy and avoid discussing embarrassing issues
    4. Include the adolescent's parent in all discussions

21. The nurse is working with a group of parents getting ready to send their children to day care for the first time. The nurse should instruct the parents that immunizations are
    1. improved and stronger, so "booster" shots are no longer required.
    2. safe and without risks.
    3. an improved part of health promotion.
    4. available in oral form if the client does not like injections.

22. A child is receiving an immunization before starting preschool. Which of the following assessments is a priority for the nurse to make at this time?
    1. The child's general state of health
    2. Preexisting diseases the client has
    3. The child's immunization history
    4. Recent exposure to infectious diseases

23. Which of the following drugs should the nurse use in the treatment of a child with *Giardia*?
    1. Penicillin G
    2. Furazolidone (Furoxone)
    3. Mebendazole (Vermox)
    4. Ceftriaxone (Rocephin)

24. The nurse assesses which of the following to be a clinical manifestation of human papillomavirus (HPV)?
    1. Soft papules in the anogenital area
    2. Nocturnal anal itching
    3. Erythematous and macular rash on the ankles and wrists
    4. Painful raised vesicles

25. Which of the following drugs should the nurse administer to a child with tetanus who is experiencing muscle spasms and seizures?
    1. Methocarbamol (Robaxin)
    2. Cyclobenzaprine (Flexeril)
    3. Tizanidine (Zanaflex)
    4. Diazepam (Valium)

26. The registered nurse is preparing the clinical assignments for an infectious and communicable disease unit. Which of the following assignments should the nurse delegate to a licensed practical nurse?
    1. Teach an immunization class to a group of parents
    2. Provide comfort measures for a child with mumps
    3. Counsel the parents of a child with herpes genitalis (HSV-2) about the potential for recurrent outbreaks
    4. Monitor a child with hepatitis B for progressive liver disease

27. Which of the following is the priority nursing intervention for the nurse to include in the plan of care for a child with rotavirus presenting with severe stomach cramps and explosive diarrhea?
    1. Provide a high-calorie diet
    2. Encourage the child to rest

3. Monitor the serum electrolytes
4. Administer normal saline bolus at a rate of 50 ml/kg

28. The nurse suspects a diagnosis of measles (rubeola) in a child who comes to a clinic with which of the following clinical manifestations?
    Select all that apply:
    [ ] 1. Red maculopapular disrete rash
    [ ] 2. High fever for 3–5 days
    [ ] 3. Koplik spots
    [ ] 4. Coryza spots
    [ ] 5. Hepatosplenomegaly
    [ ] 6. Conjunctivitis

29. A parent suspects a child has measles and asks the nurse how many days the incubation period is. The nurse responds that the incubation period is how many days?_____

30. The nurse assesses which of the following clinical manifestations to be present in a child with erythema infectiosum (Fifth disease)?
    Select all that apply:
    [ ] 1. Red facial rash giving a "slapped cheek" appearance
    [ ] 2. Gradual onset of membranous nasopharyngitis
    [ ] 3. Circumoral pallor
    [ ] 4. Paroxysms of cough
    [ ] 5. Symmetric lacy rash on the trunk and limbs
    [ ] 6. Arthralgia

31. Which of the following is the appropriate nursing intervention when a child develops a reactive purified protein derivative (PPD)?
    1. Refer the child to the physician for immediate treatment
    2. Obtain a full health and immunization history
    3. Reassess the site in 5 days
    4. Don personal protective equipment

ANSWERS AND RATIONALES

1. 4. Infectious diseases continue to account for many serious illnesses, and prevention of infection is a major goal of the World Health Organization.

2. 3. Modern sanitation and our ability to sanitize surfaces and instruments used in daily activities have had a huge impact on reducing the spread of infectious diseases. Infections such as sexually transmitted diseases have

played a part in reducing fertility and birth rates. Steroid-enhanced protein sources have no direct role in the spread of infectious or communicable diseases. The Immunization Act of 1986 is a legal act of Congress protecting individuals harmed by vaccines.

3. 2. Infectious or communicable diseases occur in humans of all ages. Certain infectious illnesses occur in specific age or developmental groups.

Most infectious diseases are transmitted by direct or indirect contact, and isolation categories are assigned accordingly. Many infectious diseases have total systemic involvement or sequelae. Many infectious diseases develop slowly after a prolonged incubation period.

4. 4. A local infection is limited to one locality of the body but may have some systemic repercussions, such as fever and malaise. An infection occurring in a geographic area is an endemic outbreak. Local infections are not always treated easily; treatment is dependent on the causative agent. Local infections can become severe. Local infections are not usually contagious.

5. 7–14 days

6. 4. An acute infection develops rapidly and resolves in a short period of time, but if not treated completely or with the appropriate pharmaceuticals, an acute infection could become chronic.

7. 4. Antibiotics, isolation, and ethyl alcohol have roles in preventing the spread of disease, but the simplest and most effective weapon against the spread of disease is hand washing.

8. 1. In 2002, the CDC guidelines for isolation of clients with infectious or communicable diseases were revised to align according to methods of transmission. The extent of illness is not a useful indication of communicability. Many infectious diseases are spread because the infected individual feels well enough to be out and about. Appropriate personal protective equipment should be readily available to all health care workers in America, so lack of such equipment is not a justifiable reason to employ isolation. A client's ability to pay should never define the appropriate treatment course.

9. 4. The chickenpox infection begins 1 to 2 days before the eruption of the rash and the contagious state ends 6 days after the onset of the lesions, when crusts have formed.

10. 4. The herpes simplex virus type 2 (HSV-2) is characterized by periods of latency between outbreaks and recurrence. The virus can be shed, and is contagious when the client is asymptomatic. There are effective treatments available, but no known cure, for HSV-2. Antibiotics are not effective against viruses.

11. 3. It would be appropriate to provide children with mumps with high-calorie diets because they frequently have nutritional problems. Spicy and irritating foods that require a lot of chewing may cause discomfort for the child. Respiratory isolation should be initiated for 4 days after the appearance of a rash with rubeola (measles). Ganciclovir (Cytovene) is an

antiviral used to treat life-threatening cytomegalovirus in immunocompromised hosts. The white blood cell count is monitored in infectious mononucleosis.

12. 1. 3. 5. The most effective methods of controlling infectious disease are drug prophylaxis, immunization, and hand washing. There is no evidence that herbal therapies are effective against infection. A general state of wellness, including good nutrition and rest, is important to general health, but is not the most effective approach to reducing the spread of infectious diseases.

13. 1. Rotavirus is the most common cause of severe diarrhea in children. It is primarily spread by the fecal-oral route.

14. 1. There is no specific treatment for hepatitis B. Treatment focuses on symptom management. Oral acyclovir (Zovirax) is an antiviral used in the treatment of herpes genitalis (HSV-2). Doxycycline (Vibramycin) and azithromycin (Zithromax) are antibiotics used in the treatment of chlamydia. Monitoring the white blood cell is important in the treatment of infectious mononucleosis.

15. 1. 4. 5. Clinical manifestations for congenital syphilis include hepatosplenomegaly, mucocutaneous lesions, and lymphadenopathy. Pain in the chest and weight loss are clinical features of tuberculosis. A generalized rash is characteristically present in varicella (chickenpox).

16. 2. Varicella (chickenpox) is a varicella zoster virus that is highly contagious through direct contact or may be airborne-spread from respiratory secretions. Severe skin pain, burning, or purulent discharge may indicate a secondary infection, and prompt medical attention is required. Clinical manifestations that are anticipated in chickenpox include a generalized pruritic rash and mild fever. A body rash that begins on the upper body and head and progresses to the lower body and Koplik's spots are clinical manifestations of rubeola (measles). A red facial (slapped cheek) rash and circumoral pallor are characteristically found in erythema infectiosum (Fifth's disease).

17. 1. Erythema infectiosum (Fifth's disease) is an infectious disorder spread through contact with respiratory secretions. The child is highly contagious before the onset of the illness. Children may return to school after the appearance of the rash because they are no longer contagious. There is no immunization for Fifth's disease. A generalized pruritic rash is characteristic of chickenpox; a child with such a rash is highly contagious. Diarrhea is not a clinical manifestation of Fifth's disease.

18. 2. Birth control pills, withdrawal method, and latex condoms and spermicidal foam are not 100% effective in preventing the spread of sexually transmitted diseases. Each method contains some risk of infection. Birth control pills simply protect individuals from pregnancy. The withdrawal method is ineffective in every way. Latex condoms and spermicidal foam are ineffective barriers in the event of tears or breakage of the device or incorrect application. Only abstinence from sexual behavior is 100% effective in protecting against sexually transmitted disease.

19.   *Enterobius* (pinworm) is the most common helminth infection in the United States. It frequently occurs in preschoolers and school-age children, in crowded conditions, institutions, and families. The classic feature is nocturnal anal itching. Weight loss is a symptom of ascariasis. Chronic or relapsing diarrhea and flatulence are symptoms of giardia.

20. 1. Adolescents frequently participate in behaviors that put them at risk for infection, and they falsely believe themselves not to be at risk. Unprotected sex, drug use, and gang relationships are behaviors that put them at risk for infection. Continuity of health care is important with all clients and not just adolescents. All clients require personal privacy, and, although embarrassing, they are encouraged to discuss personal physical concerns. Making the parents a part of a discussion of personal issues with an adolescent will actually make the adolescent uncomfortable and reluctant to discuss pertinent issues.

21. 3. Immunizations are an important part of health promotion and disease prevention. Improvements have been made, but booster shots are still required. Although a small percentage of the population, some clients have adverse reaction to immunizations. Some immunizations are available in oral forms, but not every required immunization can be taken orally.

22. 3. The child's general state of health, preexisting diseases, and any recent exposure to infectious diseases are important considerations in the general assessment of any child. The failure to collect this information may cause a delay in administration of the vaccine. It is a priority to obtain the child's immunization history. This is most important in deciding which vaccines are required and determining the appropriate schedule for immunization.

23. 2. Penicillin G is used in the treatment of tetanus. *Giardia* is a protozoan disorder transmitted by hand-to-mouth transfer of cysts from feces of an infected individual. Furazolidone (Furoxone) is the drug of choice in treatment. Mebendazole (Vermox) is used in the treatment of *Enterobius* (pinworm). Ceftriaxone (Rocephin) is used in the treatment of gonorrhea.

24. 1. Soft, fleshy single or multiple papules occur in the anogenital area (genital warts) in human papillomavirus (HPV). Nocturnal anal itching is a manifestation in *Enterobius* (pinworm). Erythematous and macular rash on the ankles and wrists is found in *Rickettsia rickettsii* (Rocky Mountain spotted fever). Painful raised vesicles are the initial lesions in herpes genitalis (HSV-2).

25. 4. Although methocarbamol (Robaxin), cyclobenzaprine (Flexeril), tizanidine (Zanaflex), and diazepam (Valium) are all skeletal muscle relaxants, Valium is the drug of choice in the treatment of tetanus to control muscle spasms and seizures.

26. 2. A licensed practical nurse may provide comfort measures to a child with mumps. Teaching, counseling, and monitoring are all nursing assignments that require the skills of a registered nurse.

27. 4. Although providing a high-calorie diet, encouraging the child to rest, and monitoring the serum electrolytes are appropriate interventions, the priority is to replace the fluid lost with the explosive diarrhea. A rate of 50 ml/kg is an appropriate fluid replacement for this child.

28. 3. 4. 6. Clinical manifestations of measles (rubeola) include Koplik's spots, coryza, and conjunctivitis. A red maculopapular discrete rash is a symptom of German measles (rubella). A high fever for 3–5 days occurs with roseola (human herpes virus 6). Hepatosplenomegaly is a clinical manifestation of cytomegalovirus (CMV).

29.   8–12 days. The incubation period is 8–12 days for measles (rubeola).

30. 1. 3. 5. Clinical manifestations of erythema infectiosum (Fifth disease) include a red facial rash giving a "slapped cheek" appearance, circumoral pallor, and a symmetrical lacy rash on the trunk and limbs. A gradual onset of membranous nasopharyngitis is a clinical manifestation of diphtheria. Severe paroxysms of cough are present in bordatella (whooping cough). A clinical manifestation of Lyme's disease is arthralgia.

31. 2. The nurse should investigate whether the child has had contact with an individual who has tuberculosis (TB). The nurse also should assess whether the child has received any treatment for TB, what clinical manifestations the child has, and whether the child received the immunization BCG, which creates a positive skin test response to the PPD injection. A positive reaction to the skin test does not indicate a need for immediate treatment. Retesting the PPD skin test is most reactive within 72 hours, and the response will begin to subside after that. A positive reaction to PPD is not a positive indication that the client is infectious.

REFERENCES

Daniels, R. (2012). *Delmar's manual of laboratory and diagnostic tests* (2nd ed.). Clifton Park, NY: Delmar Cengage Learning.

Potts, N., & Mandleco, B. (2012). *Pediatric nursing: Caring for children and their families* (3rd ed.). Clifton Park, NY: Delmar Cengage Learning.

Spratto, G. R., & Woods, A. L. (2012). *PDR nurse's drug handbook 2012.* Clifton Park, NY: Delmar Cengage Learning.

MATERNITY AND WOMEN'S HEALTH NURSING

CHAPTER 42

THE ANTEPARTAL PERIOD

I. ANATOMY AND PHYSIOLOGY

A. UTERUS

1. SMOOTH MUSCLE SHAPED LIKE AN UPSIDE-DOWN PEAR
2. MIDLINE IN THE PELVIS
3. DIVIDED INTO TWO MAJOR PARTS: UPPER TRIANGULAR PORTION CALLED THE CORPUS AND THE LOWER PORTION SHAPED LIKE A CYLINDER OR TUBE CALLED THE CERVIX
4. UTERUS HAS THREE LAYERS: ENDOMETRIUM—HIGHLY VASCULAR LINING; MYOMETRIUM—LAYERS OF SMOOTH MUSCLES; AND PART OF THE PERITONEUM.
5. UTERUS SERVES AS AN ORGAN OR AREA OF IMPLANTATION FOR THE FERTILIZED OVUM THAT BECOMES THE FETUS.
6. UTERUS IS RESPONSIBLE FOR EXPULSION OF THE FETUS DURING CHILDBIRTH FROM THE STRONG MUSCLE CONTRACTIONS AS WELL AS MENSTRUATION.
7. DURING PREGNANCY, THE UTERUS INCREASES IN SIZE, WEIGHT, AND CAPACITY.
8. INEFFECTUAL UTERINE CONTRACTIONS, CALLED BRAXTON-HICKS, SOMETIMES OCCUR DURING PREGNANCY.
9. FUNDAL HEIGHT (DISTANCE FROM THE SYMPHYSIS PUBIS TO THE TOP OF THE UTERUS OR FUNDUS) GROSSLY CORRELATES WITH GESTATIONAL AGE.
   a. At the level of the symphysis at 12–14 weeks
   b. Rises at 1 cm/week until 36 weeks of gestation
   c. At the umbilicus at 20 weeks (20 cm)

B. CERVIX

1. LOWER PORTION OF THE UTERUS IN A CYLINDER OR TUBE SHAPE
2. MADE UP OF FIBROUS CONNECTIVE AND ELASTIC TISSUE TO ALLOW FOR STRETCHING FOR CHILDBIRTH
3. THE ENDOCERVICAL CANAL CONNECTS THE UTERINE CAVITY WITH THE VAGINA; THE OPENING OF THE ENDOCERVICAL CANAL AT THE UTERUS END IS CALLED THE INTERNAL OS AND THE OPENING AT THE VAGINA IS THE EXTERNAL OS.
4. DURING PREGNANCY THE CERVIX SOFTENS (GOODELL'S SIGN), MAY HAVE A BLUISH COLOR (CHADWICK'S SIGN), HAS INCREASED VASCULARITY, AND FORMS A MUCUS PLUG.

C. VAGINA

1. COLLAPSIBLE TUBE THAT CONNECTS THE UTERUS AT THE CERVIX TO THE VULVA (EXTERNAL GENITALIA)
2. FOUND BETWEEN THE BLADDER AND THE RECTUM
3. BEFORE MENOPAUSE THE VAGINA IS LINED WITH TRANSVERSE FOLDS CALLED RUGAE, WHICH ALLOW THE VAGINA TO EXPAND DURING CHILDBIRTH.
4. SLIGHTLY ACIDIC PH (4–5) TO DECREASE RISK OF INFECTIONS
5. FUNCTIONS INCLUDE A PASSAGEWAY FOR MENSTRUAL FLOW FROM THE ENDOMETRIUM OF THE UTERUS, THE FEMALE ORGAN FOR INTERCOURSE, AND A PASSAGEWAY FOR VAGINAL CHILDBIRTH
6. DURING PREGNANCY, THE MUCOSA OF THE VAGINA MAY HAVE A BLUISH VIOLET COLOR (CHADWICK'S SIGN), INCREASED VASCULARITY, AND INCREASED VAGINAL MUCUS DISCHARGE (LEUKORRHEA).

D. EXTERNAL STRUCTURES

1. THE EXTERNAL GENITAL ORGANS, OR VULVA, INCLUDE ALL THE STRUCTURES FOUND EXTERNALLY

BETWEEN THE PUBIS AND THE PERINEUM (SKIN-COVERED MUSCULAR AREA BEFORE THE ANUS).

2. STRUCTURES INCLUDE THE MONS PUBIS, LABIA MAJORA, LABIA MINORA, PREPUCE, FRENULUM, FOURCHETTE, CLITORIS, AND VESTIBULE.

3. APPEARANCE (SIZE, SHAPE, AND COLOR) VARIES GREATLY AMONG WOMEN AND IS DETERMINED BY AGE, RACE, HEREDITY, AND NUMBER OF CHILDREN.

4. THESE STRUCTURES UNDERGO INCREASED VASCULARITY AND HYPERTROPHY DURING PREGNANCY.

E. OVARIES

1. CORPUS LUTEUM REMAINS ACTIVE EARLY IN PREGNANCY TO PRODUCE PROGESTERONE AND ESTROGEN.

2. THE PLACENTA LATER TAKES OVER THIS FUNCTION.

F. PLACENTA

1. BEGINS TO FORM AT IMPLANTATION

2. CHORIONIC VILLI (BEGINNING OF FETAL CIRCULATION) FORM AND INVADE THE LINING OF THE UTERUS WHERE ENDOMETRIAL ARTERIES FILL WITH BLOOD.

3. CHORIONIC VILLI DEVELOP LAYERS SURROUNDING SECTIONS OF THE PLACENTA CALLED COTYLEDONS, EACH CONTAINING A COMPLEX SYSTEM OF FETAL VESSELS.

4. EACH COTYLEDON IS A FUNCTIONAL UNIT AND COMBINED THEY MAKE UP THE PLACENTA.

5. EARLIEST FUNCTION IS AS AN ENDOCRINE GLAND TO EXCRETE:

   a. Human chorionic gonadotropin (hCG) that maintains the corpus luteum in order for estrogen and progesterone early in pregnancy

   b. Human placental lactogen (hPL) as a growth hormone by stimulating maternal metabolism and facilitating glucose transfer across the placenta for the fetus to use

6. METABOLIC FUNCTIONS OF THE PLACENTA:

   a. Respiration: a fetal substitution for respiration in that oxygen transfers across the placental membrane to fetal circulation and carbon dioxide diffuses in the opposite direction.

   b. Nutrition: nutrients cross the placental membrane by passive and active means.

   c. Excretion: metabolic waste products cross the placenta into maternal circulation to be excreted by the maternal kidneys.

7. MATERNAL CIRCULATION AND FETAL CIRCULATION ARE NOT DIRECTLY CONNECTED.

8. FETAL BLOOD CELLS CAN LEAK INTO MATERNAL CIRCULATION FROM OCCASIONAL BREAKS IN THE PLACENTAL MEMBRANE AND THE MOTHER MAY DEVELOP ANTIBODIES (BECOME SENSITIZED) TO THE FETAL RED BLOOD CELLS IN THE PROCESS KNOWN AS ISOIMMUNIZATION.

9. INTERFERENCE WITH THE CIRCULATION TO THE PLACENTA, SUCH AS MATERNAL VASOCONSTRICTION FROM HYPERTENSION OR COCAINE OR DECREASED MATERNAL BLOOD PRESSURE OR DECREASED MATERNAL CARDIAC OUTPUT, IMPEDES THE BLOOD SUPPLY TO THE FETUS.

G. MEMBRANES

1. AMNIOTIC "BAG" MADE UP OF TWO LAYERS (CHORION AND AMNION) CONTAINING THE FETUS, THE UMBILICAL CORD, AND AMNIOTIC FLUID

H. UMBILICAL CORD

1. TWO ARTERIES CARRY BLOOD FROM THE EMBRYO TO THE CHORIONIC VILLI (THE PLACENTA).

2. ONE VEIN RETURNS BLOOD TO THE FETUS FROM THE PLACENTA.

3. THE VESSELS IN THE CORD ARE SURROUNDED BY CONNECTIVE TISSUE CALLED WHARTON'S JELLY TO PREVENT COMPRESSION OF THE BLOOD VESSELS AND PROTECT FETAL CIRCULATION.

4. THE UMBILICAL CORD IS USUALLY LOCATED CENTRALLY AS THE PLACENTA DEVELOPS FROM THE CHORIONIC VILLI; VESSELS ARE ARRAYED OUT FROM THE INSERTION SITE OF THE CORD IN ALL DIRECTIONS TO PERFUSE ALL OF THE PLACENTA.

I. AMNIOTIC FLUID

1. FETAL URINE IS THE PRIMARY SOURCE.

2. MAINTAINED THROUGH A BALANCE OF PRODUCTION AND RESORPTION

3. CONTAINS CHLORIDE, THE PRESENCE OF WHICH IN THE VAGINA WILL BE USED TO DETERMINE IF THE MEMBRANES HAVE RUPTURED

4. FUNCTIONS INCLUDE FETAL LUNG DEVELOPMENT, PROTECTION OF THE CORD, AND ALLOWS FOR NORMAL LIMB DEVELOPMENT AND

DEVELOPMENT OF THE GASTROINTESTINAL (GI) AND RENAL SYSTEMS.

J. CARDIOVASCULAR SYSTEM
1. BLOOD VOLUME INCREASES 30–50% DURING PREGNANCY.
2. VENA CAVAL SYNDROME IS SUPINE HYPOTENSION AS BLOOD RETURNING TO THE RIGHT ATRIUM IS DIMINISHED WHEN A PREGNANT CLIENT LIES SUPINE WITH THE PRESSURE OF THE UTERUS COMPRESSING THE VENA CAVA.

K. GASTROINTESTINAL SYSTEM
1. HORMONES OF PREGNANCY ARE RESPONSIBLE FOR DECREASED GI MOTILITY AND RELAXATION/ DIMINISHED TONE, WHICH MAY RESULT IN CONSTIPATION AND GASTROESOPHAGEAL REFLUX.
2. DIMINISHED STOMACH CAPACITY FROM PRESSURE FROM THE GROWING FETUS

L. URINARY SYSTEM
1. SIMILAR RELAXATION OF THE URINARY TRACT PLACES THE PREGNANT CLIENT AT RISK FOR URINARY TRACT INFECTIONS (UTIS) OR PYELONEPHRITIS FROM BACTERIA ASCENDING FROM THE PERINEUM.
2. URINARY FREQUENCY IS NORMAL FROM PRESSURE OF THE GROWING FETUS; HOWEVER, PAIN OR BURNING ON URINATION IS NOT NORMAL WITH PREGNANCY.

M. ENDOCRINE SYSTEM
1. PANCREAS
   a. Physiologic changes in carbohydrate metabolism in pregnancy required to supply continuous nutrients to the fetus result in increased demand for insulin.
   b. Clients with borderline pancreatic reserve prior to pregnancy will not be able to meet the metabolic challenge of pregnancy and will develop gestational diabetes mellitus.
   c. Clients with diabetes mellitus prior to pregnancy will require increased insulin doses during pregnancy.
2. THYROID
   a. Gland increases in size and function.
   b. Basic metabolic rate (BMR) increases up to 25% by term.
3. PITUITARY
   a. Follicle-stimulating hormone (FSH) and luteinizing hormone (LH) production are suppressed in pregnancy.
   b. Oxytocin production increases during pregnancy.

N. RESPIRATORY SYSTEM
1. INCREASED BMR REQUIRES MORE OXYGEN FOR THE PREGNANT BODY.
2. TIDAL VOLUME AND MINUTE VENTILATION INCREASE UNTIL THE THIRD TRIMESTER WHEN THE LARGE UTERUS MAY IMPEDE LUNG EXPANSION.
3. CO_2 OUTPUT INCREASES, RESULTING IN SLIGHT RESPIRATORY ALKALOSIS.

O. HEMATOLOGIC SYSTEM
1. RED BLOOD CELLS (RBCS) INCREASE BY ONE-THIRD.
2. HOWEVER, PLASMA VOLUME INCREASE IS GREATER, RESULTING IN PHYSIOLOGIC ANEMIA OF PREGNANCY FROM HEMODILUTION OF CELLS.
3. CLOTTING FACTORS INCREASE IN PREGNANCY, WHICH INCREASE THE CLIENT'S RISK FOR BLOOD CLOTS.
4. CLIENTS WITH A PREEXISTING HYPERCOAGULOPATHY (CLOTTING DISORDER) ARE AT INCREASED RISK FOR THROMBUS FORMATION DURING PREGNANCY.

P. BREASTS
1. BREAST ENLARGEMENT AND TENDERNESS FROM ESTROGEN
2. INCREASED VASCULARITY

Q. SKIN
1. INCREASED PIGMENTATION
2. CHLOASMA IS THE BLOTCHY BROWN AREAS OF HYPERPIGMENTATION ON THE FACE AND IS KNOWN AS THE MASK OF PREGNANCY.
3. THE LINEA NIGRA IS THE DARK LINE ON THE ABDOMEN FROM THE UMBILICUS TO THE SYMPHYSIS PUBIS.
4. STRETCHING OF THE SKIN CAUSES PINK OR REDDISH STREAKS CALLED STRIAE GRAVIDARUM, USUALLY FOUND ON THE ABDOMEN, BREASTS, BUTTOCKS, OR THIGHS.

R. FETAL DEVELOPMENT
1. FERTILIZATION
   a. At the time of ovulation, the spermatozoa and ovum join and the egg is fertilized.
   b. This usually takes place in the outer third of the fallopian tube and the fertilized egg must travel to the uterus for implantation; failure to do this leaves the growing ovum in the fallopian tube (ectopic pregnancy).
2. IMPLANTATION
   a. Normal implantation is in the upper part of the uterus.
   b. It takes place approximately 1 week after fertilization.

3. PLACENTAL DEVELOPMENT
   (SEE PLACENTA IN SECTION I.)
   a. Begins to form at implantation
4. DEVELOPMENTAL LANDMARKS IN
   PREGNANCY
   a. Fetal heart tones (FHT) can be assessed
      by ultrasonic Doppler beginning
      around 8 weeks of gestation.
   b. Quickening (the first fetal movements)
      are felt by the pregnant client between
      16 and 18 weeks of gestation.
5. INFANTS AT GENETIC RISK FOR
   ABNORMALITIES
   a. African American: sickle cell
      disease
   b. Jewish ethnicity of Northern European
      descent (Ashkenazi Jews): Tay-Sachs
      disease
   c. Mediterranean: thalassemia
   d. Family history of hereditary condition
      such as cystic fibrosis or cleft lip or
      palate
   e. Born to a woman of advanced maternal
      age (considered to be 40 years for the
      purposes of this review)
   f. Parents are closely related blood
      relatives.
6. CHROMOSOMAL ABNORMALITIES
   a. Range from lethal to undetectable
      without chromosomal studies
   b. Types of transmission to the fetus
      1) Autosomal dominant: in
         chromosome pair other than sex-
         linked, the abnormal gene
         dominates, thus passing on the
         condition to the offspring.
      2) Autosomal recessive: in
         chromosome pair other than
         sex-linked, a defect will not be
         demonstrated in the offspring
         unless the abnormal gene is passed
         on by both parents; if inherited
         from only one parent, the offspring
         would be a carrier for the condition
         with one abnormal and one normal
         gene but not evidence the
         condition.
      3) Sex-linked transmission: carried on
         the sex-linked chromosome and is
         usually recessive such as color
         blindness or hemophilia; X-linked
         recessive will affect all males
         because the information is carried
         on the X chromosome and there is
         no coding on the Y chromosome to
         counteract the information.
   c. May be structurally altered, such as
      an extra "arm," or vary in number,
      such as an extra X for gender;
      examples follow.

d. Down syndrome (trisomy 21)
   1) Risk increases in women over
      35 years old and continues to
      increase with each year of age.
   2) Characteristics: low-set ears, large
      fat pads at the nape of a short neck,
      protruding tongue, small mouth
      and high palate, epicanthal folds
      and slanted eyes, small rounded
      head with flattened occiput,
      hypotonic muscles with
      hypermobility of joints, simian
      crease across the palm of hand, and
      mental retardation
e. Turner's syndrome
   1) Female with only one X
      chromosome (XO)
   2) Characteristics: usually infertile,
      small stature, cognitive functions
      unimpaired
f. Klinefelter's syndrome
   1) Male with an extra X chromosome
      (XXY)
   2) Characteristics: usually infertile,
      cognitive functions vary from
      unimpaired to mild mental
      retardation
g. Inborn errors of metabolism: enzymes
   missing at birth alter the body's
   metabolism of fat, protein, or
   carbohydrates; usually autosomal
   recessive
   1) Phenylketonuria (PKU): disorder of
      amino acid metabolism in which
      phenylalanine cannot be converted
      to tyrosine because of a missing
      enzyme, and this results in toxic
      levels of phenylalanine that cause
      mental retardation.
   2) Tay-Sachs disease: enzyme
      deficiency leads to an
      accumulation of a glycolipid,
      causing neuromuscular
      manifestations and death.
   3) Cystic fibrosis: a deletion on
      chromosome 7 is responsible
      for this exocrine disorder of
      metabolism of chloride transport;
      clinically there are viscous lung
      secretions, pancreatic deficiencies,
      and increased sodium chloride in
      sweat.
   4) Congenital adrenal hyperplasia:
      enzymes necessary for cortisol
      synthesis are lacking and there is
      overstimulation of the adrenal
      gland; this leads to overproduction
      of androgens, and infant girls will
      have ambiguous genitalia
      (virilization).

5) Congenital hypothyroidism: results in mental retardation from inadequate thyroid function after birth when brain development is occurring in infancy

II. ASSESSMENT

A. PRENATAL CARE

1. ASSESSMENT OF A POSITIVE PREGNANCY (SEE TABLE 42-1)
2. NAEGELE'S RULE
    a. To determine the estimated date of confinement (EDC) or estimated date of delivery (EDD), count back 3 months from the first day of the last menstrual cycle and then add 1 year and 7 days.
3. OBSTETRIC CLASSIFICATIONS
    a. Gravida: total number of pregnancies, including the present pregnancy; a multigravida has been pregnant before this pregnancy, a primigravida is experiencing the first pregnancy, and a nulligravida has never been pregnant; represented by the letter G.
    b. Para or parity: the number of pregnancies that have progressed past 20 weeks; it can be subdefined as a series of numbers representing the number of term deliveries (T), preterm deliveries (P), abortions (elective or spontaneous) (A), and number of living children (L) as G:T-P-A-L.
4. FREQUENCY AND ELEMENTS OF MATERNAL AND FETAL ASSESSMENTS
    a. Initial visit
        1) Intake assessment: medical and reproductive history, family history, current pregnancy complications, psychosocial and nutritional assessment, and physical examination
        2) Lab evaluations: complete blood count (CBC), blood type and antibody screen, Pap smear, gonorrhea and chlamydia test, serology, rubella, hepatitis B screen, urinalysis and culture, group B beta strep vaginal and rectal culture

3) Client education: screenings indicated, normal pregnancy changes, and warning signs (vaginal leaking or bleeding, fever, persistent vomiting, swelling, dysuria, decreased fetal movement, epigastric pain, or headache)

b. If indicated:
1) Assessment: ask questions to determine risk for these lab tests.
2) Lab evaluations: sickle cell screen, Tay-Sachs screening, glucose challenge test, TORCH titers
3) Client education: discuss screening tests indicated.

c. Every visit
1) Assessment: ask about contractions, fetal movement, bleeding, and leaking; vital signs, urine dipstick for protein, weight, fundal height, fetal heart rate; Leopold's maneuver; examine for edema.
2) Client education: review abnormal signs and symptoms and when to call the physician.

d. Period specific evaluations in pregnancy
1) Every 4 weeks until 28 weeks
2) At 5–20 weeks of gestation: monitor maternal alpha-feto protein, begin preterm birth prevention education, and review warning signs.
3) At 20–24 weeks of gestation: provide preterm birth prevention education.
4) At 24–28 weeks of gestation: 1 hour glucose tolerance test (GTT), cervical exam if indicated by risk status, begin education and treatment if diabetic, and review preterm birth prevention and warning signs.
5) Every 2 weeks from 28 to 36 weeks of gestation
6) At 28–36 weeks of gestation: CBC for at-risk clients; blood group antibody screen and if Rh negative,

Table 42-1 Assessment of a Positive Pregnancy

Type of Assessment	Signs	Clinical Manifestation
Presumptive	Amenorrhea, breast changes and tenderness, Chadwick's sign, skin changes, abdominal enlargement	Nausea and vomiting, urinary frequency, weight gain, constipation, fatigue, feeling of fetal movement, breast tenderness
Probable	Softening of uterine isthmus (Hegar's sign), Goodell's sign, Braxton-Hicks sign, positive hCG on lab test	Same as for Presumptive assessment
Positive	Fetal heartbeat, fetal outline on sonogram, fetal movement by examiner	Same as for Presumptive assessment

give Rh immune globulin; cervical exam if indicated; follow up with a dietician if diabetic; breast assessment and educational preparation for breastfeeding if desired; review warning signs for which to contact the physician; and begin parenting classes.

    7) At 35–37 weeks of gestation: vaginal and rectal group B beta strep culture

    8) Weekly visits from 36 weeks of gestation until delivery

    9) At 36–40 weeks of gestation: CBC for clients with abnormal 28-week CBC; repeat gonorrhea, chlamydia, RPR, HIV, hepatitis B screen if indicated; educate about signs of labor and begin childbirth preparation.

5. ASSESSMENT OF PSYCHOSOCIAL ASPECTS OF PREGNANCY

  a. Economic status

  b. Marital status

  c. Age

  d. Perceived support—lack of perceived support is a risk factor for high-risk pregnancies

  e. Self-esteem

  f. Culture

  g. Religion and importance of faith beliefs to the client

  h. Stability of living conditions

  i. Assess mood—mood swings.

    1) Ambivalence about becoming a mother appears early in pregnancy.

    2) Increased sensitivity and irritability are possible throughout pregnancy.

    3) Sense of vulnerability peaks during the seventh month.

    4) Fears about the health of the baby and the ability to give birth safely are normal unless noted to be excessive.

  j. Assess developmental tasks of pregnancy.

    1) Pregnancy validation: initial ambivalence about pregnancy is common.

    2) Fetal embodiment: woman incorporates the fetus into body image.

    3) Fetal distinction: conceptualizes the fetus as a separate individual

    4) Role transitions: include preparing to separate from the fetus, anxiety about labor and delivery, exhibiting "nesting" behaviors, and feeling ready for the pregnancy to end

  k. Substance abuse

  l. Victim of domestic violence

B. ASSESSMENT OF HIGH-RISK PREGNANCY CONDITIONS

  1. HEALTH HISTORY: AS IN INITIAL INTAKE ASSESSMENT

  2. SOCIAL HISTORY: INCLUDE EDUCATION, OCCUPATION, AND PSYCHOSOCIAL ASSESSMENT

  3. PROBLEMS WITH THIS PREGNANCY: HEADACHE, BLURRED VISION, NAUSEA AND VOMITING, SWELLING, EPIGASTRIC PAIN, UPPER RIGHT QUADRANT PAIN, CONTRACTIONS, THIGH PAIN, CHANGE IN VAGINAL MUCUS, RHYTHMIC BACK PAIN, AND CERVICAL DILATION, VAGINAL BLEEDING OR LEAKING

  4. PHYSICAL EXAM

    a. Inspection: inspect for distress, level of comfort, edema, and color.

    b. Auscultation: auscultate lung sounds and bowel sounds.

    c. Palpation: palpate the abdomen and uterus for contractions or tenderness, extremities for edema, skin for temperature and capillary refill, and cervix for dilation and effacement (only when indicated).

    d. Vital signs: assess temperature, pulse, blood pressure (BP), and respirations; also include the client's weight to assess for recent or excessive weight gain.

    e. Deep tendon reflexes (DTR): assess popliteal DTRs bilaterally.

III. DIAGNOSTIC STUDIES

A. STERILE SPECULUM EXAM (SSE)

  1. DESCRIPTION

    a. A sterile speculum is introduced into the vagina by the physician or qualified examiner to open the vault for inspection of the cervix and sterile sampling of any fluid in the vagina.

    b. Indicated for suspected ruptured membranes

    c. Amniotic fluid will turn Nitrazine paper blue because of the alkaline pH—urine is usually acidic; you can perform this test on any vaginal fluid that has wet the client's garments.

    d. Free flow of fluid may be seen coming through the cervix when the client is asked to cough or perform a Valsalva maneuver.

    e. A fern pattern is seen under a microscope once the amniotic fluid is dried on a slide.

  2. PREPROCEDURE

    a. Client is assisted into the lithotomy position.

      b. Gather supplies—sterile speculum, sterile gloves, exam light, Nitrazine paper or Amnioswabs, sterile Q-tips, and slide.

   3. POSTPROCEDURE

      a. No special care is required.

B. URINALYSIS WITH REAGENT STRIPS (URINE DIPSTICK)

   1. DESCRIPTION

      a. Urine is tested with a reagent strip to test for the presence of components in the urine such as WBC, blood, protein, bilirubin, leukocytes, ketones, glucose, specific gravity, pH, urobilinogen, and nitrite.

      b. Urine should not be standing for more than 1–2 hours for an accurate test.

      c. The reagent strip is dipped into the urine specimen and results are read by holding the strip alongside the color-coded legend on the side of the bottle.

   2. PREPROCEDURE

      a. Instruct the client not to discard urine.

   3. POSTPROCEDURE

      a. Compare the results with the legend on the side of the bottle to determine normal or abnormal findings.

      b. Discard the urine and record the results.

C. 24-HOUR URINE

   1. DESCRIPTION

      a. The client's total urine output for 24 hours is collected and analyzed for amount, specific gravity, pH, presence and amount of protein, and creatinine clearance.

      b. It is useful in clients being evaluated for severity of pregnancy-induced hypertension (PIH).

      c. Greater than 300 mg proteinuria in 24 hours as well as decreased urine output evidences worrisome kidney involvement in PIH.

   2. PREPROCEDURE

      a. Instruct the client not to discard any urine for 24 hours.

      b. Obtain special collection jugs and keep specimen on ice for the duration of the test.

      c. Have the client empty the bladder and record the start time.

      d. Post signs in the bathroom to remind the client, family, and all staff that the test is in progress (one missed void will invalidate the test).

   3. POSTPROCEDURE

      a. Send the entire specimen to the lab.

      b. Record the end time.

D. URINALYSIS AND CULTURE

   1. DESCRIPTION

      a. Urinalysis is a laboratory evaluation of a specimen of urine appearance, specific gravity, pH, and presence of and quantity of substrates or components.

      b. Urine culture is a laboratory test in which a specimen of urine found to be positive for the presence of bacteria is allowed to grow the bacteria for 48 hours in order to identify the organism and the drugs to which it is sensitive and resistive.

      c. They are useful in determining the presence of a UTI, which during pregnancy can result in preterm labor (PTL)

   2. PREPROCEDURE

      a. Obtain the specimen as ordered (clean catch or indwelling catheter specimen).

      b. Label the specimen and send it to the lab.

   3. POSTPROCEDURE

      a. No special care is required.

E. LABORATORY SERUM EVALUATIONS

   1. DESCRIPTION

      a. CBC is used to determine infection, anemia, and thrombocytopenia.

      b. Metabolic panel indicates the level of metabolic products and electrolytes in the blood.

      c. Liver profile reveals the quantity of liver enzymes in the circulating serum.

      d. D-dimer and fibrinogen are laboratory indices of bleeding that are used in evaluating placental abruption.

      e. Kleinhauer-Betke identifies fetal blood cells in maternal circulation and is drawn after maternal trauma to determine if RhoGAM is necessary for the Rh-negative client to avoid isoimmunization.

      f. C-reactive protein (CRP) is a test of generalized inflammatory reaction and is used in addition to the CBC to determine infection as the CBC is influenced by giving antenatal steroids for fetal lung maturity.

      g. Beta hCG can be found in the urine or the blood of the pregnant client as it is produced by the placental trophoblasts; considered a positive pregnancy test; high levels are found with multiple gestations, hyperemesis, and hydatiform mole.

      h. Maternal serum alpha-fetoprotein (AFP or MS-AFP) is a protein in fetal serum and is found in low levels in maternal serum; elevations may mean multiple gestation, neural tube defect, or fetal chromosomal problem.

    i. OB panel includes maternal rubella status (immune or nonimmune), presence of hepatitis B antibodies, blood group, and Rh status.

    j. TORCH titers: T represents toxoplasmosis, which is a protozoan infection the pregnant client can acquire from handling cat litter without proper hand washing or ingesting infested undercooked meat; it can pass to the fetus and cause serious or lethal neurologic complications. Other infections included in TORCH are hepatitis, rubella, cytomegalovirus, and herpes simplex virus.

  2. PREPROCEDURE

    a. Instruct the client on the reason for obtaining the specimen.

  3. POSTPROCEDURE

    a. No special care is required.

F. FETAL FIBRONECTIN

  1. DESCRIPTION

    a. A protein found in amniotic fluid, the placental tissue itself, and following injury to the membranes—either mechanical or inflammatory

    b. A special swab is used to obtain a cell specimen at the cervix.

    c. If the test is negative, the chance for delivery in the next 14 days is less than 5%.

    d. Used to gauge the risk of preterm birth for the client hospitalized with PTL

  2. PREPROCEDURE

    a. Assist the client in assuming the lithotomy position for the test.

    b. Gather the equipment similar to that required for an SSE but substitute the Q-tip and slides for the special swab used to collect fetal fibronectin.

  3. POSTPROCEDURE

    a. No special care is provided.

G. ORAL GLUCOSE TOLERANCE TEST (OGTT OR GTT)

  1. DESCRIPTION

    a. The pregnant client's pancreas is challenged by giving an oral glucose load in order to evaluate the pancreatic response (insulin production); this is done by measuring blood glucose levels per testing protocols.

    b. The client is given 50 grams of glucose to drink in a liquid form in 5 minutes and the client is to fast for 1 hour and have her serum glucose measured by a peripheral blood draw at precisely 1 hour.

    c. Blood glucose greater than or equal to 140 indicates an abnormal screen, and the 3-hour GTT is indicated.

    d. 3-hour GTT: 100 grams of glucose is given to the client to drink in a liquid form in 5 minutes; fasting is now required for 12 hours before the test as well as for 3 hours after; serum glucose levels are evaluated at 1, 2, and 3 hours after drinking the glucose solution.

    e. Elevations are used to diagnose diabetes mellitus in pregnancy.

  2. PREPROCEDURE

    a. Obtain the glucose solution (usually Glucola) and arrange for the blood draw on schedule.

  3. POSTPROCEDURE

    a. No special care is required.

H. DAILY FETAL MOVEMENT COUNT

  1. DESCRIPTION

    a. Also known as kick counts

    b. Gross measurement of fetal well-being that can be done at home

    c. The client is to eat a snack or meal, turn off all distractions such as radio and TV, lie down (with the hand on the abdomen), and count the number of fetal movements.

    d. Advised to do daily or twice daily in high-risk pregnancies

    e. Counting 10 movements in 1 hour is a reassuring kick count.

    f. Less than 10 movements is not reassuring and the client should call the physician to be evaluated for decreased fetal movement.

  2. PREPROCEDURE

    a. Supply the client with a sheet for daily record keeping.

  3. POSTPROCEDURE

    a. No special care is required.

I. ELECTRONIC FETAL MONITORING (EFM)

  1. DESCRIPTION

    a. Noninvasive method of fetal heart rate (FHR) monitoring

    b. Part of fetal assessment

    c. Purpose is identification of the fetus experiencing well-being and the fetus experiencing compromise.

    d. Minimal assessment is done with an external ultrasonic Doppler in which the nurse dopples the FHR for 1 full minute and records the audible rate.

    e. Richer data are obtained by using a machine known as an electronic fetal monitor for a minimum of 20 minutes.

    f. Same technology is employed to make audible and also record the FHR with the machine's Doppler ultrasound transducer; this is secured over the pregnant uterus with a stretchable, soft belt.

g. Also used for uterine assessment: the tocodynamometer or tocotransducer placed externally on the abdomen will detect the pressure change in the uterus as it contracts and hardens.

h. Internal FHR monitoring yields the most sensitive FHR assessment as the device (a spiral electrode) is attached directly to the fetal head; this is used in select situations for labor management.

2. PREPROCEDURE
   a. Apply conducting gel to the ultrasound component.

3. POSTPROCEDURE
   a. Interpret findings (ongoing evaluation if on electronic fetal monitor) and record findings.
   b. Wipe off the abdomen and equipment of conducting gel.
   c. Key points of EFM interpretation:
      1) Baseline: sustained rate for 10 minutes; 110–160 is normal.
      2) Variability: change in heart rate from beat to beat over a 1-minute interval; should be average
      3) Acceleration: abrupt rise in baseline of at least 15 beats/min
      4) Variable deceleration: abrupt decline in heart rate in response to cord compression
      5) Early deceleration: gradual decrease in heart rate, which begins and ends with a contraction; benign periodic change from head compression
      6) Late deceleration: gradual decrease in heart rate beginning at the peak of a contraction; sign of fetal hypoxia and requires intervention
      7) Contraction: gradual rise and fall in muscle tone registered by tocodynameter

8) Nonstress test (NST): a positive or reactive test is two or three (interpretation varies) periods of FHR accelerations without contractions in 20 minutes.

9) Contraction stress test (CST): a positive test is heart rate decelerations with contractions and is not reassuring.

J. ULTRASOUND
   1. DESCRIPTION
      a. Uses sound waves undetected by the human ear
      b. Obstetric ultrasound scanning can be either transvaginally or transabdominally.
      c. Indications for antepartum care include estimation of fetal age, fetal weight, and fetal presentation, placental position and integrity, or a follow-up of fetal anomalies or well-being (biophysical profile).
      d. May be screening and routine or be selective and targeted to search for fetal anomalies
   2. PREPROCEDURE
      a. Client should have a full bladder for better visualization of the pregnant uterus up to 20 weeks of gestation for abdominal viewing.
   3. POSTPROCEDURE
      a. No special care is required.

K. BIOPHYSICAL PROFILE (BPP) (SEE TABLE 42-2)
   1. DESCRIPTION
      a. Used in addition to the NST to evaluate the dynamic functions that reflect the integrity of the fetal central nervous system via ultrasound
      b. Fetal well-being is determined scoring components of the BPP as 0 or 2 points each to total 10 points.
      c. Delivery is indicated for a score of 4 or below.

Table 42-2 Biophysical Profile Scores

Variable	Score 2	Score 0
Fetal breathing movements	The presence of sustained fetal breathing movements for at least 30 seconds in 30 minutes of observation	Less than 30 seconds of fetal breathing movements in 30 minutes of observation
Fetal movements	Three or more gross body movements in 30 minutes of observation	Less than three gross body movements in 30 minutes of observation
Fetal tone	At least one episode of motion of a limb from position of flexion to extension and rapid return to flexion	Semilimb extension or full-limb extension without return or slow return to flexion; or absence of movements
Fetal reactivity	Two or more fetal heart rate accelerations of at least 15 beats per minute lasting at least 15 seconds; associated with fetal movement	No acceleration or less than two accelerations of fetal heart rate in 20 minutes of observation
Amniotic fluid volume or index	Pocket of amniotic fluid that measures at least 2 cm in two perpendicular planes	Largest pocket of amniotic fluid measures < 2 cm in two perpendicular planes

L. UMBILICAL ARTERY DOPPLER VELOCIMETRY
   1. DESCRIPTION
      a. There is a difference or "shift" from the sound waves that are sent out via ultrasound and the waves that are returned.
      b. This shift is noted in Doppler velocimetry and recorded as a wave form that reflects placental blood flow resistance.
      c. Resistance is measured during fetal systole (S) and fetal diastole (D), yielding an S/D ratio.
      d. Certain pregnancy conditions are associated with increased S/D ratios that evidence poor placental perfusion.
      e. The ratio can be absent (equal resistance) or reversed, which is usually associated with poor perinatal outcome.
      f. Noninvasive test is done via ultrasound, examining the umbilical artery.
      g. Test is done when placental/fetal perfusion compromise is suspected.

M. AMNIOCENTESIS
   1. DESCRIPTION
      a. Needle is inserted into the amniotic cavity through the abdomen with aseptic technique by the physician guided by ultrasound to find amniotic fluid pocket.
      b. Amniotic fluid is then removed for the following indications: genetic screening, diagnostic for isoimmunization, follow-up after an abnormal ultrasound, to evaluate fetal lung maturity, to evaluate for subclinical infection, or to aspirate amniotic fluid to reduce volume in problematic polyhydramnios.
      c. Not a risk-free procedure; complications include isoimmunization, umbilical cord laceration, fetal hemorrhage, emergency cesarean section, amniotic fluid leakage, fetal injury, and infection.
      d. Dye can be inserted through the needle after amniotic fluid sampling is done and will stain the amniotic fluid blue.
      e. This can be useful to confirm the client has rupture of the membranes (ROM) if this diagnosis is suspected in spite of negative or equivocal SSE; blue amniotic fluid will escape into the vagina and be captured on the tampon the client temporarily places in her vagina.

   2. PREPROCEDURE
      a. Written consent discussion must take place between the client and the physician.
      b. Educate the client about the procedure.
   3. POSTPROCEDURE
      a. EFM for minimum of 30 minutes
      b. Give Rh immune globulin or RhoGAM as ordered for women who are Rh negative.

N. GROUP B BETA STREPTOCOCCUS (GBBS) CULTURE
   1. DESCRIPTION
      a. Vaginal and rectal culture to test for GBBS
      b. Universal screening at 35–37 weeks of gestation
      c. Antibiotic treatment during labor for positive cultures
      d. Treated with PCN if not allergic
      e. Indicated for clients hospitalized preterm with high-risk pregnancy conditions
      f. Untreated GBBS disease in neonates is the leading cause of infectious mortality in the neonate.

IV. **NURSING DIAGNOSES**
   A. DEFICIENT KNOWLEDGE
   B. ACUTE PAIN
   C. RISK FOR CONSTIPATION
   D. DISTURBED BODY IMAGE
   E. INEFFECTIVE COPING
   F. RISK FOR DEFICIENT FLUID VOLUME
   G. NONCOMPLIANCE
   H. ANXIETY
   I. IMBALANCED NUTRITION: LESS THAN BODY REQUIREMENTS

Nursing Diagnoses: Definitions and Classification 2012–2014.
Copyright © 2012, 1994–2012 by NANDA International.
Used by arrangement with John Wiley & Sons Limited.

V. **NORMAL PREGNANCY**
   A. **CHARACTERISTICS**
      1. 40 LUNAR WEEKS OF GESTATION
      2. A TERM PREGNANCY IS FROM THE BEGINNING OF THE 38TH WEEK UNTIL THE COMPLETION OF 42 WEEKS.
   B. NORMAL CONCERNS OF PREGNANCY
      1. NAUSEA AND VOMITING
      2. BREAST TENDERNESS
      3. URINARY FREQUENCY
      4. CONSTIPATION AND HEMORRHOIDS
      5. LIGHTHEADEDNESS OR DIZZINESS
      6. LEG CRAMPS
      7. FATIGUE
      8. HEARTBURN
      9. BACKACHE
      10. EMOTIONAL REACTIONS
      11. SEXUALITY AND INTIMACY

VI. HIGH-RISK PREGNANCY CONDITIONS

A. PRETERM LABOR (PTL)

1. DESCRIPTION
   a. Progressive dilation or effacement of the cervix with uterine contractions or cervical dilation greater than or equal to 2 cm or cervical effacement of greater than 80% between 20 and 37 weeks of gestation with intact membranes
   b. It is not the same as low birth weight, which is less than or equal to 2500 grams at birth, which can occur with prematurity but also from other conditions causing intrauterine growth restriction (IUGR) such as PIH.
   c. Complications include premature rupture of membranes and preterm birth (PTB). Complications from PTB result in 60–85% of fetal and neonatal deaths and are the single greatest cause of neonatal morbidity and mortality.
   d. Risk factors for PTL: African-American race, young or advanced maternal age, low socioeconomic status, history of previous PTB, multiple pregnancy losses or abortions, uterine or cervical anomalies, infection, incompetent cervix, bleeding during pregnancy, multiple pregnancy, premature rupture of membranes, smoking, or substance use

2. ASSESSMENT
   a. Careful history
   b. Uterine contractions
   c. Feeling that the baby is balling up and relaxing
   d. Rhythmic back pain, thigh pain, and change in vaginal mucus

3. DIAGNOSTIC TESTS
   a. Electronic fetal monitoring: for uterine contractions and to assess for fetal well-being by evaluation of FHR
   b. Vaginal ultrasound: to evaluate cervical change
   c. Fetal fibronectin

4. MEDICAL-SURGICAL MANAGEMENT
   a. Hospitalization
   b. Antenatal glucocorticoids for promotion of fetal lung maturity
   c. Tocolytic therapy (see Table 42-3)
   d. Prophylactic IV antibiotics (PCN or clindamycin if PCN allergy) if group B beta strep infection intravaginally

5. NURSING INTERVENTIONS
   a. Encourage hydration.
   b. Monitor for contractions with EFM and by hand palpation.
   c. Monitor maternal vital signs.
   d. Provide comfort measures and emotional support.
   e. Report the changes to the physician.
   f. Obtain lab specimens as ordered.
   g. Encourage bed rest and side-lying position.
   h. Prepare the client and family for possible diagnostic procedures and tests.
   i. Instruct the client about the early clinical manifestations to report.
   j. Perform kick counts daily or twice daily.
   k. Palpate the uterus for contraction.
   l. Perform a digital cervical exam to evaluate for cervical change.

Table 42-3 Tocolytic Therapy

Drug	Dose	Adverse Reactions	Contraindications
Terbutaline (Brethine)	0.25 mg s.q.; may repeat after 15–20 minutes; maximum 0.5 mg in 4 hours	Tachycardia, palpitations, nervousness or drowsiness, tremors, headache, pulmonary edema, cardiac arrhythmia, hyperglycemia	Cardiac arrhythmia, poorly controlled diabetes, hypertension, hyperthyroidism
Magnesium sulfate	4–6 g IV bolus over 20 minutes; then 2–4 g/hr infusion	Flushing, lethargy, headache, muscle weakness, dry mouth, diplopia, pulmonary edema, cardiac arrest, respiratory insufficiency	Myasthenia gravis, respiratory depression
Nifedipine (Procardia)	20 mg p.o. loading dose; then 10–20 mg p.o. every 4–6 hours, or 30 mg p.o. every 6 hours	Flushing, headache, dizziness, nausea, transient hypotension	Cardiac disease, use caution with renal disease, maternal hypotension, avoid concomitant use with magnesium sulfate
Indomethacin	Loading dose: 50 mg per rectum or 50–100 mg p.o. then 25–50 mg p.o. every 4 hours for 48 hours	Nausea, heartburn Fetal: renal insufficiency, premature closure of ductus arteriosus, oligohydramnios	ASA allergy, significant renal or hepatic impairment

B. INCOMPETENT CERVIX
1. DESCRIPTION
    a. May result in spontaneous abortion or preterm delivery
    b. Clients at risk include those with uterine or cervical anomalies, previous cervical surgery, cervical infection or inflammation, maternal DES (diethylstilbestrol) exposure.
    c. Must be differentiated from PTL
    d. Complications include PTB, premature rupture of membranes, and intrauterine infection or chorioamnionitis.
2. ASSESSMENT
    a. Effacement and dilation of the cervix not associated with pain or uterine contractions
3. DIAGNOSTIC TESTS
    a. Similar to PTL, excluding fetal fibronectin
4. MEDICAL-SURGICAL MANAGEMENT
    a. Similar to PTL but may involve the surgical placement of a cervical cerclage (a looping stitch through the cervix) to hold the cervix closed; the stitch must be removed during labor or the client is at risk for cervical or uterine rupture.
5. NURSING INTERVENTIONS
    a. Similar to PTL
    b. Evaluate for contractions—palpate with your hand and use an electronic fetal monitor.
    c. Evaluate cervical change through a digital exam or vaginal sonogram.
    d. Assess lab values and clinical picture for infectious process.
C. PREMATURE RUPTURE OF MEMBRANES (PROM)
1. DESCRIPTION
    a. Occurs in approximately 10% of all pregnancies
    b. One in 10 PROM occurs before term; preterm PROM is discussed in this chapter as a high-risk pregnancy condition requiring hospitalization.
    c. Clients with PROM at term need to be hospitalized for delivery.
    d. Complications include risks to the mother and risks to the fetus.
        1) Risks to the mother include sepsis secondary to chorioamnionitis, postpartum endometritis, placental abruption (decompression of the bag can tear the placenta away from the uterine wall), and death.
        2) Risks to the fetus include umbilical cord prolapse, meconium aspiration, infection or sepsis, skeletal compression deformities, abruption, death, onset of labor/prematurity, and possibly cerebral palsy secondary to chorioamnionitis.
2. ASSESSMENT
    a. Premature rupture of membranes before the onset of labor
3. DIAGNOSTIC TESTS
    a. SSE
    b. Ultrasound for amniotic fluid index (AFI); fluid volume is likely to be down if the client has PROM.
    c. BPP to determine fetal well-being
    d. Serial lab tests (complete blood count [CBC] and C-reactive protein [CRP]) to monitor for infection
    e. Amniocentesis to determine presence of subclinical (subtle) infection (chorioamnionitis) is sometimes necessary.
4. MEDICAL-SURGICAL MANAGEMENT
    a. Hospitalize the client.
    b. Prophylactic antibiotic regimen currently ampicillin IV and erythromycin orally
    c. Antenatal glucocorticoids for fetal lung maturity
    d. Induction of labor for early signs of infection if the fetus is in cephalic position (otherwise surgical delivery is indicated)
    e. Emergency cesarean section for fetal distress and placental abruption
    f. Close observation for complications in the hospital until 34–36 weeks of gestation when the goal of treatment becomes delivery
5. NURSING INTERVENTIONS
    a. Medicate as prescribed.
    b. Encourage bed rest in the Trendelenburg position to minimize leaking of amniotic fluid.
    c. Encourage hydration.
    d. Monitor maternal vital signs.
    e. Monitor intake and output.
    f. Provide comfort measures and support.
    g. Encourage side-lying position.
    h. Report any changes to the physician.
    i. Monitor the vital signs for signs of infection, such as fever and tachycardia.
    j. Assess for contractions, which could be onset of labor.
    k. Palpate the abdomen and uterus for tenderness.
    l. Ask the client about pain such as uterine infection or abruption,

contractions indicating labor, vaginal leaking, vaginal bleeding that may indicate abruption, and fetal movements as well as complaints of malaise.

  m. Monitor FHR pattern for fetal well-being and consider chorioamnionitis (infection in the amniotic bag) if fetal tachycardia is present.

D. DIABETES IN PREGNANCY
  1. DESCRIPTION
    a. Pregestational diabetes mellitus: type 1 and type 2 are diagnosed before pregnancy.
    b. Gestational diabetes mellitus (GDM) is impaired glucose tolerance with pregnancy; also referred to as diabetes mellitus (DM) type 3.
    c. Diabetes in pregnancy is further classified by the time of onset as well as organ involvement known as White's classification.
    d. Oral hypoglycemics are contraindicated in pregnancy; if medication is required, the client is managed with insulin.
    e. Maternal complications include increased risk for the mother developing DM later in life if GDM and fetal complications include risks to pregnancy such as macrosomia, stillbirth, organ malformations, pre-eclampsia, and increased chance of operative delivery
  2. ASSESSMENT (SEE CHAPTER 6, ENDOCRINE DISORDERS, DIABETES MELLITUS)
  3. DIAGNOSTIC TESTS
    a. A 50-g oral glucose challenge is administered, with blood drawn 1 hour after, and if the client fails the 1-hour test, a 100-g glucose challenge is given with blood draws at 1, 2, and 3 hours after drinking the glucose.
    b. Screen at first prenatal if client has any risk factors.
    c. Otherwise screen at 24 to 28 weeks.
  4. NURSING INTERVENTIONS
    a. Provide the client with an appropriate diet if hospitalized.
    b. Instruct the client on the nature of the disease.
    c. Encourage hydration.
    d. Encourage side-lying.
    e. Blood glucose readings are taken fasting, before meals, 1 hour postprandial (pp) and at bedtime: glycemic goals are less than 95 fasting, less than 120 1 hour pp, and less than 100 before meals.

    f. Administer insulin as ordered or instruct the client on self-administration.
    g. Encourage the client to monitor fetal movement.
    h. Ask about risk factors: overweight, family history of DM, previous GDM, ethnic predisposition, and prior birth of infant over 9 pounds (macrosomia), polyhydramnios, or stillbirth.

E. VAGINAL BLEEDING FROM ABRUPTIO PLACENTAE
  1. DESCRIPTION
    a. Placental abruption is found in 13% of cases of vaginal bleeding after 20 weeks; 7% of these cases are placenta previa and the other 80% are thought to be early labor, local bleeding lesions in the lower genital tract, or no source can be identified.
    b. Placental abruption is premature separation of the normally implanted placenta from the uterine wall.
    c. The separation creates a hemorrhage at the site of separation, causing a hematoma; as the hematoma grows, there is further separation.
    d. The amount of placenta detached from the uterine wall is the amount of surface area lost for the exchange of respiratory gases and nutrients for the fetus.
    e. Associated causes and risks include cocaine use, trauma, sudden decompression of the uterine cavity as in PROM, maternal hypertension, cigarette smoking, advanced maternal age, and multiparity.
    f. Maternal complications include hemorrhage, disseminated intravascular coagulation (DIC), and death, and fetal complications include intrauterine growth restriction, congenital abnormalities, neonatal anemia, fetal distress, and death.
  2. ASSESSMENT
    a. Severe abdominal pain with or without vaginal bleeding as the growing hematoma creates pressure inside the uterine cavity
    b. Painful hard abdomen
    c. Fetal distress
  3. DIAGNOSTIC TESTS
    a. D-dimer and fibrinogen
    b. Ultrasound
  4. NURSING INTERVENTIONS
    a. Monitor vital signs for cardiovascular stability and the abdomen for signs of abruption.
    b. Assess fetal status with EFM.

c. Assess the client's blood type and Rh factor, gestational age, amount of bleeding, painful or painless bleeding, and presence of other medical conditions such as bleeding disorders.

d. Obtain IV access with a minimum 18-gauge needle.

e. Prepare for an emergency cesarean section if the client is experiencing an acute placental abruption.

f. Administer IV fluid bolus or blood transfusions as ordered.

g. Obtain lab specimens as ordered.

h. Provide emotional support to the client and family.

i. Ask clarifying questions to help differentiate between previa and abruption; painful labor contractions may precipitate bleeding from the previa and thus confuse the clinical picture.

j. Avoid performing a vaginal exam if the client is bleeding vaginally.

k. Palpate the abdomen for hard, boardlike texture, which indicates there is trapped blood in the uterus if the abruption is in the upper uterine segment and cannot flow out the cervix.

l. Estimate blood loss—count peripads and determine how quickly the client is saturating one peripad and weigh the pads (1 g = 1 m).

F. VAGINAL BLEEDING FROM PLACENTA PREVIA

1. DESCRIPTION

a. Of cases of vaginal bleeding after 20 weeks, 7% involve documented placenta previa, as discussed previously.

b. The placenta is covering or encroaching on the internal os to varying degrees (different classifications).

1) Total placenta previa or complete previa covers the os in the third trimester.

2) Partial placenta previa covers part of the internal os.

3) Marginal placenta previa does not cover the os but lies within 2–3 cm of it.

4) Low-lying placenta is implanted in the lower uterine segment but does not lie within 2–3 cm of the os.

c. Most placentas that appear to cover the os during the second trimester will move or migrate and not cover the os at term.

d. Risk factors include advanced maternal age, multiparity, African or Asian ethnic background, prior placenta previa, smoking, one or more previous cesarean births, and cocaine use.

2. ASSESSMENT

a. Sudden onset of painless vaginal bleeding in the second or third trimester

3. DIAGNOSTIC TESTS

a. D-dimer and fibrinogen

b. Ultrasound

4. NURSING INTERVENTIONS

a. See the nursing interventions for abruptio placentae on page 828.

b. Prepare the client for an emergency cesarean section if term or the bleeding is persistent and excessive.

c. Place the client on bed rest with a bedside commode or bathroom privileges.

d. Perform intermittent EFM for onset of labor and fetal well-being.

e. Administer antenatal steroids as ordered.

f. Encourage side-lying position.

g. Provide the client and family education.

h. Maintain IV access.

G. PREGNANCY-INDUCED HYPERTENSION (PIH)

1. DESCRIPTION

a. The term *PIH* is used interchangeably with *pre-eclampsia*.

b. Occurs in 5–10% of pregnancies

c. Complex disease process with physiologic effects ranging from hypertension to multiorgan failure

d. May progress into HELLP (hemolysis elevated liver enzymes low platelets) syndrome with liver involvement and platelet destruction, which is life threatening, or seizures from cerebral edema (eclampsia)

e. Risk factors for developing PIH include first pregnancy, older than 40 years old, African-American race, DM, twin pregnancy, family history of PIH, antiphospholipid antibody syndrome, and chronic hypertension or renal problems.

2. ASSESSMENT

a. Headache

b. Visual changes

c. Right upper quadrant pain

d. Epigastric pain

e. Nausea and vomiting

3. DIAGNOSTIC TESTS

a. 24-hour urine for proteinuria

b. CBC to evaluate platelet destruction (thrombocytopenia)

c. Labs such as BUN, LDH, ALT, AST, uric acid, and serum creatinine to evaluate other organ involvement, blood type and antibody screen

d. Ultrasound to determine intrauterine growth restriction or oligohydramnios (decreased amniotic fluid)

e. Biophysical profile on the fetus via ultrasound

f. Umbilical artery Doppler studies via ultrasound

4. NURSING INTERVENTIONS

  a. Promote bed rest—encourage side-lying position.

  b. Perform frequent assessments of maternal hemodynamics, lung sounds, urine output, reflexes, symptoms or neurologic irritability, and fetal well-being.

  c. Encourage hydration.

  d. Decrease stimulus in the client's environment as the pre-eclampsia progresses.

  e. Monitor the blood pressure.

  f. Test the urine with a urine dipstick to test for protein in the urine, which indicates kidney involvement from the disease process allowing too much protein to spill into the urine.

  g. Inspect for edema: peripheral, sacral, generalized (anasarca) or facial.

  h. Perform deep tendon reflexes (DTR) for hyperreflexia from cerebral edema.

  i. Palpate for liver tenderness (right upper quadrant [RUQ]) and epigastric discomfort.

  j. Auscultate lung sounds.

  k. Measure intake and output to determine oliguria.

  l. Administer magnesium sulfate IV infusion to quiet the CNS if eclampsia is threatened.

  m. Prepare for dexamethasone dosing if thrombocytopenia is severe to abate platelet destruction if HELLP syndrome.

  n. Provide steroid prophylaxis for fetal lung maturity before 34 weeks of gestation.

  o. Inform the client that surgical delivery is likely.

H. HYPEREMESIS GRAVIDARUM

  1. DESCRIPTION

    a. Nausea and vomiting are common in pregnancy due to the hormones of pregnancy in the first 10 weeks, but excessive or persistent vomiting is hyperemesis gravidarum.

    b. Criteria for the disorder are met with 5% weight loss along with dehydration, electrolyte imbalance, ketosis, and acetonuria (nitrogen compounds like urea in urine).

    c. Risk factors include young maternal age (less than 20 years old), obese,

nonsmoker, multifetal pregnancy, and molar pregnancy.

    d. Maternal complications include decreased maternal weight gain and electrolyte imbalances, and fetal complications include decreased fetal weight gain with an increased mortality rate.

  2. ASSESSMENT

    a. Excessive or persistent vomiting

  3. NURSING INTERVENTIONS

    a. Provide small, frequent meals, as tolerated, after an initial period of NPO.

    b. Administer IV hydration such as dextrose if indicated.

    c. Monitor intake and output.

    d. Administer antiemetics, as ordered, to maximize oral intake.

    e. Provide parenteral nutrition via central line, as ordered, if long-term parenteral nutrition is indicated.

    f. Monitor daily weight.

I. HEART DISEASE

  1. DESCRIPTION

    a. With the cardiac output increasing 30–50% during pregnancy, the hemodynamic changes increase the workload on the heart; a heart that is compromised by heart disease may not be able to meet the demands of pregnancy.

    b. The prognosis for the pregnancy and the plan of care depend on the degree of cardiac compromise.

    c. The cardiac disease is classified by the level of functional capacity.

    d. The most common complication is heart failure.

  2. ASSESSMENT

    a. Edema: pedal, pitting, pulmonary, and generalized (anasarca)

    b. Poor oxygenation: dyspnea at rest or with exertion, excessive fatigue, nailbed cyanosis, circumoral cyanosis, basilar rales, and moist cough

    c. Tachycardia, murmurs, chest pain, and irregular pulse

  3. DIAGNOSTIC TESTS

    a. None

  4. NURSING INTERVENTIONS

    a. Monitor the client for signs of cardiac overload throughout pregnancy.

    b. Evaluate fetal well-being throughout pregnancy.

    c. Instruct the client as follows: avoid excessive weight gain and emotional stress, report any signs of infection promptly, and avoid anemia with adequate nutrition and supplements.

    d. Avoid anemia with Fe supplementation.

    e. Administer prophylactic antibiotics such as penicillin (unless allergic) for invasive procedures to prevent bacterial endocarditis.

    f. Administer prescribed diuretics.

    g. Treat dysrhythmias and use cardiac glycosides (digitalis) to slow the heart rate and strengthen contractions, making the heart more effective.

J. SUBSTANCE ABUSE

  1. DESCRIPTION

    a. Substances include alcohol, tobacco, marijuana, cocaine, and heroin.

    b. Many clients use substances in combination.

  2. ASSESSMENT

    a. Clinical manifestations depend on the type of drug abused.

  3. DIAGNOSTIC TEST

    a. Toxicology screening of urine for drugs

  4. NURSING INTERVENTIONS

    a. Support all the client's efforts to decrease substance use.

    b. Monitor the fetus for complications such as spontaneous abortion, intrauterine growth restriction (IUGR), placental abruption, stillbirth, PTL, PROM, fetal alcohol syndrome (FAS), PIH, and neonatal addiction.

    c. Screen the client for use of substances.

    d. Encourage the client to disclose all substances and amount used as well as patterns of use and previous efforts to quit.

    e. Monitor for maternal complications such as anemia, inadequate nutrition, maternal risks of PROM and PIH, and social implications including surrendering custody of the infant to authorities for certain substances.

    f. Promote a slow withdrawal during pregnancy; clients addicted to heroin may be put on methadone hydrochloride during withdrawal to block severe symptoms.

K. HUMAN IMMUNODEFICIENCY VIRUS (HIV)

  1. DESCRIPTION

    a. Acquired immunodeficiency syndrome (AIDS) is caused by HIV where the classic symptoms surround the severely impaired immune system and devastating opportunistic infections.

    b. The disease is transmitted through blood and body fluids, sharing of contaminated needles by IV drug users, vertical transmission from vaginal childbirth, through the placenta, and through breast milk.

    c. Antiretroviral drugs that control replication of the virus are given to the client throughout pregnancy or initiated during labor and delivery if newly diagnosed or noncompliant.

    d. The newborn will test positive for the maternal HIV antibodies that cross the placenta until up to 18 months; antiretrovirals are continued for the infant to promote this process of seroconversion when the maternal antibodies are depleted from the infant's body.

    e. Complications for uncontrolled AIDS are fatal for the client and infant.

  2. ASSESSMENT

    a. Flu-like syndrome

    b. Night sweats

    c. Chronic diarrhea

    d. Recurrent headaches

    e. Extreme fatigue

    f. Oral hairy leukoplakia

  3. DIAGNOSTIC TESTS

    a. ELISA

    b. Western blot

  4. NURSING INTERVENTIONS

    a. Maintain a nonjudgmental attitude.

    b. Offer emotional support and counseling as needed.

    c. Monitor the client for presence of infections.

    d. Implement universal precautions.

    e. Instruct the client about the need for antiretroviral medications during pregnancy and for the infant once born.

    f. Prepare the client for the need to formula feed the infant (breastfeeding is contraindicated).

    g. Monitor for fetal well-being.

    h. Evaluate for other sexually transmitted diseases and hepatitis B.

    i. Monitor the progress of viral status or disease state with lab tests: viral load and CD4 count.

L. ECTOPIC PREGNANCY

  1. DESCRIPTION

    a. The fertilized ovum implants outside the uterus.

    b. The most common site is the fallopian tube.

    c. Risk factors include tubal surgery leading to scarring and narrowing, infections in the tubes, pelvic inflammatory disease (PID), and intrauterine device (IUD) contraceptive device.

    d. Positive pregnancy clinical manifestations

    e. If the ovum has grown enough to cause pressure, the client will exhibit unilateral lower abdominal pain, which may build gradually or have sudden onset.

    f. No pregnancy is revealed in the uterus by ultrasound.

    g. Ovum must be destroyed with medication or removed surgically.

2. ASSESSMENT
  a. Vaginal bleeding
  b. Abdominal pain
  c. Hypotensive
3. DIAGNOSTIC TESTS
  a. B-hCG
  b. Ultrasound
4. NURSING INTERVENTIONS
  a. Monitor for signs of hemodynamic instability and shock with ruptured ectopic pregnancy.
  b. Start an 18-gauge IV, have oxygen available, and prepare the client for surgery (whenever possible the fallopian tube will be left intact for future fertility).
  c. Allow the client and her family to grieve the lost pregnancy.
  d. Administer RhoGAM for appropriate clients.
M. HYDATIFORM MOLE
  1. DESCRIPTION
    a. Also called gestational trophoblastic disease, as it is an abnormal growth of trophoblastic tissue (early placenta)
    b. Chorionic villi tissue of the placenta grows into grapelike cluster of fluid-filled sacs.
    c. It may have a partial embryo that will usually spontaneously abort in the first trimester.
    d. It can develop into choriocarcinoma or into malignant trophoblastic disease.
  2. ASSESSMENT
    a. The client will have positive pregnancy clinical manifestations but abnormal lab values; B-hCG is very high and maternal alpha-fetoprotein is very low.
    b. Excessive nausea and vomiting are common with high B-hCG levels.
    c. Ultrasound has a classic "snowstorm" pattern.
    d. May have vaginal bleeding or pass parts of the mole, which looks similar to grapes
  3. DIAGNOSTIC TESTS
    a. B-hCG and alpha-fetoprotein
    b. Ultrasound
  4. NURSING INTERVENTIONS
    a. Assess clients with very high B-hCG levels for molar pregnancy.
    b. Once determined, monitor for PIH, bleeding, or DIC.
    c. Assist with the evacuation of the mole.
    d. Allow the client and family to grieve the loss of the pregnancy.
    e. Administer RhoGAM for appropriate clients.
    f. Instruct the client on the importance of follow-up in the next year for early detection of cancer.

Table 42-4 Clinical Classifications of Abortion

Classification	Description
Threatened abortion	Vaginal bleeding through a closed cervix; possible cramping.
Inevitable abortion	Vaginal bleeding and uterine cramping are accompanied by cervical dilation.
Incomplete abortion	Vaginal bleeding and uterine cramping result in expulsion of part of the products of conception.
Complete abortion	Vaginal bleeding and uterine cramping result in expulsion of all the products of conception.
Missed abortion	Fetus died in utero but has not been expelled.

© Cengage Learning 2015

  g. Instruct the client on contraception for the next year; conception is discouraged in case chemotherapy is indicated for the development of cancer.
N. SPONTANEOUS ABORTION
  1. DESCRIPTION
    a. Unplanned pregnancy loss before 20 weeks of gestation
    b. Also referred to as a miscarriage
    c. Clinical classifications vary (see Table 42-4).
  2. ASSESSMENT
    a. Vaginal bleeding
    b. Passage of clots or tissue
    c. Uterine cramping
    d. Declining B-hCG levels
    e. Absence of fetal heart tones or absence of fetal movement
  3. DIAGNOSTIC TESTS
    a. FHR Doppler
    b. Possibly ultrasound
    c. Lab values such as CBC to monitor maternal blood loss
    d. B-hCG level
  4. NURSING INTERVENTIONS
    a. Monitor for maternal blood loss and hemodynamic status—estimate the amount of bleeding, monitor vital signs, and be prepared for shock with a minimum 18-gauge needle IV.
    b. Prepare the client for surgery if products of conception are retained; dilation and curettage (D&C) is indicated for incomplete abortion.
    c. Medicate for pain as indicated.
    d. Allow the client and family to grieve the pregnancy loss.
    e. Administer RhoGAM to appropriate clients.
    f. Advise bed rest for threatened abortions.
    g. Evacuate the uterus for incomplete and missed abortions.

PRACTICE QUESTIONS

1. During a prenatal visit, the nurse evaluates the fundal height of the uterus to be at the umbilicus. The nurse should estimate the gestation at
   1. 16 weeks.
   2. 20 weeks.
   3. 24 weeks.
   4. 28 weeks.

2. A client is receiving education about preterm labor during a prenatal visit. Which of the following is a priority for the nurse to instruct the client to report?
   1. Nausea and vomiting
   2. Back pain that radiates down into the buttocks and legs
   3. Feeling that the baby is balling up and relaxing
   4. Vaginal spotting after a vaginal exam

3. A client asks the nurse what is the purpose of the placenta. Based on the understanding of the metabolic functions of the placenta, which of the following would be the most appropriate response by the nurse? The purposes of the placenta for the baby include which of the following?
   Select all that apply:
   [ ] 1. Cushion
   [ ] 2. Protects the skin
   [ ] 3. Respiration
   [ ] 4. Excretion
   [ ] 5. Pancreatic function
   [ ] 6. Nutrition

4. The nurse evaluates a vaginal and rectal group B beta strep culture at how many weeks of gestation? _____

5. A client is 24 weeks pregnant and has just been told at her prenatal visit that her amniotic fluid volume has decreased. She is confused and asks the nurse, "What does that mean for my baby?" Which of the following is the appropriate response by the nurse?
   1. "The amniotic fluid is important for the baby. You should ask your doctor about that."
   2. "The less amniotic fluid, the more your baby is at risk for complications. The fluid protects the baby from trauma and helps the baby develop."
   3. "Your membranes may have ruptured, which heralds the beginning of labor. I think it would be a good idea to notify your labor support person."

   4. "You need to ask the doctor that question. In the meantime, I will notify the hospital you will be coming."

6. A pregnant client is admitted to the hospital for preterm labor. The nurse's first intervention is to
   1. obtain a complete history and update the physician.
   2. initiate IV hydration and begin tocolytic medication.
   3. obtain a fetal fibronectin and a complete blood count.
   4. monitor for contractions and fetal well-being.

7. After a routine screening ultrasound, a pregnant client in her third trimester asks the nurse to explain where all the fluid comes from that surrounds her baby. The nurse's response should be based on the understanding that the amniotic fluid is
   1. fluid from the maternal serum that diffuses passively across the membranes.
   2. primarily fetal urine maintained by a balance of production and reabsorption.
   3. produced primarily by the placenta and remains static unless rupture of the membranes has occurred.
   4. fluid from the fetal serum that diffuses actively across the membranes.

8. A pregnant client who is 28 weeks pregnant and is taking an exercise class calls the prenatal clinic to ask if there are any maneuvers that should be avoided. Which of the following should the nurse instruct the client to avoid?
   1. Lifting the arms over the head
   2. Pelvic rocking
   3. Sitting with the knees tucked up against the chest
   4. Lying supine

9. Admitting a pregnant client to the hospital from the prenatal clinic for preterm premature rupture of membranes, the nurse includes in the client teaching which of the following treatment expectations?
   1. Drugs will include antibiotic coverage
   2. Activity will be restricted to ambulating in the hospital room
   3. Blood pressure will need to be continuously monitored
   4. Amniotic fluid volume will need to be continuously monitored

10. The nurse working in a triage clinic should return which one of the following clients' telephone messages first? A woman who is at
    1. 37 weeks of gestation with shortness of breath.
    2. 10 weeks of gestation with breast tenderness.
    3. 35 weeks of gestation with feet that swell at the end of the day.
    4. 12 weeks of gestation with darkening blotches of skin over her cheekbones.

11. A pregnant client asks the nurse about gestational diabetes mellitus. The nurse responds based on the understanding that gestational diabetes in pregnancy is
    1. an impaired glucose tolerance.
    2. beta cell failure in pregnancy.
    3. type 1 DM undetected prior to pregnancy.
    4. type 2 DM undetected prior to pregnancy.

12. A client of Mediterranean descent tells the nurse that her mother told her she was at greater risk for which of the following blood disorders?
    1. Sickle-cell disease
    2. Tay-Sachs disease
    3. Thalassemia
    4. Phenylketonuria

13. Which of the following is the appropriate pregnancy classification for a client pregnant for the third time, whose first pregnancy ended in a miscarriage at 9 weeks and second pregnancy was a vaginal delivery at 39 weeks of gestation and the child is 3 years old now?
    1. Gravida 3 para 1-0-1-1
    2. Gravida 2 para 2-1-1-0
    3. Gravida 3 para 3-2-0-1-0
    4. Gravida 2 para 2-1-0-0

14. Which of the following health indicators for a client does the nurse evaluate as a risk factor for diabetes mellitus in pregnancy?
    Select all that apply:
    [ ] 1. History of ovarian tumors
    [ ] 2. Caucasian
    [ ] 3. Prior stillbirth
    [ ] 4. Polyhydramnios
    [ ] 5. History of DES exposure
    [ ] 6. Overweight

15. The nurse has implemented education about HIV in pregnancy. Which statement illustrates that the pregnant HIV-positive client understood the nurse's teaching about HIV and pregnancy?
    1. "My baby will not have AIDS."
    2. "I will need to take a drug throughout my pregnancy."
    3. "They will start giving me a drug for HIV when I come in to deliver."
    4. "I will need to continue taking the HIV drug the entire time I breastfeed."

16. A pregnant client is African American and had a baby with a birth weight of 10 lb 2 oz with her last pregnancy. Based on this information, the nurse expects that the oral glucose tolerance test should be done
    1. at the first prenatal appointment.
    2. at 28 weeks of gestation.
    3. at the end of the first trimester.
    4. when the client evidences glucose in the urine.

17. During a prenatal visit, a client approaching term asks many questions about labor and delivery. The nurse's response should be based on the understanding of normal adaptation to pregnancy because
    1. anger and confusion often follow initial ambivalence as the client nears term.
    2. a client has fears for safe laboring and delivery as the end of pregnancy approaches.
    3. it is typical for a client to only have questions as the end of the pregnancy approaches.
    4. pregnant clients will enter a phase of trust at term and ask questions only as they near term.

18. The nurse informs a client that quickening or the first fetal movements are felt between how many weeks of gestation? _____

19. The nurse emphasizes the importance of good glycemic control during pregnancy to a client. Which of the following potential fetal complications does the nurse include in the education?
    Select all that apply:
    [ ] 1. Intraventricular hemorrhage (IVH)
    [ ] 2. Organ malformations
    [ ] 3. Placenta previa
    [ ] 4. Pre-eclampsia
    [ ] 5. Pancreatic tumors
    [ ] 6. Macrosomia

20. During pregnancy, the client experiences infrequent, nonpainful, uterine contractions. The nurse documents this as _____.

21. After delivering a newborn infant, a client asks about the appearance of the umbilical cord. Based on an understanding of anatomy and physiology, which of the following responses by the nurse would be appropriate?
    1. "There is protective tissue called chorionic villi, which surround the vessels in the cord."
    2. "The umbilical cord is normally coiled with three vessels evident from any side of the cord."
    3. "The umbilical cord normally develops one to two knots during pregnancy from fetal movement."
    4. "The vessels in the cord are surrounded by a connective tissue called Wharton's jelly."

22. Based on the understanding of the physiologic adaptations of pregnancy, the nurse understands the client may have complications because of which of the following?
    1. Blood volume increases 30–50% during pregnancy
    2. Thyroid function decreases 10–25% during pregnancy
    3. Respiratory rate increases by one-third during pregnancy
    4. Follicle-stimulating hormone (FSH) and luteinizing hormone (LH) production is stimulated and overproduced during pregnancy

23. Which of the following interventions should the nurse include in the plan of care for a client who has diabetes in pregnancy?
    Select all that apply:
    [ ] 1. Monitor vital signs for cardiovascular stability
    [ ] 2. Encourage the client to monitor fetal movement
    [ ] 3. Place the client on bed rest with a bedside commode
    [ ] 4. Provide the client with an appropriate diet if hospitalized
    [ ] 5. Encourage side-lying position
    [ ] 6. Monitor 24-hour urine for proteinuria

24. A pregnant client is hospitalized for vaginal bleeding from suspected abruptio placentae. The nurse bases the appropriate interventions on which understanding of the pathology?
    1. Placenta tears away from the cervical os during dilation and results in fetal hemorrhage
    2. Placental abruption is umbilical cord hemorrhage from trauma

    3. Placental abruption is premature separation of the normally implanted placenta from the uterine wall
    4. Abruptio placentae is the rupturing of membranes along the uterine wall and the resulting loss of fetal blood and amniotic fluid

25. The registered nurse is delegating client assignments on a maternity unit. Which of the following assignments should the nurse delegate to a licensed practical nurse?
    1. Provide the care to a client suspected of having abruptio placentae
    2. Provide the care to a woman in her 37th week of gestation experiencing dyspnea
    3. Teach a pregnancy class to a group of women
    4. Document the characteristics of a woman's lochia

26. Which of the following risk factors should the nurse include in a class for clients with diabetes in pregnancy?
    Select all that apply:
    [ ] 1. Prior birth of an infant over 9 pounds
    [ ] 2. Twin pregnancy
    [ ] 3. Polyhydramnios
    [ ] 4. Having a stillbirth infant
    [ ] 5. Cocaine use
    [ ] 6. Young maternal age (less than 20 years old).

27. A pregnant client asks the nurse when the stretch marks will disappear. The most appropriate response by the nurse is
    1. "They will disappear with the birth of the infant."
    2. "They will take up to 6 months to disappear."
    3. "They will fade but do not totally disappear."
    4. "They will disappear with a nutritionally balanced diet and exercise."

ANSWERS AND RATIONALES

1. 2. The fundal height rises 1 cm/week until the 36th week of gestation and is at the umbilicus (20 cm) at 20 weeks of gestation.

2. 3. A feeling that the baby is balling up and relaxing is a classic clinical manifestation of preterm labor. Nausea, vomiting, and back pain that radiates down the buttocks and legs should be reported if they continue, but are not indications of preterm labor. Vaginal spotting after a vaginal exam is a normal finding.

3. 3. 4. 6. The placenta is responsible for the gas exchange (respiration), for nutrients that actively and passively cross the placental

membrane for the fetus (nutrition), and for removal of metabolic waste for the fetus (excretion).

4. 35–37 weeks. At 35–37 weeks of gestation, a vaginal and rectal group B beta strep culture is performed.

5. 2. Telling the client that less amniotic fluid places the baby at risk for complications, and that the fluid protects the baby from trauma and helps the baby develop, answers the client's question using as much information as the nurse has at the time, without assuming the fluid is low from ruptured membranes. Although telling the client that the amniotic fluid is good for the

baby is true, it does not answer the client's question. Telling the client that the membranes may have ruptured and labor has started informs the client that she will be hospitalized for labor and delivery of a 24-week infant; there is no information in the question to indicate that. Telling the client that she will need to ask the doctor her question puts the client off, and there may be no need for the client to go to the hospital.

6. 4. The first information the nurse should assess in a case of suspected preterm labor is to determine the labor pattern and if the fetus is evidencing any distress. This information will drive the rest of the plan of care.

7. 2. After the first trimester, the amniotic fluid is almost entirely fetal urine and is continually recycled via fetal swallowing and urinating.

8. 4. Lifting the arms over the head, pelvic rocking, and sitting with the knees tucked up against the chest do not need to be avoided because of pregnancy. Lying supine should be avoided because it will cause compression of the vena cava by the gravid uterus and result in supine hypotension, which will impair uterine blood flow and possibly cause the pregnant woman to faint.

9. 1. The client is at risk for an intrauterine infection and infection of the membranes called chorioamnionitis once there has been a rupture of membranes. Antibiotic coverage is the standard of care. Ambulation is restricted to prevent further loss of fluid. Blood pressure is not affected by loss of amniotic fluid. Amniotic fluid will need to be regularly monitored, but not continuously.

10. 1. Darkening blotches of skin over the cheekbone describes chloasma and is a normal finding called the mask of pregnancy. Breast tenderness from early pregnancy and hormonal changes are common. The swelling of feet at the end of the day is benign, as long as the swelling is resolved by morning. This can also indicate pre-eclampsia, a concern that should be investigated further. However, the first call should be made to the woman who is complaining of dyspnea. A woman who is in her 37th week can have dyspnea from the term gravid uterus pushing up on her diaphragm, but she may also be experiencing a respiratory emergency such as pulmonary embolus.

11. 1. Impaired glucose tolerance in pregnancy is the definition of gestational diabetes mellitus. Beta cell failure is the hallmark of type 1 diabetes mellitus.

12. 3. Thalassemia is an autosomal recessive genetic condition that causes an inadequate production of normal hemoglobin. It occurs in clients of Mediterranean descent. Sickle-cell disease is genetically linked to clients of African descent. Tay-Sachs disease is linked to Ashkenazi Jews. Phenylketonuria is an inborn error of metabolism.

13. 1. This client has conceived three times and has delivered a term infant and has one living child. A 9-week miscarriage is a spontaneous abortion.

14. 3. 4. 6. Risk factors include overweight, family history of diabetes mellitus, previous gestational diabetes mellitus, ethnic predisposition (African American, Native American, Hispanic), prior birth of infant over 9 lb, polyhydramnios, and stillbirth.

15. 2. Drugs (antiretrovirals) should be taken throughout pregnancy and not started at the onset of labor. The newborn will be considered infected with maternal antibodies and will be medicated until 18 months of age, when the infant can seroconvert to negative status. It is unknown if the infant will develop AIDS. Breastfeeding is prohibited to lower the risk of transmission to the newborn.

16. 1. A history of macrosomia is a positive finding in the client's medical history indicating early screening for gestational diabetes mellitus with this pregnancy. Macrosomia is a cause of cephalopelvic disproportion.

17. 2. Expressing fears of a safe delivery for the infant and self is a normal part of adaptation to pregnancy.

18. 16–18 weeks. Quickening, the first fetal movements, is felt by the pregnant client between 16 and 18 weeks of gestation.

19. 2. 4. 6. Fetal complications from diabetes mellitus in pregnancy include macrosomia, stillbirth, organ malformations, pre-eclampsia, and increased chance of operative delivery.

20. Braxton-Hicks contractions are ineffectual uterine contractions from uterine stretching during pregnancy.

21. 4. The umbilical cord is usually straight and the vessels are surrounded by a protective connective tissue called Wharton's jelly.

22. 1. Blood volume increases to perfuse the placenta and can cause complications for clients with cardiac disease or hypertension. Thyroid function increases to meet the demands of pregnancy. Other compensatory mechanisms in the respiratory system negate the need for tachypnea during pregnancy. Production of follicle-stimulating hormone (FSH) and luteinizing hormone (LH) is suppressed once their role in fertilization is completed.

23. 2. 3. 5. Nursing interventions for a client with diabetes in pregnancy include encouraging the client to monitor fetal movement, encouraging side-lying, and providing the client with an appropriate diet if hospitalized. An intervention for vaginal bleeding from abruption placentae is monitoring vital signs for cardiovascular stability. Placing a client on bed rest with a beside commode is an intervention for bleeding for placenta previa. Monitoring a client's urine for proteinuria is an intervention for a client with pregnancy-induced hypertension.

24. 3. Abruptio placentae is a premature separation of the normally implanted placenta from the uterine wall.

25. 4. Providing the care to a woman suspected of abruptio placentae and a woman in her 37th week of gestation experiencing dyspnea both require the skills of a registered nurse. A woman in her 37th week of gestation experiencing dyspnea may have a pulmonary embolus and requires the critical thinking skills of the registered nurse. Teaching a pregnancy class should be done by a registered nurse. A licensed practical nurse may document a woman's lochia.

26. 1. 3. 4. Risk factors for diabetes in pregnancy include having an infant over 9 pounds, polyhydramnios, or having a stillbirth infant. Vaginal bleeding from placenta previa occurs in a client who uses cocaine. Pregnancy-induced hypertension may occur in a twin pregnancy.

27. 3. The stretch marks a pregnant woman experiences will fade after the birth of the infant, but will not totally disappear.

REFERENCES

Daniels, R. (2010). *Delmar's manual of laboratory and diagnostic tests* (2nd ed.). Clifton Park, NY: Delmar Cengage Learning.

Garite, T. J. (2002). Intrapartum fetal evaluation. In S. G. Gabbe, J. R. Niebyl, & J. Simpson (Eds.), *Obstetrics: Normal and problem pregnancies* (4th ed., pp. 395–430). New York: Churchill Livingstone.

Iams, J. D. (2002). Preterm birth. In S. G. Gabbe, J. R. Niebyl, & J. Simpson (Eds.), *Obstetrics: Normal and problem pregnancies* (4th ed., pp. 755–826). New York: Churchill Livingstone.

Littleton, L., & Engebretson, J. (2002). *Maternal, neonatal, and women's health nursing*. Clifton Park, NY: Thomson Delmar Learning.

CHAPTER 43

THE INTRAPARTAL PERIOD

I. **ANATOMY AND PHYSIOLOGY**
   A. PELVIS (SEE FIGURE 43-1 AND TABLE 43-1)
      1. THE LAXITY OF THE SYMPHYSIS PUBIS INCREASES UNDER THE INFLUENCE OF RELAXIN.
   B. UTERUS
      1. IN PREGNANCY, THE SIZE OF THE UTERUS INCREASES TO 20 TIMES ITS NONPREGNANT SIZE, ITS WALLS THIN TO 1.5 CM, ITS WEIGHT INCREASES FROM 50 TO 1000 GRAMS, AND ITS CAPACITY INCREASES FROM LESS THAN 10 ML TO 4–8 LITERS.
   C. CERVIX
      1. THE CERVIX IS COMPOSED PRIMARILY OF FIBROUS CONNECTIVE TISSUE (COLLAGEN), AND ONLY 15% SMOOTH MUSCLE.
      UNDER THE INFLUENCE OF PROSTAGLANDINS, COLLAGEN DEGRADES AND THE CERVIX SOFTENS AND "RIPENS."
   D. VAGINA
      1. HYPERTROPHY AND HYPERPLASIA OF EPITHELIUM AND ELASTIC TISSUES IN PREPARATION FOR DELIVERY
   E. VULVA
      1. INCREASED VASCULARITY
      2. HYPERTROPHY AND FAT DEPOSITS CAUSE THE LABIA MAJORA TO COVER THE INTROITUS.
      3. THE OBSTETRICAL PERINEUM IS THE AREA BETWEEN THE FOURCHETTE (POSTERIOR ASPECT OF THE INTROITUS) AND THE ANUS.
   F. NEUROLOGIC SYSTEM
      1. PAIN IMPULSES FROM THE UTERUS, UTERINE LIGAMENTS, FALLOPIAN TUBES, AND BONY PELVIS ARE CARRIED ALONG SYMPATHETIC NERVE FIBERS ENTERING THE NEURAXIS BETWEEN THE 10TH AND 12TH THORACIC AND 1ST LUMBER SPINAL SEGMENTS.
      2. PAIN IMPULSES FROM THE PELVIC FLOOR MUSCLES, VAGINA, BLADDER, URETHRA, AND RECTUM ARE CARRIED ALONG SYMPATHETIC NERVE FIBERS ENTERING THE NEURAXIS BETWEEN THE 2ND AND 4TH SACRAL SPINAL SEGMENT.
      3. SENSORIAL CHANGES OCCUR AS THE CLIENT PROGRESSES THROUGH THE PHASES AND STAGES OF LABOR. ENDOGENOUS ANALGESICS (ENDORPHINS) DECREASE PAIN PERCEPTION AND CAUSE SEDATION.
   G. HEMATOLOGIC SYSTEM (SEE CHAPTER 42, SECTION I.)

Figure 43-1 Pelvic types.

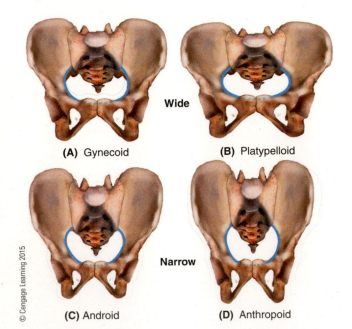

(A) Gynecoid   Wide   (B) Platypelloid

(C) Android   Narrow   (D) Anthropoid

© Cengage Learning 2015

Table 43-1 Pelvic Anatomy

Type	Incidence	Inlet	Midpelvis	Outlet	Implications for Birth
Gynecoid	50%	Round, adequate diameters	Round, adequate diameters and long posterior (AP) diameter	Wide transverse	Occiput anterior most common, normal spontaneous delivery favorable
Android	20%	Heart shaped, angulated	Short AP diameter	Short AP diameter	Slow descent, arrest of labor, forceps/vacuum delivery more common
Anthropoid	25%	Ovoid, long AP diameter	Rounded, adequate diameters	Narrow transverse	Occiput A or P, normal spontaneous vaginal delivery (NSVD) favorable
Platypelloid	5%	Ovoid, wide transverse	Rounded, wide transverse	Wide transverse, short AP	OP more common, unfavorable for labor

© Cengage Learning 2015

Table 43-2 Cardiac Output During Labor

Stage	Cardiac Output
Early first trimester	15%
Late first trimester	30%
Second trimester	45%
5 minutes after delivery	65%
60 minutes after delivery	40%

During contractions, cardiac output increases an additional 15%

Contractions may increase systolic pressure by 30 mm Hg and diastolic by 25 mm Hg

© Cengage Learning 2015

H. CARDIOVASCULAR SYSTEM (SEE TABLE 43-2)
   1. MATERNAL POSITION CAN GREATLY INFLUENCE CARDIAC OUTPUT. IN THE SUPINE POSITION, PRESSURE EXERTED ON THE INFERIOR VENA CAVA BY THE GRAVID UTERUS DECREASES VENOUS RETURN, AND THEREFORE RESULTS IN DECREASED CARDIAC OUTPUT. THIS MAY LEAD TO SUPINE HYPOTENSION SYNDROME WITH DIAPHORESIS AND POSSIBLE SYNCOPE. CHANGING FROM THE SUPINE POSITION TO THE LATERAL POSITION CAN INCREASE CARDIAC OUTPUT 25–30%, WITH RESULTANT INCREASE IN UTERINE AND RENAL BLOOD FLOW.
I. RESPIRATORY SYSTEM (SEE CHAPTER 42, SECTION I.)
J. ENDOCRINE SYSTEM
   1. INCREASES IN HUMAN CHORIONIC GONADOTROPIN, HUMAN PLACENTAL LACTOGEN, ESTROGEN, PROGESTERONE, RELAXIN, PROSTAGLANDINS, AND PROLACTIN
   2. PITUITARY (SEE CHAPTER 42, SECTION I.)
   3. THYROID (SEE CHAPTER 42, SECTION I.)
   4. PARATHYROID
      a. Glandular activity increases, and blood levels of parathyroid hormone increase due to increased requirement for calcium and vitamin D; increase is greatest in the second half of pregnancy.
   5. PANCREAS (SEE CHAPTER 42, SECTION I.)
   6. ESTROGEN (FROM THE ADRENAL CORTEX AND PLACENTA) CAUSES:
      a. Enlargement of the breasts, uterus, and genitals (weight of the uterus increases from 70 gm to 1–2 kilos)
      b. Changes in sodium and water retention, fat deposits
      c. Hematological and vascular changes
      d. Alterations in thyroid function, increase in melanocyte-stimulating hormone, leading to hyperpigmentation
   7. PROGESTERONE (FROM THE PLACENTA)
      a. Decreasing uterine contractility, smooth muscle tone, and gastric motility
      b. Development of the lobular-alveolar system and ducts of the breasts
      c. Increased sensitivity of the respiratory system to CO_2
   8. RELAXIN
      a. Promotes softening of the cervix
      b. Alters collagen to promote the softening of the articulation of the bones of the pelvis—allows for increased space for the developing fetus, contributes to maternal joint instability
K. RENAL SYSTEM
   1. DURING LABOR, DIAPHORESIS, RESTRICTIONS ON ORAL FLUID INTAKE, AND INCREASE IN INSENSIBLE WATER LOSS DUE TO

INCREASED RESPIRATORY RATE LEAD TO DECREASED HYDRATION.

2. DURING LABOR AND AFTER DELIVERY, EDEMA, ANESTHESIA, PRESSURE, AND PAIN MAY MAKE VOIDING DIFFICULT.

3. PROTEINURIA IS NORMAL DURING LABOR, AS A RESULT OF BREAKDOWN OF MUSCLE FROM EXERTION.

L. MUSCULOSKELETAL SYSTEM
   1. INCREASED MUSCLE ACTIVITY DURING LABOR CAUSES DIAPHORESIS, FATIGUE, PROTEINURIA, AND POSSIBLY INCREASE IN TEMPERATURE. JOINT LAXITY IS INCREASED DUE TO RELAXIN, LEADING TO JOINT PAIN (E.G., SYMPHYSIS PUBIS).

M. GASTROINTESTINAL SYSTEM (SEE CHAPTER 42, SECTION I.)

II.   ASSESSMENT

A. ADMISSION ASSESSMENT
   1. REVIEW OF PRENATAL RECORD
      a. Gravida (number of times the client has been pregnant)
      b. Para (number of deliveries after 20 weeks—each delivery is para 1 regardless of whether singleton or multiple birth, and whether liveborn or stillborn)
      c. Term (37 completed weeks or more)
      d. Preterm (deliveries after 20 weeks, prior to 37 completed weeks)
      e. Abortions (elective or spontaneous)
      f. Living children
   2. CLINICAL ASSESSMENTS
   3. FUNDAL HEIGHT: HEIGHT IN CENTIMETERS FROM THE SYMPHYSIS PUBIS TO THE TOP OF THE FUNDUS; NORMAL MEASUREMENT ABOUT 38 CM AT 40 WEEKS
   4. FETAL LIE
   5. LEOPOLD'S MANEUVERS (SEE FIGURE 43-2)
   6. STATUS OF FETAL MEMBRANES (AMNION/CHORION)
   7. SPONTANEOUS RUPTURE
   8. AMNIOTOMY (ARTIFICIAL RUPTURE)
   9. MECONIUM STAINING (ASSOCIATED WITH INCREASED RISK OF FETAL HYPOXIA OR ASPHYXIA)
   10. BLOODY DISCHARGE (ASSOCIATED WITH ABRUPTIO PLACENTAE)
   11. ODOR (FOUL ODOR ASSOCIATED WITH INFECTION—CHORIOAMNIONITIS)
   12. FERNING: A SAMPLE OF FLUID FROM THE CERVICAL OS IS DRIED ON A GLASS SLIDE, THEN VIEWED UNDER A MICROSCOPE FOR CHARACTERISTIC SODIUM CHLORIDE CRYSTAL

Figure 43-2 Leopold's maneuver

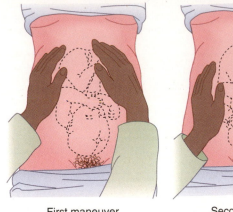
First maneuver

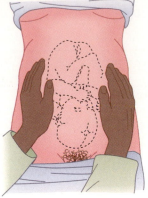
Second maneuver

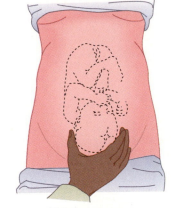
Third maneuver

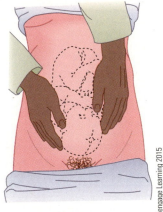
Fourth maneuver

© Cengage Learning 2015

PATTERN (ARBORIZATION) OF AMNIOTIC FLUID.

13. ULTRASOUND STUDIES: FOR FETAL POSITION, PLACENTA LOCATION, FETAL WELL-BEING

14. BIOCHEMICAL ASSESSMENTS (SEE CHAPTER 42, SECTION III, LABORATORY SERUM EVALUATIONS SUBSECTION.)

B. MATERNAL ASSESSMENT DURING THE INTRAPARTUM PERIOD
   1. GENERAL SYSTEMS ASSESSMENT (SEE CHAPTER 42, SECTION II.)
      a. Cardiovascular: blood pressure, pulse, capillary refill
      b. Respiratory: breath sounds, SaO_2 (oxygen saturation), shortness of breath, particularly for the client with pre-eclampsia
      c. Endocrine: monitor blood glucose, insulin as ordered for the client with diabetes.
      d. Renal: monitor urine output, particularly for the client with pre-eclampsia.

e. Gastrointestinal (GI): nausea and vomiting, right upper quadrant pain, particularly for the client with pre-eclampsia

f. Central nervous system (CNS): headache, changes in mentation in the client with pre-eclampsia (seizure precautions); deep tendon reflexes: hyperreflexia may indicate CNS irritability from pre-eclampsia.

2. VITAL SIGNS

  a. Heart rate: tachycardia may reflect blood loss.

  b. Respiratory rate: tachypnea or respiratory distress may be a sign of pulmonary embolism or pulmonary edema.

  c. Blood pressure: hypertension may reflect pre-eclampsia or pain. Drastic blood loss may occur before hypotension develops; monitor heart rate, capillary refill, respiratory rate for earlier signs.

  d. Temperature: elevation may be a sign of infection.

C. CERVIX FOR EFFACEMENT AND DILATATION

D. THE FOUR "PS"

  1. POWER: CONTRACTIONS

  2. PASSAGE: PELVIS, UTERUS, CERVIX, AND VAGINA

  3. PASSENGER: FETUS (BELOW)

  4. PSYCHE: MATERNAL BELIEFS, ANXIETY, SUPPORT SYSTEM

    a. Some add a fifth "P" position, the influence of maternal position and movement on labor progress.

  5. FETAL LIE: THE RELATIONSHIP OF THE LONG AXIS OF THE FETUS TO THAT OF THE MOTHER

    a. Longitudinal (either cephalic or breech)

    b. Transverse (crosswise): cannot deliver vaginally

    c. Oblique (diagonal): cannot deliver vaginally

  6. PRESENTATION: THE PART OF THE FETUS ENTERING THE PELVIC INLET FIRST; THREE POSSIBLE PRESENTATIONS ARE:

    a. Shoulder

    b. Breech

    c. Cephalic

  7. POSITION: THE RELATIONSHIP OF THE PRESENTING PART TO A SPECIFIC AREA OF THE MOTHER'S PELVIS

    a. The denominator is the fetal landmark used to describe position relative to the mother's pelvis. In cephalic presentation these are the fetal vertex, sinciput, occiput, mentum; in breech presentation, the sacrum; and in shoulder presentation, the scapula or acromial process.

    b. Right or left occiput transverse anterior or posterior

    c. Occiput posterior or anterior (straight, with no rotation to the right or left)

    d. Face presentations are rare so examples using the mentum are not given.

    e. Right or left sacrum transverse anterior or posterior

    f. Sacrum posterior or anterior

  8. ATTITUDE: THE RELATIONSHIP OF THE FETAL PARTS (CHEST, CHIN, ARMS) TO EACH OTHER

    a. In cephalic presentation, the fetal neck can be flexed or extended.

    b. Full flexion presents (points) the vertex (crown, smallest diameter) of the head into the pelvis (normal position). The occiput is the denominator.

    c. "Military," or sincipital, attitude means the neck is in neutral position, neither flexed nor extended.

    d. Brow means the neck is partially extended and the fetal forehead (sinciput) presents.

    e. In "face" presentation the neck is fully extended and the mentum (chin) is the denominator (a fetus in this position cannot be delivered vaginally).

    f. Asynclitic: head is tilted to one side; synclitic: head is aligned correctly.

E. IDENTIFICATION OF MATERNAL AND FETAL RISK FACTORS

  1. FETAL AND MATERNAL RISK FACTORS ASSOCIATED WITH INTRAPARTAL FETAL HYPOXEMIA AND ASPHYXIA

  2. ANTEPARTAL FACTORS

    a. Prior stillbirth or neonatal death

    b. Fetal anomalies

    c. Prematurity

    d. Oligohydramnios

    e. Polyhydramnios

    f. Maternal medical complications, for example, diabetes, cardiac disease

    g. Maternal obstetric complications, for example, hemorrhage, intrauterine fetal death

    h. Regular painful contractions that spontaneously ceased 24 hours prior to the onset of active labor (associated with an increase in arrest of labor disorders and cesarean section)

  3. INTRAPARTAL FACTORS

    a. Maternal hypoxia

    b. Uterine artery occlusion

    c. Umbilical vessel occlusion

    d. Fetal anemia

     e. Preterm or postterm labor

     f. Meconium

     g. Abnormal labor (prolonged, unfavorable progress)

     h. "Major" malpresentation

F. PAIN

  1. FIRST STAGE OF LABOR

     a. Uterine muscle hypoxia; lactic acid accumulation; stretching of the cervix and lower uterine segment; traction on the ovaries, fallopian tubes, uterine ligaments; and pressure on the bony pelvis produce afferent pain impulses that are carried along sympathetic nerve fibers entering the neuraxis between the 10th and 12th thoracic and 1st lumber spinal segments.

  2. SECOND STAGE OF LABOR

     a. Distention of pelvic floor muscles, vagina, perineum, and vulva; and pressure on the urethra, bladder, and rectum produce afferent pain impulses that are carried along sympathetic nerve fibers entering the neuraxis between the second and the fourth sacral spinal segment.

     b. Some women report a decrease in pain during the second stage (possibly due to focus on pushing), whereas others experience an increase in painful sensations.

     c. Gate control theory

     d. Based on three physiologic processes:

       1) Large fibers (those carrying sensory impulses from the skin) are myelinated and small, thinly myelinated or unmyelinated fibers carry pressure and pain impulses from the uterus, cervix, and pelvic joints. Because large, myelinated fibers transmit impulses to the CNS more quickly than do small fibers, cutaneous stimulation can block or alter pain impulses (sensations).

       2) The reticular activating system in the brainstem interprets auditory, visual, and painful sensory stimuli. When the cerebral cortex focuses on auditory or visual stimulation, painful stimuli are less able to pass through the gate (partially or completely stopped at the "gate"). Memory and cognitive processes affect the perception of pain. A sense of confidence and control can decrease painful sensations. Therefore, prenatal education and labor support, which enhance maternal confidence and sense of control, are effective labor support strategies.

       3) Pain causes increased production of catecholamines (such as norepinephrine), which leads to increased cardiac output, increased peripheral vascular resistance, increased maternal oxygen consumption and blood pressure, and decreased uterine blood flow. Catecholamines also decrease the strength, duration, and coordination of uterine contractions and produce nonreassuring changes in the fetal heart rate pattern.

G. COMFORT (NONPHARMACOLOGIC STRATEGIES)

  1. USE OF CUTANEOUS STIMULI TO RELIEVE PAIN

     a. Massage

     b. Touch

     c. Back rub

     d. Counterpressure

     e. Movement

     f. Positioning

     g. Application of heat or cold

     h. Acupuncture

     i. Hydrotherapy (shower, jet tub)

     j. Effleurage

  2. USE OF AUDITORY OR VISUAL STIMULI

  3. FOCAL POINT, FOCUSED ATTENTION

  4. BREATHING TECHNIQUES

  5. DISTRACTION

  6. HYPNOSIS

  7. MUSIC

  8. USE OF MEMORY OR COGNITIVE PROCESSES

     a. Prenatal education

     b. Relaxation

  9. LABOR SUPPORT (E.G., DOULA, A TRAINED LABOR SUPPORT PERSON)

H. PROGRESS OF LABOR

  1. VAGINAL EXAMINATION FOR CERVICAL DILATION AND EFFACEMENT, AND FETAL DESCENT

  2. INTEGRITY OF FETAL MEMBRANES

  3. SPONTANEOUS RUPTURE

  4. AMNIOTOMY

  5. MECONIUM STAINING (ASSOCIATED WITH INCREASED RISK OF FETAL HYPOXIA/ASPHYXIA)

  6. CLEAR DISCHARGE

  7. BLOODY DISCHARGE (ASSOCIATED WITH ABRUPTIO PLACENTAE)

  8. ODOR (FOUL ODOR ASSOCIATED WITH INFECTION)

  9. FERNING: A SAMPLE OF FLUID FROM THE CERVICAL OS IS DRIED ON A GLASS SLIDE, THEN VIEWED UNDER A MICROSCOPE FOR CHARACTERISTIC CRYSTAL PATTERN OF AMNIOTIC FLUID.

10. FRIEDMAN'S CURVE (PARTOGRAM) GRAPH OF CERVICAL DILATATION AND DESCENT OF PRESENTING PART IN NULLIPAROUS AND MULTIPAROUS LABOR

I. PSYCHOSOCIAL AND CULTURAL ASPECTS OF LABOR
   1. RELIGIOUS BELIEFS AND PRACTICES
   2. PRESCRIPTIVE PRACTICES: EXPECTED BEHAVIORS; THINGS THE MOTHER SHOULD DO TO HAVE A HEALTHY BABY AND PREGNANCY
   3. RESTRICTIVE PRACTICES: THINGS THE MOTHER SHOULD AVOID TO HAVE A HEALTHY BABY AND PREGNANCY
   4. TABOO PRACTICES: RESTRICTIONS INVOLVING SUPERNATURAL CONSEQUENCES
   5. CULTURAL NORMS REGARDING:
      a. Presence and role of support persons; many cultures have prohibitions against male partners or health care providers seeing a woman's body.
      b. Expression of labor pain: some cultures consider crying out during labor shameful; others expect the woman to cry and scream. In many cultures, labor pain is to be endured; women refuse analgesia or anesthesia.
   6. DIETARY PRACTICES
      a. Heat and cold: in many cultures pregnancy is considered a "hot" state; the birth process is thought to cause the loss of much heat, leaving the postpartum woman in a "cold" state.
   7. DOMESTIC ABUSE: ASK THE WOMAN PRIVATELY ABOUT HER SAFETY AND THAT OF HER BABY; OBSERVE FOR INJURIES; BE SUSPICIOUS IF THE MALE PARTNER REFUSES TO LEAVE THE WOMAN'S ROOM AND ANSWERS QUESTIONS FOR HER.
      a. Desired birthing plan: elicit information on admission, and advocate for the woman whenever possible.
      b. Family interaction and support: foster inclusion of the support person(s) by teaching or assisting with comfort measures. If support person(s) is(are) not helpful or disrespectful to the woman, advocate for her.
      c. If history of sexual assault or childhood sexual abuse, be aware that aspects of the labor process and procedures (e.g., exams) may have painful associations for the client. Client may respond with dissociation ("out of body" sensation), regression (fetal position, childlike behavior), overcontrolling (detailed plans, may

express rage or panic if actual labor and birth are not as planned), or may "fight" labor contractions and urge to push.
      d. Assist the client with dissociation to reconnect with her body through massage, position change, movement, and so on. Interventions for regression include addressing the client, asking questions, encouraging participation in decisions about her care. If the client "fights" labor, assist with identification and relax tense muscles. The controlling client will benefit from choices among options.

J. FETAL WELL-BEING
   1. FETAL ASSESSMENT DURING THE INTRAPARTUM PERIOD
   2. FETAL HEART RATE MONITORING, INCLUDING INTERPRETATION
      a. Electronic
      b. Auscultation
      c. Fetal scalp blood sampling
   3. ELECTRONIC FETAL MONITORING (EFM)
      a. Baseline variability
      b. Long-term variability: slow, rhythmic fluctuations above and below an average baseline rate
      c. Short-term variability (beat-to-beat variability [BTBV]): the fluctuation in intervals between consecutive R to R intervals of fetal QRS complexes (heartbeats)
      d. Baseline rate (recorded either as range or average): the fetal heart rate over a period of time, not including accelerations or decelerations
   4. PERIODIC CHANGES
      a. Accelerations
         1) Definition: increase in the fetal heart rate above the baseline level
         2) Etiology: fetal movement, head compression
         3) Interventions: none
      b. Early decelerations
         1) Definition: a uniform (consistent in shape) deceleration which is caused by compression of the fetal head and characterized by a gradual onset at the beginning of a contraction and a slow return, gradual offset, or gradual recovery to the baseline soon after the contraction ends
         2) Etiology: head compression
         3) Interventions: none
      c. Late deceleration
         1) Definition: deceleration caused by uteroplacental insufficiency (low oxygen delivery to the fetus) and characterized by a gradual, slanted

onset after the contraction begins, and usually a slow return to baseline, after the contraction ends. The nadir (lowest point) is always after the contraction peak. Late decelerations tend to be consistent (uniform) in shape.

2) Etiology: uteroplacental insufficiency

3) Interventions: turn the mother to the lateral position; assess blood pressure; administer oxygen (per orders or protocol); increase IV fluids (per orders or protocol); turn off oxytocin infusion (if applicable); notify the physician or nurse-midwife; anticipate diagnostic procedure(s): fetal scalp sampling, insertion of internal electronic fetal monitoring devices (if applicable), operative delivery.

d. Variable

1) Definition: deceleration of the fetal heart rate caused by umbilical cord compression or head compression (especially in the second stage of labor with pushing), characterized by a rapid onset and return to baseline, and a variable relationship to the contraction (may occur at any time in the contraction phase)

2) Etiology: umbilical cord or head compression, or both

3) Interventions: perform vaginal examination to assess for prolapsed cord; change maternal position (attempt to relieve cord compression); administer oxygen (per orders or protocol); increase IV fluids (per orders or protocol); turn off oxytocin infusion (if applicable); notify the physician or nurse-midwife; anticipate procedure(s): fetal scalp sampling, insertion of internal EFM devices (if applicable), amnioinfusion, and operative delivery.

e. Contractions

1) Tocodynamometer: pressure-sensing instrument applied externally to the maternal abdomen to assess uterine contractions

2) Intrauterine pressure catheter (IUPC): a catheter inserted transvaginally into the uterus. Intrauterine pressure is conducted through the catheter, exerted on a pressure transducer, and transformed to an electronic signal, then printed on the tracing.

3) Palpation: examiner's hands feel the uterine fundus to detect increment (onset to acme), acme (high point), and decrement (acme to end) of contractions, and relaxation between contractions.

f. Uterine resting tone: lowest pressure between contractions

III. **DIAGNOSTIC STUDIES (SEE CHAPTER 42, SECTION III, ELECTRONIC FETAL MONITORING [EFM].)**

IV. **NURSING DIAGNOSES**
   A. ANXIETY
   B. INEFFECTIVE BREATHING PATTERN
   C. DEFICIENT KNOWLEDGE
   D. ACUTE PAIN
   E. RISK FOR DEFICIENT FLUID VOLUME
   F. INEFFECTIVE TISSUE PERFUSION

Nursing Diagnoses: Definitions and Classification 2012–2014. Copyright © 2012, 1994–2012 by NANDA International. Used by arrangement with John Wiley & Sons Limited.

V. **LABOR AND SPONTANEOUS VAGINAL DELIVERY (SVD)**
   A. LABOR INITIATION THEORIES
      1. INCREASE IN MYOMETRIAL SENSITIVITY TO OXYTOCIN
      2. WITHDRAWAL OF PROGESTERONE AND INCREASED SYNTHESIS OF PROSTAGLANDIN
      3. FETAL CORTISOL
      4. UTERINE DISTENTION
   B. LABOR
      1. DEFINED AS CERVICAL EFFACEMENT AND DILATATION
      2. PREMONITORY SIGNS OF LABOR
      3. EXPULSION, LOSS, OR PASSAGE OF MUCUS PLUG (OPERCULUM), MUCORRHEA
      4. LIGHTENING: DESCENT OF THE FETUS INTO THE PELVIS
      5. BRAXTON-HICKS CONTRACTIONS: IRREGULAR, INTERMITTENT, USUALLY PAINLESS UTERINE CONTRACTIONS
      6. CERVICAL RIPENING: SOFTENING AND EFFACEMENT
      7. SOFTENING AND ANTERIOR MOVEMENT OF THE CERVIX
      8. BLOODY SHOW: PINK OR RED MUCUS REFLECTING BLEEDING FROM THE CAPILLARIES DUE TO CERVICAL DILATATION OR EFFACEMENT
      9. RUPTURE OF MEMBRANES
   C. MECHANISMS OF LABOR (CARDINAL MOVEMENTS)
      1. ENGAGEMENT: PRESENTING PART AT STATION 0; WIDEST PART OF THE FETAL HEAD HAS PASSED THROUGH THE PELVIC INLET
      2. DESCENT: DOWNWARD PROGRESS OF THE FETUS INTO THE PELVIS

3. FLEXION: OF THE FETAL NECK
4. INTERNAL ROTATION: ROTATION OF THE FETAL HEAD TO ALIGN THE ANTEROPOSTERIOR (LARGEST) DIAMETER OF THE FETAL HEAD WITH THE (LONG) ANTEROPOSTERIOR DIAMETER OF THE MATERNAL PELVIS
5. EXTENSION: OF THE FETAL NECK AS IT COMES UNDER THE SYMPHYSIS PUBIS AND EMERGES FROM THE VAGINA
6. RESTITUTION: FETAL HEAD TURNS TO REALIGN THE HEAD WITH THE LONG AXIS OF THE FETUS (RETURN TO NEUTRAL POSITION)
7. EXTERNAL ROTATION: TURNING OF THE FETAL HEAD TO ALIGN THE LATERAL DIAMETER OF THE FETAL SHOULDERS WITH THE ANTEROPOSTERIOR DIAMETER OF THE MATERNAL PELVIS

D. NORMAL LABOR PATTERNS
  1. FIRST STAGE
     a. Latent phase
        1) Definition: 0–3 cm
        2) Average length: nullipara, 8.6 hours; multipara, 5.3 hours
        3) Contractions
        4) Frequency may be irregular; every 5–10 minutes
        5) Duration: 30–45 seconds
        6) Intensity: mild, 25–40 mm Hg by IUPC
        7) Cervix: posterior, moving to anterior, 0–3 cm, effacement 0–40%
     b. Active phase
        1) Definition: 4–7 cm
        2) Average length: nullipara, 4.6 hours; multipara, 2.4 hours. Generally, expect 1.2 cm/hr progress for primipara, 1.5 cm/hr for multipara
        3) Contractions
        4) Frequency: every 2–5 minutes
        5) Duration: 45–60 seconds
        6) Intensity: moderate to strong, 50–70 mm Hg by IUPC
        7) Cervix: 4–7 cm, effacement 40–80%, station 22 to 0
     c. Transition phase
        1) Definition: 8–10 cm (complete dilatation)
        2) Average length: nullipara, 3.6 hours; multipara, 30 minutes
        3) Contractions
        4) Frequency: every 2–3 minutes
        5) Duration: 60–90 seconds
        6) Intensity: strong, 70–90 mm Hg by IUPC
        7) Cervix: 8–10 cm, 80–100%, station 21 to 11

  2. SECOND STAGE
     a. Definition: time from complete cervical dilatation to delivery of the fetus
     b. Length varies
     c. Contractions
     d. Frequency: every 2–3 minutes
     e. Duration: 60–90 seconds
     f. Intensity: strong, 80–100 mm Hg by IUPC
     g. Cervix: 10 cm (complete), effacement 100%, station 0 to 12
     h. Bearing down efforts, assisted delivery (forceps or vacuum)
     i. Ends with expulsion of fetus
     j. Bloody show
     k. Nausea and vomiting
     l. Trembling limbs
     m. Decrease in coping abilities
     n. Urge to push or involuntary pushing
     o. Pushing
     p. Closed glottis (closed-glottis pushing, using the Valsalva maneuver, increases intrathoracic pressure, decreases venous return, increases venous pressure, and may cause fetal hypoxia). Open glottis: client exhales during pushing; may vocalize. Less effect on vascular and intrathoracic pressures
     q. Episiotomy: surgical incision of the perineum to enlarge the vaginal opening; may be performed to hasten delivery if fetal distress is present, or to avoid laceration of the perineal tissues
     r. Mediolateral: oblique incision from the vagina (fourchette) toward one hip
     s. Medial or midline: straight incision from the vagina (fourchette) toward the rectum, may extend to third- or fourth-degree laceration
     t. Lacerations
        1) First degree: involves only epidermal layers
        2) Second degree: epidermal and muscle or fascia; requires repair (sutures)
        3) Third degree: extends into the rectal sphincter
        4) Fourth degree: extends through the rectal mucosa

  3. THIRD STAGE
     a. Expulsion of the placenta
     b. Change in shape of the uterus, gush of blood, lengthening of the cord when the placenta detaches from the uterine wall
     c. Definition: time from delivery of the baby to delivery of the placenta
     d. Length: varies, 5–20 minutes is usual
     e. Contractions: decreased
     f. Cervix: approximately 4 cm after delivery of the fetus

4. **FOURTH STAGE**
   a. Definition: time from delivery of the placenta; no specific endpoint
   b. Immediate postpartum
   c. Length: mother is usually observed closely for the first 4 hours, then every 4–8 hours until discharge, more often if antepartum, intrapartum, or postpartum complications.
   d. Nursing interventions specific to the fourth stage
      1) Assessment of:
         a) Uterine involution: firmness, fundal height and position
         b) Lochia
         c) Bladder
         d) Perineum
         e) Emotional status/bonding
         f) Vital signs

E. **NURSING INTERVENTIONS DURING LABOR**
   1. **ONGOING ASSESSMENT**
      a. Assessment of labor progress
      b. Vaginal examination for cervical dilatation and effacement and fetal descent (avoid performing vaginal examination in the presence of bleeding other than bloody show)
      c. Friedman's curve: a standard graph of cervical dilatation and fetal descent for multigravidas and primigravidas (nulliparas), to which a client's labor progress may be compared
   2. **ASSESSMENT FOR RUPTURE OF MEMBRANES**
      a. Presence of bloody show
      b. Evaluation of contractions (uterine activity)
      c. Intake and output
      d. Deep tendon reflexes
   3. **NURSING INTERVENTIONS**
      a. The priority of nursing care for a laboring client is fetal well-being.
      b. Promote hygiene, particularly skin, perineal, and oral.
      c. Encourage fluid intake.
      d. Maintain elimination.
      e. Provide psychoprophylaxis and coping support.
   4. **BREATHING TECHNIQUES**
   5. **RELAXATION TECHNIQUES**
   6. **EFFLEURAGE AND MASSAGE**
   7. **COUNTERPRESSURE (PRESSURE TO THE SACRUM TO ALLEVIATE "BACK LABOR" DISCOMFORT)**
   8. **OFFER HEAT AND COLD THERAPY**

F. **OBSTETRIC ANALGESIA AND ANESTHESIA**
   1. **PARENTERAL MEDICATION**
      a. Medication: narcotics, narcotic or narcotic antagonists, anxiolytics, antiemetics
      b. Indications: pain, anxiety, nausea, and vomiting
      c. Contraindications: nonreassuring fetal status, anticipated delivery
      d. Effect of medication on:
         1) Client: analgesia, sedation, alleviation of nausea and vomiting
         2) Fetus: sedation; if delivered soon after medication is given, respiratory depression
         3) Labor: may slow labor progress if it causes contractions to decrease in frequency or intensity; may improve progress if it promotes relaxation and decreases anxiety
         4) Regional anesthesia and analgesia
         5) Pudendal block
      e. Advantages: rapid onset of action
      f. Disadvantages: does not relieve the pain of uterine contractions
      g. Indications: anesthesia for second stage
      h. Contraindications: infection at the site of puncture (transvaginal or perineal)
      i. Effect on the client: complete anesthesia of the posterior portions of the perineum and labia majora; partial anesthesia of the anterior portions. Effect on the fetus: none if correctly performed, fetal bradycardia if the anesthetic enters circulation.
      j. Labor: (usually performed in second stage) no effect on uterine contractions
      k. Adverse reactions and interventions: inadvertent intravascular administration of anesthetic; may require resuscitation
         1) Epidural (usually done at the L2–5 levels)
         2) Advantages: slow onset of hypotension; no postpuncture headache with correct technique; variable density of block
         3) Disadvantages: slow onset of anesthesia
         4) Indications: labor; cesarean delivery when slow onset of vasodilatation or hypotension is desirable or vital, as with pre-eclampsia
         5) Contraindications: infection at the site of planned puncture, sepsis, coagulopathy, acute CNS disease
         6) Effect on the client: variable level of anesthesia from approximately T10 caudal for labor and vaginal delivery or T4 caudal for cesarean delivery
         7) Fetus: uteroplacental insufficiency if maternal hypotension occurs

8) Labor: decreased uterine activity; may interfere with maternal pushing efforts

9) Adverse reactions and interventions: maternal cerebral hypoxia (manifests as nausea), maternal hypotension, inadvertent intravascular injection of anesthetic (a test dose with epinephrine will identify intravascular placement), urinary retention, postdural puncture headache. To avoid hypotension, hydration with 1500–2000 ml of IV fluid just prior to the procedure

l. Spinal (usually done at the L2–5 levels)

1) Advantages: rapid onset of dense block

2) Disadvantages: single dose, fixed duration; continuous spinal anesthesia is not suitable for obstetric anesthesia.

3) Indications: cesarean delivery

4) Contraindications: same as epidural

5) Effect on the client: same as epidural

6) Fetus: same as epidural

7) Labor: not applicable

8) Adverse reactions and interventions: maternal cerebral hypoxia (manifests as nausea), maternal hypotension, inadvertent intravascular injection of anesthetic (a test dose with epinephrine will identify intravascular placement), urinary retention, postdural puncture headache to avoid hypotension, hydration with 1500–2000 ml of IV fluid just prior to the procedure. If done above the L2 level, spinal cord injury (rare)

9) Note: caudal is similar to epidural and spinal but is done at the level of the sacrum.

m. Local infiltration

1) Advantages: no interference with labor

2) Disadvantages: perineal anesthesia only

3) Indications: anesthesia for an episiotomy or repair of an episiotomy or lacerations

4) Contraindications: true allergy to agents

5) Effect on the client: anesthesia of the perineum

6) Fetus: none, unless toxicity

7) Labor: not applicable

8) Adverse reactions and interventions toxicity: (related to the total dose, not volume, of the medication); CNS toxicity (manifests as maternal or fetal seizures); cardiovascular toxicity produces initial bradycardia in the fetus, increased arterial pressure and heart rate in the mother

VI. **SPECIAL INTRAPARTAL SITUATIONS**

A. INDUCTION AND AUGMENTATION

1. DESCRIPTION: CAUSE LABOR TO BEGIN (INDUCTION) OR BECOME MORE INTENSE (AUGMENTATION)

2. ASSESSMENT

a. Maternal readiness: Bishop score (see Table 43-3)

3. DIAGNOSTIC TESTS

a. Fetal maturity: L:S ratio, phosphatidylglycerol (PG) tests on amniotic fluid sample

4. MEDICAL-SURGICAL MANAGEMENT

a. Methods

1) Prostaglandin (medical induction)

2) Prostaglandin analogue (misoprostol)

3) Oxytocin (medical induction) side effects include water intoxication from antidiuretic effect.

4) Amniotomy (artificial rupture of membranes, also called surgical induction)

5. NURSING INTERVENTIONS

a. Monitor frequency and intensity of uterine contractions for hyperstimulation.

b. Monitor fetal response to labor.

c. Provide labor support.

B. DYSFUNCTIONAL LABOR PATTERN

1. DESCRIPTION: DYSFUNCTIONAL LABOR

a. Nulliparous women are more subject to conditions that occur in early labor.

1) Hypertonic uterine dysfunction

2) Primary inertia

3) Prolonged latent phase

Table 43-3 Bishop Score

Bishop	0	1	2	3
Dilation	Closed	1–2 cm	3–4 cm	5 cm
Effacement	30%	40–50%	60–70%	80%
Station	23	22	21/0	11
Cervical consistency	Firm	Medium	Soft	
Cervical position	Posterior	Middle	Anterior	

      b. Multiparous women more often demonstrate problems that occur in the active phase.
         1) Hypotonic uterine dysfunction
         2) Secondary inertia
         3) Arrest or protraction of the active phase
      c. Friedman's terminology lists prolonged latent phase, protraction disorders, and arrest disorders.
      d. Complications include failure to progress and cesarean delivery.
  2. ASSESSMENT
      a. Friedman's curve
  3. DIAGNOSTIC TESTS
      a. None
  4. MEDICAL-SURGICAL MANAGEMENT
      a. Augmentation of labor with oxytocin, cesarean delivery
  5. NURSING INTERVENTIONS
      a. Promote movement.
      b. Provide hydrotherapy (if medically safe).
      c. Maintain position change.
      d. Promote relaxation (massage, breathing techniques).
      e. Specific maternal positions facilitate proper position of the fetus.

C. PRECIPITOUS DELIVERY
  1. DESCRIPTION
      a. Rapid (faster than 5 cm/hour in nulliparas or 10 cm/hour in multiparas), unexpected labor progress resulting in delivery in the absence of a health care provider
      b. Complications include hematoma of the vagina or perineum, uterine atony (failure to contract and control bleeding), laceration, and ecchymosis petechiae of the newborn.
  2. ASSESSMENT
      a. Labor progress
         1) Maternal behaviors such as involuntary bearing down, nausea, and retching
         2) Increased bloody show or bulging of the perineum or anus
  3. DIAGNOSTIC TESTS
      a. None
  4. MEDICAL-SURGICAL MANAGEMENT
      a. Oxytocin for management of uterine atony
  5. NURSING INTERVENTIONS
      a. Prepare equipment and supplies for delivery.
      b. Reassure the client.
      c. Maintain continuous observation of the perineum.

      d. Place the client in a comfortable position.
      e. Open the delivery pack and don sterile gloves; cleanse and drape the perineum (if time allows).
      f. If the client is in a delivery bed, lower but do not remove the lower (foot) section. Position the client so the perineum is just beyond the break in the table to allow room for extension and delivery of the fetal head.
      g. As the head crowns, support the perineum with the thumb and index finger of one hand and use the other to maintain flexion of the fetal neck and control delivery of the head.
      h. After the head delivers, sweep your fingers around the neck to check for the nuchal cord (loop of the cord around the neck of the fetus). If present, attempt to slip the loop over the head; if not possible, clamp the cord in two places and cut between the clamps, then unwind the loop.
      i. After the head rotates, gently lower the head to deliver the anterior shoulder, then lift to deliver the posterior shoulder.
      j. After the body delivers, clamp the cord in two places and cut.
      k. Provide delivery room care or resuscitation of the newborn.
      l. Monitor maternal vital signs, lochia, fundus, and perineum.

D. FETAL DISTRESS (NONREASSURING FETAL STATUS)
  1. DESCRIPTION
      a. Late decelerations (uteroplacental insufficiency), fetal seizures; fetal arrhythmias are not usually an indication for cesarean delivery.
      b. Complications include intrauterine fetal death, and hypoxia resulting in encephalopathy.
  2. ASSESSMENT
      a. Interpretation of EFM tracing
      b. Clinical manifestations of maternal hypotension, such as nausea, pallor, presyncope ("light-headed" sensation)
  3. DIAGNOSTIC TESTS
      a. Fetal scalp sampling (emerging technology: fetal pulse oximetry)
  4. MEDICAL-SURGICAL MANAGEMENT
      a. Attempt in utero resuscitation (support maternal blood pressure with fluids, medications [e.g., ephedrine]; change position; oxygen, medications to stop contractions [tocolytics]).
      b. If unsuccessful, cesarean delivery

5. NURSING INTERVENTIONS
   a. Place the client in lateral position.
   b. Assess for hypotension.
   c. Administer oxygen, IV fluids, medications as ordered.
E. PLACENTA PREVIA (SEE CHAPTER 42, SECTION VI.)
F. ABRUPTIO PLACENTAE (SEE CHAPTER 42, SECTION VI.)
G. PREGNANCY-INDUCED HYPERTENSION (PRE-ECLAMPSIA, "TOXEMIA" IN OLD TERMINOLOGY) (SEE CHAPTER 42, SECTION VI.)
H. PREMATURE RUPTURE OF MEMBRANES (SEE CHAPTER 42, SECTION VI.)
I. CORD PROLAPSE
   1. DESCRIPTION
      a. The umbilical cord drops past the presenting part into the cervix or vagina and becomes trapped, causing severe cord compression.
      b. Complications include fetal asphyxia and death.
   2. ASSESSMENT
      a. Vaginal examination
   3. DIAGNOSTIC TESTS
      a. None
   4. MEDICAL-SURGICAL MANAGEMENT
      a. Cesarean delivery
      b. Administer oxygen.
   5. NURSING INTERVENTIONS
      a. Elevate the presenting part of the cord with your fingers (maintain elevation until delivery); avoid touching the cord (may cause spasm of vessels).
      b. Place the client in knee-chest (preferred) or Trendelenburg position, and transport to surgery immediately.
J. SHOULDER DYSTOCIA
   1. DESCRIPTION
      a. Anterior shoulder os wedged beneath the symphysis pubis
      b. Complications include fractured clavicle, palsy, fetal asphyxia, and fetal death.
   2. ASSESSMENT
      a. Turtle sign—head delivers, then draws back like a turtle pulling its head into its shell.
   3. DIAGNOSTIC TESTS
      a. None
   4. MEDICAL-SURGICAL MANAGEMENT
      a. Maneuvers to deliver the shoulders (e.g., screw maneuver)
   5. NURSING INTERVENTIONS
      a. Perform McRobert's procedure (flexion and external rotation of maternal hips).
      b. Apply suprapubic pressure.
      c. Avoid using fundal pressure.

K. OPERATIVE DELIVERY (INCLUDES CESAREAN DELIVERY)
   1. DESCRIPTION
      a. Use of a device to supplement or replace maternal bearing-down efforts in the second stage
         1) Forceps
         2) Vacuum
      b. Complications include injury to the fetal head or breech, and lacerations of the vagina or cervix.
   2. ASSESSMENT
      a. Inadequate or ineffective pushing efforts
      b. Maternal exhaustion
      c. Friedman's curve
   3. DIAGNOSTIC TESTS
      a. None
   4. MEDICAL-SURGICAL MANAGEMENT
      a. If forceps or vacuum extractor fails, cesarean delivery
   5. NURSING INTERVENTIONS
      a. Assist with positioning.
L. VAGINAL BIRTH AFTER A CESAREAN
   1. DESCRIPTION
      a. Vaginal birth after a cesarean (uterine incision must be transverse in the lower uterine segment)
      b. Two previous cesarean deliveries is the usual maximum.
      c. Indication for previous cesareans must be nonrecurring.
      d. Complications include uterine rupture or fetal or maternal death due to hemorrhage.
   2. ASSESSMENT
      a. History (indication for previous cesarean delivery)
      b. Progress of labor
   3. DIAGNOSTIC TESTS
      a. None
   4. MEDICAL-SURGICAL MANAGEMENT
      a. Pitocin and epidural anesthesia acceptable
      b. Cesarean delivery if indicated
   5. NURSING INTERVENTIONS
      a. Maintain venous access.
      b. Assess for pain not typical of normal labor, change in or an abnormal contour of the uterus or abdomen, and fetal distress, which may indicate uterine rupture (requires immediate surgery).
M. SURGICAL DELIVERY (CESAREAN SECTION)
   1. DESCRIPTION
      a. Surgical abdominal incision through which the fetus and placenta are removed
      b. Complications as with any abdominal surgery, such as hemorrhage or GI, pulmonary, thromboembolic events

2. ASSESSMENT
  a. Indications relate to the "3 Ps"—passage (e.g., too narrow), passenger (e.g., malpresentation), and power (contractions).
  b. In some cases, for example, maternal cardiac disease, the fetus or mother, or both, cannot tolerate the stress of labor.
3. DIAGNOSTIC TESTS
  a. Ultrasound for fetal lie, presentation, position
4. NURSING INTERVENTIONS
  a. Provide preoperative teaching and support.
  b. Provide perioperative care.

N. EXTERNAL BREECH VERSION
1. DEFINITION
  a. Manipulation of a fetus in breech presentation through the abdominal wall to turn to cephalic presentation
  b. Done approximately 37 weeks of gestation so the fetus is not as large as it will be at term, but would be mature if delivery were necessary due to nonreassuring fetal status
  c. One or two operators
2. ASSESSMENT
  a. Fetal well-being: verify prior to the procedure (reassuring fetal monitor tracing)
  b. Ultrasound for fetal position
3. MEDICAL-SURGICAL MANAGEMENT
  a. Breech is lifted from the pelvis while pressure is applied to the fetal head to turn the fetus to vertex presentation.
  b. Personnel and facilities for emergency cesarean delivery must be immediately available before, during, and after the procedure.
4. NURSING INTERVENTIONS
  a. Tocolytics such as terbutaline (Brethine) are sometimes used prior to the procedure to relax the uterus and decrease the likelihood of contractions (uterine contractility).
  b. Provide preprocedure teaching.
  c. Administer medication(s) as ordered.
  d. Verify fetal well-being after the procedure.
  e. Monitor for uterine contractions after the procedure.
  f. Prepare for emergency cesarean delivery if nonreassuring fetal status.
  g. If the mother is Rh negative, administer Rh immune globulin.
  h. Maintain venous access.

VII. IMMEDIATE RECOVERY AND NEWBORN CARE
A. UTERINE INVOLUTION (SEE FOURTH STAGE OF LABOR ON PAGE 846.)
B. POSTPARTUM COMPLICATIONS
1. UTERINE ATONY AND POSTPARTUM HEMORRHAGE
  a. Normally, the uterus contracts after delivery, clamping off blood vessels and minimizing bleeding. Uterine atony allows the bleeding to continue, eventually leading to shock.
    1) Fundal massage and medications to increase uterine contractility
    2) Support of blood volume and blood pressure, intravenous fluids, medications, and, possibly, transfusion
2. AMNIOTIC FLUID EMBOLISM
  a. Amniotic fluid or vernix or fetal hair enters the maternal circulation (embolus) and causes cardiopulmonary collapse.
  b. Resuscitation
3. HEMATOMA
  a. Collection of blood in the tissues of the vulva or vagina, causing intense pain and, possibly, shock
C. POSTSURGICAL RECOVERY
1. SAME AS IN THE FOURTH STAGE OF LABOR, PLUS ASSESSMENT OF THE INCISION AND DRESSING, PAIN, BREATH SOUNDS, RETURN OF SENSATION AND MOTION (REGIONAL ANESTHESIA); AIRWAY, RETURN OF CONSCIOUSNESS (GENERAL ANESTHESIA)
D. NEONATAL CARE (SEE CHAPTER 45, NEWBORN CARE.)
1. ASSESSMENTS AT DELIVERY
  a. Neonatal resuscitation
  b. Apgar score
  c. Evaluation of umbilical vessels (two arteries, one vein; single artery may signal anomalies)
  d. Evaluation of cord blood gases, if applicable
  e. Physical assessment
  f. Gestational age assessment
  g. Adaptation to extrauterine life
2. ADAPTATION OF FETAL CIRCULATION TO EXTRAUTERINE LIFE
  a. With expansion of the lungs, pulmonary capillary resistance falls and pulmonary blood flow increases; pulmonary capillaries and lymphatic vessels remove remaining lung fluid.
  b. As pulmonary blood flow increases, the increasing pressure in the left side of the heart begins to close the two

remaining fetal circulatory shunts: the foramen ovale closes almost immediately; the ductus arteriosus functionally closes at about 12 hours.

3. ADAPTATION OF RESPIRATORY SYSTEM TO EXTRAUTERINE LIFE
   a. Compression and release of the chest during vaginal delivery draws air into the lungs.
   b. Chemical: decreased O_2 concentration, increased CO_2 concentration, or decreased pH stimulates carotid and aortic chemoreceptors, triggering initiation of respirations.
   c. Thermal (cold stress stimulates breathing) and tactile stimuli (uterine contractions, descent through the pelvis and birth canal, drying after delivery) stimulate the brain to trigger respiratory efforts.

4. THERMOREGULATION
   a. Heat is generated by the metabolism of brown fat.
   b. Unable to shiver

5. IDENTIFICATION OF THE NEWBORN

6. INITIAL PARENT–CHILD ATTACHMENT

7. INITIAL FEEDING

8. PROPHYLAXIS
   a. Eye
   b. Vitamin K

9. ANTIVIRAL THERAPY, IF APPLICABLE

VIII. PERINATAL BEREAVEMENT
A. LOSS AND GRIEF
   1. LOSS OF PREGNANCY AND FETUS OR LOSS OF EXPECTED OR HOPED-FOR CHILD OR BIRTH
      a. Grief varies with acceptance of the pregnancy, religious or spiritual beliefs, and prior experience of death or grief; not necessarily with gestational age.
   2. SOMATIC MANIFESTATIONS OF GRIEF MAY INCLUDE NAUSEA AND ANOREXIA, HYPERVENTILATION, PALPITATIONS OR HEAVY FEELING IN THE CHEST, VERTIGO, AND HEADACHES.
   3. BEHAVIORAL MANIFESTATIONS MAY INCLUDE GUILT; ANGER AT GOD, HEALTH CARE PERSONNEL, SELF, AND/OR PARTNER; APATHY; HELPLESSNESS; NIGHTMARES.
   4. OFFER THE CLIENT THE OPTION TO VIEW, BATHE, AND DRESS THE FETUS (PREPARE THE FETUS FOR VIEWING BY BATHING, DRESSING, AND DRAPING IT). OFFER KEEPSAKES SUCH AS PHOTOGRAPHS, FOOTPRINTS OR HAND PRINTS, LOCK OF HAIR, CLOTHING, BLANKET.
   5. OFFER MEMORIAL SERVICE AND FUNERAL OPTIONS.
   6. ASSESS THE SUPPORT SYSTEM.
   7. FOSTER CONTACT BETWEEN THE CLERGY AND THE CLIENT AND FAMILY, AS REQUESTED.

PRACTICE QUESTIONS

1. When caring for the mother with premature rupture of the membranes, the nurse monitors the mother and fetus for indications of
   1. chorioamnionitis.
   2. placenta previa.
   3. hemorrhage.
   4. arrest of descent.

2. The nurse should monitor for which of the following fetal life-threatening emergencies when the fetal head is not engaged and the membranes rupture?
   1. Uterine hyperstimulation
   2. Placenta previa
   3. Cord prolapse
   4. Abruptio placentae

3. When observing a mother receiving oxytocin (Pitocin) for induction of labor, which of the following should the nurse assess for?
   1. Maternal hypotension
   2. Uterine hyperstimulation
   3. Maternal hyperthermia
   4. Placenta previa

4. After observing variable decelerations of the fetal heart rate on the fetal monitor tracing, the nurse should plan to care for a possible
   1. head compression.
   2. uteroplacental insufficiency.
   3. cord compression.
   4. cardiac conduction defect.

5. A nullipara client asks the nurse what the average length of the active phase of labor in the first stage is. What is the most appropriate response by the nurse? _____

6. The nurse observes early decelerations of the fetal heart rate on the fetal monitor tracing of a mother who has an epidural anesthesia and denies pain with the contractions. Which of the following is the intervention the nurse should take?
   1. Perform a sterile vaginal examination
   2. Assist the mother to change positions from side to side
   3. Anticipate starting an amnioinfusion
   4. Administer oxygen

7. The nurse should monitor for complications of disseminated intravascular coagulation (DIC) after observing which of the following decelerations of the fetal heart rate on the fetal monitor tracing? Decelerations that are
   1. uniform in shape and timing.
   2. variable in shape and timing.
   3. uniform in shape and variable in timing.
   4. variable in shape and consistent in timing.

8. A client presents with a 1-cm dilation, 40% effacement, −2 station, a medium consistency, and a middle cervical position. The nurse evaluates this client to have what Bishop score? _____

9. Which of the following fetal heart rate patterns would the nurse anticipate seeing from a fetus with anencephaly?
   1. Early-onset decelerations
   2. Absent long-term variability
   3. Accelerations
   4. Late-onset decelerations

10. After noting early decelerations on the fetal monitor tracing, the nurse should
    1. prepare for emergency cesarean section.
    2. administer an IV fluid bolus.
    3. administer oxygen to the mother.
    4. continue to observe the tracing.

11. In planning the care for the following four clients, which of the clients is a priority for the nurse to begin preoperative instructions and preparation for cesarean section?
    1. A client with a complete placenta previa
    2. A client who has a placenta abruptio
    3. A client experiencing variable decelerations on the fetal monitor
    4. A client with a fever

12. A mother in labor is admitted with profuse, bright red vaginal bleeding and late decelerations on the fetal monitor. Which of the following questions is a priority for the nurse to ask the client to determine whether the source of the bleeding is placenta previa or abruptio placentae?
    1. "Are you having pain?"
    2. "Do you have a fever?"
    3. "Is this your first baby?"
    4. "Do you have a headache or blurred vision?"

13. The nurse is caring for a mother at 32 weeks of gestation who thinks her "water broke" about 1 hour prior to arrival at the hospital. The nurse should prepare the client for which procedure to evaluate the status of the membranes?
    1. Digital vaginal exam
    2. Ultrasound
    3. Fern test
    4. Group B beta strep culture

14. The nurse is reviewing the laboratory results of a mother in labor. Which of the following nursing actions should the nurse implement with a white blood cell count of 14,000?
    1. Notify the physician
    2. Repeat the test in 2 hours
    3. Continue to monitor the client
    4. Prepare the client for a cesarean delivery

15. Which of the following nursing interventions should the nurse take after assessing slight respiratory alkalosis on the arterial blood gas analysis of a pregnant client?
    1. Notify the physician
    2. Repeat the test in 1 hour
    3. No action needed
    4. Consult respiratory therapy

16. The nurse is admitting a mother in labor who reports a small amount of dark red, mucoid vaginal discharge. The nurse should
    1. prepare for immediate cesarean delivery.
    2. proceed with the admission.
    3. obtain a specimen for coagulation studies.
    4. notify the physician.

17. The nurse is caring for a mother in labor whose membranes spontaneously rupture. The amniotic fluid is wine-colored. The appropriate action is to
    1. continue to observe the mother and fetus.
    2. test the fluid with Nitrazine paper to determine the pH.
    3. notify the physician and review the fetal monitor tracing.
    4. obtain a group B beta strep culture.

18. After a mother receives epidural anesthesia for labor and vaginal delivery, the nurse should evaluate the expected outcome of
    1. a decrease in sensation and motor control of lower extremities, bladder, and vasomotor tone.
    2. a heaviness in the legs and numb feet bilaterally.

3. a postdural epidural headache and a decrease in blood pressure.

4. sedation and a decrease in the mother's ability to push.

19. The nurse is caring for a newly delivered Asian mother and notes the family has piled blankets on the mother and brought her hot water and soup. The nurse understands this behavior is
   1. to prevent the mother from experiencing fever and chills.
   2. an indication of the cultural beliefs about birth.
   3. to compensate for a cool room temperature.
   4. to prevent exposure and preserve the modesty of the mother.

20. The nurse should prepare for a forceps and vacuum delivery after determining which of the following pelvis types to be present? Select all that apply:
   [ ] 1. Gynecoid
   [ ] 2. Android
   [ ] 3. Platypelloid
   [ ] 4. Anthropoid

21. The nurse assesses a multiparous woman to be more prone to which of the following dysfunctional labor patterns in the active phase of labor? Select all that apply:
   [ ] 1. Hypertonic uterine dysfunction
   [ ] 2. Secondary inertia
   [ ] 3. Arrest or protraction of the active phase
   [ ] 4. Primary inertia
   [ ] 5. Prolonged latent phase
   [ ] 6. Hypotonic uterine dysfunction

22. The nurse should perform which of the following hourly assessments when a pregnant woman is receiving magnesium sulfate for pre-eclampsia and eclampsia?
   1. Romberg sign
   2. Deep tendon reflexes

3. Temperature
4. Maternal heart rate

23. Which of the following is a priority for the nurse to assess in a mother receiving magnesium sulfate?
   1. Loss of patellar reflex
   2. Diaphoresis
   3. Respiratory rate less than 16
   4. Flushing

24. When the nurse notes an absent patellar reflex in a client receiving magnesium sulfate, the correct action is
   1. increase the rate of infusion per protocol.
   2. discontinue the infusion per protocol.
   3. administer an IV fluid bolus without medication.
   4. administer oxygen.

25. A client who is pre-eclamptic complains of blurred vision and scotomata to the nurse. The nurse should report this as indicating which of the following?
   1. Glaucoma
   2. Cerebral edema
   3. Spinal cord injury
   4. Hydrocephalus

26. The registered nurse is preparing clinical assignments for a maternity unit. Which of the following assignments should the nurse delegate to a licensed practical nurse?
   1. Administer oxytocin (Pitocin) IV to a woman in labor
   2. Instruct a mother on the clinical manifestations of eclampsia
   3. Initiate prescribed magnesium sulfate to a mother experiencing toxemia
   4. Walk a woman in labor to the delivery room

ANSWERS AND RATIONALES

1. 1. Loss of the protective barrier provided by the membranes increases the risk of infection (chorioamnionitis). The likelihood of placenta previa, hemorrhage, and arrest of descent are not increased by rupture of the membranes.

2. 3. Although uterine hyperstimulation, placenta previa, and abruptio placentae all pose a threat to the fetus, only cord prolapse is the direct result of rupture of membranes. Although the other conditions pose a threat to the mother as well as the fetus, cord prolapse threatens only fetal well-being.

3. 2. Oxytocin (Pitocin) is an oxytocic drug used in the treatment of induction or stimulation of labor at term. Excessive use of oxytocin is associated with uterine hyperstimulation.

4. 3.   Variable decelerations are caused by cord compression. Head compression, uteroplacental insufficiency, and cardiac conduction defect are associated with other types of periodic changes in fetal heart rate.

5.   4.6 hours. The average length of active labor for a nullipara client in the first stage of labor is 4.6 hours.

6. 1.   Early decelerations of the fetal heart rate may indicate the cervix is dilated and the labor may have progressed to the second stage. Changing the position of the mother from side to side is the intervention if umbilical cord compression is suspected. An amnioinfusion is the instillation of an isotonic glucose-free solution into the uterus to form a cushion for the umbilical cord or to thin out the meconium. It is also used when cord compression is present. Administration of oxygen is also performed when cord compression is suspected, because the oxygen will saturate the mother's blood, with the goal of supplying an adequate oxygen source to the fetus when the cord compression is relieved.

7. 2.   Variable decelerations most frequently occur after rupture of the membranes. They are variable in shape and timing.

8.   2. A 1- to 2-cm dilation, 40–50% effacement, -2 station, a medium cervical consistency, and a middle cervical position result in a Bishop Score of 2.

9. 2.   Absent long-term variability seen on the fetal heart monitor is present in congenital brain anomalies such as anencephaly. Anencephaly is a fatal condition in which the infant is born with a severely underdeveloped brain and skull. The infant most certainly dies shortly after birth.

10. 4. Early decelerations do not reflect fetal jeopardy. Observation for the source of head compression (e.g., possible descent of fetal head) is all that is indicated.

11. 1. Although a client with a complete placenta abruptio, a client experiencing variable decelerations, or a client with a fever *may* require a cesarean birth, complete placenta previa *always* mandates a cesarean birth.

12. 1. Both placenta previa and abruptio placentae can lead to uteroplacental insufficiency and threaten fetal well-being. The bleeding of placenta previa is usually painless and different from that with abruptio placentae. Questions regarding fever and gravida or para can be asked later. Headache and blurred vision are clinical manifestations of pre-eclampsia.

13. 3. A sterile speculum exam is performed to obtain a sample of vaginal fluid for a fern test to evaluate the status of the membranes. In the fern test, a sample of fluid is obtained from the vagina with a cotton-tipped applicator during a speculum exam. The fluid-soaked applicator is swabbed over a glass slide and examined under the microscope. A frondlike pattern indicates the presence of amniotic fluid. A digital exam should be deferred until the status of the membranes is determined. Ultrasound would not detect the leakage of a small amount of fluid. The nurse might obtain a vaginal group B beta strep culture after rupture of the membranes is confirmed by the fern test.

14. 3. During labor, a white blood cell count of 14,000 is normal, due to the physical stress of labor. No further action is necessary.

15. 3. During pregnancy, a slight respiratory alkalosis occurs, resulting from the 30–40% increase in tidal volume. The increased PaO_2 and the decreased PCO_2 of the maternal circulation facilitate the removal of the carbon dioxide from the fetal circulation. The decreased PCO_2 of the mother is compensated by the increased renal excretion of the bicarbonate permitting the arterial pH to remain in the normal range. No action is necessary.

16. 2. The mother is describing "bloody show," a normal finding in a mother in labor. This does not reflect coagulopathy, so no laboratory studies are indicated. Notifying the physician, obtaining coagulation studies, and preparing for a cesarean section apply to bright red vaginal bleeding, which is an abnormal finding.

17. 3. The "port wine" staining of the fluid is associated with abruptio placentae. Continuing to observe could place the mother and fetus in jeopardy. Obtaining a culture or testing with Nitrazine paper is not indicated. The nurse should notify the physician and monitor the fetus for evidence of abruptio placentae.

18. 1. Epidural anesthesia for labor and delivery produces anesthesia from T10 caudal to block both first- and second-stage pain. The block is usually higher for cesarean delivery. Correctly administered, regional anesthesia does not produce sedation or loss of consciousness. A postdural epidural headache results from an accidental puncture of the dura, which creates a larger hole and increases the incidence of postdural epidural headache. An epidural may lengthen the second stage of labor, resulting in a decreased ability of the mother to push. A heaviness in the legs and numb feet indicate the epidural catheter has gone into the subarachnoid space and should be withdrawn.

19. 2. Many cultures consider the postpartum mother to be in a "cold" state, and keep the mother warm to help regain the heat lost in childbirth. Although the family may have concerns about

room temperature or modesty, drinking warm liquids is a cultural practice. To prevent fever is not correct because the practice of drinking hot liquids is cultural, not medical.

20. 2. 4. The narrow dimensions of the android pelvis and the anthropoid pelvis cause slow descent of the fetal head, making the likelihood of forceps and vacuum delivery greater. The gynecoid pelvis has wider suprapubic arches and is favorable for a vaginal delivery. A platypelloid pelvis is present in only 3% of women, but a vaginal delivery may be performed.

21. 2. 3. 6. A multiparous woman may demonstrate dysfunctional labor patterns in the active phase of labor, such as hypotonic uterine dysfunction, secondary inertia, and arrest or protraction of the active phase. Dysfunctional labor patterns such as hypertonic uterine dysfunction, primary inertia, and a prolonged latent phase may occur in a nulliparous woman in the early phase.

22. 2. Magnesium sulfate decreases neuromuscular transmission of impulses; thus, reflexes would be affected. Also, loss of the patellar reflex is the first sign of magnesium sulfate toxicity. Urine output and respiratory status are also assessed hourly or more often.

23. 1. Adverse reactions to magnesium sulfate include diaphoresis, flushing, and decreased respirations. Loss of deep tendon reflexes, including the patellar reflex, is a sign of impending toxicity and is the priority assessment.

24. 2. Because an absent patellar reflex is an early sign of toxicity, the magnesium sulfate infusion should be discontinued and the physician notified. Administering IV fluids or oxygen would not treat the toxicity. Increasing the rate would increase toxicity.

25. 2. Visual disturbances may reflect cerebral edema in the pre-eclamptic client.

26. 4. Administering oxytocin (Pitocin), instructing a mother on the clinical manifestations of eclampsia, and initiating magnesium sulfate to a mother experiencing toxemia should all be performed by a registered nurse. A licensed practical nurse may walk a woman in labor to the delivery room.

REFERENCES

Daniels, R. (2010). *Delmar's manual of laboratory and diagnostic tests* (2nd ed.). Clifton Park, NY: Delmar Cengage Learning.

Littleton, L., & Engebretson, J. (2002). *Maternal, neonatal, and women's health nursing.* Clifton Park, NY: Delmar Cengage Learning.

Littleton, L., & Engebretson, J. (2013). *Maternity nursing care* (2nd ed.). Clifton Park, NY: Delmar Cengage Learning.

CHAPTER 44

THE POSTPARTAL PERIOD

I. **ANATOMY AND PHYSIOLOGY**
   A. UTERUS (SEE TABLE 44-1)
      1. INVOLUTION IS THE PROCESS WHEREIN THE REPRODUCTIVE ORGANS RETURN TO THEIR NONPREGNANT STATE.
      2. INVOLUTION OF THE UTERUS INVOLVES TWO MAJOR PROCESSES.
      3. THE FIRST PROCESS INVOLVES THE AREA WHERE THE PLACENTA WAS ATTACHED.
      4. CONTRACTIONS OF THE UTERUS AFTER DELIVERY PINCH OFF THESE VESSELS TO PREVENT BLEEDING.
      5. THE SECOND PROCESS INVOLVES THE UTERUS RETURNING TO ITS NONPREGNANT SIZE BY CONTRACTION OF THIS MUSCLE.
      6. IMMEDIATELY AFTER DELIVERY, THE UTERINE FUNDUS MAY BE PALPATED HALFWAY BETWEEN THE UMBILICUS AND THE SYMPHYSIS PUBIS.
      7. ONE HOUR LATER, THE FUNDUS WILL RISE TO THE LEVEL OF THE UMBILICUS, WHERE IT WILL REMAIN FOR THE NEXT 24 HOURS.
      8. AFTER 24 HOURS, THE UTERUS WILL DECREASE 1 CM/DAY IN SIZE.
      9. BY DAY 9 OR 10, THE UTERUS WILL HAVE WITHDRAWN INTO THE PELVIS TO THE POINT WHERE IT IS NO LONGER PALPABLE.
      10. BY 4 WEEKS, THE UTERUS RETURNS TO ITS NONPREGNANT SIZE.
      11. WEIGHT OF THE UTERUS IS 1000 GRAMS IMMEDIATELY AFTER DELIVERY AND 50–100 GRAMS AFTER INVOLUTION IS COMPLETED, APPROXIMATELY 6 WEEKS POSTPARTUM.
   B. LOCHIA
      1. UTERINE DISCHARGE OF BLOOD, MUCUS, AND TISSUE AFTER CHILDBIRTH
      2. SLOUGHING OFF OF DECIDUAL TISSUES, INCLUDING ERYTHROCYTES, EPITHELIAL CELLS, AND BACTERIA
      3. ASSESSED ACCORDING TO AMOUNT, COLOR, AND CHANGE WITH ACTIVITY
      4. DURATION IS NOT AFFECTED BY BREAST FEEDING OR THE USE OF ORAL CONTRACEPTIVES.
      5. BY 48 HOURS POST DELIVERY, FLOW SHOULD BE LIGHT TO MODERATE.
      6. NORMAL INCREASE IN FLOW IN THE MORNING AND WITH BREAST FEEDING
      7. STAGES:
         a. Lochia rubra: bright red in color, lasting first 3–4 days postpartum
         b. Lochia serosa: light pink in color, days 3–4 until day 10 postpartum
         c. Lochia alba: white and yellow discharge lasting up to 6 weeks
      8. AMOUNT OF FLOW:
         a. Scant flow: less than 1-inch stain/1 hour
         b. Light flow: less than 4-inch stain/1 hour
         c. Moderate flow: less than 6-inch stain/1 hour
         d. Heavy flow: saturated pad in 1 hour
   C. CERVIX
      1. FOLLOWING DELIVERY, THE CERVIX IS SOFT AND FLEXIBLE, AND THE INTERNAL AND EXTERNAL OS ARE OPEN.

Table 44-1 Size of the Uterus Following Delivery

Time After Delivery	Size
Post delivery (1–6 days)	1000 grams
7 days postpartum	300–350 grams
14 days postpartum	100 grams
End of sixth week (involution)	50 grams

© Cengage Learning 2015

2. THE CERVIX CLOSES TO 2–3 CM AFTER SEVERAL DAYS, OPENING THE SIZE OF A PENCIL AT 1 WEEK POSTPARTUM.

3. IF VAGINAL DELIVERY, THE INTERNAL OS WILL CLOSE COMPLETELY BUT THE EXTERNAL OS WILL REMAIN SLITLIKE COMPARED TO THE NULLIPAROUS ROUND SHAPE.

D. VAGINA

1. AFTER VAGINAL DELIVERY, THE VAGINA IS DISTENDED BEYOND ITS NORMAL SIZE.

2. THE RUGAE, OR SKIN FOLDS THAT LINE THE VAGINA, ARE ABSENT BUT REAPPEAR AROUND 3 WEEKS POSTPARTUM.

3. INVOLUTION IS AFFECTED BY ESTROGEN STIMULATION AND WILL TAKE LONGER IF THE MOTHER IS BREAST FEEDING.

4. WITH THE ONSET OF OVULATION, MUCUS PRODUCTION RETURNS TO THE VAGINA.

E. EXTERNAL STRUCTURES

1. DEPENDENT ON DELIVERY FACTORS, THE WOMAN MAY HAVE ECCHYMOSIS, EDEMA, OR SWELLING OF THE PERINEAL AREA.

2. THE WOMAN MAY HAVE AN EPISIOTOMY OR LACERATION REPAIR.

3. LACERATION MAY BE FIRST, SECOND, THIRD, OR FOURTH DEGREE.

   a. First degree: superficial through the skin and muscle layer
   b. Second degree: extends through the perineal muscle layer
   c. Third degree: continues through the anal sphincter
   d. Fourth degree: also involves the anterior rectal wall

4. LABIA MAJORA AND LABIA MINORA REMAIN ATROPHIC AND SOFTENED, NEVER RETURNING TO THEIR PREPREGNANT STATE.

F. BREASTS AND NIPPLES

1. BREASTS INCREASE IN SIZE DUE TO ESTROGEN AND PROGESTERONE INFLUENCE.

2. COLOSTRUM IS THE EARLY MILK.

3. COLOSTRUM IS RICH IN ANTIBODIES.

4. CALORIC CONTENT OF COLOSTRUM IS SIMILAR TO BREAST MILK.

5. BREAST MILK IS USUALLY PRODUCED BY 72 HOURS POSTPARTUM.

6. BREAST SIZE DOES NOT PREDICT THE ABILITY TO PRODUCE MILK.

7. BREAST CHANGES DUE TO PREGNANCY REGRESS IN 1–2 WEEKS IF NOT BREAST FEEDING.

8. AS LONG AS MILK DUCTS WERE NOT SEVERED, WOMEN WHO HAD BREAST AUGMENTATION SHOULD BE ABLE TO BREAST FEED.

9. BREAST REDUCTION SURGERY RELATED TO BREAST FEEDING SUCCESS IS DEPENDENT ON THE AMOUNT OF FUNCTIONAL TISSUE REMOVED AND THE TYPE OF PROCEDURE PERFORMED.

G. EXTREMITIES

1. EDEMA OF THE LOWER EXTREMITIES IS VERY COMMON AFTER DELIVERY.

2. THIS IS DUE TO EXTRA FLUIDS AND HORMONE CHANGES AFTER DELIVERY.

3. AS LONG AS THE EDEMA IS SYMMETRICAL THERE IS NO CAUSE FOR CONCERN.

4. IF THE EDEMA IS UNILATERAL, INVOLVES REDNESS, WARMTH, OR TENDERNESS, EVALUATE FOR A DEEP VEIN THROMBUS.

5. EDEMA MAY GET WORSE AFTER DISCHARGE DUE TO INCREASED TIME A CLIENT IS UP ON HER FEET.

H. CARDIOVASCULAR SYSTEM

1. BLOOD VOLUME INCREASES 40–50% DURING PREGNANCY.

2. BY 1 WEEK POSTPARTUM, BLOOD VOLUME RETURNS TO NORMAL.

3. USUAL BLOOD LOSS IS 300–500 ML AFTER A VAGINAL BIRTH AND 500–1000 ML FOLLOWING A CESAREAN BIRTH.

4. DECREASE IN HEMATOCRIT OF 4 POINTS AND A 1-GRAM DROP IN HEMOGLOBIN OCCUR FOR EACH 250 ML BLOOD LOSS.

5. HEMOGLOBIN AND HEMATOCRIT USUALLY RETURN TO NORMAL LEVELS BY 4–6 WEEKS POSTPARTUM.

6. INCREASED FIBRINOGEN LEVELS THROUGH THE FIRST POSTPARTUM WEEK ALLOW A PROTECTIVE EFFECT AGAINST HEMORRHAGE.

7. THIS INCREASED LEVEL ALSO INCREASES THE RISK OF THROMBUS FORMATION.

8. LEUKOCYTOSIS IS ALSO A PROTECTIVE MECHANISM AGAINST INVADING ORGANISMS, ALONG WITH AN AID WITH HEALING.

I. GASTROINTESTINAL (GI) SYSTEM

1. MANY COMMON GI COMPLAINTS EXPERIENCED DURING PREGNANCY RESOLVE DUE TO A DROP IN PROGESTERONE LEVELS.

2. DIGESTION AND ABSORPTION RESUME AFTER DELIVERY.

3. INCREASED HUNGER AND THIRST AFTER DELIVERY IS DUE TO THE GLUCOSE USED DURING LABOR AND FROM RESTRICTED FLUIDS, ALONG WITH BEGINNING OF THE DIAPHORESIS STAGE.

4. CLIENT MAY HAVE DELAY IN RETURN TO NORMAL BOWEL FUNCTION AFTER DELIVERY, LEADING TO CONSTIPATION DUE TO THE LINGERING EFFECTS OF ESTROGEN AND PROGESTERONE.

5. HEMORRHOIDS ARE THE RESULT OF VENOUS DILATION, PRESSURE OF THE GRAVID UTERUS, AND SLOWED PERISTALSIS DURING PREGNANCY.

6. HEMORRHOIDS USUALLY DISAPPEAR A FEW WEEKS AFTER DELIVERY.

J. URINARY SYSTEM

1. INCREASED BLADDER CAPACITY AND DECREASED TONE LEAD TO DECREASED SENSATION AFTER DELIVERY.

2. UTERINE LIGAMENTS ARE STRETCHED FROM THE DELIVERY PROCESS, ALLOWING A FULL BLADDER TO MOVE THE UTERUS.

3. AS THE BLADDER FILLS, IT DISPLACES THE UTERUS TO THE RIGHT.

4. HYDRONEPHROSIS, OR THE INCREASED SIZE OF THE URETERS DUE TO PREGNANCY EFFECTS, REMAINS PRESENT FOR UP TO 4 WEEKS POSTPARTUM.

5. THE INCREASED SIZE OF THESE STRUCTURES ALONG WITH DECREASED SENSATION INCREASE THE POSSIBILITY OF URINARY STASIS AND URINARY TRACT INFECTION IN THE POSTPARTUM PERIOD.

6. NORMAL URINE OUTPUT MAY REACH 2000–3000 ML/24 HOURS.

7. THIS IS A RESULT OF DECREASED ALDOSTERONE PRODUCTION AND REDUCED SODIUM RETENTION.

8. MILD PROTEINURIA IS COMMON AND MAY PERSIST DUE TO CATABOLIC EFFECTS OF THE INVOLUTION PERIOD.

K. ENDOCRINE SYSTEM

1. PANCREAS

a. The increased insulin resistance from the hormones of pregnancy resolves after delivery.

b. Pancreas should return to the prepregnancy state with decreased production of insulin needed.

2. THYROID

a. Clinical manifestations of postpartum thyroiditis may manifest up to 1 month postpartum.

b. Of women who develop thyroiditis, 10–30% develop permanent hypothyroid.

c. Thyrotoxic storm is a life-threatening emergency.

d. Clinical manifestations include increased temperature, weakness, restlessness, and wide emotional mood swings leading to confusion, psychosis, and possible coma.

e. This condition is due to excessive release of thyroid hormones.

3. PITUITARY

a. Serum prolactin levels rise dramatically during the first 2 weeks postpartum and rapidly decline to prepregnant levels if the mother is not breast feeding.

b. Follicle-stimulating hormone (FSH) and luteinizing hormone (LH) are absent in the early postpartum period.

4. PLACENTAL

a. Human chorionic gonadotropin (hCG) is undetected by 1 week postpartum.

b. Human chorionic somatomammotropin (HCS) is undetected by 24 hours postpartum.

c. Plasma progesterone levels are undetected by 3 days postpartum.

d. Estrogen levels decrease to 10% of the prenatal value within 3 hours after delivery and reach their lowest level by 7 days postpartum.

L. RESPIRATORY SYSTEM

1. DIAPHRAGM DESCENDS AND ABDOMINAL ORGANS REVERT TO NORMAL POSITION.

2. ACID-BASE BALANCE RETURNS TO PREPREGNANT LEVELS BY 3 WEEKS POSTPARTUM.

3. BASAL METABOLIC RATE REMAINS ELEVATED FOR UP TO 14 DAYS POSTPARTUM.

M. MUSCULOSKELETAL SYSTEM

1. MUSCLE STRAINS AND ACHES ARE COMMON DUE TO THE EXERTION OF LABOR.

2. EFFECTS FROM RELAXIN, THE HORMONE THAT RELAXES CARTILAGE AND LIGAMENTS DURING PREGNANCY, GRADUALLY DECLINE AND JOINTS RETURN TO NONPREGNANT POSITION.

3. THERE MAY BE SEPARATION OF THE DIASTASIS RECTI, THE LONGITUDINAL MUSCLES OF THE ABDOMEN.

4. PELVIC FLOOR MUSCLES STRETCH AND THIN DUE TO PREGNANCY AND DELIVERY EFFECTS AND MAY LACK TONE AFTER DELIVERY.

N. SKIN

1. PIGMENT CHANGES THAT COMMONLY OCCUR ON THE SKIN DURING PREGNANCY USUALLY FADE DURING THE POSTPARTUM PERIOD.

2. STRIAE GRAVIDARUM WILL FADE TO A PALE WHITE DURING THE FIRST 6 MONTHS POSTPARTUM.

3. IN DARKER-SKINNED CLIENTS, THE STRIAE GRAVIDARUM MAY TURN DARKER BEFORE FADING TO A MORE NEUTRAL SKIN COLOR.

O. IMMUNE SYSTEM
   1. MOTHER WITH RH-NEGATIVE BLOOD TYPE AND RH-POSITIVE INFANT MUST RECEIVE RHOGAM WITHIN 72 HOURS POSTPARTUM.
   2. IT PREVENTS SENSITIZATION TO THE RH FACTOR AND PREVENTS HEMOLYTIC DISEASE IN THE NEWBORN IN SUBSEQUENT PREGNANCIES.
   3. AMOUNT OF RHOGAM NEEDED IS DETERMINED BY THE CORD BLOOD.
   4. RHOGAM IS A BLOOD PRODUCT AND GIVEN AS AN INTRAMUSCULAR (IM) INJECTION.
   5. APPROXIMATELY 7000 PREGNANCIES EACH YEAR ARE AFFECTED BY HIV INFECTION.
   6. PERINATAL TRANSMISSION IS ESTIMATED AT 14–40% UNLESS TREATED WITH ANTIVIRAL DRUGS.
   7. ANTIVIRAL DRUGS GIVEN ORALLY DURING PREGNANCY AND GIVEN INTRAVENOUSLY (IV) DURING LABOR AND DELIVERY HAVE DECREASED NEONATAL TRANSMISSION TO LESS THAN 7% WITH A VAGINAL DELIVERY, AND LESS THAN 1% WITH A SURGICAL DELIVERY.
   8. ALL NEWBORNS WILL TEST POSITIVE AT BIRTH DUE TO ANTIBODIES RECEIVED BY THE MOTHER BUT WILL SEROCONVERT BETWEEN 15 AND 18 MONTHS OF AGE AFTER DEPLETION OF THESE ANTIBODIES.
   9. BREASTFEEDING IS PROHIBITED DUE TO THE VIRUS BEING PRESENT IN BREAST MILK.
   10. PREGNANCY DOES NOT CAUSE A FASTER PROGRESSION OF HIV.

II. **ASSESSMENT**
   A. CLIENT'S SUBJECTIVE OPINION
      1. MUST TAKE ATTITUDES AND BELIEFS OF CULTURE INTO CONSIDERATION REGARDING BASIC CARE ISSUES.
      2. PAIN IS AS THE CLIENT PERCEIVES IT.
   B. HEALTH HISTORY
      1. IDENTIFY ANY PREEXISTING CONDITIONS.
      2. PREVIOUS RELEVANT OBSTETRIC INFORMATION
      3. ADDRESS PERSONAL CONCERNS AND QUESTIONS.
   C. SOCIAL HISTORY
      1. CULTURE
      2. SOCIAL SUPPORT

3. EDUCATION LEVEL
4. OCCUPATION
5. RISK FOR DOMESTIC VIOLENCE
6. COPING MECHANISMS
7. HEALTH PATTERNS

D. BONDING AND FAMILY ADJUSTMENT
   1. BONDING IS THE ATTRACTION FELT BY THE PARENTS FOR THE INFANT.
   2. MANY FACTORS AFFECT THIS, SUCH AS AGE, MATERNAL AND NEWBORN HEALTH, CULTURE, BIRTH EXPERIENCE, AND DESIRE TO HAVE A CHILD.
   3. REVA RUBIN, A NURSING THEORIST, IDENTIFIED THREE STAGES IN ATTAINING THE MOTHERING ROLE:
      a. Taking-in stage: first postpartum day characterized by the woman being more concerned with her own physical and emotional needs and demonstrating little initiative for infant care or decision making
      b. Taking-hold stage: 2nd to 10th postpartum days characterized by the woman assuming greater responsibility toward the infant and self; often referred to as the "teachable, reachable, and referable moment"
      c. Letting-go stage: attainment of mothering role by readjustments of previously held roles and relationships

E. PHYSICAL EXAM
   1. VITAL SIGNS
      a. A temperature over 38°C (100.4°F) after 48 hours postdelivery may indicate infection.
      b. Pulse: relative bradycardia is not unusual due to increased blood volume.
      c. After delivery of the placenta, women experience as much as 1000 ml autotransfusion.
      d. Tachycardia may indicate hypovolemia.
      e. Blood pressure should be back to normal level within 4 days postpartum.
      f. Orthostatic hypotension may indicate hemorrhage or inadequate fluid intake.
      g. Pain is the fifth vital sign.
      h. Assess and provide p.r.n. medications as ordered.
   2. INSPECT BREASTS FOR SIZE, CONTOUR, ASYMMETRY, ENGORGEMENT, AND AREAS OF WARMTH REGARDLESS IF BREAST OR BOTTLE FEEDING.
   3. INSPECT NIPPLES FOR TISSUE INTEGRITY, CRACKS, BLISTERS, OR FISSURES.
   4. LISTEN TO THE LUNGS; ASSESS FOR COUGH OR SPUTUM PRODUCTION.

5. CHECK THE UTERINE FUNDUS FOR POSITION AND FIRMNESS.
6. MONITOR THE LOCHIA FOR COLOR AND AMOUNT.
7. ASSESS THE PERINEUM FOR REDNESS, EDEMA, ECCHYMOSIS, DRAINAGE, AND APPROXIMATION (REEDA).
8. ASSESS FOR PASSAGE OF FLATUS AND BOWEL MOVEMENT.
9. AUSCULTATE BOWEL SOUNDS AND ASSESS FOR SIGNS OF ABDOMINAL DISTENTION.
10. ASSESS FOR HEMORRHOIDS.
11. PALPATE FOR BLADDER DISTENTION.
12. CHECK THE LOWER EXTREMITIES FOR REDNESS, EDEMA, WARMTH, AND DISCOMFORT.
13. CHECK HOMAN'S SIGN.
    a. Dorsiflexion of each foot
    b. A positive sign is pain with this maneuver.
14. MONITOR FOR BONDING BEHAVIOR BETWEEN THE FAMILY AND THE INFANT.

III. DIAGNOSTIC STUDIES

A. COMPLETE BLOOD COUNT (CBC)
   1. DESCRIPTION
      a. Laboratory test on the client's serum
      b. The CBC is obtained routinely after delivery to evaluate for presence of infection or anemia.
      c. An elevated white blood cell (WBC) count above expected values is indicative of infection in the postpartum period.
      d. However, elevation above normal, called leukocytosis, may represent an early infectious state or the body's stress reaction to childbirth.
      e. WBC measurement of 14,000 to 16,000/mm^3 is normal in the immediate postpartum period; it may be as high as 20,000/mm^3.
      f. The WBCs are separated and counted on the CBC; this categorization is called the differential.
      g. The differential is used to determine infection based on the increase of the immature types of WBCs in the serum (circulating blood).
      h. Anemia is the state of deficient red blood cells (RBCs) or hemoglobin to meet the body's requirement for oxygen.
      i. Low hemoglobin in the postpartum period is often due to the blood loss of delivery following physiologic anemia of pregnancy.
      j. Those clients with iron deficiency anemia prior to delivery are a concern even with normal blood loss at delivery (< 500 ml for a vaginal delivery).

2. PREPROCEDURE
   a. Instruct the client about the blood draw and the reason for obtaining the specimen.
3. POSTPROCEDURE
   a. No special care is required.
B. CONTRAST VENOGRAPHY OR CONTRAST PHLEBOGRAPHY
   1. DESCRIPTION
      a. For diagnosis of deep vein thrombus or thrombosis (DVT)
      b. Radiographic contrast dye is injected into the distal, dorsal foot vein while the client is in 40% reversed Trendelenburg position, and x-rays are taken of the blood flow.
      c. Two views of intraluminal filling defects are diagnostic for DVT.
      d. Accurate technique is difficult to perform, and interpretation requires considerable experience.
      e. The test is not without risks, which include foot pain during injection or 1–2 days afterward, superficial phlebitis, DVT, hypersensitivity to the dye, or local skin reaction.
   2. PREPROCEDURE
      a. Assess the client for a hypersensitivity to any contrast dye or if there are renal problems.
      b. Unless the test is done in an emergency, the client will fast or drink only clear liquids.
      c. Inform the client that a catheter is inserted to inject the dye, which may cause a flushing feeling or nausea, and that she will be required to keep her leg still.
   3. POSTPROCEDURE
      a. A solution is injected to help clear the contrast.
      b. The client is to drink a large amount of fluids to flush the remaining dye from the body.
      c. Observe and report the following to the physician: any signs of local irritation, swelling, fever, superficial vein thrombosis, DVT, or complaints of pain.
C. IMPEDANCE PLETHYSMOGRAPHY (IPG)
   1. DESCRIPTION
      a. Noninvasive test that uses electrical pulses to measure blood flow in the veins of the legs to diagnose DVT.
      b. IPG measures the resistance (or impedance) to the electric impulse that is normally seen with adequate blood flow.
      c. Electrodes are placed on the calf with conductive jelly and connected to a plethysmograph, which records changes in electrical resistance.

2. PREPROCEDURE
   a. Inform the client that the test requires the leg be raised 30 degrees of the level of the heart while a blood pressure (BP) cuff is inflated and deflated on the thigh.
   b. Instruct the client that this procedure will be repeated several times in both legs.
3. POSTPROCEDURE
   a. No special care is required.

D. DUPLEX ULTRASONOGRAPHY
1. DESCRIPTION
   a. Noninvasive ultrasound imaging of venous blood flow
   b. Useful in determining disruptions of blood flow that can be occlusions from clots
   c. Portable ultrasound on both lower legs is done when a client has clinical manifestations of DVT or pulmonary embolism (PE).
2. PREPROCEDURE
   a. No preparation is required.
3. POSTPROCEDURE
   a. No special care is required.

E. VENTILATION/PERFUSION (V/Q) SCAN
1. DESCRIPTION
   a. Nuclear medicine test to detect pulmonary emboli by scanning the lungs for ventilation (the ability to take in air) and perfusion (blood flow to the lungs)
   b. The client breathes in a combination of air and radioactive gas and is given intravenous radioisotope; a special camera takes images that demonstrate the distribution of air in the lungs and blood flow to the lungs.
   c. Areas absent of blood flow seen as areas absent of injected radioactive marker suggest occlusion by blood clots (emboli).
   d. The diagnosis is only suggestive and not definite because the test does not visualize the clot.
2. PREPROCEDURE
   a. No special preparation is required and the procedure is often done on an emergency basis.
3. POSTPROCEDURE
   a. No special care is required.

F. SPIRAL COMPUTERIZED TOMOGRAPHY (CT) SCAN
1. DESCRIPTION
   a. CT using spiral (helical) scans allows for the central pulmonary arteries to be visualized following IV contrast medium injected through a peripheral IV.
   b. Used for the detection of pulmonary emboli in the main, lobar, or segmental pulmonary arteries
   c. Newer form of CT scanning, which scans in continuous motion (not slices) and allows for three-dimensional re-creation of images
   d. Greater than 95% sensitivity and specificity
   e. Noninvasive, but does require tolerance to radiopaque dye
   f. Does not require personnel qualified to cannulate the pulmonary arteries
   g. May be the initial diagnostic test or a follow-up test if the V/Q scan is not diagnostic
2. PREPROCEDURE
   a. Educate the client about the test.
   b. Remove all metal and jewelry from the client.
   c. Gather requested information from the client, such as her experience with contrast dye and general health status; inquire about pregnancy or claustrophobia.
3. POSTPROCEDURE
   a. The client is immediately observed in the scanning area for possible adverse contrast reactions—particularly respiratory difficulty.

G. PULMONARY ANGIOGRAM
1. DESCRIPTION
   a. Accepted diagnostic reference to diagnose pulmonary embolus; thought of as the gold standard test
   b. The pulmonary arteries are catheterized with repeated injections of small amounts of radiopaque dye, which can be visualized on x-ray.
   c. The brachial or the femoral artery is most often used for this procedure; a catheter is threaded into the pulmonary artery.
   d. May be used as a follow-up test if the V/Q scan is not diagnostic
2. PREPROCEDURE
   a. Similar to any surgical procedure
   b. Verify that the consent form is signed by the client and physician.
   c. Instruct the client to be NPO status for 12 hours.
   d. Prep the catheter insertion site by shaving it.
   e. Ensure IV access.
   f. Administer preoperative medications as ordered; antihistamines or steroids to prevent allergic reactions.
   g. Instruct the client that a warm or flushed feeling when the dye is injected may be experienced.

3. POSTPROCEDURE
   a. Apply manual pressure to the site for 5–15 minutes, followed by a pressure dressing.
   b. Monitor the client for the signs of bleeding at the site or concealed bleeding in the upper leg (discoloration, increase in size, and decreased pulses).
   c. Apply a cold compress to the site if ordered.
   d. Observe for signs of delayed allergic reaction (hives, fainting, bronchospasm, laryngeal edema, hypotension, pulmonary edema, and respiratory arrest).

H. URINALYSIS AND CULTURE (SEE CHAPTER 42, SECTION III, SUBSECTION D.)
I. ORAL GLUCOSE TOLERANCE TEST (OGTT OR GTT) (SEE CHAPTER 42, SECTION III, SUBSECTION G.)

IV. NURSING DIAGNOSES
A. DEFICIENT KNOWLEDGE
B. SELF-CARE DEFICIT
C. IMPAIRED URINARY ELIMINATION
D. ACUTE PAIN
E. RISK FOR CONSTIPATION
F. INTERRUPTED FAMILY PROCESSES
G. INEFFECTIVE ROLE PERFORMANCE

Nursing Diagnoses: Definitions and Classification 2012–2014.
Copyright © 2012, 1994–2012 by NANDA International.
Used by arrangement with John Wiley & Sons Limited.

V. NORMAL POSTPARTUM RECOVERY
A. SYSTEMS RETURN TO THEIR PREPREGNANT STATE.
B. PHYSIOLOGIC AND PSYCHOLOGICAL CHANGES OCCUR AS THE CLIENT TRANSITIONS TO A FAMILY FOCUS.
C. BONDING AND FAMILY ADJUSTMENT IS EVIDENT.

VI. POSTPARTUM COMPLICATIONS
A. POSTPARTUM HEMORRHAGE
   1. DESCRIPTION
      a. Blood loss greater than 500 ml in the first 24 hours after delivery; may be greater amount of blood loss with cesarean delivery
      b. Significant cause of morbidity and mortality
      c. One-third of maternal deaths attributed to this complication
      d. Most common cause (75%) is uterine atony
      e. Other causes include lacerations, uterine rupture, uterine inversion, and altered clotting factors, anesthesia, previous history, high parity, prolonged labor, and coagulation disorders.
      f. Each 500 ml blood loss leads to a 1–1.5 g/dl drop in hemoglobin, 2–4% drop in hematocrit.

   2. ASSESSMENT
      a. At term, 600 ml of blood perfuse the uterus each minute.
      b. Blood loss can happen very quickly after delivery.
      c. Subjective report of excessive bleeding, "gushing" of blood from vaginal area
   3. DIAGNOSTIC TESTS
      a. CBC to verify hemoglobin and hematocrit levels
      b. Blood gases to rule out acidosis or hypoxia
   4. NURSING INTERVENTIONS
      a. Take frequent vital signs.
      b. Perform frequent assessments.
      c. Obtain oxygen saturation levels.
      d. Assess vaginal blood flow.
      e. Weigh and count pads.
      f. Massage the uterus if boggy.
      g. Insert a urinary catheter.
      h. Provide adequate hydration and start an IV.
      i. Monitor intake and output.
      j. Instruct the client on how to self-massage the uterus.
      k. Provide support.
      l. Administer oxytocin medications ordered to increase contractility of the uterus.
      m. Administer vasoconstrictive medications to decrease the blood flow to the uterus.
      n. Prepare the client for surgical intervention if uterine massage and pharmacological therapies are ineffective.
      o. Monitor the client for complications such as hypovolemia, shock, disseminated intravascular coagulation (DIC), anoxic brain injury, and death (see Table 44-2).
      p. Prepare the client for a dilation and curettage (D&C) if she retained placental parts.
      q. Monitor for adverse effects of oxytocic medications such as hypotension after rapid infusion of IV bolus of pitocin (Oxytocin), or hypertension with methylergonovine (Methergine) and ergotrate.

B. HEMATOMA
   1. DESCRIPTION
      a. A collection of blood, often vulvar or vaginal, that occurs as a result of injury to a blood vessel during spontaneous delivery
      b. In an assisted delivery, the most common site is the lateral wall of the vagina in the ischial spine area.
      c. Incidence: 1:300–1:500 births
      d. Predisposing factors include prolonged pressure of the fetal head on the vaginal mucosa, operative delivery, prolonged

Table 44-2 Signs of Shock

	Mild	Moderate	Severe	Irreversible
Respiration	Rapid but still deep	Rapid and becoming shallow	Rapid and shallow; may be irregular	Irregular; may be barely perceptible
Blood pressure	Normal or increased	60–90 mm Hg systolic	Less than 60 mm Hg systolic	No palpable blood pressure
Pulse	Rapid with normal tone or tone growing weaker	Rapid and irregular	Very rapid	Irregular apical pulse
Skin	Pale and cool	Cool, pale, and moist	Cold and clammy; cyanosis of the nail beds and lips	Cold, clammy, and cyanotic
Urinary output	No change	Decreased; 10–22 ml/hr	Less than 10 ml/hr; may be anuric (none)	Anuric
Level of consciousness	Alert and oriented; some anxiety	Oriented; may have difficulty thinking	Lethargic; responds to painful stimuli	Comatose; does not respond to painful stimuli

© Cengage Learning 2015

Table 44-3 Common Postpartum Infections

Wound Infection	Uterus	UTI	Breast
Bacterial invasion of a perineal wound or surgical incision	Bacteria ascend up the genital tract or exposure during surgery.	Bacteria ascend up the urethra.	Backwash of bacteria from the infant's mouth while nursing into the mother's breast tissue
Redness and drainage at the site, fever, malaise, and increasing pain	Increasing pain, fever, tender uterus, prolonged and severe cramping, and malodorous discharge	Frequency and burning on urination, fever, or evidence of infection on urinalysis (UA)	Localized area of pain, redness, and warmth; fever, chills, and malaise
All wound contact should be aseptic; teach the client to wipe the perineum front to back to avoid cross-contamination.	Teach good handwashing technique.	Encourage a high fluid intake (up to 3 L/day) and foods that increase the acidity of urine (cranberry juice, apricots, plums, or prunes).	Avoid missed feedings (nurse frequently); prevent cracked nipples if possible.

© Cengage Learning 2015

second stage of labor, precipitous delivery, or macrosomia.
  e. Complications include inability to void due to excessive size and placement of hematoma and postpartum hemorrhage.
2. ASSESSMENT
  a. Hypotension
  b. Tachycardia
  c. Extreme perineal or pelvic pain, which is a cardinal sign
  d. Firm uterus with bright red blood
  e. Bluish bulging area just under the skin surface
  f. Difficulty in voiding
3. DIAGNOSTIC TEST
  a. CBC for anemia
4. MEDICAL-SURGICAL MANAGEMENT
  a. If hematoma is large, or with excessive bleeding, may need to be surgically opened and drained, with the blood vessel ligated.
5. NURSING INTERVENTIONS
  a. Monitor vital signs frequently.
  b. Observe for signs of blood loss and shock.

  c. Check the fundus and observe the perineal area frequently.
  d. Check oxygen saturation.
  e. Monitor IV fluids.
  f. Monitor urine output.
  g. Insert a Foley catheter if indicated.
  h. Monitor pain control.
  i. Apply ice to the perineal area after delivery.
  j. Offer reassurance and support.
C. BACTERIAL INFECTIONS
  1. DESCRIPTION
    a. Presence of bacteria that causes tissue damage
    b. Generalized and cardinal signs are elevated temperature, tachycardia, and pain.
    c. Common sites of infection in the postpartum period include urinary tract (UTI), breast (mastitis), wound (perineal laceration, episiotomy, or surgical incision), or of the uterus or lining of the uterus (metritis/endometritis) (see Table 44-3).

    d. Nonsteroidal anti-inflammatory drugs (NSAIDs) such as ibuprofen and other pain relievers such as Tylenol, which are commonly used in the postpartum period, are antipyretics and may mask fever as a clinical sign of infection.

    e. Complications include metritis, which may progress to pelvic cellulitis manifested by absent bowel sounds, abdominal distention, and nausea and vomiting, bacteremia or septicemia, and pyelonephritis.

2. ASSESSMENT

    a. Pain

    b. Difficulty voiding

    c. Lochia

3. DIAGNOSTIC TESTS

    a. CBC

    b. Wound culture

    c. Blood cultures if bacteremia is suspected

4. NURSING INTERVENTIONS

    a. Instruct the client in proper perineal hygiene and the clinical manifestations of infection to report.

    b. Ensure infection prevention strategies.

    c. Notify the physician of the clinical manifestations of infection.

    d. Obtain wound culture or arrange for lab tests as ordered.

    e. Administer antibiotics, pain medications, and antipyretics as ordered.

    f. Raise the head of the bed to Fowler's position to promote lochia drainage in the client who has a uterine infection.

D. DEEP VEIN THROMBUS (DVT)

1. DESCRIPTION

    a. "Thrombus" is clot formation.

    b. Clients are at risk in the postpartum period for thrombus because of increased clotting factors.

    c. A thrombus in the deep venous circulation is a concern because it can migrate to the pulmonary arteries.

    d. A thrombus is generally found in the leg, thigh, or pelvis.

    e. Thrombophlebitis is the inflammation of the lining of the blood vessel from a thrombus; symptoms include pain, tenderness, edema, and positive Homan's sign.

    f. Complications include pulmonary emboli and septic pelvic thrombophlebitis.

2. ASSESSMENT

    a. Leg pain

3. DIAGNOSTIC TESTS

    a. Contrast venography or contrast phlebography

    b. IPG

    c. Duplex ultrasonography

4. NURSING INTERVENTIONS

    a. Encourage the client to wear pneumatic compression stockings if ordered.

    b. Encourage early ambulation.

    c. Discourage the client from crossing the legs.

    d. Instruct the client on prevention strategies and the manifestations to report promptly.

    e. Administer heparin, as ordered, for prevention in high-risk clients or for treatment of thrombus.

    f. Avoid massaging the legs.

    g. Instruct the client about the clinical manifestations of pulmonary embolus and actions to take if the manifestations develop.

    h. Regularly inspect the legs in the postpartum period for manifestations of thrombophlebitis (the inflammation of the lining of the blood vessel), which indicate deep vein thrombosis.

E. PULMONARY EMBOLI (PE)

1. DESCRIPTION

    a. Leading cause of pregnancy-related death in the United States

    b. Thrombus travels through the deep venous system (usually from the lower extremities) and gets stuck in the pulmonary vessels, occluding blood flow.

    c. Manifestations depend on the size of the vessel occluded.

    d. Most manifestations present are subtle or ambiguous, and the onset is always sudden.

    e. Complications include death or morbidity from anoxic brain injury.

2. ASSESSMENT

    a. Tachypnea (most common)

    b. Dyspnea

    c. Cough

    d. Pleuritic chest pain

    e. Tachycardia

    f. Pleural friction rub

    g. Diaphoresis

    h. Cyanosis

    i. Hemoptysis

3. DIAGNOSTIC TESTS

    a. V/Q scan

    b. Spiral CT

    c. Pulmonary angiogram

    d. Electrocardiogram (ECG)

    e. Chest x-ray

    f. Arterial blood gases (ABGs) to evaluate oxygenation status

4. NURSING INTERVENTIONS
   a. Promptly notify the physician of clinical manifestations.
   b. Provide supportive care.
   c. Apply oxygen.
   d. Provide IV access.
   e. Instruct the client and family, if appropriate, of possible condition and what to expect.
   f. Perform respiratory and cardiac resuscitation as required.
   g. Assess the client for anxiousness, acute respiratory distress, restless, or cyanosis.
   h. Monitor vital signs.
   i. Auscultate lung sounds.
   j. Administer heparin if prescribed.

F. POSTPARTUM BLUES
  1. DESCRIPTION
    a. Transient depression lasting up to 2 weeks postpartum
    b. Affects 50–80% of postpartum women
    c. May be related to rapid hormone changes, stress, and fatigue
    d. Usually resolves spontaneously
    e. May lead to postpartum depression
  2. ASSESSMENT
    a. Irritability
    b. Tearfulness
    c. Let-down feelings
    d. Insomnia
    e. Labile moods
    f. Sleeplessness
    g. Anger toward family
    h. Anxiety
  3. DIAGNOSTIC TESTS
    a. None needed
  4. NURSING INTERVENTIONS
    a. Instruct the client regarding postpartum blues.
    b. Encourage the client to verbalize feelings.
    c. Provide support and reassurance

G. POSTPARTUM DEPRESSION (PPD)
  1. DESCRIPTION
    a. Develops in 10–15% of postpartum women
    b. May develop any time during the first year after delivery
    c. Most commonly starts 4–6 weeks postpartum
    d. Most common cause due to lack of support from significant other or family
    e. Other risk factors include primiparity, history of depression in self or family, recent life changes, and stressors.
    f. Socialized from childhood that motherhood is "happiest time of your life"
    g. Unprepared for all the lifestyle changes that occur with a newborn
    h. Rapid hormonal changes after delivery may potentiate mood swings and feelings of inadequacy.
    i. Complications include an interference with bonding, suicide, and infanticide.
  2. ASSESSMENT
    a. Tearfulness
    b. Despondency
    c. Feeling unable to cope
    d. Feelings of inadequacy
    e. Difficulty concentrating
    f. Problems with sleep
    g. Lack of interest in activities and appearance
    h. Loss of appetite
  3. DIAGNOSTIC TESTS
    a. Psychosocial profile to identify risk factors
    b. Hormonal level determinations
    c. Self-administered depression scale
  4. NURSING INTERVENTIONS
    a. Instruct the client regarding postpartum depression, risk factors, clinical manifestations, and interventions.
    b. Encourage frequent rest periods.
    c. Provide reading material on the subject.
    d. Talk with the significant other regarding need for support.
    e. Encourage exercise, a healthy diet, and self-care.
    f. Encourage attendance at local support group.
    g. Refer to the physician for evaluation.
    h. Administer selective serotonin reuptake inhibitors (SSRIs) such as sertraline (Zoloft), paroxetine (Paxil), or fluoxetine (Prozac).

H. POSTPARTUM PSYCHOSIS
  1. DESCRIPTION
    a. Usually clinical manifestations initiated around 3 months postpartum
    b. Incidence 1–2:1000 postpartum women
    c. Up to 25% recurrence rate
    d. Increased risk with history of mental illness or depression, family history of mood disorder, or with identified stressors
  2. ASSESSMENT
    a. Agitation
    b. Insomnia
    c. Moodiness
    d. Poor judgment
    e. Delusions
    f. Hallucinations
  3. DIAGNOSTIC TEST
    a. Psychiatric testing

4. NURSING INTERVENTIONS
   a. Identify risk factors before discharge from the hospital.
   b. Instruct the client on the clinical manifestations and need for frequent evaluation.
   c. Place the infant in a safe environment until resolution.
   d. Administer drugs such as antipsychotics and sedatives, or electroconvulsive therapy and psychotherapy.
I.   PREGNANCY-INDUCED HYPERTENSION (PIH) (SEE CHAPTER 42, SECTION V.)
J.   DIABETES MELLITUS (DM) (SEE CHAPTER 42, SECTION VI.)

PRACTICE QUESTIONS

1. Twelve hours after delivery, the nurse assesses a client's vital signs. Which of the following findings should be reported?
   1. Temperature of 37.8°C, or 100.2°F
   2. Respiratory rate of 18 bpm
   3. Blood pressure of 120/80
   4. Pulse of 96

2. The nurse assesses which of the following clinical manifestations to be present in a client with pulmonary emboli associated with pregnancy?
   Select all that apply:
   [ ] 1. Leg pain
   [ ] 2. Difficulty voiding
   [ ] 3. Tachypnea
   [ ] 4. Dyspnea
   [ ] 5. Problems with sleep
   [ ] 6. Pleural friction rub

3. After assessing a postpartum client's breast, diagnosed with mastitis, the nurse notices a red streak and tenderness around the right areola. Which of the following is the most important nursing intervention?
   1. Apply cold soaks to the area
   2. Avoid administering pain medication
   3. Instruct the client to empty the breasts frequently
   4. Instruct the client to avoid breast feeding due to pain

4. During the 24-hour postpartum assessment, the nurse anticipates the uterine fundus to be in which of the following positions?
   1. U/3
   2. U/4
   3. Unable to palpate, too low in the pelvic cavity
   4. U/U

5. The nurse is giving a client who is postpartum the discharge instructions from the hospital. The nurse should instruct the client to return immediately for evaluation if which of the following occurs?
   1. Temperature of 37.2°C, or 99°F
   2. Slight swelling in the lower legs without pain or redness
   3. Bleeding becomes heavier than a heavy period
   4. Small hemorrhoids

6. A client phones the nurse to express concern about having intercourse 6 weeks after delivery. She is breast feeding and reports that intercourse is uncomfortable. Which of the following is the appropriate response by the nurse?
   1. "Excess abdominal fat after delivery leads to painful intercourse."
   2. "Your estrogen levels are low and there is decreased mucus production and dryness."
   3. "Your vaginal walls are smooth and have not redeveloped rugae, making intercourse uncomfortable."
   4. "Intercourse is uncomfortable because of the distention of the vaginal canal."

7. A client who had a vaginal delivery the previous day asks the nurse what it meant when she was informed that she had a third-degree laceration. The nurse's response should be based on the understanding that a third-degree laceration is characterized by a tear
   1. through the skin and into the muscle.
   2. that extends through the anal sphincter.
   3. that involves the anterior rectal wall.
   4. that extends through the perineal muscle layer.

8. A client who had breast augmentation 1 year ago asks the nurse after delivery if she will be able to breast feed. Based on knowledge of breast feeding, the nurse provides which of the following responses?
   1. "Yes, you will be able to breast feed without any problems."
   2. "You will be unable to breast feed only if the milk ducts were severed."
   3. "No, you will be unable to breast feed because the implants will chemically alter the milk."
   4. "No, you will be unable to breast feed due to the risk of infection."

9. The nurse caring for a client who delivered 1 hour ago assesses the uterine fundus to be displaced to the right. Which of the following is the priority intervention the nurse should implement?
   1. Take the client's vital signs
   2. Check the client's perineal area
   3. Reevaluate the client after assisting to the bathroom to void
   4. Check the client's legs for swelling

10. The nurse informs a graduate nurse on a postpartum unit that the human chorionic gonadotropin (hCG) would no longer be detected in the client's blood at
    1. 1 week postpartum.
    2. 2 days postpartum.
    3. 4 weeks postpartum.
    4. 1 hour postpartum.

11. A postpartum client delivered a baby 24 hours ago. The client's blood type is O2. The baby's blood type has come back O1. The nurse evaluates the need for RhoGam and concludes that RhoGam is
    1. not needed because they both have type O blood.
    2. needed because the baby has a positive antibody.
    3. not needed until the infant is 3 months old.
    4. given to all infants to prevent an antibody reaction.

12. A client who is HIV positive has just given birth to her first child by cesarean section. The client received an antiviral medication during pregnancy and received the same medication through an IV during the delivery process. The client asks the nurse what is the risk of giving the baby HIV. Which of the following is the appropriate response by the nurse?
    1. "10%."
    2. "35%."
    3. "50%."
    4. "1%."

13. A client who is postpartum is complaining of perineal pain. The nurse should implement which of the following interventions? Select all that apply:
    [ ] 1. Apply an ice pack to the perineal area
    [ ] 2. Administer a pain medication
    [ ] 3. Change position
    [ ] 4. Apply a warm pack to the perineal area
    [ ] 5. Administer a smooth muscle relaxant
    [ ] 6. Increase fluids

14. Which of the following is the most appropriate consideration to include in the plan of care for an Asian postpartum client who delivered 3 days ago and refuses to drink ice water or use ice packs on her perineum?
    1. The client does not like water
    2. It is an important cultural belief
    3. The ice feels uncomfortable
    4. The client is in too much pain

15. A client delivered an infant 12 hours ago and has lots of questions regarding care, but shows little initiative in caring for the newborn. According to Rubin's theory, the nurse identifies this as which stage the client is exhibiting?
    1. Taking-in phase
    2. Taking-hold phase
    3. Letting-go phase
    4. Good bonding behavior

16. A postpartum client's complete blood count reflects a white blood cell count immediately after delivery of 14,000 per cubed mm. The nurse reports this as
    1. abnormal and indicating an infection is present.
    2. an atypically low level.
    3. elevated but normal following delivery.
    4. within the normal range.

17. The nurse is reviewing physician orders for a client in the postpartum period in the hospital who is exhibiting clinical manifestations of pulmonary emboli (PE). Which of the following procedures should the nurse ensure is done first?
    1. Pulmonary angiogram
    2. Spiral CT scan
    3. V/Q scan
    4. Duplex ultrasonogram

18. When preparing a client who is not pregnant for an oral glucose tolerance test (OGTT or GTT), it is essential for the nurse to explain that the client must drink what amount of glucose?
    1. 25 grams
    2. 50 grams
    3. 75 grams
    4. 100 grams

19. A client after a vaginal delivery is at risk for postpartum hemorrhage. Nursing education to prevent postpartum hemorrhage is based on the knowledge that priority explanation for the cause is
   1. laceration of the perineal area.
   2. uterine rupture.
   3. high parity.
   4. uterine atony.

20. While assessing a client who just delivered a baby weighing 9 lb and 6 oz, the nurse assesses a firm fundus that is midline at U/U. There is also a constant trickle of blood from the vaginal area. Which of the following is the priority nursing intervention?
   1. Suspect postpartum hemorrhage and massage the uterus
   2. Question the client regarding a history of hemorrhoids
   3. Notify the physician of a possible laceration
   4. Document this as a normal finding

21. A client with a history of hypertension had an oxytocin drug ordered due to increased bleeding after delivery. The nurse appropriately administers which of the following drugs?
   1. Oxytocin (Pitocin)
   2. Methylergonovine maleate (Methergine)
   3. Ergonovine (Ergotrate)
   4. Acetylsalicylic acid (aspirin)

22. Following giving birth, a client complains of excruciating pain around her labial area. Upon assessment, the nurse observes a bluish, bulging area just under the skin on the left labia majora. The nurse reports this as a(n)
   1. hemorrhage.
   2. indication of infection.
   3. hematoma.
   4. laceration.

23. A client who delivered an infant 3 days ago is complaining of pain, frequency of urination, and nausea. The nurse takes the client's temperature and it is 38.9°C, or 102°F. Which of the following is the priority intervention?
   1. Call the physician to obtain an order for a urine specimen for culture
   2. Increase fluids and reassess the temperature in 4 hours
   3. Tell the client that this is a normal finding and not to worry
   4. Administer prescribed pain medication

24. A nurse is discharging a postpartum client who has anemia. The nurse instructs the client that which of the following food selections are iron-rich?
   Select all that apply:
   [ ] 1. Red meats
   [ ] 2. Milk
   [ ] 3. Cheese
   [ ] 4. Fish
   [ ] 5. Poultry
   [ ] 6. Yogurt

25. The nurse is caring for a client postoperatively following a cesarean section. It is a priority for the nurse to monitor the client for
   1. postpartum depression.
   2. infection.
   3. dehydration.
   4. blood clots.

26. The registered nurse is delegating nursing tasks on a postpartum maternity unit. Which of the following tasks should the nurse delegate to a licensed practical nurse?
   1. Assess the postdelivery fundus
   2. Administer oxytocin (Pitocin) IV after delivery of the placenta
   3. Maintain an accurate intake and output
   4. Report lochia rubra 10 days after delivery

ANSWERS AND RATIONALES

1. 4. Relative bradycardia is normal after delivery due to an increased maternal blood volume. The presence of tachycardia warrants exploration. Temperature of 37.8°C or 100.2°F, respiratory rate of 18 bpm, and blood pressure of 120/80 are all normal variants of vital signs.

2. 3. 4. 6. Clinical manifestations of pulmonary emboli associated with pregnancy include tachypnea, dyspnea, and pleural friction rub. Leg pain is a clinical manifestation of deep vein thrombosis. Difficulty voiding occurs with

bacterial infections. A clinical manifestation of postpartum depression is problems with sleep.

3. 3. It is important to empty the breasts frequently to prevent milk stasis. Warm soaks would be warranted for an infection. Pain medication is appropriate and will help during breast feeding. The milk stasis allows the infection a warm medium to continue to grow and proliferate.

4. 4. U/U is a normal involution of the uterus and indicates a normal process of healing. U/3, U/4, and a uterus that is unable to palpate because it

is too low in the pelvic cavity all indicate that the uterus is further along in the involution process.

5. 3. Bleeding heavier than a period after discharge indicates hemorrhage and warrants evaluation. A temperature under 38°C, or 100.4°F, is insignificant. Slight swelling in the lower legs without redness or pain is a normal variant after delivery, due to excess fluids. The development of small hemorrhoids is a normal finding during the postpartum period.

6. 2. Estrogen allows for the production of mucous in the vaginal area. The estrogen levels return at a slower pace if a woman is breast feeding exclusively. Abdominal fat has no effect on intercourse. Vaginal rugae reappear 3 weeks after delivery. Distention would not lead to discomfort.

7. 2. A third-degree laceration goes through the perineal muscle layer with involvement of the anal sphincter. A tear through the skin and into the muscles defines a first-degree laceration. A tear that involves the anterior rectal wall defines a fourth-degree laceration. A tear that extends through the perineal muscle layer defines a second-degree laceration.

8. 2. If the milk ducts were severed during breast augmentation surgery, breast feeding will not be possible due to the lack of a functioning ductal system. Surgery alters the breast's collection system. Implants have not been found to alter milk composition. Breast surgery does not lead to an increased risk of infection.

9. 3. Excessive bleeding can occur with bladder distention because the uterus cannot fully contract. Frequent voiding is therefore important to prevent this from happening and putting the postpartum client at risk for hemorrhage. Although taking the client's vitals, checking the client's perineal area, and checking the client's legs for swelling are all important to assess, they are not the priority with the findings observed.

10. 1. hCG is produced by the placenta and is nonexistent by the first week postpartum.

11. 2. The Rh-negative client who delivers an Rh-positive infant receives RhoGam to prevent the formation of antibodies that might complicate future pregnancies. The nurse should look at Rh factor, not blood type. RhoGam must be given within 72 hours of delivery. The only clients who need RhoGam are those with an Rh-negative blood type who have an Rh-positive infant.

12. 4. Current treatment with antiviral medications has greatly reduced the transmission to 1% after a surgical delivery through this prophylactic treatment plan.

13. 1. 2. 3. Administering an ice pack to the perineal area, administering a pain medication, and changing the client's position are comfort measures that should help decrease pain. Warm packs cause vasodilation and increase inflammation.

14. 2. Cultural values influence personal self-care. The Asian culture believes that exposure to cool air leads to infection; therefore, Asian mothers will not put themselves at risk for this through oral fluids or ice packs.

15. 1. The taking-in stage usually occurs during the first 24 hours postpartum. This is a time when the client is concerned about her own needs and illustrates little initiative in performing infant care.

16. 3. An increase in the white blood count is a protective mechanism after delivery. It helps to protect the client from infection and is in response to the stress associated with the labor process.

17. 1. A pulmonary angiogram is considered the definitive test because x-rays can visualize the emboli after catheterization and contrast dye is injected. A spiral CT scan is the test used if the V/Q scan is not diagnostic. The V/Q scan is only suggestive and not a definitive test for PE. A duplex ultrasonogram is a test that shows a disruption of blood flow in the lower legs.

18. 3. Drinking 25 or 50 grams of glucose is not enough to challenge the pancreas when evaluating for diabetes mellitus; 100 grams is widely used to screen for gestational diabetes mellitus; 75 grams of glucose is the recommended glucose load to screen the nonpregnant pancreas for diabetes mellitus or impaired glucose tolerance.

19. 4. About 75% of all hemorrhages are due to uterine atony, which is the lack of uterine tone. Laceration of the perineal area, uterine rupture, and high parity are other causes of hemorrhage, but they are not as likely.

20. 3. The bleeding from a laceration is not due to uterine atony but to a lacerated area in the perineal, vaginal, or cervical area. It is a priority to notify the physician of a possible laceration. The uterus is firm midline and at an appropriate level.

21. 1. Oxytocin (Pitocin) may cause hypotension, but this would not be of much concern in a client who is hypertensive. Hypertension is an adverse reaction to both methylergonovine maleate (Methergine) and ergonovine (Ergotrate). These drugs would be contraindicated for the client with hypertension. Aspirin inhibits the synthesis of clotting factors and can increase the risk of bleeding.

22. 3. Extreme pain is a classic indication of a hematoma. This pain is caused by pressure from the swelling of tissues in the pelvic area from damage to a vessel wall.

23. 1. Pain, frequency of urination, and nausea are all common clinical manifestations of a urinary tract infection. The postpartum client is at risk due to decreased tone and sensation of the bladder after delivery. Because the ureters are enlarged after delivery due to the effects of pregnancy, infection may travel up to the kidneys. It is therefore very important to have prompt intervention and treatment started immediately. It is important to notify the physician of any deviations.

24. 1. 4. 5. Foods high in iron include red meats, fish, and poultry.

25. 2. The nurse should closely monitor a client postoperatively for infection, which has an incidence ranging from 4–12% due to increased tissue trauma. Postpartum depression, dehydration, and blood clots are possible complications, but they occur at a lower incidence.

26. 3. Assessing the postdelivery fundus, administering oxytocin (Pitocin), and reporting abnormal lochia are all skills that should be performed by a registered nurse. Maintaining an accurate intake and output is a task that can be delegated to a licensed practical nurse. The client experiences diuresis after delivery.

REFERENCES

Bartnick, D. (2003). The normal postpartal period. In M. Hogan & R. Glazebrook (Eds.), *Maternal-newborn nursing* (pp. 217–234). Upper Saddle River, NJ: Prentice Hall.

Daniels, R. (2010). *Delmar's manual of laboratory and diagnostic test* (2nd ed.). Clifton Park, NY: Delmar Cengage Learning.

Harkey, A. (2003). The complicated postpartal period. In M. Hogan & R. Glazebrook (Eds.), *Maternal-newborn nursing* (pp. 235–260). Upper Saddle River, NJ: Prentice Hall.

Littleton, L., & Engebretson, J. (2002). *Maternal, neonatal, and women's health nursing.* Clifton Park, NY: Delmar Cengage Learning.

Littleton, L., & Engebretson, J. (2013). *Maternity nursing care* (2nd ed.). Clifton Park, NY: Delmar Cengage Learning.

CHAPTER 45

NEWBORN CARE

I. ANATOMY AND PHYSIOLOGY

A. SKIN

   1. OPACITY: FROM NEARLY TRANSPARENT IN THE VERY PRETERM NEWBORN TO ALMOST OPAQUE IN THE TERM AND POSTTERM NEWBORN

   2. COLOR VARIES WITH RACE. DARKER-SKINNED NEWBORNS USUALLY HAVE HEAVIER PIGMENTATION OF THE GENITALS, LINEA NIGRA, SKIN AROUND NAILS, AND LIPS.

   3. ACROCYANOSIS: BLUISH COLOR OF THE HANDS, FEET, AND, SOMETIMES, DISTAL EXTREMITIES, DUE TO VASOMOTOR INSTABILITY, CAPILLARY STASIS, AND HIGH HEMOGLOBIN LEVEL; APPEARS INTERMITTENTLY OVER THE FIRST WEEK TO 10 DAYS

   4. VARIATIONS

     a. Milia: distended sebaceous glands, usually on the nose, due to influence of maternal hormones

     b. Mongolian spots: bluish-black areas of pigmentation, more common in dark-skinned newborns, most often on the back or buttocks (differentiate from ecchymosis)

     c. Petechiae: localized petechiae are usually due to pressure applied to an area of the skin (such as the scalp). Generalized petechiae may be an indication of thrombocytopenia or sepsis.

     d. Forceps or vacuum extraction marks: swelling and ecchymosis may occur at the site of application of the forceps or vacuum extractor cup.

     e. Scalp electrode sites: electrode penetrates the skin 1.5 mm, causes puncture wound on the presenting part.

     f. Jaundice: yellow color to the skin and sclera caused by bilirubin

     g. Lanugo: fine, downy hair present from 20 weeks of gestation, gradually decreasing toward term

     h. Vernix: mixture of sebum (oil) and shed skin cells; protects fetal skin from maceration and promotes temperature stability

   5. TRAUMATIC INJURY DUE TO DIFFICULT BIRTH

     a. Ecchymosis from extraction, lacerations from caesarean birth

B. NEUROLOGIC SYSTEM

   1. REFLEXES

     a. Grasp: the newborn will grasp an object placed against the palm.

     b. Root: the newborn will turn toward the cheek that is stroked by a finger or nipple.

     c. Suck: the newborn will suck on a nipple or finger placed in the mouth.

     d. Moro: abduction and extension of the arms and fanning of the fingers, then adduction and flexion of the arms, clenching of the fingers in "C" position

     e. Babinski: stroking the lateral plantar surface causes fanning of the toes (positive Babinski).

     f. Tonic neck (fencer position): when head is turned to one side, the ipsolateral extremities extend and the contralateral extremities flex.

     g. Newborn's brain is one-quarter the size of an adult's. Myelination of nerve fibers is incomplete.

     h. Movements uncoordinated, startles easily, tremors of extremities

C. CARDIOVASCULAR SYSTEM

   1. FIBROSIS OF THE DUCTUS ARTERIOSUS OCCURS WITHIN 3 WEEKS; FIBROSIS OF THE UMBILICAL VEIN AND ARTERIES AND DUCTUS VENOSUS OCCURS IN 3 TO 7 DAYS.

D. GASTROINTESTINAL SYSTEM
1. MECONIUM IS THE FIRST STOOL, COMPOSED OF BILE, EPITHELIAL CELLS, AND AMNIOTIC CELLS.
2. LITTLE SALIVA IS PRODUCED FOR THE FIRST 3 MONTHS.
3. FAT DIGESTION IS POOR DUE TO ABSENCE OF THE PANCREATIC ENZYMES AMYLASE AND LIPASE.

E. URINARY SYSTEM
1. DEVELOPMENT OF NEPHRONS IS COMPLETE BY 34–36 WEEKS, BUT RENAL FUNCTION DOES NOT MATURE UNTIL AFTER THE FIRST YEAR.
2. DECREASED ABILITY TO EXCRETE DRUGS
3. LOW GLOMERULAR FILTRATION RATE RENDERS THE NEWBORN PRONE TO SODIUM REABSORPTION AND EXCESSIVE WATER LOSS.

F. RESPIRATORY SYSTEM
1. NEWBORN IS AN OBLIGATE NOSE BREATHER.

G. ENDOCRINE SYSTEM
1. THYROID, PANCREAS, AND ADRENAL CORTEX ARE FUNCTIONAL.

H. HEMATOLOGIC SYSTEM
1. BLOOD VOLUME OF THE TERM NEWBORN IS 80–85 ML/KG.
2. HEMOGLOBIN, 15–20 G/DL
3. HEMATOCRIT, 43–61%
4. WHITE BLOOD CELLS (WBCS), 10,000–30,000
5. PLATELETS, 100,000–280,000

I. GENITALIA
1. APPEARANCE VARIES WITH GESTATION; FEMALES ARE AFFECTED BY MATERNAL HORMONES.

II. **ASSESSMENT**
A. GENERAL APPEARANCE
1. PROPORTIONS
   a. Head is relatively large, approximately one-quarter of body length.
   b. Hands, genitals, and feet are relatively large.
2. POSTURE
   a. General flexion; extension may indicate prematurity, illness, or neurologic problem.

B. VITAL SIGNS
1. RESPIRATIONS
   a. Rate: 30–60 per minute, irregular; tachypnea may follow activity, or may indicate respiratory distress, hyperthermia.
   b. Character: chest and abdomen both rise with inspiration.
   c. Seesaw breathing, nasal flaring, grunting, and retractions (drawing in of tissue between the ribs, below the sternum, or above the suprasternal notch) are signs of respiratory distress.
   d. Nose breathing
2. HEART
   a. Rate around 140 beats per minute (bpm); may fall below 100 bpm during sleep, or reach 180 bpm with crying
   b. Sinus arrhythmia common
   c. Murmurs: may be due to patent ductus arteriosus; if so will usually resolve around 12 hours of age
   d. Point of maximum impulse (PMI) at the fourth intercostal space and just lateral to the midclavicular line
   e. Blood pressure: varies with gestation and age
3. TEMPERATURE
   a. Axillary readings; the practice of taking one rectal reading to assess patency is outdated.
   b. Range: 36.4°C (97.6°F) to 37.6°C (99.7°F)

C. HEAD AND NECK
1. SCALP
   a. Fontanelles
      1) Anterior (bregma) is diamond shaped and located at the junction of the coronal and sagittal sutures.
      2) Posterior is triangular and located at the junction of the lambdoidal and sagittal sutures.
      3) Caput succedaneum is edema of the scalp noted at birth and crosses suture lines.
      4) Cephalhematoma is a collection of blood between the periosteum and skull that appears within 2 days and does not cross suture lines.
2. FACE
   a. Symmetry of features
   b. Mouth
   c. Lips: assess for cleft.
   d. Symmetry of motion
   e. Tongue
   f. Palate: assess for cleft.
   g. Nose
   h. Patency of nares
   i. Assess by passing a suction catheter (if indicated) or by occluding each naris while holding the mouth closed and observing whether the newborn can breathe through the other.
   j. Auricles
   k. Placement
   l. Top of the auricle should be at or above the line drawn from the inner to the outer canthus of the eye.
   m. Appearance: malformation or anomalies are sometimes associated with renal anomalies.
   n. Preauricular sinus, tags, and so on

3. NECK
   a. Clavicles
   b. Crepitus: associated with fracture
   c. Supple and rigid
   d. Nuchal fold
D. THORAX
   1. SYMMETRY
   2. EXCURSION OF CHEST WALL WITH RESPIRATION
   3. BREAST
      a. Breast tissue (bud)
      b. Nipple or areola
      c. Supernumerary nipples
E. ABDOMEN
   1. INSPECTION
   2. UMBILICUS
   3. AUSCULTATION: BOWEL SOUNDS AUDIBLE BY 1 HOUR AFTER BIRTH
   4. PALPATION
   5. HEPATIC MARGIN: BELOW COSTAL MARGIN
   6. SPLENIC MARGIN
   7. PERCUSSION
F. BACK
   1. SPINE
      a. Palpation of vertebrae (to detect occult spina bifida)
      b. Presence of pilonidal sinus
G. ANUS
   1. PATENCY
   2. ANAL WINK
H. GENITALIA
   1. MALE
      a. Scrotum
      b. Rugae: vary with gestation
      c. Descent of testes: varies with gestation
      d. Meatus should be at the end of the penis, not ventral (hypospadias) or dorsal (epispadias).
   2. FEMALE
      a. Relative sizes of the labia majora, labia minora, and clitoris vary with gestation.
      b. Discharge mucus
      c. Pseudomenstruation: small amount blood-streaked discharge due to maternal hormones
I. EXTREMITIES
   1. SYMMETRY
   2. RANGE OF MOTION
   3. TONE
   4. HIPS
   5. ORTOLANI'S MANEUVER: CHECK FOR SUBLUXATION OF THE FEMORAL HEAD.
   6. BARLOW'S MANEUVER: CHECK FOR SUBLUXATION OF THE FEMORAL HEAD.
   7. SYMMETRY OF GLUTEAL FOLDS
   8. BOW-LEGGED
   9. FEET FLAT (NO ARCH)
   10. PLANTAR CREASES (ASSESS IMMEDIATELY AFTER BIRTH)
   11. REFLECT GESTATIONAL AGE
J. REFLEXES (SEE CHAPTER 7, SECTION II, "ASSESS REFLEXES" SUBSECTION.)
K. GESTATIONAL AGE ASSESSMENT
   1. TERM
   2. PRETERM (PREMATURE)
   3. POSTTERM (POSTMATURE)
   4. SMALL FOR GESTATIONAL AGE
   5. APPROPRIATE FOR GESTATIONAL AGE
   6. GESTATIONAL AGE
   7. BALLARD/DUBOWITZ
      a. The examiner evaluates the newborn on six neuromuscular and six physical characteristics shortly after birth.
      b. Each characteristic is assigned a score of 1 to 5; total score correlates to a gestational age. Newborn's weight, length, and head circumference are plotted on graphs with the gestational age. A rating below the 10th percentile indicates small for gestational age, one between the 10th and 90th percentile indicates appropriate for gestational age, and one above the 90th percentile indicates large for gestational age.
   8. TERM: 37 COMPLETED WEEKS TO 41 6/7 WEEKS
   9. PRETERM (PREMATURE): LESS THAN 37 WEEKS
   10. POSTTERM (POSTMATURE): 42 WEEKS OR MORE
   11. SMALL FOR GESTATIONAL AGE: AT RISK FOR PERINATAL ASPHYXIA, MECONIUM ASPIRATION SYNDROME, HYPOGLYCEMIA, AND HEAT LOSS (COLD STRESS)
   12. APPROPRIATE FOR GESTATIONAL AGE
   13. LARGE FOR GESTATIONAL AGE: AT RISK FOR HYPOGLYCEMIA, BIRTH TRAUMA, AND OPERATIVE BIRTH (VACUUM- OR FORCEPS-ASSISTED BIRTH, CESAREAN BIRTH)
   14. INTRAUTERINE GROWTH RETARDATION
      a. Symmetric: growth retardation, which affects all aspects of fetal growth; due to conditions occurring in the first trimester such as infection, teratogens, and chromosomal abnormalities
      b. Asymmetric: weight less than or equal to the 10th percentile, head circumference greater than or equal to the 10th percentile; asymmetric growth retardation is due to placental insufficiency (inadequate oxygen and nutrients) and begins in later stages of pregnancy. These infants may achieve normal growth and development.

L. MEASUREMENTS
1. WEIGHT
2. LENGTH
3. HEAD CIRCUMFERENCE (SOMETIMES CALLED FRONTAL-OCCIPITAL CIRCUMFERENCE)
   a. Measured from the occiput to just above the eyebrows
   b. 32–37 cm (average 33–35), usually 2 cm greater than chest circumference
4. CHEST CIRCUMFERENCE (MEASURED AT THE LEVEL OF THE NIPPLES)
5. LABS
   a. Complete blood count (CBC): suspected infectious disease
   b. WBC count of up to 30,000 is normal in the newborn.
   c. Bands (10 or greater) are significant.
   d. Bilirubin: trend is more significant than a single elevated value. Elevated bilirubin before 24 hours suggests hemolysis.
   e. Cord blood pH and gases: pH of venous and arterial cord blood samples reflects fetal acid-base and oxygenation status.
6. CONGENITAL MALFORMATIONS
   a. Anomalies resulting from absent or abnormal development such as anencephaly
7. CONGENITAL DEFORMATIONS
   a. Anomalies in which structures formed correctly and were later deformed, often by position or pressure, such as talipes equinovarus ("club foot")

M. ADAPTATION TO EXTRAUTERINE LIFE
1. ADAPTATION OF FETAL CIRCULATION TO EXTRAUTERINE LIFE
   a. Normal: with expansion of the lungs, pulmonary capillary resistance falls and pulmonary blood flow increases; pulmonary capillaries and lymphatic vessels remove remaining lung fluid. As pulmonary blood flow increases, the increasing pressure in the left side of the heart begins to close the two remaining fetal circulatory shunts: the foramen ovale closes almost immediately; the ductus arteriosus functionally closes at about 12 hours.
   b. Abnormal: possible causes include hypoxemia or acidemia, congenital abnormalities, pulmonary hypoplasia, hypoplastic left heart, and anomalies of great vessels.
2. ADAPTATION OF RESPIRATORY SYSTEM TO EXTRAUTERINE LIFE
   a. Normal: compression and release of the chest during vaginal delivery draws air into the lungs; chemical (decreased O_2 concentration, increased CO_2 concentration, or decreased pH stimulate carotid and aortic chemoreceptors, triggering initiation of respirations); thermal (cold stress stimulates breathing); and tactile stimuli (uterine contractions, descent through the pelvis and birth canal, drying after delivery) stimulate the brain to trigger respiratory efforts.
   b. Abnormal: possible causes include prematurity or immaturity, aspiration, and pneumonia usually group B beta strep.
      1) Clinical manifestations include grunting, retractions, use of accessory muscles, decreased SaO_2, abnormal blood gas studies, and abnormal chest radiogram.
3. THERMOREGULATION
   a. Heat is generated by the metabolism of brown fat.
   b. Inability to shiver
   c. Abnormal: possible causes include heat loss due to convection, evaporation, radiation, or conduction.
      1) Clinical manifestations include acidemia, hypoxemia, and hypoglycemia (depletion of glycogen stores).
4. RESUSCITATION
5. APGAR SCORE (SEE TABLE 45-1)
   a. Perform at 1 and 5 minutes after birth.
   b. The 1-minute score is a transitional result.
   c. The 5-minute score is most often used to determine the direction of the infant's care.
   d. A score of 7 or above indicates a healthy newborn, a score of 5–7 indicates the infant needs intensive treatment, and a score of 0–4 indicates a grave prognosis.
6. CORD VESSELS (TWO ARTERIES, ONE VEIN; SINGLE UMBILICAL ARTERY MAY INDICATE ANOMALY[IES])
7. CORD BLOOD SPECIMEN
   a. For type and Rh (of baby)
   b. Some parents may wish to "bank" cord blood.
      1) Private services store cord blood for possible future use for the baby only.
      2) Registries store cord blood for stem cell transplants for any possible recipient.
8. CORD CLAMP
9. EYE PROPHYLAXIS: SILVER NITRATE OR ERYTHROMYCIN OINTMENT. BOTH PROTECT AGAINST OPHTHALMIA NEONATORUM (GONORRHEA) BUT

Table 45-1 Apgar Score

Category	0	1	2	Score
Heart rate	Absent	Less than 100 bpm	Greater than 100 bpm	
Respiratory rate	Absent	Slow and irregular	Strong cry	
Muscle tone	Absent or limp	Some flexion	Active motion	
Reflex irritability	No response	Grimace	Cry	
Color	Blue and pale	Pink body but blue extremities	Pink body and extremities	
				Total Score

ONLY ERYTHROMYCIN PROTECTS AGAINST CHLAMYDIA. BECAUSE CHLAMYDIA IS MORE PREVALENT THAN GONORRHEA, ERYTHROMYCIN IS MORE WIDELY USED.

10. VITAMIN K PROTECTS AGAINST CEREBRAL HEMORRHAGE. THE NEWBORN CANNOT MAKE VITAMIN K UNTIL SEVERAL DAYS AFTER BIRTH WHEN THE GUT IS COLONIZED WITH BACTERIA THAT PRODUCE VITAMIN K.

11. EVERY HOSPITAL HAS IDENTIFICATION PROCEDURES TO IDENTIFY MOTHER-BABY "SETS" (AND SOMETIMES A SECOND ADULT).

12. INFANT SECURITY
    a. An alarm device (bracelet) may be used to prevent infant abduction.

13. INITIAL PARENT–CHILD ATTACHMENT: IF THE NEWBORN'S CONDITION PERMITS, FOSTER THE DEVELOPMENT OF THE PARENT–CHILD BOND BY ENCOURAGING TOUCHING, AND BY POINTING OUT THE NEWBORN'S SENSORY CAPABILITIES.

N. INFANT FEEDING AND ELIMINATION
  1. FEEDING
     a. Infants should be fed formula or breast milk for the first year of life.
     b. Nipple
     c. Breast: breast milk is the ideal food for infants.
        1) Composition varies during a feeding, through the day, and with the age of the infant.
        2) Decreases allergies and protects against infection
        3) Always ready, warm, and clean
        4) Milk supply is related to frequency of feeding for the first 3 to 4 weeks. Thereafter, supply is based on breast emptying.

5) Positions: assist the mother to assume a comfortable position, using pillow for support as needed.
   a) Cradle (Madonna): the baby's abdomen touches the mother's abdomen, the baby's head is in line with the body (not rotated).
   b) Football: the baby's abdomen is in contact with the mother's midriff (side), with the mother's arm around the baby's back and the hand supporting the head.
   c) Side-lying: the mother and baby are in side-lying position facing each other. It may be more comfortable for the cesarean-birth mother.

6) The mother supports the breast with her hand, with the thumb on top and fingers beneath the breast. The nipple touches the baby's cheek to elicit the rooting reflex. When the baby opens the mouth, it draws the baby to the breast.

7) Latch-on: nipple and approximately 1 inch of the areola should be drawn into the baby's mouth. Baby's lips should be flanged (turned out). Tongue should be troughed, just visible over the lower lip. Cheeks should look full, not sucked in. Bursts of sucking followed by brief rest periods. Audible swallowing verifies milk transfer. If latch-on is not correct, break suction and repeat.

8) Breastfeeding on demand: when the baby displays hunger cues such as rooting, sucking on fists, or clenched fists

d. Duration of feedings varies. Signs of satiation are slowing of swallowing, relaxation, release of the nipple, and sleep.

e. Bottle: follow instructions for formula preparation exactly. Hold the infant close, keeping the head elevated. Tip the bottle so the nipple remains full of formula.

   1) Never prop the bottle or put the infant to bed with a bottle. Propping can cause aspiration or otitis media.

   2) Discard the formula remaining in the bottle after feeding.

f. Gavage: when sucking, swallowing, or breathing is problematic, continuous or intermittent feedings through the tube passed via the nose or mouth to the stomach or intestines may be performed.

g. Parenteral: supplemental or total nutrition by vascular route

2. URINE

a. Newborns usually urinate within 24 hours after birth.

b. May contain uric acid crystals, which appear as a salmon or peach color in the diaper. May be mistaken for blood; reassure parents the crystals are normal in the first few days of life.

3. STOOLS

a. The first stool is usually passed within 48 hours after birth.

b. Meconium: dark green or black, tarry, composed of epithelial and amniotic cells, bile

c. Transitional: brown or olive color, may contain "seeds" of yellow stool

d. The stools of breastfed babies are mustard yellow, unformed, and do not irritate skin. Frequency varies from every feeding to every few days.

e. Bottle-fed babies have brown, formed, malodorous stools.

III. DIAGNOSTIC STUDIES

A. HEARING SCREENING

1. DESCRIPTION: NATIONAL INSTITUTES OF HEALTH RECOMMENDS, AND MANY STATES REQUIRE, NEWBORN SCREENING FOR HEARING LOSS. METHODS VARY.

a. Automated otoacoustic device

b. Auditory brain-evoked response

2. PREPROCEDURE

a. Have the newborn calm, preferably asleep.

3. PROCEDURE

a. Attach earphones and electrodes (specific to each device); run the program.

4. POSTPROCEDURE

a. Carefully remove the device.

b. Follow protocol for referral of newborns who fail.

B. BLOOD GAS ANALYSIS

1. DESCRIPTION

a. pH: reflects acid-base status

b. PaO_2: reflects oxygenation of arterial blood

c. PCO_2: accumulation of carbon dioxide; reflects ventilation

d. Oxygen saturation: reflects oxygenation of arteriolar blood

e. Bicarbonate: compensatory mechanisms

f. Base excess: compensatory mechanisms (report may include other parameters)

2. PREPROCEDURE

a. If radial artery puncture is planned, verify collateral circulation using Allen's test for ulnar artery.

3. PROCEDURE

a. Locate the radial pulse.

b. Perform an arterial puncture and obtain a specimen in a heparinized syringe.

c. Send to the lab immediately for analysis.

4. POSTPROCEDURE

a. Apply firm pressure for at least 5 minutes until bleeding is controlled.

C. PULSE OXIMETRY

1. DESCRIPTION

a. Noninvasive measurement of oxygen saturation of arteriolar blood

b. May be continuous or intermittent

2. PREPROCEDURE

a. Select a site with intact skin.

3. PROCEDURE

a. Apply the probe (sensor) to the hand, wrist, foot, or ear. Be sure the extremity is still; motion causes artifact.

b. Observe for pulsatile motion of display, indicating a good signal.

c. Read and record oxygen saturation.

4. POSTPROCEDURE

a. Remove the probe gently.

b. Assess the site.

D. METABOLIC SCREEN

1. DESCRIPTION: TESTING FOR INBORN ERRORS OF METABOLISM, CONGENITAL ENDOCRINE DISORDERS, AND HEMOGLOBINOPATHIES (VARIES WITH THE STATE OR PROVINCE)

2. PREPROCEDURE

a. No special care is required.

3. PROCEDURE

a. Verify the correct client and proper age.

b. Locate the correct site for heel puncture (capillary sample); intact skin, avoid skin overlying calcaneus.

c. Thoroughly clean and dry the skin.

d. Perform heel puncture, using a device designed for newborns.

e. Obtain a sample per laboratory instructions.

E. INBORN ERRORS OF METABOLISM (TESTING VARIES BY STATE)

1. COMMON TESTS INCLUDE: PHENYLKETONURIA, GALACTOSEMIA, CONGENITAL HYPOTHYROIDISM, CONGENITAL ADRENAL HYPERTROPHY, G6PD DEFICIENCY, SICKLE CELL DISEASE, AND CYSTIC FIBROSIS IN SOME STATES.

IV. NURSING DIAGNOSES

A. NURSING DIAGNOSES MAY AFFECT ANY BODY SYSTEM DEPENDENT ON THE NEWBORN'S TRANSITIONAL PERIOD AND THE FIRST FEW DAYS OF LIFE.

B. INEFFECTIVE DISORGANIZED INFANT BEHAVIOR

C. INEFFECTIVE FEEDING PATTERN

Nursing Diagnoses: Definitions and Classification 2012–2014. Copyright © 2012, 1994–2012 by NANDA International. Used by arrangement with John Wiley & Sons Limited.

V. COMMON NEWBORN PROCEDURES

A. CIRCUMCISION

1. DESCRIPTION: SURGICAL REMOVAL OF THE PREPUCE (FORESKIN)

2. PREPROCEDURE

a. Review the family history for bleeding disorders.

b. Monitor vital signs.

3. PROCEDURE

a. Anesthesia

1) Dorsal penile block: injections of local anesthetic at the right and left dorsal penile nerves, good anesthesia

2) EMLA cream, music, swaddling, and sugar water have also been studied; efficacy varies.

3) Analgesia: newborn may receive acetaminophen (Tylenol) just before or after the procedure.

b. Technique

1) For each technique, the normal adhesions between the foreskin and glans must first be disrupted.

2) Gomco: metal bell, which fits inside the foreskin, inserts into a metal ring on the outside of the foreskin. Trapped foreskin is cut away.

3) Ring and ligature: plastic bell fits into the foreskin, the ligature is tied tightly over the foreskin, the bell is snapped off, leaving the ring with the ligature. Foreskin distal to the ligature falls off (sometimes trimmed).

4) Mogen: foreskin is drawn between two sides of a clamp, which is closed tightly, and the foreskin is cut away.

4. POSTPROCEDURE

a. Monitor for bleeding, infection.

b. Ensure that the newborn is voiding after the procedure.

B. VITAMIN K INJECTION

1. DESCRIPTION: TO SUPPLY VITAMIN K UNTIL THE GUT IS COLONIZED WITH FLORA THAT PRODUCE VITAMIN K (OCCURS AT 3–4 DAYS OF AGE)

2. PREPROCEDURE

a. Select a site (vastus lateralis) where no other injections have been given and skin is intact.

3. PROCEDURE

a. Administer by intramuscular (IM) injection.

4. POSTPROCEDURE

a. Apply pressure to the site until bleeding is controlled; apply a bandage.

C. EYE PROPHYLAXIS

1. DESCRIPTION: ANTIBIOTIC THERAPY TO PREVENT OPHTHALMIA NEONATORUM

2. PROCEDURE

a. Instill silver nitrate drops into the conjunctival sac, or apply a ribbon of erythromycin ointment to the inner aspect of the lower lids, bilaterally, to treat gonorrhea.

b. Administer erythromycin ophthalmic ointment to treat gonorrhea and chlamydia.

3. POSTPROCEDURE

a. Monitor for eye drainage.

D. CAR SEAT TEST FOR OXYGENATION

1. DESCRIPTION: USED TO VERIFY THAT THE NEWBORN CAN TOLERATE POSITIONING IN A CAR SEAT WITHOUT COMPROMISE TO OXYGENATION

2. PROCEDURE

a. Preterm newborn is placed in a car seat and oxygen saturation is monitored for a period of time to detect decreased oxygenation. If this occurs, the car seat must be modified (or must use a car bed) so the newborn can maintain oxygenation during use.

3. POSTPROCEDURE

a. Report desaturation (decrease in oxygen saturation) to the physician.

VI. HIGH-RISK NEWBORN CONDITIONS
A. INADEQUATE ORAL INTAKE (POOR FEEDER)
  1. DESCRIPTION: PRETERM INFANTS AT GREATER RISK
  2. ASSESSMENT
    a. Weight loss greater than or equal to 7% (10%)
  3. DIAGNOSTIC TEST
    a. Diagnostic imaging if anomalies are suspected
  4. MEDICAL-SURGICAL MANAGEMENT
    a. Nasogastric/orogastric feedings
    b. Parenteral feedings
  5. NURSING INTERVENTIONS
    a. Instruct the parents on feeding techniques and procedures.
    b. Assess the infant's interest in feeding.
    c. Evaluate the anatomy of the mouth.
    d. Evaluate the infant's ability to coordinate sucking, swallowing, and breathing.
    e. Evaluate the feeding technique of the mother.
B. COLD STRESS
  1. DESCRIPTION
    a. Due to the large ratio of body surface to mass, and limited thermogenesis, newborns are susceptible to cold stress.
    b. Complications increase oxygen requirements and lead to hypoxemia and acidemia, leading to pulmonary hypertension and worsening hypoxemia or acidemia.
  2. ASSESSMENT
    a. Temperature instability
  3. DIAGNOSTIC TESTS
    a. May be indicated for suspected cause of temperature instability such as sepsis
  4. NURSING INTERVENTIONS
    a. Maintain a neutral thermal environment.
    b. Place on a radiant warmer.
    c. Wrap in warm blankets.
    d. Monitor temperature.
C. NEONATAL RESPIRATORY DISTRESS SYNDROME (FORMERLY CALLED HYALINE MEMBRANE DISEASE)
  1. DESCRIPTION
    a. Serious lung disorder in which there is an insufficient pulmonary surfactant, causing the alveoli to collapse on expiration, and greatly increasing the work of breathing
    b. High-risk groups include preterm newborns and infants of mothers with diabetes.
    c. Complications include pneumothorax and persistent pulmonary hypertension

that may develop if hypoxemia and acidemia are not treated early and adequately.
  2. ASSESSMENT
    a. Tachypnea
    b. Expiratory grunting
    c. Flaring nares
    d. Retractions
    e. Apnea
    f. Pallor
    g. Cyanosis
    h. Decreased breath sounds
  3. DIAGNOSTIC TESTS
    a. Chest x-ray
    b. Blood gas (capillary or arterial)
    c. Pulse oximetry
    d. Silverman-Anderson Index of respiratory status scores newborns on intercostal retractions, nasal flaring, expiratory grunt, xiphoid retractions, and synchrony of chest and abdominal movements on inspiration.
  4. NURSING INTERVENTIONS
    a. Hold breastfeedings.
    b. Nasogastric or orogastric tube (gavage) feedings may be given if the newborn has mild tachypnea.
    c. Newborn may be NPO and receives IV fluids.
    d. Auscultate for air entry, adventitious sounds, and asymmetry of sounds.
    e. Monitor arterial blood gases (ABGs).
    f. Place the newborn on the back or in a side-lying position with the neck slightly extended.
    g. Prepare the newborn to receive surfactant replacement through an endotracheal tube.
    h. Administer the lowest oxygen concentration possible.
    i. Facilitate respiratory therapy.
D. INFECTION AND SEPSIS
  1. DESCRIPTION
    a. Infection (viral or bacterial) acquired in utero or during vaginal birth
    b. TORCH: toxoplasmosis, other (varicella), rubella, cytomegalovirus, herpes
    c. Bacterial: group B beta strep, *E. coli*
    d. Complications may include death or developmental delays from septic shock, meningitis, hypoxemia, and acidemia from pneumonia.
  2. ASSESSMENT
    a. Respiratory distress
    b. Shock or acidemia
    c. Temperature instability
    d. Gastrointestinal clinical manifestations, including ileus, diarrhea, abdominal distention, vomiting, or poor feeding

    e. Lethargy
    f. Omphalitis (infection of the umbilical cord stump)
    g. Seizures (central nervous system infection)
    h. Hepatomegaly
    i. Petechiae or purpura

  3. DIAGNOSTIC TESTS
    a. Chest x-ray, if pneumonia
    b. CBC
    c. C-reactive protein
    d. Blood culture

  4. NURSING INTERVENTIONS
    a. Monitor vital signs.
    b. Perform infection control measures.
    c. Maintain hydration.
    d. Administer prescribed IV antibiotics and fluids.

E. TRANSIENT TACHYPNEA OF THE NEWBORN (TTN)
  1. DESCRIPTION
    a. Self-limiting tachypnea due to retained lung fluid in the first 6 hours after birth
    b. Risk factors include cesarean birth.
    c. Generally, there are no complications.

  2. ASSESSMENT
    a. Tachypnea

  3. DIAGNOSTIC TESTS
    a. Chest x-ray
    b. Blood gas

  4. NURSING INTERVENTIONS
    a. Monitor for resolution of transitional tachypnea vs. developing neonatal respiratory distress syndrome.
    b. Evaluate the most appropriate feeding method based on respiratory rate and effort.
    c. Administer prescribed oxygen.
    d. Ensure continuous positive airway pressure (CPAP).
    e. Provide supportive care.

F. INFANT OF A MOTHER WITH DIABETES
  1. DESCRIPTION
    a. Newborn whose mother had preexisting or acquired diabetes mellitus during pregnancy
    b. Poorly controlled maternal diabetes or hyperglycemia causes the fetus to produce increased insulin.
    c. After delivery, maternal glucose is no longer available, and this excess insulin causes neonatal hypoglycemia.
    d. Complications include seizures.

  2. ASSESSMENT
    a. Large size and weight of the newborn
    b. Clinical manifestations of hypoglycemia
    c. Clinical manifestations of respiratory distress
    d. Hyperbilirubinemia

  3. DIAGNOSTIC TESTS
    a. Blood glucose
    b. Electrolytes
    c. Maternal hemoglobin A1C

  4. NURSING INTERVENTIONS
    a. Monitor blood glucose and electrolytes.
    b. Monitor neurological and respiratory status.
    c. Assess for neurological manifestations such as tremors, eye rolling, and lip smacking.
    d. Administer intravenous (IV) glucose if needed.
    e. Monitor weight.

G. HEMOLYTIC DISEASE OF THE NEWBORN
  1. DESCRIPTION
    a. ABO blood group incompatibility
    b. Rh factor incompatibility
    c. Caused by maternal antibodies
    d. Complications include anemia and kernicterus (neurological damage).

  2. ASSESSMENT
    a. Jaundice due to hyperbilirubinemia
    b. Pallor due to hemolytic anemia

  3. DIAGNOSTIC TESTS
    a. Cord blood studies
    b. CBC
    c. Reticulocyte count
    d. Bilirubin

  4. NURSING INTERVENTIONS
    a. Provide phototherapy (lights or phototherapy blankets, or both).
    b. Monitor labs.
    c. Assist with exchange transfusion.

H. SURGICAL DELIVERY
  1. DESCRIPTION
    a. Abdominal delivery or cesarean birth: delivery through a surgical incision in the uterine and abdominal walls
    b. Complications are related to specific indication for cesarean delivery, such as macrosomia, nonreassuring fetal status, and anomalies.

  2. ASSESSMENT
    a. Birth through the abdomen
    b. Transient tachypnea
    c. Birth injury

  3. DIAGNOSTIC TESTS
    a. Based on assessment criteria

  4. NURSING INTERVENTIONS
    a. Based on newborn assessment

I. HYPERBILIRUBINEMIA
  1. DESCRIPTION
    a. Physiologic jaundice: results from hemolysis of RBCs that were necessary in utero (low oxygen environment) but are no longer needed when the newborn begins breathing
    b. Hemolytic: results from destruction of RBCs, usually by maternal antibodies

such as ABO incompatibility or a sensitized Rh-negative mother.

c. Complications include lethargy leading to poor feeding, kernicterus.

2. ASSESSMENT
   a. Jaundice, a yellow-to-bronze coloration of the skin, sclera, and mucous membranes, which reflects bilirubinemia
   b. Jaundice proceeds in the cephalocaudal direction (first appears in the nose, sclera, and sublingual mucosa).
   c. Poor sucking reflex
   d. Lethargy
   e. Poor muscle tone

3. DIAGNOSTIC TESTS
   a. Total and direct bilirubin
   b. Reticulocyte count
   c. Hemoglobin and hematocrit

4. NURSING INTERVENTIONS
   a. Provide phototherapy (ultraviolet light to break down bilirubin in the skin).
   b. Administer intravenous immune globulin if prescribed.
   c. Rarely, exchange transfusion to replace RBCs and correct antigen-antibody interaction is needed.
   d. Monitor for jaundice.
   e. Maintain adequate hydration.
   f. Encourage early frequent feedings to pass meconium that encourages excretion of bilirubin.

J. INFANTS BORN TO HIV-POSITIVE MOTHERS

1. DESCRIPTION
   a. Vertical transmission of HIV occurring during pregnancy or delivery
   b. Antiviral medication during pregnancy greatly reduces transplacental transmission.
   c. Mothers with HIV infection usually deliver by cesarean section to minimize intrapartum transmission of infection.
   d. Breastfeeding can transmit infection and is therefore contraindicated.
   e. Complications include AIDS in newborns, and HIV that may progress rapidly to AIDS and death; average survival time is 9 months from diagnosis to death.

2. ASSESSMENT
   a. Hypothermia
   b. Signs of sepsis
   c. Poor feeding
   d. Skin lesions

3. DIAGNOSTIC TESTS
   a. Since the newborn will usually test positive for HIV antibody due to transfer of maternal antibody, he must

be tested for the virus (usually polymerase chain reaction).

4. NURSING INTERVENTIONS
   a. Avoid circumcision on the male newborn until HIV status is determined.
   b. Anticipate testing.
   c. Bathe thoroughly as soon as possible and before performing any injections, heel sticks, or other invasive procedures.
   d. Administer zidovudine (AZT) during the first 6 weeks of life.
   e. Monitor for manifestations of immune deficiency.
   f. Instruct the parents to have the newborn seen by the physician at birth and at 1 week, 2 weeks, 1 month, and 12 months of life.
   g. Maintain nutrition.

K. MECONIUM ASPIRATION SYNDROME

1. DESCRIPTION
   a. Most common of the aspiration syndromes
   b. Of births, 10–15% have meconium-stained fluid.
   c. Of those infants with 3–4+ meconium fluid, 56% will have meconium below the cords on endotracheal intubation.
   d. Asphyxia or other stress causes passage of meconium in utero; if this meconium-stained fluid is aspirated either before or after delivery, meconium aspiration syndrome results.
   e. Complications include air leak, pulmonary interstitial emphysema, pulmonary hemorrhage, persistent pulmonary hypertension of the newborn, pneumonia, asphyxia, infection, and thrombocytopenia.

2. ASSESSMENT
   a. Mechanical obstruction by particles of meconium (ball-valve effect), air trapping
   b. Chemical pneumonitis due to irritation by meconium, causing thickening of the alveoli
   c. Meconium fosters the growth of pathogens; provides medium for bacterial growth.

3. DIAGNOSTIC TESTS
   a. Chest x-ray
   b. CBC
   c. C-reactive protein
   d. Blood cultures

4. NURSING INTERVENTIONS
   a. Monitor for fetal distress.
   b. Administer intrauterine resuscitation per protocol.

  c. Prepare for immediate endotracheal intubation on delivery.
  d. Anticipate need for ventilatory support.
  e. Administer prescribed oxygen.
  f. Administer prescribed antibiotics.
L. DRUG-EXPOSED NEWBORN
  1. DESCRIPTION
    a. Newborns exposed in utero to narcotics
    b. Newborns exposed in utero to cocaine
    c. Newborns exposed in utero to alcohol (fetal alcohol syndrome)
    d. Newborns exposed in utero to marijuana do not experience abstinence syndrome nor require special care (effects are similar to those of cigarette smoking).
  2. ASSESSMENT
    a. Newborns exposed to narcotic(s) in utero may be born with acute intoxication, and may experience abstinence syndrome.
    b. Newborns exposed to cocaine, PCP, or methamphetamine in utero do not experience an abstinence syndrome but have neurodevelopmental and (later) behavioral problems.
    c. Newborns exposed to alcohol in utero may experience abstinence syndrome, may be small for gestational age, and may have characteristic abnormal facial features.
  3. DIAGNOSTIC TESTS
    a. Urine or stool tests for drugs of abuse

  4. NURSING INTERVENTIONS
    a. Assess for signs of acute drug intoxication—decreased level of consciousness, respiratory depression, tachycardia, elevated blood pressure, or seizures.
    b. Assess for signs of narcotic abstinence syndrome—shrill cry, vomiting, diarrhea, tremulousness, perianal excoriation from acidic stools, tachypnea, yawning, or seizures.
    c. Assess for signs of fetal alcohol syndrome—characteristic facies, irritability, shrill cry.
    d. Assess for signs of cocaine exposure—inability to "tune out" stimuli such as other babies crying, lights, or voices as a normal newborn can.
    e. For all drug-exposed newborns, minimize sensory stimulation (dimly lit quiet room, swaddling) and stimulate only one sense at a time. Either talk or sing to the newborn, or hold or touch the newborn, or look at the newborn—only one sensory stimulus at a time.
    f. Administer sedatives for tremulousness or irritability.
    g. Fetus or neonate cannot tolerate "cold turkey" withdrawal and must be weaned slowly and gradually on medication.

PRACTICE QUESTIONS

1. Which of the following is a priority for the nurse to monitor in an infant born to a mother who has diabetes mellitus?
   1. Hypoglycemia
   2. Rh sensitization
   3. ABO incompatibility
   4. Hypothermia

2. Based on an understanding of maternal hyperglycemia, which of the following is a priority to assess in the newborn?
   1. Cardiac anomalies
   2. Group B beta-hemolytic strep pneumonia
   3. Group B beta-hemolytic strep meningitis
   4. Inborn errors of metabolism

3. The nurse is preparing to administer vitamin K to an infant when the mother asks why her newborn is receiving a vitamin K injection. Which of the following is the most appropriate response? "Vitamin K is administered to
   1. "prevent excessive bleeding from heel sticks."
   2. "prevent petechiae that may occur from routine cares."
   3. "prevent excessive bleeding from IM injection sites."
   4. "protect against intracranial hemorrhage."

4. When preparing the delivery room to care for the newborn, which of the following should the nurse obtain?
   1. A radiant warmer
   2. Formula
   3. Cool washcloths
   4. Clothing and blankets

5. The nurse assesses which of the following
   clinical manifestations to be present in an
   infant born to an HIV positive mother?
   Select all that apply:
   [ ] 1. Diarrhea
   [ ] 2. Large size and weight of the infant
   [ ] 3. Poor feeding
   [ ] 4. Hypothermia
   [ ] 5. Chemical pneumonitis
   [ ] 6. Skin lesions

6. The nurse caring for a large-for-gestational-age
   newborn monitors blood glucose to detect
   hypoglycemia as the result of
   1. limited glycogen stores.
   2. hyperinsulinemia.
   3. large ratio of body surface to weight.
   4. excessive brown fat stores.

7. The nurse admitting a preterm newborn to the
   nursery should assess the newborn for which of
   the following?
   1. Respiratory distress
   2. Shoulder dystocia
   3. Clavicle fracture
   4. Palsies

8. The nurse evaluates a newborn with a heart rate
   of less than 100 bpm, slow and irregular
   respiratory rate, some flexion of muscle tone, a
   grimace, and a pink body but blue extremities
   to have an Apgar score of what number?

   _____

9. The nurse caring for a newborn of an
   Rh-negative mother determines the newborn
   may be at risk for which of the following?
   1. Hemolytic disease
   2. Sepsis
   3. Cardiac anomalies
   4. Petechiae

10. After reviewing the medical record of a mother,
    the nurse evaluates a type A fetus to be at risk
    of ABO incompatibility from the mother
    because she has a blood type of
    1. A.
    2. B.
    3. AB.
    4. O.

11. The nurse reviewing a newborn's chart informs
    the parents that ABO incompatibility is not
    possible in their newborn because the mother's
    blood type is
    1. A.
    2. B.
    3. AB.
    4. O.

12. Based on an understanding of plantar creases in
    the newborn, the nurse assesses plantar creases
    immediately after birth because
    1. after footprinting, creases will be obscured
       by residual ink.
    2. fluid loss may give the appearance of more
       plantar creases.
    3. they will fade as the skin dries in the first
       hours after birth.
    4. as acrocyanosis resolves, creases will be
       more difficult to see.

13. The parents of a newborn ask why their
    newborn is undergoing testing for inborn errors
    of metabolism, congenital adrenal hyperplasia,
    and hypothyroidism. The nurse informs the
    parents that the priority reason that all
    newborns are tested is to
    1. prepare them for complex medical care
       for life.
    2. detect conditions that require special diet
       and drugs.
    3. permit them to prepare advance directives.
    4. prepare them for the child's illness.

14. When admitting a newborn to the nursery,
    the nurse prepares to administer
    erythromycin ointment to the newborn's
    eyes to prevent blindness caused by which
    of the following?
    Select all that apply:
    [ ] 1. Gonorrhea
    [ ] 2. Syphilis
    [ ] 3. Herpes simplex virus
    [ ] 4. Hepatitis
    [ ] 5. Chlamydia
    [ ] 6. Human immunodeficiency
          virus (HIV)

15. The nurse is performing a newborn
    assessment and evaluates a collection of
    blood beneath the newborn's scalp that does
    not cross suture lines. The nurse documents
    this as
    1. caput succedaneum.
    2. cephalohematoma.
    3. occiput.
    4. sinciput.

16. The nurse is assessing a newborn following
    delivery. Which of the following assessments
    is abnormal and determines that further
    evaluation is needed?
    1. Rosy skin color
    2. Heart rate of 138 beats per minute
    3. Noisy breath sounds
    4. An axillary temperature of 36.5°C,
       or 97.7°F

17. The nurse is assessing the reflexes of a newborn. The nurse assesses which of the following reflexes by placing a finger in the newborn's mouth?
    1. Moro reflex
    2. Sucking reflex
    3. Rooting reflex
    4. Babinski reflex

18. The nurse assesses a newborn with neonatal respiratory distress syndrome to have which the following clinical manifestations? Select all that apply:
    [ ] 1. Tachypnea
    [ ] 2. Shock
    [ ] 3. Jaundice
    [ ] 4. Expiratory grunting
    [ ] 5. Retractions
    [ ] 6. Skin lesions

19. The nurse assesses which of the following reflexes by lifting the newborn's body slightly above the crib, followed by suddenly lowering the body and observing for bilateral arm extension and leg flexion?
    1. Moro reflex
    2. Gallant reflex
    3. Palmar grasp
    4. Babinski reflex

20. The nurse documents which of the following reflexes as being responsible for an infant incurving the toes with uncurling and fanning out of the toes when the lateral plantar surface is stroked?
    1. Moro reflex
    2. Gallant reflex
    3. Rooting reflex
    4. Babinski reflex

21. The parents of a newborn ask the nurse why their infant must be tested for phenylketonuria. The appropriate response by the nurse is "to
    1. prevent mental retardation."
    2. prevent chronic lung infections."
    3. treat conductive deafness effectively."
    4. treat hematuria and proteinuria before complications develop."

22. The parents of a newborn ask the nurse why the doctor said the infant must be tested for galactosemia. The nurse should inform the parents that galactosemia is an inborn error of metabolism, in which the newborn cannot metabolize which of the following?
    1. Phenylalanine
    2. Lactose
    3. Saccharine
    4. Ketones

23. The nurse evaluates a newborn to have which of the following STORCH (syphilis, toxoplasmosis, rubella, cytomegalovirus, and herpes) diseases because the newborn's mother handled cat feces and ate raw or undercooked meat during pregnancy?
    1. Cytomegalovirus
    2. Herpes
    3. Rubella
    4. Toxoplasmosis

24. The nurse should inform a mother that which of the following occupations during pregnancy puts the infant at risk for developing cytomegalovirus?
    1. Veterinary assistant
    2. Waitress
    3. Day care worker
    4. Cook

25. The nurse evaluates a newborn with a heart rate of greater than 100 bpm, a strong cry, active motion, crying, and a pink body and extremities to have an Apgar score of what number? _____

26. The registered nurse is preparing clinical assignments for a newborn care unit. Which of the following clinical assignments should the nurse delegate to a licensed practical nurse?
    1. Assess an infant for cephalohematoma
    2. Monitor an infant for tachypnea
    3. Administer vitamin K to an infant
    4. Instruct the parents of an infant on normal nutrition

27. The nurse is teaching a well-baby class to a group of pregnant clients on the characteristics of the feces of newborns and toddlers. Which of the following should the nurse include?
    1. Infants who are breastfed have dark yellow or tan, formed feces
    2. During the first week of life, the feces of the newborn are brown, formed, and firm
    3. For the first 24 hours, the feces passed by the newborn are black, tarry, and sticky
    4. Infants who are formula-fed have bright yellow or golden-colored feces

ANSWERS AND RATIONALES

1. 1. Maternal hyperglycemia causes the fetus to produce more insulin. After delivery, when maternal glucose is suddenly withdrawn, this excessive insulin produces neonatal hypoglycemia. Although Rh sensitization, ABO incompatibility, and hypothermia may be appropriate to assess in any newborn, they are not associated with maternal diabetes.

2. 1. Maternal hyperglycemia has a teratogenic effect. Infants born to mothers with insulin dependence are at greater risk for cardiac anomalies.

3. 4. An injection of prophylactic vitamin K is administered by intramuscular (IM) injection into the newborn's thigh during the first hour of life to stimulate the production of vitamin K by the bacteria in the newborn's intestine. Because the newborn's intestinal tract is considered to be sterile at birth, serious consequences, such as central nervous system hemorrhages, may result if vitamin K is not administered. Deficiencies rapidly occur within the first 2 to 3 days of life. Heel sticks and IM injections do not cause excessive bleeding in the normal newborn. Petechiae are associated with abnormalities of coagulation, not with adaptation to extrauterine life.

4. 1. Due to the high ratio of a newborn's body surface to weight and the inability to shiver, newborns are at risk for hypothermia. Newborns lose heat to the environment through conduction, radiation, evaporation, and convection. A radiant warmer decreases these losses. Applying cool washcloths would increase heat loss. Clothing would prevent warmth from reaching the skin. Formula is not indicated immediately after delivery.

5. 3. 4. 6. Clinical manifestations of infants born to HIV-positive mothers include poor feeding, hypothermia, and signs of sepsis. Diarrhea occurs in infection and sepsis. Infants of a mother with diabetes are of large size and weight. Chemical pneumonitis if a clinical manifestation of meconium aspiration syndrome.

6. 2. Large-for-gestational-age newborns are likely to develop hyperinsulinemia in order to adapt to elevated maternal blood glucose. When the delivery of maternal glucose ceases with the clamping of the cord, the newborn's blood sugar may plummet. Large-for-gestational-age newborns do not have limited glycogen stores.

Although they may have excessive fat stores, this does not cause hypoglycemia. A large ratio of body surface to weight ratio is true of all newborns.

7. 1. Preterm newborns may not have adequate pulmonary surfactant. This increases the work of breathing and may cause respiratory distress and failure. Shoulder dystonia, clavicle fractures, and palsies are complications associated with larger newborns.

8. 1 An Apgar score of 1 includes a heart rate of less the 100 bpm, slow and irregular respiratory rate, some flexion in muscle tone, a grimace, and a pink body but blue extremities.

9. 1. Rh sensitization is the most common cause of maternal immunization and hemolysis (destruction of the red blood cells) in the newborn. The sensitized Rh-negative mother produces antibodies to the Rh factor. In the Rh-positive fetus and newborn, these antibodies cause hemolysis. Petechiae, sepsis, and cardiac anomalies are not associated with hemolytic disease of the newborn.

10. 4. Type O persons produce both anti-A and anti-B antibodies. Type AB persons produce no antibodies. Type A and type B persons produce the antibody to the opposite type. For example, a type B person would produce anti-A antibodies. ABO incompatibility occurs when a type O mother is pregnant with a type A or type B fetus. The mother may develop antibodies that may result in hemolysis in the fetus and newborn. The infants may go on to develop hyperbilirubinemia, requiring phototherapy.

11. 3. Type O persons produce both anti-A and anti-B antibodies. Type AB persons produce no antibodies. Type A and type B persons produce the antibody to the opposite type. For example, a type B person would produce anti-A antibodies. No ABO incompatibility occurs with a type AB mother regardless of the fetus's blood type.

12. 2. Newborns lose fluid in the first few days, which may produce the appearance of more plantar creases. The process of footprinting does not obscure the crease. Acrocyanosis and drying of the surface of the skin do not affect the creases.

13. 2. Early detection and treatment of inborn errors of metabolism, congenital adrenal hyperplasia, and hypothyroidism will prevent complications and disabilities, such as mental retardation and developmental delays. These conditions are preventable.

14. 1. 5. Erythromycin prevents blindness due to gonorrhea and chlamydia. Erythromycin does not treat syphilis, herpes simplex virus, hepatitis, and human immunodeficiency virus. None of these illnesses causes blindness in the newborn.

15. 2. Cephalohematoma is the collection of blood between a cranial bone and its periosteum. Because it is contained by the periosteum, the cephalohematoma does not cross suture lines. Caput succedaneum is a soft tissue swelling that does cross the suture line. Occiput and sinciput are anatomical points on the head.

16. 3. A newborn's skin should be pink or rosy as circulation improves. An infant's heart rate should decrease from a high of 150 to 160 beats per minute to a rate of between 130 and 140 beats per minute. Noisy breath sounds may indicate an obstruction of the air flow through the nares and oropharynx. Suctioning with a bulb syringe may clear the nasal passage of fluid and debris. As a result, the breath sounds would become quiet. Axillary infant temperature should be between 36.5°C and 37.6°C, or 97.7°F and 99.7°F.

17. 2. The sucking reflex is tested by placing something, such as a finger, in the infant's mouth and seeing if the infant begins to suck on the object. The Moro reflex is tested by suddenly lowering the newborn's body. The infant should demonstrate a bilateral arm extension and leg flexion. The rooting reflex is tested by stroking the cheek. The infant may open the mouth. The Babinski reflex is tested by firmly stroking the plantar surface. The anticipated response is the incurving of the toes as in plantar the grasp, with uncurling and fanning out.

18. 1. 4. 5. Clinical manifestations of neonatal respiratory distress syndrome include tachypnea, expiratory grunting, and retractions. Shock is a clinical manifestation of infection and sepsis. Jaundice occurs in hyperbilirubinemia. Skin lesions are a clinical manifestation of infants born to HIV-positive mothers.

19. 1. The Moro reflex is assessed by lifting the newborn's body slightly above the crib, followed by suddenly lowering the body and observing for bilateral arm extension and leg flexion. The Babinski reflex is tested by firmly stroking the plantar surface. The palmar grasp is assessed by watching the infant wrap fingers around an object placed across the palm.

The Gallant reflex is performed by holding an infant prone and stroking the lateral aspect of the leg from below the knee superiorly to the buttocks.

20. 4. The Babinski reflex is tested by firmly stroking the plantar surface. The anticipated outcome is the incurving of the toes with uncurling and fanning out of the toes. The Moro reflex is tested by suddenly lowering the newborn's body. The expected outcome is bilateral arm extension and leg flexion. The rooting reflex is tested by stroking the cheek. The anticipated outcome is the infant turning the head in the direction of the stroking and opening the mouth. The Gallant reflex is performed by holding an infant prone and stroking the lateral aspect of the leg from below the knee superiorly to the buttocks. The infant reacts by moving the buttocks toward the side that is stroked in a curving movement.

21. 1. Phenylketonuria is deficiency of phenylalanine hydroxylase, which results in failure to metabolize phenylalanine. A deficiency of phenylalanine may result in mental retardation. Cystic fibrosis is a chronic lung disease in which recurrent infections occur, resulting from the inability of the ciliated epithelium to secrete mucus. Osteogenesis imperfecta type I involves osteoporosis and recurrent fractures of the long bones. It is characterized by blue sclera, conductive deafness, and discolored teeth. Polycystic kidney disease causes cysts in the kidneys, liver, pancreas, and spleen. Hematuria and proteinuria result.

22. 2. Galactosemia is a deficiency in beta galactosidase, which results in failure to properly metabolize lactose.

23. 4. Toxoplasmosis is a STORCH disease transmitted by handling cat feces or eating raw and undercooked meat. Cytomegalovirus, herpes, and rubella are diseases that are transmitted by humans.

24. 3. Cytomegalovirus is transmitted in the urine of infected persons. Individuals who work in day care during pregnancy put the infant at risk for developing cytomegalovirus. Toxoplasmosis is transmitted by cat feces and by eating raw or undercooked meat.

25. 2 A newborn with a heart rate of greater than 100 bpm, active motion, a cry, and a pink body and extremities has an Apgar score of 2.

26. 3. A licensed practical nurse may administer vitamin K to an infant. Assessing an infant for cephalohematoma, monitoring an infant for tachypnea, and instructing the parents of an infant on normal nutrition are nursing tasks that require the skills of a registered nurse.

27. 3. For the first 24 hours of life, the feces of the newborn are called meconium stools and are black, tarry, and sticky. Generally by the third day of life, the stools become greenish brown to yellowish brown, thin, and less sticky than the meconium stool. Infants who are breastfed have stools that are bright yellow or golden colored and pasty. Infants who are bottle-fed have stools that are pale yellow to tan colored and formed.

REFERENCES

Daniels, R. (2010). *Delmar's manual of laboratory and diagnostic tests* (2nd ed.). Clifton Park, NY: Delmar Cengage Learning.

Littleton, L., & Engebretson, J. (2002). *Maternal, neonatal, and women's health nursing.* Clifton Park, NY: Delmar Cengage Learning.

Littleton, L., & Engebretson, J. (2013). *Maternity nursing care* (2nd ed.). Clifton Park, NY: Delmar Cengage Learning.

CHAPTER 46

REPRODUCTIVE DISORDERS

I. **ANATOMY AND PHYSIOLOGY (SEE FIGURE 46-1)**
   A. VAGINA
      1. TUBE CONNECTING THE EXTERNAL GENITALIA WITH THE CERVIX OF THE UTERUS
      2. LIES BETWEEN THE BLADDER AND THE RECTUM
      3. LINING PROTECTED FROM INFECTION BY:
         a. Thickness
         b. Presence of Doderlein's bacilli
         c. Acidic environment—pH of 3.5–4.5
   B. UTERUS
      1. PEAR-SHAPED, HOLLOW, AND MUSCULAR ORGAN
      2. LIES IN FRONT OF THE RECTUM AND BEHIND THE SYMPHYSIS PUBIS AND URINARY BLADDER
      3. USUALLY TILTS FORWARD AND IS SLIGHTLY ANTEFLEXED
      4. FUNDUS—UPPER, WIDER PORTION
      5. CERVIX—LOWER, NARROWER PART CONNECTING THE VAGINA WITH THE UTERUS
      6. ENDOMETRIUM—INNER LINING WHICH UNDERGOES CYCLIC CHANGES DURING MENSTRUATION AND IMPLANTATION OF THE FERTILIZED EGG
   C. FALLOPIAN TUBES
      1. TUBES CONNECTED TO THE UPPER PORTION OF THE UTERUS ON THE RIGHT AND LEFT SIDES
      2. TRANSPORT EGG INTO THE UTERINE CAVITY
   D. OVARIES
      1. TWO GLANDS IN THE PELVIC CAVITY THAT PRODUCE OVA AND SEX HORMONES
      2. SIZE AND SHAPE OF ALMONDS
      3. SUSPENDED IN THE PELVIS BY LIGAMENTS
      4. THE HORMONES PRODUCED GOVERN THE ACTIVITY OF THE ENDOMETRIUM OF THE UTERUS, SUCH AS CYCLIC MENSTRUATION.
      5. HORMONES RELEASE UNDER THE INFLUENCE OF HORMONES RELEASED FROM THE ANTERIOR PITUITARY GLAND.
      6. OVA ARE DEVELOPED FROM THE PRIMARY OVARIAN FOLLICLES.
      7. WHEN ALL FOLLICLES ARE GONE FROM THE OVARY BY ATRESIA OR OVULATION, OVARIAN ACTIVITY CEASES (MENOPAUSE).

II. **ASSESSMENT**
   A. HEALTH HISTORY
      1. MENSTRUAL HISTORY
      2. OBSTETRICAL HISTORY
      3. DOUCHING HISTORY
      4. CONTRACEPTIVE HISTORY
      5. INFERTILITY
      6. SEXUALITY
      7. SUBSTANCE ABUSE
      8. PAST GYNECOLOGICAL HISTORY
      9. FAMILY HISTORY AFFECTING THE REPRODUCTIVE SYSTEM
      10. CURRENT GYNECOLOGICAL PROBLEMS (E.G., ABNORMAL BLEEDING, MENSTRUAL DYSFUNCTION, AMENORRHEA, VAGINAL DISCHARGE, URINARY TRACT SYMPTOMS, PAIN, PRURITUS, AND POSTMENOPAUSAL PROBLEMS)
   B. PHYSICAL EXAMINATION
      1. PELVIC EXAMINATION
         a. Client should void prior to the examination.
         b. Client is placed in the lithotomy position.
         c. External genitalia is inspected.
         d. Pelvic support and muscle tone are palpated.

Figure 46-1 The female reproductive system.

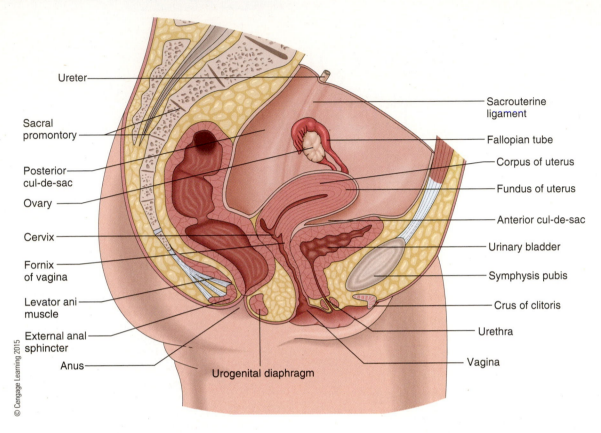

Ureter

Sacral promontory

Posterior cul-de-sac

Ovary

Cervix

Fornix of vagina

Levator ani muscle

External anal sphincter

Anus

Urogenital diaphragm

Sacrouterine ligament

Fallopian tube

Corpus of uterus

Fundus of uterus

Anterior cul-de-sac

Urinary bladder

Symphysis pubis

Crus of clitoris

Urethra

Vagina

© Cengage Learning 2015

2. SPECULUM EXAMINATION
   a. Speculum is wet with warm water prior to insertion.
   b. Lubricants are not used as they interfere with cultures and Pap smear results.
   c. Smears and cultures are obtained in the following order: Pap smears, gonococcal specimen, chlamydial specimen, wet prep.
3. BIMANUAL PELVIC EXAMINATION
   a. Uterus, cervix, ovaries, and fallopian tubes are palpated to determine their location, position, size, shape, contour, consistency, and mobility.
4. RECTOVAGINAL EXAMINATION
   a. Assesses sphincter tone and rectovaginal septum thickness and tone
   b. Enables the posterior aspect of the uterus and anterior and posterior rectal wall to be assessed
   c. Guaiac test is performed on stool if applicable.

III. **DIAGNOSTIC TESTS**
   A. ULTRASONOGRAPHY
      1. DESCRIPTION
         a. High-frequency sound waves, which provide three-dimensional image of an organ

   b. Does not use contrast media or radiation
   c. Can distinguish between a cyst and a solid mass but cannot distinguish whether the solid mass is benign or malignant.
   d. Useful for identifying masses in the pelvis, breasts, and abdomen
      2. PREPROCEDURE
         a. Day of the test
            1) Preparation varies according to the organ to be scanned.
            2) A full bladder is necessary to visualize the uterus and adnexa.
      3. POSTPROCEDURE
         a. None
   B. COMPUTERIZED TOMOGRAPHY (CT) SCANS AND MAGNETIC RESONANCE IMAGING (MRI)
      1. DESCRIPTION
         a. Radiographic studies (CT scans) and electromagnetic studies (MRI) providing three-dimensional cross-sectional images that distinguish between benign and malignant tumor masses
         b. Contrast media may be used to identify vascular structures.

    c. Useful for breast, uterine, ovarian, or retroperitoneal tumors and disorders of the pelvic organs

    d. Contraindicated in pregnancy, obesity (over 300 pounds), allergies to iodine and shellfish, and implanted metal devices such as intrauterine devices, pacemakers, orthopedic metal insertions, and metal clips used in repair of abdominal aortic aneurysms

  2. PREPROCEDURE

    a. Day of the test

      1) Inform the client that there are no food or fluid restrictions unless contrast medium is used.

      2) If contrast medium is to be given, the client should be NPO at least 4 hours prior to the test.

      3) Instruct the client to remove all metal objects.

      4) Instruct the client to void just prior to the test.

      5) Instruct the client to lie still during the entire procedure.

      6) If the client has claustrophobia, a sedative may be ordered prior to the test.

  3. POSTPROCEDURE

    a. None

C. PAPANICOLAOU SMEAR

  1. DESCRIPTION

    a. Laboratory study of cells collected from the cervix and vagina to determine presence of premalignant or malignant conditions

    b. Cells are collected by swab and applied to a clean slide; fixative is applied before sending to the lab.

  2. PREPROCEDURE

    a. Day before the test

      1) Client should not be menstruating.

      2) Instruct the client to avoid douching or taking a tub bath for 24 hours prior to the exam.

    b. Day of the test

      1) Instruct the client to empty the bladder prior to the exam.

  3. POSTPROCEDURE

    a. None

D. DILATATION AND CURETTAGE (D & C)

  1. DESCRIPTION

    a. A surgical procedure in which the cervix is dilated and the uterine wall is scraped with an instrument (curet)

    b. Used for diagnostic and therapeutic purposes to detect uterine malignancy, evaluate dysfunctional uterine bleeding, treat heavy uterine bleeding, treat dysmenorrhea, remove products of incomplete abortion, remove polyps, and perform elective abortion

  2. PREPROCEDURE

    a. Prior to the procedure

      1) NPO for 12 hours prior to the procedure

    b. Day of the procedure

      1) Instruct the client to empty the bladder prior to the procedure.

  3. POSTPROCEDURE

    a. Monitor the client for signs of infection, lacerations, and uterine perforation.

    b. Instruct the client not to use tampons or douches and to refrain from sexual intercourse for 2 weeks.

E. ENDOSCOPY PROCEDURES

  1. DESCRIPTION

    a. Procedures that permit direct visualization of hollow organs and body cavities by means of a lighted instrument

    b. Laparoscopy visualizes the abdominal organs and is used for diagnostic and therapeutic purposes, for example, assessment of endometriosis, assessment of stage of cancer, removal of ovarian tumors and cysts, lysis of pelvic adhesions, to perform tubal ligation, removal of intrauterine device (IUD), and removal of biopsy specimens.

    c. Colposcopy visualizes the vagina and cervix with a binocular microscope and is used to rule out invasive cancer of the cervix and to monitor the status of precancerous tissue.

    d. Hysteroscopy visualizes the uterine cavity with an endoscope to detect abnormal uterine bleeding, malignancies, and fallopian tube competency, and to evaluate infertility.

    e. Hysterosalpingography permits study of the uterus and fallopian tubes by fluoroscopic examination with introduction of a dye to assess fertility, confirm tubal ligation, and evaluate competency of the uterus, and to detect anomalies of the uterus.

  2. PREPROCEDURE

    a. Day before the procedure

      1) Instruct the client to be NPO after midnight prior to the procedure.

    b. Day of the procedure

      1) Instruct the client to void prior to the procedure.

  3. POSTPROCEDURE

    a. Instruct the client to refrain from drinking carbonated beverages for 48 hours, which may react with the

carbon dioxide used in the procedure, causing the client to vomit.
  b. Instruct the client that she may experience mild pain in the shoulder and abdomen due to the insufflation of carbon dioxide during the procedure. The pain should dissipate in 24–48 hours.
  c. Monitor the client for infection, severe pain, and unusual bleeding following all endoscopic procedures.
  d. Following some of the procedures, the client may have a vaginal packing or tampon in place. Physician's instructions should be followed regarding removal.
F. CERVICAL BIOPSY
  1. DESCRIPTION
    a. A sample of atypical cervical tissue obtained with biopsy forceps to confirm a diagnosis of cancer after an abnormal Pap smear or to diagnose abnormal cervical secretions
    b. Acetic acid applied to the cervix helps to identify abnormal areas for biopsy.
    c. Should be performed 1 week after menses begins to minimize the possibility of the client being pregnant
  2. PREPROCEDURE
    a. Prior to the procedure
      1) NPO 12 hours prior to the procedure
      2) Instruct the client to avoid douching or having sexual intercourse for 48 hours prior to the procedure.
    b. Day of the procedure
      1) Instruct the client to void prior to the procedure.
  3. POSTPROCEDURE
    a. Instruct the client to leave the vaginal packing or tampon in place for several hours.
    b. Assess for excessive bleeding and complaints of pain.
    c. Instruct the client to maintain bed rest for 24 hours.
    d. Instruct the client to avoid strenuous exercise for 24 hours.
    e. Instruct the client to avoid sexual intercourse for at least 72 hours until the biopsy site has healed.
G. CONE BIOPSY (CERVICAL CONIZATION)
  1. DESCRIPTION: A COLD KNIFE OR LASER IS USED TO CUT AN INCISION AROUND THE EXTERNAL OS OF THE CERVIX, AFTER WHICH TISSUE IS EXCISED FROM THE CERVIX FOR BIOPSY.
  2. PREPROCEDURE
    a. None

  3. POSTPROCEDURE
    a. Monitor the client for excessive bleeding and infection.
    b. Instruct the client that the next menstrual bleeding may be heavier, with brownish premenstrual discharge.
H. ENDOMETRIAL BIOPSY
  1. DESCRIPTION
    a. Excision of endometrial tissue by means of a curet for laboratory examination
    b. Used to monitor precancerous and ovulatory abnormalities
  2. PREPROCEDURE
    a. Prior to the procedure:
      1) Discontinue antibiotic creams 1 month before the procedure.
      2) Instruct the client not to douche or have sexual intercourse for 48 hours prior to the procedure.
      3) Performed 1 week after menses to minimize risk that the client is pregnant
    b. Day before the procedure
      1) NPO for 12 hours prior to the procedure
    c. Day of the procedure
      1) Instruct the client to void prior to the procedure.
  3. POSTPROCEDURE
    a. See the postprocedure for cervical biopsy on page 890.
I. CULTURES AND SMEARS
  1. DESCRIPTION: EXAMINATION OF A SAMPLING OF TISSUE OR BODY SECRETIONS TO IDENTIFY MICROORGANISMS CAUSING INFECTION OR INFLAMMATION
  2. PREPROCEDURE
    a. Instruct the client to avoid douching 2 hours before a culture is taken.
  3. POSTPROCEDURE
    a. None

IV. **NURSING DIAGNOSES**
  A. DEFICIENT KNOWLEDGE
  B. INEFFECTIVE HEALTH MAINTENANCE
  C. ACUTE PAIN
  D. RISK FOR DEFICIENT FLUID VOLUME
  Nursing Diagnoses: Definitions and Classification 2012–2014. Copyright © 2012, 1994–2012 by NANDA International. Used by arrangement with John Wiley & Sons Limited.

V. **NORMAL PHYSIOLOGICAL PROCESS OF AGING**
  A. MENOPAUSE
    1. DESCRIPTION
      a. A normal physiological process in which menstruation ceases. It is considered complete after amenorrhea for 1 year.

b. Occurs gradually with declining ovarian function, resulting in the loss of function of estrogen-dependent tissue

c. Increased risk of heart disease, osteoporosis, and urinary tract dysfunction

d. If estrogen hormone replacement therapy is used after menopause, there is an increased risk for breast cancer and dysfunctional uterine bleeding.

2. ASSESSMENT
a. Hot flashes
b. Irregular menses progressing to amenorrhea
c. Tenderness in the breasts
d. Difficulty sleeping
e. Mood changes
f. Night sweats
g. Vaginal dryness
h. Decreased bone density (osteoporosis)
i. Urinary incontinence
j. Dyspareunia

3. MEDICAL MANAGEMENT
a. Water-soluble lubricants or estrogen creams for vaginal dryness
b. Hormone replacement therapy with estrogen
c. Progesterone may be included as part of hormone replacement therapy to decrease risk of uterine cancer.
d. Treatment of osteoporosis by pharmacotherapy if at risk

4. NURSING INTERVENTIONS
a. Instruct the client in changes that occur in menopause to decrease anxiety.
b. Instruct the client in a diet of decreased calories and fats and increased whole grains, fiber, fruit, vegetables, and foods high in calcium.
c. Support the client in developing positive coping mechanisms to improve body image, sexual functioning, and feelings of wellness.
d. Instruct the client in need for regular exercise to improve bone mass and sense of well-being.
e. Instruct the client in need for periodic bone density studies to monitor development of osteoporosis.

VI. MENSTRUAL DISORDERS

A. AMENORRHEA
1. DESCRIPTION
a. Cessation of menstruation at any time between menarche and menopause when one is not pregnant
b. Primary amenorrhea is delayed menarche in adolescents.
c. Secondary amenorrhea is absence of menstrual periods for 3 consecutive months or 6 months after a normal menstrual cycle.

d. Secondary amenorrhea can be due to psychological factors, oversecretion of prolactin from the anterior pituitary gland, lack of ovarian production of estrogens, and nutritional factors (dieting or obesity).

e. Obesity can result in anovulation, which may be a contributing factor to the development of amenorrhea.

f. Clients with eating disorders, for example anorexia nervosa and bulimia, or those on crash diets often have complaints of anemorrhea due to a decline in body fat and caloric intake, which causes a hormonal imbalance.

g. Thin women who engage in heavy athletic activity frequently experience amenorrhea due to reduced body fat.

B. DYSMENORRHEA
1. DESCRIPTION
a. Pelvic pain or cramping that occurs usually during the first 72 hours of menstruation
b. Factors contributing to dysmenorrhea include an excessive production of prostaglandins, psychological factors (anxiety and stress), and pelvic disorders (tumors, endometriosis, infections).
c. Low-dose treatment with contraceptives often is effective in clients who are sexually active but do not wish to become pregnant.

2. ASSESSMENT
a. Abdominal cramping
b. Nausea and vomiting
c. Fatigue
d. Low back pain
e. Diarrhea
f. Headaches

3. NURSING INTERVENTIONS
a. Instruct the client in the use of nonsteroidal anti-inflammatory drugs (NSAIDs), prostaglandin antagonists, or hormonal therapy for treatment for pain.
b. Advise the client to increase physical activities for relief of pain.

C. PREMENSTRUAL SYNDROME (PMS)
1. DESCRIPTION
a. The onset of a number of physical and emotional changes that occur prior to the beginning of menstruation and cease when menses begin
b. Cause not known but may be due to fall in levels of estrogen and progesterone, which causes an increase in aldosterone production, resulting in sodium retention and edema

2. ASSESSMENT
   a. Edema or swelling
   b. Feeling of fullness in the abdomen
   c. Headache
   d. Low back pain
   e. Painful breasts
   f. Emotional outbursts
   g. Mood swings
   h. Facial acne
3. NURSING INTERVENTIONS
   a. Perform a detailed health history that includes description of the pain and symptoms in relation to beginning of menses and include a nutritional history related to salt intake, caffeine or alcohol use, and dietary habits.
   b. Instruct the client in measures to control pain and edema with diet, such as using natural diuretics (asparagus and parsley) and small frequent meals high in protein and complex carbohydrates.
   c. Instruct the client to limit intake of coffee, tea, chocolate, cola, and other caffeine substances, which contribute to depression and breast discomfort.
   d. Support the client in establishing positive coping strategies such as exercise, meditation, and imagery for stress reduction.
   e. Instruct the client in the use of prescribed medications for pain, edema, pelvic pressure, or hormonal imbalance.
   f. Assess the client's ability to cope, and make referral for psychological or psychiatric consultation if the client exhibits abnormal behavior.

D. DYSFUNCTIONAL UTERINE BLEEDING
   1. DESCRIPTION
      a. Excessive, frequent, or prolonged painless bleeding from the uterus usually occurring in anovulatory cycles
      b. Amount varies from spotting to hemorrhaging with the passage of clots.
      c. Can be caused by decrease in production of ovarian hormones, cysts, obesity, and benign or malignant tumors of the uterus
      d. Anemia can occur if persistent.
      e. Menorrhagia is prolonged or excessive bleeding with menses.
      f. Metrorrhagia is vaginal bleeding between regular menstrual periods.
      g. Postmenopausal bleeding that occurs 1 year or more after menses cease is significant and needs to be evaluated for possible malignancy.

2. DIAGNOSTIC TESTS
   a. Endometrial biopsy
   b. D & C
   c. Vaginal ultrasound
3. NURSING INTERVENTIONS
   a. Monitor vital signs, fluid and blood loss, and laboratory values, especially hemoglobin (Hgb) and hematocrit (Hct).
   b. Assess vaginal bleeding (pad count and description of flow).
   c. Administer fluids and blood products as ordered.
   d. Instruct the client to report any future recurrences of bleeding.

VII. **STRUCTURAL DISORDERS**
   A. FISTULAS
      1. DESCRIPTION
         a. An abnormal opening between two organs or between an organ and the external body
         b. Usually caused by tissue damage occurring during childbirth, pelvic surgery, radiation therapy to the pelvis, trauma, or spreading malignant lesion
         c. A vesicovaginal fistula is an abnormal opening between the bladder and vagina resulting in the leakage of urine continuously through the vagina.
         d. A rectovaginal fistula is an abnormal opening between the rectum and vagina resulting in the passage of fecal material and flatus through the vagina.
         e. A ureterovaginal fistula is an abnormal opening between a ureter and the vagina resulting in a constant drip of urine seeping through the vagina.
         f. Methylene blue dye is instilled into a body cavity or injected intravenously to identify the bodies abnormally connected.
      2. ASSESSMENT
         a. Fecal material in the vagina
         b. Perineal fecal or urine odor
         c. Vaginal urinary incontinency
      3. MEDICAL AND SURGICAL MANAGEMENT
         a. Goals of care are to eliminate the fistula, prevent or treat infection, and relieve discomfort.
         b. Medically treated with low-residue diet, cleansing douches and enemas, perineal heat lamp applications, perineal irrigations, and antibiotics
         c. Surgical closure is sometimes possible but recurrences are common. Client is monitored for 2 years postoperatively.

4. NURSING INTERVENTIONS
   a. Provide comfort measures for vaginal discharge and related odors.
   b. Provide meticulous skin care measures for cleanliness and prevention of skin irritation.
   c. Instruct the client in procedures for sitz baths and perineal irrigations.
   d. Apply heat lamp to the perineum as ordered.
   e. Instruct the client in the procedure for deodorizing douche using 1 tablespoon of white vinegar to 1 quart of warm water.
   f. If enemas are ordered, instruct the client to carefully direct the catheter tip beyond the fistula on the side opposite the fistula.
   g. Instruct the client not to restrict her diet and fluids to control bowel action, as eventually will cause pressure that may aggravate the condition and increase the size of the fistula.

B. CYSTOCELE AND RECTOCELE
   1. DESCRIPTION
      a. Cystocele is a condition in which the bladder herniates downward into the vagina.
      b. Cystocele is repaired surgically in a procedure called anterior colporrhaphy.
      c. Rectocele is a condition in which the rectum herniates into the vagina.
      d. Rectocele is repaired surgically in a procedure called posterior colporrhaphy.
      e. Both are caused by trauma during childbirth or by injury.
   2. ASSESSMENT
      a. Dragging pain in the back and pelvis that may worsen when standing or walking
      b. Stress incontinence when laughing, walking, or lifting (cystocele)
      c. Difficulty in voiding (cystocele)
      d. Constipation (rectocele)
      e. Hemorrhoids (rectocele)
   3. NURSING INTERVENTIONS
      a. Administer preoperative cleansing douche the morning of surgery.
      b. Instruct the client in administration of cathartic or enema, or both, preoperatively (rectocele).
      c. Implement measures to attain postoperative goals to prevent pressure on the vaginal suture line and prevent infection.
      d. If a urinary catheter is not inserted in surgery, monitor voiding every 4 hours to ensure that no more than 100 ml of

urine accumulates in the bladder—bladder must be kept essentially empty to prevent tension.
      e. Perform perineal care at least two times per day and after each voiding and defecation.
      f. Instruct the client to cleanse the perineum away from the vagina toward the rectum.
      g. Apply a heat lamp for 15–20 minutes two to three times per day and after perineal care to dry the area and encourage healing.
      h. Apply an ice pack to the perineum to decrease swelling and provide comfort.
      i. Instruct the client in the use of sitz baths when sutures are removed.
      j. Instruct the client in the procedure of vaginal douches with normal saline to begin 1 week postoperatively.
      k. Administer daily laxatives or mineral oil to prevent constipation during the postoperative period.
      l. Advise the client that the physician will notify her when sexual intercourse can be resumed.
      m. If posterior colporrhaphy, instruct the client in a clear liquid diet for 5 days post-op.
      n. Advise the client to refrain from straining to have a bowel movement.
      o. Advise the client to avoid jarring activities, heavy lifting, and standing for long periods of time for 6 weeks.
      p. Instruct the client in the procedure for Kegel exercises (contracting the perivaginal muscles and anal sphincter for 10 seconds and relaxing for 10 seconds), which should be done 30–80 times per day.
      q. Instruct the client to report any pelvic pain, vaginal pain, or vaginal bleeding.

C. UTERINE PROLAPSE
   1. DESCRIPTION
      a. Marked downward displacement of the uterus into the vagina due to stretching of the ligaments supporting the uterus and stretching of the muscles of the perineum
      b. As the uterus descends, circulation to the cervix may become impaired, resulting in ulcerations.
      c. Weakened ligaments and muscles result from unrepaired lacerations during childbirth; ill-advised bearing down during labor; and repeated, close pregnancies.
      d. As the uterus descends, it may pull the bladder and rectum downward with it.

2. ASSESSMENT
   a. Chronic backache
   b. Pelvic pressure
   c. Fatigue
   d. Leukorrhea
   e. Stress incontinence when laughing, walking, or lifting
   f. Difficulty in voiding
   g. Dysmenorrhea
3. MEDICAL AND SURGICAL MANAGEMENT
   a. Treated medically with insertion of a pessary (usually older clients)
   b. Surgery is treatment of choice and consists of suturing the uterus back in place and strengthening the pelvic ligaments.
   c. A hysterectomy may be performed if the client is postmenopausal.
4. NURSING INTERVENTIONS
   a. Instruct the client in the correct procedure for insertion and care of a pessary if ordered.
   b. Vaginal hysterectomy or uterine suspension postoperative interventions are the same as for cystocele and rectocele (see page 893).
   c. Abdominal hysterectomy postoperative interventions are the same as for any abdominal surgery.

VIII. INFECTIOUS DISORDERS
A. VULVOVAGINAL INFECTIONS
   1. DESCRIPTION
      a. The vulva and vagina are relatively resistant to infection due to an acid pH (3.5–4.5), presence of Doderlein's bacilli, and thickness of the vaginal epithelium from the effects of estrogen.
      b. Infections generally reveal inflammation of tissues, abnormal discharge, and itching (pruritus).
      c. Risk of infection increases if resistance is lowered by stress, illness, aging, malnutrition, introduction of pathogens, or altered pH.
      d. Clients most at risk include those who douche frequently; use hormonal contraceptives; use broad-spectrum antibiotics; are perimenopausal; have diabetes, allergies, HIV infection, or intercourse with an infected partner; or use poor hygiene practices.
      e. Infectious disorders include candidiasis, a fungal or yeast infection caused by *Candida albicans;* bacterial vaginosis, a bacterial infection; and trichomoniasis, a protozoan infection of the vagina. All may be transmitted sexually.

2. ASSESSMENT
   a. Vaginal discharge (each organism has a specific type of discharge)
      1) Watery or thick with cottage cheese–like particles—candidiasis
      2) Grey to yellow white discharge with a fishlike odor—bacterial vaginosis
      3) Thin, yellow or brown, malodorous—trichomoniasis
   b. Pruritus
   c. Burning
   d. Erythema of the vagina and cervix (trichomoniasis)
   e. Dysuria
3. DIAGNOSTIC TEST
   a. Microscopic identification of causative organisms
4. MEDICAL MANAGEMENT
   a. Antifungal medication is prescribed to treat candidiasis, antibiotics to treat bacterial vaginosis, and antiprotozoal medication to treat trichomoniasis.
   b. Treatment focuses on goals to relieve pain and discomfort, reduce anxiety, prevent reinfection and spread of organisms to sexual partner(s), and teach measures for self-care.
   c. Douching as a general practice is not recommended but therapeutic douching may be ordered for treatment of vaginal infections to lessen odor, remove vaginal discharge, change the pH of the vagina, or as an antiseptic irrigation.
5. NURSING INTERVENTIONS
   a. Instruct the client in administration of prescribed medications—antifungal pills or vaginal suppositories, ointments, or creams (candidiasis); antibiotic pills (bacterial vaginosis); or antiprotozoal pills (trichomoniasis).
   b. Stress with the client the need to treat her sexual partner (trichomoniasis).
   c. Instruct the client to keep the perineal area clean and dry, especially after voiding and defecation, as organisms grow in dark, moist areas.
   d. Instruct the client in the procedure for warm perineal irrigations and sitz baths.
   e. Discuss with the client the need to prevent reinfection and ways to protect oneself from reinfection (use of condoms for sexual intercourse).
   f. Instruct the client to wear loose-fitting, cotton underwear to allow circulation of air to the perineum and to absorb moisture.

g. Instruct the client in the procedure for douching (if prescribed) and proper care and cleaning of equipment.

h. Instruct the client to use 1 tablespoon of white vinegar to 1 quart of warm water for a deodorizing douche.

i. Instruct the client to wash and then soak the douching equipment in diluted bleach for approximately 30 minutes after each use.

B. INFECTION INVOLVING THE CERVIX, VAGINA, AND EXTERNAL GENITALIA

1. HERPESVIRUS TYPE 2 (HERPES SIMPLEX VIRUS)

   a. Description

      1) An incurable viral infection that infects the mucosal or surface lining of the vagina, cervix, and vulva, forming single or multiple vesicles that rupture

      2) Ruptured vesicles may become secondarily infected with bacteria and create small, painful ulcers.

      3) Multiple lesions cause a significant local tissue reaction.

      4) If vesicles do not become infected, they will heal spontaneously but the virus remains in the body in latent form in the nervous system.

      5) First episode is usually the worst, with symptoms beginning 2–20 days after exposure to the virus.

      6) Recurrent infections frequently occur but are less severe.

      7) Recurrent infections are associated with a variety of stressful life events, including illnesses, fever, menses, and emotional crises.

      8) Transmission occurs when mucous membranes, genitalia, or skin breaks directly contact the virus from a person who has active herpes.

      9) The virus from herpesvirus type 1 (cold sores) can be transmitted to the genitalia (herpesvirus type 2) and vice versa by kissing, touching the sore with the hands, or oral sex.

      10) Herpesvirus requires darkness, moisture, and warmth to survive.

   b. Assessment

      1) Tingling or burning sensation in the vagina that changes to intense itching and then becomes extremely painful

      2) Multiple vesicles on the cervix, vagina, and external genitalia that rupture

      3) Erythema and edema at the infected site

      4) Headache

      5) Achiness

      6) Fever

      7) Tender, swollen inguinal lymph nodes

      8) Painful urination

      9) Vaginal discharge

      10) Anxiety as to the diagnosis

   c. Nursing interventions

      1) Instruct the client to have own set of towels and launder them after using them to dry the perineum or other areas where active lesions are present.

      2) Inform the client that towels are safe for others to use after laundering.

      3) Instruct the client to wash the toilet seat with soap and water if any of the fluid-filled vesicles break open while using the toilet.

      4) Instruct the client to avoid kissing while infectious.

      5) Instruct the client that it is extremely important that she wash her hands carefully after any contact with the lesion(s)—otherwise she can infect another part of her body.

      6) Instruct the client to restrict sexual activity that would involve contact with the lesions from the first moment she feels twinges or tingling sensations (prodromal symptoms), as viruses are shed throughout this time.

      7) Instruct the client that lesions should be kept clean and dry.

      8) Advise the client to wear soft, absorbent, loose undergarments.

      9) Instruct the client in the procedure for sitz baths for perineal comfort and comfort in voiding.

      10) Advise the client to get sufficient rest and increase fluid intake to enhance recovery.

      11) Provide the client with information regarding available community resources.

C. INFECTIONS OF THE CERVIX
  1. CHLAMYDIA AND GONORRHEA
    a. Description
      1) Sexually transmitted diseases that cause inflammation of the endocervix
      2) Frequently seen in young clients who have more than one sex partner and who have had a prior history of sexually transmitted diseases
      3) If untreated, may progress to disorders such as pelvic inflammatory disease, sterility, and ectopic pregnancy
      4) Clients often do not have symptoms.
      5) Chlamydial infections can be transmitted to infants during delivery, causing conjunctivitis and pneumonia in many.
      6) A pregnant client with chlamydia may deliver a stillborn child or experience premature labor.
      7) Gonorrhea is caused by the gonococcus bacteria.
      8) Males and females who have rectal or oral sex can develop gonorrheal infections in those areas.
    b. Assessment
      1) Purulent discharge (thick, yellow, or bloody)
      2) Endocervical mucus
      3) Spotting after intercourse
      4) Spotting between periods
      5) Vague lower abdominal pain
      6) Infertility
      7) Pain during sexual intercourse
      8) Dysuria
      9) Pruritus
      10) Urethritis (males)
      11) Epididymitis (males)
    c. Diagnostic tests
      1) Cervical cultures (females) or urethral smears (males)
      2) Rectal or oral cultures, or both
    d. Nursing interventions
      1) Instruct the client in the need to take the prescribed antibiotic, as ordered, and to return for repeat culture in 2 weeks.
      2) Instruct the client to avoid sexual intercourse until she and her partner(s) have completed their medication and follow-up cultures or smears are done and reported as negative. The client needs weekly cultures until two are negative.
      3) Instruct the client in safe sex practices.
      4) Stress to the client the importance of treating all sex partners to prevent reinfection and complications.

D. PELVIC INFLAMMATORY DISEASE (PID)
  1. DESCRIPTION
    a. An infectious process involving the fallopian tubes, ovaries, pelvic peritoneum, pelvic veins, or pelvic connective tissue
    b. May be confined to one structure, or widespread and involve all pelvic structures
    c. Usually caused by bacteria but could also be viral, fungal, or from parasites
    d. Organisms from chlamydia and gonorrhea are the most common causative agents.
    e. Inflammation of the fallopian tubes is called salpingitis.
    f. Inflammation of the ovary is called oophoritis.
    g. Pathogens are usually introduced from outside the body and pass up the cervical canal into the uterus.
    h. Pathogens invade the pelvic organs during sexual intercourse, childbirth, or the postpartum period, or when an abortion is done.
    i. PID is common in women who have IUDs.
    j. Pathogens do not cause difficulty in the uterus but pass into the pelvis by way of the fallopian tubes through thrombosed uterine veins or through the lymphatics of the uterus.
    k. Invaded structure develops an acute or chronic inflammatory process.
    l. Most of the pathogens lodge in the fallopian tubes, giving off a purulent discharge that collects in the tubes and forms adhesions and strictures that frequently result in sterility.
    m. Complications include generalized peritonitis, abscess formation, and strictures or complete obstruction of the fallopian tubes, leading to infertility.
    n. Obstruction of tubes may be partial or complete. If complete, conception is impossible.
    o. Partial obstruction predisposes to ectopic pregnancy because the fertilized ovum cannot reach the uterus although the sperm has been able to pass the stricture and produce conception.

p. Women at risk are those who have their first intercourse at an early age, have multiple sex partners, have frequent intercourse, do not use protection in sexual intercourse, have intercourse with partners who have sexually transmitted diseases (STDs), and have a history of previous STDs.

2. ASSESSMENT
   a. Severe abdominal pain
   b. Feeling of pressure and fullness in the abdomen
   c. Lower abdominal cramps and tenderness
   d. Dyspareunia (pain during intercourse)
   e. Spotting between menses
   f. Fever
   g. Chills
   h. Malaise
   i. Nausea and vomiting
   j. Foul-smelling purulent vaginal discharge

3. DIAGNOSTIC TESTS
   a. Smears from the vagina and cervix for culture and sensitivity
   b. Laparoscopy
   c. Hysterosalpingography

4. SURGICAL MANAGEMENT
   a. Salpingectomy if tubal abscess
   b. Total hysterectomy if severe case of chronic inflammation

5. NURSING INTERVENTIONS
   a. Maintain bed rest in semi-Fowler's position to facilitate dependent drainage during the acute phase (helps to prevent abscesses from forming high in the abdomen, where they might rupture and cause generalized peritonitis).
   b. Administer antibiotics and intravenous fluids as ordered.
   c. Note the amount, color, consistency, and odor of any vaginal drainage.
   d. Monitor vital signs frequently to detect changes in condition.
   e. Apply heat to the abdomen to increase circulation and promote comfort.
   f. Administer analgesics for pain.
   g. Instruct the client in measures to prevent spread of infection and protect from reinfection.
   h. Instruct the client in safe sex practices.
   i. Stress that the client's sex partner(s) need to receive treatment.
   j. Instruct the client of clinical manifestations of ectopic pregnancy as incidence is high in clients with PID.

E. TOXIC SHOCK SYNDROME
   1. DESCRIPTION
      a. An acute bacterial infection caused by *Staphylococcus aureus*
      b. Frequently associated with use of super-absorbency tampons
      c. Occurs where there is a breakdown of skin or mucous membrane, or both
      d. Clinical manifestations may become life threatening, with loss of consciousness, disorientation, fall in blood pressure, and impaired renal functioning.
      e. Potential complications may include disseminated intravascular coagulopathy (DIC) and septic shock.
      f. Risk factors include previous infections of the reproductive system, surgical wound infections, postpartum, and use of intravenous drugs.
   2. ASSESSMENT
      a. Sudden high fever (over 38.8°C [102°F])
      b. Chills
      c. Muscle pain
      d. Vomiting and diarrhea
      e. Red, macular rash that looks like a sunburn
      f. Hypotension
   3. MEDICAL MANAGEMENT
      a. Extensive fluid replacement
      b. Treatment for shock
   4. NURSING INTERVENTIONS
      a. Monitor intake and output.
      b. Assess for fluid volume deficit.
      c. Monitor weight.
      d. Monitor closely for changes in vital signs and level of consciousness.
      e. Assess for signs of DIC, such as bleeding, oozing from needle and infusion sites, cyanosis, and cold skin.

IX. BENIGN TUMORS
   A. FIBROID TUMORS OF THE UTERUS
      1. DESCRIPTION
         a. Benign masses of muscle and connective tissue that grow in the uterus and are found in the lining, muscle wall, and outer surface of the uterus
         b. Because the mass growth is stimulated by ovarian hormones, it tends to disappear spontaneously with the advent of menopause.
         c. Most fibroids are found in the body of the uterus.
         d. The size of tumors varies—some clients have no change in the size of their uterus, whereas others have a large increase in uterine size and may appear as if they were pregnant.
         e. If fibroids impinge on blood vessels, vaginal bleeding will be present.

f. If fibroids are growing at the opening of the fallopian tubes, the client will be sterile.

g. If fibroids are growing in the body of the uterus, they may cause spontaneous abortion.

h. Some fibroids cause no symptoms.

2. ASSESSMENT
   a. Menorrhagia (excessive bleeding with menses)
   b. Low abdominal pressure and pain
   c. Backache
   d. Constipation
   e. Dysmenorrhea

3. DIAGNOSTIC TESTS
   a. Ultrasonography
   b. D & C
   c. CT scan and MRI

4. MEDICAL AND SURGICAL MANAGEMENT
   a. Treatment depends on the size and location of the fibroids, the severity of symptoms, the age of the client, whether the client desires more children, and how near the client is to menopause.
   b. Conservative treatment (watch closely) if the client desires to have children.
   c. Myomectomy (surgical removal of the tumor) is done if the fibroid is near the outer wall and is not embedded in musculature.
   d. Hysterectomy (surgical removal of uterus abdominally or vaginally) is done if severe bleeding or obstruction is present.
   e. Radiation therapy is used if surgery is contraindicated—it reduces the size of the tumor and controls vaginal bleeding.

5. NURSING INTERVENTIONS FOR HYSTERECTOMY
   a. Assess for hemorrhage by observing dressing and vaginal discharge every 15 minutes, progressing to every 1 hour during the first 8 hours postoperatively.
   b. Monitor output from the suction apparatus that drains the surgical site (remains for 3–5 days) and change the dressing at the site as needed.
   c. Foley catheter to continuous drainage until the client is ambulating well; bladder atony is common and temporary.
   d. Monitor urinary output and assess the abdomen for distention when the Foley catheter is removed to ensure the client is emptying the bladder sufficiently.
   e. Monitor the abdomen for distention and monitor the bowel sounds for complication of paralytic ileus.
   f. Encourage early ambulation to prevent thrombophlebitis and advise the client not to sit with legs crossed or to sit in the same position for long periods of time.
   g. Apply antiemboletic stockings and encourage the client to move her legs when in bed.
   h. Monitor the client for complaints of low back pain or lessened urinary output, which could indicate that a ureter was accidentally ligated during surgery.
   i. Attend to the emotional needs of the client, who may have concerns about femininity, lost ability to bear children, or grief and depression over losing a body part.
   j. Instruct the client to avoid heavy lifting and jarring movements for 2 months postoperatively.
   k. Instruct the client that the physician will advise as to when sexual intercourse may be resumed.

B. OVARIAN CYSTS OR TUMORS
   1. DESCRIPTION
      a. Benign neoplasms arising from a variety of ovarian tissues
      b. Follicle cysts are thin walled and translucent and arise during the evolution or involution of the graafian follicles.
      c. Corpus luteum cysts are derived from ruptured follicles resulting in an abnormal resorption of the corpus luteum, leaving a distended cavity with hemorrhagic or clear fluid.
      d. Simple cysts are thin-walled structures containing serous fluid.
      e. Effects of cysts often are not noted unless there is compression of a neighboring organ, obstruction of blood supply, twisting of the cyst at its attachment to the ovary, a menstrual disorder, or infertility.
   2. ASSESSMENT
      a. Increase in abdominal size
      b. Fatigue
      c. Sensation of weight, fullness, or pressure in the pelvis
      d. Pain (only occurs when the cyst twists at the site of attachment)
      e. Pressure complaints (urinary frequency, backache, constipation)
      f. Menstrual irregularities
      g. Ovarian mass felt on palpation

3. DIAGNOSTIC TESTS
   a. Laparoscopy
   b. Ultrasonography
   c. CT scan and MRI
4. SURGICAL MANAGEMENT
   a. Oral contraceptives
   b. Oophorectomy
   c. Hysterectomy with salpingo-oophorectomy
5. NURSING INTERVENTIONS (SEE "NURSING INTERVENTIONS FOR HYSTERECTOMY" ON PAGE 898.)

C. ENDOMETRIOSIS
1. DESCRIPTION
   a. Benign condition in which endometrial cells that normally line the uterus are seeded throughout the pelvis and occasionally extend to as far as the umbilicus
   b. With each menstrual period the endometrial cells are stimulated by ovarian hormones and bleed into the surrounding areas, causing inflammation.
   c. Subsequent adhesions may be so severe that pelvic organs may become fused together, occasionally causing a stricture of the bowel or interference with bladder function.
2. ASSESSMENT
   a. Pain and general discomfort accompanying menstruation that appears 1–2 days before menstruation and lasts for 2–3 days
   b. Feeling of fullness in the lower abdomen
   c. Dyspareunia (pain during intercourse)
   d. Menorrhagia (excessive bleeding with periods)
   e. Irregular menstrual cycles
   f. Infertility
3. DIAGNOSTIC TESTS
   a. Laparoscopy
4. MEDICAL AND SURGICAL MANAGEMENT
   a. Oral contraceptives to create endometrial atrophy and lessen endometrial flow into the peritoneal cavity
   b. Use of synthetic androgens, which cause atrophy of endometrium with resultant amenorrhea
   c. Pregnancy alleviates symptoms.
   d. Laparoscopy with or without laser surgery
   e. Hysterectomy, oophorectomy, or bilateral salpingo-oophorectomy
5. NURSING INTERVENTIONS
   a. Instruct the client in measures to minimize pain that occurs

with dysmenorrhea and dyspareunia.
   b. See "Nursing interventions for hysterectomy" on page 898.

X. **INFERTILITY, ECTOPIC PREGNANCY, CONTRACEPTION, AND ABORTION**
A. INFERTILITY
1. DESCRIPTION
   a. A couple's inability to achieve pregnancy after 1 year of unprotected intercourse
   b. For conception, a female needs to be able to develop and release a normal, fertilizable ovum; provide an environment in which conception can take place; and provide a place where the fertilized ovum can develop and mature.
   c. For conception, males need to be able to provide a sufficient number of viable, motile sperm (more than 20 million/ml) and be able to ejaculate the sperm into the female.
   d. The entire pathway from the vagina to the oviduct must be patent for conception to occur.
   e. Factors that influence fertility include age of the couple, frequency of intercourse, presence of infection, abnormalities of the reproductive tract, endocrine and immune system disorders, and lifestyle.
   f. Finding causes of infertility involves evaluation of the functioning of the ovaries, fallopian tubes, cervix, and uterus, and adequacy of the seminal fluid.
2. DIAGNOSTIC TESTS
   a. Basal body temperature for a minimum of four cycles (ovary)
   b. Endometrial biopsy (ovary)
   c. Serum progesterone level (ovary)
   d. Hysteroscopy (uterus)
   e. Hysterosalpingography (fallopian tubes and uterus)
   f. Laparoscopy (fallopian tubes)
   g. Postcoital cervical mucus test (cervix)
   h. Examination of ejaculate (seminal fluid)
   i. Culdoscopy (pelvic organs in general)
   j. Serum testosterone, follicle-stimulating hormone (FSH), leutinizing hormone (LH), and antisperm antibodies (male)
3. MEDICAL MANAGEMENT
   a. Drugs to induce ovulation
   b. Artificial insemination (partner or donor)
   c. In vitro fertilization
   d. Embryo or egg donor

4. NURSING INTERVENTIONS
   a. Administer specific medications as prescribed and instruct the client in self-administration.
   b. Instruct the couple in basic principles of reproduction, menstruation, ovulation, and optimum times for intercourse.
   c. Encourage both individuals to discuss their feelings about infertility.
   d. Prepare the couple for a battery of diagnostic tests—both laboratory and surgical.
   e. Make referrals to appropriate community agencies for support group.

B. ECTOPIC PREGNANCY
  1. DESCRIPTION
   a. The implantation of a fertilized ovum in an area outside the uterus
   b. The most common site is the fallopian tube.
   c. Clients with risk factors include those with previous pelvic infections with resultant adhesions or strictures, ectopic pregnancies, and induced abortions, use of IUDs, and tumor injury to reproductive organs.
   d. Mortality increases if the fallopian tube ruptures, as the client goes into shock.
  2. ASSESSMENT
   a. Severe pain
   b. Dizziness, fainting
   c. Nausea and vomiting
   d. Hypotension
   e. Pallor
   f. Rapid, thready pulse
   g. Excessive vaginal bleeding
  3. DIAGNOSTIC TESTS
   a. Ultrasound
   b. Serum beta portion of human chorionic gonadotropin levels
   c. Laparoscopy
  4. MEDICAL AND SURGICAL MANAGEMENT
   a. Conservative therapy using methotrexate to halt the pregnancy
   b. Salpingostomy (opening into the fallopian tube)
   c. Salpingo-oophorectomy
  5. NURSING INTERVENTIONS
   a. Provide measures for relief of pain.
   b. Monitor for complications of shock and hemorrhage.
   c. Maintain bed rest during the acute phase.
   d. Provide psychological support.
   e. Instruct the client to report any abnormal menstrual cycle in the future (may indicate another ectopic pregnancy).

C. CONTRACEPTION
  1. DESCRIPTION
   a. The prevention of fertilization or implantation of a fertilized ovum in the uterus
   b. Methods of contraception include abstinence; use of oral contraceptives; surgical sterilization of the female by tubal ligation and the male by vasectomy; skin implant contraception; use of long-acting hormone therapy by injection; use of mechanical barriers such as diaphragms, cervical caps, female or male condoms; use of chemical spermicides in foams, creams, and jellies; coitus interruptus; natural rhythm method; and intrauterine devices.
   c. Method selected is a personal choice—each method has its own side effects and long-term risks.
   d. No method is 100% satisfactory in preventing a pregnancy.
  2. NURSING INTERVENTIONS
   a. Discuss contraceptive choices and describe the benefits and possible side effects and risks for the method selected.
   b. Provide specific instructions for application of the method chosen.
   c. Instruct the client that if using a chemical or barrier method, the spermicide is only effective for 1 hour after applying.
   d. Stress that use of condoms decreases the risk of sexually transmitted diseases.

D. ABORTION
  1. DESCRIPTION
   a. Termination of a pregnancy with expulsion of the products of conception
   b. Fetus is considered viable after the fifth month of gestation.
   c. Abortion may be spontaneous (miscarriage) or an elective procedure.
   d. Method chosen for elective procedure is determined by the length of the pregnancy.
   e. Ideal time for abortion is the first 8 weeks of pregnancy.
   f. A progesterone antagonist will prevent implantation of the ovum if administered 10 days before menstruation.
   g. Vacuum aspiration or dilation and curettage are methods used for first-trimester abortion (first 12 weeks from

the first day of the last menstrual period).

h. Hypertonic saline and prostaglandins are used for abortion after the 13th week.

i. Risks of abortion include hemorrhage, infection, and injury to reproductive organs.

2. NURSING INTERVENTIONS

a. Explain options to the client, including appropriate procedures and expected outcomes.

b. Discuss with the client alternative methods of contraception for future reference.

c. Instruct the client to report excessive vaginal bleeding, temperature elevation, and severe pain.

d. Instruct the client on the need for a follow-up appointment 2 weeks following the procedure.

e. Provide psychological support to the client.

PRACTICE QUESTIONS

1. The nurse is preparing a client for an ultrasound of her uterus. Which of the following nursing interventions should the nurse perform prior to sending the client for the examination?
   1. Ask the client if she has any allergies to iodine
   2. Have the client drink two glasses of water
   3. Ask the client to remove all metal jewelry and hair clips
   4. Have the client void before she leaves the nursing unit

2. Which of the following statements by the nurse should be included in the instructions for a client with endometriosis who is scheduled for a laparoscopy?
   1. "Do not drink carbonated beverages for 48 hours after the procedure."
   2. "The dressing should be removed the next day and the incision left open to air."
   3. "The dye that is used will color your urine blue for the first few voidings."
   4. "Notify your physician if you experience any pain in the shoulder area."

3. Which of the following should the nurse include in the instructions for a client who is to have a cervical biopsy?
   1. Food and fluids are to be restricted for 4 hours before the procedure
   2. A cleansing douche should be done the morning of the procedure
   3. Sexual intercourse may be resumed the day after the procedure
   4. The procedure must be scheduled for 1 week after menses begin

4. A client beginning menopause asks the nurse, "What can I expect if I don't go on hormone replacement therapy?" The best response of the nurse should be which of the following?
   1. "You will eventually be symptom-free once your body adjusts to the withdrawal of estrogen from your ovaries."
   2. "You may be more prone to fracturing a bone if you fall or injure yourself, so you will need to be very careful."
   3. "You will have occasional periods of spotting, which is normal for the first few years, and then it will stop."
   4. "You will be free of your monthly periods and won't have to worry about getting pregnant from now on."

5. The nurse instructs a client in menopause to eat foods that are high in calcium. The nurse includes which of the following foods that has the highest calcium content in these instructions?
   1. Low-fat plain yogurt
   2. Egg omelet
   3. Ice cream
   4. Eggnog

6. Which of the following nursing diagnoses would be most important for the nurse to include in the nursing care plan for a 55-year-old client who has had amenorrhea for 1 year?
   1. High risk for sexual dysfunction
   2. Self-care deficit
   3. Impaired skin integrity
   4. Risk for impaired physical mobility

7. The nurse instructs the client with premenstrual syndrome (PMS) that, prior to starting her menses when she notices fluid retention, she should eat which of the following?

Select all that apply:
[ ] 1. Asparagus
[ ] 2. Cranberry juice
[ ] 3. Brussels sprouts
[ ] 4. Celery
[ ] 5. Bananas
[ ] 6. Parsley

8. The nurse should instruct the client with premenstrual syndrome (PMS) to avoid which of the following?
Select all that apply:
[ ] 1. Exercise
[ ] 2. Coffee
[ ] 3. Chocolate
[ ] 4. Applications of heat
[ ] 5. Vitamin B supplements
[ ] 6. Tea

9. The nurse assesses a client with a vesicovaginal fistula to have which of the following?
1. Fecal material passing into the vagina
2. Urine passing from the urethra into the vagina
3. Urine leaking continuously from the bladder into the vagina
4. Passage of urine from the ureter to the vagina

10. Which of the following diets should the nurse include in the teaching plan for a client who has a rectovaginal fistula?
1. Low fat
2. Low residue
3. Bland
4. Clear liquid

11. The nurse includes which of the following in the discharge instructions for a client with a rectovaginal fistula?
1. Do not douche until the area is healed
2. Use antifungal vaginal suppositories to prevent infection
3. Limit fluid intake until the vaginal discharge ceases
4. Avoid straining to have a bowel movement

12. The client who had a rectovaginal fistula surgically repaired a year ago asks the nurse, "Why does the surgeon want to see me again in 6 months?" The best response of the nurse would be, "The surgeon
1. has to write a new prescription for the paregoric every 6 months."
2. wants to be sure you're adhering to the diet and not gaining weight."
3. wants to monitor the site to be sure the fistula hasn't returned."
4. needs to be sure that the perineal area has healed completely."

13. The nurse monitors the urinary output every 4 hours of a postoperative client who had a cystocele and rectocele repair (anterior and posterior colporrhaphy). Which of the following measurements is the maximum amount of urine that should accumulate in the bladder?
1. 150 ml
2. 100 ml
3. 200 ml
4. 250 ml

14. Which of the following assessment findings is an anticipated finding for the client with a rectocele?
1. Difficulty in voiding
2. Hemorrhoids
3. Tarry stools
4. Stress incontinence

15. The nurse suspects a diagnosis of ectopic pregnancy in a client with which of the following assessments?
Select all that apply:
[ ] 1. Dyspareunia
[ ] 2. Severe pain
[ ] 3. Dizziness
[ ] 4. Menorrhagia
[ ] 5. Increase in abdominal size
[ ] 6. Nausea and vomiting

16. Which of the following statements by the nurse should be included in the instructions for a client receiving treatment for vaginitis?
1. "The vagina needs to be acidic to decrease your chance of another infection."
2. "Douching more frequently will help to rid the vagina of organisms."
3. "Sexual intercourse is permitted as long as your partner uses protection."
4. "A water-soluble lubricant should be used until your symptoms are gone."

17. The nurse should monitor which of the following clients for a potential vaginal infection?
1. A menstruating client who uses sanitary napkins
2. A menopausal client who is sexually active
3. A client treated with Bactrim for a urinary tract infection
4. A client given broad-spectrum antibiotics for a wound infection

18. The nurse should include which of the following in the discharge instructions for a client with herpesvirus type 2?
1. Sexual activity is permitted as long as the partner wears protection
2. The lesions should be covered when they break open
3. The antibiotic therapy should be sufficient to prevent recurrence
4. Abstinence from sex is necessary when the prodromal symptoms are noticed

19. Which of the following assessment findings would indicate to the nurse that a client with a history of gonorrhea is experiencing a complication of the disease?
    1. Inability to conceive
    2. Cottage cheese–like vaginal discharge
    3. Multiple ruptured vesicles on vagina and perineum
    4. Heavy vaginal bleeding after several missed periods

20. The nurse should include which of the following questions in a nursing history from a client admitted with pelvic inflammatory disease (PID)?
    1. "When did you first notice the heavy bleeding with clots?"
    2. "When did you start to have the sudden high fever?"
    3. "Have you ever used an intrauterine device?"
    4. "Do you have spotting after intercourse?"

21. The nurse should report which of the following client assessments as consistent with a diagnosis of toxic shock syndrome?
    Select all that apply:
    [ ] 1. Menorrhagia
    [ ] 2. Sudden temperature elevation of 39.2°C, or 102.6°F
    [ ] 3. Complaints of headache and dizziness
    [ ] 4. Muscle pain
    [ ] 5. Red, macular rash
    [ ] 6. Hemoglobin of 12 gm/dl

22. The nurse develops a plan of care for the immediate postoperative period for a client who had an abdominal hysterectomy. The plan should include measures to
    1. assess intake and output every shift.
    2. clamp wound suction catheter in the morning.
    3. assess for abdominal distention.
    4. maintain bed rest until the morning, followed by assisted ambulation.

23. The nurse performs an assessment on a client diagnosed with endometriosis. Which of the following assessment findings would be indicative of this disorder?
    Select all that apply:
    [ ] 1. Spotting after intercourse
    [ ] 2. Pain prior to menstruation

[ ] 3. Dyspareunia
[ ] 4. Menorrhagia
[ ] 5. Mass felt on palpation
[ ] 6. Yellow purulent discharge

24. The nurse is collecting a nursing history from a client admitted with an ectopic pregnancy. Which of the following questions should the nurse ask?
    1. "Has your partner's sperm been examined?"
    2. "Do you have frequent miscarriages?"
    3. "Do you have a family history of ectopic pregnancies?"
    4. "Have you ever had an infection in your pelvis?"

25. The nurse should include which of the following in the instructions to the client who has selected a barrier method of contraception?
    1. Spermicides lose effectiveness after 1 hour
    2. A condom can be used a second time if washed with soap and water
    3. Condoms are the safest form of contraception
    4. A diaphragm should not be removed for 24 hours post coitus

26. The registered nurse is preparing the clinical assignments on a women's health unit. Which of the following assignments would be appropriate to delegate to a licensed practical nurse?
    1. Perform an admission assessment of a woman admitted with vaginitis
    2. Conduct a health history on a woman suspected of having endometriosis
    3. Develop a plan of care for a woman following a hysterectomy
    4. Ask a woman about an allergy prior to a diagnostic test

27. A client asks the nurse "How many days after exposure to the herpes simplex virus does the first episode occur?" The appropriate response of the nurse is how many days? _____

ANSWERS AND RATIONALES

1. 2. An ultrasound uses high-frequency sound waves to provide an image of an organ. An ultrasound of the uterus requires that the bladder be full in order to visualize the uterus; thus, the client needs to drink fluids prior to the examination. An ultrasound does not use contrast media, such as iodine preparations, and metal objects, such as jewelry and hair clips, are not contraindicated for an ultrasound. Having the client void before the examination would prevent the visualization of the uterus.

2. 1. Clients having a laparoscopy should refrain from drinking carbonated beverages for 48 hours after the procedure because the beverages may react with the carbon dioxide used in the procedure, causing vomiting. The laparoscope is inserted through a stab wound, thus eliminating the necessity of a surgical incision and dressing. A blue dye is not used for assessment of endometriosis. Clients having laparoscopy normally have mild pain in the shoulder area due to the insufflation of carbon dioxide during the procedure.

3. 4. A cervical biopsy must be scheduled for 1 week after menses begin to minimize the possibility that the client might be pregnant. The client should be NPO after midnight for the procedure. The client should not douche or have intercourse for 48 hours before the procedure. The client should not have sexual intercourse until the biopsy site has healed, which is at least 72 hours after the procedure.

4. 2. Menopausal women who do not take estrogen replacement therapy are at risk for developing osteoporosis and will be more prone to fractures. Some of the manifestations of menopause do not disappear, such as vaginal and urethral atrophy. Women going through menopause will have irregular menses, not spotting. Women beginning menopause are still ovulating irregularly and may get pregnant if contraception is not used.

5. 3. Calcium is present in all of the food groups, but is highest in dairy products. Ice cream contains 1406 mg per serving. Low-fat plain yogurt contains 415 mg per serving. Eggnog contains 330 mg per serving and an egg omelet contains 47 mg per serving.

6. 4. Menopause is considered complete after amenorrhea for 1 year in the older adult woman. A menopausal client is at risk for impaired mobility due to osteoporosis in the spine. Menopausal women can continue to function sexually and perform self-care measures. Although the skin becomes dryer in menopause, it is not of major consequence.

7. 1. 4. 6. Asparagus, celery, and parsley are natural diuretics, which are recommended when the client experiences fluid retention. Cranberry juice, brussels sprouts, and bananas are fruits and vegetables that are high in water content and would promote fluid retention rather than alleviate it.

8. 2. 3. 6. Clients with premenstrual syndrome (PMS) should limit foods with caffeine, such as coffee, tea, cola, and chocolate, to decrease breast discomfort and prevent depression. Exercise should be encouraged to reduce stress. Applications of heat are effective in relieving the abdominal and pelvic cramping symptoms of PMS. Vitamin B supplements, especially B complex and vitamin B_6, are helpful in treating the depression that accompanies PMS.

9. 3. A fistula is an abnormal opening between two organs or between an organ and the external body. The name of the fistula identifies the two areas of the body that are connected by the abnormal opening. Therefore, a vesicovaginal fistula connects the bladder with the vagina, resulting in urine from the bladder leaking continuously out the vagina. Fecal material in the vagina would be a rectovaginal fistula and urine passing from the urethra into the vagina would be a urethrovaginal fistula. The passage of urine from the ureter to the vagina is a ureterovaginal fistula.

10. 2. A low-residue diet is prescribed for the client with a rectovaginal fistula to decrease the stool bulk and slow the transit time. A low-fat diet would be ordered for clients having gastrointestinal symptoms related to fat intolerance. A bland diet is ordered for disorders of the stomach and eliminates foods that may be irritating to the stomach mucosa. A clear liquid diet is a short-term, very restrictive diet that would not provide the necessary calories and protein needed for tissue repair.

11. 4. Clients with rectovaginal fistulas are advised not to strain to have a bowel movement, because the increase in pressure aggravates the fistula and usually increases the size of the opening. Clients are advised to use either cleansing or deodorizing douches during the course of treatment. Clients with rectovaginal fistulas are prone to bacterial infections rather than fungal infections. Fluid intake should not be limited as this would cause constipation, which in turn puts pressure on the site of the fistula when one strains to have a bowel movement.

12. 3. Rectovaginal fistulas that are surgically repaired may recur within 2 years after the repair, necessitating follow-up care for a 2-year period. Paregoric is prescribed to inhibit bowel action and would be contraindicated for a rectovaginal fistula. Weight gain would not be a consequence of this type of surgery and would not be a contributing factor for a recurrence of the fistula. A rectovaginal fistula is repaired internally and any related perineal irritation should have healed shortly after the surgery.

13. 2. The client who has a cystocele and rectocele repair should not have more than 100 ml of urine accumulating in the bladder to prevent tension on the suture line. Amounts of 150 ml, 200 ml, and 250 ml enlarge the bladder sufficiently to put pressure on the operative site.

14. 2. A rectocele is herniation of the rectum into the vagina. As a rectocele enlarges, the client has difficulty having a bowel movement, becomes constipated, and begins to strain to have a bowel movement, resulting in hemorrhoids. A rectocele does not affect the urinary tract. Tarry stools would occur with gastrointestinal bleeding at a site remote from the rectum.

15. 2. 3. 6. Assessment findings in a client with ectopic pregnancy include severe pain, dizziness, and nausea and vomiting. Dyspareunia and menorrhagia are assessment findings of endometriosis. An increase in abdominal size is found in ovarian cysts.

16. 1. The normal pH of the vagina is approximately 3.5 to 5.5 and it is the acidic nature of the vaginal discharge that protects the vagina from infection by bacteria. Douching decreases the amount of normal vaginal discharge, which alters the acid nature of the vagina. Sexual intercourse, with or without protection, should not be done when a vaginal infection is present. A water-soluble lubricant has no therapeutic value in the treatment of vaginitis.

17. 4. Broad-spectrum antibiotics decrease the quantity of helpful bacteria as well as harmful bacteria, so a client on broad-spectrum antibiotics for a period of time may develop vaginitis due to a decrease in the normal vaginal flora. Use of sanitary napkins has not been related to vaginal infections, but tampon use is the suspected cause of toxic shock syndrome, a bacterial infection. A sexually active menopausal client would not normally be at risk for vaginitis. Trimethoprim-sulfamethoxazole (Bactrim), an antibacterial prescribed for urinary tract infections, does not normally alter the flora in the vagina and rectum.

18. 4. The client with herpesvirus type 2 is considered infectious when the prodromal clinical manifestations occur, as the virus is being shed throughout this time. Wearing protection for sexual intercourse will not totally prevent contact with the virus, as any break in the mucous membranes or skin that comes into contact with an active lesion may become infected. Lesions should not be covered, but should be left open to the air to dry. Herpesvirus type 2 is a viral infection with no known cure. Antibiotics will not prevent a recurrence.

19. 1. One of the complications of gonorrhea is sterility, caused by scarring of the fallopian tubes during the course of the disease and resulting in strictures. A cottage cheese–like vaginal discharge would occur with the client with candidiasis, a fungal infection. Multiple ruptured vesicles on the vagina and perineum occur when the client has herpesvirus type 2. A client having heavy vaginal bleeding after several missed periods is probably experiencing a miscarriage, which indicates that the conceived ovum was transported through the fallopian tube to the uterus.

20. 3. Clients who use or have used intrauterine devices are at risk for developing pelvic inflammatory disease (PID). The discharge for PID is foul smelling and purulent, not bloody with clots. Clients with PID may have fever and chills, but the temperature elevation is not sudden, and they do not normally have spotting after intercourse.

21. 2. 4. 5. One of the most pronounced clinical manifestations of toxic shock syndrome is a sudden temperature elevation above 38.9°C, or 102°F. Other clinical manifestations include chills; muscle pain; vomiting and diarrhea; red, macular rash that looks like a sunburn; and hypotension. The condition is not known to affect menses or to give rise to complaints of headache and dizziness. A hemoglobin of 12 gm/dl is within the normal range of 12 to 16 gm/dl for a female.

22. 3. Abdominal distention in a postoperative client who had an abdominal hysterectomy could be an indication of the complication of a paralytic ileus. Intake and output should be assessed more frequently than every shift to detect postoperative complications of urinary retention and paralytic ileus. Wound suction catheters should remain open to prevent abscess formation. Clients should be ambulated the evening of surgery to prevent thrombophlebitis.

23. 2. 3. 4. Pain in endometriosis occurs 1 to 2 days before menstruation and lasts for 2 to 3 days after menses begins. Other clinical manifestations include dyspareunia (pain during intercourse), menorrhagia (excessive bleeding with periods), heavy feeling in the lower abdomen, irregular menstrual cycles, and infertility. Clients with endometriosis do not spot after intercourse or have an infection noted by a yellow purulent discharge. The endometrial cells, which are seeded in the pelvis, cannot be palpated.

24. 4.   Clients who have had previous pelvic infections, such as chlamydia, gonorrhea, or pelvic inflammatory disease, are at risk for having an ectopic pregnancy, due to the strictures and adhesions created by these conditions. The cause of an ectopic pregnancy is not related to a problem with the male partner. Women at risk for an ectopic pregnancy are women who have had induced abortions, not miscarriages. Ectopic pregnancies are not genetic.

25. 1.   Spermicides in the form of gels, foams, creams, or tablets kill sperm and should be used a few minutes before intercourse by placing on condoms, diaphragms, or inserting into the vagina. Their effectiveness lasts for approximately 1 hour. Condoms should be used once and discarded, as slippage, breaks, or tears in the condom are possible. Condoms have a 10% to 15% failure rate, which is more than other forms of contraception. Diaphragms should not be left in place for more than 24 hours.

26. 4.   A registered nurse may delegate asking a woman about an allergy prior to a diagnostic test. Performing an admission assessment, conducting a health history, and developing a plan of care involve the skills of a registered nurse.

27.   2–20. The first episode of herpes simplex virus is the worst, with symptoms beginning 2 to 20 days after exposure to the virus.

REFERENCES

Daniels, R. (2010). *Delmar's manual of laboratory and diagnostic tests* (2nd ed.). Clifton Park, NY: Delmar Cengage Learning.

Littleton, L., & Engebretson, J. (2002). *Maternal, neonatal, and women's health nursing.* Clifton Park, NY: Delmar Cengage Learning.

Littleton, L., & Engebretson, J. (2013). *Maternity nursing care* (2nd ed.). Clifton Park, NY: Delmar Cengage Learning.

PSYCHIATRIC NURSING

CHAPTER 47

ANXIETY DISORDERS

I. ANXIETY

  A. DESCRIPTION: ANXIETY IS AN EVOLVED ADAPTIVE MECHANISM THAT:

    1. HELPS SURVIVAL IN A DANGEROUS WORLD

    2. CAN BE PRODUCED BY EITHER AN INTERNAL OR EXTERNAL STIMULUS

    3. IS EXPERIENCED AS AN UNCOMFORTABLE AND APPREHENSIVE TENSION

    4. MANIFESTS PHYSIOLOGICAL CLINICAL MANIFESTATIONS THROUGH THE ACTIVATION OF THE HYPOTHALAMIC-PITUITARY-ADRENAL AXIS

    5. THE RELEASE OF ADRENOCORTICAL HORMONES ACTIVATES THE SYMPATHETIC NERVOUS SYSTEM, PRODUCING THE PHYSIOLOGICAL CLINICAL MANIFESTATIONS OF THE "FIGHT-OR-FLIGHT" REACTION, INCLUDING:

      a. Increased pulse rate and blood pressure

      b. Dry mouth

      c. Sweating

      d. Muscle tension

      e. Rapid, shallow respiration

      f. Tremor

      g. Tightness in the throat and chest

      h. Frequent urination

      i. Dizziness

      j. Queasy stomach

    6. THE MOST PRONOUNCED PSYCHOLOGICAL (COGNITIVE OR EMOTIONAL) MANIFESTATION OF ANXIETY IS A SENSE OF IMPENDING DANGER OR DOOM.

II. LEVELS OF ANXIETY

  A. MILD

    1. PROMPTED BY THE ORDINARY TENSIONS EXPERIENCED IN DAILY LIFE

    2. SENSES ARE HEIGHTENED, AND INDIVIDUALS ARE ALERT, FOCUSED, AND ABLE TO BOTH LEARN NEW INFORMATION AND PROBLEM SOLVE.

    3. APPEAR CALM AND FEEL IN CONTROL

    4. PERFORM MORE COMPETENTLY AT THIS LEVEL OF ANXIETY THAN IF RELAXED

    5. MOST PEOPLE WOULD DESCRIBE THIS STATE AS BEING "ON" RATHER THAN LABEL IT AS ANXIETY.

  B. MODERATE

    1. MOTIVATION TO LEARN CONTINUES.

    2. ABLE TO PROBLEM SOLVE BUT FUNCTIONAL ABILITY BEGINS TO DECREASE

    3. THE RELEASE OF ADRENOCORTICAL HORMONES PRODUCES A LOW LEVEL OF SYMPATHETIC AROUSAL.

    4. BECOMES AWARE OF SOME MOTOR TENSION

    5. THE PERCEPTUAL FIELD NARROWS.

    6. THE FOCUS OF ATTENTION IS MORE EXCLUSIVELY THE CONCERN.

    7. BECOMES AWARE OF BEING SOMEWHAT ANXIOUS

    8. SPEECH PRODUCTION, RATE, AND VOLUME BEGIN TO INCREASE.

  C. SEVERE

    1. PRODUCES WHAT IS COMMONLY LABELED THE "FIGHT-OR-FLIGHT" RESPONSE

    2. ADRENOCORTICAL HORMONE LEVELS CONTINUE TO INCREASE.

    3. SENSORY INPUT BEGINS TO DISORGANIZE.

    4. PERCEPTIONS CAN BECOME DISTORTED.

    5. ATTENTION IS VERY NARROWLY FOCUSED AND DIFFICULT TO REFOCUS.

    6. CONCENTRATION AND PROBLEM-SOLVING ABILITIES BECOME OBVIOUSLY IMPAIRED.

7. MOTOR ACTIVITY INCREASES, OFTEN WITH PACING AND HAND WRINGING.
8. ALL ACTIVITY IS DIRECTED AT RELIEVING THE ANXIETY.
9. EMOTIONAL DISTRESS IS VERBALIZED.

D. PANIC
1. PERCEPTIONS BECOME EVEN MORE DISTORTED AND THE ABILITY TO DISTINGUISH REALITY IS IMPAIRED.
2. THE INABILITY TO CONCENTRATE OR THINK LOGICALLY AND RATIONALLY RESULTS IN AN INABILITY TO PROBLEM SOLVE.
3. THE EXPERIENCE IS OF BEING OVERWHELMED, HELPLESS, OUT OF CONTROL AND UNABLE TO FUNCTION ADEQUATELY.
4. A SENSE OF DREAD AND TERROR PREDOMINATES.
5. EGO INTEGRITY BEGINS TO DISINTEGRATE.
6. LOSS OF CONTROL OVER BEHAVIOR MAY BE DISPLAYED AS ANGER, AGGRESSION, WITHDRAWAL, CLINGING, OR WEEPING.

III. **THEORIES OF ANXIETY**
A. PSYCHOBIOLOGICAL
1. ALL INDIVIDUALS RESPOND PHYSIOLOGICALLY WHEN ANXIOUS.
2. THOSE INDIVIDUALS WHO ARE PREDISPOSED TO ANXIETY DISORDERS APPEAR TO HAVE BODY SYSTEMS THAT FUNCTION IMPROPERLY IN RESPONSE TO STRESS.
3. THE AUTONOMIC NERVOUS SYSTEM OF THE INDIVIDUAL WITH AN ANXIETY DISORDER RESPONDS TO A WIDER VARIETY OF STIMULI THAN NORMAL, TO A GREATER DEGREE THAN NORMAL, AND FOR A LONGER TIME THAN NORMAL.
4. THE NEUROTRANSMITTERS RESPONSIBLE FOR MEDIATING THE RESPONSE TO STRESSFUL SITUATIONS ARE BELIEVED TO FUNCTION IMPROPERLY IN INDIVIDUALS WITH ANXIETY DISORDERS.
   a. Gamma-aminobutyric acid (GABA) is an inhibitory neurotransmitter that may either exist in low levels or function inadequately.
   b. Norepinephrine dysregulation may be responsible for sympathetic hyperarousal.
   c. Serotonin helps the amygdala to attach appropriate emotional arousal to internal and external events, and its imbalance may be responsible for the emotional overreaction to some stimuli.

5. GENETIC FACTORS ARE BELIEVED AT LEAST PARTLY RESPONSIBLE FOR THESE PHYSIOLOGICAL ABERRATIONS.

B. COGNITIVE
1. COGNITION, OR INFORMATION PROCESSING, IS A CENTRAL PROCESS IN SUCCESSFUL HUMAN ADAPTATION TO VARIED AND CHALLENGING ENVIRONMENTS.
2. ANXIOUS INDIVIDUALS ARE MORE LIKELY THAN OTHERS TO:
   a. Interpret ambiguous stimuli or situations as threatening
   b. Spend more time attending to threatening stimuli
   c. Demonstrate enhanced memory for threatening information
   d. Overestimate the likelihood of future threatening events
3. BIASED OR DISTORTED COGNITIVE PROCESSING LEADS TO AN UNDUE RELIANCE ON DISTRACTION AND AVOIDANCE AS COPING MECHANISMS.
4. THE USE OF AVOIDANCE AND DISTRACTION LIMITS THOSE EXPERIENCES THAT MIGHT CHALLENGE THE COGNITIVE DISTORTIONS PRESENT AND THUS PERPETUATES THE ANXIETY.

C. DEVELOPMENTAL
1. ALTHOUGH CERTAIN OBJECTS OR SITUATIONS, SUCH AS THE DARK, HEIGHTS, AND BEING LOST, UNIVERSALLY PRODUCE SOME DEGREE OF FEAR OR ANXIETY IN THE YOUNG, THESE ANXIETIES ARE GENERALLY MASTERED AS THE INDIVIDUAL DEVELOPS.
2. ANXIETY DISORDER OFTEN EVOLVES GRADUALLY WHEN ANXIOUS TEMPERAMENT AND NORMAL CHILDHOOD FEARS INTERACT WITH OTHER PREDISPOSING FACTORS.
3. THE MAIN FACTORS RESPONSIBLE FOR THE DEVELOPMENT AND MAINTENANCE OF ANXIETY DISORDERS IN THE DEVELOPING INDIVIDUAL ARE:
   a. Excessive reliance on coping responses involving cognitive or behavioral avoidance
   b. Incompetence with regard to social, emotional regulation, and academic skills
   c. Cognitive biases and distorted belief
   d. Punishment and failure experience
   e. Behavior by others that protects against exposure to anxiety-provoking situations, or rewards anxiety-related behavior

4. TRAUMATIC EPISODES (EITHER DIRECTLY OR INDIRECTLY EXPERIENCED) APPEAR TO PRODUCE ANXIETY DISORDER ONLY WHEN OTHER FACTORS SUCH AS ANXIOUS TEMPERAMENT OR COGNITIVE BIASES ARE ALSO PRESENT.

IV. NURSING DIAGNOSES
A. ANXIETY
B. FEAR
C. POWERLESSNESS
D. INEFFECTIVE COPING
E. DISTURBED THOUGHT PROCESSES
F. SLEEP DEPRIVATION

Nursing Diagnoses: Definitions and Classification 2012–2014. Copyright © 2012, 1994–2012 by NANDA International. Used by arrangement with John Wiley & Sons Limited.

V. THE ANXIETY DISORDERS
A. GENERALIZED ANXIETY DISORDER (GAD)
  1. DESCRIPTION
    a. For 6 months or more the individual has experienced unrealistic, excessive or persistent anxiety about two or more life concerns, events, or activities.
    b. The individual realizes these worries are out of proportion to any real threat.
    c. The anxiety is difficult to control, causes significant distress, and impairs functioning.
    d. The key cognitive features of this disorder are:
      1) Intolerance of uncertainty
      2) A belief that worry serves a protective function
      3) Lack of confidence in one's ability to control or solve problems
      4) Avoidance of threatening mental imagery associated with past trauma
    e. Also prominent are:
      1) Somatic clinical manifestations of shakiness, restlessness, fatigue, jumpiness, and motor tension
      2) Cognitive clinical manifestations of vigilance and scanning
      3) Difficulty in sleeping and concentrating
    f. The lifetime prevalence of this disorder is 5.1%.
    g. Women are affected twice as often as men.
    h. The onset of the disorder tends to be gradual.
    i. The course is chronic.
    j. The severity of clinical manifestations tends to fluctuate with the current level of stress.
  2. ASSESSMENT
    a. Somatic: autonomic hyperactivity such as palpitations, tachycardia, hyperventilation, difficulty breathing, gastrointestinal distress, urinary frequency, weakness, fatigue, chills, and shakiness, difficulty falling asleep, and decreased appetite often with nausea or weight loss, or both
    b. Cognitive: impaired concentration, obsessive rumination about concerns, and impaired probability estimation (overestimates the probability of negative life events)
    c. Affective: irritability, sense of foreboding, impending doom or dread
    d. Behavioral: hypervigilant, restless, edgy
  3. MEDICAL MANAGEMENT
    a. The main treatment used for GAD is cognitive behavioral therapy (CBT).
      1) Because the client with GAD perceives the world as a dangerous place, his cognitive, behavioral, and physiological systems interact maladaptively.
      2) The client's intolerance of uncertainty, attentional bias toward threat cues, and avoidance of negative images through worry are the targets for CBT intervention.
      3) This intervention includes education about the process of thinking in GAD, reevaluation of beliefs about the advantages of worry, problem-solving skills, and relaxation and time management training.
    b. Pharmacotherapy for GAD
      1) Is typically accomplished with the selective serotonin reuptake inhibitors (SSRIs) such as fluoxetine (Prozac), paroxetine (Paxil), sertraline (Zoloft), and citalopram (Celexa)
      2) The anti-anxiety agent of choice is buspirone (BuSpar) because it can be taken over extended periods of time without fear of tolerance or addiction.
  4. NURSING INTERVENTIONS
    a. Instruct the client and family about the disorder.
    b. Assist the client to recognize and label clinical manifestations as expressions of anxiety.
    c. Assist the client to establish a connection between stressors, life concerns, and clinical manifestations.
    d. Assist the client to reevaluate beliefs about the advantages of worrying.
    e. Provide opportunities for learning and practicing new coping strategies such as problem solving, time management, thought stopping, reframing, and visualization.

f. Instruct the client relaxation techniques such as meditation and progressive muscle relaxation.

g. Encourage a diet with small, frequent meals, excluding caffeine and refined carbohydrates.

h. Encourage regular exercise.

i. Explore with the client what has provided relief from anxiety in the past.

j. Provide a calm and reassuring environment and talk with the client using short, simple sentences.

B. PANIC DISORDER
  1. DESCRIPTION
    a. A disorder affecting 1.5% to 3.5% of the population with onset typically in early adulthood
    b. Approximately one-third to one-half of those with panic disorder also have agoraphobia.
    c. Characterized by discrete episodes of intense anxiety that begin abruptly and usually peaks within a few minutes
    d. The effects of a panic attack can last for hours.
    e. Clinical manifestations typically experienced are both physiological and psychological (cognitive and emotional).
    f. Panic attacks typically happen unexpectedly, although in later stages of panic disorder they often become associated with certain trigger events or situations.
    g. Little or no residual anxiety between attacks
    h. Often a constant fear of future attacks
    i. Frequently a history of thyroid disease, hypoglycemia, mitral valve prolapse, concussion, mononucleosis, encephalitis, or recurrent ear infection
  2. ASSESSMENT
    a. Somatic: autonomic hyperactivity such as palpitations, sweating, trembling, shortness of breath, sensation of choking, chest pain or tightness, nausea, dizziness, numbness or tingling, and chills or hot flashes
    b. Cognitive: fear of dying, losing control, or going crazy; an altered sense of reality; anticipatory anxiety; impaired probability estimation; and preoccupation with escape
    c. Affective: sense of impending doom and helplessness
    d. Behavioral: take safety precautions such as being with a "safe" person or avoid places and situations associated with panic attacks. The degree of avoidance associated with panic attacks defines the overlap with agoraphobia.

  3. MEDICAL MANAGEMENT
    a. The common treatment for panic disorder is a combination of CBT and pharmacotherapy.
    b. CBT encompasses a number of strategies and typically consists of:
      1) Psychoeducation about genetic vulnerabilities, physiological arousal mechanism, and cognitive behavioral treatment strategies
      2) Coping skills training that involves both cognitive self-control (identifying feared outcomes and negative imagery, questioning their validity, and identifying logical alternatives) and physiological self-control (recognizing early signs of anxiety and applying relaxation strategies such as progressive muscle relaxation and diaphragmatic breathing)
      3) Exposure to both sensations associated with anxious responding (to test faulty perceptions regarding the dangerousness of these sensations) and to panic-producing situations in a planned, hierarchical way (in order to desensitize to them)
    c. Pharmacotherapy
      1) The significant adverse reactions of the tricyclics such as imipramine (Tofranil) and amitriptyline (Elavil) are often troublesome, and they have generally been replaced with the SSRIs such as fluoxetine (Prozac) and citalopram (Celexa).
      2) Benzodiazepines such as alprazolam (Xanax) and diazepam (Valium) are also sometimes used for panic disorder.
      3) Although all three classes of medications reduce anxiety and may make clients more available for CBT, there is a concern that clients should taper off these medications before the CBT is complete to prevent future relapse.
      4) The addictive nature of benzodiazepines and the rebound anxiety experienced during withdrawal are also a concern.
      5) Benzodiazepines are not suitable for clients with concurrent substance abuse.
  4. NURSING INTERVENTIONS
    a. Instruct the client and family about the disorder and its treatment.
    b. Review the physiological arousal mechanism and cognitive distortions about the meaning of the bodily sensations produced by it.

c. Identify triggers for attacks.

d. Review usual coping strategies and discuss alternatives such as thought stopping, reframing, deep breathing, and desensitization.

e. Assist the client to structure a plan for approaching avoided situations.

f. Instruct the client on relaxation techniques such as progressive muscle relaxation, visualization, and meditation.

g. Encourage regular exercise.

h. Recommend eliminating caffeine, nicotine, and refined carbohydrates from the diet.

i. Encourage small, frequent meals to maintain stable blood glucose levels.

C. OBSESSIVE-COMPULSIVE DISORDER (OCD)

   1. DESCRIPTION

     a. The onset of OCD is typically between 19 and 26 years. The course of the disease is chronic, with acute exacerbations during stressful times.

     b. The lifetime prevalence is 1–1.5%, it is equally distributed between men and women, and it displays an inherited pattern.

     c. The diagnosis of OCD requires the occurrence of either or both:

       1) Recurrent thoughts, images, or impulses that are inappropriate, intrusive, perceived as beyond one's control, and cause significant distress (obsessions)

       2) Repetitive behaviors or mental acts ritualistically performed in order to reduce the anxiety that is generated by the expectation of harm attributed to the obsessional thought (compulsions)

     d. The individual realizes that the thoughts and behaviors are unreasonable.

     e. The content of thoughts, images, or impulses clusters around several themes:

       1) Aggression, religiosity, and sex

       2) Contamination and cleaning

       3) Order, symmetry, and counting

       4) Collecting and hoarding

     f. The compulsive behaviors may or may not be logically related to the obsessional content, but if logically related they are performed excessively.

   2. ASSESSMENT

     a. Somatic: autonomic hyperarousal such as palpitations, sweating, trembling are especially acute during and after the obsessive thought and before the compulsive act that reduces the anxiety.

b. Cognitive: several cognitive distortions are apparent:

   1) Being unable to accept making mistakes, however small

   2) Being intolerant of uncertainty

   3) Overestimating the likelihood of catastrophic events

   4) Believing one's thoughts can influence the outcome of events

   5) Believing that controlling one's thoughts is generally possible

   6) Bearing an inflated sense of responsibility for preventing the harm caused by not controlling one's thoughts

c. Affective

   1) Perceives anxiety to be dangerous and thus cannot tolerate experiencing it

   2) Anxiety is particularly acute if compulsive ritual performance is prevented.

d. Behavioral: reduces the anxiety of obsessive thoughts through compulsive rituals such as cleaning, checking, counting, hoarding, requesting assurances, and escape and avoidance

3. MEDICAL MANAGEMENT

   a. Pharmacotherapy, cognitive therapy, and behavioral therapy appear to be equally effective in the treatment of OCD.

   b. The pharmacotherapy agents currently used are clomipramine (Anafranil), tricyclic antidepressants, and the SSRIs.

   c. The behavior therapy commonly employed is exposure and response prevention (ERP).

   d. In ERP, the client is exposed to the feared stimulus and is prevented from responding with the accustomed rituals in order to break the association between ritual performance and anxiety reduction.

   e. ERP is most effective with:

     1) Therapist-assisted rather than self-assisted exposure

     2) Complete rather than partial response prevention

     3) Combined imagined and actual exposure rather than only actual exposure

   f. Cognitive therapy to identify and challenge irrational beliefs about the power and feared consequences of obsessive thoughts and the efficacy of compulsive behaviors to affect these consequences has been shown to be as effective a treatment as ERP.

4. NURSING INTERVENTIONS
   a. Instruct the client and family about the disorder and its treatment.
   b. Assist the client to identify situations that increase anxiety and lead to intrusive thoughts.
   c. Expose the client to anxiety-producing situations or prevent anxiety-reducing ritual performance only as part of a planned ERP program.
   d. Assist the client to reevaluate faulty beliefs such as:
      1) Giving inflated importance to the occurrence of obsessive thoughts
      2) Overestimating dangerousness
      3) Overestimating the consequences of thoughts or behaviors
      4) Assuming personal responsibility for the feared consequences of thoughts
      5) Needing to be certain
      6) Needing to maintain perfect control over own thoughts
   e. Instruct the client on relaxation techniques such as deep breathing, warm baths, calming music, meditation, and progressive muscle relaxation, both as alternative coping skills for anxiety-producing obsessions and to decrease overall physiological arousal.
   f. Encourage regular exercise.
   g. Instruct the client to avoid caffeine, nicotine, and refined carbohydrates in the diet.
   h. Instruct the client on small, frequent meals to stabilize blood glucose levels.

D. AGORAPHOBIA
   1. DESCRIPTION
      a. Persistent, unreasonable fear of being in any physical setting from which summoning help or escaping may be difficult
      b. While in a physical setting, usually public, the individual fears either doing something embarrassing or humiliating, assaulting, or hurting someone.
      c. Approximately one-third to one-half of those with panic disorder also have agoraphobia.
      d. Agoraphobia occurs both with and without panic attack.
      e. Approximately half of those with agoraphobia have a history of separation anxiety, such as fear of leaving familiar people and places in childhood.
   2. ASSESSMENT
      a. Somatic: no somatic clinical manifestations outside of feared situations unless a panic disorder is also present
      b. Cognitive
         1) Fears being away from safe places or people, or both, or being alone
         2) Worries will do something embarrassing or harmful in public and awful consequences will result
         3) Realizes these fears are unrealistic or excessive
      c. Affective: often feels very isolated and as if he is a burden to family and friends
      d. Behavioral: reduces anxiety by avoiding those places associated with fears or taking safe people or talisman (lucky charm) with him
   3. MEDICAL MANAGEMENT
      a. The treatment for agoraphobia without panic attack is planned, gradual, systematic exposure to feared settings while managing anxiety levels (systematic desensitization).
      b. Pharmacotherapy may not be very helpful in the desensitization process.
      c. If panic attack is also present, treatment is a combination of CBT and pharmacotherapy.
   4. NURSING INTERVENTIONS
      a. Instruct the client and family about the disorder and its treatment.
      b. Help structure a plan for approaching avoided situations.
      c. Encourage and reward any gains made.
      d. Instruct the client on relaxation techniques such as progressive muscle relaxation, visualization, and meditation.
      e. Encourage regular exercise.
      f. Instruct the client to avoid caffeine, nicotine, and refined carbohydrates in the diet.
      g. Encourage small, frequent meals to maintain stable blood glucose levels.

E. SPECIFIC PHOBIA
   1. DESCRIPTION
      a. Excessive or unreasonable fear of an object, such as a dog, needle, heights, or blood; or a situation, such as flying, riding an elevator, stepping over cracks, or being injured
      b. Exposure to the object or situation provokes an immediate anxiety response.
      c. The object or situation is either avoided or endured with intense anxiety or distress.
      d. Avoidance interferes with interpersonal, social, or occupational functioning or causes marked distress.

2. ASSESSMENT
   a. Somatic: autonomic arousal is restricted to objects or situations involving phobic stimuli.
   b. Cognitive: realizes fear is unreasonable or out of proportion to actual danger posed by an object or situation
   c. Affective: often feels embarrassed by and ashamed of phobic reactions and the inability to control them
   d. Behavioral: manages anxiety by avoiding feared objects and situations and attempts to decrease the negative impact of this avoidance on interpersonal, social, and occupational functioning

3. MEDICAL MANAGEMENT
   a. Because the individual is only anxious in the presence of the phobic stimulus, it is usually possible to avoid medication and treat phobias with CBT and graduated exposure or desensitization.
   b. For phobic stimuli that are both infrequently encountered and can be planned for such, as plane flights or blood drawing, the use of a benzodiazepine or relaxation techniques, or both, may be the preferred approach.

4. NURSING INTERVENTIONS (SEE "NURSING INTERVENTIONS FOR AGORAPHOBIA" ON PAGE 913.)

F. SOCIAL PHOBIA
  1. DESCRIPTION
    a. A significant, persistent fear of being in social or performance situations, either involving unfamiliar people or where the scrutiny of others is likely
    b. This may occur in one or a few particular settings or situations, such as public speaking, eating in front of others, or writing in public, or it may include many or most social or performance situations.

   c. The lifetime prevalence is approximately 13%, with females slightly more likely than males to suffer from the disorder.
   d. The age of onset is typically early to midadolescence.
   e. Without treatment, the disorder can be expected to persist throughout life.

2. ASSESSMENT
   a. Somatic: many demonstrate no greater somatic arousal than the nonphobic person in social or performance situations.
   b. Cognitive
    1) Worries that will be embarrassed or humiliated, including appearing anxious in certain social or performance situations and that the consequences of this will be catastrophic
    2) Recognizes that these fears are unreasonable or excessive
   c. Affective: often feels isolated, inept, and depressed as a consequence of few social-skill-building opportunities
   d. Behavioral: manages anxiety by avoiding situations that produce phobic reaction and often by using alcohol

3. MEDICAL MANAGEMENT
   a. Typically involves cognitive, behavioral, and pharmacological treatments
   b. May be most effective when tailored to the individual's particular deficits
   c. Pharmacological treatment with the MAO inhibitors phenelzine (Nardil) and tranylcypromine (Parnate) or SSRIs, notably paroxetine (Paxil), has been effective.

4. NURSING INTERVENTIONS (SEE "NURSING INTERVENTIONS FOR AGORAPHOBIA" ON PAGE 913.)

PRACTICE QUESTIONS

1. A client diagnosed with social phobia asks the nurse about the likelihood of children inheriting this disorder from their parents. Which of the following is the most appropriate response by the nurse?
  1. "It is only inherited if the child's father carries the trait."

2. "There is no research supporting the heritability of social phobia."
3. "The child of a parent with a social phobia has a 25% chance of inheriting it."
4. "The chances of developing social phobia increase about 10% if a parent has the disorder."

2. Which of the following should be the priority consideration for the nurse caring for a client performing overt rituals?
   1. The ritual should be interrupted every time it is observed
   2. The client should be asked what the rationale is for performing the ritual
   3. Performing the ritual serves to decrease the client's anxiety
   4. A less disruptive ritual should be substituted

3. Which of the following instructions should the nurse give a client about relaxation techniques?
   1. Relaxation techniques are most effective when practiced regularly
   2. Heart rate should be carefully monitored when relaxing
   3. Avoid teaching these techniques to children under 12
   4. To avoid dependence, these techniques should be used only when really needed

4. While educating a client who has a social phobia about the use of a selective serotonin reuptake inhibitor (SSRI), the nurse assesses the client's knowledge about the drug. The client tells the nurse the physician explained that the drug will correct a "chemical imbalance" but states being unsure about what that means. Which of the following is the appropriate response by the nurse?
   1. "You should ask the physician to explain the purpose of your medication again."
   2. "Sometimes the brain produces too little of a chemical called serotonin and the SSRI corrects this."
   3. "What do you think chemical imbalance means?"
   4. "I'm also unsure what chemical imbalance means."

5. A client with a dog phobia has undergone desensitization to this stimulus. The nurse evaluates which of the following client behaviors that indicates the treatment was successful?
   1. The client recounts how the fear of dogs began, stating this fear is both unreasonable and excessive
   2. The client visits caged dogs in the pet shelter for 10 minutes three times a week
   3. The client states the fear of dogs is greatly diminished
   4. The client can pet the neighbor's dog without undue anxiety

6. Which of the following characteristics should the nurse include when teaching a class on the developmental theory of anxiety? Select all that apply:
   [ ] 1. Individuals respond physiologically when anxious
   [ ] 2. Anxiety disorder often evolves gradually when anxious temperament and normal childhood fears interact with other predisposing factors
   [ ] 3. Excessive reliance on coping responses involving cognitive or behavioral avoidance
   [ ] 4. Interpret ambiguous stimuli or situations as threatening
   [ ] 5. Biased or distorted cognitive processing leads to an undue reliance on distraction and avoidance as coping mechanisms
   [ ] 6. Incompetence with regard to social and emotional regulation and academic skills

7. While preparing a client for surgery the next day, the nurse observes that the client is having trouble paying attention to instructions, is trembling, and has sweaty palms, a rapid heart rate, and rapid respirations. The client states, "All I can think about is this surgery tomorrow, and whether everything will go all right. The nurse notifies the physician that the client's level of anxiety is
   1. mild.
   2. moderate.
   3. severe.
   4. panic.

8. Which of the following client assessments on the use of a benzodiazepine would be a priority concern to the nurse?
   1. A history of alcohol or substance abuse
   2. A lack of adequate coping skills
   3. A history of closed head injury
   4. A diet high in tyramine-rich foods

9. Which of the following would be the most appropriate statement for the nurse to make to a client found pacing in the hall?
   1. "The ballgame is on in the dayroom. Perhaps you'd like to watch it."
   2. "I noticed you've been pacing. Can you tell me how you're feeling?"
   3. "I think you'd be much more comfortable in your room."
   4. "I can tell something is wrong. What is it?"

10. When a client has panic-level anxiety, plans for nursing intervention should include
    1. darkening the room and offering warm blankets.
    2. having the client describe how he or she usually copes with anxiety.
    3. staying with the client.
    4. alerting security to the situation.

11. The nurse caring for a client with a somatic panic disorder includes which of the following manifestations?
Select all that apply:
[ ] 1. Fear of dying
[ ] 2. Palpitations
[ ] 3. Sense of impending doom and helplessness
[ ] 4. Sensation of choking
[ ] 5. Takes safety precautions such as being with a "safe" person or avoiding places and situations associated with panic attacks
[ ] 6. Numbness or tingling

12. A client diagnosed with generalized anxiety disorder reports feeling increasingly ineffective at work and at home states, "I'm letting everyone down. I don't know what to do anymore." Which of the following diagnoses should the nurse select as most appropriate?
1. Thought processes, disturbed
2. Conflict, decisional
3. Adjustment, impaired
4. Role performance, ineffective

13. While assessing a new client, the nurse asks the client about any fears. The client states, "Well, I've been afraid to go up and down the basement steps since my hip replacement last fall. I let my children do the laundry." The nurse should evaluate this response as
1. manipulative behavior.
2. normal anxiety.
3. a phobic reaction.
4. chronic anxiety.

14. A client being assessed for anxiety disorder relates to the nurse a concern with many physical clinical manifestations. The client states, "My heart races, my chest gets tight, and I can't breathe. I must be having a heart attack." Which of the following is the nurse's most appropriate response?
1. "Those clinical manifestations, although frightening, are very common with anxiety."
2. "Has anyone in your family had a heart attack?"
3. "Maybe we should ask the doctor to run some tests on your heart."
4. "Those are the clinical manifestations I get when I too am anxious."

15. The nurse is reviewing the care plan for a client diagnosed with generalized anxiety disorder. Which of the following is an appropriate client goal? The client will
1. describe the traumatic event in detail.
2. report no dissociative episodes.
3. be able to confront the phobic stimulus if accompanied.
4. report tolerating the presence of mild anxiety during activities.

16. A new client in a mental health center program asks the nurse about the purpose of an assigned cognitive reframing group. Which of the following explanations should the nurse give?
1. "This group will help you with your short-term memory."
2. "This group will help you socialize more effectively with others."
3. "All new clients are assigned to this group for assessment."
4. "This group will help you change your faulty beliefs."

17. The nurse is assessing an obviously anxious client. Which of the following approaches should the nurse use?
1. Avoid any questioning about the anxiety until it has subsided
2. Ask specific, direct questions about the anxiety
3. Don't mention the anxiety unless the client does
4. Teach the client a relaxation exercise

18. A client reports having stopped the buspirone (BuSpar) prescribed for generalized anxiety disorder because, after taking it for a week, it did not seem to be helping. Which of the following explanations should the nurse give?
1. Buspirone is not indicated for anxiety disorder
2. It is likely that the dosage is too low
3. Buspirone takes 2 to 3 weeks to become effective
4. Buspirone must be taken on an empty stomach

19. The nurse evaluates a client to have which of the following characteristics of severe anxiety?
Select all that apply:
[ ] 1. Prompted by the ordinary tensions experienced in daily life
[ ] 2. Produces what is commonly labeled the "fight-or-flight" response
[ ] 3. Becomes aware of some motor tension
[ ] 4. Sensory input begins to disorganize
[ ] 5. Senses are heightened, and individuals are alert, focused, and able to both learn new information and problem solve
[ ] 6. Emotional distress is verbalized

20. A client with agoraphobia tells the nurse in the outpatient clinic, "Now that my medication is working, I don't think I need to come here for therapy anymore." The most therapeutic response by the nurse is which of the following?
1. "Your medicine will only work if you continue with therapy."
2. "You need to tell the doctor you want to quit therapy."

3. "You made a commitment to stay in therapy for at least six sessions."

4. "Combining medicine and therapy gives better, more lasting results."

21. The spouse of a client with a phobia of water has planned a sailing vacation to the islands and says to the nurse, "I think the best way to overcome these silly fears is to confront them head on." The nurse's most helpful response is which of the following?
   1. "That kind of exposure may well do more harm than good."
   2. "I agree. I think a vacation would be a good idea."
   3. "For a plan like that to work, I think it would have to be a surprise."
   4. "Have you discussed this plan with other family members?"

22. During an assessment interview, a client replies to the nurse's question about work relationships, "Oh no. I don't go to lunch with anyone at work. I've never been able to eat in front of other people." Which of the following disorders should the nurse consider?
   1. Generalized anxiety disorder
   2. Obsessive-compulsive disorder
   3. Social phobia
   4. Xenophobia

23. A client recently diagnosed with obsessive-compulsive disorder says to the nurse, "I know the doctor said this was just an anxiety problem, but I think I must really be crazy. I keep thinking that people are mad at me, and then I have to keep telling them I'm sorry." Which of the following is the most appropriate response by the nurse?
   1. "Be careful. You might offend someone by using the word 'crazy.'"
   2. "Very often, people's obsessive ideas seem rather bizarre to them."
   3. "This is serious. We must let the doctor know."
   4. "What makes you think someone is angry with you?"

24. The registered nurse is preparing to delegate clinical assignments for a psychiatric unit. Which of the following assignments should the nurse delegate to a licensed practical nurse?
   1. Encourage a client with a generalized anxiety disorder to verbalize personal feelings
   2. Develop a plan of care for a client with obsessive-compulsive disorder
   3. Monitor the laboratory tests of a client admitted to a psychiatric unit
   4. Take a detailed social history from a client admitted with a social phobia

25. A client approaches the nurse and says, "I don't know what's going on, but I have this terrible feeling that something awful is going to happen." The nurse's best response is which of the following?
   1. "Don't worry, you're very safe here."
   2. "Can you tell me what you think is going to happen?"
   3. "It sounds like you're having some anxiety."
   4. "Would you like some anxiety medication?"

26. An inpatient behavioral health unit employs some unlicensed assistive personnel. Which of the following activities may the nurse appropriately delegate to unlicensed assistive personnel?
Select all that apply:
   [ ] 1. Document the response of a client with social phobia to a cinema field trip
   [ ] 2. Evaluate the effect of a client's relaxation practice on the level of anxiety reported
   [ ] 3. Monitor a client's blood pressure after a new drug is given
   [ ] 4. Plan the weekly current events for a client discussion group
   [ ] 5. Teach the client about dietary restrictions
   [ ] 6. Inform the client on the visiting hours

ANSWERS AND RATIONALES

1. 4. Although the precise mechanism of inheritance is unknown, developing a social phobia is 11% more likely if a family member has the disorder.

2. 3. The purpose served by rituals is anxiety reduction. A ritual should only be interrupted as part of a carefully crafted program of exposure response prevention. The rationale the client gives for the ritual is seldom helpful in decreasing the behavior. The substitution of a less disruptive behavior only prolongs the treatment process.

3. 1. The ability to effectively use relaxation techniques takes significant practice. Although heart rate often decreases during relaxation, monitoring it is unnecessary. Very young children can effectively use relaxation techniques. Relaxation can be safely and effectively used on most occasions.

4. 2. The nurse should tell the client that a SSRI produces the chemical serotonin in the brain of a client who naturally produces too little. This is a simple but accurate explanation that makes sense of why this particular drug will help. The nurse, along with the physician, is responsible for medication education. This client already admitted to knowing about it. The nurse is responsible for knowing what a chemical imbalance means.

5. 4. Success in phobic desensitization is shown when the client is able to do what the average person can do without undue anxiety. Clients with phobias routinely believe their fears are unreasonable before treatment begins. A client visiting a dog shelter three times a week and stating that fears are greatly diminished are both steps in the overall desensitization process, but they are not the end result.

6. 2. 3. 6. Characteristics of the developmental theory of anxiety include anxiety disorder often evolves gradually when anxious temperament and normal childhood fears interact with other predisposing factors, excessive reliance on coping responses involve cognitive or behavioral avoidance, and incompetence with regard to social, emotional regulation, and academic skill. Characteristics of the cognitive theory of anxiety include interpreting ambiguous stimuli or situations as threatening and biased or distorted cognitive processing leads to an undue reliance on distraction and avoidance as coping mechanisms. All individuals respond physiologically when anxiety occurs in the psychobiological theory of anxiety.

7. 3. When the client begins to display frank sympathetic arousal clinical manifestations and verbalize distress, the level of anxiety is severe.

8. 1. Because benzodiazepines have a serious abuse potential, they are generally contraindicated for clients with a history of alcohol or substance abuse. A lack of adequate coping skills, a closed head injury, and a diet high in tyramine-rich foods are not factors in prescribing benzodiazepines.

9. 2. What the nurse needs to do is assess what is happening with the client. Distraction is unlikely to resolve this degree of agitation. Being alone tends to increase anxiety. It is assumed the client can explain the agitation.

10. 3. Staying with the client reduces the anxiety and helps assure safety. Darkening the room may increase anxiety for a client whose perceptions may already be distorted. When in a panic level of anxiety, a client can focus only on the present and cannot think clearly enough to describe usual behaviors. Security would only be necessary if the client loses behavioral control.

11. 2. 4. 6. Somatic manifestations of a panic disorder include palpitations, sensation of choking, and numbness or tingling. A sense of impending doom and helplessness is an affective manifestation of a panic disorder. Taking safety precautions such as being with a "safe" person or avoiding places and situations associated with panic attacks is a manifestation of a behavioral panic attack.

12. 4. A client who has a generalized anxiety disorder expresses difficulty in performing usual roles in work and family environments. There is no evidence that the client's thinking is not reality based. There is no particular decision with which the client is wrestling. There is no indication that the client is facing any change in circumstances.

13. 2. It is adaptive and normal for people to be afraid to trust the reliability of a recently repaired joint. There is no indication that the client's motive is to avoid work. The client is not afraid of the stairs themselves but is afraid of getting hurt. There is no indication that this fear has persisted for a long time.

14. 1. Accurate information about the physical clinical manifestations of anxiety can be reassuring. Telling the client that the clinical manifestations are frightening and common in anxiety not only reassures the client but lets the client know the etiology of the clinical manifestations. Asking a client if anyone in the family has had a heart attack will likely increase anxiety and will not help to address the client's main concern. Telling a client that the doctor should run some tests only reinforces the concern with physical manifestations. It is inappropriate to self-disclose and will not likely comfort the client.

15. 4. It is an unrealistic goal for clients with generalized anxiety disorder to be anxiety-free. Being able to tolerate mild anxiety so the client can perform activities is a realistic goal. Describing a traumatic event, reporting no dissociative episodes, and confronting a phobic stimulus are not goals for a general anxiety disorder.

16. 4. Cognitive reframing and restructuring can help clients change maladaptive beliefs that negatively affect emotions and behavior. Helping a client with short-term memory and socializing more effectively with others occurs in other groups. Psychosocial assessment is not typically done in groups.

17. 2. Specific, direct questions will help the client become aware of the anxiety and give pertinent information about it. Not questioning the client until the anxiety has subsided or not mentioning the anxiety unless the client does avoids assessing the client's anxiety, which

must be done for the assessment to proceed. Teaching a client a relaxation exercise is an intervention, without adequate assessment and premature.

18. 3. The full effect of buspirone (BuSpar) takes at least 2 to 3 weeks to become apparent. BuSpar is routinely used for chronic anxiety. The adequacy of the dose cannot be assessed until after the drug has been taken for at least 2 to 3 weeks. There is no evidence that food or the absence of it has any effect on absorption.

19. 2. 4. 6. Characteristics of a severe panic disorder include producing what is commonly labeled the "fight-or-flight" response, sensory input begins to disorganize, and emotional distress is verbalized. Characteristics of mild anxiety include those that are prompted by the ordinary tensions experienced in daily life, the senses are heightened, and individuals are alert, focused, and able to learn new information and problem solve. A client becomes aware of some motor tension with moderate anxiety.

20. 4. Research demonstrates a better outcome with combination therapy when treating a client with agoraphobia. A drug will decrease clinical manifestations on its own. Telling the client to tell the doctor about wanting to quit therapy passes off the nurse's responsibility to address this issue presently. Reminding a client about the commitment to stay in therapy for six sessions tries to keep the client in therapy by inducing guilt.

21. 1. Intense exposure to feared stimuli without careful planning and the agreement of the client is likely to increase clinical manifestations and decrease trust. Affirming the spouse's comments shows the nurse's lack of understanding of the dynamics of phobia. Telling the spouse that such a plan should be a surprise demonstrates a lack of respecting the need for client involvement in the treatment planning. Asking the client's spouse if other family members' opinions have been sought is not pertinent.

22. 3. One of the variants of social phobia is being unable to perform some common activity, such as eating, speaking, or writing, in the presence of others. Individuals with a general anxiety disorder worry about a number of things. A client with a social phobia does not report either obsessive thoughts or compulsive behaviors. Xenophobia is a fear of strangers, and this client reports a phobic reaction with associates.

23. 2. Obsessive thoughts are commonly considered to be odd, foreign, and shameful to those who have them. Telling a client that using the word "crazy" may be offensive to someone may well prompt the client to feel the nurse and others will be angry. It would be inappropriate to tell a client with an obsessive-compulsive disorder that it is serious. The doctor would know that these kinds of thoughts are typical in obsessive-compulsive disorders. Clients pose no particular danger to self or others. It would be inappropriate to ask why the client thinks someone is angry, because the client has no idea why this is believed and this question will just increase the client's anxiety.

24. 1. Developing a plan of care, monitoring laboratory tests, and taking a detailed social history are all assignments that should be performed by a registered nurse. It would be appropriate to delegate to a licensed practical nurse talking to a client and encouraging the verbalization of feelings.

25. 3. Saying that the client may be having some anxiety encourages the client to become aware of and explore the anxiety. Telling the client not to worry, for whatever what reason, cuts off an exploration of the client's concern. It would be inappropriate to ask a client to anticipate what might happen, because the client has already indicated having only a general sense of impending doom. Offering the client some medication is incorrect because such an intervention is premature.

26. 1. 3. 6. Unlicensed assistive personnel are trained to document behavior accurately. Monitoring vital signs and informing the client about visiting hours are within the capabilities and job description of unlicensed assistive personnel. Only a registered nurse (RN) can evaluate the effect of a treatment, such as relaxation techniques. The RN is the only one who can be responsible for planning therapeutic activities or teaching clients.

REFERENCES

Antai-Otong, D. (2008). *Psychiatric nursing, biological and behavioral concepts* (2nd ed.). Clifton Park, NY: Delmar Cengage Learning.

Frisch, N. C., & Frisch, L. E. (2011). *Psychiatric mental health nursing* (4th ed.). Clifton Park, NY: Delmar Cengage Learning.

CHAPTER 48

SOMATOFORM DISORDERS

I. SOMATOFORM DISORDERS
  A. DESCRIPTION
    1. PSYCHOLOGICAL STRESS EXHIBITED THROUGH PHYSICAL MANIFESTATIONS
    2. PHYSICAL COMPLAINTS NOT VERIFIED BY PHYSIOLOGICAL TESTS
    3. INDUCED AND PRECIPITATED BY STRESS
    4. NOT UNDER VOLUNTARY CONTROL
    5. CLINICAL MANIFESTATIONS ARE REAL AND NOT INTENTIONALLY PRODUCED.
    6. CREATES IMPAIRMENT IN SOCIAL, OCCUPATIONAL, OR OTHER AREAS OF FUNCTIONING

II. THEORIES OF SOMATOFORM DISORDERS
  A. BIOLOGICAL FACTORS
    1. CLINICAL MANIFESTATIONS HYPOTHESIZED TO BE PRODUCED BY COGNITIVE DEFICITS OR ATTENTION DEFICITS WITH INCREASED DISTRACTIBILITY
    2. SOMATIZATION DISORDER MANIFESTED BY NUMEROUS PHYSICAL COMPLAINTS NOT CONFIRMABLE BY LAB TESTS
    3. HYPOCHONDRIASIS WITH INTENSE FEAR OF AND PREOCCUPATION WITH DISEASE
    4. PAIN DISORDER UNRELATED TO MEDICAL DISEASE HYPOTHESIZED TO BE ATTRIBUTED TO LIMBIC SYSTEM OR CHEMICAL IMBALANCE OF SEROTONIN
    5. BODY DYSMORPHIC DISORDER MANIFESTED BY A DISTORTED PERCEPTION OF BODY IMAGE
    6. CONVERSION DISORDER WITH LOSS OF SENSORY AND VOLUNTARY MOTOR FUNCTION
  B. GENETIC FACTORS
    1. SOMATOFORM DISORDERS TEND TO OCCUR IN FAMILIES; 10–20% IN FIRST-DEGREE RELATIVES.
    2. PAIN DISORDER SHOWS INCREASED PREVALENCE IN IMMEDIATE FAMILY MEMBERS.
  C. CULTURAL FACTORS
    1. CONVERSION DISORDER REPORTED MORE COMMONLY IN LOWER SOCIOECONOMIC GROUPS AND LOWER EDUCATIONAL LEVELS
    2. MAY BE CULTURALLY INFLUENCED
    3. RELIGION AND HEALING RITUALS OFTEN USED CONCURRENTLY WITH OR IN LIEU OF MODERN MEDICINE
    4. TRADITIONAL HEALERS OFTEN USED TO REMOVE SPELLS THAT ARE UNEXPLAINED BY THE MODERN MEDICAL PROFESSIONALS
  D. PSYCHOSOCIAL FACTORS
    1. PSYCHOANALYTICAL THEORY
      a. Pain, illness, or loss of function related to repression of conflict, usually aggressive or sexual conflict
      b. Forbidden wishes or urges sufficiently repressed to hide their source
      c. A means to communicate need for special treatment
      d. Anger, aggression, and hostility have origins in losses and appear as hypochondriasis.
      e. Pain disorder perceived as a deserved punishment
      f. Body dysmorphic disorder manifests when a body part is felt as unacceptable.
    2. BEHAVIORAL THEORY
      a. Communication style that is learned conveys helplessness
      b. Allow manipulation of others
      c. Rewarded with secondary gain of attention
    3. COGNITIVE THEORY
      a. Focuses on body sensations that are misrepresented and given erroneous meaning

III. NURSING DIAGNOSES
   A. INEFFECTIVE COPING
   B. DISTURBED BODY IMAGE
   C. CHRONIC PAIN
   D. INTERRUPTED FAMILY PROCESSES
   E. SOCIAL ISOLATION
   F. INEFFECTIVE ROLE PERFORMANCE
   G. DISTURBED SLEEP PATTERN
   H. POWERLESSNESS
   I. CHRONIC LOW SELF-ESTEEM

Nursing Diagnoses: Definitions and Classification 2012–2014.
Copyright © 2012, 1994–2012 by NANDA International.
Used by arrangement with John Wiley & Sons Limited.

IV. TYPES OF SOMATOFORM DISORDERS
   A. SOMATIZATION DISORDER
   1. DESCRIPTION
      a. History of multiple physical complaints without physiological cause
      b. Begins before the age of 30 years
      c. Occurs over a period of years
      d. Results in treatment for significant impairment in occupation and social areas
      e. Clinical manifestations cannot be explained by medical conditions unintentionally produced.
   2. TYPES
      a. Undifferentiated type
         1) One or more physical complaints such as fatigue, loss of appetite, gastrointestinal or urinary problems
         2) If accompanied by a medical condition, the distress or impairment exceeds what would be expected.
         3) Duration of disturbance at least 6 months
   3. ASSESSMENT
      a. History of pain clinical manifestations in at least four different sites or functions, such as the head, abdomen, back, joints, extremities, chest, rectum, during menstruation, or during sexual intercourse or urination
      b. Two gastrointestinal clinical manifestations other than pain, such as nausea, bloating, vomiting, diarrhea, or food intolerance
      c. One sexual or reproductive clinical manifestation, such as erectile or ejaculatory dysfunction, irregular menses, or excessive bleeding and vomiting throughout pregnancy
      d. One pseudoneurological clinical manifestation, such as impaired coordination, imbalance, paralysis, localized weakness, difficulty swallowing or lump in the throat, aphonia, urinary retention, hallucinations, loss of touch, loss of pain sensation, double vision, blindness, deafness, or seizures; dissociative symptoms of amnesia or loss of consciousness
   4. MEDICAL MANAGEMENT
      a. Establishing the diagnosis through screening
      b. Be alert to the possibility of undiagnosed physical illness.
   5. NURSING INTERVENTIONS
      a. Rule out an organic cause for physical clinical manifestations.
      b. Display an understanding attitude that the undiagnosed physical complaints seem real to the client.
      c. Provide consistent reassurance to the client.
      d. Investigate the psychological benefit that comes from having physical complaints.
      e. Avoid reinforcing the sick role and discussions over physical clinical manifestations.
      f. Encourage the client to verbalize her feelings.
      g. Assist the client to develop ways to increase self-esteem.
      h. Assist the client to identify feelings that come from the presence of physical manifestations.
      i. Encourage relaxation therapy to decrease anxiety.
      j. Establish a firm therapeutic alliance.
      k. Redirect the client's focus on her physical clinical manifestations by encouraging diversional activities.
      l. Ensure to the client that a physical condition has been ruled out.
   B. HYPOCHONDRIASIS
   1. DESCRIPTION
      a. Unwarranted belief or fear with having a serious disease based on the misinterpretation of one or more bodily signs or clinical manifestations
      b. Theories exist that a repetition of rewards of attention encourages a reporting of physical complaints.
      c. Learned behavior with increased sensitivity to normal bodily sensations that increases anxiety
      d. Duration of disorder at least 6 months
      e. Significant impaired social functioning
   2. ASSESSMENT
      a. Anxiety
      b. Complaints of physical ailments
      c. Preoccupation with physical illness that causes clinically significant distress or impairment in social occupational functioning

    d. Unwarranted fear and visits to the physician despite medical reassurance that there is no organic cause

    e. Not restricted to circumscribed concern about appearance, such as body dysmorphic disorder

  3. MEDICAL MANAGEMENT

    a. Physical examination to rule out a physical cause

    b. Treatment of any medical condition

    c. Treatment of any concurrent psychiatric disorder such as anxiety or depression

  4. NURSING INTERVENTIONS (SEE "NURSING INTERVENTIONS FOR SOMATIZATION DISORDER" ON PAGE 921.)

C. PAIN DISORDER

  1. DESCRIPTION

    a. Pain is the predominant focus of clinical presentation, with severity to warrant clinical attention.

    b. Pain is not intentionally produced.

    c. It results in significant social and occupational impairment.

    d. Chronic pain is 6 months or longer.

    e. Acute pain is less than 6 months.

    f. Pain is associated with both psychological factors and general medical condition.

  2. ASSESSMENT

    a. Pain in one or more anatomical sites

    b. Psychological factors judged to play a significant role in onset, severity, exacerbation

  3. MEDICAL MANAGEMENT

    a. If the major portion of pain is attributable to a medical condition, emphasize medical treatment and support with psychotherapy.

    b. If the major portion of pain is due to psychological etiology, emphasize psychotherapy and support medically.

  4. NURSING INTERVENTIONS

    a. Refer to a pain clinic.

    b. Encourage visual imaging and relaxation.

    c. Refer to physical therapy.

    d. Encourage pain management.

D. BODY DYSMORPHIC DISORDER

  1. DESCRIPTION

    a. Preoccupation with a slight or imagined defect in appearance

    b. If slight defect appears, the concern is markedly excessive.

    c. Significant distress or impairment in social and occupational functioning

    d. Not accounted for by mental illness

  2. ASSESSMENT

    a. Clinical manifestations involve imagined or slight flaws of the face,

head, and hair, such as acne, wrinkles, scars, vascular markings, paleness or redness of complexion, swelling, facial asymmetry or disproportion, or excessive facial hair; as well as the nose, eyes, eyelids, eyebrows, ears, mouth, lips, teeth, jaw, chin, cheeks, or genitals, breasts, buttocks, abdomen, arms, hands, feet, legs, hips, shoulders, spine, larger body regions, or overall body size.

    b. Described as intensely painful, tormenting, or devastating

    c. Excessive grooming behaviors such as hair combing, hair removal, ritualized makeup application, or skin picking and excessive mirroring or avoidance of mirroring may try to camouflage the defect.

    d. Social isolation

  3. MEDICAL MANAGEMENT

    a. History to make a diagnosis

  4. NURSING INTERVENTIONS

    a. Develop a therapeutic relationship.

    b. Refer to a mental health specialist.

    c. Develop interventions for social isolation, low self-esteem, and ineffective coping.

E. CONVERSION DISORDER

  1. DESCRIPTION

    a. Presence of one or more clinical manifestations that appear of neurologic origin but not explained by tests

    b. Psychological factors precipitate usual stress or conflict.

    c. Not intentionally produced

    d. Results in clinically significant impairment in occupational or social functioning

    e. Not limited to pain or sexual dysfunction and occurs outside of the somatization disorder

  2. ASSESSMENT

    a. Characterized by the client's indifference, termed la belle indifférence, to the clinical manifestations that may be a result of psychological or central nervous system (CNS) inhibition of sensory input

  3. MEDICAL MANAGEMENT

    a. Often resolve by themselves

    b. Explanation and prolonged therapy with a mental health specialist

  4. NURSING INTERVENTIONS

    a. Establish a supportive relationship.

    b. Instruct the client about the disorder.

    c. Avoid providing secondary gain by paying too much attention to the client.

    d. Encourage the client to focus on anxiety reduction and not physical clinical manifestations.

e. Encourage diversional activities.

f. Implement matter-of-fact approach with the client.

g. Encourage the client to verbalize feelings.

F. FACTITIOUS DISORDER

1. DESCRIPTION

a. Physical or psychological clinical manifestations that are intentionally produced to gain attention

b. Clinical manifestations may be real or feigned; also known as Munchausen's syndrome.

c. Munchausen's by proxy is a form of child abuse, where a child is reported as ill with fabrication of clinical manifestations, or an attempt is made to have the child appear ill.

d. The motivation for the behavior is to assume the sick role.

e. External incentives for the behavior, such as economic gain, avoiding legal responsibility, or improving physical well-being, may occur.

f. May manifest with psychological signs and clinical manifestations or physical signs and manifestations

g. Only present when the individual is being observed

h. Disruptive behavior toward nurses or doctors

i. Develops new pathology after the initial workup proves to be negative

j. Extensive knowledge of medical terminology and hospital routines

2. ASSESSMENT

a. Fabrication of subjective complaints

b. Intentionally produced physical or psychological signs

3. MEDICAL MANAGEMENT

a. Difficult to treat because the client will seek attention elsewhere

4. NURSING INTERVENTIONS

a. Refer to a mental health specialist.

G. MALINGERING

1. DESCRIPTION

a. Malingering is the fabrication of clinical manifestations to achieve objectives such as financial compensation or attention.

b. Clients are unable to see the relationship between clinical manifestations and conflicts.

c. Clinical manifestations may be used to manipulate others.

d. Clinical manifestations are exaggerated.

e. History of clinical manifestations are usually poor and vague.

2. ASSESSMENT

a. Distorted body perception of functions and clinical manifestations

b. Chronic pain of psychological origin

c. Diminished family interaction

d. Self-care may be compromised.

e. Ability to perform usual tasks is diminished.

f. Difficulty in continuing employment

g. Family roles altered

h. Difficulty with communications

i. Excessive anxiety and obsessive attention to detail

3. MEDICAL MANAGEMENT

a. Diagnostic workup to rule out a medical etiology

4. NURSING INTERVENTIONS

a. Assist the client to build her self-esteem.

b. Reinforce the client's strengths.

c. Monitor for dependence on anxiolytic agents.

d. Avoid the misuse of medications and prescription seeking.

e. Assist the client to find new and more effective ways for coping.

PRACTICE QUESTIONS

1. Which of the following assessment findings does the nurse make before a diagnosis of body dysmorphic disorder can be made? Select all apply:

[ ] 1. Pain in one or more anatomical sites

[ ] 2. Client's indifference (la belle indifférence)

[ ] 3. Imagined flaw of some part of the body

[ ] 4. Fabrication of subjective complaints

[ ] 5. Excessive grooming behaviors

[ ] 6. Intensely painful, tormenting, or devastating

2. The nurse informs another nurse that stress is an essential component of somatoform disorders because stress

1. is the only feature of this disorder.

2. exacerbates the illness.

3. is a positive force in overcoming the illness.

4. is not a precursor to the development of this disorder.

3. Which of the following is the most critical component leading to the client's ability to adapt to a somatoform disorder?
   1. The client's psychological makeup
   2. The etiology of the stress
   3. The nurse's ability to manipulate the environment
   4. The establishment of a medical etiology

4. When interviewing a client with a somatoform disorder, which of the following factors is important for the nurse to understand?
   1. The client is able to remember the precipitating event
   2. Somatoform disorder is not usually within the awareness of the client
   3. Somatoform disorder is generally within the awareness of the client
   4. The client's behavior is an attempt to manipulate the nurse

5. The nurse should assess a client suspected of having a somatoform disorder for which of the following clinical manifestations?
   Select all that apply:
   [ ] 1. A decreased ability for motor function
   [ ] 2. The absence of pain
   [ ] 3. Intense localized pain in one identified site
   [ ] 4. Two or more gastrointestinal clinical manifestations
   [ ] 5. A sexual abnormality
   [ ] 6. A pseudoneurological manifestation

6. Which of the following assessments are essential for the nurse to make before a diagnosis of hypochondriasis can be made for a client?
   Select all that apply:
   [ ] 1. The presence of an elaborate delusional process
   [ ] 2. The preoccupation of a medical malady is not better accounted for by another psychological disorder
   [ ] 3. Absence of a fear that something is wrong medically
   [ ] 4. A 3-month duration of the disorder
   [ ] 5. The medical malady causes significant social and occupational impairment
   [ ] 6. The absence of a delusional process

7. When assessing a client for hypochondriasis, which of the following questions should the nurse ask the client?
   1. "Is your pain localized in one identifiable anatomical site?"
   2. "Do you have multiple pain sites?"
   3. "You are not feeling pain, are you?"
   4. "Do you understand the cause of your pain?"

8. The nurse suspects a diagnosis of malingering when which of the following assessment findings are present?
   Select all that apply:
   [ ] 1. Distorted body perception of functions and clinical manifestations
   [ ] 2. Intentionally produced physical or psychological signs
   [ ] 3. Anxiety
   [ ] 4. Chronic pain of psychological origin
   [ ] 5. Ability to perform usual tasks is diminished
   [ ] 6. Preoccupation with physical illness

9. Somatoform disorders tend to occur in families in what percent in first-degree relatives?

   _____

10. The nurse assesses which of the following for a client with a conversion disorder?
    Select all that apply:
    [ ] 1. One or more sensory or motor manifestations
    [ ] 2. Intentionally produced clinical manifestations
    [ ] 3. Minimal distress or impairment
    [ ] 4. Clinical manifestations not limited to pain or sexual dysfunction
    [ ] 5. Condition not caused by a medical problem
    [ ] 6. Absence of causative psychological factors

11. The nurse is caring for a client who is complaining of a headache that cannot be confirmed by diagnostic tests. Which of the following factors would be critical before making a diagnosis of somatoform disorder?
    1. The client has feelings of guilt
    2. There is an absence of other physical complaints
    3. The manifestations occurred at age 40 years
    4. Laboratory tests showed an abnormal electroencephalogram (EEG)

12. When planning to care for the client with hypochondriasis, the nurse should include which of the following?
    1. Avoid focusing on the preoccupation with the disease
    2. Attempt to identify the sources of anxiety
    3. Inform the client about normal sensations
    4. Discourage the client from making frequent visits to health care specialists

13. The nurse is caring for a client with somatization disorder. Which of the following nursing measures should be included in this client's plan of care?
    1. Encourage the use of pain relievers or anxiolytics
    2. Support medical intervention
    3. Discourage social interactions
    4. Identify somatic clinical manifestations as coping strategies

14. A nurse is caring for a client with body dysmorphic disorder. The client asks the nurse about the disorder. Which of the following would be an appropriate response by the nurse?
    1. "There is no medical cause for your disorder."
    2. "Because of your disorder, you will be exceptionally needy."
    3. "Significant distress in social functioning is a result of your disorder."
    4. "The defects you are experiencing are real."

15. A client is admitted to the psychiatric unit with sudden unexplained blindness. Which of the following conditions does the nurse need to establish before making a diagnosis of conversion disorder?
    1. Establish where the clinical manifestation is prominent
    2. The client is indifferent to the condition
    3. The clinical manifestations are produced for secondary gain
    4. The clinical manifestations are unrelated to unresolved conflict

16. The nurse is assessing a client with factitious disorder. Which of the following information is a priority for the nurse to understand before making a diagnosis?
    1. The clinical manifestations are real
    2. The clinical manifestations are feigned
    3. There is a secondary gain
    4. The clinical manifestations are unintentionally produced

17. When establishing a diagnosis of malingering, the nurse should assess the client for which of the following features of the disorder?
    1. The clinical manifestations are confirmed with lab tests
    2. The client attempts to hide the clinical manifestations
    3. The client actively seeks attention
    4. The client has a tendency to withdraw

18. The registered nurse is delegating the clinical assignments on a psychiatric unit. Which of the following assignments should the nurse delegate to a licensed practical nurse?
    1. Notify the physician of a child being admitted who has a mother suspected of Munchausen's syndrome by proxy
    2. Assess a client for the diagnostic criteria of a somatization disorder
    3. Empathize with a client who has a somatoform disorder by understanding the client's pain
    4. Establish the nursing diagnoses for a client with a somatization disorder

19. Which of the following information would the nurse consider significant when assessing a client for a somatoform disorder?
    1. The clinical manifestations are under the client's voluntary control
    2. The client fails to see the relationship between clinical manifestations and conflicts
    3. The client's ability to perform usual tasks is unaltered
    4. The client is unaware of the clinical manifestations

20. Which of the following interventions should the nurse include in the plan for the client with a somatoform disorder?
    1. Assist the client to recognize somatic clinical manifestations
    2. Avoid focusing on the client's secondary gains
    3. Confront the client's defenses
    4. Administer drug therapy

21. When teaching a client with a somatoform disorder how to deal with the clinical manifestations, the nurse should
    1. instruct the client to ignore the clinical manifestations.
    2. encourage the client to minimize the number of health care visits.
    3. instruct the client about alternative medicine.
    4. caution the client about dependence on drugs.

22. The nurse administers which of the following drugs to a client with somatoform disorder?
    1. Benzodiazepines
    2. Anxiolytics
    3. Selective serotonin reuptake inhibitor
    4. Antipsychotics

23. A client is admitted with a body dysmorphic disorder. Which of the following clinical manifestations does the nurse interpret as indicative of an exacerbation? The client will
    1. exhibit an increased preoccupation with appearance of an imagined defect.
    2. display an excessive need for social contact.
    3. exhibit a decrease in grooming behaviors.
    4. emotionally disengage.

24. The nurse is caring for a client on benzodiazepines for a pain disorder. Which of the following observations is a priority for the nurse to immediately report?
    1. Agitation
    2. An abrupt rise in temperature
    3. Restlessness
    4. Excessive sleeplessness

25. When the nurse monitors the client diagnosed with hypochondriasis, it is important that the nurse assesses for which of the following behaviors?
    1. The client's increased ability to cope with anxiety
    2. The client's clinical manifestations move from the primary site to a secondary site
    3. The client asks for more medication
    4. The client reports additional clinical manifestations

26. Which of the following instructions should the nurse include in the plan of care for a client with a body dysmorphic disorder?
    1. Encourage a well-balanced diet
    2. Encourage the client to achieve control over family dynamics
    3. Instruct the client to avoid social interaction
    4. Educate the client that binging and purging are methods to control weight

ANSWERS AND RATIONALES

1. 3. 5. 6. Assessments of body dysmorphic disorder include any imagined flaw of the body, excessive grooming, and described as intensely painful, tormenting, or devastating. The client's indifference or la belle indifférence is characteristic of a conversion disorder. Fabrication of subjective complaints is an assessment finding of a factitious disorder.

2. 2. Stress is one of the key components that exacerbates and intensifies the somatoform clinical manifestations. Stress is not the only feature, however, because there are psychological, neurobiological, and familial components as well. Stress does not contribute to overcoming the illness. The presence of stress actually makes the condition worse. Stress is a precursor to developing somatoform disorders.

3. 1. A psychological makeup determines the client's ability to recognize the dysfunctional manifestations of a somatoform disorder and take corrective action. The etiology of the stress is outside the nurse's control. The ability to manipulate the environment also depends on external sources for control. The somatoform disorder does not have a medical etiology.

4. 2. The cure for somatoform disorder lies in the client being able to identify the etiology of the disorder. The client may not be able to link the precipitating event to the disorder. The disorder is not within the awareness of the client. Unlike malingering, the primary goal is not manipulation.

5. 4. 5. 6. Clinical manifestations of a somatoform disorder include at least four pain manifestations, two gastrointestinal manifestations other than pain, one sexual manifestation, and one pseudoneurological manifestation. Somatoform disorders manifest with numerous physical complaints in multiple sites in the body, including the head, abdomen, back, joints, extremities, chest, and rectum. Motor function is not impaired by the disorder. The pain is not localized to a single site.

6. 2. 5. 6. Hypochondriasis is the fear of having a medical malady based on the incorrect interpretation of the body's function. There is no delusional process involved. The preoccupation with a medical malady is not better accounted for by another psychological disorder. The disorder generally has a duration of at least 6 months. The medical malady causes significant social or occupational impairment.

7. 2. Hypochondriasis manifests itself in at least four sites to meet the diagnostic criteria. Pain is manifested in multiple sites. The client does not recognize the etiology of the pain.

8. 1. 4. 5. Assessment findings of malingering include distorted body perception of functions and clinical manifestations, chronic pain of psychological origin, and a decreased ability to perform usual tasks. A clinical manifestation of factitious disorder is intentionally produced physical or psychological signs. Anxiety and preoccupation with physical illness are clinical manifestations of hypochondriasis.

9. 10–20%. Somatoform disorders tend to occur in families; 10–20% in first-degree relatives.

10. 1. 4. 5. Conversion disorder is not within the control of the client. One or more clinical manifestations affect the sensory or motor function, suggesting a medical or neurologic disorder. The clinical manifestations are not intentionally produced. There is significant distress or impairment in the client's functioning that may bring the client to the health care provider. The clinical manifestations are not limited to pain or sexual dysfunction. Conversion disorders are not caused by a medical disorder, and there are always psychological manifestations present.

11. 1. An unresolved guilt is a major contributor to somatoform disorder. Once the guilt is cleared up, the disorder abates. Somatoform disorder is accompanied by multiple physical complaints before the age of 30 years. Physiologic laboratory tests fail to show any physical abnormalities in somatoform disorder.

12. 2. The major treatment objective of hypochondriasis is to identify the source of anxiety and treat it. Ignoring the client's preoccupation with illness will escalate the behavior. Acknowledgment of the client's concern with a redirection toward the source of anxiety is more therapeutic. Telling the client about normal sensations does not help the client deal with personal manifestations. Health care visits should be encouraged at routine times to discourage overuse for the purpose of gaining attention.

13. 4. The priority intervention for a client with a somatization disorder is that the client recognizes that the pain is a coping strategy. The use of pain relievers or anxiolytics should be discouraged to avoid dependence. The primary source of a pain disorder is psychological, so medical interventions are not effective. The need for social interaction is important, because the consequence of diminished social interaction is social isolation.

14. 3. Social isolation is a major contributor to a body dysmorphic disorder. It is a cyclical process in which the more withdrawn the client becomes, the more the dysmorphic belief will contribute to more withdrawal. The disorder will become even more pronounced. There may be a minor problem, but the response to it is beyond reasonable. Clients tend to avoid social contact because of self-consciousness concerning the imagined defect. Any defects the client is experiencing are not real.

15. 2. One of the classic signs of conversion disorder is the client's indifference to sudden and severe impairment, "la belle indifférence." The site of the clinical manifestations is not as important as the precipitating factors. The disorder is not to achieve secondary gain and is out of the client's control. Conversion disorder is directly related to underlying conflict.

16. 3. Factitious disorder is well within the awareness of the client, and clinical manifestations may be real or feigned. It is the secondary gain, for attention or financial reward, that is the priority feature for diagnosis of factitious disorder. Clinical manifestations are intentionally produced for personal gain.

17. 3. Malingering is characterized by the client's deliberate attempt to gain attention. The clinical manifestations are not confirmed by lab tests. The client will bring the clinical manifestations to the attention of others for secondary gain. The client does not withdraw but becomes demanding of health care providers and others.

18. 3. Notifying the physician of a client being admitted with a suspected condition, assessing the client for the diagnostic criteria, and establishing the nursing diagnoses are assignments that should be performed by a registered nurse. Any nurse working with a client with a somatization disorder should be prepared to empathize with the client by understanding the client's pain. Empathizing would be appropriate to delegate to a licensed practical nurse.

19. 2. Somatoform disorder is characterized by the client's inability to link the clinical manifestations with unresolved conflicts. This link is a key to overcoming the disorder. The client has no voluntary control over the clinical manifestations. The client's ability to perform tasks is highly diminished. The client is very aware of the clinical manifestations and only unaware of their etiology.

20. 1. The key to treatment of a client with a somatoform disorder is to recognize when the clinical manifestations are somatic in nature and when they are of a medical origin. The secondary gains must be addressed so that the client can make more healthy adaptation to meet personal needs. Confrontation of defenses will increase the client's fixation. Administering a drug is not a cure and will only complicate the treatment.

21. 4. Somatoform disorder is characterized by the risk that the client may become addicted to either pain medications or anxiolytics. Careful client teaching is necessary to help the client avoid an overdependence on drugs. The client will need to understand the purpose of the clinical manifestations before relinquishing them. Routine health care visits are essential to not encourage anxiety or overuse. Shifting treatment to alternative medicine does not address the etiology of the disorder, but merely shifts the dependence to another substance.

22. 3. Selective serotonin reuptake inhibitors are the drugs recommended in the treatment of somatoform disorders, because they have relatively few adverse effects and a good response. The benzodiazepines are addictive. There is a high potential for dependence on the anxiolytics as well. The antipsychotics are inappropriate, because the client is not psychotic.

23. 1. The primary clinical manifestation of a body dysmorphic disorder is an increased preoccupation with the appearance of the

imagined defect. Social withdrawal is common. There is an increase in grooming behaviors. The client does not disengage but becomes increasingly anxious.

24. 2. Neuromalignant syndrome is characterized by a high fever, 39.4°C (103°F) or higher, and can be fatal. The client's agitation may be from sources other than a drug. The client's restlessness may be from a drug; however, the clinical manifestations need to be observed over a period of time. The client may be sleeping due to factors other than drugs.

25. 1. The reduction in clinical manifestations is manifested in the ability to appropriately deal with psychological anxiety. The client's clinical manifestations need to abate rather than move. The need for an additional drug is not a sign of dealing with hypochondria. The clinical manifestations should diminish rather than increase.

26. 1. Even the client who complains about being too heavy must maintain life-sustaining nutrition. The client's core struggle is over family dynamics and it is expressed in eating disorders. Avoiding social interaction exacerbates the disorder. Binging and purging are dysfunctional means of coping.

REFERENCES

Antai-Otong, D. (2008). *Psychiatric nursing, biological and behavioral concepts* (2nd ed.). Clifton Park, NY: Delmar Cengage Learning.

Frisch, N. C., & Frisch, L. E. (2011). *Psychiatric mental health nursing* (4th ed.). Clifton Park, NY: Delmar Cengage Learning.

CHAPTER 49

DISSOCIATIVE DISORDERS

I. DISSOCIATIVE DISORDERS
A. DESCRIPTION
1. DISRUPTION IN USUAL MENTAL FUNCTIONS, MEMORY IDENTITY, OR PERCEPTIONS OF ENVIRONMENT IN RESPONSE TO EXTREME INTERNAL OR EXTERNAL EVENTS OR STRESS
2. ATTEMPTS TO USE REPRESSION TO BLOCK TRAUMATIC EVENTS, PROVIDING A PSYCHOLOGICAL ESCAPE
3. CLIENT HAS AMNESIA, IS DYSFUNCTIONAL, AND IS UNABLE TO WORK.
4. MEMORY LOSS IMPAIRS RELATIONSHIPS.
5. CLIENT IS FEARFUL AND HAS A DISTORTED CONCEPT OF PERSONAL APPEARANCE.

II. THEORIES OF DISSOCIATIVE DISORDERS
A. BIOLOGICAL FACTORS
1. THE LIMBIC SYSTEM MAY PROCESS TRAUMATIC MEMORIES AND STORE THEM IN THE HIPPOCAMPUS.
2. EARLY TRAUMA PREVENTS ATTACHMENT OF MEMORY AND STRESS THAT MAY PRECIPITATE DISSOCIATION.
3. THERE MAY BE A NEUROLOGICAL LINK. SUCH DISEASES AS BRAIN TUMORS AND EPILEPSY, AS WELL AS DRUG ABUSE, CAN INFLUENCE DEPERSONALIZATION EXPERIENCE.
B. GENETIC FACTORS
1. MORE COMMON AMONG FIRST-DEGREE RELATIVES
C. CULTURAL FACTORS
1. DIFFERENT VERSIONS OF TRANCELIKE STATE SEEN IN NAVAJO AND ARCTIC POPULATIONS
2. POSSESSION IS A TRANCELIKE STATE WHERE INDIVIDUALS BELIEVE THEY SEE DEMONS OR DEITIES, OR BOTH.
D. PSYCHOSOCIAL FACTORS
1. AVOIDANCE OF STRESS THAT IS LEARNED
2. INTOLERABLE STRESS OR PAIN IS DISSOCIATED TO AVOID REMEMBERING.

III. NURSING DIAGNOSES
A. DISTURBED PERSONAL IDENTITY
B. INEFFECTIVE COPING
C. ANXIETY
D. INEFFECTIVE ROLE PERFORMANCE
E. RISK FOR SELF-DIRECTED VIOLENCE
F. SOCIAL ISOLATION
G. DISTURBED BODY IMAGE
H. CHRONIC LOW SELF-ESTEEM DISTURBANCE
I. POWERLESSNESS
J. DISTURBED SLEEP PATTERN

Nursing Diagnoses: Definitions and Classification 2012–2014. Copyright © 2012, 1994–2012 by NANDA International. Used by arrangement with John Wiley & Sons Limited.

IV. TYPES OF DISSOCIATIVE DISORDERS
A. DEPERSONALIZATION DISORDER
1. DESCRIPTION
a. Persistent or recurrent alterations in perception of the self so that one's own reality is temporarily lost while reality-testing ability remains intact
b. Incidence declines after 20 years of age.
c. Does not occur exclusively during the course of another mental disorder and is not due to substance abuse or medical condition
2. ASSESSMENT
a. Persistent or recurrent feelings of being detached from one's body or mental processes similar to a dream
b. Reality testing remains intact.

c. Significant distress or impairment in social, occupational, or other important areas of functioning
d. Feels a sense of deadness of the body
e. Limbs may feel larger or smaller.
f. Elusive sensation of not being human or alive and disconnected from the body

3. MEDICAL MANAGEMENT
   a. Counseling offering emotional support during recall of painful experience, providing a sense of safety and an optimal level of functioning
   b. Psychotherapy creating a therapeutic alliance, feelings of conflict, and situations that can be explored
   c. Hypnotherapy for advanced practice clinicians trained with the integration of personality
   d. Behavioral therapy
   e. Cognitive restructuring
   f. Family therapy
      1) Involve family members in client therapy to support, not pressure, the client to remember.
   g. Milieu therapy
      1) Provide a safe environment—quiet, simple, structured, and supportive.
      2) Decrease confusion and noise that increase anxiety.
      3) Group therapy with opportunity for self-expression

4. NURSING INTERVENTIONS
   a. Rule out substance use, medical and neurological etiology.
   b. Admit the client to the hospital if suicidal.
   c. Assess ability to identify self or change in behavior, voice, and dress.
   d. Assess the client's use of the third-person pronouns such as "we" instead of "I."
   e. Evaluate the client's memory.
      1) Is recent memory available to recall?
      2) Is the memory clear and complete?
      3) Is the client aware of gaps in memory?
      4) Do memories have a context in school or work?
      5) Is the client disoriented from time, place, as well as person?
      6) Presence of blackouts or loss of time
      7) Does the client find himself in places without any idea of how he got there?
   f. Evaluate the client's history. Gather information about the client's life events such as recent injuries, epilepsy, temporal lobe damage, or sexual abuse.

g. Evaluate the client's mood.
   1) Is the client depressed, anxious, or detached?
   2) Are there mood shifts or predominant moods different from primary personality?
   3) Is there an indifference, unconcern, or anxiousness?
h. Evaluate potential drug use.
   1) May be due to recent alcohol use
   2) May be marijuana use in depersonalization
i. Assess the impact on family
   1) Is the client's ability to function impaired?
   2) Are the family interactions impaired?
   3) Are there evident secondary gains?
   4) Are family members highly distressed over the client's behavior?
j. Evaluate the potential suicide risk—expressions of suicide and hopelessness, helplessness, worthlessness, and self-mutilating or self-destructive behaviors.
k. Establish a relationship.
l. Establish a trusting relationship—give simple explanations of what the client can expect.
m. Assist the client with self-care activities.
   1) Give simple directions to assist in grooming and activities of daily living (ADLs).
   2) Observe and document sleep loss and fatigue.
   3) Provide for good nutrition.
n. Psychobiological interventions
   1) Administer drugs such as clonazepam (Klonopin), lorazepam (Ativan), selective serotonin reuptake inhibitors (SSRIs), tricyclic antidepressants, or antipsychotics.
   2) Narcotherapy, sodium pentothal, may be given for amnesia or fugue states by the physician.
o. Health teaching
   1) Prevent dissociative episodes by becoming aware of triggers.
   2) Engage in behavioral interventions such as playing an instrument, singing, or physical activity to foster cooperation and socialization.
   3) Encourage client to maintain a daily journal.

B. DISSOCIATIVE AMNESIA
   1. DESCRIPTION
      a. An inability to recall personal information usually of a traumatic or stressful nature not due to common forgetfulness
      b. Disturbance does not occur exclusively during the course of other mental disorders and is not due to substance abuse or medical condition.
   2. ASSESSMENT
      a. Inability to recall important personal information of a traumatic event
      b. Causes significant distress or impairment in social, occupational, or other important areas of functioning
      c. Generalized amnesia results in an inability to remember the entire events of one's life.
      d. Memory involves certain features of an event but with the elimination of some traumatic details.
   3. NURSING INTERVENTIONS (SEE "NURSING INTERVENTIONS FOR DEPERSONALIZATION DISORDER" ON PAGE 930.)
C. DISSOCIATIVE FUGUE
   1. DESCRIPTION
      a. Individual experiences an unexpected and sudden traveling away from customary places while in the dissociated state.
      b. Client demonstrates confusion about personal identity or assumes a new identity.
      c. To meet criteria, does not occur in context of dissociative identity disorder and not due to substance use or medical condition
      d. If memory returns, the fugue state is forgotten.
      e. Can experience rapid and complete recovery
   2. ASSESSMENT
      a. Sudden unexpected travel away from customary location
      b. Inability to recall how one arrived there
      c. Confusion of own identity/may assume a new identity.
      d. Clinical manifestations cause clinically significant distress or impairment in social, occupational, or other important areas of functioning.
   3. NURSING INTERVENTIONS (SEE "NURSING INTERVENTIONS FOR DEPERSONALIZATION DISORDER" ON PAGE 930.)

D. DISSOCIATIVE IDENTITY DISORDER
   1. DESCRIPTION
      a. Loss of sense
      b. Also known as multiple personality disorder
      c. Presents with two or more distinct identities or personality states with enduring patterns. At least two must take recurrent control of the person's behavior.
      d. Too severe to be accounted for by normal forgetting and not due to the effects of substances or general medical conditions
      e. Precipitated by severe sexual, physical, or psychological trauma in childhood
         1) Child is confronted with intolerable terror event.
         2) Child dissociates and splits off the memory.
   2. ASSESSMENT
      a. Presence of two or more distinct alternate personality or subpersonality states
      b. Alternating control of the client's behavior
      c. Inability to recall important personal information beyond ordinary forgetfulness
      d. Dissociated part takes on an existence of its own
      e. Alternate personality learns to deal with feelings that are overwhelming.
      f. Each personality is its own unit with individual memories, behavior, and social relations.
      g. Primary personality may be religious and moralistic and alternate personalities may be aggressive, pleasure seeking, nonconforming, or sexually promiscuous.
      h. Personalities may differ in race, gender, religion, or sexual orientation.
      i. May differ in intelligence, voice, and emotional disturbances
      j. Primary personality is usually not aware of others.
      k. Alternate personalities may be aware of each other and interact.
      l. Transitions may occur when stressed.
      m. May be chronic and continuous or episodic
      n. Not due to direct physiological effects of substances or general medical conditions
   3. NURSING INTERVENTIONS (SEE "NURSING INTERVENTIONS FOR DEPERSONALIZATION DISORDER" ON PAGE 930.)

PRACTICE QUESTIONS

1. The nurse is assessing a client suspected of having a dissociative disorder. Which of the following describes a dissociative disorder? Dissociative disorders
   1. are produced by extreme anxiety.
   2. appear only in schizophrenia.
   3. are fixed and chronic.
   4. are voluntary.

2. When assessing a client who is experiencing dissociative fugue, the nurse should assess for which of the following clinical manifestations?
   Select all that apply:
   [ ] 1. Travel away from common locations
   [ ] 2. Chronic long-term state
   [ ] 3. Recollection of the fugue after an acute phase
   [ ] 4. Not preceded by a stress event
   [ ] 5. Unable to recall past identity
   [ ] 6. Assumes new identity

3. The nurse admitting a client suspected of dissociative amnesia would report which of the following manifestations?
   1. The client's inability to recall personal information
   2. The amnesia has its etiology in a medical condition
   3. The amnesia is the result of prolonged substance abuse
   4. The client exhibits common forgetfulness

4. The nurse identifies which of the following as the primary feature of dissociative identity disorder (DID)?
   1. The presence of alternating control by two or more personalities
   2. The personalities are always unaware of each other
   3. The condition is unique to schizophrenia
   4. All of the personalities possess similar sexual, racial, and intellectual characteristics

5. Which of the following is the priority goal for a client with dissociative identity disorder?
   1. Meet safety and security needs
   2. Reorient the client to the true identity
   3. Assist the client to forget the stress-producing events
   4. Avoid discussing stress-producing subjects

6. When establishing a diagnosis of a dissociative disorder for a client, what information is a priority for the nurse to assess?

   1. Conduct an interview until all lost information is available
   2. Rule out the use of substances or the existence of a medical condition
   3. The client has been treated for depression
   4. The client's ability to recall the precipitating event

7. When treating a client with a dissociative disorder, which of the following is a priority intervention that the nurse should implement for early intervention?
   1. Establish a therapeutic alliance
   2. Complete the history that the client cannot recall
   3. Suggest hypnosis to uncover repressed information
   4. Try to establish the triggering events

8. Which of the following clinical manifestations should the nurse assess in a client with depersonalization disorder?
   1. Anger
   2. A loss of reality testing ability
   3. Mechanical dreamy or detached feelings
   4. Ambivalence

9. The nurse assesses a client with dissociative amnesia to have which of the following clinical manifestations?
   Select all that apply:
   [ ] 1. Sudden unexpected travel away from customary location
   [ ] 2. Alternating control of the client's behavior
   [ ] 3. Inability to recall important personal information of a traumatic event
   [ ] 4. Cause significant distress or impairment in social, occupational, or other important areas of functioning
   [ ] 5. Primary personality is usually not aware of others
   [ ] 6. Memory involves certain features of an event but eliminating some traumatic details

10. Which of the following is the goal of therapy that is a priority when treating a client with a dissociative disorder?
    1. Behavioral therapy
    2. Cognitive restructuring
    3. Family therapy
    4. Safety

11. The nurse is recording the history of a client with a dissociative disorder. Which of the following events would most likely contribute to the diagnosis? History of
    1. brain tumor.
    2. substance abuse.
    3. child abuse.
    4. seizures.

12. Which of the following interventions is appropriate for the nurse to include in a plan of care for a client with a dissociative disorder?
    1. Avoid confirming the identity of the client
    2. Recall past events for the client
    3. Assist the client to understand the benefits of dissociation to cope
    4. Avoid letting the client make decisions

13. The nurse is assessing the client with dissociative amnesia. Which of the following clinical manifestations is most indicative of the disorder?
    1. The inability to recall important personal information, usually of a traumatic nature
    2. Disturbance occurs exclusively during the course of other mental disorders
    3. Existence of two or more subpersonalities
    4. Memory is retrievable at the will of the client

14. A client is admitted to the psychiatric ward of a hospital with complaints of a loss of a sense of self. The nurse treating the client anticipates which of the following clinical manifestations?
    1. The presence of a change in voice and mannerism when under stress
    2. The presence of active hallucinations
    3. The inability of the client to follow simple directions
    4. A history of substance abuse

15. When planning the care of a client with a dissociative disorder, the nurse should include which of the following interventions?
    1. Aid the client to learn to deal constructively with stress
    2. Instruct the client to suppress anxiety-producing thoughts
    3. Encourage the client to ignore the personalities
    4. Assist the client to maintain occupational pursuits

16. The nurse is working with a client who has a dissociative disorder. Which of the following would indicate to the nurse that the client's condition is deteriorating?
    1. Expressions of suicide and hopelessness
    2. Expressions of forgetfulness
    3. The presence of substance abuse
    4. The inability to take care of basic needs

17. The nurse evaluating the progress of a client with a dissociative disorder should consider which of the following behaviors as significant?
    1. The client can voluntarily call up all of the subpersonalities
    2. The client successfully suppresses feelings about events in the past
    3. The client has difficulty recognizing the environment
    4. The client identifies significant others

18. The client with clinical manifestations of a dissociative disorder may develop secondary manifestations. Which of the following behaviors should be a priority for the nurse to consider?
    1. The client's confusion clears after identity is reestablished
    2. The client decreases assaultive behavior
    3. The client controls panic during a depersonalization experience
    4. The client attempts self-harm from alternate personalities

19. The nurse is caring for a client with a dissociative disorder. Which of the following is a priority to include in the client's health teaching?
    1. Prevent dissociative episodes by becoming aware of triggers
    2. Avoid outside activities that divert the focus of care from the disorder
    3. Avoid focusing on delusional processes
    4. Delegate stressful tasks away from the client and to other family members

20. The registered nurse is preparing to delegate nursing assignments to various team members in a psychiatric unit. Which of the following assignments is appropriate for the nurse to delegate?
    1. A licensed practical nurse establishes the nursing diagnoses for a client with a dissociative disorder
    2. Unlicensed assistive personnel provide a safe environment for a client with a dissociative disorder
    3. A licensed practical nurse assesses a client for clinical manifestations of dissociative fugue
    4. Unlicensed assistive personnel encourage a client with a dissociative disorder to verbalize feelings of suicide

21. The nurse assesses which of the following clinical manifestations in a client suspected of depersonalization disorder?
    Select all that apply:
    [ ] 1. Thoughts of being someone else
    [ ] 2. Sensations of not being human
    [ ] 3. Intact reality testing

[ ] 4. Impaired social and occupational
functioning
[ ] 5. Indifference to personal condition
[ ] 6. Onset before the age of 20 years

22. The nurse is caring for a client who has
amnesia related to a traumatic event. Which of
the following nursing diagnoses would be most
appropriate for the client?
1. Disturbed body image
2. Ineffective coping
3. Anxiety
4. Disturbed personal identity

23. The nurse is teaching a client with dissociative
identity disorder about the disorder. Which of
the following interventions would be a priority?
1. Make a suicide contract with the client
2. Explain the client's behavior to other clients
3. Inform the client of the forgotten material
4. Encourage anxiety-producing activities to
bring out subpersonalities

24. The nurse should include which of the
following interventions in the plan of care for a
client with a dissociative disorder?
1. Avoid placing the client in group therapy
2. Provide the client with complex instructions
for maintenance of activities of daily living

3. Decrease the confusion and noise in the
environment
4. Avoid social interaction with other clients

25. Following a serious car accident, a client is
admitted to the psychiatric unit of the hospital
with memory loss. Which of the following
behaviors would the nurse assess that would
support a diagnosis of dissociative amnesia?
The client
1. has an inability to recall important
information of the event.
2. experienced a flashback while high on PCP,
which resulted in the accident.
3. has a seizure disorder, which precipitated
the accident.
4. is not concerned about the accident.

26. The nurse understands which of the following
to be a manifestation of dissociative identity
disorder?
1. The personalities are all aware of one
another
2. The disorder is never chronic
3. The recall of traumatic events is intact
4. The client was confronted with an
intolerable terror event

ANSWERS AND RATIONALES

1. 1. Dissociative disorders are produced by extreme
anxiety, when circumstances become
overwhelming and the traditional coping
mechanism cannot contain the anxiety.
Dissociative disorders are not confined to
schizophrenia but are a diagnostic category by
themselves. Dissociative disorders are not fixed
and chronic but change and can be temporary.
Dissociative disorders are not voluntary.

2. 1. 5. 6. Clinical manifestations of dissociative
fugue include travel away from common
locations, inability to recall past identity, and
assuming a new identity. Dissociative fugue is
not long term and can remit spontaneously.
There is no recollection of the fugue state.
Dissociative fugue is precipitated by stress.

3. 1. A client with dissociative amnesia is unable to
recall familiar personal information. The
amnesia is not associated with a medical
condition, such as brain injury, trauma, or
toxicity of substances. The amnesia is beyond
common forgetfulness.

4. 1. The presence of multiple personalities is a
classic feature of dissociative identity disorder.
The personalities are sometimes aware of each
other but often out of the awareness of the

primary personality. Dissociative identity
disorder is a condition in a diagnostic category
by itself and is not necessarily tied to
schizophrenia. The personalities may possess
different sexual, racial, and intellectual
characteristics.

5. 1. Ensuring the safety and security needs of the
client are the priority goals for a client
experiencing dissociative identity disorder,
because the normal protective processes for the
client are impaired. Reorientation of the client
to the identity is done with a therapist at the
appropriate time in the therapy. The client will
need to understand the stress-producing events
in the course of therapy in order to deal with
the anxiety. The client will need to discuss
stress-producing subjects to help develop
methods of dealing appropriately with the
stress.

6. 2. It is essential that the use of substances and
the existence of a medical condition are ruled out,
because they may cause the same type
of clinical manifestations. The client cannot recall
all lost information. The client may
or may not be depressed, which is not a
precondition for a dissociative disorder.

The client may not remember what precipitated the dissociative event.

7. 1. The nurse must establish a therapeutic alliance, so that trust may develop and the client may be able to reveal traumatic events with reduced anxiety. The nurse should not fill in the history for the client, because the client may find it frustrating and because mobilizing the memory is healing for the client. Hypnosis has been used with mixed success and is now considered much less effective than initially thought. Establishing the triggering event is the work of the client and the psychotherapist at the appropriate time in the therapy.

8. 3. A client with depersonalization disorder has a mechanical dreamy or detached feeling. Client anger is not a cardinal sign. The client does not lose the ability to perform reality tests. Ambivalence is not a criterion for the diagnosis of depersonalization disorder.

9. 3. 4. 6. Assessments for dissociative amnesia include inability to recall important personal information of a traumatic event, causes significant distress or impairment in social, occupational, or other important areas of functioning, and memory involves certain features of an event but eliminating some traumatic details. Sudden unexpected travel away from customary location is clinical manifestation of dissociative fugue. Alternating control of the client's behavior is an assessment finding for dissociative identity disorder.

10. 4. Safety is the priority goal when caring for a client with a dissociative disorder, because the client's natural protective instincts have been compromised. Behavioral therapy is inappropriate for a dissociative disorder, because it involves cognitive restructuring. Family therapy may be appropriate at a later date but is not usually indicated.

11. 3. Traumatic events are often precipitating factors in dissociative disorders because they result in the individual's attempt to protect the self from remembering traumatic events. Brain tumors, substance abuse, and epilepsy have not been established as positive links to dissociative disorders.

12. 3. The nurse should assist the client who has a dissociative disorder to understand the benefits of the dissociation to cope. The client should be reoriented to person, place, and time. The nurse should encourage and assist the client to make personal decisions.

13. 1. The inability to recall important personal information is paramount in dissociative amnesia, because the memory does not selectively block information when attempting to suppress traumatic events. Disturbances

occur outside the course of other mental disorders. The clinical manifestations create great distress. Memory is not voluntarily retrievable. The existence of two distinct subpersonalities is a feature of dissociative identity disorder.

14. 1. The presence of alternate personalities with different affective states and changes in mannerisms, voice, and gender may appear under stress in a client with a dissociative disorder. There is no presence of hallucinations as there is in schizophrenia. The client can follow directions because the ability to understand instructions is not impaired. The etiology of the disorder is not due to substance abuse or a medical condition.

15. 1. Stress precipitates the splitting off of personalities in a client with a dissociative disorder. Constructive reintegration relies on the ability to deal with stress. The client should not suppress anxiety, because it will reemerge in the subpersonality. Clients cannot ignore the alternative personalities, even though they lie outside of the client's control. Clients are often unable to maintain occupational functioning due to the intensity of the disorder.

16. 1. Expressions of suicidal ideation and feelings of hopelessness and worthlessness are critical markers for impending suicide attempts in a client who has a dissociative disorder. They indicate that the client's condition is deteriorating and that intervention is imperative. Forgetfulness is not in itself a dangerous risk. Substance abuse may preclude the diagnosis of a dissociative disorder because the substance masks the disorder. The client with a dissociative disorder maintains the ability to conduct activities of daily living.

17. 4. As personality disturbances clear with a dissociative disorder, the client will regain the ability to identify and recognize significant others. There will be an absence of subpersonalities. Feelings will not be suppressed but will become available for recall. The client can identify and recognize the environment.

18. 4. The client's attempt of self-harm is a secondary manifestation in a dissociative disorder. The client's confusion and assaultive behavior may worsen. The client is likely to experience an escalation in panic.

19. 1. Awareness of the triggers of the dissociative process allows the client the control to reduce the occurrence of episodes. Outside activities are encouraged, such as music, physical activity, and socialization. Therapy involves the free exchange of communication, including any existence of delusions. The client's recovery depends on the ability of the client to deal with the stressors in life.

20. 2.   Unlicensed assistive personnel may provide a safe environment for a client with a dissociative disorder. Only a registered nurse should write nursing diagnoses to direct a plan of care. A registered nurse should assess a client for clinical manifestations. It is inappropriate for unlicensed assistive personnel to encourage a client to verbalize feelings of suicide.

21. 2. 3. 4.   Sensations of not being human or alive are common in depersonalization disorders. The thought of being someone else is not characteristic. The incidence of depersonalization disorder decreases as the client ages. There is great distress associated with a depersonalization episode.

22. 4.   The appropriate nursing diagnosis for a client who is experiencing amnesia related to a traumatic event would be disturbed personal identity.

23. 1.   One-to-one supervision and making a suicide contract with a client who has a dissociative disorder are priorities to meet the safety needs of the client under distress. Confidentiality is of the utmost importance. Never try to force recall of information the client is not prepared to know. Reduction of anxiety helps avoid the emergence of subpersonalities.

24. 3.   Nursing interventions appropriate for a client with a dissociative disorder include decreasing confusion and noise in the environment. This will decrease anxiety. Group therapy is recommended. Simple instructions for grooming and activities of daily living are recommended. Social interaction is encouraged to avoid withdrawal and isolation.

25. 1.   Inability to recall important personal information of the event is a diagnostic criterion for dissociative amnesia. It is not precipitated by substances or a medical condition. The amnesia causes great distress to the client.

26. 4.   The initial event of a dissociative disorder was an event the client confronted and found so intolerable that the client's memory split off into another personality. The personalities are often out of the awareness of the primary personality. The disorder can be episodic or chronic. Recall of the traumatic event is not available to the primary personality.

REFERENCES

Antai-Otong, D. (2008). *Psychiatric nursing, biological and behavioral concepts* (2nd ed.). Clifton Park, NY: Delmar Cengage Learning.

Frisch, N. C., & Frisch, L. E. (2011). *Psychiatric mental health nursing* (4th ed.). Clifton Park, NY: Delmar Cengage Learning.

CHAPTER 50

PERSONALITY DISORDERS

I. PERSONALITY DISORDERS
A. DESCRIPTION
   1. EXTREME SET OF PERSONALITY TRAITS, BEYOND THE RANGE FOUND IN MOST PEOPLE
   2. PERSONALITY TRAITS ARE INFLEXIBLE AND MALADAPTIVE.
   3. ONSET IN ADOLESCENCE OR EARLY ADULTHOOD
   4. STABLE OVER TIME
   5. LEAD TO DISTRESS OR IMPAIRMENT IN FUNCTIONING
   6. MALADAPTIVE, ESPECIALLY IN INTERPERSONAL CONTEXTS
   7. DISTRESSES THOSE CLOSE TO THEM
   8. PERSONALITY CHANGE IS NOT RELATED TO A MEDICAL CONDITION.
   9. LACK INSIGHT INTO SELF-BEHAVIOR
   10. STAY IN TOUCH WITH REALITY
   11. CLUSTER A PERSONALITY DISORDERS ARE MORE COMMON IN BIOLOGICAL RELATIVES OF CLIENTS WITH SCHIZOPHRENIA.
   12. CLUSTER B PERSONALITY DISORDERS ARE MORE COMMON IN BIOLOGICAL RELATIVES OF CLIENTS WITH DEPRESSION, BIPOLAR DISORDER, AND SUBSTANCE ABUSE.
   13. CLUSTER C PERSONALITY DISORDERS ARE MORE COMMON IN BIOLOGICAL RELATIVES OF CLIENTS WITH OBSESSIVE-COMPULSIVE DISORDER OR DEPRESSION, OR BOTH.
   14. LOW SEROTONIN LEVELS ARE RELATED TO SUICIDE, DEPRESSION, IMPULSIVENESS, AND AGGRESSION.

II. THEORIES OF PERSONALITY DISORDERS
A. ENVIRONMENTAL INFLUENCES
   1. CHILD ABUSE
   2. REPEATED TRAUMA RESULTS IN THE CLIENT FEELING VICTIMIZED OR POWERLESS TO PREVENT IT FROM HAPPENING AGAIN.
   3. THE CLIENT MAY UNCONSCIOUSLY DISCONNECT FROM HER FEELINGS, RESULTING IN HER FAILURE TO CONNECT ADAPTIVELY TO OTHERS.
B. BIOLOGICAL INFLUENCES
   1. HEREDITARY
   2. LIFE WITH A FAMILY MEMBER WITH A SIMILAR PERSONALITY DISORDER RESULTS IN FEELINGS OF EMPATHY, FAMILIARITY, AND BEING UNDERSTOOD.
   3. LIFE WITH A FAMILY MEMBER WHO HAS A DIFFERENT TYPE OF PERSONALITY DISORDER RESULTS IN FEELINGS OF ISOLATION AND MISUNDERSTANDING.
   4. SCHIZOTYPAL PERSONALITY DISORDER IS FOUND IN NONPSYCHOTIC CLIENTS WITH SCHIZOPHRENIA.
C. PSYCHOLOGICAL INFLUENCES
   1. COMBINED DEVELOPMENTAL OR ENVIRONMENTAL FACTORS

III. NURSING DIAGNOSES
A. RISK FOR OTHER-DIRECTED VIOLENCE
B. RISK FOR SELF-DIRECTED VIOLENCE
C. RISK FOR SELF-MUTILATION
D. INEFFECTIVE COPING
E. IMPAIRED PARENTING
F. IMPAIRED SOCIAL INTERACTION

Nursing Diagnoses: Definitions and Classification 2012–2014. Copyright © 2012, 1994–2012 by NANDA International. Used by arrangement with John Wiley & Sons Limited.

IV. CLUSTER A PERSONALITY DISORDERS
A. SCHIZOID PERSONALITY DISORDER
   1. DESCRIPTION
      a. Lacks social skills and a desire for intimacy
      b. Detached from interpersonal relationships
   2. ASSESSMENT
      a. Pervasive pattern of detachment from society

b. Restricted range of emotion and expression

c. Lacks desire for intimacy

d. Lacks satisfaction from being part of a family or social group

e. Socially isolated, loner

f. Reduced sense of pleasure

g. Behaves inappropriately in social settings

h. Prefers intellectually involved tasks

3. NURSING INTERVENTIONS

a. Provide information to the client in a task-oriented manner.

b. Limit large-group social interactions.

c. Be clear in identifying what the client can expect and what is expected of her.

d. Attempt to prevent the client from self-destructive behaviors.

e. Inform the client about the consequences of her behavior.

f. Encourage the client to be as independent as possible.

g. Instruct the client to keep a daily journal of her feelings.

h. Set limits for the client's behavior.

i. Offer the client praise for positive behavior exhibited in social settings.

j. Administer psychotropic drugs as prescribed.

B. PARANOID PERSONALITY DISORDER

  1. DESCRIPTION

    a. Distrustful and suspicious

    b. Believes that others' motives are underhanded

  2. ASSESSMENT

    a. Generalized, unwarranted suspiciousness

    b. Misinterprets actions of others to be a direct threat

    c. Hypersensitivity to criticism

    d. May be hypervigilant, angry, or hostile when feeling taken advantage of or humiliated

    e. Often feel there is a "hidden meaning" to being approached

  3. NURSING INTERVENTIONS (SEE "NURSING INTERVENTIONS FOR SCHIZOID PERSONALITY DISORDER" ON PAGE 938.)

C. SCHIZOTYPAL PERSONALITY DISORDER

  1. DESCRIPTION

    a. Eccentric behavior shows cognitive or perceptual distortions.

    b. Feels uncomfortable in close relationships

  2. ASSESSMENT

    a. Deficits in interpersonal relationships

    b. Cognitive distortions

c. Often has ideas of reference, giving special meaning or power to objects or people

d. Superstitious or preoccupied with paranormal phenomena

e. May believe she has magical powers or controls others

f. Lacks few close friends

g. Speech may be odd or idiosyncratic

3. NURSING INTERVENTIONS (SEE "NURSING INTERVENTIONS FOR SCHIZOID PERSONALITY DISORDER" ON PAGE 938.)

V. CLUSTER B PERSONALITY DISORDERS

A. HISTRIONIC PERSONALITY DISORDER

  1. DESCRIPTION

    a. Exhibits excessive emotionality

    b. Behavior is attention seeking.

  2. ASSESSMENT

    a. Excessive emotional expression and attention-seeking behavior

    b. Views relationships as closer than they actually are

    c. Appearance is very important.

    d. Vulnerable to suggestion of others

    e. If not the center of attention, the client will do something dramatic to be in the center of attention.

    f. Sexually provocative in dress and behavior

    g. Excessive grooming and expensive clothes

    h. Seek out compliments

    i. Crave novelty, stimulation, and excitement

  3. NURSING INTERVENTIONS (SEE "NURSING INTERVENTIONS FOR SCHIZOID PERSONALITY DISORDER ON PAGE 938.)

B. ANTISOCIAL PERSONALITY DISORDER

  1. DESCRIPTION: HAS A DISREGARD FOR, AND VIOLATION OF, THE RIGHTS OF OTHERS

  2. ASSESSMENT

    a. Guiltless, exploitative, and irresponsible behavior

    b. Disregards the rights of others

    c. Failure to conform to social norms

    d. Unlawful behavior

    e. Deceitful and manipulative in order to profit or gain pleasure

    f. Blames the victim for being foolish

    g. Self-centered

    h. Unable to tolerate frustration and things that do not go her way

    i. Lacks a sense of shame

    j. Reports a poor work history

  3. NURSING INTERVENTIONS (SEE "NURSING INTERVENTIONS FOR SCHIZOID PERSONALITY DISORDER" ON PAGE 938.)

C. BORDERLINE PERSONALITY DISORDER
1. DESCRIPTION
   a. Unstable in interpersonal relationships
   b. Unstable self-image
   c. Incongruent affect and marked impulsivity
2. ASSESSMENT
   a. Unstable mood
   b. Unstable affect
   c. Unstable self-image
   d. Borders between neurosis and psychosis
   e. Abandonment is frantically avoided.
   f. Suicide threats and attempts are made.
   g. Self-mutilation is common.
   h. Describes feeling empty inside
   i. Depersonalization
   j. May idealize others only to then devalue them
   k. May have paranoid ideation
   l. Self-destructive relationships
   m. Past physical, emotional, or sexual abuse
3. NURSING INTERVENTIONS (SEE "NURSING INTERVENTIONS FOR SCHIZOID PERSONALITY DISORDER" ON PAGE 938.)
D. NARCISSISTIC PERSONALITY DISORDER
1. DESCRIPTION
   a. A pattern of grandiosity
   b. Need for admiration while possessing a lack of empathy for others
2. ASSESSMENT
   a. Grandiosity
   b. Lack of empathy for others
   c. Need for admiration
   d. Has fantasies about unlimited success, brilliance, and beauty with few accomplishments
   e. Arrogant
   f. Manipulative
   g. Envious of others
   h. Condescending attitude
   i. Hypersensitivity to criticism
   j. Readily blames others
3. NURSING INTERVENTIONS (SEE "NURSING INTERVENTIONS FOR SCHIZOID PERSONALITY DISORDER" ON PAGE 938.)

VI. **CLUSTER C PERSONALITY DISORDERS**
A. AVOIDANT PERSONALITY DISORDER
1. DESCRIPTION: A PATTERN OF SOCIAL INHIBITION, FEELING OF INADEQUACY, AND OVERSENSITIVITY TO REJECTION
2. ASSESSMENT
   a. Fear of rejection
   b. Feelings of inadequacy

   c. Avoids activities
   d. Limits relationships with others
   e. Expects to be criticized
   f. Low self-view
   g. Exaggerates minor failures or disappointments
   h. Shyness
   i. Outwardly disinterested, inwardly hypersensitive
3. NURSING INTERVENTIONS (SEE "NURSING INTERVENTIONS FOR SCHIZOID PERSONALITY DISORDER" ON PAGE 938.)
B. DEPENDENT PERSONALITY DISORDER
1. DESCRIPTION: A PATTERN OF SUBMISSIVE AND CLINGING BEHAVIOR THAT IS RELATED TO AN EXCESSIVE NEED TO BE TAKEN CARE OF
2. ASSESSMENT
   a. Excessive need for nurturance and emotional support
   b. Has others assume responsibility for major areas of life
   c. Decision making is difficult.
   d. Lacks motivation
   e. Fears being left to care for self
   f. Lacks self confidence
   g. Expresses emotional pain as physical complaints
   h. Most common in youngest child out of siblings
3. NURSING INTERVENTIONS (SEE "NURSING INTERVENTIONS FOR SCHIZOID PERSONALITY DISORDER" ON PAGE 938.)
C. OBSESSIVE-COMPULSIVE PERSONALITY DISORDER
1. DESCRIPTION: A PATTERN OF BEHAVIOR CHARACTERIZED BY PREOCCUPATION WITH ORDERLINESS, PERFECTIONISM, AND CONTROL
2. ASSESSMENT
   a. Rigid
   b. Perfectionistic
   c. Orderliness
   d. Indecisiveness
   e. Interpersonal control
   f. Preoccupied with details, rules, plans, and organization
   g. Reluctant to delegate tasks
   h. Frugal
   i. Inflexible
   j. Lacks spontaneity
   k. Controls others due to her unconscious dependency
3. NURSING INTERVENTIONS (SEE "NURSING INTERVENTIONS FOR SCHIZOID PERSONALITY DISORDER" ON PAGE 938.)

PRACTICE QUESTIONS

1. At what stage of life does the nurse anticipate the clinical manifestations of personality disorders to become evident in the client's behaviors and actions?
   1. Childhood
   2. Adolescence or early adult
   3. Middle age
   4. Old age

2. The nurse should include which of the following interventions in the plan of care for a client with dependent personality disorder?
   1. Limit the client's opportunity to make decisions
   2. Ask the client's family to make important decisions for the client
   3. Acknowledge the client's situation with empathy while encouraging independence
   4. Withhold feedback regarding the client's situation until the client has made decisions

3. The nurse assesses a client suspected of having histrionic personality disorder for which of the following behaviors?
   Select all that apply:
   [ ] 1. Dissatisfaction associated with being in a group
   [ ] 2. Concerned about appearance
   [ ] 3. Idealizes the nurse and then devalues the nurse
   [ ] 4. Verbalizations of grand things done or planned
   [ ] 5. Compliment-seeking behavior
   [ ] 6. Has rapid shifts of emotion

4. Which of the following should the nurse include when planning to provide education to a client with schizoid personality disorder?
   1. Provide education in a large-group setting to encourage socialization
   2. Deliver education individually in a clear and concise manner
   3. Present the information in a theoretical format
   4. Engage the client in a therapeutic relationship before providing education

5. The nurse concludes which of the following to be characteristics of personality disorders?
   Select all that apply:
   [ ] 1. Is unstable over time
   [ ] 2. Leads to distress or impairment in functioning
   [ ] 3. Is adaptive in interpersonal contexts
   [ ] 4. Has insight into self-behavior
   [ ] 5. Distresses those close to them
   [ ] 6. Onset in adolescence

6. Which of the following assessments would provide the nurse with the most accurate information regarding a low serotonin level in a client with a personality disorder?
   1. Psychosis and hallucinations
   2. Delusions and paranoia
   3. Depression and impulsiveness
   4. Restlessness and agitation

7. During an initial interview with a client who has a personality disorder, the nurse evaluates which of the following to be present in the client's personality traits?
   1. Changes in the personality that have come about because of a stressful event
   2. Personality traits that are beyond the range found in most people
   3. Personality traits that have changed with advanced age
   4. Changes in personality that differ to fit the situation

8. The nurse is caring for a client with schizoid personality disorder. In determining what the plan of care should consist of, which of the following should the nurse consider? The client
   1. quickly becomes attached to the group leader.
   2. displays behavior lacking social tact or grace in a group.
   3. becomes overly emotional in the group setting.
   4. attempts to build intimate relationships with other group members.

9. The nurse evaluates a client with schizoid personality disorder to exhibit which of the following behaviors?
   Select all that apply:
   [ ] 1. Irresponsibility with intentional deceit of others
   [ ] 2. Grandiosity and a lack of empathy for others
   [ ] 3. Peculiar, with exaggerated social anxiety
   [ ] 4. Social isolation
   [ ] 5. Restricted range of emotion
   [ ] 6. Appears indifferent to praise

10. The nurse suspects a narcissistic personality disorder in a client when which of the following clinical manifestations are present?
    Select all that apply:
    [ ] 1. Grandiosity
    [ ] 2. Excessive need for nurturance and emotional support
    [ ] 3. Rigid behavior
    [ ] 4. Lacks empathy for others
    [ ] 5. Arrogant
    [ ] 6. Unlawful behavior

11. Which of the following interventions should the nurse include in the plan of care for a client with schizoid personality disorder?
    1. Empathize with the situation and avoid validating the distortions
    2. Promote trust by recognizing the distortions
    3. Use reality orientation whenever possible
    4. Dispel the distortions by identifying their bizarre nature

12. The nurse is planning the care of a client with borderline personality disorder based on which of the following behaviors?
    Select all that apply:
    [ ] 1. Chronic feelings of emptiness
    [ ] 2. Unstable interpersonal relationships
    [ ] 3. Suicidal gestures or self-mutilation
    [ ] 4. Excessive attention to appearance
    [ ] 5. Holding of grudges for long periods of time
    [ ] 6. Submissive behaviors

13. The nurse is caring for a client who is seeing UFOs and asks if the nurse is also afraid of the UFOs. Which of the following would be an appropriate response from the nurse?
    1. "I don't know what you are talking about; I don't see any UFOs."
    2. "I can tell that what you're seeing frightens you; how can I help to make you more comfortable?"
    3. "I see the UFOs too, and they scare me; what are we going to do?"
    4. "I don't see the UFOs; are you ready to come to group?"

14. A client comes to group provocatively dressed and is dramatic in conversation, often straying from the topic. The nurse should use which of the following approaches to maintain a therapeutic environment in the group?
    1. Allow the client to express him- or herself and encourage independence
    2. Address the client with closed-ended questions and permit only responses that are relevant
    3. Avoid acknowledging the client and speak only to group members who remain on track
    4. Reprimand the client for unacceptable behavior and inappropriate dress

15. The nurse assesses which of the following behaviors to be present in a client who has antisocial personality disorder?
    Select all that apply:
    [ ] 1. Disregards the rights of others
    [ ] 2. Shows a dramatic emotion to situations
    [ ] 3. Self-blames for situations
    [ ] 4. Avoids engaging in interactions with the nurse

    [ ] 5. Voices a lack of responsibility for situations
    [ ] 6. Demonstrates impulsivity

16. Which of the following should the nurse consider when planning the care of a client who has antisocial personality disorder?
    1. The client's lack of ability to engage with the nurse
    2. The client's attempts to manipulate the nurse
    3. The client's hindered ability to justify actions
    4. The client's openness and honesty about past experiences

17. In planning care for a client with borderline personality disorder, the nurse should consider which of the following?
    1. The client's desire for outward perfection
    2. The client's fear of abandonment
    3. The client's lack of ability to show affection
    4. The client's desire to be the center of attention

18. The nurse assesses which of the following characteristics to be present in obsessive-compulsive personality disorder?
    Select all that apply:
    [ ] 1. Need for admiration
    [ ] 2. Perfectionistic
    [ ] 3. Indecisiveness
    [ ] 4. Hypersensitivity to criticism
    [ ] 5. Lacks spontaneity
    [ ] 6. Self-centered

19. Which of the following is an appropriate goal for the nurse caring for a client who has a diagnosis of borderline personality disorder?
    1. To identify irrational thoughts and beliefs that the client's decision making is founded on
    2. To eliminate boundaries between the client and nurse so the client can more easily share problems
    3. To eliminate the immediate focus on the client by encouraging the client to focus on relationships with others
    4. To eliminate the client's involvement in treatment planning because of the accompanying irrational thoughts and beliefs

20. The nurse is collecting a nursing history on a client suspected of having narcissistic personality disorder. Which of the following assessments would the nurse expect to find?
    1. A style of speech that lacks detail
    2. An unconscious dependency on others
    3. A lack of empathy for others
    4. Attempts to promote self-esteem in others

21. The registered nurse is preparing to make clinical assignments on a psychiatric unit. Which of the following assignments does the nurse appropriately delegate to a licensed practical nurse?
   1. Report the empathy that a client with a narcissistic personality has
   2. Assist a client with borderline personality disorder to the dayroom for group therapy
   3. Develop a plan of care for a client with schizoid personality disorder
   4. Assess a client suspected of having paranoid personality disorder

22. Because a client has narcissistic personality disorder, plans for nursing intervention should include
   1. promoting a rapport by showing interest in personal stories.
   2. making interactions limited in time and technical in nature.
   3. decreasing the tendency for embellishment by acknowledging that the client is better than others.
   4. using reality focus, which occurs by challenging the client's misrepresentations.

23. When planning the care for a client with avoidant personality disorder, the nurse understands that the best intervention is to
   1. allow the client to stay in the room until feeling comfortable with people.
   2. avoid acknowledging goals achieved by the client.
   3. enable the client to set and drive the goals independent of the nurse.
   4. promote self-esteem by praising the client's success.

24. The nurse anticipates finding which of the following characteristics in a client who has a diagnosis of obsessive-compulsive personality disorder?
   Select all that apply:
   [ ] 1. Is rigid and inflexible
   [ ] 2. Avoids details
   [ ] 3. Is indecisive
   [ ] 4. Delegates tasks
   [ ] 5. Is envious of others
   [ ] 6. Is excessively devoted to work and productivity

25. Which of the following behaviors in a client suspected of obsessive-compulsive personality disorder validates the diagnosis and should be reported?
   1. Fantasies about unlimited success
   2. Looks for hidden meanings from others
   3. Task completion hampered by perfectionism
   4. Task completion hampered by lack of confidence

26. Based on an understanding of obsessive-compulsive personality disorder, which of the following should be considered before planning the care?
   1. The client is eager to become involved in a therapeutic relationship because there is a sense of attachment
   2. The client is eager to tell personal stories and have others admire what has been accomplished in the past
   3. The client views the therapeutic relationship as a waste of time because the client doesn't see a personal behavior problem
   4. The client may vacillate between wanting the therapeutic relationship and pushing it away, depending on what threat is seen

ANSWERS AND RATIONALES

1. 2. Adolescence or early adulthood is the time of onset. Personalities are formed during childhood. Therefore, dysfunctional pathology will not appear until the client's personalities have been tested by the trials of life. These life events begin in adolescence or early adulthood.

2. 3. Clients with dependent personality disorder feel inadequate to make decisions for themselves. By acknowledging their difficulties, confidence is built. In turn, the confidence will facilitate independence from care providers and others they may be dependent on.

3. 2. 5. 6. Although the person with histrionic personality disorder seeks attention and craves novelty, stimulation, and excitement, the satisfaction for this person comes from attention given by others, not from within the self. The dialect of first valuing and then devaluing the nurse is indicative of borderline personality disorder. People with histrionic personality disorder seek out groups or other people to validate themselves.

4. 2. The client with schizoid personality disorder is technically minded. Attempting to draw the client into a personal or therapeutic relationship or to participate in a group or social setting may push the client to withdraw and become isolated.

5. 2. 5. 6. Personality traits include an early onset in adolescence, leads to distress or impairment in functioning, and distresses those close to them.

Personality disorders are maladaptive, especially in interpersonal contexts. Clients lack insight into self-behavior and the disorder is stable over time.

6. 3. Serotonin is believed to maintain mood stability and control impulsivity, rage, aggression, and depressive clinical manifestations. Delusions result from a faulty thought structure and are related to thought disturbances such as paranoia and grandiose beliefs. Restlessness and agitation are symptomatic of increased serotonin levels.

7. 2. Personality characteristics are formed in childhood to early teens. The characteristics are set and stable over time. Events and situations may make characteristics more apparent, but these characteristics do not change. Changes in personality in advanced age are potentially related to a medical condition. The prolonged stability of the personality structure makes treating personality disorders a difficult and long process.

8. 2. Individuals with schizoid personality disorder have difficulty showing and sharing their emotions. They lack the desire to be part of a group or have intimacy in their relationships. This leads to inappropriate behaviors and a lack of social tact and grace in a group or social setting.

9. 4. 5. 6. Irresponsibility and intentional deceit are descriptive of antisocial personality disorder. Grandiosity and lack of empathy are behaviors of narcissistic personality disorder. A client with schizotypal personality disorder would have peculiar behaviors and show exaggerated social anxiety. Schizoid personality disorder behaviors are described as social isolation, restricted range of emotion, and indifferent to praise.

10. 1. 4. 5. Characteristics of a narcissistic personality disorder include grandiosity, lacks empathy for others, and arrogant. An excessive need for nurturance and emotional support is found in dependent personality disorder. A characteristic of antisocial personality disorder is unlawful behavior.

11. 1. Schizoid personality disorder is a personality disorder characterized by a marked detachment from people and events. Such clients lack close friends, spend most of their time alone, and show little emotion. Empathizing with the client and not endorsing the distortions that validate the client is the appropriate approach. This will allow the client to trust the nurse as the caregiver. Statements should be used that validate a client's response and feelings to the distortions, such as "I can see this is upsetting to you." Challenging the client's reality will push away the client and may elicit an aggressive reaction.

12. 1. 2. 3. Suicidal gestures, self-mutilation, chronic feelings of emptiness, and unstable interpersonal relationships are behaviors found in persons with borderline personality disorder. The client with histrionic personality disorder will pay excessive attention to appearance. A client with paranoid personality disorder will hold grudges for long periods of time. Submissive behaviors are descriptive of dependent personality disorder.

13. 2. Telling the client who complains of seeing UFOs that "I can tell that what you're seeing frightens you; how can I help to make you more comfortable?" validates the client's feelings without agreeing with or challenging the client's irrational beliefs.

14. 2. Histrionic personality disorder is a personality disorder in which the client seeks attention and has excessive emotionality. The client with histrionic personality disorder needs to know from the group leader what the boundaries of the group are. This learning may need to be shown by example. Simply ignoring the client will only escalate the behavior, and allowing or endorsing the behavior will be maladaptive to the group and the individual. For clients with personality disorders, this is how they have learned to have their needs met in the past. They need to relearn appropriate behavior. Reprimanding the client may lead to the client's lack of investment in therapy.

15. 1. 5. 6. Antisocial personality is a personality disorder in which classic features include blatant disregard for others, verbalization of a lack of responsibility for situations, and impulsivity. Dramatic emotion is descriptive of histrionic personality disorder. Self-blaming would be a behavior exhibited by a client with dependent personality disorder. Avoiding interactions with the nurse would be descriptive of avoidant personality. Clients with antisocial personality disorder engage easily with others on a superficial level, often in an attempt to exploit them. They lack insight and responsibility for their behavior and are deceitful.

16. 2. Clients with antisocial personality disorder engage in relationships easily and need to have rapport built to engage in therapeutic relationships. Clients with antisocial personality disorder misrepresent themselves in an effort to meet their needs above all else. Their behavior is manipulative. Clients with this disorder also embellish or exaggerate experiences in an effort to appear different from those around them.

17. 2. Clients with borderline personality disorders have an extreme instability in their relationships with a great fear of being abandoned. Their behaviors are maladaptive but they attempt to keep people close to them.

They have a poor sense of self, which leads to their behaviors causing problems for others so that they feel secure. Outward perfection and the desire to be the center of attention are descriptions of histrionic personality disorder. Lack of ability to show affection is found in schizoid and schizotypal personality disorders.

18. 2. 3. 5. Characteristics of obsessive-compulsive personality disorder include perfectionistic behavior, indecisiveness, and lacks spontaneity. A need for admiration is found in narcissistic personality disorder. Being self-centered is a characteristic of antisocial personality disorder.

19. 1. An appropriate goal for helping a client with borderline personality disorder is to focus on the client and the client's belief system in order to encourage an understanding of how those beliefs affect relationships. The client with borderline personality disorder is already focused on relationships with others, which continues the chaotic relationship. The client focuses on others and fails to focus on oneself. Once the client can distinguish between rational and irrational thoughts, the client can begin to evaluate surrounding relationships.

20. 3. Lack of empathy, arrogance, and a need for admiration are key characteristics of narcissistic personality disorder. Persons with this disorder want to feel better or more important than others, and so would not promote self-esteem in another person. Their dependency is outwardly expressed in the need for admiration, so they focus on surrounding themselves with "special" people, those who are considered to be important or influential. A style of speech that lacks detail is characteristic of histrionic personality disorder.

21. 2. Skills that involve reporting, developing a plan of care, and assessing a client are all assignments that should be performed by a registered nurse. A licensed practical nurse may assist a client to a dayroom for group therapy.

22. 1. Engaging, listening, and connecting with the client will build rapport with a client who has narcissistic personality disorder. The nurse should never encourage the grandiosity but must remain nonjudgmental to what the client says. Approaching the client in a cold, technical manner will stop the grandiosity but will also impair the therapeutic relationship.

23. 4. A client with avoidant personality disorder disregards and violates the rights of others. Classic features are social inhibition and feelings of inadequacy. The client may never feel comfortable enough on his or her own to join the group, so the client remains isolated and fosters avoidance behaviors. The client needs encouragement to participate along with acknowledgment of vulnerability. Any successes and accomplishments by the client should be praised. Goal setting should be a combined effort by the nurse and client. The nurse needs to drive the advancement of the goals for the client to make progress.

24. 1. 3. 6. The client with obsessive-compulsive personality disorder does not like to relinquish control for fear something may go wrong. Such clients are rigid and inflexible. Their constant drive for perfection leads to indecisiveness, because they fear making the wrong decision. They are not envious of others; in fact, they often pity others for not being more like themselves. They are reluctant to delegate tasks and are often excessively devoted to work and productivity.

25. 3. A client with obsessive-compulsive disorder likes to hoard money and finds it hard to discard worn-out possessions. Such a client is preoccupied with details, aspires to perfection, is excessively devoted to work, is overconscientious, is rigid, and is reluctant to delegate tasks. Aspirations for perfection may hamper task completion. Fantasies of unlimited success are related to narcissistic personality disorder. Clients with paranoid personality disorder look for hidden meanings in the actions of others. Task completion hampered by lack of confidence is indicative of dependent personality disorder.

26. 3. A client with obsessive-compulsive personality disorder views a therapeutic relationship as a waste of time, because personal behavior is not recognized as a problem. A client with dependent personality disorder is eager to start any kind of relationship. Such a client will go anywhere at any time for the sense of attachment and security. A client eager to be admired falls into the category of narcissistic personality disorder. The vacillation between wanting a relationship and then pushing it away is indicative of borderline personality disorder.

REFERENCES

Antai-Otong, D. (2008). *Psychiatric nursing, biological and behavioral concepts* (2nd ed.). Clifton Park, NY: Delmar Cengage Learning.

Frisch, N. C., & Frisch, L. E. (2011). *Psychiatric mental health nursing* (4th ed.). Clifton Park, NY: Delmar Cengage Learning.

CHAPTER 51

MOOD DISORDERS

I. MOOD DISORDERS
A. DESCRIPTION
   1. CHRONIC MOOD DISORDER THAT RECURRENTLY MANIFESTS ITSELF THROUGHOUT AN INDIVIDUAL'S LIFE
   2. INCIDENCE IS TWO TIMES GREATER IN WOMEN DUE TO HORMONAL VARIANCES, EFFECTS OF CHILDBIRTH, VARYING PSYCHOSOCIAL STRESSORS, AND THEORY OF LEARNED HELPLESSNESS.
   3. INCIDENCE OF MAJOR DEPRESSIVE DISORDER IS INCREASING AMONG PEOPLE LESS THAN 20 YEARS OLD DUE TO INCREASING USE OF ALCOHOL AND MOOD-ALTERING SUBSTANCES IN THIS AGE GROUP.

II. THEORIES OF MOOD DISORDERS
A. BIOLOGICAL FACTORS
   1. DECREASED LEVELS OF NOREPINEPHRINE AND SEROTONIN ARE THE MOST IMPLICATED FACTORS IN THE PATHOPHYSIOLOGY OF MOOD DISORDERS.
   2. POSSIBILITY OF AN UNDERLYING AUTOIMMUNE DISORDER
   3. ABNORMAL ELECTROENCEPHALOGRAMS (DELAYED SLEEP ONSET–INITIAL INSOMNIA), SHORTENED RAPID EYE MOVEMENT (REM) LATENCY, INCREASED LENGTH OF FIRST REM PERIOD
   4. DYSREGULATION OF CIRCADIAN RHYTHMS
   5. CLIENTS WITH MAJOR DEPRESSIVE DISORDER HAVE SMALLER FRONTAL LOBES AND SMALLER CAUDATE NUCLEI.
B. GENETIC FACTORS
   1. GENETIC COMPONENT PLAYS A LARGER ROLE IN BIPOLAR I DISORDER THAN IN MAJOR DEPRESSIVE DISORDER.
   2. APPROXIMATELY 50% OF CLIENTS WITH BIPOLAR I DISORDER HAVE A PARENT WITH A MAJOR DEPRESSIVE ILLNESS.
   3. THERE IS A 25% CHANCE OF DEVELOPING A MOOD DISORDER IF ONE PARENT HAS BIPOLAR I DISORDER.
   4. THERE IS A 50–75% CHANCE OF DEVELOPING A MOOD DISORDER IF BOTH PARENTS HAVE BIPOLAR I DISORDER.
C. PSYCHOSOCIAL FACTORS
   1. LASTING CHANGES IN THE BRAIN'S BIOLOGY OCCUR WHEN STRESS ACCOMPANIES THE FIRST MOOD EPISODE.
   2. THESE INDIVIDUALS ARE AT HIGH RISK FOR REOCCURRING MOOD EPISODES DUE TO ABSENCE OF AN EXTERNAL STRESSOR.
   3. LOSS OF A PARENT PRIOR TO AGE 11 IS A MOST SIGNIFICANT LIFE EVENT THAT PRECLUDES DEVELOPMENT OF MOOD DISORDER.
   4. LOSS OF SPOUSE IS THE MOST SIGNIFICANT ENVIRONMENTAL STRESSOR PRECLUDING THE DEVELOPMENT OF DEPRESSED MOOD EPISODE.
   5. FAMILY PSYCHOPATHOLOGY MAY AFFECT RATE OF RECOVERY, MAY PRECIPITATE SYMPTOM RETURN, AND MAY AFFECT ADJUSTMENT TO POSTRECOVERY.
D. COGNITIVE AND BEHAVIORAL FACTORS
   1. UNREALISTIC THOUGHTS AND BELIEFS LEAD TO NEGATIVE FEELINGS, RESULTING IN ABHORRENT BEHAVIORS.

2. THERE IS A LEARNED HELPLESSNESS SUCH AS A PESSIMISTIC VIEW OF LIFE AND A BELIEF THAT NO MATTER WHAT ONE DOES, IT IS NO USE.

E. DEVELOPMENTAL FACTORS
   1. DEPRESSION MAY ARISE DUE TO THE EARLY LOSS OF A PARENTAL FIGURE THROUGH SEPARATION, DEATH, OR INSUFFICIENT EMOTIONAL PARENTING.

III. DIAGNOSTIC TESTS
A. PHOTOTHERAPY
   1. DESCRIPTION
      a. Utilized in clients with a seasonal component to depression
      b. Depressive clinical manifestations occur primarily in the winter months and rarely in summer months.
      c. Bright, white light, with strength of the light source at least 2500 lux
      d. Provide therapy in early morning hours to produce maximum benefit.
      e. Ultraviolet rays are blocked.
   2. PREPROCEDURE
      a. Instruct the client to begin using phototherapy in August or September on through April.
      b. Instruct the client to sit at least 3 feet in front of a phototherapy light for 30 minutes initially on up to 2 hours.
   3. POSTPROCEDURE
      a. Beginning antidepressant response occurs within 4 days.
      b. Maximum antidepressant benefit occurs in 2 weeks of therapy.
      c. Full antidepressant benefit is maintained with 30-minute daily sessions.

B. ELECTROCONVULSIVE THERAPY (ECT)
   1. DESCRIPTION
      a. Utilized in clients whose clinical manifestations are refractory to antidepressant medication.
      b. Utilized in clients who require rapid intervention in the treatment of major depressive disorder with clinical manifestations such as malnutrition, thoughts of suicide, and catatonia
      c. Produces rapid improvement in the client's depression due to increase in serotonin
      d. Administration of treatments three times per week for 4–6 weeks, then assess for additional treatments
   2. PREPROCEDURE
      a. Unilateral or bilateral placement of electrodes
      b. Unilateral placement is on the nondominant side of the brain, which assists with decreased memory loss; this may be less effective.
      c. Conduct memory assessment.
      d. Obtain medical clearance for procedure.
      e. Obtain written consent.
      f. Instruct the client that memory loss may occur for a short time before and after treatments.
      g. Ensure the client is NPO after midnight prior to the procedure.
      h. Have the client wear a gown during the procedure.
      i. Intravenous line is inserted; ensure emergency medical equipment is readily available during the procedure.
   3. POSTPROCEDURE
      a. Ensure an open airway.
      b. Prevent aspiration.
      c. Provide reassurance to the client.
      d. Orient to surroundings.
      e. Evaluate response to ECT.
      f. Memory loss may occur for months and possibly years in some clients.

IV. NURSING DIAGNOSES
A. RISK FOR INJURY
B. INEFFECTIVE COPING
C. DISTURBED THOUGHT PROCESSES
D. RISK FOR OTHER-DIRECTED VIOLENCE
E. RISK FOR SELF-DIRECTED VIOLENCE
F. INTERRUPTED FAMILY PROCESSES
G. SELF-CARE DEFICIT
H. DISTURBED SLEEP PATTERN

Nursing Diagnoses: Definitions and Classification 2012–2014. Copyright © 2012, 1994–2012 by NANDA International. Used by arrangement with John Wiley & Sons Limited.

V. DEPRESSION ASSESSMENT TOOLS
A. BECK DEPRESSION INVENTORY (BDI)
B. GERIATRIC DEPRESSION SCALE
C. HAMILTON DEPRESSION SCALE

VI. SUICIDE ASSESSMENT (SAD PERSONS SUICIDE ASSESSMENT SCALE)
A. GENDER—MALES ARE AT A HIGHER RISK FOR COMMITTING SUICIDE AND USE MORE LETHAL MEANS.
B. AGE—ADOLESCENCE, MIDDLE AGE, OVER 65)
C. DEPRESSION—MOOD DISORDER IS PREVALENT IN 25–30% OF INDIVIDUALS WHO ATTEMPT SUICIDE.
D. PREVIOUS ATTEMPTS—COMPLETED SUICIDES OCCUR IN 50–80% OF INDIVIDUALS WHO HAVE ATTEMPTED SUICIDE PREVIOUSLY.
E. ALCOHOL OR DRUG USE— COMPLETED SUICIDES ARE CONNECTED WITH HEAVY ALCOHOL OR DRUG USE, OR BOTH, IN 20–90% OF CASES.
F. RATIONAL THOUGHT LOSS—THE RISK OF SUICIDE INCREASES WITH PSYCHOTIC THOUGHT PROCESSES.
G. LACK OF SOCIAL SUPPORT, —LACK MINIMAL TO NO SUPPORT FROM FRIENDS, RELATIVES, RELIGIOUS PRACTICES, OR MINIMAL TO NO

OCCUPATIONAL SATISFACTION INCREASES THE RISK FOR SUICIDE.
   H. ORGANIZED PLAN—LETHALITY OF METHOD; TIME, DATE, PLACE, AND FANTASIES, INCLUDING WHO WOULD FIND THEM, FUNERAL AND GRIEF OF SIGNIFICANT OTHERS
   I. NO SIGNIFICANT OTHERS—THOSE WHO ARE SINGLE, DIVORCED, WIDOWED, OR SEPARATED ARE AT HIGHER RISK FOR SUICIDE.
   J. SICKNESS—THOSE WITH DEBILITATING, PAINFUL, CHRONIC, OR TERMINAL ILLNESSES ARE AT INCREASED RISK FOR SUICIDE.
   K. SCORING OF SAD PERSONS SCALE
      1. 0–2 POINTS: CLIENT MAY STAY AT HOME WITH ASSISTANCE OF SIGNIFICANT OTHERS, FRIENDS, OUTPATIENT TREATMENT.
      2. 3–4 POINTS: SUPPORT OF SIGNIFICANT OTHERS, MORE INTENSE OUTPATIENT TREATMENT, POSSIBLE HOSPITALIZATION
      3. 5–6 POINTS: STRONG CONSIDERATION OF HOSPITALIZATION
      4. 7 POINTS: HOSPITALIZATION WARRANTED

VII. **CATEGORIES OF MOOD DISORDERS**
   A. DESCRIPTION
      1. MOOD EPISODE
         a. A new or worsening experience of depression or mania, or both, nearly every day for most of the day within a 2-week period of time
         b. Mood disorder is diagnosed based on the pattern of the mood episodes.
   B. UNIPOLAR (DEPRESSIVE) DISORDER
      1. INCLUDES THE DOWNWARD SWING OF EMOTIONS
      2. FEELINGS OF SADNESS, LOSS OF ENERGY, WITH ACCOMPANYING IRRITABILITY
      3. ISOLATION, LOW SELF-ESTEEM, SELF-DEROGATORY THOUGHTS
      4. FOUND IN MAJOR DEPRESSIVE ILLNESS AND DYSTHYMIA
   C. BIPOLAR (MANIA) DISORDER
      1. INCLUDES THE UPWARD SWING OF EMOTIONS
      2. FEELINGS OF ELATION, HIGH ENERGY, AND NEED FOR LITTLE REST, SLEEP, OR FOOD
      3. INFLATED SENSE OF SELF-IMPORTANCE, SELF-ESTEEM
      4. GRANDIOSE BEHAVIORS OF EXCESSIVE SPENDING, PLEASURE SEEKING, HIGH-RISK BEHAVIOR
      5. EXAGGERATED SOCIALIZATION FOUND IN BIPOLAR I AND BIPOLAR II DISORDERS

VIII. **DEPRESSIVE DISORDERS**
   A. MAJOR DEPRESSIVE DISORDER
      1. DESCRIPTION
         a. A change from previous level of functioning
         b. At least four clinical manifestations occurring predominantly during a 2-week period of time
         c. Individuals with a severe or chronic medical illness are at 20–25% greater risk of developing a major depressive disorder.
      2. ASSESSMENT
         a. Depressed mood
         b. Decreased concentration
         c. Decreased interest or pleasure in all or most activities
         d. Fatigue
         e. Feelings of worthlessness, guilt
         f. Insomnia or hypersomnia
         g. Psychomotor retardation
         h. Recurrent thoughts of suicide, with or without a plan; suicide attempt or plan to attempt suicide
         i. Significant weight loss or weight gain
      3. NURSING INTERVENTIONS (SEE TABLE 51-1)
         a. Administer antidepressant drugs such as fluoxetine (Prozac), paroxetine (Paxil), sertraline (Zoloft), venlafaxine (Effexor), and bupropion (Wellbutrin) as prescribed.
         b. Refer the client to psychotherapy, if appropriate.
   B. DYSTHYMIC DISORDER
      1. DESCRIPTION
         a. A milder but more chronic form of major depression
         b. Experience of depressed mood
         c. At least two clinical manifestations during most days for a 2-year period of time
      2. ASSESSMENT
         a. Difficulty with decision making
         b. Fatigue
         c. Feelings of hopelessness
         d. Low self-esteem
         e. Poor concentration
      3. NURSING INTERVENTIONS (SEE TABLE 51-1)
         a. Administer antidepressant drugs as prescribed.
         b. Refer the client to psychotherapy if appropriate.
   C. DEPRESSIVE DISORDER NOT OTHERWISE SPECIFIED
      1. DESCRIPTION
         a. Experience of mood clinical manifestations
         b. Does not meet criteria for a specific mood disorder

Table 51-1 Nursing Interventions for Mood Disorders Based on Clinical Manifestations

Clinical Manifestations	Nursing Interventions
Depressed, or dysthymic, mood	Administer medication as prescribed. Instruct the client on the importance of taking the prescribed medication. Facilitate a physical exam. Obtain blood levels of complete blood count (CBC) with differential, thyroid function tests (T3 , T4 , TSH), vitamin B$_{12}$, and folate to assess for general medical problems that may be causing depressive manifestations. Assess food intake. Encourage the intake of foods that will lead to alertness, motivation, and "up" mood state, such as fish, salmon, tuna, sardines, chicken, lean beef, shellfish, and veal. Encourage intake of foods that can increase serotonin levels, such as pumpkin, milk, sunflower seeds, turkey, bananas, red plums, tomatoes, pineapple, avocados, dates, eggplant, and passion fruit. Instruct the client regarding the effects of anger turned inward. Assist the client in identifying the cause of depression. Encourage discussion of grief and loss issues. Assist the client in relating how thoughts impact one's feelings and behaviors. Assist the client in counteracting negative, unhelpful thoughts with positive, helpful thoughts. Ascertain from the client movies, books, comics, and entertainers that have assisted in improving her mood in the past. Suggest that the client rent and watch a movie or read a book that has been pleasurable in the past.
Anhedonia	Explore with the client activities that were enjoyed in the past and encourage participation in these activities. Encourage activities with others to decrease isolation and decrease feelings of self-pity.
Hopelessness	Encourage the client to explore thoughts and feelings regarding hopelessness. Spend time with the client to increase trust. Explore prior coping mechanisms that have and have not worked for the client. Facilitate a discussion regarding the client's purpose in life, spiritual belief system. Explore the client's strengths and past successes. Place focus on the client's strengths.
Low self-esteem	Facilitate a discussion regarding the client's origin of low self-esteem. Assist the client in identifying positive characteristics of self.
Increased appetite and weight gain	Clinical manifestations may be targeted with a higher dose of selective serotonin reuptake inhibitor (SSRI) if behavior is obsessive and compulsive. Encourage exercise, as tolerated, to facilitate weight loss.
Decreased appetite and weight loss	Encourage intake of water, juice, and milk to maintain hydration. Encourage the client to drink a high-calorie supplement, such as Ensure. Lower doses of mirtazapine (Remeron) may be considered because it can increase appetite.
Increased libido	Ascertain from the client and, if possible, significant other, to see if this is a problem or not.
Decreased libido	Generally, a stimulant such as yohimbine is given.
Decreased ability to sleep	Instruct the client on sleep hygiene techniques. • Avoid daytime napping. • Avoid caffeine within 12 hours of retiring to bed (caffeine has a 12-hour half-life). • Snack on cottage cheese, yogurt, or other dairy products and turkey sandwiches, as they contain L-tryptophan (a natural sedative). Take a warm bath or have the significant other give a massage. Encourage listening to soft, relaxing music.
Hypersomnia	Encourage the client to get out of bed at a set time each morning and establish a routine for the day. Encourage exercise, such as walking, to stimulate endorphins. Set limits for time spent in the bedroom. Plan diversionary activities to keep the client occupied.
Poor concentration, indecisiveness	Encourage the client to eat foods that can lead to increased concentration and alertness, such as skim or low-fat milk, low-fat or nonfat yogurt, low-fat mozzarella or ricotta cheese, eggs (poached or scrambled), peanuts, almonds, beans, and peas. Encourage the client not to make any major decisions while feeling depressed. Explore support systems that the client can rely on until the client's mood becomes euthymic.

Clinical Manifestations	Nursing Interventions
Psychomotor agitation	Allow the client to have space.
	Decrease stimuli in the environment.
	Provide calming music or sounds (ocean waves, sound of nature, brook) as tolerated.
	Provide limits for the client. If agitation continues or is severe, administer lorazepam (Ativan) 0.5 mg–2 mg p.o. or IM.
Psychomotor retardation	Encourage exercise such as walking.
	In severe catatonia, ECT would be the treatment of choice.
	Fluoxetine (Prozac), an SSRI, may be considered, as it can be excitatory.
Recurrent suicidal thoughts	Provide a suicide assessment. Assess risk for suicide—method, date, time, means. Assess age, chronicity of medical illness, and previous attempts.
Manic or hypomanic mood	Administer mood-stabilizing medication such as divalproex (Depakote), gabapentin (Neurontin), carbamazepine (Tegretol), or lithium.
Inflated mood, grandiosity	Attempt to avoid grandiose statements and reinforce content that is reality based.
	Decrease environmental stimuli.
	Set limits on behavior.
Distractibility, flight of ideas, racing thoughts	Instruct the client in deep-breathing technique if appropriate.
	Encourage a warm bath, or listening to soft, soothing music.
	Encourage the client to slow down.
	Explore stressors that precipitate manic behavior.
	Assist the client to connect behavior to feelings of increased anxiety.
Increased goal-directed activity; excessive indulgence in pleasurable activities	Instruct the client on techniques to reduce anxiety.
	Provide constructive feedback regarding self-destructive behavior.
	Explore thoughts and feelings that occur prior to increased, excessive indulgence in activity.
	Assist the client in identifying negative consequences of behavior.
	Explore with the client alternative behaviors to utilize when feeling anxious or hyperactive.

© Cengage Learning 2015

c. Given when it is difficult to choose between this diagnosis and bipolar disorder, not otherwise specified
2. TYPES
  a. Premenstrual dysphoric disorder
    1) Description
      a) Occurred during most menstrual cycles in the past year during the last week of the luteal phase
      b) Abates within several days of onset of menses
    2) Assessment
      a) Depressed mood
      b) Irritability
      c) Decreased interest in activities
    3) Nursing interventions
      a) Instruct the client to monitor mood, sleep, and appetite during the month.
      b) Administer vitamin B$_6$ 100 mg per day 2 weeks prior to the menstrual cycle as prescribed.
      c) Encourage intake of water and juice.

      d) Instruct the client to avoid caffeine-containing beverages and chocolate.
      e) Decrease sodium intake.
  b. Minor depressive disorder
    1) Description
      a) Mood episodes lasting at least 2 weeks
      b) Recurrent brief depressive disorder
      c) Postpsychotic depressive disorder of schizophrenia
    2) Assessment
      a) Less than the five clinical manifestations that are required for major depressive disorder
    3) Nursing interventions (see Table 51-1)
      a) Administer antidepressant medication as ordered by the physician.
  c. Recurrent brief depressive disorder
    1) Description
      a) Mood episodes occur once per month for 12 months.

b) Mood episodes last 2 days to 2 weeks.

c) Diagnosis is given when there is a depressive disorder, but it is difficult to differentiate if mood episodes are primary, substance induced, or due to a general medical condition.

2) Assessment

a) Same as for major depressive disorder with clinical manifestations lasting from 2 days to 2 weeks (see page 947)

3) Nursing interventions (see Table 51-1)

d. Postpsychotic depressive disorder of schizophrenia

1) Description: mood occurring during the residual phase of schizophrenia

2) Assessment

a) Same as the clinical manifestations in major depressive disorder (see page 947)

3. NURSING INTERVENTIONS (SEE TABLE 51-1)

IX. TYPES OF BIPOLAR DISORDERS

A. BIPOLAR I DISORDER

1. DESCRIPTION: CLINICAL MANIFESTATIONS OF MANIA, HYPOMANIA, MIXED MOOD EPISODES, OR MAJOR DEPRESSIVE EPISODE

2. TYPES

a. Mania

1) Description: extreme elevation of mood lasting for at least 1 week

2) Assessment

a) Three of the following clinical manifestations (four if mood is irritable):

1. Distractibility

2. Exaggerated self-importance, self-esteem

3. Flight of ideas, racing thoughts

4. Grandiose behaviors (excessive pleasure seeking, buying sprees)

5. Increased goal-directed behavior (business deals, socially, sexually)

6. Little need for sleep, rest, or food

3) Nursing interventions (see Table 51-1)

b. Hypomania

1) Description

a) Elevated mood episode not severe enough to create significant alteration in social or occupational functioning

b) Lasts at least 4 days

2) Assessment

a) Two manic clinical manifestations (three if irritable mood) (See assessment section under Mania on page 950.)

3) Nursing interventions (see Table 1-1)

c. Mixed mood episode

1) Description

a) Includes both a major depressive episode and manic episode for most days within a 1-week period of time

b) Creates a severe impairment with lack of ability to function in occupational, social, or interpersonal settings

c) May need to be hospitalized

d) There may be psychotic features.

2) Assessment

a) Both depressive clinical manifestation and manic-type clinical manifestations for most days during a 1-week period of time

3) Nursing interventions

a) See Table 51-1.

b) Administer mood-stabilizing medication such as lithium, divalproex (Depakote), gabapentin (Neurontin), or carbamazepine (Tegretol).

B. BIPOLAR II DISORDER

1. DESCRIPTION

a. Current or past depressive episodes

b. Current or past hypomanic episodes

c. Clinical manifestations create great impairment in social, occupational, and other necessary areas of functioning.

d. No history of mixed mood episode

2. ASSESSMENT

a. Rapid cycling of mood

b. Impulse difficulties

c. Interpersonal sensitivity

d. Depression

e. Instability of mood

3. NURSING INTERVENTIONS

a. See Table 51-1.

b. Administer mood-stabilizing medication, such as lithium, divalproex (Depakote), gabapentin (Neurontin), or carbamazepine (Tegretol).

c. Administer antidepressant drugs, such as fluoxetine (Prozac), paroxetine (Paxil), sertraline (Zoloft), venlafaxine (Effexor), and bupropion (Wellbutrin) as prescribed.

    d. If the client has seasonal affective depression superimposed, administer phototherapy in late afternoon. Light therapy needs to be utilized in late afternoon hours to avoid triggering a manic phase.

  C. CYCLOTHYMIC DISORDER

    1. DESCRIPTION

      a. Numerous, chronic, vacillating mood states between hypomania and depression for a 2-year period

      b. Mood states are insufficient for meeting full criteria for either a manic episode or major depressive episode.

      c. Client has not been without clinical manifestations for more than a 2-month period

      d. Significant distress in areas of functioning as a result of the unpredictable mood changes

    2. ASSESSMENT

      a. Alternating periods of hypomania and mania

    3. NURSING INTERVENTIONS

      a. See Table 51-1.

      b. Administer mood-stabilizing medication, such as lithium, divalproex (Depakote), gabapentin (Neurontin), or carbamazepine (Tegretol).

  D. BIPOLAR DISORDER NOT OTHERWISE SPECIFIED

    1. DESCRIPTION: INCLUDES DISORDERS WITH BIPOLAR CHARACTERISTICS BUT DOES NOT MEET FULL CRITERIA FOR A PARTICULAR BIPOLAR DISORDER

    2. TYPES

      a. Reoccurring hypomanic episodes without accompanying depressive clinical manifestations

      b. Hypomanic episodes, along with persistent depressive clinical manifestations, that are too infrequent to be diagnosed with cyclothymic disorder

      c. Situations in which it is felt a bipolar disorder is present but is difficult to determine if it is primary, substance induced, or due to a general medical condition

    3. ASSESSMENT (SEE ASSESSMENT SECTIONS UNDER BIPOLAR I DISORDER ON PAGE 950 AND BIPOLAR II DISORDER ON PAGE 950.)

    4. NURSING INTERVENTIONS

      a. See Table 51-1.

      b. Administer mood-stabilizing medication such as lithium, divalproex (Depakote), gabapentin (Neurontin), or carbamazepine (Tegretol).

X. **OTHER MOOD DISORDERS**

  A. MOOD DISORDERS DUE TO A GENERAL MEDICAL CONDITION

    1. DESCRIPTION

      a. Depressed, elevated, or irritable moods as a direct result of physiological changes created by a general medical condition such as hypothyroidism, hyperthyroidism, or multiple sclerosis

      b. Mood states create significant problems in social, occupational, and other important areas of functioning.

    2. ASSESSMENT (SEE ASSESSMENT SECTIONS UNDER BIPOLAR I DISORDER ON PAGE 950 AND BIPOLAR II DISORDER ON PAGE 950.)

    3. NURSING INTERVENTIONS

      a. See Table 51-1.

      b. Encourage yearly physical examination.

      c. Administer prescribed medication to treat the medical condition.

      d. Provide clinical manifestations relief based on clinical manifestations of the medical condition.

  B. SUBSTANCE-INDUCED MOOD DISORDER

    1. DESCRIPTION

      a. A distinct change in mood that is directly the result of the physiological consequences of a substance, such as alcohol, or medication, such as benzodiazepines

      b. May be related to a somatic treatment for depression such as mania due to light therapy or electroconvulsive therapy

    2. ASSESSMENT

      a. Clinical presentation is similar to that of major depressive disorder, mania, hypomania, or mixed mood episodes.

      b. Mood symptoms create serious distress within social, occupational, and other significant areas of functioning.

    3. NURSING INTERVENTIONS

      a. See Table 51-1.

      b. Instruct the client on the effects of substance use on mood and functioning levels.

      c. Instruct on coping skills to manage stress, feelings of anger, or anxiety.

  C. SCHIZOAFFECTIVE DISORDER

    1. DESCRIPTION

      a. Presence of hallucinations or delusions for at least 2 weeks without any mood symptoms

      b. Hallucinations or delusions are noted for at least 1 month, with full criteria being met for a mood disorder superimposed at some point during the illness.

Table 51-2 Nursing Interventions Based on Clinical Manifestations of Schizoaffective Disorder

Clinical Manifestations	Nursing Interventions
Delusional thinking	Administer psychotropic drugs such as risperidone (Risperdal) or olanzapine (Zyprexa).
	Assess for neuroleptin malignant syndrome, extrapyramidal clinical manifestations, sedation, and increased weight.
	Develop trust with the client.
	Identify difficult experiences and assist to decrease anxiety.
	Inform the client about the consequences of delusions.
	Provide reality testing.
	Ensure the safety of the client.
	Set realistic goals.
Hallucinations	Cross reference interventions for delusional thinking.
	Determine type and dangerousness of hallucinations.
	Assist the client in scheduling routines.
	Instruct the client in sleep hygiene techniques.
	Instruct the client in positive coping strategies.
Anhedonia and flat affect	Instruct the client on socialization techniques.
	Encourage the client to socialize with others.
Decreased energy	Encourage exercise.
	Encourage the client to be adequately nourished.
Difficulty making decisions	Develop a regular schedule with the client.
	Encourage family members to assist the client with decisions regarding housing and finances.

© Cengage Learning 2015

2. ASSESSMENT
   a. Positive clinical manifestations
      1) Hallucinations, visual, auditory, tactile, olfactory, gustatory
      2) Delusional thinking
   b. Negative clinical manifestations
      1) Anhedonia
      2) Decreased energy
      3) Difficulty making decisions
      4) Flat affect
      5) Limited ability to say anything new
      6) Decreased ability in carrying on a conversation
3. NURSING INTERVENTIONS
   (SEE TABLE 51-2)

PRACTICE QUESTIONS

1. The nurse is assessing the client who is suicidal. Which of the following is the priority nursing intervention?
   1. Ask the client, "Do you have a plan to kill yourself?"
   2. Get the client to the hospital for further evaluation
   3. Assess the client for suicidal risk, method, and ability to carry the plan out
   4. Assess for past suicide attempts

2. The nurse should instruct a client that of the following, which would be an expected clinical manifestation for up to 2 months following an electroconvulsive therapy treatment?
   1. Dizziness
   2. Heartburn
   3. Nausea and vomiting
   4. Short-term memory loss

3. When assessing a client for a bipolar disorder, the nurse should include which of the following in the mental status exam to make a positive diagnosis of a bipolar disorder? Assessment of
   1. gait.
   2. mood.
   3. emotional developmental level.
   4. nutritional status.

4. The parents of a client diagnosed with major depression and who attempted suicide ask the nurse what the difference is between major depression and a bipolar disorder. The most appropriate response by the nurse is which of the following?
   1. "Major depression and bipolar disorder are two different mood disorders, but the treatment is the same."
   2. "Bipolar disorder is an upswing of mood, whereas major depression is a downward mood swing. They require very similar treatment modalities."
   3. "Major depression is a downward swing of mood with treatment, including mood stabilizers, whereas bipolar depression is an upward swing of mood with antidepressants given to bring the mood down."
   4. "Major depression is a depressed mood state that requires antidepressant medication, whereas bipolar disorder is an upward swing of mood that requires mood stabilizers for treatment."

5. During an admission interview, which of the following clinical manifestations should the nurse report as indicative of hypomania? Select all that apply:
   [ ] 1. Decreased delusions of grandeur
   [ ] 2. Decreased self-esteem
   [ ] 3. Pressured speech
   [ ] 4. Talkativeness
   [ ] 5. Decreased motivation
   [ ] 6. Flight of ideas

6. A female client expresses that she has had difficulties with irritability, depressed mood, and decreased interest during the last week of luteal phase during most of her menstrual cycles in the past year. Which of the following nursing interventions is most appropriate when planning nursing care for this client with premenstrual dysphoric disorder?
   1. Instruct the client to avoid focusing on mood, sleep, and appetite during the month
   2. Administer vitamin B_6 100 mg per day for 2 weeks prior to the menstrual cycle
   3. Encourage intake of water and juice
   4. Instruct the client to consume caffeine-containing beverages and chocolate

7. The nurse is planning the care of a client with cyclothymia. Currently, the client has a hypomanic mood episode. Which of the following nursing interventions would be a priority when caring for this client?
   1. Set limits with the client if the client is getting into the personal space of others
   2. Increase stimuli in the environment to prevent the client from becoming depressed
   3. Ask the client about issues related to self-esteem
   4. Encourage the client to decrease physical activity

8. The nurse is preparing to care for a client with major depression. The priority nursing intervention is to assess the client's
   1. response to medication administration.
   2. current mood and activity level.
   3. appetite and weight.
   4. risk of suicide.

9. A client has been making derogatory remarks about herself and states, "I'm not able to get a boyfriend because I am worthless." Which of the following cognitive nursing interventions would be most appropriate at this time?
   1. Encourage the client to explore feelings of worthlessness
   2. Instruct the client not to feel that way
   3. Encourage the client to explore positive thoughts about self
   4. Instruct the client to take an antidepressant drug as prescribed

10. A client scheduled to receive phototherapy asks the nurse what phototherapy is. The nurse should respond with which of the following statements?
    1. "It is a camera that takes pictures of your brain to see why you are becoming depressed."
    2. "It is a bright white light that is used to help treat depression in the winter months."
    3. "It assists in decreasing stress and will help you function better at work in the winter months."
    4. "It is used to treat depression that is resistant to electroconvulsive therapy."

11. The client asks the nurse how long phototherapy should be used each day. Which of the following is the appropriate response by the nurse?
    1. "If you get a headache, then you have sat in front of the light for too long."
    2. "Each individual is different. Sit in front of the light just long enough so that you do not get a headache."
    3. "Sit in front of the light while reading, preferably in the evening."
    4. "You may sit in front of the light as long as you are comfortable doing so."

12. Which of the following is the priority intervention to encourage a client who is depressed to discuss any suicidal thoughts, plan, or intent?
    1. Instruct the client about the consequences of hidden anger
    2. Focus on the need to keep the client safe
    3. Avoid discussion of depressing topics
    4. Encourage the client to verbalize feelings

13. While assessing a client in the emergency room after an attempted suicide, the priority question the nurse should ask the client is which of the following?
    1. "What is happening in your life that would cause you to attempt to kill yourself?"
    2. "How are you feeling since you have awakened after your overdose?"
    3. "Where is the pill bottle of the medications that you had taken?"
    4. "What can be done to make your life better?"

14. The priority intervention for an outpatient nurse to perform for a client who is depressed and has told the nurse that "I am worthless and there is nothing to live for" would be
    1. immediately seek a psychiatric hospitalization for the client.
    2. explore feelings of worthlessness and hopelessness.
    3. encourage the client to identify self-deprecating thoughts.
    4. remove all potentially dangerous objects from the immediate area.

15. The nurse who is caring for a client who is manic and exhibiting psychomotor agitation implements which of the following interventions as the priority?
    1. Explore alternative behaviors with the client for use when feeling anxious or hyperactive
    2. Provide limits for the client while allowing the client space
    3. Explore stressors that precipitate manic behavior
    4. Assist the client in identifying negative consequences of behavior

16. When completing an admissions assessment of a client with schizoaffective disorder, the nurse should assess for the presence of which of the following clinical manifestations?
    Select all that apply:
    [ ] 1. Increased use of substances
    [ ] 2. Decreased libido
    [ ] 3. Hallucinations
    [ ] 4. Feelings of entitlement
    [ ] 5. Decreased energy
    [ ] 6. Anhedonia

17. A client diagnosed with a bipolar disorder and who has a superimposed seasonal affective depression is using phototherapy as a treatment to lift the depression. The client calls the nurse at the outpatient mental health clinic, reporting, "My mood, libido, and interest in shopping have improved dramatically." Based on this information, which of the following is the priority to assess first?
    1. Explore energy level and level of appetite
    2. Ascertain how much money the client is spending
    3. Identify the time of day the client is utilizing the phototherapy treatment
    4. Encourage the client to explore thoughts of improved self-worth

18. Discharge plans are being made for a client hospitalized for depression. Which of the following is the priority outcome for a diagnosis of depression?
    1. Share more realistic expectations of the client and the situation
    2. Identify negative, unrealistic thoughts about oneself and ways to counteract those thoughts
    3. Discuss reasons why the client has turned the anger inward
    4. Openly express thoughts and feelings of depression

19. The nurse evaluates a client who stays at home with the assistance of significant others and friends and is undergoing outpatient treatment to have how many points on the Sad Persons Suicide Assessment Scale? _____

20. The nurse receives a report on a client with dysthymia. It would be most important for the nurse to make which of the following assessments?
    Select all that apply:
    [ ] 1. Chronic feelings of low self-esteem
    [ ] 2. Poor concentration
    [ ] 3. Flight of ideas
    [ ] 4. Hallucinations
    [ ] 5. Depressed mood
    [ ] 6. Increased libido

21. Which of the following interventions should the nurse implement when treating delusional thinking in a schizoaffective disorder?
    Select all that apply:
    [ ] 1. Instruct the client on socialization techniques
    [ ] 2. Identify difficult experiences and assist to decrease anxiety
    [ ] 3. Provide reality testing
    [ ] 4. Develop a regular schedule with the client
    [ ] 5. Set realistic goals
    [ ] 6. Encourage exercise

22. The nurse assesses which of the following to be negative clinical manifestations in a client with a schizoaffective disorder?
    Select all that apply:
    [ ] 1. Auditory hallucinations
    [ ] 2. Anhedonia
    [ ] 3. Difficulty making decisions
    [ ] 4. Delusional thinking
    [ ] 5. Decreased ability in carrying on a conversation
    [ ] 6. Tactile hallucinations

23. The nurse is caring for a client who is in the manic state of a bipolar disorder. Which of the following should the nurse prioritize as the most appropriate nursing outcome?
    1. The client will be free of agitation, hyperactivity, and restless behavior
    2. The client will appropriately verbalize feelings of anger
    3. The client will be free of aggression and threatened behavior toward others
    4. The client will demonstrate lessened buying sprees and grandiosity

24. The nurse is caring for a client with a mood disorder caused by a medical condition. Which of the following are most important for the nurse to assess?

    1. Serum drug screen
    2. Electrocardiogram (ECG)
    3. Bowel sounds
    4. Dental hygiene

25. Which of the following clinical manifestations of schizoaffective disorder should the nurse assess the client for?
    Select all that apply:
    [ ] 1. Flat affect
    [ ] 2. Hallucinations
    [ ] 3. Decreased energy
    [ ] 4. Delusional thinking
    [ ] 5. Anhedonia
    [ ] 6. Anorexia

26. The registered nurse is preparing to delegate clinical assignments on a psychiatric unit. Which of the following assignments should the nurse delegate to a licensed practical nurse?
    1. Develop a plan of care for a client with hypomania
    2. Ensure a client is NPO for electroconvulsive therapy
    3. Teach a class on bipolar disorders
    4. Organize the care to be provided to a client with a bipolar disorder

ANSWERS AND RATIONALES

1. 3. Assessing the client is necessary before determining if the client needs to be hospitalized or not. Assessing for past suicide attempts is very important, but the priority is to determine if the client has a plan.

2. 4. Short-term memory loss would be an expected clinical manifestation post electroconvulsive therapy (ECT), occurring after treatment and lasting for 1 week to 2 months or more. Unilateral placement of the electrodes may decrease the amount of short-term memory loss, because the current passes through only the nondominant side of the brain. Unilateral placement is less effective in treating depression than bilateral placement. Although dizziness, heartburn, and nausea and vomiting may be experienced post ECT, they would not be expected clinical manifestations for 1 week to 2 months post ECT.

3. 2. Although it is necessary to assess the client's gait, emotional developmental level, and nutritional status, these are not part of a mental status exam. Assessing the client's mood (either

mania, hypomania, or depression) would provide the information needed to assist in verifying a diagnosis of a bipolar disorder.

4. 4. Major depression and bipolar disorder are two different mood disorders with different treatment regimens. Major depression is a downward swing of mood, and bipolar disorder is an upward swing of mood (mania) and a downward swing of mood (hypomania). Major depression is treated with an antidepressant, whereas bipolar disorder is treated with a mood stabilizer such as gabapentin (Neurontin) or divalproex sodium (Depakote).

5. 3. 4. 6. Hypomania is a form of mania in which the clinical manifestations are less severe than those of mania. Clinical manifestations of hypomania include pressured speech, talkativeness, flight of ideas, delusions of grandeur, inflated self-esteem, and increased motivation.

6. 2. Instructing a client to monitor mood, sleep, and appetite during the month is an appropriate nursing intervention to assist the nurse in

knowing when the client is having difficulty with clinical manifestations. Encouraging the intake of fluids will increase water retention and will increase irritability. Administering vitamin B$_6$ 100 mg per day for 2 weeks prior to the menstrual cycle is the most appropriate intervention. Vitamin B$_6$ is a precursor to serotonin, which can assist in decreasing clinical manifestations of depressed mood and irritability. Instructing the client to consume caffeine-containing beverages and chocolate would not be appropriate because it would increase fluid retention and therefore increase clinical manifestations of irritability and depression.

7. 1. Cyclothymia is a mood disorder that is generally chronic, lasting at least 2 years, and involves hypomanic and dysthymic mood swings. Setting limits for a client with hypomania is a priority nursing intervention, because the client is unaware of the intrusiveness and the annoyance of this behavior to other clients. The client who is hypomanic presents an inflated self-esteem or grandiosity but is using it to cover chronic feelings of low self-esteem. Asking about issues related to self-esteem would be an appropriate nursing intervention but is not the priority at this time. Encouraging the client to perform relaxation techniques during the hypomanic state is also appropriate but not a priority. Increasing stimuli in the environment will not prevent the client who is hypomanic from becoming depressed and would not be an appropriate nursing intervention, because it would further increase the irritable or elevated mood.

8. 4. Although it is important for the nurse to assess the client's areas of functioning, current mood, and fluid/electrolyte balance, assessing the suicide risk of the client with major depression takes priority.

9. 1. Instructing a client who is feeling worthless not to feel that way and exploring positive thoughts about herself minimizes and discourages the exploration of the client's thoughts and feelings about feeling worthless. Instructing the client to take an antidepressant drug disregards the comment made by the client. By exploring feelings of worthlessness, the client will more easily identify the source of the feelings. The client will also feel a sense of having been heard by the nurse, thus increasing trust.

10. 2. Phototherapy is a bright white light that is used to treat seasonal affective depression in the winter months, generally between September and March. The light (approximately 2500 to 10,000 lux) can be used from 30 minutes to 2 hours each day during the winter months. It

does not decrease stress and most likely would be used prior to or after electroconvulsive therapy treatments.

11. 2. If a client sits in front of the phototherapy light for too long, the client will develop a headache. The length of time is different for each individual. Some individuals may experience a headache within 30 minutes. Sitting in front of the light while reading or comfortable are statements of when, not how long, the client should use phototherapy each day. During the first one or two treatments, the client may get a headache because the period of treatment has not yet been established and the client does not yet know yet what reaction he or she will have to the treatment.

12. 4. The best plan for a nursing intervention for the client who may be contemplating suicide is to encourage the client to discuss feelings, because this will allow the nurse to understand the client's emotional state and the client's mood. Although instructing the client about the consequences for hidden anger and talking to the client about the need to keep safe are important, neither of these is a priority nursing intervention. Avoiding depressing topics is not the priority nursing intervention, because there may be depressing topics or situations that may be contributing to the depression.

13. 1. Although asking a client how he or she is feeling after an overdose, where the pill bottle is, and what can be done to make life better are appropriate interventions, the priority is to ask the client what has led to the attempted suicide. This gets at the heart of the matter of a suicide attempt and encourages the building of the nurse–client relationship. This encouragement will allow the client to further express personal thoughts and feelings.

14. 2. Although it is important to encourage the client to identify self-defeating thoughts, it is not the most appropriate intervention in the outpatient setting. While exploring the client's feelings of worthlessness and hopelessness, the nurse can assist the client in exploring a sense of worth, value, and hope. There are numerous clients living in the community who are chronically suicidal and can be managed on an outpatient basis. Removing all potentially dangerous objects from the immediate area and seeking immediate psychiatric hospitalization are premature.

15. 2. A client who is manic and exhibiting the clinical manifestation of psychomotor agitation is only minimally able to have insight into those behaviors or ways to change the behaviors. This client requires limits within provided structure and space.

16. 3. 5. 6. Schizoaffective disorder is characterized by elements of schizophrenia and manic-depressive disorder. Clinical manifestations include hallucinations, decreased energy, and anhedonia (lack of interest in pleasure or daily activities).

17. 3. A client with a bipolar disorder and a superimposed seasonal affective depression needs to be careful about the time of day that the phototherapy is utilized. Because of circadian rhythms, it has been found that bipolar clients with seasonal depression do best if they utilize the phototherapy treatment in the later afternoon. If the phototherapy is used in the morning, manic manifestations may result. Exploring appetite, energy level, feelings of self-worth, and how much money the client is spending may all be important interventions, but determining the time of day the client is using the phototherapy allows the nurse to obtain the information that may be causing the dramatic change and elevation in mood.

18. 4. The priority outcome for a client with depression would be to openly express thoughts and feelings of depression. Although not the priority, it may prove beneficial to share a more realistic expectation of the client, to help the client identify negative and unrealistic thoughts about him- or herself, and discuss reasons why the client has turned the anger inward.

19. 0–2 0–2. A client who stays at home with assistance of significant others, has friends, and is undergoing outpatient treatment would score 0–2 points.

20. 1. 2. 5. Dysthymia is a chronic depressive disorder lasting for several years. Clinical manifestations of dysthymia include chronic feelings of low self-esteem, poor concentration, and depressed mood. Flight of ideas and increased libido are clinical manifestations found in the manic phase of a bipolar affective disorder. Hallucinations can be found in schizoaffective disorder.

21. 2. 3. 5. Nursing interventions for delusional thinking based on the clinical manifestations of schizoaffective disorder include the following: identify difficult experiences and assist to decrease anxiety, provide reality testing, and set realistic goals. Instructing the client on socialization techniques is an intervention for anhedonia and flat affect. Encouraging exercise is an intervention for decreased energy. Developing a regular schedule with the client is an intervention in the treatment for difficulty making decisions.

22. 2. 3. 5. Negative clinical manifestations for schizoaffective disorder include anhedonia, difficulty making decisions, and a decreased ability in carrying on a conversation. Positive clinical manifestations for schizoaffective disorder include auditory and tactile hallucinations and delusional thinking.

23. 3. The priority nursing outcome for a client in the manic state of a bipolar disorder is that the client will be free from aggression and threatened behavior toward others.

24. 2. Approximately 20% to 25% of clients with certain medical conditions, such as myocardial infarction, cancer, stroke, and diabetes mellitus, will develop a major depressive disorder. An electrocardiogram (ECG) would assess the client's cardiac status.

25. 1. 3. 5. Schizoaffective disorder is a disorder characterized by a major depressive, manic, or mixed episode that coincides with a diagnosis of schizophrenia. The clinical manifestations must not be the result of abuse or a medical condition. The main clinical manifestations are flat affect, decreased energy, and anhedonia.

26. 2. A licensed practical nurse may ensure a client is NPO for electroconvulsive therapy. Developing a plan of care, teaching a class, and organizing care to be provided to a client should be performed by a registered nurse.

REFERENCES

Antai-Otong, D. (2008). *Psychiatric nursing, biological and behavioral concepts* (2nd ed.). Clifton Park, NY: Delmar Cengage Learning.

Frisch, N. C., & Frisch, L. E. (2011). *Psychiatric mental health nursing* (4th ed.). Clifton Park, NY: Delmar Cengage Learning.

CHAPTER 52

SCHIZOPHRENIA AND PSYCHOTIC DISORDERS

I. SCHIZOPHRENIA

A. DESCRIPTION
1. DEVASTATING DISEASE AFFECTING ONE'S ABILITY TO THINK AND PERCEIVE REALITY
2. THE EFFECTS OF THE DISEASE AFFECT LANGUAGE, EMOTIONS, AND SOCIAL BEHAVIOR.
3. THE AVERAGE AGE OF ONSET IS IN LATE ADOLESCENCE AND EARLY ADULTHOOD.
4. ONE-THIRD OF THE HOMELESS POPULATION HAS SCHIZOPHRENIA. THE FACT THAT THEY ARE HOMELESS IS SECONDARY TO DEINSTITUTIONALIZATION OF CLIENTS WITH MENTAL HEALTH DISORDERS.
5. HIGHER RATES IN URBAN AREAS VERSUS RURAL AREAS

B. THEORIES OF SCHIZOPHRENIA
1. GENETIC FACTORS
   a. Incidence increases among first-degree relatives. Relatives have 10 times greater risk than the general population.
   b. Incidence increases among monozygotic twins versus dizygotic twins.
   c. Genetic locations on the human chromosome
2. BIOLOGICAL FACTORS
   a. Neurodevelopment during the perinatal period results in an injury or trauma that causes schizophrenia to manifest in the later years of adolescence or early adulthood.
   b. Brain abnormalities: specifically, possible enlarged ventricles and prominent cortical sulci
   c. The dopamine hypothesis supports an increased level of dopamine in the brain.
   d. Diathesis-stress model: a client's biological predisposition is exacerbated by personal, social, and environmental stressors, resulting in schizophrenia.

C. ASSESSMENT
1. POSITIVE CLINICAL MANIFESTATIONS ARE EXCESS OR DISTORTED NORMAL FUNCTIONS SUCH AS HALLUCINATIONS, DELUSIONS, IDEAS OF INFLUENCE, IDEAS OF REFERENCE, AND ALTERED THOUGHT AND SPEECH (SEE TABLE 52-1).

Table 52-1 Positive Clinical Manifestations of Schizophrenia

Persecutory	Belief or paranoia that the client or loved ones are singled out for being victimized such as by the Federal Bureau of Investigation (FBI) or being followed and spied on, or that others are plotting against them. These people often take their cases to court or to the government.
Jealous	Belief that one's intimate partner is disloyal. This is associated with paranoia.
Ideas of reference	Belief that personal or environmental cues are directed at the client, such as: Gestures / TV shows or commercials / Radio shows or announcements / Comments / Book passages or readings / Songs or lyrics
Ideas of influence	Belief that the client's thoughts are controlled by external forces: Thought insertion: the belief that the client's thoughts are coming from elsewhere and are not her own / Thought broadcasting: the belief that the client's thoughts are readable, or can be heard, by other people / Thought control: the belief that someone or something controls the client's thoughts
Magical thinking	The belief that the client's own thoughts can control others' thoughts and behavior

2. NEGATIVE CLINICAL MANIFESTATIONS ARE A LOSS OF NORMAL FUNCTIONS, INCLUDING:
   a. Flat affect (difficulty expressing emotions)
   b. Ambivalence (indecisiveness)
   c. Avolition (lack of motivation, passive)
   d. Anhedonia (lack of pleasure or interest in activities)
   e. Alogia (limited ability to converse)
   f. Isolation (emotional and social)
3. HALLUCINATIONS (SEE TABLE 52-2)
4. DELUSIONS (SEE TABLE 52-3)
5. DISORGANIZED SPEECH
6. ALTERED THOUGHT AND SPEECH (SEE TABLE 52-4)

7. DISORGANIZED OR CATATONIC BEHAVIOR
8. DISTURBED ABILITY TO ACHIEVE EDUCATION, MAINTAIN WORK, AND MAINTAIN RELATIONSHIPS
D. ASSESSMENT POINTS
   1. HALLUCINATION ASSESSMENT
      a. Auditory: time of occurrence, precipitating factors, number of voices, gender of voices, what voices say, whether voices are recognizable
         1) Do you hear voices when you cannot see people?
         2) How many different voices speak to you?
         3) What do they say?
         4) Do you recognize the voices?
         5) When did you first hear voices?
         6) What else was going on in your life at that time?
         7) How do you respond to the voices?
         8) What gives you relief?
      b. Visual: what do they see, any particular time of day?
      c. Olfactory: this often has organic implications.
      d. Gustatory: this often has organic implications.
      e. Tactile: organic or drug related
   2. HISTORY OF PRESENT ILLNESS
      a. Health history can be obtained from client, family, or significant other.
      b. History of psychiatric illness, treatment, hospitalization, and medication use
      c. Family history

Table 52-2 Types of Hallucinations

Auditory	Most common
	Perceived as distinct from the person's own thoughts
	Hearing familiar or unfamiliar voices
	Hearing one or many voices
	Hearing voices talking to each other or talking to the person
	Voices may be intelligible or unintelligible
	Hearing commands—demanding that the person perform a specific behavior, which generally is harmful to self or others
	Must occur separately from the time of sleep onset or awakening
Visual	Seeing something or someone who is not really there
Olfactory	Smelling something that is not really there
	Often has organic implications
Gustatory	Tasting something that is not really there
	Often has organic implications
Tactile	Feeling something on the skin or body that is not really there
	Often organic or drug related

© Cengage Learning 2015

Table 52-3 Delusions Types

Definition	Fixed false beliefs
Somatic	The client's belief that she has a physical illness or medical problem such as disease or cancer. The focus is on bodily functions and perceived sensations. Nonmedical conditions, such as infections, parasites, and nonfunctioning body systems, cause this belief.
Nihilistic	Belief that the world is ending, death is certain, or there is impending disaster
Grandiose	Belief that the client is famous; has extra powers, talent, or knowledge; or has a special relationship with a famous person or God; inflated sense of self
Erotomaniac	Belief that someone, usually of greater status and who is unattainable, is in love with her (the client)

© Cengage Learning 2015

Table 52-4 Altered Thought and Speech

Circumstantial	Gets to the point but digresses (speech that takes a circuitous route)
Tangential	There is a link between thoughts but the conversation detours
Loose associations	Thoughts, ideas, and topics are not related
Flight of ideas	Rapid and abrupt changes of the topic follow sentence or phrase
Perseverative	Persistent, repetitive expression of a single idea
Blocking	Speech or thought flow is stopped or slowed due to emotions
Mutism	Refusal to speak for conscious or unconscious reasons
Word salad	Words are not connected
Neoglisms	Unrecognizable, made-up words
Verbigeration	Repetition of words or phrases
Clang association	Repetition of words or phrases that rhyme

© Cengage Learning 2015

d. Identification of stressors that could trigger a relapse

e. History of medication, past or present, prescribed or over the counter

3. HISTORY AND PHYSICAL

a. Rule out medical causes for disturbance.

b. Identify comorbid illnesses and diseases.

c. Decreased activity, sleep, and poor hygiene generally are found.

d. Assess physical adverse reactions to medication.

e. Recognize that the client's family, caregivers, significant other, or representative may need to provide the majority of the information.

4. BIOLOGICAL FINDINGS

a. Possible enlarged ventricles and prominent cortical sulci

b. Increased levels of dopamine in the brain

5. FUNCTIONAL ASSESSMENT

a. Independence level in activities of daily living (ADLs)

b. Bizarre habits such as odd eating behaviors

c. Support system and activity level

d. Living status such as homelessness or group home

6. PSYCHOLOGICAL TESTING

a. Identifies cognitive impairment

7. TRANSCULTURAL CONSIDERATIONS

a. Delusions and psychotic states may appear unusual in one culture and normal in another; for example, religious beliefs may support visions or hearing voices from a spiritual figure.

E. DIAGNOSTIC TESTS

1. POSITRON EMISSION TOMOGRAPHY (PET)

2. MAGNETIC RESONANCE IMAGING (MRI)

3. PSYCHOLOGICAL TESTING

4. NEUROPSYCHOLOGICAL EVALUATION

F. NURSING DIAGNOSES

1. DISTURBED THOUGHT PROCESSES

2. DISTURBED SENSORY PERCEPTIONS SUCH AS AUDITORY, GUSTATORY, KINESTHETIC, OLFACTORY, AND VISUAL

3. DISTURBED PERSONAL IDENTITY

4. IMPAIRED VERBAL COMMUNICATION

5. SELF-CARE DEFICIT

6. SOCIAL ISOLATION

7. INEFFECTIVE COPING

8. POWERLESSNESS

9. LOW SELF-ESTEEM

Nursing Diagnoses: Definitions and Classification 2012–2014. Copyright © 2012, 1994–2012 by NANDA International. Used by arrangement with John Wiley & Sons Limited.

G. MEDICAL COMPLICATIONS

1. PSYCHOGENIC POLYDIPSIA: DISTURBED WATER AND ELECTROLYTE BALANCE; MAY OCCUR RELATED TO TOXIC AMOUNTS OF WATER THAT ARE COMPULSIVELY CONSUMED BY AN INDIVIDUAL WHO HAS BEEN DIAGNOSED WITH SCHIZOPHRENIA AND OTHER POSSIBLE MAJOR MENTAL ILLNESSES; THE AMOUNT OF WATER CONSUMED IS GENERALLY GREATER THAN 3 L OF WATER PER DAY (RANGE OF 4–10 L/DAY).

a. Chronic clinical manifestations

1) Weight gain

2) Generalized edema

3) Serum sodium decreased (hyponatremia)

4) Nocturia

5) Irritability

6) Headache

7) Decreased appetite

8) Restlessness

b. Acute clinical manifestations of water intoxication by self-induced consumption of large amounts of water (polydipsia) with rapid physiologic changes are a major cause of death in institutionalized clients.

1) Hyponatremia: rapid shift

2) Increased urinary output (polyuria)

3) Decreased urinary concentration (osmolality)

4) Decreased urine specific gravity (hyposthenuria)

5) Decreased serum concentration (osmolality)

6) Muscle twitches

7) Weakness and lethargy

8) Nausea and vomiting

9) Confusion

10) Neurological changes such as ataxia, seizures, and coma

11) Urine characteristics such as urinary incontinence, urinary urgency, urine odor, and frequent changes of bedding and clothing

H. BARRIERS TO ASSESSMENT

1. DECREASED ABILITY FOR THE CLIENT TO ESTABLISH A TRUSTING RELATIONSHIP

2. DECREASED ABILITY FOR THE CLIENT TO COMMUNICATE DUE TO HALLUCINATIONS AND DELUSIONS

3. SOCIAL ISOLATION OF THE CLIENT, RESULTING IN THE LACK OF A SUPPORT SYSTEM FOR TREATMENT

I. BARRIERS TO TREATMENT
1. "DEINSTITUTIONALIZATION," WHICH CREATED LARGE CASELOADS FOR COMMUNITY MENTAL HEALTH WORKERS
2. DECREASED NATIONAL AND STATE FUNDING FOR COMMUNITY MENTAL HEALTH CENTERS
3. DECREASED REIMBURSEMENT FOR MENTAL HEALTH BY INSURANCE COMPANIES
4. MANAGED CARE WITH LIMITED ACCESSIBILITY TO SERVICES
5. SHORTER LENGTHS OF STAY FOR INPATIENT HOSPITALIZATIONS

J. TYPES OF SCHIZOPHRENIA
1. PARANOID SCHIZOPHRENIA
   a. Frequent auditory hallucinations
   b. Preoccupation with one or more delusions (see Table 52-2)
   c. Often have delusions of persecution
   d. Social isolation
   e. Unable to establish trust
   f. Argumentative
   g. Anger and potential violence
   h. Threatened safety of self and others
   i. Anxiety
2. CATATONIC SCHIZOPHRENIA
   a. Least common type of schizophrenia
   b. Slowed or lacking motor activity
      1) Waxy flexibility: posture held in bizarre positions for an extended period of time
      2) Catatonia: immobility
      3) Mutism: not speaking
      4) Vegetative
      5) Negativism: does not follow instructions with no known reason
      6) Voluntary movements
         a) Posturing: voluntary bizarre positions that are resistant to being moved by another
         b) Distinctive mannerisms and grimacing
         c) Stereotypical movements: continuously repeating one movement
      7) Childlike (regressed behavior)
      8) Impulsive episodes
      9) Social isolation
   c. Agitated motor activity
      1) Purposeless movements
      2) Activity is unrelated to external stimuli.
      3) Decreased reaction to the environment
      4) Stereotypy: repetitive movements without purpose

      5) Echolalia: imitation of another's words
      6) Echopraxia: involuntary imitation of another's movements
      7) Word salad: string of spoken words that do not have a meaningful connection
3. DISORGANIZED SCHIZOPHRENIA
   a. Incoherent speech
   b. Uninhibited behavior
   c. Flat affect
   d. Socially withdrawn
   e. Poor personal hygiene
   f. Altered personality
4. UNDIFFERENTIATED SCHIZOPHRENIA
   a. All characteristic clinical manifestations present but not enough clinical manifestations to be classified as paranoid, disorganized, or catatonic schizophrenia
5. RESIDUAL SCHIZOPHRENIA
   a. Has had, in the past, an acute episode of schizophrenia
   b. Now has continuing negative clinical manifestations, or has achieved total remission
   c. Continuation of two or more positive clinical manifestations

K. SUBTYPES OF SCHIZOPHRENIC-LIKE DISORDERS
1. SCHIZOAFFECTIVE
   a. A mood disorder such as depression or mania, or both, accompanied with negative clinical manifestations of schizophrenia such as anhedonia, avolition, and anergia
   b. If there are no mood disorder clinical manifestations, and there are two or more positive clinical manifestations of schizophrenia present, such as delusions, hallucinations, disorganized speech, disorganized behavior, and catatonic behavior
   c. The mood clinical manifestations and clinical manifestations of schizophrenia are present independently of the other.
   d. Behaviors that may be present include poor occupational functioning, lesser range of social contacts, deficient self-care, and greater suicide risk.
2. SCHIZOPHRENIFORM
   a. Features of schizophrenia for greater than 1 month and less than 6 months
   b. Social or occupational impairment is not necessarily evident.

L. NURSING INTERVENTIONS (SEE TABLE 52-5)

Table 52-5 Nursing Interventions for Thought Disorders

Delusion management	Orient the client to date, time, place, and situation.
	Avoid confronting the client about the delusional content.
	Decrease anxiety—avoid whispering or laughing in front of the client.
	Actively listen by offering verbal and nonverbal responses.
	Allow the client personal space without appearing distant.
	Provide attentive eye contact without staring.
	Avoid touching the client without asking for permission.
	Explain all procedures and answer questions.
Hallucination management	Decrease environmental stimulation with low lighting, low noise level, and decreased activity surrounding the client.
	Identify the client's stressors that precede hallucinations.
	Administer antipsychotic medications as scheduled and p.r.n. for breakthrough hallucinations and delusional content.
	Administer anxiolytic medications to reduce anxiety related to hallucinations and paranoia.
	Monitor command hallucinations of self-harm or harm directed toward others.
Psychotropic medication management	Monitor for extrapyramidal (parkinsonian) adverse reactions such as hand tremors, masklike facies, akathesia, and cogwheeling.
	Monitor for abnormal involuntary movements such as oculogyric crisis, retrocollis, torticollis, tongue tremor, dystonia, pill rolling, and athetoid or myokymic movements.
	Monitor for pain related to abnormal involuntary movements.
Environmental management	Initiate cognitively motivating activities.
	Provide animal-assisted recreation.
	Encourage milieu (surroundings) management.
	Decrease stimuli in the environment such as noise or activities.
	Prepare a structured schedule to prevent unoccupied time.
	Enhance sleep with decreased stimuli, routines, sleep aids.
Communication enhancement	Orient the client to date, time, place, and situation.
	Initiate behavioral techniques using physical space, eye contact, and nonthreatening gestures.
	Establish a trusting relationship by providing respect. Avoid criticizing the client.
	Respond neutrally to potentially emotional content.
	Utilize alternative methods of communication such as written communication and visual aids.
	Provide short, simple instructions to increase comprehension and cooperation.
	Involve the client in care planning, especially goal setting, review of progress, and adjustment of the treatment plan.

© Cengage Learning 2015

II. OTHER PSYCHOTIC DISORDERS

A. BRIEF PSYCHOTIC DISORDER
  1. AT LEAST ONE POSITIVE CLINICAL MANIFESTATION OF SCHIZOPHRENIA FOR AT LEAST 1 DAY AND LESS THAN 1 MONTH
  2. SUDDEN ONSET
  3. INTENSE CONFUSION AND EMOTIONAL LABILITY
  4. INDIVIDUAL GENERALLY MAKES A FULL RECOVERY.
  5. ONSET USUALLY OCCURS IN EARLY ADULTHOOD.
B. SHARED PSYCHOTIC DISORDER, ALSO KNOWN AS FOLIE A' DEUX (DSM)
  1. AN INDIVIDUAL WHO IS DELUSIONAL DEVELOPS A CLOSE RELATIONSHIP WITH ANOTHER INDIVIDUAL WHO IS NOT INITIALLY DELUSIONAL.
  2. THE SECOND PERSON DEVELOPS THE SAME DELUSION AS THE FIRST PERSON.

C. SUBSTANCE-INDUCED PSYCHOTIC DISORDER
  1. THEORIES
    a. Genetic
    b. Cultural influence (religion, family, nationality)
    c. Individuals who have a history of abuse usually have also experienced depression or anxiety.
  2. THE HALLUCINATIONS OR DELUSIONS BECOME EVIDENT WITHIN 1 MONTH OF THE SUBSTANCE USE OR WITHDRAWAL.
  3. THE HALLUCINATIONS OR DELUSIONS ARE THE DIRECT PHYSIOLOGICAL RESULT OF THE CONSUMPTION OF SUBSTANCES.
    a. Hallucinogens
      1) Lysergic acid diethylamide (LSD)
      2) Phencyclidine (PCP)
      3) Cannabis (marijuana)

b. Dextromethorphan: common ingredient in cold medicines
c. Alcohol
   1) Alcoholic hallucinosis
   2) Korsakoff's syndrome
d. Amphetamine psychosis
e. Medical treatment
   1) Digitalis toxicity
4. THE HALLUCINATIONS OR DELUSIONS ARE THE DIRECT PHYSIOLOGICAL RESULT OF SUBSTANCE WITHDRAWAL.
   a. Alcohol: beer, wine, liquor
   b. Sedatives or barbiturates

D. PSYCHOTIC DISORDER DUE TO A MEDICAL CONDITION
   1. HALLUCINATIONS OR DELUSIONS ARE THE RESULT OF THE PHYSICAL EFFECTS OF A MEDICAL CONDITION.
      a. Sleep or sensory deprivation
      b. Endocrine imbalance
         1) Steroid psychosis
         2) Thyrotoxicosis
      c. Neurologic diseases
      d. Infection
      e. Fever
      f. Toxins

E. PSYCHOSIS RELATED TO MAJOR DEPRESSIVE EPISODE
   1. PRESENCE OF DELUSIONS OR (USUALLY) PERSECUTORY AUDITORY HALLUCINATIONS
   2. DELUSIONS AND HALLUCINATIONS (USUALLY) CONSISTENT WITH DEPRESSION (E.G., GUILT, PUNISHMENT, ILLNESS, DESTRUCTION)

F. PSYCHOSIS RELATED TO MANIC EPISODE
   1. PRESENCE OF DELUSIONS OR GENERALLY PERSECUTORY AUDITORY HALLUCINATIONS
   2. DELUSIONS AND HALLUCINATIONS GENERALLY CONSISTENT WITH MANIC THEMES SUCH AS SPECIAL MISSION FROM GOD, PERSECUTION RELATED TO HAVING SPECIAL GIFTS OR RELATIONSHIP

G. DELUSIONAL DISORDER
   1. DESCRIPTION
      a. Disorder that involves nonbizarre delusions for a period of at least 1 month
      b. Most common among 40- to 55-year-olds
      c. Onset is any time during adolescence to old age.
      d. Etiology is not clearly identified.
   2. ASSESSMENT
      a. Delusions are nonbizarre.
      b. There are no other psychiatric clinical manifestations.
      c. Individuals display normal behavior except when they are focusing on their delusion.
      d. When the delusion is affecting the individual, she displays an irritable mood, anger, potentially violent behavior, and social and marital problems.
      e. The delusion is usually not eliminated, but the individual is able to contain the effects of the delusion in her personal life.
   3. NURSING INTERVENTIONS (SEE TABLE 52-5)
      a. Initiate cognitive therapy.
      b. Provide supportive therapy.
      c. Discuss the impact of the delusion on the client's life.
      d. Promote coping enhancement.
      e. Assist in setting realistic goals.
      f. Instruct the client on the effects of the delusion on life and on others.

PRACTICE QUESTIONS

1. Because a hospitalized client is disoriented and actively psychotic, plans for nursing intervention should include
   1. requests that the client interact with peers.
   2. encouraging the client to participate in unit programs.
   3. reality orientation.
   4. involvement in the milieu.

2. Which of the following interventions should the nurse include when caring for a client with delusions?
   Select all that apply:
   [ ] 1. Orient the client to date, time, place, and situation
   [ ] 2. Avoid whispering or laughing in front of the client

[ ] 3. Decrease environmental stimulation with low lighting, low noise level, and decrease activity around the client

[ ] 4. Avoid touching the client without asking for permission

[ ] 5. Initiate cognitively motivating activities

[ ] 6. Provide animal-assisted recreation

3. A client diagnosed with schizophrenia is displaying a flat affect, slowed thinking, and a lack of motivation. The nurse interprets these as which of the following?
   1. Delusions
   2. Positive symptoms
   3. Hallucinations
   4. Negative symptoms

4. Which of the following descriptions of the dopamine hypothesis should the nurse include when educating another nurse about the causes of schizophrenia?
   1. The kidneys cause excessive amounts of dopamine in the body that the kidneys do not readily excrete
   2. There is an excess of dopamine found at the synaptic clefts in the brain
   3. Too little dopamine in the brain causes hallucinations
   4. Abnormal levels of dopamine cause structural brain abnormalities

5. The family of a client with schizophrenia asks the nurse what the brain imaging study ordered for the client is most likely to find. The most appropriate response by the nurse is which of the following?
   1. "It would most likely find an absent frontal cortex."
   2. "It would most likely find abnormal auditory and optical nerves."
   3. "It would most likely find overactivity in the center of creativity."
   4. "It would most likely find enlarged lateral and third ventricles."

6. The family of a 25-year-old female client asks the nurse if any of the family members are at risk to get schizophrenia. The nurse anticipates that which of the following individuals is most likely to also suffer from schizophrenia?
   1. The younger brother
   2. The older sister
   3. The monozygotic twin
   4. The 50-year-old maternal aunt

7. Which of the following is the priority nursing intervention in the plan of care for a client with catatonic schizophrenia?
   1. Introduce the client to the other clients
   2. Begin obtaining the client's history
   3. Give the client the prescribed drugs
   4. Settle the client in the room

8. A public health nurse is providing case management for a client who has chronic paranoid schizophrenia. Which of the following is the most appropriate goal for this client? The client will
   1. take public transportation to go shopping.
   2. obtain and hold down a steady job.
   3. attend appointments with health care providers.
   4. socialize with neighbors on a daily basis.

9. A client recently hospitalized for schizophrenia has just returned back to a group home. Although the client's hallucinations have resolved, negative symptoms of schizophrenia continue. Based on this assessment, the nurse should monitor the client for which of the following negative clinical manifestations? Select all that apply:
   [ ] 1. Anhedonia
   [ ] 2. Failure to socialize
   [ ] 3. Smiling
   [ ] 4. Strong desire to resume work
   [ ] 5. Alogia
   [ ] 6. Daily hygiene practices

10. A client with acute psychosis is being evaluated in the emergency room to determine the need for hospitalization. During the initial interview, the client became mute and unable to move out of the chair. The nurse appropriately documents this behavior as what type of schizophrenia?
   1. Catatonic schizophrenia
   2. Disorganized schizophrenia
   3. Disorganized schizophrenia
   4. Residual schizophrenia

11. What are the chronic clinical manifestations for the medical complications of schizophrenia? Select all that apply:
   [ ] 1. Weight gain
   [ ] 2. Immobility
   [ ] 3. Generalized edema
   [ ] 4. Hyponatremia
   [ ] 5. Purposeless movements
   [ ] 6. Activity that is unrelated to external stimuli

12. The nurse caring for a client with schizophrenia evaluates which of the following behaviors as an idea of influence?
   1. The belief that a radio can control someone's thoughts
   2. Inability to identify person, place, and time
   3. Confusion that worsens to the point of delirium
   4. Interpreting a shadow as a person

13. The nurse administers which of the following prescribed drugs for the purpose of relieving

both the positive and negative clinical manifestations of schizophrenia?
1. Selective serotonin reuptake inhibitor
2. Dopaminergic
3. Anxiolytic
4. Sedative

14. The nurse is reviewing the chart of a client who was recently diagnosed with schizophrenia following graduation from college and notices that the date coincides with the date of the client's mother's diagnosis of schizophrenia. The nurse evaluates the major risk factor contributing to the development of schizophrenia in this client as
1. a recent search for employment.
2. being from a low socioeconomic class.
3. the mother's genetics at the time of diagnosis.
4. being recently divorced.

15. The nurse is caring for a client with schizophrenia who is experiencing delusions. Which of the following nursing diagnoses would be appropriate?
1. Impaired verbal communication
2. Ineffective role performance
3. Disturbed thought processes
4. Disturbed sensory perception

16. A newly married client is delusional and believes that his partner is having an affair with the next door neighbor. Which of the following is the priority that will lead the nurse to expect that these delusions will incapacitate this man?
1. He will be consumed by his thoughts
2. He will predominantly be affected at work
3. These beliefs will not have any effect on him
4. These beliefs will affect his social relationships

17. A well-known substance user is brought to the emergency department at 0200 by the probation officer (P.O.). The P.O. is concerned because the client has been threatening peers with a knife and accusing them of having an affair with the client's partner. While making the assessment, the nurse understands that psychosis is most likely related to
1. using methamphetamine tonight.
2. marijuana use 2 days ago.
3. use of alcohol over the last week.
4. use of a friend's tranquilizers.

18. A nurse using the downtown transportation system in a large city sees a homeless woman sitting on a park bench. The woman is talking to herself and frequently looks over to the empty space on the bench beside her. What is the best explanation for this situation?
1. The woman is experiencing auditory and visual hallucinations

2. The woman is lonely because she is homeless
3. She was speaking on her cell phone by using the headset
4. She was calling to her friend down the street

19. The nurse working in an adult inpatient psychiatric unit is admitting a client recently diagnosed with schizophrenia. The nurse notices that this client is constantly drinking water. Which of the following interventions is a priority for this client?
1. Monitor intake and output
2. Obtain serum sodium and potassium levels
3. Restrict the client's oral intake
4. Educate the client about a low-sodium diet

20. A client with chronic schizophrenia is experiencing polydispia and polyuria and begins to complain of nausea and muscle cramps. The nurse should report this as a clinical manifestation of psychogenic polydipsia when the client drinks greater than how many liters a day? _____

21. A client who belongs to a familial religious sect reports seeing "visions." Neither the client nor the family are concerned. The nurse understands that which of the following explanations accounts for the lack of concern about this visualization?
1. The client is not convinced of the religious sect
2. The family believes that the client made it up
3. Cultural variations of spiritual beliefs exist
4. This is the first time "visions" have been seen

22. Knowing that it is difficult to establish trust with a client experiencing delusions, the nurse who is taking care of a client with delusional disorder should initiate conversation by saying which of the following?
1. "What happened to make you come here?"
2. "What is bothering you right now?"
3. "I'm your nurse; tell me if you need something."
4. "The other clients want to meet you."

23. The registered nurse on a psychiatric unit is making clinical assignments. Which of the following assignments should the nurse delegate to a licensed practical nurse?
1. Plan the medication schedule for a client with schizophrenia
2. Instruct a client with schizophrenia on the anxiolytic
3. Document the description of the hallucinations a client is experiencing
4. Discuss with a client's family the treatment plan for the client

24. A client's family asks the nurse what the primary reason is for conducting a physical exam as part of the diagnostic process for a psychiatric client. Which of the following is the most appropriate response? "The physical exam is performed to
    1. "rule out any medical causes for the psychiatric clinical manifestations."
    2. "determine functional status."
    3. "replace the mental status exam."
    4. "test the client's perception of what is happening."

25. A client is admitted to a medical-surgical unit with an infection of the right great toe and temperature of 38.9°C (102°F). The client appears to be becoming psychotic. In determining what action to take next, which of the following factors should the nurse consider?

    1. The client is having an acute onset of dementia
    2. The client was postictal
    3. The client's circadian rhythm is unsynchronized
    4. The client is psychotic because of the infection

26. A client with a bipolar disorder is brought to the emergency department by the spouse after the client pointed a steak knife at the spouse and yelled, "I know that you are jealous of my special gifts from God!" The nurse informs the spouse that this behavior is most likely explained by which of the following? The client
    1. cannot handle the marital discord.
    2. is becoming demented.
    3. became psychotic during a manic phase.
    4. wants to kill the spouse.

ANSWERS AND RATIONALES

1. 3. Requesting a client who is disoriented and psychotic to interact with peers, participate in unit programs, or encourage involvement in the milieu would agitate the client. Reality orientation would orient the client to the surroundings.

2. 1. 2. 4. Interventions for a client in the treatment of delusions include orienting the client to date, time, place, and situation. Decrease the client's anxiety by avoiding whispering or laughing in front of the client, and avoid touching the client without permission. In hallucination management, an intervention is to decrease environmental stimulation with low lighting, low noise level, and decreased activity surrounding the client. Interventions for environmental management are to initiate cognitively motivating activities and provide animal-assisted recreation.

3. 4. Negative clinical manifestations of schizophrenia are much harder to detect and describe than are positive clinical manifestations. The negative clinical manifestations, such as flattened affect, slowed thinking, and lack of motivation, are observed and in many ways are more debilitating. Unlike positive clinical manifestations, negative clinical manifestations are behaviors not fundamentally different from behaviors exhibited by many people. They are more common and severe in schizophrenia. They are particularly obvious when contrasted to how the client was before the onset of the disorder. Delusions and hallucinations are positive clinical manifestations because they must be self-reported by the client.

4. 2. Although the etiology of schizophrenia remains unknown, there is research suggesting the validity of the dopamine hypothesis—that the functional abnormalities in schizophrenia are the result of excessive amounts of the dopamine in the brain. Normally dopamine is produced in the brain and functions as a neurotransmitter.

5. 4. Computerized tomography scanning may be used to evaluate brain structure in schizophrenic clients. The results have shown that clients with schizophrenia have larger lateral ventricles than nonschizophrenic individuals. This is a well-documented fact, but the meaning behind this finding remains unclear. It remains unknown as to whether the enlargement is the cause or a consequence of the schizophrenia. It also has no bearing on the severity of the clinical manifestations. Some data demonstrate that the ventricular enlargement is related to cerebral atrophy. Although speculative, there is some research suggesting that schizophrenia may be a degenerative neurological disorder.

6. 3. Schizophrenia is a disorder that has a large genetic component. This conclusion has been reached based on the close incidence of schizophrenia in twins and particularly monozygotic twins, which have a higher concordance rate than any other biological relationship. Although genetics plays a role in the development of schizophrenia, the relationship remains unclear. Some studies indicate that this relationship may be as high as 50%, but other studies indicate that a monozygotic twin has less than a 10% chance of developing schizophrenia when the other twin is affected.

7. 4. Catatonic schizophrenia is a type of schizophrenia in which there is a marked decrease in reactivity to the environment. The client will not likely be able to socialize or adequately communicate secondary to the catatonia. Although administering prescribed drugs may be appropriate, it is not the priority. Decreasing the stimuli in the client's environment is the priority. The client with catatonia will be less stimulated in the client's room.

8. 3. A function of case management is to coordinate the client's health care needs. The priority goal for a client with paranoid schizophrenia is to encourage the client to regularly attend all the scheduled appointments with health care providers. Although taking public transportation, maintaining a steady job, or socializing with the neighbors may be appropriate interventions, they are not the priority. Clients with paranoid schizophrenia are likely to be socially isolated and have few trusting relationships.

9. 1. 2. 5. Anhedonia, alogia, and a failure to socialize are all negative clinical manifestations seen in schizophrenia. Anhedonia is the inability to find enjoyment in daily activities. Alogia is a tendency to speak very little or use short, empty phrases.

10. 1. Catatonia is a state in which there is a large decrease in reactivity to the environment. An extreme degree of immobility and unawareness may result.

11. 1. 3. 4. Chronic clinical manifestations of the medical complications of schizophrenia include weight gain, generalized edema, and hyponatremia. Catatonic schizophrenia clinical manifestations include immobility. Clinical manifestations of agitated motor activity are purposeless movements and activity that is unrelated to external stimuli.

12. 1. An idea of influence is a client's false impression that outside activities have a unique meaning for the client. It is an internal thought regarding some content in which the client's thoughts are controlled by an external entity. The client's inability to identify person, place, and time, as well as the client's confusion to the point of delirium, is related to the client's orientation. Interpreting a shadow as a person is an illusion that is an incorrect perception of a sensory stimulus.

13. 2. Dopamine has been specifically identified as having an influence on both the positive and negative clinical manifestations of schizophrenia. Selective serotonin reuptake inhibitors treat depression. Anxiolytics treat anxiety, and sedatives are calming agents.

14. 3. The mother's genetics at the time of diagnosis of schizophrenia is the major risk factor for the client diagnosed with schizophrenia. Being recently divorced, from a lower socioeconomic status, and a recent search for employment are all environmental influences.

15. 3. Delusions are false ideas that an individual believes to be real despite evidence to the contrary. They are disturbed thought processes, so a nursing diagnosis of disturbed thought processes would be appropriate. A nursing diagnosis of disturbed role performance would be appropriate with a loss of function. Impaired verbal communication would be an appropriate nursing diagnosis for a clinical manifestation of incomprehensible language. Hallucinations are a sensory perception for which there is no reality, and disturbed sensory perception would be an appropriate nursing diagnosis.

16. 4. Paranoid delusions are disturbances in thought processes that generally affect only an individual's social relationships. They do not predominantly impact the work environment or daily functioning.

17. 1. Methamphetamine causes psychosis and is the most recent drug that was abused by the client, so it would be the most plausible explanation for the behavior. Current use of alcohol may cause psychosis but not alcohol taken a week ago. Marijuana used 2 days ago and use of tranquilizers are both unlikely to cause psychosis.

18. 1. About 30% of the homeless suffer from schizophrenia. The woman is showing signs of responding to internal stimuli. Auditory and visual hallucinations are precipitated by internal stimuli. Speaking on a cell phone and calling to a friend down the street are both external stimuli.

19. 2. Although monitoring the intake and output may be an appropriate intervention, it is not the priority intervention, because the client is a new admission and the electrolyte levels need to be monitored first to determine if any other nursing interventions are necessary. Educating the client about a low-sodium diet may also be an appropriate intervention but is not the priority. The client's oral intake should not be restricted unless there is a medical reason to do so.

20.   3. Psychogenic polydipsia is a major cause of death among clients who have schizophrenia. Polyuria, polydipsia, nausea, and muscle cramps are classic features of psychogenic polydipsia.

21. 3. Culture variations that exist among spiritual beliefs in family and friends are the most plausible explanation for a lack of concern over seeing "visions."

22. 3. Telling a client who is experiencing delusions that you are the nurse provides the least

threatening approach to initiate conversation. The client is most likely experiencing some paranoia along with the delusional content. Asking a client what happened to cause the visit to the hospital has an accusatory tone. Asking what is bothering the client is too intrusive for an initial stage of establishing trust. Telling the client that the other clients want to meet the client is perceived as a socially uncomfortable situation for someone who is experiencing paranoia.

23. 3. A licensed practical nurse may document the hallucinations a client is experiencing. Planning a medication schedule, instructing a client on a drug, and discussing a treatment plan with a client's family are all activities that should be performed by a registered nurse.

24. 1. A physical examination is a necessary part of the initial assessment for a client diagnosed to be a psychiatric client, because many clinical manifestations that appear to be psychiatric in nature may in actuality have a medical etiology. Any medical cause must be ruled out before making a definitive psychiatric diagnosis. A physical exam cannot determine functional status. A physical exam cannot replace the mental status exam. Testing the client's perception of what is happening is not the primary reason for conducting a physical exam.

25. 4. An infection may contribute to a client's distortion of perceptual reality. Dementia does not have an acute onset. There is no evidence that the client had a seizure. It is unlikely that an infection would make someone psychotic.

26. 3. A client may become psychotic during a manic phase of a bipolar disorder. Not handling marital discord and wanting to kill one's spouse do not most likely correlate with a manic episode. Dementia has a slow onset and usually appears in an older client.

REFERENCES

Antai-Otong, D. (2008). *Psychiatric nursing, biological and behavioral concepts* (2nd ed.). Clifton Park, NY: Delmar Cengage Learning.

Frisch, N. C., & Frisch, L. E. (2011). *Psychiatric mental health nursing* (4th ed.). Clifton Park, NY: Delmar Cengage Learning.

CHAPTER 53

PARANOID DISORDERS

I. **PARANOID DISORDERS**
   A. DESCRIPTION
      1. DISORDERS IN WHICH THE CLIENT EXHIBITS A MISTRUST AND A SUSPICIOUSNESS OF OTHERS
      2. THE CLIENT IS OFTEN MISUNDERSTOOD AND JUDGED TO BE OBSTINATE, DEFENSIVE, AND HOSTILE.
   B. ASSESSMENT
      1. FEELINGS OF GRANDIOSITY
      2. PERSECUTORY BEHAVIOR
      3. DISTORTED REALITY
   C. NURSING DIAGNOSES
      1. ANXIETY
      2. INEFFECTIVE DENIAL
      3. DEFENSIVE COPING
      4. RISK FOR VIOLENCE OTHER-DIRECTED
      5. INEFFECTIVE COPING
      6. SOCIAL ISOLATION
      7. IMPAIRED ADJUSTMENT

   Nursing Diagnoses: Definitions and Classification 2012–2014.
   Copyright © 2012, 1994–2012 by NANDA International.
   Used by arrangement with John Wiley & Sons Limited.

   D. TYPES OF PARANOID DISORDERS
      1. PARANOID SCHIZOPHRENIA
         a. Description
            1) Devastating disorder affecting an individual's thinking, language, emotions, ability to perceive reality, and social behavior
            2) Predominant features are delusions and hallucinations.
            3) The average age of onset is in late adolescence or early adulthood.
         b. Theories (See Chapter 52.)
         c. Assessment
            1) Persecutory delusions: preoccupation with one or more untrue beliefs
            2) Auditory hallucinations
            3) Disturbed ability to achieve education, work, and maintain relationships
            4) Social isolation
            5) Unable to establish trust
            6) Argumentative
            7) Anger and potential violence
            8) Threatened safety of self and others
            9) Anxiety
         d. Assessment (See Chapter 52, Section I.)
         e. Nursing interventions (See Chapter 52, Table 52-5.)
      2. PARANOID DELUSIONAL DISORDER
         a. Description: disorder in which there is paranoia or persecutory delusions (fixed false beliefs)
         b. Assessment
            1) Belief or paranoia that the person or loved ones are singled out for being victimized, such as being watched by the Federal Bureau of Investigation (FBI), being followed, or being plotted against
            2) Feelings of being conspired against, spied or cheated on, poisoned or drugged, and harassed
            3) Often ends up in court to rectify issues that are caused by the person's belief that others are intentionally harassing him
            4) No hallucinations
            5) Uses denial as a defense mechanism
            6) Ideas of reference (things in the environment are taken personally)
            7) Lack of trust
            8) Irritable
            9) Angry or violent
         c. Nursing interventions
            1) Instruct the client on relaxation techniques, such as visual imagery, deep breathing, and progressive muscle relaxation.

2) Instruct the client on calming techniques, such as soothing music, warm milk, prayer, meditation, or going for a walk.

3) Encourage recreational games or cooperative sports.

4) Encourage individual counseling.

5) Identify stressors and responses to those stressors.

6) Use distractions.

7) Assist the client to develop a self-awareness of delusional thoughts.

8) Encourage identification of feelings.

9) Assist the client to develop new ways to change problematic behavior.

10) Encourage the client to journal feelings.

11) Promote resiliency such as connectedness to a trusted adult or a spiritual belief system.

12) Provide emotional support.

13) Actively listen to the client's concerns.

14) Enhance coping by facilitation of meditation and relaxation.

15) Assist the client to develop a support system.

16) Ensure safety for the client and others.

17) Provide opportunity for the development of problem-solving skills.

18) Promote a sense of trust by maintaining eye contact with the client.

3. PARANOID PERSONALITY DISORDER
  a. Description
    1) A sense of distrust and suspiciousness in others; perceive their motives as malevolent
    2) More common in men
    3) Develops early in adolescence and early adulthood
  b. Theories
    1) Biological
      a) Genetic predisposition: more common in families with persecutory delusional disorders and chronic schizophrenia; excess of limbic and sympathetic system reactivity with an acceleration of synaptic activity; not a result of a medical condition
    2) Environmental
      a) One's experiences contribute to its development.

c. Assessment
  1) Is highly suspicious of others and finds hidden meanings
  2) Mistrusts others, including friends and relatives
  3) Believes others are exploiting him
  4) Extreme jealousy over his partner
  5) Doubts the fidelity of his partner
  6) Questions the loyalty of others
  7) Suspects others' motives
  8) Hypersensitive and hypervigilant
  9) Misperceives criticism from others
  10) Blames others for his difficulties
  11) Unable to confide in others
  12) Becomes easily angered or has a lack of humor
  13) Holds grudges persistently
  14) Avoids relationships, especially those in which he feels lack of control
  15) Rigid, with a need to be in control
  16) Sense of self-importance
  17) Nervousness
  18) Lack of social support systems
  19) Delusional thinking
  20) Uses projection as a defense mechanism
  21) Very private

d. Nursing interventions
  1) Remove dangerous objects from the client's environment.
  2) Identify stressors and the responses to those stressors.
  3) Provide counseling.
  4) Foster trust with the client.
  5) Actively listen to the client's concerns.
  6) Provide assistance in utilizing anger control techniques.
  7) Encourage anxiety reduction and relaxation exercises.
  8) Identify impulsive thoughts and behaviors.
  9) Encourage new coping strategies.

4. PARANOIA FROM SUBSTANCE WITHDRAWAL
  a. Assessment
    1) Amphetamines
      a) Paranoia
      b) Restlessness and agitation
      c) Decreased or increased sleep
      d) Exhaustion
      e) Disorientation
      f) Depression and suicidal thoughts
    2) Cocaine and crack cocaine
      a) See assessment section for amphetamines.

b) Increased appetite
c) Drug cravings
3) Alcohol
   a) Tremors or seizures, or both
   b) Tachycardia and hypertension
   c) Decreased appetite
   d) Disorientation
   e) Decreased sleep
   f) Delusions
   g) Visual hallucinations

b. Nursing interventions for substance withdrawal
1) Monitor vital signs.
2) Monitor for suicidal thoughts.
3) Ensure a nonstimulating environment.
4) Encourage rest and sleep, if possible.
5) Remain with the client if disoriented.
6) Promote reality orientation.

PRACTICE QUESTIONS

1. The wife of a client with paranoid personality disorder asks the nurse why the client keeps blaming her for plotting against him. Which of the following is the appropriate response by the nurse?
   1. "A client with paranoid personality disorder suspects others' motives."
   2. "A client with paranoid personality disorder prefers solitary activities."
   3. "A client with paranoid personality disorder lacks interests or hobbies."
   4. "A client with paranoid personality disorder is emotionally detached."

2. A client diagnosed with paranoid personality disorder has been hospitalized because of his suspicions and threats toward the company boss. While in the hospital, the client continues to be suspicious of the nursing staff. The primary goal for this client would be which of the following?
   1. Inform the client that the boss has no harmful intentions
   2. Promote the development of trust with the nursing staff
   3. Educate the client about the legal risks of harming the boss
   4. Convince the client of the true motives of the nurses

3. Two staff members are talking and laughing about their weekend activities in the hall outside the room of a client diagnosed with paranoid personality disorder. The client appears annoyed and is suspicious of them while they are talking. Which of the following is the most appropriate intervention?
   1. Encourage the client to engage in the conversation
   2. Report the staff members' inappropriate behavior
   3. Inform the staff members that the talking can be misinterpreted as secretiveness
   4. Close the door to the client's room

4. An important role of the nurse is to facilitate social interactions between a client who is paranoid and the client's peers. The nurse implements this intervention based on the understanding that a client with paranoid personality disorder
   1. is gregarious and outgoing in socialization style.
   2. tends to exhibit loose boundaries when sharing feelings.
   3. likes to be around large groups of people.
   4. tends to be isolated and lacks social skills.

5. The nurse monitors for which of the following assessment findings in a client with paranoid personality disorder?
   Select all that apply:
   [ ] 1. Is highly suspicious of others and finds hidden meanings
   [ ] 2. Persecutory delusions
   [ ] 3. Belief or paranoia that the person or loved ones are singled out or being victimized, such as being watched by the FBI, being followed, or being plotted against
   [ ] 4. Mistrusts others, including friend and relatives
   [ ] 5. Feelings of being conspired against, spied or cheated on, poisoned or drugged, or harassed
   [ ] 6. Believes others are exploiting him

6. Which of the following assessment finds are common in paranoia from substance withdrawal from amphetamines?
   Select all that apply:
   [ ] 1. Increased appetite
   [ ] 2. Paranoia
   [ ] 3. Tremors or seizures
   [ ] 4. Tachycardia or hypertension
   [ ] 5. Restlessness and agitation
   [ ] 6. Disorientation

7. The nurse assesses for what characteristics in a client suspected of having paranoid schizophrenia?
   Select all that apply:
   [ ] 1. A sense of distrust and suspiciousness in others; perceives their motives to be malevolent
   [ ] 2. Devastating disorder affecting an individual's thinking, language, emotions, ability to perceive reality, and social behavior
   [ ] 3. Predominant features are delusions and hallucinations
   [ ] 4. Ideas of reference
   [ ] 5. Average age of onset is late adolescence or early adulthood
   [ ] 6. Angry or violent

8. When planning the care of a client who is paranoid, the nurse should include which of the following interventions to increase the sense of trust?
   1. Give the client the nurse's home phone number for support
   2. Spend more time with this client than with other clients
   3. Solicit the client's participation in the development of the treatment plan
   4. Fulfill all of the client's requests to provide assurance of active listening

9. Which of the following interventions would be most appropriate for the nurse to implement for a client in a paranoid state who is having difficulty falling asleep and has tried reading, taking a warm bath, and drinking warm milk, all of which have been unsuccessful?
   1. Instruct the client to try all of these again but for a longer time
   2. Administer a prescribed drug for relaxation
   3. Offer the client a back rub
   4. Encourage the client to listen to the radio

10. A client experiencing paranoid behavior believes that the drugs are poisonous and doesn't want to take them. Which of the following nursing interventions should the nurse include in this client's plan of care?
    1. Administer the drugs intravenously if the client refuses to take them orally
    2. Tell the client that taking the drugs are a part of the treatment
    3. Restrict the client to the room until the client agrees to take the drugs
    4. Inform the client that the doctor ordered the drugs and they are necessary

11. The nurse should instruct a client with paranoid delusions to avoid which of the following beverages?

Select all that apply:
   [ ] 1. Coffee
   [ ] 2. Ginger ale
   [ ] 3. Lemonade
   [ ] 4. Whole milk
   [ ] 5. Cola
   [ ] 6. Chocolate milkshake

12. Which of the following does the nurse evaluate as a disturbance in the activities of daily living for a client who is paranoid? The client
    1. goes to the grocery store only when more food is needed.
    2. signs up for the Meals on Wheels service.
    3. refuses to eat any food item that is not prepackaged and can be self-opened.
    4. goes over to the neighbor's house for dinner once a week on Friday evenings.

13. A client who has been diagnosed with paranoid delusions frequently takes issues to the legal system, resulting in court hearings. This is most likely due to the fact that
    1. the client initiates legal action due to the persecutory content of the delusions.
    2. other individuals are taking the client to court because of the client's poor decisions.
    3. the client has often been taken advantage of by other individuals.
    4. the client doesn't know how else to get the attention of individuals who hurt the client.

14. A client who has paranoid delusional disorder has been having spousal difficulties but is making good progress at work during this quarter. The nurse identifies which of the following as the most likely cause of the client's behavior?
    1. The client is projecting frustrated energy into work
    2. The client would rather be at work than at home
    3. The client's paranoia causes worry about the work situation
    4. The client's delusions mainly affect relationships

15. A client who has been diagnosed with paranoid delusional disorder is developing healthier interpersonal relationships. During this development, the nurse encourages the client to
    1. identify people with whom it is safe to talk.
    2. talk about the delusions whenever they occur.
    3. remember the paranoid thoughts until the next therapy session.
    4. seek feedback regarding the realistic nature of the delusion.

16. A client is diagnosed with paranoid schizophrenia and has been hospitalized due to auditory hallucinations resulting in verbal threats. These hallucinations are of a persecutory nature. Which of the following is the most appropriate nursing diagnosis?
    1. Noncompliance
    2. Health maintenance, ineffective
    3. Personal identity, disturbed
    4. Sensory perception, disturbed

17. A nurse teaching a class on paranoid personality disorder correctly describes the client as appearing angry and argumentative, but in reality the client feels
    1. shy and awkward.
    2. vulnerable and powerless.
    3. depressed and suicidal.
    4. secure and confident.

18. A client is being evaluated for headaches and paranoid delusions. A computerized tomography (CT) scan reveals a brain tumor. The diagnosis of paranoid delusional disorder is in question at this point because the
    1. clinical manifestations present along with a medical condition.
    2. client is only suspicious of the physician.
    3. client is not experiencing any hallucinations.
    4. clinical manifestations really aren't delusions.

19. A nurse has worked to establish a relationship with a client who has been diagnosed with paranoid personality disorder. It has been difficult to make any progress based on what classic features of the client's thought pattern?
    Select all that apply:
    [ ] 1. Auditory hallucinations
    [ ] 2. Social isolation
    [ ] 3. Sense of distrust
    [ ] 4. Suspiciousness in others
    [ ] 5. Argumentative
    [ ] 6. Perceives other's motives are malevolent

20. A client with paranoid schizophrenia has been seeing a public health nurse every week for drug administration and compliance. The current drugs have been effective in decreasing positive clinical manifestations. The nurse anticipates that the client will report
    1. a decrease in motivation to go to church.
    2. a week without hearing voices.
    3. seeing his dead grandmother.
    4. a schedule that has become very busy with social outings.

21. Which of the following interventions should the nurse include in a plan of care for a client with paranoid personality disorder?
    Select all that apply:
    [ ] 1. Remove dangerous objects from the client's environment
    [ ] 2. Identify impulsive thoughts and behaviors
    [ ] 3. Instruct the client on relaxation techniques such as visual imagery, deep breathing, and progressive muscle relaxation
    [ ] 4. Encourage recreational games or cooperative sports
    [ ] 5. Provide assistance in utilizing anger control techniques
    [ ] 6. Provide opportunity for the development of problem-solving skills

22. The registered nurse is preparing to delegate nursing tasks to a licensed practical nurse. Which of the following tasks should the nurse delegate to a licensed practical nurse?
    1. Evaluate a client suspected of having paranoid schizophrenia for delusions
    2. Document a client's paranoid behavior
    3. Assess a client with paranoia for auditory hallucinations
    4. Instruct a client's family on the clinical features of paranoid schizophrenia

23. Which of the following is a priority goal for the nurse to plan in the care of a client who experiences paranoid delusions?
    1. Absence of delusions
    2. Establishment of trust
    3. Participation in all unit activities
    4. Independent activities of daily living

24. A client who suffers from paranoid delusions utilizes denial as a defense mechanism. The nurse wants to foster other ways of dealing with the anxiety that the client experiences. The nurse could best do this by planning for the client to be involved in which of the following activities?
    1. Community mental health support group
    2. Psychodynamic group therapy
    3. Adult education class on emotions
    4. Individualized relaxation therapy

25. A client who has been diagnosed with paranoid delusional disorder is getting ready for an evening discharge. This client has a history of expressing anger by threatening to hurt family members with household objects. In preparation for discharge, the nurse should instruct the family that which of the following is a priority if the client becomes threatening?

1. Call the client's health care provider in the morning
2. Encourage the client to go to a quiet room to cool down
3. Remove any potential weapons from the home
4. Administer an extra dose of a prescribed drug when the anger surfaces

26. In preparation for practicing new coping skills, the nurse assists the client with paranoia in
   1. asking for the physician's methods.
   2. copying other clients' techniques.
   3. learning by reading books.
   4. identifying personal manifestations of anxiety.

ANSWERS AND RATIONALES

1. 1. Suspicion of others is a hallmark of paranoid personality disorder. Preferring solitary activities, lacking interest in hobbies or other interests, and becoming emotionally detached are all clinical manifestations of an individual with schizoid personality disorder.

2. 2. Promoting the development of trust with the nursing staff is the best goal for a client who is experiencing paranoia. This will support and encourage the client to make better progress in treatment and begin to trust the staff.

3. 3. Behavior that can be interpreted as secretive by a client who is paranoid will reinforce the client's feelings of suspiciousness. A client who is paranoid may interpret seeing two staff members talking outside the client's room as being secretive.

4. 4. A client with paranoid personality disorder often becomes socially isolated because of suspiciousness toward others. This client would not be gregarious or outgoing. Such clients do not feel that they have a problem. A client who suffers from paranoia would not have social skills that would be enhanced by being around or sharing with others.

5. 1. 4. 6. Assessment findings for paranoid personality disorder include highly suspicious of others; finds hidden meanings; mistrusts others, including friends and relatives; and believes others are exploiting him. Assessment findings include belief or paranoia that the person or loved ones are singled out for being victimized, such as being watched by the FBI, being followed, or being plotted against. Assessment findings for paranoid schizophrenia include persecutory delusions.

6. 2. 5. 6. Assessment findings in amphetamine withdrawal include paranoia, restlessness and agitation, and disorientation. Increased appetite is an assessment finding for cocaine and crack cocaine withdrawal. Tremors or seizures and tachycardia and hypertension are assessment finding for alcohol withdrawal.

7. 2. 3. 5. Features of paranoid schizophrenia include that it is a devastating disorder affecting an individual's thinking, language, emotions, ability to perceive reality, and social behavior. Paranoid schizophrenia has an average age of onset in late adolescence or early adulthood and is characterized by delusions and hallucinations. Features of paranoid personality disorder include a sense of distrust and suspiciousness toward others and perceiving the motives of others as malevolent. Ideas of reference and being angry or violent are features of paranoid delusional disorder.

8. 3. Soliciting a client's participation in the development of the treatment plan is an effective way to get a client who is paranoid to improve communication and participation in the treatment plan and to develop a trusting relationship. Giving a client a home phone number or spending more time with this client than with other clients violates professional boundaries. Fulfilling all of the client's requests can cause the client to become more suspicious.

9. 2. After unsuccessful attempts to sleep, as evidenced by reading, drinking milk, or taking a warm bath, the next appropriate intervention would be to offer a prescribed drug for relaxation. It would be inappropriate to instruct the client to try these measures for a longer time period, to give the client a back rub, or to encourage the client to listen to the radio because the client has already tried nondrug-related measures and continues to be frustrated.

10. 2. The most appropriate intervention for a client who thinks the drugs are poisonous is to be direct with the client and tell the client that the drugs are an important part of the treatment. Forcing the client to take the drugs, restricting the client to the room until the drugs are taken, or informing the client that the doctor ordered the drugs would not work, because this is a suspicious client who will not respond to reason.

11. 1. 5. 6. A client who has paranoid delusions should be instructed to avoid caffeine-containing beverages because the stimulating effects of caffeine may contribute to feelings of paranoia and anxiety. Coffee, cola, and a chocolate milkshake all contain caffeine.

12. 3. A disturbance in the activities of daily living for a client who is paranoid is to refuse to eat any food that is not prepackaged and can be self-opened. A client with paranoia would not sign up for Meals on Wheels or go to a neighbor's house for dinner because the client did not prepare the food and may believe it is contaminated. Going to the grocery store when more food is needed is not an impairment to the activities of daily living.

13. 1. A client with persecutory delusions frequently initiates legal action because of the belief that others are attacking him. It is through the court actions that the client attempts to remedy these beliefs about the other individuals. Other individuals taking the client to court because of the client's poor decisions is focusing on the thoughts and actions of someone other than the client. The client being taken advantage of also focuses on the other individual's thoughts and actions, rather than the client's. A client with persecutory delusions is not trying to get attention; instead, the issue is about rectification for the perceived wrongs done to the client.

14. 4. Clients with delusional disorders can generally function adequately when they do not focus on their delusional belief system, which usually affects social and marital relationships. Because of this, the client would be able to manage adequately in the work environment.

15. 1. Establishment of trust and a safe relationship is important and difficult for the client who has paranoid delusions. Talking about the client's delusions whenever they occur, remembering the paranoid thoughts until the next therapy session, and seeking feedback regarding the realistic nature of the delusion all focus on the delusional thoughts.

16. 4. Hallucinations are, by definition, perceptual distortions and are not the result of deliberate choices. Therefore, the most appropriate nursing diagnosis is disturbed sensory perception. Nursing diagnoses of Noncompliance, Ineffective health maintenance, and Disturbed personal identity would all involve deliberate choices.

17. 2. Clients who have paranoid personality disorder use denial and projection as their main defense mechanisms, because in reality they feel vulnerable and powerless. Shy, awkward, depressed, suicidal, secure, and confident may co-occur with paranoia, although they do not explain the projection of insecurity into anger.

18. 1. Medical issues must be diagnosed and evaluated as a potential cause of clinical manifestations that may also appear psychiatric in nature.

19. 3. 4. 6. Mistrust and suspiciousness toward others and perceiving their motives as malevolent accompanies the paranoia found in paranoid personality disorder and becomes a barrier to establishing a client–provider relationship. Features of paranoid schizophrenia include auditory hallucinations, social isolation, and argumentative.

20. 2. A client who reports a week without hearing voices demonstrates a decrease in positive clinical manifestations. Lack of motivation is a negative clinical manifestation, and a decrease in the motivation to go to church would indicate no improvement in the client's condition. A client who sees his dead grandmother is having a positive clinical manifestation, clearly demonstrating that the client is still in the throes of paranoid schizophrenia. More social activities is a negative clinical manifestation, indicating an improvement in the client's condition.

21. 1. 2. 5. Nursing interventions for paranoid personality disorder include removing dangerous objects from the client's environment, providing assistance in utilizing anger control techniques, and identifying impulsive thoughts and behavior. Interventions for paranoid delusional disorder include instructing the client on relaxation techniques such as visual imagery, deep breathing, and progressive muscle relaxation; encouraging recreational games or cooperative sports; and providing opportunity for the development of problem-solving skills.

22. 2. Nursing tasks that involve the skills of evaluating, assessing, and instructing are reserved for the registered nurse. A licensed practical nurse may document a client's paranoid behavior.

23. 2. As with many psychiatric disorders, establishing trust is paramount to the success of the nurse–client therapeutic relationship.

24. 4. A client with paranoid delusions is most likely to deal with the anxiety in situations by getting involved in relaxation therapy. Attempting to get clients involved in group therapy or an education class would foster further paranoia because of the group environment.

25. 3. The first action to take when discharging a client who in the past threatened to hurt family members with household items would be to remove any potential weapons from the home. It would not be appropriate to wait to call the health care provider in the morning because the call is too delayed. It would not be particularly helpful for an agitated client to go to a quiet room to cool down. The client should not be unsupervised. Although an extra dose of a drug may be administered, it is not the priority.

26. 4. Before planning interventions for new coping skills for a client, the nurse needs to consider the client's manifestations of anxiety. Anxiety is a common emotion with paranoia. Asking the physician for other coping methods, copying other clients' techniques, and reading books all focus on sources other than the client. The focus should be on the client and the client's needs.

REFERENCES

Antai-Otong, D. (2008). *Psychiatric nursing, biological and behavioral concepts* (2nd ed.). Clifton Park, NY: Delmar Cengage Learning.

Frisch, N. C., & Frisch, L. E. (2011). *Psychiatric mental health nursing* (4th ed.). Clifton Park, NY: Delmar Cengage Learning.

CHAPTER 54

POST-TRAUMATIC STRESS DISORDERS

I. POST-TRAUMATIC STRESS DISORDERS

A. DESCRIPTION
1. DISORDER IN WHICH THE CLINICAL MANIFESTATIONS OCCUR AFTER WITNESSING A PERCEIVED OR ACTUAL TRAUMATIC EVENT TO SELF OR OTHERS, SUCH AS AN ACCIDENT, SHOOTING, FIRE, SEXUAL ASSAULT, EXPLOSION, BOMBING (E.G., 9/11/2001 TRAGEDY, OKLAHOMA CITY BOMBING)
2. CLASSIFIED AS AN ANXIETY DISORDER
3. RESPONSE IS FEAR, HELPLESSNESS, OR HORROR.
4. MAY BE EXPERIENCED BY CHILDREN, ADOLESCENTS, ADULTS, AND OLDER ADULTS
5. EXPERIENCED REGARDLESS OF RACE, SEX, AGE, CULTURE, OR SOCIOECONOMIC CLASS
6. CLINICAL MANIFESTATIONS MUST BE EXPERIENCED FOR GREATER THAN 1 MONTH.
7. MAY BE ASSOCIATED WITH ADDITIONAL RISK FACTORS SUCH AS SUBSTANCE ABUSE, DEPRESSION, SUICIDAL IDEATION, ANXIETY, AND PANIC ATTACKS

B. ASSESSMENT
1. REEXPERIENCING OF TRAUMATIC EVENT
   a. Flashbacks, illusions, or hallucinations of an event
   b. Nightmares
   c. Vivid memories or images
2. FEELINGS OF AVOIDANCE OF TRAUMATIC EVENT
   a. Feelings of numbness
   b. Inability to recall event
   c. Withdrawal from friends, family, and events
   d. Avoidance of events associated with the traumatic event
   e. Depression
3. BEHAVIORAL RESPONSES
   a. Difficulty staying or falling asleep
   b. Irritability
   c. Outbursts of anger
   d. Poor impulse control
   e. Difficulty concentrating
   f. Unpredictable behavior

C. TYPES
1. ACUTE POST-TRAUMATIC STRESS DISORDER: CLINICAL MANIFESTATIONS OCCUR GREATER THAN 1 MONTH AND LESS THAN 3 MONTHS AFTER THE EVENT.
2. CHRONIC POST-TRAUMATIC STRESS DISORDER: CLINICAL MANIFESTATIONS LAST 3 MONTHS OR MORE.
3. DELAYED POST-TRAUMATIC STRESS DISORDER: ONSET OF CLINICAL MANIFESTATIONS IS AT LEAST 6 MONTHS AFTER THE EVENT.

D. NURSING DIAGNOSES
1. ANXIETY
2. INEFFECTIVE COPING
3. DISTURBED THOUGHT PROCESSES
4. POWERLESSNESS
5. RISK FOR POST-TRAUMA SYNDROME
6. FEAR
7. DYSFUNCTIONAL GRIEVING
8. RISK FOR SELF-DIRECTED VIOLENCE
9. RAPE-TRAUMA SYNDROME

Nursing Diagnoses: Definitions and Classification 2012–2014. Copyright © 2012, 1994–2012 by NANDA International. Used by arrangement with John Wiley & Sons Limited.

E. MEDICAL MANAGEMENT
1. COGNITIVE BEHAVIORAL THERAPY (CBT)
2. DESENSITIZATION
3. PLAY THERAPY (FOR CHILDREN)

4. PSYCHOEDUCATION
5. PARENTAL INVOLVEMENT (FOR CHILDREN AND ADOLESCENTS)
6. RELAXATION TRAINING
7. GROUP THERAPY
8. PSYCHOPHARMACOLOGY
   a. Selective serotonin reuptake inhibitors (SSRIs)
   b. Tricyclic antidepressants
   c. Monoamine oxidase inhibitors (MAOs)
   d. Benzodiazepines
F. NURSING INTERVENTIONS
   1. DEVELOP A TRUSTING RELATIONSHIP WITH THE CLIENT.
   2. UTILIZE EFFECTIVE COMMUNICATION SKILLS.
   3. ENCOURAGE EXPRESSION OF THOUGHTS AND FEELINGS OF THE EVENT.
   4. MAINTAIN A CALM ENVIRONMENT.
   5. ASSESS THE CLIENT FOR SUICIDAL IDEATION.
   6. ASSESS THE CLIENT FOR CHANGES IN BEHAVIOR.
   7. ASSESS DRUG AND ALCOHOL USE.
   8. ASSESS CLIENT SUPPORT SYSTEMS IN THE FAMILY AND COMMUNITY.
   9. MAINTAIN CLIENT SAFETY.

II. **RAPE-TRAUMA SYNDROME**
   A. DESCRIPTION
      1. A VARIATION OF POST-TRAUMATIC STRESS DISORDER
      2. A SERIES OF PHYSICAL AND EMOTIONAL RESPONSES EXPERIENCED BY CLIENTS WHO HAVE BEEN ASSAULTED SEXUALLY
      3. MAY LAST FROM A FEW DAYS TO SEVERAL WEEKS
      4. ADDITIONAL RISK FACTORS MAY BE ASSOCIATED WITH ANXIETY, DEPRESSION, ANGER, DISSOCIATIVE REACTION, SEXUAL DYSFUNCTION, AND SUBSTANCE ABUSE.
   B. ASSESSMENT
      1. EXPRESSED STYLE: RESPONSE EASILY OBSERVABLE
         a. Confusion
         b. Restlessness
         c. Agitation
         d. Crying
         e. Anger
         f. Laughing
         g. Pacing
      2. CONTROLLED STYLE: RESPONSE NOT EASILY OBSERVED
         a. Calm
         b. Confused
         c. Numb
         d. Difficulty making decisions
         e. Moodiness
         f. Disorientation
      3. SOMATIC REACTION: PHYSICAL RESPONSE TO TRAUMA
         a. Bruises
         b. Soreness
         c. Headache
         d. Changes in appetite
         e. Changes in sleep patterns
         f. Insomnia
         g. Nausea
         h. Vomiting
         i. Diarrhea
         j. Constipation
         k. Vaginal pain or discharge
      4. REORGANIZATION PHASE: OCCURS 2 OR MORE WEEKS AFTER THE RAPE; CLIENT RESPONSES MAY BE SIMILAR TO THOSE OF POST-TRAUMATIC STRESS DISORDER.
         a. Flashbacks
         b. Nightmares
         c. Insomnia
         d. Mood swings
         e. Crying
         f. Depression
         g. Fear of being alone
         h. Fear of sexual encounters
   C. NURSING INTERVENTIONS
      1. MAINTAIN CLIENT CONFIDENTIALITY.
      2. DEVELOP A TRUSTING RELATIONSHIP WITH THE CLIENT.
      3. ENCOURAGE THE CLIENT TO EXPRESS THOUGHTS AND FEELINGS FREELY.
      4. APPROACH THE CLIENT WITH A NONJUDGMENTAL ATTITUDE.
      5. AVOID "WHY" QUESTIONS.
      6. ASSESS THE CLIENT'S LEVEL OF ANXIETY.
      7. ASSESS AVAILABLE FAMILY AND COMMUNITY SUPPORT SYSTEMS.
      8. ASSESS THE CLIENT FOR SUICIDAL IDEATION.
      9. EVALUATE FOR INDICATIONS OF PHYSICAL TRAUMA.
      10. EVALUATE FOR INDICATIONS OF EMOTIONAL TRAUMA.
      11. ASSESS THE CLIENT'S CURRENT LEVEL OF COPING.
      12. DOCUMENT PHYSICAL TRAUMA ON A BODY MAP.
      13. DOCUMENT THE CLIENT'S STATEMENT WORD FOR WORD.
      14. OFFER EMOTIONAL SUPPORT.
      15. OBTAIN GYNECOLOGIC HISTORY AND RISK FOR PREGNANCY.
      16. OBTAIN NECESSARY SAMPLES OF BODY FLUIDS, HAIR, AND SEMEN FOR DNA TESTING.

PRACTICE QUESTIONS

1. A client has been experiencing irritability, difficulty concentrating, difficulty sleeping, and withdrawal for the past 8 weeks since her house burned to the ground after an explosion. The nurse assesses that this client is experiencing
   1. depression.
   2. a panic attack.
   3. post-traumatic stress disorder.
   4. generalized anxiety disorder.

2. A client experiencing post-traumatic stress disorder was started on a monoamine oxidase inhibitor (MAOI). Which of the following should the nurse include in the medication teaching? Select all that apply:
   [ ] 1. Sit up slowly when taking an MAOI
   [ ] 2. Report signs of nausea and vomiting
   [ ] 3. Avoid foods such as cheese, salami, and smoked fish
   [ ] 4. Take on an empty stomach
   [ ] 5. Restrict extra fluids
   [ ] 6. Monitor for weight loss

3. A client recently started on a monoamine oxidase inhibitor (MAOI) is experiencing severe headache, tachycardia, and cold, clammy skin. Which of the following is the priority nursing intervention?
   1. Assess the client's blood pressure
   2. Instruct the client to lie down
   3. Notify the client's physician
   4. Offer the client a high-carbohydrate snack

4. The nurse assesses which of the following clients to be at the highest risk of developing post-traumatic stress disorder?
   1. A client who recently moved to a new city
   2. A client who witnessed a fatal shooting
   3. A client with a family history of depression
   4. A client who has a panic disorder

5. A client reports experiencing nightmares and constant worry about the weather since a tornado destroyed the client's house 1 year ago. The nurse assesses that this client is experiencing
   1. delusions.
   2. panic attacks.
   3. flashbacks.
   4. hallucinations.

6. The nurse assesses a client of rape-trauma syndrome for which of the following expressed style features? Select all that apply:
   [ ] 1. Flashbacks
   [ ] 2. Nightmares
   [ ] 3. Crying
   [ ] 4. Restlessness
   [ ] 5. Mood swings
   [ ] 6. Laughing

7. A client scheduled to begin relaxation therapy as part of treatment for post-traumatic stress disorder asks the nurse what the purpose is of the relaxation therapy. Which of the following is the appropriate response by the nurse?
   1. "It will help you not to be frightened anymore."
   2. "It will help produce effects that are the opposite of those produced by anxiety."
   3. "It will help you learn about your illness."
   4. "It will help you learn calming self-talk."

8. The nurse is caring for a client working at a high school who witnessed a bombing at the school and is experiencing sadness, sleeplessness, and lack of energy, and appears to be withdrawn. Which of the following interventions should the nurse include in the plan for this client?
   1. Allow the client to talk about the traumatic event in a safe, supportive environment
   2. Assist the client to look at other career choices and work environments
   3. Instruct the client that physical exercise may improve the quality of sleep
   4. Encourage the client to avoid focusing on the event and to make plans for the future

9. When planning the care of a client who is experiencing post-traumatic stress disorder, the nurse identifies which of the following as an appropriate goal? The client will report
   1. spending less time on ritualistic behavior.
   2. a decrease in flashbacks and nightmares.
   3. having more energy.
   4. a decrease in hearing voices.

10. A client tearfully reports having been sexually attacked by a spouse during an argument. The nurse evaluates this situation as
    1. an emotional reaction but not a rape, because the couple is married and has had sexual relations.
    2. the right of the partner to expect sex because they are married.
    3. a rape because sex against one's will is rape.
    4. a reaction to the couple's argument that will most likely not happen again.

11. The client who has been raped tells the nurse, "I am not pressing charges and I'm afraid of seeing my attacker because we live in the same

town." Which of the following should the nurse include in the plan of care for this client?
1. Assess the client's safety and develop a safety plan
2. Encourage the client to change jobs to avoid future encounters with the perpetrator
3. Instruct the client not to worry about safety because perpetrators don't attack twice
4. Support the client's desire to move to a new town and assume a new identity

12. During an interview, the nurse observes a client becoming increasingly defensive. The client states, "You wouldn't understand what I've been through." Which of the following is the most appropriate response by the nurse?
1. "You're right, I probably won't understand what you've been through."
2. "Why are you becoming so defensive?"
3. "Sometimes it feels like no one else can understand, but I would like to try."
4. "Maybe you will feel better if you concentrate on something else."

13. Which of the following should the nurse include when teaching a class on recognizing post-traumatic stress in children?
1. Post-traumatic stress disorder is not diagnosed until the age of 18
2. Only physically and sexually abused children and adolescents will experience clinical manifestations of post-traumatic stress disorder
3. School-age children do not experience clinical manifestations of post-traumatic stress disorder because of their developmental level
4. Children and adolescents can develop clinical manifestations of post-traumatic stress disorder after experiencing any traumatic event

14. The nurse is talking with a client who just had a beautiful bouquet of roses delivered. Suddenly the client becomes tearful and stares out the window. The client has a history of sexual abuse. Which of the following should the nurse include in the plan of care for this client?
1. Tell the client that the sexual abuse was in the past
2. Tell the client to relax and enjoy the roses
3. Give the client some alone time and return later
4. Assess if the client is having a flashback

15. A client currently taking fluoxetine (Prozac) to decrease clinical manifestations of post-traumatic stress disorder asks the nurse if continuing to take dietary supplements such as Saint John's wort, ginseng, and kava kava is acceptable. The most appropriate response by the nurse is which of the following?
1. "If it makes you feel better, continue to take the dietary supplements."
2. "Dietary supplements may interact negatively with your prescribed drugs; check with your care provider."
3. "Make sure you take the dietary supplements at a different time."
4. "Dietary supplements are harmless and won't make any difference in how you feel."

16. The registered nurse is preparing the clinical assignments for team members on a psychiatric unit. Which of the following assignments indicates that the nurse has appropriately delegated assignments?
1. Unlicensed assistive personnel attend group therapy with a client
2. A licensed practical nurse assesses a client suspected of having a post-traumatic stress disorder
3. Unlicensed assistive personnel sit with a client who is tearful
4. A licensed practical nurse develops a plan of care for a client who experienced a rape trauma

ANSWERS AND RATIONALES

1. 3. Clients may experience clinical manifestations of post-traumatic stress disorder after experiencing a traumatic event, such as a house burning down. Clinical manifestations need to be present for at least 1 month for a diagnosis of post-traumatic stress disorder. The client's clinical manifestations begin abruptly after a traumatic event and last for a period greater than a month.

2. 1. 2. 3. MAOIs are a classification of drugs used for post-traumatic stress disorder. They act by blocking an enzyme (monoamine oxidase). Clients taking MAOIs should be instructed to sit up slowly to prevent orthostatic hypotension. Nausea, vomiting, and weight gain are all adverse reactions. An MAOI should be administered with food to prevent gastrointestinal upset. Fluids are generally

encouraged because constipation is an adverse reaction. Clients must avoid foods that contain tyramine when taking an MAOI. Foods containing tyramine include aged cheese, salami, sauerkraut, beer and wine containing yeast, smoked fish, avocados, fava beans, and caviar. Eating foods containing tyramine when taking an MAOI can lead to a hypertensive crisis, making this the priority intervention.

3. 1. A toxic and serious adverse reaction to MAOIs is a hypertensive crisis. Clinical manifestations of a hypertensive crisis include severe headache, tachycardia, hypertension, and cold, clammy skin. The nurse's priority would be to assess for an increase in blood pressure. A hypertensive crisis can begin abruptly after taking a contraindicated food or drug. Immediate medical intervention is indicated when a hypertensive crisis is suspected. It is only after assessing the blood pressure and confirming the diagnosis that interventions can begin.

4. 2. Experiencing a traumatic event such as a shooting is an event likely to trigger a post-traumatic stress disorder in a person.

5. 3. A client who repeatedly experiences nightmares and constantly worries about the weather since a tornado destroyed the client's house 1 year ago is experiencing flashbacks. Clients who have flashbacks have recurrent intrusive recollections of the traumatic event. Clients with delusions, hallucinations, and panic attacks would not reexperience the traumatic event in this way.

6. 2. 3. 6. Expressed style assessment findings for rape-trauma syndrome are those in which a response is easily observable and include crying, restlessness, and laughing. Assessment findings of the reorganization of rape-trauma syndrome occur 2 or more weeks after the rape and include flashbacks, nightmares, and mood swings.

7. 2. Relaxation therapy helps the client learn ways to relax the body and reduce the tension produced by anxiety. Relaxation therapy does not guarantee that the client will not be frightened anymore. Helping a client learn about personal illness is the definition of psychoeducation. Helping the client learn calming self-talk defines cognitive restructuring.

8. 1. Allowing clients to talk about traumatic events such as bombings, explosions, and fires enables them to acknowledge their feelings and begin to take control of difficult situations. Assisting the client to consider other career choices, to increase physical exercise, to avoid focusing on the event, and to make plans for the future all discourage the client from acknowledging personal feelings.

9. 2. The target clinical manifestation for a client with post-traumatic stress disorder is flashbacks. Ritualistic behavior is associated with obsessive-compulsive disorder. Having a decreased energy level is associated with depression. Hearing voices is associated with schizophrenia.

10. 3. Acquaintance rape and marital rape are currently recognized by the court system. The current law allows a person to bring charges against a spouse for rape. Awareness continues to be raised that women are individuals with rights and privileges and not property.

11. 1. The client may very well be at risk for future attacks if the perpetrator is known. The nurse needs to make a thorough assessment of the client's safety and assist the client in developing a safety plan in the event the perpetrator is encountered. Moving to a new town or changing jobs places the blame and responsibility on the client.

12. 3. Frequently, clients have experienced things that the nurse has not. By using therapeutic communication skills such as reflecting and empathizing, the nurse can encourage the client to share experiences and begin to understand and develop a therapeutic relationship.

13. 4. Many children and adolescents have experienced natural and man-made disasters in their lives, such as kidnapping, rape, school shootings, peer suicides, fires, and floods. Clinical manifestations of post-traumatic stress disorder may develop in children and adolescents after experiencing these types of traumatic events.

14. 4. Clients who have experienced a traumatic event such as sexual abuse may experience flashbacks. The triggers for these flashbacks may be visual, auditory, tactile, or olfactory.

15. 2. Current studies have shown that dietary supplements may have beneficial uses in decreasing clinical manifestations of mild depression, anxiety, and insomnia when not used in conjunction with prescription drugs. Dietary supplements are not controlled by the Food and Drug Administration (FDA). Studies have shown that taking dietary supplements along with prescription drugs may cause adverse reactions. The client should be encouraged to discuss the amount and type of supplements being taken with the person who is prescribing the drugs.

16. 3.   Unlicensed assistive personnel may sit with a client who is tearful. A licensed practical nurse should not perform the skills of assessing a client or developing a plan of care. These are tasks reserved for the registered nurse. It is not appropriate for unlicensed assistive personnel to attend group therapy with a client.

REFERENCES

Antai-Otong, D. (2008). *Psychiatric nursing, biological and behavioral concepts* (2nd ed.). Clifton Park, NY: Delmar Cengage Learning.

Frisch, N. C., & Frisch, L. E. (2011). *Psychiatric mental health nursing* (4th ed.). Clifton Park, NY: Delmar Cengage Learning.

CHAPTER 55

SUBSTANCE DISORDERS

I. **SUBSTANCE DISORDERS**
   A. DESCRIPTION
      1. MALADAPTIVE USAGE PATTERNS OF ONE OR MORE MOOD-ALTERING SUBSTANCES OR CHEMICALS
      2. OVER 50% OF INDIVIDUALS WITH A SERIOUS MEDICAL OR MENTAL CONDITION ARE ADDICTED TO AN ILLICIT DRUG.
      3. ALCOHOL IS THE MOST COMMON SUBSTANCE THAT OCCURS IN SUBSTANCE ABUSE.
   B. THEORIES
      1. BIOLOGICAL
         a. Substance abuse problems tend to occur in families.
         b. Children of alcoholic parents have a greater incidence of developing alcoholism than children of nonalcoholic parents.
      2. PSYCHOLOGICAL
         a. There is no addictive personality, but certain factors—such as an intolerance to frustration or pain, failure to establish a meaningful or loving relationship, low self-esteem, or a lack of success in one's life—may predispose a client to a substance addiction.
      3. SOCIOCULTURAL
         a. Certain cultures may have a higher incidence of substance abuse.
         b. Substance abuse tends to be more common in certain socioeconomic cultures; individuals my abuse substances in an attempt to develop an identity and a sense of belonging.
         c. Women tend to have a low rate of substance abuse.
   C. TERMS
      1. SUBSTANCE ABUSE
         a. Maladaptive usage pattern of a mood-altering substance

         b. Usage causes significant distress or impairment in numerous areas within a period of time.
         c. Unable to fulfill major responsibilities at home, work, or school
         d. Persistent substance use in situations where it is physically dangerous
         e. Persistent legal problems related to use of a mood-altering substance
         f. Substance use continues, with ongoing disregard of the social and interpersonal problems created or made worse by the effects of the substance, such as physical fights or loss of family relationships or job.
      2. SUBSTANCE INTOXICATION
         a. Syndrome that is specific to the abused substance
         b. Caused by recent ingestion of a mood-altering substance that has an effect on the central nervous system (CNS)
         c. Maladaptive psychological and behavioral changes caused by mood-altering substances are experienced, such as mood lability and belligerence.
         d. May develop shortly after the use of the substance
      3. SUBSTANCE DEPENDENCE
         a. Maladaptive usage pattern of a mood-altering substance, leading to significant distress or impairment
         b. Characterized by three or more of the following within 12 months of time:
            1) Tolerance to the substance is developed and either increased or smaller amounts are needed to achieve intoxication.
            2) Withdrawal clinical manifestations occur on discontinuation of usage of the substance.
            3) Client requires the consumption of the same or a similar substance to

relieve or avoid withdrawal clinical manifestations.

4) Larger amounts of the substance are consumed over a longer period of time than was intended.

5) There is a desire to cut down or control the substance intake, with or without successful efforts to do so.

6) Large amounts of time are spent obtaining the substance.

7) Important occupational, social, or recreational activities are unfulfilled due to substance use.

8) Substance use continues, with disregard of knowledge of the physiological and psychological problems caused by it.

4. SUBSTANCE WITHDRAWAL

a. Substance-specific syndrome develops due to decrease or cessation of heavy and prolonged substance use.

b. Clinically significant impairment or distress in occupational, social, or other significant areas of functioning occurs.

c. Clinical manifestations are not caused by a general medical condition or other mental disorder.

d. Withdrawal clinical manifestations vary depending on:

1) Length of use
2) Dosage
3) Other mood-altering substances taken simultaneously
4) Type of drug taken and half-life of the drug or substance

II.   NURSING DIAGNOSES

A. HOPELESSNESS
B. INEFFECTIVE COPING
C. CHRONIC LOW SELF-ESTEEM
D. SOCIAL ISOLATION
E. DISTURBED SENSORY PERCEPTION
F. DISTURBED THOUGHT PROCESSES
G. INEFFECTIVE HEALTH MAINTENANCE
H. IMBALANCED NUTRITION: LESS THAN BODY REQUIREMENTS
I. DEFICIENT FLUID VOLUME
J. SELF-CARE DEFICIT
K. RISK FOR SUICIDE
L. ANXIETY
M. DISTURBED SLEEP PATTERN
N. INTERRUPTED FAMILY PROCESSES

Nursing Diagnoses: Definitions and Classification 2012–2014. Copyright © 2012, 1994–2012 by NANDA International. Used by arrangement with John Wiley & Sons Limited.

III.   ALCOHOL ABUSE

A. DESCRIPTION: MALADAPTIVE PATTERN OF ALCOHOL USE, CAUSING SIGNIFICANT IMPAIRMENT IN NUMEROUS AREAS, INCLUDING THE JOB, HOME LIFE, OR SCHOOL

B. ASSESSMENT

1. JOB OR SCHOOL PERFORMANCE IS NEGATIVELY IMPACTED.

2. LEGAL DIFFICULTIES OCCUR DUE TO THE EFFECTS OF ALCOHOL, SUCH AS AN ARREST DUE TO DRIVING WHILE UNDER THE INFLUENCE.

3. INTERPERSONAL AND SOCIAL ISSUES ARISE DUE TO ALCOHOL USE, SUCH AS FIGHTS WITH SIGNIFICANT OTHERS OR FAILURE TO ATTEND SCHEDULED SOCIAL ACTIVITIES.

C. NURSING INTERVENTIONS

1. INSTRUCT THE CLIENT TO ABSTAIN FROM ALCOHOL AND OTHER MOOD-ALTERING SUBSTANCES.

2. INSTRUCT THE CLIENT TO ATTEND ALCOHOLICS ANONYMOUS.

3. INSTRUCT THE CLIENT AND THE FAMILY ABOUT THE MEDICAL CONSEQUENCES OF LONG-TERM ALCOHOL USAGE.

IV.   ALCOHOL INTOXICATION

A. DESCRIPTION

1. AN ALCOHOL-SPECIFIC SYNDROME CAUSED BY RECENT INGESTION OF ALCOHOL BECAUSE OF ITS EFFECT ON THE CNS

2. MALADAPTIVE PSYCHOLOGICAL AND BEHAVIORAL CHANGES CAUSED BY ALCOHOL ARE EXPERIENCED, SUCH AS MOOD LABILITY, BELLIGERENCE, AND IMPAIRED JUDGMENT.

3. DEVELOPS WITHIN 8–12 HOURS OF LAST USAGE OF ALCOHOL ON UP TO 5 DAYS

B. ASSESSMENT

1. BLOOD PRESSURE DECREASED
2. PULSE INCREASED
3. RESPIRATIONS DECREASED
4. TEMPERATURE DECREASED
5. DROWSINESS
6. SLURRED SPEECH
7. GASTROINTESTINAL (GI) TRACT SLOWED
8. SLOWED THOUGHT PROCESSES
9. SLOWED REFLEXES

C. NURSING INTERVENTIONS

1. PROMOTE SAFETY, SUCH AS PREVENTING FALLS AND MANAGING BLOOD PRESSURE.

2. ASSESS NEUROLOGICAL FUNCTIONING.

3. ENCOURAGE REST.

V.   ALCOHOL WITHDRAWAL

A. DESCRIPTION: AN ALCOHOL-SPECIFIC SYNDROME DEVELOPING WITHIN 8–12 HOURS AFTER THE DECREASE OR CESSATION OF HEAVY AND PROLONGED USE OF ALCOHOL

B. ASSESSMENT
1. BLOOD PRESSURE INCREASE
2. PULSE INCREASE
3. RESPIRATION INCREASE
4. TEMPERATURE INCREASE
5. ANXIETY, RESTLESSNESS
6. GASTROINTESTINAL HYPERACTIVITY
7. HYPERACTIVE THOUGHT PROCESS
8. HYPERREFLEXIC
9. INSOMNIA
10. SKIN DIAPHORETIC, PALE

C. MEDICAL MANAGEMENT
1. IF WITHDRAWAL CLINICAL MANIFESTATIONS ARE NOTED, MEDICATE THE CLIENT WITH THE SAME OR A SIMILAR CNS DEPRESSANT, SUCH AS A BENZODIAZEPINE CHLORDIAZEPOXIDE (LIBRIUM), CLORAZEPATE (TRANXENE), OR DIAZEPAM (VALIUM).
2. ADMINISTER PRESCRIBED THIAMINE FOR CLIENTS IN ALCOHOL WITHDRAWAL DUE TO VITAMIN DEFICIENCY.
3. ADMINISTER PRESCRIBED DISULFIRAM (ANTABUSE).
   a. Antabuse produces an unpleasant reaction when taken with alcohol, including palpitations, vomiting, perspiration, dyspnea, and thirst.
   b. Alcohol must be abstained from for at least 12 hours before starting the Antabuse.
   c. The Antabuse reaction starts within minutes after the ingestion of alcohol and may last for hours.
   d. The client should be informed of the Antabuse reaction that results from the ingestion of alcohol.
   e. Inform the client of other sources of alcohol, such as cough syrup and mouthwash.
   f. Initial dose of Antabuse is 500 mg daily for 1 to 2 weeks followed by a maintenance dose of 250 mg daily.

D. NURSING INTERVENTIONS
1. ASSESS VITAL SIGNS EVERY 2–4 HOURS.
2. ENCOURAGE FLUID INTAKE SUCH AS WATER OR JUICE.
3. INFORM THE CLIENT ABOUT THE WITHDRAWAL PROCESS.
4. ASSIST WITH ACTIVITIES OF DAILY LIVING AS NEEDED.

VI. **ALCOHOL DEPENDENCE**
A. DESCRIPTION
1. DEVELOPMENT OF TOLERANCE TO ALCOHOL AND SUBSEQUENT PHYSIOLOGICAL WITHDRAWAL CLINICAL MANIFESTATIONS
2. LEADS TO SIGNIFICANT DISTRESS OR IMPAIRMENT ON THE JOB AND IN SOCIAL AND INTERPERSONAL RELATIONSHIPS

B. ASSESSMENT
1. ASSESSMENT OCCURS THROUGH A VARIETY OF METHODS:
   a. Information received from the significant other, family, coworkers, boss, or friends
   b. Serum and urine drug screens
   c. Blood alcohol levels (BALs)
   d. Michigan Alcohol and Drug Screening Test
   e. CAGE questionnaire
   f. Criteria met based on the *Diagnostic and Statistical Manual of Mental Disorders*, Fourth Edition, Text Revision (DSM-IV-TR)
   g. The following criteria occur at any time within a 12-month period:
      1) Tolerance to alcohol is developed and is either increased or smaller amounts are needed to achieve intoxication.
      2) Withdrawal clinical manifestations occur on discontinuation of use of alcohol.
      3) Client requires the consumption of alcohol or a benzodiazepine to relieve or avoid withdrawal clinical manifestations.
      4) Larger amounts of alcohol are consumed or are consumed over a longer period of time than was intended.
      5) There may be a desire to cut down or control the alcohol intake with or without successful efforts to do so.
      6) Large amounts of time are spent obtaining alcohol.
      7) Use causes lack of fulfillment of important occupational, social, or recreational activities.

C. MEDICAL COMPLICATIONS
1. BRAIN ATROPHY
2. WERNICKE-KORSAKOFF SYNDROME
   a. One of the most commonly found conditions in the alcoholic
   b. Caused primarily from deficiency in thiamine (vitamin B_1)
   c. Clinical manifestations include marked confusion, which occurs suddenly, unsteady gait, double vision, and uncoordinated movement.
      1) Medical management
         a) Prompt treatment with large amounts of thiamine is required within the first few hours to the first few days of onset of clinical

manifestations (if thiamine is not given within this time period, death may result or the client may develop marked impairment of memory; disorientation to person, place, date, and time; an inability to retain memory of ongoing events; and short-term memory loss).

3. CHRONIC SUBDURAL HEMATOMA
  a. May develop due to frequent falls to which the alcoholic individual is very prone

4. GASTRITIS
  a. Due to alcohol causing an increase in production of stomach acid
  b. Clinical manifestations include upper abdominal pain, indigestion, nausea, and decreased appetite.
  c. Infrequent vomiting of blood may result due to the erosion of the stomach lining.

5. PANCREATITIS
  a. Inflammation of the pancreas with clinical manifestations, including acute abdominal pain, nausea, and vomiting

6. DIARRHEA
  a. Results as alcohol causes the retention of water and salt in the intestine and encourages strong movements within the intestine

7. FATTY LIVER
  a. Fat accumulates on the liver because the fat is not burned or metabolized due to the high levels of alcohol consumed

8. ALCOHOLIC HEPATITIS
  a. Inflammation of the liver due to the toxic effects of alcohol on the liver
  b. Occurs between the development of a fatty liver and liver cirrhosis
  c. Flulike clinical manifestations develop.

9. ASCITES
  a. Fluid accumulation in the abdominal cavity

10. ALCOHOLIC LIVER CIRRHOSIS
  a. Liver becomes inactive due to severe damage to and scar development on it.
  b. Liver will atrophy and may become rock hard or nodular.
  c. Clinical manifestations include jaundice (a yellow coloring of the skin and eyes) or a palmar erythema (a reddening of the palms of the hands).

11. ESOPHAGEAL VARICES
  a. Pockets of blood that accumulate in the varicose veins in the esophagus

12. PORTAL HYPERTENSION
  a. Blood is blocked in the liver and cannot flow freely through it, requiring finding another route to the heart, causing undue pressure on the already vulnerable vein systems such as the esophagus and stomach.
  b. Portal hypertension is not associated with high blood pressure.

13. CARDIAC ARRHYTHMIAS
  a. May result from consumption of small to moderate amounts of alcohol
  b. Drinking alcohol along with caffeinated beverages will predispose an individual to developing an arrhythmia.

14. CORONARY ARTERY DISEASE
  a. Narrowing of the blood vessels due to accumulation of fatty substances

15. ALCOHOLIC CARDIOMYOPATHY
  a. Heart muscle damage
  b. Clinical manifestations include shortness of breath, peripheral edema, decreased tissue perfusion to the nail beds, fatigue, and palpitations.

16. PERIPHERAL NEUROPATHY
  a. Occurs due to a decrease of thiamine in the nerves of the arms and legs of the individual
  b. Clinical manifestations include prickling, tingling, or a burning sensation in the fingers and feet.

17. DIMINISHED SEXUAL DESIRE
  a. Initially increased in women and men, or at least the perception of their performance is increased
  b. Diminished sexual desire and potency is a frequent complaint of chronic alcoholics.

18. GYNECOMASTIA (ENLARGEMENT OF THE BREAST AREA)
  a. Can result in men due to the alcohol increasing the amount of estrogen in the male

19. ATROPHY OF THE TESTICLES

20. FETAL ALCOHOL SYNDROME
  a. Excessive maternal alcohol consumption during pregnancy, which may cause one or more of the following birth defects:
    1) Small head, low weight, short body length, and slow growth after birth
    2) Narrowed eye slits
    3) Underdeveloped facial structure
    4) Flattened cheekbones
    5) An abnormally thin upper lip

21. SLEEP DISTURBANCES
  a. During the sobering-up period, there is an increase in rapid eye movements.
  b. Restless sleep, along with vivid dreams or nightmares, or both

c. Within weeks to months after cessation of the alcohol, sleep may be restless, and there can be frequent, yet unremembered, awakenings.

D. NURSING INTERVENTIONS
1. MONITOR THE CLIENT EVERY 2–4 HOURS TO ASSESS FOR ALCOHOL WITHDRAWAL.
2. IF WITHDRAWAL CLINICAL MANIFESTATIONS ARE OBSERVED, INSTRUCT THE CLIENT ABOUT THE NECESSITY FOR DETOXIFICATION.
3. DETOXIFY THE CLIENT WITH A PRESCRIBED CNS DEPRESSANT.
4. INSTRUCT THE CLIENT REGARDING LONG-TERM EFFECTS OF ALCOHOL USAGE.
5. INSTRUCT THE CLIENT ABOUT THE CONSEQUENCES OF BEHAVIOR, SUCH AS PROVIDING FEEDBACK REGARDING LIVER FUNCTION TESTS.
6. PROVIDE INTRAPERSONAL SKILLS TRAINING, SUCH AS PROBLEM SOLVING, COPING SKILLS, AWARENESS AND MANAGEMENT OF NEGATIVE SELF-TALK, INCREASING PLEASANT ACTIVITIES, AND RELAXATION TRAINING.
7. ASSIST THE CLIENT WITH INTERPERSONAL SKILLS SUCH AS STARTING CONVERSATIONS, ASSERTIVENESS TRAINING, NONVERBAL COMMUNICATION, HOW TO REFUSE OFFERS OF ALCOHOL AND DRUGS, AND STRENGTHENING SOCIAL SUPPORT NETWORKS.

VII. **SEDATIVE-, HYPNOTIC-, OR ANXIOLYTIC-RELATED USE DISORDERS**
A. SEDATIVE, HYPNOTIC, OR ANXIOLYTIC ABUSE
1. DESCRIPTION: MALADAPTIVE PATTERN OF SEDATIVE, HYPNOTIC, OR ANXIOLYTIC USE THAT CAUSES SIGNIFICANT IMPAIRMENT IN A NUMBER OF AREAS, INCLUDING JOB, HOME LIFE, AND SCHOOL
2. ASSESSMENT (SEE ASSESSMENT SECTION FOR ALCOHOL ABUSE ON PAGE 984.)
3. NURSING INTERVENTIONS
a. Instruct the client regarding the necessity to abstain from sedative-, hypnotic-, or anxiolytic-induced disorders and other mood-altering substances.
b. Encourage the client to attend Narcotics Anonymous.
c. Inform the client and the family about the medical consequences of long-term sedative, hypnotic, or anxiolytic usage.

B. SEDATIVE, HYPNOTIC, OR ANXIOLYTIC INTOXICATION
1. DESCRIPTION
a. A sedative-, hypnotic-, or anxiolytic-specific syndrome
b. Caused by recent ingestion of a sedative, hypnotic, or anxiolytic because of its effect on the CNS
c. Maladaptive psychological and behavioral problems caused by the sedative, hypnotic, or anxiolytic are experienced, such as mood lability, belligerence, or impaired judgment.
d. Develops within the time period of the half-life of the drug up to the half-life of the drug multiplied by 5.
2. ASSESSMENT
a. One or more of the following clinical manifestations occur shortly after usage of the sedative, hypnotic, or anxiolytic:
1) Nystagmus
2) Slurred speech
3) Impaired memory or attention
4) Incoordination
5) Unsteady gait
6) Coma or stupor
3. NURSING INTERVENTIONS
a. Ensure safety of the client, such as preventing falls.
b. Monitor the client's vital signs.
c. Assess cardiac and respiratory status.
d. Assess neurological status by completing a cranial nerve exam.

C. SEDATIVE, HYPNOTIC, OR ANXIOLYTIC WITHDRAWAL
1. DESCRIPTION: A SEDATIVE-, HYPNOTIC-, OR ANXIOLYTIC-SPECIFIC SYNDROME WITH CLINICAL MANIFESTATIONS DEVELOPING WITHIN SEVERAL HOURS TO SEVERAL DAYS AFTER PROLONGED USAGE
2. ASSESSMENT
a. Hyperactivity of the autonomic nervous system, such as elevated pulse or diaphoresis
b. Nausea or vomiting
c. Anxiety
d. Psychomotor agitation
e. Increased hand tremors
f. Insomnia
g. Occasional auditory, visual, or tactile hallucinations or illusions
3. MEDICAL MANAGEMENT
a. Administer a benzodiazepine, per detoxification protocol, followed by tapered dosages.
b. Administer a barbiturate for detoxification if the client is using and withdrawing from it.

4. NURSING INTERVENTIONS
 a. Monitor vital signs every 4 hours.
 b. Assess for clinical manifestations of benzodiazepine or barbiturate withdrawal.
 c. Provide comfort and management of the clinical manifestations measures to reduce distress.
 d. Encourage rest.
 e. Provide adequate fluid and food intake.

D. SEDATIVE, HYPNOTIC, OR ANXIOLYTIC DEPENDENCE
 1. DESCRIPTION: DEVELOPMENT OF TOLERANCE AND PHYSIOLOGICAL WITHDRAWAL CLINICAL MANIFESTATIONS DUE TO MALADAPTIVE USAGE PATTERN OF SEDATIVE, HYPNOTIC, OR ANXIOLYTIC, LEADING TO SIGNIFICANT DISTRESS OR IMPAIRMENT ON THE JOB OR IN SOCIAL AND INTERPERSONAL RELATIONSHIPS
 2. ASSESSMENT
  a. Assessment occurs through a variety of methods:
   1) Information received from the significant other, family, coworkers, boss, or friends
  b. Serum and urine drug screens
  c. Criteria met based on the DSM-IV-TR
  d. Presence of physiological dependence or withdrawal clinical manifestations along with increased or decreased tolerance for the substance
 3. MEDICAL MANAGEMENT
  a. Detoxify the client with a prescribed CNS depressant in tapering dosages.
 4. NURSING INTERVENTIONS
  a. Monitor the client every 2–4 hours to assess for sedative, hypnotic, or anxiolytic withdrawal.
  b. If withdrawal clinical manifestations are observed, instruct the client about the necessity for detoxification.
  c. Inform the client regarding the long-term effects of sedative, hypnotic, or anxiolytic use.
  d. Inform the client about the consequences of chemical use, such as providing feedback about the effect of chemical use on family relationships and medical complications as a result of use.
  e. Assist the client to develop interpersonal skills, such as assertiveness training, skills in refusing offers of chemicals, and strengthening social support networks.
  f. Inform the client regarding clinical manifestations that could precipitate a relapse.

VIII. OPIOID (NARCOTIC) USE DISORDERS
A. OPIOID ABUSE
 1. DESCRIPTION
  a. Maladaptive pattern of opioid use that causes significant impairment in a number of areas, including job, home life, or school
  b. Includes drugs such as meperidine (Demerol), morphine sulfate, hydromorphone (Dilaudid), opium, and heroin
 2. ASSESSMENT (SEE THE ASSESSMENT SECTION FOR ALCOHOL ABUSE ON PAGE 984.)
 3. MEDICAL COMPLICATIONS
  a. Abscesses
  b. Transmission of human immunodeficiency virus (HIV) and hepatitis through the use of contaminated needles by more than one person
  c. Death from an overdose of an opiate or an opioid is generally due to respiratory arrest from the respiratory depressant effects of the drug.
 4. NURSING INTERVENTIONS
  a. Instruct the client to abstain from opioids and other mood-altering substances.
  b. Instruct the client regarding benefits of attending Narcotics Anonymous meetings and participating in recreational activities.
  c. Instruct the client on socialization skills.
  d. Instruct the client and family about the medical consequences of long-term opioid use.
B. OPIOID INTOXICATION
 1. DESCRIPTION
  a. An opioid-specific syndrome caused by recent ingestion of an opioid
  b. Maladaptive psychological and behavioral problems caused by the opioid are experienced, such as mood lability, belligerence, or impaired judgment.
 2. ASSESSMENT
  a. Analgesia
  b. Apathy
  c. Drooling
  d. Drowsiness
  e. Euphoria
  f. Flushing of skin
  g. Itching
  h. Nodding
  i. Peripheral vasodilation
  j. Slowed speech
  k. Spontaneous orgasm
  l. Respiratory depression

3. NURSING INTERVENTIONS
   a. Promote a safe environment for the client.
   b. Monitor vital signs.
   c. Assess for respiratory depression.
   d. Administer naloxone (Narcan) as the antidote for an opioid overdose.
   e. Provide comfort measures based on clinical manifestations.

C. OPIOID WITHDRAWAL
   1. DESCRIPTION
      a. An opioid-specific syndrome that develops within 24–62 hours after prolonged and heavy usage of an opioid
      b. Clinical manifestations generally subside after 5–7 days.
   2. ASSESSMENT
      a. Three or more of the following clinical manifestations develop within 24–72 hours after prolonged and heavy use:
         1) Abdominal spasms
         2) Anorexia, weight loss
         3) Chills
         4) Depression
         5) Diarrhea
         6) Elevated temperature
         7) Elevated pulse
         8) Flushing of the skin
         9) Gooseflesh
         10) Irritability
         11) Lacrimation
         12) Lower back pain
         13) Muscle cramps
         14) Rhinorrhea
         15) Sneezing
         16) Vomiting
         17) Yawning
   3. MEDICAL MANAGEMENT
      a. Administer clonidine (Catapres), an opioid antagonist that assists in blocking the opioid receptor sites to prevent or alleviate withdrawal clinical manifestations.
      b. Administer a nonsteroidal anti-inflammatory medication p.r.n. to relieve discomfort or pain.
      c. Administer antidiarrheal medication p.r.n.
   4. NURSING INTERVENTIONS
      a. The goal of opiate withdrawal treatment is to focus on the alleviation of discomfort and to provide management of the clinical manifestations.
      b. Monitor vital signs.
      c. Provide comfort measures.
      d. Encourage warm whirlpool baths.
      e. Provide the client with warm blankets to assist in alleviating chills.

f. Provide reassurance to the client.
g. Promote adequate hydration.
h. Provide interventions to alleviate nausea and vomiting.
i. Inform the client about the medical consequences of opiate abuse.

D. OPIOID DEPENDENCE
   1. DESCRIPTION
      a. Maladaptive usage pattern of an opioid, leading to significant distress or impairment
      b. Characterized by three or more of the following within 12 months of time:
         1) Tolerance to the opioid is developed or increased after smaller amounts are needed to achieve intoxication.
         2) Withdrawal clinical manifestations occur on discontinuation of usage of the opioid.
         3) Consumption of the same or a similar opioid is necessary to relieve or avoid withdrawal clinical manifestations.
         4) Larger amounts of the opioid are consumed or consumed over a longer period of time than was originally intended.
         5) There is a desire to cut down or control the opioid intake with or without successful efforts to do so.
         6) Large amounts of time are spent obtaining the opioid.
         7) Opioid use causes an inability to fulfill important occupational, social, or recreational activities.
         8) Opioid consumption continues, with disregard of knowledge of the physiological and psychological problems caused by the substance.
   2. NURSING INTERVENTIONS
      a. Assess the client for opioid withdrawal.
      b. Inform the client about opioid withdrawal.
      c. Instruct the client about the importance of attending Narcotics Anonymous.
      d. Explore with the client alternatives to opioid use, such as exercise.
      e. Promote social support.
      f. Inform the client about medical complications that may result from opioid use.
      g. Instruct the client regarding relapse prevention, such as behaviors and attitudes to be aware of that may precipitate a relapse.

IX. STIMULANT USE DISORDERS
  A. AMPHETAMINE AND COCAINE USE
     DISORDERS
     1. AMPHETAMINE AND COCAINE ABUSE
        a. Description: maladaptive pattern of
           amphetamine or cocaine use that
           causes significant impairment in a
           number of areas, including job, home
           life, or school
        b. Assessment (See the assessment
           section for alcohol abuse on page 984.)
        c. Medical complications due to
           amphetamine abuse:
           1) Use of amphetamines with needles
              is associated with HIV, hepatitis, and
              the development of lung abscesses
              and endocarditis (inflammation of
              the lining of the heart).
           2) Impotence and sexual
              dysfunctions can occur with
              long-term use and high doses.
        d. Medical complications due to
           cocaine abuse:
           1) Acute dystonia, tics
           2) Acquired immune deficiency
              syndrome (AIDS) from
              IV cocaine use
           3) Cardiac arrhythmias
           4) Cerebral infarctions
           5) Embolisms
           6) Infection
           7) Migrainelike headaches
           8) Myocardial infarctions
           9) Nasal congestion
           10) Transient ischemic attacks (TIAs)
           11) Respiratory depression
           12) Seizures
           13) Ulceration of the nasal mucosa
     2. AMPHETAMINE AND COCAINE
        INTOXICATION
        a. Description: amphetamine- and
           cocaine-specific syndrome that
           occurs during, or shortly after, usage
           of amphetamine or cocaine
        b. Assessment
           1) Increased sense of alertness
           2) Anxiety; psychomotor agitation or
              retardation
           3) Blood pressure increase or decrease
           4) Cardiac arrhythmias
           5) Chest pain
           6) Chills or perspiration
           7) Confusion
           8) Diarrhea
           9) Dyskinesias, dystonias, coma
           10) Insomnia
           11) Muscular weakness
           12) Nausea and vomiting
           13) Panic attacks
           14) Psychomotor agitation or
               retardation

           15) Pulse increase or decrease
           16) Pupillary dilation
           17) Respiratory depression
           18) Decreased urine production
           19) Weight loss
           20) Clinical manifestations at toxic
               levels include compulsive
               behaviors, hallucinations
               (auditory, visual, tactile),
               hypertension, looseness of
               associations, overly suspicious or
               paranoia, preoccupation, and
               touching and picking of the
               extremities and face.
        c. Nursing interventions
           1) Promote safety for the client.
           2) Provide symptomatic comfort
              measures.
           3) Manage clinical manifestations.
           4) Instruct the client on sleep
              hygiene techniques.
           5) Promote abstinence from
              amphetamines and cocaine.
     3. AMPHETAMINE AND COCAINE
        WITHDRAWAL
        a. Description: an amphetamine- and
           cocaine-specific syndrome that
           develops during or shortly after usage
           of either amphetamine or cocaine
        b. Assessment
           1) Depression
           2) Drug craving
           3) Fatigue
           4) Increased appetite
           5) Psychomotor agitation or
              retardation
           6) Unpleasant, vivid dreams
        c. Nursing interventions
           1) Instruct the client on sleep
              hygiene measures.
           2) Provide distraction technique to
              keep the client's mind off drug
              cravings.
           3) Encourage a well-balanced diet.
           4) Provide a quiet and
              nonstimulating environment for
              the client.
     4. AMPHETAMINE AND COCAINE
        DEPENDENCE
        a. Description: maladaptive usage pattern
           of amphetamine or cocaine, leading to
           significant distress or impairment
        b. Assessment
           1) Characterized by three or more of
              the following within 12 months
              of time:
              a) Tolerance to amphetamine or
                 cocaine is developed or
                 increased and smaller amounts
                 are needed to achieve
                 intoxication.

b) Withdrawal clinical manifestations occur on discontinuation of usage of amphetamine or cocaine.

c) Consumption of amphetamine or cocaine is necessary to relieve or avoid withdrawal clinical manifestations.

d) Larger amounts of amphetamine or cocaine are consumed or consumed over a longer period of time than was originally intended.

e) There may be a desire to cut down or control amphetamine or cocaine intake with or without successful efforts to do so.

f) Large amounts of time are spent obtaining amphetamine or cocaine.

g) Amphetamine or cocaine use causes inability to fulfill important occupational, social, or recreational activities.

h) Amphetamine or cocaine consumption continues, with disregard of knowledge of the physiological and psychological problems caused by the stimulant.

c. Nursing interventions

1) Assess the client for amphetamine or cocaine intoxication and withdrawal.

2) Monitor vital signs.

3) Treat any respiratory or cardiac distress.

4) Perform a cranial nerve exam to assess neurological functioning.

5) Orient the client, if needed, to surroundings.

6) Administer an antidiarrheal for diarrhea.

7) Provide comfort measures for nausea and vomiting such as providing ice chips, cool cloth to the back of the neck and forehead.

8) Provide adequate food and fluid intake.

9) Instruct the client regarding relapse prevention and behaviors and attitudes that would indicate a possible relapse.

10) Instruct the client about the medical complications of amphetamine or cocaine consumption and other negative consequences that can result due to their use, such as impaired social and interpersonal relationships.

X. **CAFFEINE USE DISORDERS**

A. CAFFEINE INTOXICATION

1. DESCRIPTION: CAFFEINE-SPECIFIC SYNDROME WITH CLINICAL MANIFESTATIONS DEVELOPING AFTER PROLONGED, HEAVY (IN EXCESS OF 250 MG) CONSUMPTION OF CAFFEINE

2. ASSESSMENT

a. Clinical manifestations (five or more) that develop during or shortly after caffeine use:

1) Cardiac arrhythmias or tachycardia

2) Diuresis

3) Endurance and energy

4) Excitement

5) Flushed face

6) Increased blood sugar

7) Gastric reflux

8) Hand tremors

9) Increased bowel motility

10) Insomnia

11) Muscle twitching

12) Nervousness

13) Psychomotor agitation

14) Rambling of speech and thoughts

15) Ringing in the ears, flashes of light

3. NURSING INTERVENTIONS

a. Instruct the client on the importance of abstinence or moderation of use of caffeine.

b. If the client desires to cut down usage of caffeine, instruct the client to cut down gradually so as to decrease withdrawal clinical manifestations of fatigue, headaches, irritability, and tremulousness.

c. Instruct the client on the medical complications of prolonged excessive (more than 250 mg per day) usage of caffeine.

d. Instruct the client to abstain from caffeine 12 hours prior to retiring to bed (caffeine has a 12-hour half-life).

XI. **NICOTINE USE DISORDERS**

A. NICOTINE WITHDRAWAL

1. DESCRIPTION: CLINICAL MANIFESTATIONS PRODUCED DUE TO THE CESSATION OF NICOTINE AFTER ITS DAILY USE

2. ASSESSMENT

a. Four or more of the following clinical manifestations develop within 24 hours of nicotine use:

1) Agitation

2) Increased cravings for nicotine

3) Decreased concentration

4) Decreased judgment

5) Decreased psychomotor performance

6) Drowsiness

7) GI disturbance

8) Increased appetite and weight gain

9) Labile emotions

10) Mental dullness

11) Nervousness

12) Sleep disturbance

3. MEDICAL MANAGEMENT

   a. Administer a nicotine patch or bupropion (Zyban) to manage withdrawal clinical manifestations.

4. NURSING INTERVENTIONS

   a. Instruct the client about the medical complications of nicotine usage, such as bronchitis, lung cancer, coronary disease, and obstructive pulmonary disease.

   b. Instruct the client about the use of a nicotine patch or the use of bupropion (Zyban) for managing withdrawal clinical manifestations.

   c. Assist the client in identifying triggers to nicotine use and explore alternative coping strategies.

   d. Instruct the client on relaxation techniques such as deep breathing and guided imagery.

B. NICOTINE DEPENDENCE

1. DESCRIPTION: TOLERANCE TO NICOTINE INCLUDES EXPERIENCING A GREATER EFFECT OF NICOTINE ON THE FIRST TIME IT IS USED DURING THE DAY AND THE ABSENCE OF NAUSEA AND DIZZINESS AFTER PROLONGED USAGE.

2. ASSESSMENT

   a. Withdrawal clinical manifestations occur on discontinuation of usage of nicotine.

   b. Nicotine use is necessary to relieve or avoid withdrawal clinical manifestations.

   c. The supply of cigarettes is used up more quickly than was intended.

   d. Chain-smoking

   e. Use of nicotine continues despite knowledge of the physiological problems caused by the substance.

3. NURSING INTERVENTIONS

   a. Inform the client on the medical complications of nicotine usage and the negative consequences of secondhand smoke to family members.

   b. Inform the client of the benefits of smoking cessation.

   c. Instruct the client on smoking cessation such as the use of a nicotine patch or bupropion (Zyban).

   d. Instruct the client on ways to distract self when cravings for nicotine emerge, such as eating sunflower seeds or carrot sticks and use of relaxation techniques.

XII. HALLUCINOGEN USE DISORDERS

A. HALLUCINOGEN ABUSE

1. DESCRIPTION

   a. Maladaptive pattern of hallucinogen use that causes significant impairment in a number of areas, including job, home life, or school

   b. Examples of hallucinogenics include lysergic acid diethylamide (LSD), psilocybine (from various mushrooms), dimethyltryptamine (DMT), mescaline, and peyote.

2. ASSESSMENT (SEE ASSESSMENT SECTION FOR ALCOHOL ABUSE ON PAGE 984.)

3. MEDICAL COMPLICATIONS

   a. The effects are unique to each individual.

   b. Mild or severe depression

   c. Flashbacks can occur at any time.

   d. Death can occur from toxic drug levels, suicide, driving under the influence, and convulsions.

4. NURSING INTERVENTIONS

   a. Instruct the client to abstain from hallucinogen use.

   b. Encourage the client to participate in a 12–step program.

   c. Inform the client and family about medical complications that can result from hallucinogen abuse.

B. HALLUCINOGEN INTOXICATION

1. DESCRIPTION

   a. A hallucinogen-specific syndrome with behavioral or psychological problems, or both, such as paranoia or impaired judgment, that results due to recent hallucinogen use

   b. Perceptual changes such as hallucinations and illusions occur shortly after hallucinogen use.

2. ASSESSMENT

   a. Two or more of the following clinical manifestations develop during or shortly after hallucinogen use:

      1) Labile affect

      2) Anorexia

      3) Anxiety

      4) Blurred vision

      5) Body image changes

      6) Diaphoresis

      7) Dizziness

      8) Euphoria

      9) Floating feeling

      10) Hallucinations

      11) Hypertension

      12) Hyperthermia

      13) Incoordination

      14) Nausea and vomiting

      15) Palpitations

      16) Paresthesia

17) Pupils, dilated
18) Suspiciousness
19) Tachycardia
20) Tremors
3. NURSING INTERVENTIONS
a. Educate the client on anxiety reduction.
b. Talk calmly with the client.
c. Reassure client safety.
d. Provide management of clinical manifestations.
C. HALLUCINOGEN-PERSISTING PERCEPTION DISORDER (FLASHBACKS)
1. DESCRIPTION: CHARACTERIZED BY OCCASIONAL RECURRENCE OF PERCEPTUAL DISTURBANCES REMINISCENT OF THOSE EXPERIENCED DURING ONE OR MORE PREVIOUS HALLUCINOGEN INTOXICATIONS
2. ASSESSMENT
a. Reexperiencing of one or more perceptual disturbances experienced during previous hallucinogen intoxications, such as trails of images of moving objects, halos, and flashes of color
b. The clinical manifestations create significant distress or impairment in relational, occupational, social, and other areas of functioning.
3. NURSING INTERVENTIONS
a. Ensure safety of the client.
b. Provide reassurance to the client.
c. Assist the client with reducing anxiety, such as through decreased lighting and environmental stimuli and deep-breathing techniques.

XIII. CANNABIS (MARIJUANA) USE DISORDERS
A. CANNABIS ABUSE
1. DESCRIPTION: MALADAPTIVE PATTERN OF CANNABIS USE THAT CAUSES SIGNIFICANT IMPAIRMENT IN A NUMBER OF AREAS, INCLUDING JOB, HOME LIFE, OR SCHOOL
2. ASSESSMENT (SEE ASSESSMENT SECTION FOR ALCOHOL ABUSE ON PAGE 984.)
3. MEDICAL COMPLICATIONS
a. Cerebral atrophy
b. Susceptibility to seizures
c. Birth defects
d. Chromosomal damage
e. Alterations in concentrations of testosterone
f. Disruption in the menstrual cycle
g. Impaired immune system
4. NURSING INTERVENTIONS
a. Instruct the client regarding the physical, social, and legal effects of cannabis use.

b. Inform the client about the benefits of cessation.
c. Encourage the client to attend 12–step group meetings.
B. CANNABIS INTOXICATION
1. DESCRIPTION: A CANNABIS-SPECIFIC SYNDROME THAT CREATES BEHAVIORAL AND PSYCHOLOGICAL CHANGES CAUSED BY RECENT INGESTION OF CANNABIS
2. ASSESSMENT
a. Urine drug screens can be positive for cannabis for 7–10 days after use.
b. Heavy use of cannabis can be detected in urine for up to 2–4 weeks.
c. Anxiety
d. Conjunctival injection
e. Dry mouth
f. Euphoria
g. Impaired judgment
h. Impaired motor coordination
i. Increased appetite
j. Sensation of slowed time
k. Social withdrawal
l. Tachycardia
3. NURSING INTERVENTIONS
a. Promote environmental safety.
b. Provide adequate hydration and nutrition.
c. Encourage rest.
d. Encourage use of relaxation techniques, if needed, such as deep breathing and listening to soothing music.
C. CANNABIS DEPENDENCE
1. DESCRIPTION: MALADAPTIVE PSYCHOLOGICAL AND BEHAVIORAL PROBLEMS CAUSED BY CANNABIS ARE EXPERIENCED, SUCH AS EUPHORIA, SOCIAL WITHDRAWAL, AND IMPAIRED MOTOR COORDINATION.
2. ASSESSMENT
a. Compulsive use of cannabis
b. Decreasing or giving up important occupational, recreational, or social activities in order to use cannabis
c. Larger amounts of the drug are taken and for longer amounts of time than was originally planned.
d. Large amounts of time spent using and recovering from the effects of the substance
e. Substance use continues despite knowledge of physical and psychological problems that can result from its use.
f. There may be a desire to cut down or control cannabis intake with or without successful efforts to do so.

3. NURSING INTERVENTIONS
   a. Encourage participation in a 12–step program.
   b. Explore with the client relapse triggers and coping strategies to manage those triggers.
   c. Provide interpersonal skills training, such as problem solving, coping skills, awareness and management of negative self-talk, increasing pleasant activities, and relaxation training.
   d. Provide education on interpersonal skills, such as starting conversations, assertiveness training, nonverbal communication, refusing offers of alcohol and drugs, and strengthening social support networks.
   e. Encourage the use of relaxation techniques such as deep breathing and listening to soothing music.

XIV. INHALANT AND PHENCYCLIDINE USE DISORDERS

A. INHALANT AND PHENCYCLIDINE ABUSE
   1. DESCRIPTION
      a. Maladaptive pattern of inhalant and phencyclidine use that causes significant impairment in a number of areas, including job, home life, or school
      b. Examples of inhalants include gasoline, glue, adhesives, rubber cement, lighter fluid, paint thinners, varnish, typewriter correction fluid, and spray can propellants.
   2. ASSESSMENT
      a. Job or school performance is negatively impacted.
      b. Interpersonal and social problems due to inhalant abuse, such as fights with significant others
      c. Decreasing or giving up important occupational, recreational, or social activities
      d. Larger amounts of the inhalant and phencyclidine are taken and for longer amounts of time than was originally planned.
      e. Large amounts of time are spent using and recovering from the effects of inhalant and phencyclidine use.
      f. Substance use continues despite knowledge of physical and psychological problems that can result from its use.
   3. MEDICAL COMPLICATIONS
      a. Death can occur from respiratory depression, cardiac irregularity, asphyxiation, the aspiration of vomitus, or accident or injury such as driving while intoxicated.

   b. Irreversible liver or kidney damage and permanent muscle damage
   c. Seizures
   d. Coma
   4. NURSING INTERVENTIONS
      a. Encourage abstinence from inhalant use.
      b. Inform the client about medical complications that can result due to inhalant abuse.
      c. Encourage participation in Narcotics Anonymous 12–step program.
B. INHALANT INTOXICATION
   1. DESCRIPTION: AN INHALANT-SPECIFIC SYNDROME WITH BEHAVIORAL OR PSYCHOLOGICAL PROBLEMS, OR BOTH, SUCH AS ASSAULTIVENESS, IMPAIRED JUDGMENT, OR PARANOIA, THAT RESULT DUE TO RECENT INHALANT USE
   2. ASSESSMENT
      a. Two or more of the following clinical manifestations develop during or shortly after inhalant use:
         1) Blurred vision or diplopia
         2) Dizziness
         3) Euphoria
         4) Incoordination
         5) Lethargy
         6) Muscle weakness, generalized
         7) Nystagmus
         8) Psychomotor retardation
         9) Reflexes, depressed
         10) Slurred speech
         11) Stupor or coma
         12) Tremor
         13) Unsteady gait
   3. NURSING INTERVENTIONS
      a. Provide for environmental safety.
      b. Perform a neurological assessment, including a cranial nerve exam.
C. PHENCYCLIDINE INTOXICATION
   1. DESCRIPTION: A PHENCYCLIDINE-SPECIFIC SYNDROME WITH BEHAVIORAL OR PSYCHOLOGICAL PROBLEMS, OR BOTH, SUCH AS ASSAULTIVENESS, IMPAIRED JUDGMENT, OR PARANOIA, THAT RESULTS DUE TO RECENT PHENCYCLIDINE USE
   2. ASSESSMENT
      a. Within 1 hour or less if inhaled, two or more of the following clinical manifestations develop:
         1) Ataxia
         2) Dysarthria
         3) Horizontal or vertical nystagmus
         4) Hypercusis
         5) Hypertension
         6) Muscle rigidity

7) Numbness or decreased pain response
8) Seizures or coma
9) Tachycardia

3. NURSING INTERVENTIONS (SEE NURSING INTERVENTIONS SECTION FOR INHALANT INTOXICATION ON PAGE 994.)

D. INHALANT DEPENDENCE AND PHENCYCLIDINE DEPENDENCE
1. DESCRIPTION: MALADAPTIVE USAGE PATTERN OF AN INHALANT OR PHENCYCLIDINE THAT LEADS TO SIGNIFICANT DISTRESS OR IMPAIRMENT IN THE CLIENT'S OCCUPATION, INTERPERSONAL, AND SOCIAL LIFE
2. ASSESSMENT
   a. Larger amounts of the inhalant or phencyclidine are consumed or are consumed over a longer period of time than was originally intended.
   b. There may be a desire to cut down or control inhalant or phencyclidine intake with or without successful efforts to do so.
   c. Large amounts of time are spent using the substance along with experiencing the effects.
   d. Inhalant and phencyclidine use causes an inability to perform important occupational, social, or recreational activities.
   e. Inhalant or phencyclidine consumption continues, with disregard of knowledge of the physiological and psychological problems caused by the substance.
3. NURSING INTERVENTIONS
   a. Assess the client for amphetamine intoxication.
   b. Ensure the client's safety such as preventing falls due to incoordination, muscle weakness, psychomotor retardation, and unsteady gait.
   c. Instruct the client about negative consequences of inhalant or phencyclidine consumption, such as impaired social and interpersonal relationships and physical and psychological problems.
   d. Inform the client about methods of relapse prevention.

XV. IMPAIRED NURSES
A. DESCRIPTION
1. LICENSED PRACTICAL OR REGISTERED NURSES WHO ABUSE DRUGS ILLEGALLY OBTAINED FROM THE WORK ENVIRONMENT
2. RESULTS IN SUSPENSION OR REVOCATION OF NURSING LICENSE AND MAY RESULT IN A JAIL TERM
3. PLACES CLIENTS AT RISK FOR UNSAFE CARE BEING DELIVERED
4. MAY BE THE RESULT OF INCREASED STRESSORS IN THE NURSE'S LIFE AND THE EASY ACCESS TO A WIDE VARIETY OF DRUGS
B. ASSESSMENT
1. NARCOTIC COUNT BEING WRONG WHEN CHECKED
2. CLIENT FAILS TO REPORT A DECREASE IN PAIN AFTER SUPPOSEDLY RECEIVING PAIN MEDICATION.
3. POOR JUDGMENT
4. INABILITY TO CONCENTRATE
5. FREQUENTLY REPORTING TO WORK LATE OR REPEATED ABSENCES
6. ALCOHOL BREATH
C. NURSING INTERVENTIONS
1. IT IS THE RESPONSIBILITY OF A COWORKER TO REPORT A NURSE WHO IS SUSPECTED OF STEALING DRUGS FROM THE NURSING UNIT.
2. KEEP AND CHECK THE NARCOTIC COUNT AT THE END OF EVERY SHIFT.
3. DOCUMENT THE IMPAIRED NURSE'S BEHAVIOR.
4. REALIZE THAT THE IMPAIRED NURSE MAY DENY BEING IMPAIRED.
5. OFFER SUPPORT TO THE IMPAIRED NURSE.

PRACTICE QUESTIONS

1. Which of the following nursing interventions is a priority when planning nursing care for the client experiencing alcohol withdrawal?
   1. Teach techniques to reduce anxiety
   2. Administer a benzodiazepine
   3. Encourage fluid intake
   4. Provide a diet low in fat

2. Which of the following orders should the nurse question when planning the nursing care for a client beginning to experience alcohol withdrawal?
   1. Eliminate caffeine from the diet
   2. Assess vital signs every 2 to 4 hours
   3. Nothing by mouth
   4. Teach relaxation techniques

3. After collecting data on a client suspected of being in a narcotic withdrawal, which of the following should the nurse report?
Select all that apply:
[ ] 1. Slurred speech
[ ] 2. Decreased blood pressure
[ ] 3. Psychomotor retardation
[ ] 4. Diarrhea
[ ] 5. Muscle aches
[ ] 6. Rhinorrhea

4. Which of the following would provide the nurse with the most beneficial assessment data on alcohol abuse?
1. Complete blood cell count
2. Chemistry panel
3. The CAGE questionnaire
4. Beck Depression Inventory

5. The nurse should monitor which of the following for a client experiencing alcohol withdrawal?
Select all that apply:
[ ] 1. Hypertension
[ ] 2. Tinnitus
[ ] 3. Pupil constriction
[ ] 4. Tachycardia
[ ] 5. Sedation
[ ] 6. Startles easily

6. The priority nursing intervention in caring for a client experiencing flashbacks from hallucinogenic intoxication is which of the following?
1. Assisting the client with reduction of anxiety
2. Exploring with the client relapse triggers
3. Providing intrapersonal skills training
4. Teaching the client the medical consequences of hallucinogen abuse

7. The nurse is caring for a client who drank large amounts of alcohol for more than 2 years and abruptly stopped drinking alcohol 30 hours ago. Which of the following nursing measures should receive priority in this client's plan of care?
1. Perform a cranial nerve exam
2. Provide adequate nutrition
3. Encourage fluids
4. Monitor vital signs frequently

8. The nurse is admitting a client for alcohol withdrawal. The client states that the last drink of alcohol was at 0800. The nurse should begin to assess this client for clinical manifestations of alcohol withdrawal at
_____.

9. The nurse is asked to teach a class to a group of clients in a drug rehabilitation clinic on the medical complications of cocaine abuse. Which

of the following complications should the nurse include in the class?
1. Hypotension
2. Cardiac arrhythmias
3. Constipation
4. Kidney failure

10. Which of the following does a coworker notice in a fellow nurse suspected of being an impaired nurse?
Select all that apply:
[ ] 1. The narcotic count is wrong when checked
[ ] 2. Heightened ability to concentrate
[ ] 3. Promptly reports to work
[ ] 4. Inability to concentrate
[ ] 5. Client reports a decrease in pain after receiving a pain medication
[ ] 6. Alcohol breath

11. A client repeatedly returns to the hospital with an unsteady gait and slurred speech after several failed inpatient treatment attempts for alcohol dependence. Which of the following nursing interventions is appropriate for the nurse to implement for this client?
1. Promote safety and transition to the hospital
2. Administer a benzodiazepine and a barbiturate
3. Provide a diet high in protein
4. Administer a nonnarcotic analgesic

12. The nurse monitors for which of the following assessment findings in hallucinogen intoxication?
Select all of the following:
[ ] 1. Cardiac arrhythmias
[ ] 2. Labile affect
[ ] 3. Nervousness
[ ] 4. Floating feeling
[ ] 5. Anorexia
[ ] 6. Diuresis

13. Which of the following should the nurse include in the plan of care for a client experiencing a morphine sulfate withdrawal?
1. Provide a cool room
2. Administer diazepam (Valium)
3. Administer clonidine (Catapres)
4. Restrict fluids

14. The nurse documents which of the following clinical manifestations to be present in a client who is experiencing cannabis intoxication?
Select all that apply:
[ ] 1. Anorexia
[ ] 2. Dry mouth
[ ] 3. Euphoria
[ ] 4. Bradycardia
[ ] 5. Sensation of slowed time
[ ] 6. Drowsiness

15. A client admitted for cannabis intoxication asks the nurse what the average time in days is for urine drug screens to be positive for cannabis after the last use. The appropriate response by the nurse is how many days?

    _____

16. A client presents to the emergency room complaining of trails of images, moving objects, and flashes of color. The nurse notifies the physician that the client has been abusing which substance?
    1. Caffeine
    2. Hallucinogens
    3. Alcohol
    4. Sedatives

17. Which of the following should the nurse include when preparing to teach a nicotine-cessation program?
    1. Nicotine withdrawal clinical manifestations include hot flashes, decreased appetite, and muscle cramps
    2. The nicotine withdrawal syndrome lasts less than 1 week
    3. The nurse's personal experience with nicotine withdrawal
    4. Decreased psychomotor performance, mental dullness, and decreased judgment may be experienced by the client

18. The nurse is caring for a client who is experiencing cocaine intoxication. Which would indicate to the nurse that the client's condition is deteriorating?
    Select all that apply:
    [ ] 1. Dyskinesias
    [ ] 2. Chest pain
    [ ] 3. Decreased urine output
    [ ] 4. Hypertension
    [ ] 5. Anxiety
    [ ] 6. Tachycardia

19. The nurse is caring for a client admitted with cocaine intoxication who has a fever and is experiencing chest pain, palpitations, and increased blood pressure and pulse. The nursing priority action is to do which of the following?
    1. Establish a patent airway
    2. Perform a cranial nerve exam
    3. Provide comfort measures
    4. Instruct client about medical complications

20. The nurse is preparing to teach a class to a group of new graduate nurses on substance use disorders. Which of the following should the nurse include in the class?
    1. A client with substance dependence must take the same drug to relieve withdrawal symptoms

    2. Substance abuse is both a physical and psychological disorder
    3. A client with substance dependence who is motivated to do so can overcome the addiction by stopping use of the substance
    4. A substance must be abused over a long period of time before an addiction develops

21. The nurse should monitor a client who is suspected of having abused dextroamphetamine (Dexedrine) for which of the following? Select all that apply:
    [ ] 1. Constipation
    [ ] 2. Increased urine output
    [ ] 3. Chest pain
    [ ] 4. Pupil dilation
    [ ] 5. Tachycardia
    [ ] 6. Increased muscular endurance

22. The registered nurse is preparing the clinical assignments for a psychiatric unit. Which of the following assignments is appropriate for the nurse to delegate to a licensed practical nurse?
    1. Assess a client for cannabis intoxication
    2. Instruct a client on nicotine withdrawal
    3. Provide a safe environment for a client with alcohol dependence
    4. Report the clinical manifestations a client suspected of dextroamphetamine (Dexedrine) is experiencing

23. The nurse is admitting a client who has been abusing phencyclidine (PCP) for several months. In planning this client's care, which of the following should be the priority?
    1. Provide a well-balanced diet
    2. Instruct the client on the medical complications of PCP abuse
    3. Encourage the client to participate in a withdrawal program
    4. Ensure the safety of the client

24. A client who is seeing "pink elephants on the wall," hearing voices, constantly picking at the face and hands, and stating "people are out to kill me" and who has a blood pressure of 168/90 is admitted. The nurse assesses this client to be experiencing which of the following?
    1. Amphetamine toxicity
    2. Opioid withdrawal
    3. Inhalant side effects
    4. Alcohol dependence

25. A mother brings her adolescent son into a clinic and expresses concerns that the son has been experiencing blurred vision, dizziness, a sense of well-being, and slurred

speech. Which of the following questions is a priority for the nurse to ask?
1. "How long have you noticed these clinical manifestations and behavior?"
2. "Has your son's school work declined?"
3. "Has your son withdrawn and seems to spend more time alone?"
4. "Have you noticed your son inhaling paint and cleaning or aerosol products?"

26. The nurse assesses which of the following in a client with a blood alcohol concentration level of 0.10?
Select all that apply:
[ ] 1. Impaired balance and movement
[ ] 2. Slight impaired judgment
[ ] 3. Inability to make rational decisions
[ ] 4. Impaired reaction time
[ ] 5. Impaired sense of control
[ ] 6. Loss of consciousness

ANSWERS AND RATIONALES

1. 2. Because alcohol is a central nervous system (CNS) depressant, withdrawal will cause the client's CNS to be activated. Administering a benzodiazepine takes priority when caring for a client experiencing alcohol withdrawal. It will lower blood pressure and pulse, decrease anxiety, and assist in preventing seizures and death. Encouraging fluids, providing three well-balanced meals, and teaching techniques to reduce anxiety are all appropriate interventions but are not the priority.

2. 3. Fluids should be encouraged for clients experiencing alcohol withdrawal because they often experience dehydration. Fluids would never be withheld. Assessing vital signs, teaching relaxation techniques, and avoiding caffeine in the diet are all appropriate nursing interventions for a client in alcohol withdrawal.

3. 4. 5. 6. Clinical manifestations of narcotic withdrawal include diarrhea, muscle aches, and rhinorrhea. Slurred speech, decreased blood pressure, and psychomotor retardation are clinical manifestations of opiate intoxication.

4. 3. A complete blood cell count and a chemistry panel will assist the nurse in identifying medical issues that may be caused by alcohol abuse, but these tests alone will not reveal the information needed to assess for the alcohol abuse. The CAGE questionnaire is the acronym for assessing clients for alcohol abuse. The Beck Depression Inventory assesses a client's severity of depression.

5. 1. 4. 6. An increased blood pressure and an increased pulse are the most prevalent and first clinical manifestations experienced by the client in alcohol withdrawal. Other clinical manifestations include irritability, a sense of being hyperactive, startling easily, making jerky movements, anxiety, insomnia, and tremors.

6. 1. Although exploring with the client what triggers a relapse, providing intrapersonal skills, and teaching the client the medical consequences of hallucinogens are important interventions in a client experiencing hallucinogenic intoxication, they are not the priority. Reducing stimuli and the client's anxiety are the priority nursing intervention for a client experiencing flashbacks from hallucinogen intoxication.

7. 4. Although performing a cranial nerve assessment, providing adequate nutrition, and encouraging fluids are all appropriate interventions, monitoring vital signs is the priority intervention. Monitoring the vital signs frequently will determine when the client goes into alcohol withdrawal.

8. 1600 to 2000. Alcohol withdrawal clinical manifestations begin between 8 and 12 hours after the last drink of alcohol. If the client had the last drink at 0800, the nurse should begin to assess the client for clinical manifestations of alcohol withdrawal between 1600 and 2000.

9. 2. Cocaine is a stimulant that works directly on the central nervous system and produces cardiac arrhythmias. Cardiac arrhythmias can lead to death for a client who abuses cocaine. Hypertension is a complication that occurs with toxic levels of cocaine. Constipation does not occur as a result of cocaine; it is actually diarrhea that occurs. Kidney failure is also not a complication of cocaine use.

10. 1. 4. 6. The narcotic count is wrong when checked when an impaired nurse is suspected. Other features include an inability to concentrate, alcohol breath, the client fails to report a decrease in pain after supposedly receiving pain medication, and the nurse exhibits poor judgment and is frequently late to work or has repeated absences.

11. 1. A client who has an unsteady gait and slurred speech after several failed attempts at treatment for alcohol dependence is experiencing alcohol intoxication. Promoting safety and facilitating transition to the hospital is the appropriate intervention for this client. Administering a benzodiazepine, a barbiturate, or a narcotic would actually depress the central nervous system even further and is contraindicated. Increasing protein in the diet is not a standard intervention to be implemented for a client experiencing alcohol intoxication.

12. 2. 4. 5. Assessment findings in hallucinogen intoxication include labile affect, anorexia, and a floating feeling. Cardiac arrhythmias, diuresis, and nervousness are assessment findings in caffeine intoxication.

13. 3. Clonidine (Catapres) blocks opioid receptor sites more effectively than a central nervous system depressant (Valium) in the treatment of opioid withdrawal. Most likely the client would complain of being chilled and require multiple blankets or a warm whirlpool. Fluids are encouraged and not restricted.

14. 2. 3. 5. The clinical manifestations for cannabis intoxication include dry mouth, euphoria, and a sensation of slowed time. Increased appetite, tachycardia, and anxiety are also experienced.

15. 7 to 10 days. The average time frame for urine drug screens to be positive for cannabis is 7 to 10 days after the last use. Heavy use of cannabis may result in the cannabis being present in the urine for 2 to 4 weeks.

16. 2. The perceptual disturbances of experiencing trails of images, halos, and flashes of color occur with hallucinogen use.

17. 4. A decrease in psychomotor performance, mental dullness, and decreased judgment are experienced by the client in a nicotine-cessation program. Hot flashes, decreased appetite, and muscle cramps are not associated with nicotine withdrawal. Nicotine withdrawal lasts several weeks to months. The nurse should keep the focus of the class professional and on educating the participants of the nicotine withdrawal class and not on personal experiences.

18. 2. 4. 6. Clinical manifestations of cocaine intoxication include dyskinesias, decreased urine output, anxiety, agitation, chills, weight loss, and anorexia. None of these clinical manifestations is life threatening. Chest pain, palpitation, hypertension, and tachycardia are clinical manifestations that indicate the client's condition is deteriorating. These manifestations indicate that the client is toxic and may experience life-threatening complications such as an arrhythmia, stroke, or myocardial infarction if interventions are not taken.

19. Establish and ensure a patent airway. Establishing and ensuring a patent airway is the nursing priority for a client experiencing cocaine intoxication. Fever, chest pain, palpitations, and increased blood pressure and pulse are all indications that the client is toxic. If a patent airway is not established first, the client may die from a myocardial infarction, stroke, or life-threatening arrhythmia. Other interventions include performing a cranial nerve assessment, providing comfort measures, and instructing the client about medical complications.

20. 2. A substance use disorder is both physical and psychological. A client with substance dependence can take a similar substance to relieve withdrawal clinical manifestations. A client cannot overcome a substance use disorder simply by being motivated and stopping the substance. Management of substance use disorders must include professional intervention. Generally, the most effective treatments are in mental health clinics that can provide both physical and psychological assistance.

21. 3. 4. 5. Dextroamphetamine (Dexedrine) is a central nervous stimulant that has a high potential for abuse. Physiological manifestations of Dexedrine abuse include chest pain, tachycardia, pupil dilation, diarrhea, decreased urine output, and muscular weakness.

22. 3. A licensed practical nurse may provide a safe environment for a client with alcohol dependence. Assessing, instructing, and reporting are all skills reserved for a registered nurse.

23. 4. A client who has been abusing PCP experiences distorted perceptions, hallucinations, and delusions that may result in the client becoming violent. Ensuring the client's safety is the priority. The client has the potential to hurt himself or others. Eating a well-balanced diet, instructing the client on the medical complications of PCP use, and encouraging participation in a withdrawal program are all appropriate interventions, but they are not the priority.

24. 1. A client who has a toxic level of amphetamines experiences hallucinations (auditory, visual, and tactile), severe paranoia, picking at the face and extremities, and hypertension.

25. 4. The priority question to ask the mother of a child suspected of inhaling substances is if she has noticed the child inhaling paint or cleaning or aerosol products.

26. 3. 4. 5.   Inability to make rational decisions occurs with a blood alcohol concentration of 0.06. Impaired reaction time and impaired sense of control occur with a blood alcohol concentration of 0.10. A client with a blood alcohol concentration of 0.10 is legally intoxicated in most states. Slightly impaired judgment occurs with a blood alcohol concentration of 0.06. Impaired balance and movement generally appear with a blood alcohol concentration of 0.15.

REFERENCES

Antai-Otong, D. (2008). *Psychiatric nursing, biological and behavioral concepts* (2nd ed.). Clifton Park, NY: Delmar Cengage Learning.

Frisch, N. C., & Frisch, L. E. (2011). *Psychiatric mental health nursing* (4th ed.). Clifton Park, NY: Delmar Cengage Learning.

CHAPTER 56

SEXUAL AND GENDER IDENTITY DISORDERS

I. **SEXUAL AND GENDER IDENTITY DISORDERS**
   A. DESCRIPTION
      1. DISORDERS OF SEXUAL FUNCTIONING ARE CHARACTERIZED BY A DISTURBANCE IN SEXUAL DESIRE AND CHANGES IN THE SEXUAL RESPONSE CYCLE THAT CAUSES SIGNIFICANT DISTRESS AND INTERPERSONAL DIFFICULTY.
      2. THE FOUR CLASSIFICATIONS ARE SEXUAL DYSFUNCTIONS, GENDER IDENTITY DISORDER, PARAPHILIAS, AND SEXUAL DISORDER NOT OTHERWISE SPECIFIED.
      3. SEXUAL DESIRE DISORDERS ARE INFLUENCED BY A VARIETY OF FACTORS, SUCH AS AGE, AVAILABILITY OF A PARTNER, HEALTH, AND LEISURE.
   B. THEORIES OF SEXUAL DISORDERS
      1. BIOLOGICAL CAUSES
         a. General illness that may contribute
            1) Influenza
            2) Colds
            3) Fatigue
            4) Diabetes
            5) Hepatitis
            6) Multiple sclerosis
            7) Arthritis
            8) Back pain
            9) Obesity
            10) Vaginal infections
            11) Late stages of pregnancy
            12) Postmenopausal women may need lubrication.
            13) Older male responses are slowed.
      2. HORMONAL CAUSES
         a. Medications cause a decrease in androgen levels, such as hypopituitary problems.
         b. Feminizing effects of testicular tumors
         c. Alcohol, cocaine, and heroine use
         d. Use of hypertensive drugs
         e. Use of phenothiazine

         f. Selective serotonin reuptake inhibitors (SSRIs) and other antidepressants may cause sexual difficulties.
      3. PSYCHOLOGICAL CAUSES OF SEXUAL DYSFUNCTION
         a. Failure to understand the partner's desires
         b. Anxiety due to fear of failure
         c. Partner or self-demand for performance or excessive need to please
         d. Perceptual and intellectual defenses
         e. Allowing judgmental thoughts to intervene
         f. Poor relationship choices that can result in partner rejection
         g. Lack of trust
         h. Power struggles
         i. Sexual sabotage
   C. TYPES OF SEXUAL DYSFUNCTION
      1. HYPOACTIVE SEXUAL DESIRE DISORDER
         a. Recurrent or persistent deficit or absence of sexual fantasies and desire for sexual activity
         b. Not diagnosed for older adults and those who have hormonal abnormalities
         c. Primarily developed in puberty to adulthood
         d. Disturbance causes marked distress or interpersonal difficulty.
         e. Not explained by a substance abuse or medical condition
      2. SEXUAL AVERSION DISORDER
         a. Aversion to and active avoidance of genital sexual contact with a partner
         b. Anxiety, fear, or disgust with sexual encounter ranging from lack of pleasure to extreme psychological distress
         c. Criteria to meet the disorder need to cause the marked distress in interpersonal functioning.
         d. Dysfunction is not the result of another sexual disorder.

3. SEXUAL AROUSAL DISORDERS, MALE AND FEMALE
   a. May be accompanied by sexual desire disorder or female orgasmic disorder
   b. Male erectile disorder associated with sexual anxiety
   c. Fear of failure and concerns about sexual performance
   d. Decreased subjective sense of sexual excitement and pleasure
   e. Spontaneously remit 15% to 30% of the time
4. ORGASMIC DISORDERS
   a. Persistent or recurrent delay in or absence of orgasm
   b. Female orgasmic disorder: often not interested in orgasm
   c. Male orgasmic disorder: persistent or current delay or absence of orgasm after normal sexual excitement
   d. Inhibited desire could be due to an endocrinological dysfunction such as an elevation in the hormone prolactin or a small pituitary tumor that may reduce libido or sexual interest. Testosterone levels and normal aging also decrease sexual interest.
5. PREMATURE EJACULATIONS
   a. Male orgasm and ejaculation takes place with minimal physical stimulation and before expected.
   b. Disturbance causes marked distress or interpersonal difficulty.
   c. Not due exclusively to direct effect of substance abuse
6. MALE ERECTILE DISORDER
   a. Difficulty achieving or maintaining an erection
   b. Disorder causes marked distress or interpersonal difficulty.
   c. Not explained by the effects of substance abuse or medical condition
7. SEXUAL PAIN DISORDER
   a. Found in both males and females; associated with genital pain during intercourse
   b. Vaginismus consists of contraction of the peritoneal muscles surrounding the outer third of the vagina.
   c. May still experience desire and pleasure
   d. Often found in women who have been sexually abused or traumatized
D. ASSESSMENT
   1. OVERLY CONCERNED WITH PHYSICAL CHANGES OCCURRING AT PUBERTY
   2. PREFER OPPOSITE-SEX BEHAVIORS INTO ADULTHOOD
   3. DESIRE SEXUAL REASSIGNMENT

E. NURSING INTERVENTIONS
   1. PROVIDE SEXUAL COUNSELING CONSISTING OF TAKING A COMPLETE GENERAL HISTORY.
   2. PERFORM A COMPLETE PHYSICAL EXAMINATION TO RULE OUT ORGANIC CAUSES.
   3. OBTAIN THE CLIENT'S SEXUAL HISTORY.
   4. ASSESS COMMUNICATION PATTERNS AND EXPECTATIONS.
   5. ASSESS IF PRIMARY FOCUS IS SEXUAL OR PSYCHOSOCIAL IN ORIGIN.
   6. PROMOTE ANXIETY REDUCTION.
   7. ENCOURAGE COUPLE COUNSELING TO DISCUSS SEXUAL NEEDS AND DESIRES OPENLY.
   8. PROMOTE CONSTRUCTION OF A HEALTHY RELATIONSHIP.
   9. PROMOTE MUTUAL RESPECT.

II. **NURSING DIAGNOSES**
   A. ANXIETY
   B. INEFFECTIVE ROLE PERFORMANCE
   C. SOCIAL ISOLATION
   D. INEFFECTIVE COPING
   E. INTERRUPTED FAMILY PROCESSES

Nursing Diagnoses: Definitions and Classification 2012–2014. Copyright © 2012, 1994–2012 by NANDA International. Used by arrangement with John Wiley & Sons Limited.

III. **GENDER IDENTITY DISORDER**
   A. DESCRIPTION
      1. STRONG AND PERSISTENT CROSS-GENDER IDENTIFICATION
      2. PERSISTENT DISCOMFORT WITH GENDER
      3. SENSE OF INAPPROPRIATENESS IN GENDER ROLE
      4. IN ADOLESCENTS, THERE IS A PREOCCUPATION WITH GETTING RID OF PRIMARY AND SECONDARY SEX CHARACTERISTICS THROUGH HORMONES.
      5. DISTURBANCE IS NOT CONCURRENT WITH PHYSICAL INTERSEX CONDITION.
      6. DISTURBANCE CAUSES CLINICALLY SIGNIFICANT DISTRESS OR IMPAIRMENT IN SOCIAL, OCCUPATIONAL, OR OTHER AREAS OF FUNCTIONING.
      7. ETIOLOGY IS UNKNOWN BUT CHILDHOOD PATTERNS SEEM TO BE FAIRLY CONSISTENT.
      8. CHILDREN AS EARLY AS 2–4 YEARS OF AGE HAVE CROSS-GENDER INTERESTS AND ACTIVITIES.
      9. CHILDHOOD HISTORY OF GENDER IDENTITY DISORDER; MAY REPORT A HOMOSEXUAL OR BISEXUAL ORIENTATION
     10. MAY NOT CONSIDER HERSELF TO BE HOMOSEXUAL AND ONLY WANTS GENDER REASSIGNMENT

B. ASSESSMENT
1. REPEATEDLY STATED DESIRE TO BE THE OPPOSITE SEX
2. IN MALES, PREFERENCE FOR CROSS-DRESSING OR SIMULATING FEMALE ATTIRE
3. GIRLS' INSISTENCE ON WEARING ONLY MASCULINE CLOTHING
4. STRONG AND PERSISTENT PREFERENCES FOR CROSS-SEX ROLES IN PLAY OR FANTASY
5. INTENSE DESIRE TO PARTICIPATE IN THE STEREOTYPICAL GAMES AND PASTIMES OF THE OTHER SEX
6. STRONG PREFERENCE FOR PLAYMATES OF THE OPPOSITE SEX
7. BOYS PREFER FEMININE DRESS AND GRAVITATE TOWARD FEMALE FRIENDS AND ACTIVITIES.
8. GIRLS EXHIBIT MASCULINE BEHAVIOR.
9. ANXIETY WITH BODY CHANGES FURTHER DEFINING GENDER

C. MEDICAL MANAGEMENT
1. HORMONE THERAPY IS THE FIRST STEP.
   a. Changes bodily characteristics
   b. May require the client to live in cross-gender mode for 1–2 years before reassignment is made

D. NURSING INTERVENTIONS
1. ENCOURAGE THE CLIENT TO VERBALIZE FEELINGS.
2. ENCOURAGE COUNSELING FOR COPING SOLUTIONS.
3. SURGICAL REASSIGNMENT
4. RECOGNIZE THAT LEGAL, SOCIAL, FAMILIAL, AND EMPLOYMENT ADJUSTMENTS MAY BE A FACTOR.
5. ACCEPT THE CLIENT WHO IS HAPPY AND PRODUCTIVE WITHOUT UNDERGOING SURGERY.
6. ACCEPT THE CLIENT WHO FEELS UNABLE TO FUNCTION WITHOUT SURGICAL REASSIGNMENT.

IV. **PARAPHILIAS**
A. DESCRIPTION
1. CONSIST OF SEVERAL FEATURES
   a. Recurrent and intense sexually arousing fantasies, sexual urges, or behaviors involving inanimate objects
   b. Can involve suffering or humiliation of oneself or one's partner
   c. Can involve use of children or other nonconsenting individuals, often triggered by stress
2. HISTORY, CULTURE, AND EXPERIENCE PLAY A ROLE.
3. DIAGNOSTIC CRITERIA MUST BE PRESENT FOR AT LEAST 6 MONTHS.
4. FANTASIES, SEXUAL URGES, OR BEHAVIORS ARE CAUSING SIGNIFICANT DISTRESS OR IMPAIRMENT IN SOCIAL OCCUPATIONAL OR OTHER AREAS OF FUNCTIONING.

B. TYPES OF PARAPHILIAS
1. FETISHISM: PRESENCE OF INTENSE SEXUAL AROUSAL INVOLVING INANIMATE OBJECTS; SEXUAL AROUSAL OCCURRING FROM CONTACT WITH A NONLIVING OBJECT SUCH AS AN ARTICLE OF CLOTHING
2. PEDOPHILIA INVOLVES SEXUAL INTEREST DIRECTED PRIMARILY OR EXCLUSIVELY TOWARD CHILDREN 13 YEARS OR YOUNGER.
   a. May only be recurrent fantasies or urges
   b. Pedophile generally conservative married male but must be at least 16 years old and at least 5 years older than the child
   c. Often occurs in families with older male and younger female
   d. When it occurs in families, it is called incest.
3. EXHIBITIONISM IS THE INTENTIONAL DISPLAY OF GENITALS IN PUBLIC PLACES, OFTEN ACCOMPANIED BY MASTURBATION, TO ELICIT SHOCK, RESULTING IN SEXUAL AROUSAL OCCURRING FROM EXPOSING GENITALS TO STRANGERS.
   a. Typical profile is a sedate middle-class male.
4. VOYEURISM IS VIEWING IN INTIMATE SITUATIONS OR FANTASIZING ABOUT OBSERVING OTHERS DISROBING, NAKED, OR INVOLVED IN SEXUAL ACTIVITY.
   a. Called "peeping tom" and peeping becomes compulsive and preferable to other sexual activity
   b. Usually heterosexual male who wishes no contact with those he is watching
   c. Typically shy, socially unskilled, and without close friends
5. TRANSVESTITISM IS SEXUAL SATISFACTION BY MEANS OF DRESSING IN THE CLOTHING OF THE OPPOSITE GENDER.
   a. Usually develops early in life
   b. Not related to sexual orientation issues and there is no desire for sex change
   c. Heterosexuals often receive the cooperation and support of partners.

6. FROTTEURISM INVOLVES THE SEXUAL TOUCHING, RUBBING AGAINST, OR FONDLING OF A NONCONSENTING INDIVIDUAL, USUALLY A STRANGER, TO ACHIEVE SEXUAL SATISFACTION.
   a. Usually occurs in public places where there is an easy escape after the behavior
7. SEXUAL SADISM AND MASOCHISM
   a. Giving (sadism) and receiving (masochism) psychological or physical pain, or both
   b. Domination to achieve sexual gratification occurs.
   c. Treatment is usually cognitive and behavioral therapy with an attempt to help the individual learn a new sexual response pattern.
   d. Positive reinforcement is given for appropriate object choices.
   e. Aversion techniques in which mild electric shock may be used for inappropriate choices
   f. Psychodynamic techniques to help the client understand the etiology of the disorder
C. MEDICAL MANAGEMENT FOR PARAPHILIAS
   1. PHARMACOLOGICAL
   2. COGNITIVE THERAPY
   3. BEHAVIORAL THERAPY
   4. PSYCHODYNAMIC THERAPY

5. COMBINATION THERAPY IS USUALLY EFFECTIVE OVER AN EXTENDED PERIOD OF TIME.

V. **SEXUAL ADDICTIONS**
A. DESCRIPTION: SEXUAL ADDICTIONS OCCUR WHEN SEX AND SEXUAL ENCOUNTERS BECOME THE PRIMARY WAY OF ATTEMPTING TO FILL EMPTINESS.
B. ASSESSMENT
   1. COMPELLED TO HAVE FREQUENT SEX
   2. BEWILDERED BY OWN SEXUAL BEHAVIOR
   3. PATTERN OF UNSUCCESSFUL LOVE RELATIONSHIPS
   4. CHAOS AND DRAMA ARE OFTEN PRESENT.
   5. SEXUAL ENCOUNTERS INVOLVE ALCOHOL, DRUGS, OR COMPULSIVE EATING.
   6. NEED TO ESCAPE AFTER SEX
   7. ENGAGE IN ACTIVITIES THAT ARE REPULSIVE OR UNCOMFORTABLE TO PLEASE A PARTNER
C. NURSING INTERVENTIONS
   1. ENCOURAGE THE CLIENT TO SEEK OUT A SAFE, CARING, AND UNDERSTANDING COMMUNITY.
   2. PROVIDE THE CLIENT WITH INDIVIDUAL COUNSELING.
   3. ENCOURAGE SUPPORT GROUPS OR FRIENDS.

PRACTICE QUESTIONS

1. The nurse is assessing a client with a diagnosis of hypoactive sexual desire. Which of the following characteristics is important for the nurse to assess from the history and physical?
   1. Traumatic brain injury
   2. Hormonal abnormalities
   3. An absence of sexual fantasies
   4. History of substance abuse

2. Which of the following findings would provide the nurse with the most accurate information regarding a client with sexual aversion disorder?
   1. Substance abuse problems
   2. Preoccupation with sexual encounters
   3. Gratification with sexual activity
   4. Marked distress in interpersonal functioning

3. Which of the following assessments would provide the nurse with the most accurate information regarding a client with sexual pain disorder?

Select all that apply:
[ ] 1. The disorder does not create distress in the client
[ ] 2. The client is void of sexual desire
[ ] 3. The disorder is found in females who have been sexually abused
[ ] 4. The pain is imagined
[ ] 5. The client may experience orgasm without penetration
[ ] 6. The client may experience vaginismus

4. The nurse should instruct a client with a sexual dysfunction about drugs that have a pharmacologic influence on sexual functioning. Which of the following drugs impact sexual functioning and should be included in this discussion?
   1. Antidepressants
   2. Antibiotics
   3. Analgesics
   4. Anti-inflammatories

5. A client with orgasmic disorder may have contributing hormonal problems. The nurse should counsel the client that which of the following factors may contribute to the disorder?
   1. Normal aging
   2. Overexercise
   3. Increase in testosterone
   4. Decrease in prolactin

6. The nurse is collecting a nursing history from a client admitted with a sexual dysfunction. Which of the following questions is a priority for the nurse to ask?
   1. "What is your age?"
   2. "What medications do you take?"
   3. "Do you have anxiety about sexual performance?"
   4. "What is your exercise regime?"

7. The nurse is teaching a client with a sexual dysfunction. Which of the following elements would be the most critical for the nurse to teach the client about the disorder?
   1. Mutual respect between partners is crucial
   2. Gender preference influences sexual dysfunction
   3. Avoiding drugs will alleviate sexual dysfunction
   4. Power struggles between partners do not influence sexual dysfunction

8. Which of the following assessments would provide the nurse with the most accurate information regarding a client with gender identity disorder? Assess and evaluate if the client
   1. is homosexual.
   2. has been sexually abused.
   3. had an early feeling of being trapped in the wrong gender.
   4. has a strong aversion to same-sex individuals.

9. When the nurse is assessing a client for the possibility of gender identity disorder, which of the following clinical manifestations would support the diagnosis?
   Select all that apply:
   [ ] 1. Having playmates of the same sex
   [ ] 2. No particular preference for cross-sex role play
   [ ] 3. Anxiety that accompanies puberty
   [ ] 4. Development of secondary sex characteristics
   [ ] 5. Unconcerned about the disorder
   [ ] 6. Preoccupation with the client's sex

10. A client is admitted to the psychiatric unit with a possible diagnosis of paraphilia. When conducting an assessment, which clinical manifestations would indicate to the nurse that the diagnosis was correct?
   1. A disorder with a 3-month duration
   2. Recurrent fantasy triggered by stress
   3. A persistent disinterest in sex
   4. A significant loss of libido

11. The nurse assessing a client with the diagnosis of voyeurism should note which of the following characteristics?
   1. Socially skilled individual
   2. Peeping becomes compulsive
   3. Usually not heterosexual
   4. Has many close friends

12. Which of the following assessments would provide the nurse with the most accurate information about a client with transvestitism?
   1. A desire for a sex change
   2. Enjoyment in watching others disrobe
   3. Homosexual orientation
   4. Develops early in life

13. The nurse treating a client with paraphilia would include which of the following in the care plan?
   1. Alternative medicine
   2. Residential treatment
   3. Short-term therapy
   4. Combination therapy

14. The nurse treating a client with sexual addictions should assess for which of the following clinical manifestations when formulating the nursing assessment?
   1. The client understands the behavior
   2. Patterns of unsuccessful love relationships
   3. Need to develop relationship after sexual contact
   4. Is not a compulsion

15. When working with the client who has a sexual addiction, the nurse should include which of the following in the nursing care plan?
   1. Recommendation for individual therapy
   2. Avoid groups with similar diagnosis
   3. Limit number of friends to small, close unit
   4. Community support is not a priority

16. The nurse planning care for the client with a sexual addiction understands that the client is at risk for sexually transmitted disease. What is a priority to include in this client's care plan?
   1. Educate the client about sexual addiction
   2. Offer diversional activities to sex
   3. Educate the client about safe sex
   4. Offer support to the client

17. The nurse evaluates which of the following disorders to contribute to the severity of a sexual disorder?
   1. Schizophrenia
   2. Bipolar disorder
   3. Diabetes
   4. Anorexia

18. Which of the following drugs does the nurse evaluate to contribute to the development of a sexual disorder?
Select all that apply:
[ ] 1. Hypertensives
[ ] 2. Phenothiazines
[ ] 3. Antidepressants
[ ] 4. Antibiotics
[ ] 5. Cholinergics
[ ] 6. Histamine H_2 antagonists

19. The nurse planning for the discharge of a client with sexual dysfunction would take into consideration which of the following measures?
1. The client will have trusting relationships
2. The client's judgment may be clouded by perceptual defenses
3. Judgmental thoughts are crucial for recovery
4. Power struggles are inevitable and are a key to cure

20. The most effective treatment tool the nurse should use when working with a client with sexual disorders is
1. the complete general history.
2. the sexual disorders history.
3. drug management.
4. family therapy.

21. When working with a client with hypoactive sexual desire disorder, the nurse should include which of the following recommendations in the treatment plan?
1. Substance abuse counseling
2. Treatment for a medical condition
3. Encourage the client to focus on the disorder
4. Establish a therapeutic alliance

22. The nurse planning the treatment for a client with aversion disorder considers which of the following in the care plan?

1. Medical conditions are the etiology
2. Interpersonal functioning is a low priority
3. Anxiety and disgust contribute to distress
4. Aversion is not a part of the disorder

23. The nurse developing a treatment plan for a client with gender identity disorder would include which of the following measures?
1. Short-term therapy
2. Drugs to control dysphoria
3. Counseling for coping solutions
4. Legal counseling

24. Which of the following clinical manifestations would the nurse assess as most prevalent in a client suspected of having contracted chlamydia?
1. Discharge from the genitals
2. Generalized body aches
3. Intermittent discomfort when urinating
4. Spontaneous remission

25. When assessing a client suspected of having hepatitis B, which of the following clinical manifestations supports the diagnosis?
1. Unprotected sexual contact
2. Malnutrition
3. Fecal-oral route
4. Sexual addiction

26. The registered nurse is preparing clinical assignments for a psychiatric unit. Which of the following clinical assignments should the nurse delegate to a licensed practical nurse?
1. Perform a complete general history on a client with gender identity disorder
2. Assess a client with aversion disorder for distress
3. Develop a plan of care for a client with gender identity disorder
4. Document the behavior exhibited by a client with gender identity disorder

ANSWERS AND RATIONALES

1. 3. The diagnostic criterion for hypoactive sexual drive is the absence of sexual fantasies. Hypoactive sexual desire is diagnosed if there is no substance abuse or medical condition.

2. 4. Marked distress in interpersonal functioning is a criterion for the diagnosis of sexual aversion disorder. Substance abuse alone can cause sexual dysfunction; however, it does not meet the criteria for sexual aversion disorder. Avoidance, rather than preoccupation, with sexual encounters is a characteristic. Frustration, instead of gratification, is seen with sexual aversion disorder.

3. 3. 5. 6. The disorder occurs most frequently in females with a sexual abuse history. The client may experience orgasm without penetration. Vaginismus is a common clinical manifestation. The disorder creates great anxiety and distress for the client. The client is not void of desire for sexual contact. The client avoids a sexual encounter because it is a painful experience. The pain is real.

4. 1. Antidepressants have a direct effect on sexual performance and result in loss of libido. Antibiotics, analgesics, and anti-inflammatories do not have an effect on sexual functioning.

5. 1.   Normal aging can contribute to the slowing of an orgasm in orgasmic disorder. Exercise is not a factor in orgasmic disorder. Decreases in testosterone may contribute to orgasmic disorder. Increase in prolactin may contribute to orgasmic disorders.

6. 3.   Anxiety is the factor that most dramatically affects sexual dysfunction, so it would be a priority to ask if the client has anxiety about sexual performance. The client's age, drugs that the client takes, and the client's exercise regime may contribute to a sexual dysfunction but do not qualify as the priority.

7. 1.   Establishing mutual respect is critical between partners being treated for sexual dysfunctions. Preferences of gender do not contribute to sexual dysfunctions. Drugs may precipitate sexual dysfunctions, but they are not the priority. Power struggles between partners do contribute to sexual dysfunctions.

8. 3.   An early feeling of being trapped in the wrong gender is the diagnostic criterion for establishing the diagnosis of gender identity disorder. The sexual preference of the individual does not contribute to the disorder. The client's history of abuse also is not a diagnostic criterion for the disorder. Aversion to individuals who are of the same sex is also not a criterion for gender identity disorder.

9. 3. 4. 6.   Puberty and secondary sex characteristics often produce great anxiety in a client with gender identity disorder. Playmates of the opposite sex are preferred. There is a particular preference for cross-sex role play. Clients with gender identity disorder are preoccupied with their sex identity and highly concerned about the disorder.

10. 2.   Paraphilia is a disorder of sexual interest, arousal, and orgasm. A recurrent fantasy involving inanimate objects is triggered by stress. The disorder needs to last 6 months in order to meet the diagnostic criterion. There is a persistent interest in sex. There is no loss of libido.

11. 2.   Voyeurism is a sexual disorder that involves watching others while they disrobe, are naked, or are engaging in various sexual acts. Peeping becomes compulsive and is preferable to other sexual activities. The individual is usually heterosexual, unskilled, and socially shy. Such individuals usually have few close friends.

12. 4.   Transvestitism is a disorder that involves cross dressing or fantasies about cross dressing. It develops early in life. There is no desire for a sex change or for a change in the client's sexual orientation.

13. 4.   The recommended treatment for paraphilia is a combination of therapies. Alternative medicine

and residential treatment are not recommended. Therapy should be conducted over an extended period of time.

14. 2.   Patterns of unsuccessful love relationships are diagnostic for sexual addictions. The client is bewildered by personal behavior. The client feels a need to escape after sex and is compelled to have frequent sex.

15. 1.   Recommendations for individual and group therapy should be made for clients with sexual addictions. Group therapy is a recommendation. Friendships should not be limited but should be encouraged. A safe and supportive community is essential for client recovery.

16. 3.   Educate the client about safe sex. The priority intervention when working with a client who has a sexual addiction is to educate the client about safe sex practice. It is imperative to inform the client about the use of condoms and dental dams and the avoidance of multiple partners. The focus of nursing care should be holistic and preventive rather than disease oriented.

17. 3.   Diabetes is a physical illness that interferes with sexual functioning. Schizophrenia, bipolar disorder, and anorexia do not contribute to the severity of a sexual disorder.

18. 1. 2. 3.   Hypertensives, phenothiazines, and antidepressants are all drugs that contribute to sexual dysfunction and may result in an impairment such as impotence. Drugs that cause a decrease in androgen levels, such as these, will create problems with sexual functioning.

19. 2.   The judgment of a client with a sexual dysfunction may be clouded by perceptual as well as intellectual defenses. The client will need to develop trusting relationships. Recovery is contingent on nonjudgmental thoughts by the nurse and partner. Power struggles with the partner are to be avoided so that recovery can occur.

20. 1.   The complete general history is crucial to treatment of the whole individual dealing with a sexual disorder. The sexual disorders history will not give clues into underlying or contributing factors. Drug management is not as important as understanding of the whole person. Family therapy alone will not give a full picture.

21. 4.   The most important treatment strategy in working with a client who has hypoactive sexual desire is the establishment of a therapeutic alliance. Substance abuse precludes the client from meeting diagnostic criteria. The existence of a medical condition also precludes the diagnosis of hypoactive sexual disorder.

Focusing on the disorder increases anxiety and may exacerbate the clinical manifestations.

22. 3. Anxiety, disgust, or fear concerning the sexual encounter contributes to extreme psychological distress in a client with aversion disorder. The existence of a medical condition does not meet the diagnostic category. Interpersonal functioning is critical for the remission of the disorder. Aversion and avoidance are classic criteria.

23. 3. Counseling for coping solutions is essential for the client suffering from gender identity disorder. Therapy is long term. Therapy, rather than drugs, is recommended for control of dysphoria. Legal counseling is appropriate when gender assignment is the only option.

24. 1. Discharge from the genitals is a clinical manifestation of chlamydia. General body aches is not a clinical manifestation. Persistent burning on urination is a clinical manifestation. Treatment involves antibiotics and there is no spontaneous remission.

25. 1. Unprotected sexual contact is a route for hepatitis B. Malnutrition does not contribute to hepatitis B. The fecal-oral route relates to hepatitis A. Clients with sexual addiction may or may not contract hepatitis B.

26. 4. Documenting the behavior exhibited by a client with gender identity disorder may be delegated to a licensed practical nurse. Performing a complete general history, assessing a client, and developing a plan of care are all assignments that should be performed by a registered nurse.

REFERENCES

Antai-Otong, D. (2008). *Psychiatric nursing, biological and behavioral concepts* (2nd ed.). Clifton Park, NY: Delmar Cengage Learning.

Frisch, N. C., & Frisch, L. E. (2011). *Psychiatric mental health nursing* (4th ed.). Clifton Park, NY: Delmar Cengage Learning.

CHAPTER 57

EATING DISORDERS

I. EATING DISORDERS
A. DESCRIPTION
1. A CATEGORY OF DISORDERS CHARACTERIZED BY STARVATION, BINGE–PURGE BEHAVIOR, SELF-MUTILATION, OR SUICIDE, CAUSING A CONSIDERABLE AMOUNT OF PSYCHIC PAIN THAT HAS SERIOUS MEDICAL CONSEQUENCES AND MAY RESULT IN DEATH (TABLE 57-1)
2. GENERALLY A DISORDER OF FEMALES, ALTHOUGH THE INCIDENCE IN MALES IS INCREASING
3. CARRIES A 50–75% CHANCE OF AN ACCOMPANYING DIAGNOSIS OF DYSTHYMIA OR MAJOR DEPRESSIVE EPISODE
4. THEORY EXISTS QUESTIONING A POSSIBLE MOTHER–DAUGHTER CONNECTION
5. CORRELATION BETWEEN DEPRESSION AND EATING DISORDERS (INCREASED INCIDENCE OF DEPRESSION IN RELATIVES OF CLIENTS WITH EATING DISORDERS)
6. INCIDENCE GREATER IN WESTERNIZED CULTURES BECAUSE OF SOCIETAL PRESSURES TO BE THIN
7. MAY HAVE A HISTORY OF SEXUAL ABUSE

II. NURSING DIAGNOSES
A. INEFFECTIVE HEALTH MAINTENANCE
B. IMPAIRED ADJUSTMENT
C. INEFFECTIVE COPING
D. DISTURBED BODY IMAGE
E. RISK FOR DEFICIENT FLUID VOLUME
F. IMBALANCED NUTRITION: LESS THAN BODY REQUIREMENTS
G. POWERLESSNESS
H. RISK FOR SELF-MUTILATION

Nursing Diagnoses: Definitions and Classification 2012–2014. Copyright © 2012, 1994–2012 by NANDA International. Used by arrangement with John Wiley & Sons Limited.

III. TYPES
A. ANOREXIA NERVOSA
1. DESCRIPTION
   a. Self-induced starvation
   b. Failure to maintain body weight at a minimal normal range for age and height with a weight loss of greater than 15%
2. ASSESSMENT
   a. Weight 15% below height and age
   b. Amenorrhea
   c. Lanugo
   d. Hypothermia that is the result of dehydration or a loss of subcutaneous tissue
   e. Electrolyte imbalances (particularly potassium)
   f. Bradycardia
   g. Hypotension
   h. Intense control over eating and weight
   i. Syncope
   j. Perfectionistic tendency

Table 57-1 Complications of Eating Disorders

Cardiovascular	Metabolic	Gastrointestinal
Dysthymia	Hypokalemia	Esophagitis
Postural hypotension	Hypocalcemia	Diarrhea (laxatives)
Bradycardia	Hypomagnesemia	Constipation (starvation)
	Hyponatremia	Parotid swelling
	Dehydration	Gum erosion
	Osteopenia/ osteoporosis	Delayed gastric emptying
	Hypercholesterolemia	Pancreatitis
Endocrine	**Hematological**	**Renal**
Amenorrhea	Leukopenia	Proteinuria
	Anemia	Hematuria

© Cengage Learning 2015

1009

    k. Muscle weakness
    l. Constipation
    m. Dysrhythmias
    n. Rigorous exercise regimen
    o. Unusual practices around food, such as pushing food around the plate and cutting it into small pieces
    p. May abuse laxatives or diuretics, or both

3. DIAGNOSTIC TESTS
    a. Psychological history
    b. Height and weight measurements
    c. Laboratory tests (electrolytes and T_3 and T_4)
    d. Electrocardiograph
    e. Bone mineral density test
    f. Vital signs

4. MEDICAL MANAGEMENT
    a. Hospitalization (See Table 57-2)
    b. Psychotherapy
    c. Selective serotonin reuptake inhibitors (SSRIs) such as fluoxetine (Prozac) that improve weight gain
    d. Antipsychotics such as olanzapine (Zyprexa) that improve cooperation with treatment and decrease agitation

5. NURSING INTERVENTIONS (INPATIENT)
    a. Provide a supportive environment.
    b. Provide a highly structured setting with regard to scheduled mealtimes.
    c. Limit mealtime to 30 minutes.
    d. Observe the client for up to 1 hour after meals to prevent hoarding of food or purging.
    e. Limit exercise to a planned program only after target weight is reached.
    f. Inspect the client's clothes and belongings on return to the hospital after a pass to prevent bringing in food, laxatives, or diuretics.
    g. Weigh the client at a regularly scheduled time, generally daily then two to three times a week, wearing only a bra and underwear (client may prefer not to look at the scale to decrease anxiety).
    h. Promote a weight gain of 3 to 5 pounds a week (½ pound at each weigh-in).

Table 57-2 Criteria for Admission to the Hospital

1.	Rapid weight loss equivalent to 30% of body weight in 6 months
2.	Failure to gain weight in outpatient setting
3.	Severe hypothermia (less than 36°C [96.8°F])
4.	Severe hypokalemia (less than 3 mEq/L)
5.	Systolic blood pressure less than 70 mm Hg
6.	Severe bradycardia (less than 40 beats per minute)
7.	Dysrhythmias

© Cengage Learning 2015

    i. Implement weight-restoration program (desired goal weight is 90% of ideal body weight).
    j. Monitor vital signs, electrocardiogram (ECG), and laboratory tests.
    k. Encourage nonfood-related conversation during mealtime.
    l. Encourage verbalization of feelings.
    m. Encourage the client to participate in group therapy and nutritional counseling.
    n. Administer prescribed antidepressants (SSRIs) or antipsychotics.
    o. Monitor the client for any suicidal ideations.

6. NURSING INTERVENTIONS (OUTPATIENT)
    a. Participate in partial hospitalization or day programs.
    b. Set minimum weight on which treatment may continue in the outpatient setting (avoid negotiating the weight criteria with the client).
    c. Inform the client of the consequences of violating treatment goals such as the weight falling below the target weight.
    d. Assist the client with realistic meal planning.
    e. Encourage the client to verbalize feelings.
    f. Report any suicidal ideations.
    g. Encourage the client to keep a food diary and review it with the client.
    h. Weigh the client at the same time each week in similar clothing (ideally two to three times a week).
    i. Educate the client and the client's family about the eating disorder, such as concerning irrational thoughts about food, shape, and weight.
    j. Educate the client on meal planning, including shopping for and preparing food.
    k. Encourage the client to adhere to a long-term treatment plan (psychotherapy may range from 1 year to 6 or more years).
    l. Encourage the client's family to participate in the prescribed family therapy.
    m. Provide the client with the necessary resources such as state or federal assistance programs if needed.

B. BULIMIA
    1. DESCRIPTION
        a. Binge–purge cycle
        b. May have history of anorexia nervosa
    2. ASSESSMENT
        a. Generally a laxative or diuretic abuse, or both, is present
        b. Normally to slightly low body weight

    c. Electrolyte imbalances
    d. Muscle weakness
    e. Cardiomyopathy (ipecac toxicity)
    f. Dental erosion from repeated vomiting
    g. May have depressive clinical manifestations
    h. Risk for suicidal behaviors
    i. May exhibit chemical dependency or stealing behaviors; also incidence of self-cutting behavior

3. DIAGNOSTIC TESTS
    a. Psychological history
    b. Height and weight measurements
    c. Laboratory tests (potassium)
    d. Electrocardiograph (cardiomyopathy)
    e. Bone mineral density test

4. MEDICAL MANAGEMENT
    a. Antidepressants such as SSRIs for bulimia
    b. Antipsychotics
    c. Gastric motility enhancer such as metoclopramide (Reglan) for delayed gastric motility
    d. Hospitalization if the client becomes medically unstable
    e. Potassium supplements for hypokalemia

5. NURSING INTERVENTIONS
    a. Provide the client with a supportive environment.
    b. Monitor the client during trips to the bathroom to ensure there is no self-induced vomiting.
    c. Instruct the client on the clinical manifestations of a low potassium level (see Table 57-3).
    d. Instruct the client on the medical consequences of binge–purge behavior (vomiting, laxative, diuretic, and ipecac abuse), such as dysrhythmias, cardiomyopathy, dental erosion, and so on.
    e. Instruct the client that the binge–purge cycle is a perpetuating problem (fasting leads to binging).
    f. Encourage the client to identify foods that trigger a binge, such as pastries and fried foods.
    g. Instruct the client to avoid keeping "trigger foods" at home.
    h. Explore methods of preventing the binge–purge behavior with the client.
    i. Inform the client that there are no "forbidden foods" (thinking of some foods as forbidden foods leads to the binge–purge behavior).
    j. Educate the client on sensible, well-balanced nutrition.
    k. Instruct the client to avoid keeping medications such as laxatives, diuretics, and ipecac at home (having to go buy the laxatives, diuretics, or ipecac decreases the likelihood of binging and purging).
    l. Encourage the client to verbalize feelings.
    m. Explore with the client alternative methods to the binge–purge behavior.
    n. Encourage the client's family to participate in the prescribed family therapy.
    o. Provide the client with the necessary resources such as state or federal assistance programs if needed.

C. BINGE-EATING DISORDER (OBESITY)

1. DESCRIPTION
    a. A variation of compulsive overeating
    b. Listed as an eating disorder not otherwise specified because there are no compensatory behaviors such as use of laxatives, diuretics, or exercise
    c. Tends to be stigmatized by a large percent of society that feels obesity is the result of overeating and gluttony
      1) Research being conducted indicates that metabolic and endocrine functions rather than overeating may cause obesity.

2. ASSESSMENT
    a. Continuous rapid eating of enormous amounts of food in a short period of time (generally 2 hours)
    b. A feeling of having no control over the eating
    c. A feeling of not being able to stop eating
    d. Eating when not experiencing hunger
    e. Secretive eating
    f. Feelings of guilt or feeling ashamed with one's own overeating behavior
    g. Distressed feeling over binge behavior
    h. No association with compensatory behaviors such as use of laxatives, diuretics, or purging

Table 57-3 Clinical Manifestations of Hypokalemia

Hypotension
Weak, thready pulse
Shallow respirations
Lethargy
Confusion
Muscle weakness
Hyporeflexia
Delayed gastric motility
Constipation
ECG changes (ST depression, flat or inverted T wave, and prominent U wave)
Increased urinary output

© Cengage Learning 2015

3. DIAGNOSTIC TESTS
   a. Psychological history
   b. Height and weight measurements
4. MEDICAL MANAGEMENT
   a. Cognitive behavioral therapy
   b. SSRIs such as sertraline (Zoloft) may be used to decrease binge episodes.
5. NURSING INTERVENTIONS
   a. Encourage the client to keep both a feelings diary and a food diary.

   b. Encourage the client to plan for structured, planned meals.
   c. Instruct the client on well-balanced nutrition.
   d. Instruct the client to avoid periods of fasting or undereating (tends to lead to binging).
   e. Encourage the client to verbalize feelings.
   f. Instruct the client to weigh once a week.

PRACTICE QUESTIONS

1. The nurse is teaching a class on eating disorders to a group of nurses. Which of the following should the nurse include in the class?
   1. Eating disorders affect females and males equally
   2. There is an increased incidence of depression in clients with eating disorders
   3. There is no mother–daughter connection in eating disorders
   4. There is a 20% chance of dysthymia in clients with eating disorders

2. The nurse should monitor a client with an eating disorder for which of the following complications?
   Select all that apply:
   [ ] 1. Hypertension
   [ ] 2. Dysmenorrhea
   [ ] 3. Parotid swelling
   [ ] 4. Delayed gastric emptying
   [ ] 5. Bradycardia
   [ ] 6. Dysthymia

3. The nurse should administer which of the following drugs to a client with an eating disorder who has a delayed gastric emptying time?
   1. Esomeprazole (Nexium)
   2. Metoclopramide (Reglan)
   3. Dicyclomine (Bentyl)
   4. Diphenoxylate with atropine sulfate (Lomotil)

4. The nurse is planning the care for a client with muscle weakness, constipation, a serum potassium of 3.0 mEq/L, and a pulse of 65 bpm. What clinical manifestation should take priority in this client's plan of care?
   1. Muscle weakness
   2. Serum potassium 3.0 mEq/L
   3. Pulse of 65 bpm
   4. Constipation

5. The nurse assesses a client for which of the following findings in a client suspected of having bulimia?
   Select all that apply:
   [ ] 1. Laxative abuse
   [ ] 2. Amenorrhea
   [ ] 3. Lanugo
   [ ] 4. Dental erosion from repeated vomiting
   [ ] 5. Chemical dependency or stealing behaviors
   [ ] 6. Perfectionistic tendency

6. The nurse administers which of the following prescribed drugs to a client with anorexia nervosa for the purpose of improving weight gain?
   1. Olanzapine (Zyprexa)
   2. Sertraline (Zoloft)
   3. Fluoxetine (Prozac)
   4. Quetiapine (Seroquel)

7. Which of the following statements would provide the nurse with the most accurate information regarding how successful the treatment has been for a client with a long-standing history of bulimia?
   1. "I take my medicine when I have an urge to binge."
   2. "I try to do other things when I feel I want to eat."
   3. "I have learned to eat a variety of foods."
   4. "I no longer feel the need to see my therapist."

8. The nurse is caring for a 25-year-old client with an eating disorder who is in the hospital. The physician ordered periodic laboratory tests to monitor the client's medical status. Which of the following serum laboratory test results is abnormal and should prompt the nurse to notify the physician?
   1. Calcium of 9.2 mg/dl
   2. Magnesium of 1.8 mEq/L

3. Potassium of 3.0 mEq/L
4. Sodium of 128 mEq/L

9. The nurse is collecting data on an 11-year-old client suspected of having anorexia nervosa. Which of the following physical assessment findings should be reported to the client's physician confirming the presence of anorexia nervosa?
   1. A temperature of 37.2°C (99°F)
   2. A pulse of 72 bpm
   3. The presence of lanugo
   4. Dysmenorrhea

10. During an admission interview, a client with anorexia nervosa complains of feeling cold all the time and asks the nurse why. Which of the following is the most appropriate response by the nurse?
    1. "Let me take your temperature."
    2. "You might be getting a cold."
    3. "There is a loss of subcutaneous fat."
    4. "You probably aren't dressing warmly enough."

11. The nurse should include which of the following interventions in the plan of care for a client with a binge-eating disorder? Select all that apply:
    [ ] 1. Encourage the client to keep a food diary and a feelings diary
    [ ] 2. Encourage the client to gain ½ pound a week
    [ ] 3. Instruct the client to avoid fasting
    [ ] 4. Instruct the client that high-calorie foods are to be avoided
    [ ] 5. Encourage the client to plan for structured meals
    [ ] 6. Instruct the client on well-balanced nutrition

12. The nurse is interviewing a 46-year-old female client with a binge-eating disorder who is tearful and admits to the nurse of being depressed. The client states, "I have been fat all my life and I can't lose weight." Which of the following should be the priority response by the nurse?
    1. "In order to lose weight, you need to stop binging."
    2. "You need to eat a well-balanced diet."
    3. "Cognitive behavioral therapy offers the most success."
    4. "You will lose weight if you take your sertraline (Zoloft)."

13. The registered nurse is delegating clinical assignments on an eating disorder unit for the day. Which of the following clinical assignments would be appropriate for the nurse to delegate to a licensed practical nurse?

1. Develop a class to be taught on eating disorders
2. Instruct a client with bulimia on the prescribed medication
3. Create a meal plan for a client with anorexia nervosa
4. Monitor a client with an eating disorder after meals

14. A client with anorexia nervosa is crying and tells the nurse, "I just want to die. I can't live like this anymore." In determining what action to take next, which of the following factors is a priority for the nurse to consider?
    1. How long the client has been feeling this way
    2. The recovery rate with treatment
    3. If the client has a suicide plan
    4. If the client has a support system

15. The nurse is signing a hospitalized client with bulimia back in after a day pass at home. Which of the following should be the nurse's priority action?
    1. Ask the client about any special activities while out on pass
    2. Obtain a detailed menu of what was eaten
    3. Search the client's belonging for laxatives or diuretics
    4. Question the client about any binge–purge behavior at home

16. The nurse is collecting a health history from a 25-year-old client suspected of having an eating disorder. Which of the following questions is a priority question for the nurse to ask the client?
    1. "Is your father away from home much of the time due to his job?"
    2. "Do any siblings have issues with food?"
    3. "Does your mother have an eating disorder?"
    4. "Do you have a friend who has a body image problem?"

17. The family of a male client suspected of having an eating disorder asks the nurse how their son can have an eating disorder because eating disorders only occur in women. Which of the following is the most appropriate response by the nurse?
    1. "Your son is very slender for his height."
    2. "Your son has a poor appetite."
    3. "The incidence of eating disorders is increasing in males."
    4. "Food-related problems in males are different from eating disorders."

18. The nurse is caring for a client with anorexia nervosa. Which of the following interventions should the nurse include in this client's plan of care?

Select all that apply:

[ ] 1. Encourage the client to eat when hungry

[ ] 2. Limit mealtime to 1 hour

[ ] 3. Monitor the client for 30 minutes after eating

[ ] 4. Weigh the client two to three times a week

[ ] 5. Promote a weight gain of 3 to 5 pounds a week

[ ] 6. Restrict exercise if the target weight is not maintained

19. The nurse is admitting a client with anorexia nervosa to the hospital based on which of the following criteria?

Select all that apply:

[ ] 1. A systolic blood pressure of 90 mm Hg

[ ] 2. A loss of 20% of body weight

[ ] 3. A temperature of 35.4°C (95.8°F)

[ ] 4. A serum potassium level of 2.8 mEq/L

[ ] 5. A pulse of 60 beats per minute

[ ] 6. Failure to gain weight

20. Which of the following nursing diagnoses is appropriate for the nurse to include in the plan of care for a client with a binge disorder?

1. Ineffective thermoregulation

2. Risk for self-mutilation

3. Ineffective health maintenance

4. Anxiety

21. The nurse should administer which of the following drugs to a client with a binge-eating disorder for the purpose of decreasing the binge episodes?

1. Sertraline (Zoloft)

2. Olanzapine (Zyprexa)

3. Amitriptyline (Elavil)

4. Imipramine (Tofranil)

22. A client with anorexia nervosa who is emaciated is crying and tells the nurse, "I feel so fat when I look in the mirror." Which of the following is the priority response for the nurse?

1. "You shouldn't look in the mirror if it upsets you."

2. "You are 30% below your body weight."

3. "It must be very frightening to feel fat."

4. "Ask another person for another opinion."

23. The nurse is caring for a client with bulimia who informs the nurse of an unpleasant tingling of the hands and around the mouth, as well as muscular spasms. The nurse should notify the physician of which of the following suspected disorders?

1. Cushing's syndrome

2. Addison's disease

3. Hyperthyroidism

4. Tetany

24. The nurse is evaluating the medical records of the following four clients. It is essential that the nurse report which of the following clients immediately?

1. A client with anorexia nervosa who has a pulse of 55 beats per minute

2. A client with bulimia who has a serum potassium of 3.5 mEq/L

3. A client with anorexia who has a systolic blood pressure of 90 mm Hg

4. A client with bulimia who has a serum calcium of 8.6 mg/dl

25. The nurse should monitor a client with bulimia for which of the following clinical manifestations of hypokalemia?

Select all that apply:

[ ] 1. Hypotension

[ ] 2. Weak, thready pulse

[ ] 3. Diarrhea

[ ] 4. Hyperreflexia

[ ] 5. Decreased urinary output

[ ] 6. Shallow respirations

ANSWERS AND RATIONALES

1. 2. Although the incidence of eating disorders is increasing in male clients, the incidence is much higher in females. There is an increased incidence of depression found in clients with eating disorders. Dysthymias or major depressive episodes have a 50–75% incidence. There is a theory of a possible mother–daughter connection.

2. 3. 4. 5. 6. Clients who have eating disorders may experience postural hypotension, amenorrhea, parotid swelling, delayed gastric emptying, bradycardia, and dysthymias.

3. 2. Esomeprazole (Nexium) is a proton pump inhibitor used in the short-term management of gastroesophageal reflux (GERD). Metoclopramide (Reglan) is a gastrointestinal stimulant used in the treatment of delayed gastric emptying and gastroesophageal reflux. Dicyclomine (Bentyl) is a cholinergic-blocking drug used in the treatment of hypermotility and spasms of the gastrointestinal tract associated with irritable colon and spastic colon. Diphenoxylate with atropine sulfate (Lomotil) is an antidiarrheal used in the management of diarrhea.

4. 2. Although a client with an eating disorder may have muscle weakness, constipation, and bradycardia, it is the serum potassium of 3.0 mEq/L that should be the priority. Generally, a client with a serum potassium level of 3.0 mEq/L would be hospitalized. Severe hypokalemia may lead to dysrhythmias and subsequent death. Normal potassium is 3.5 to 5.5 mEq/L.

5. 1. 4. 5. Features of bulimia include laxative abuse, dental erosion, and chemical dependency or stealing behavior. Amenorrhea, lanugo, and perfectionistic tendency are features of anorexia nervosa.

6. 3. Olanzapine (Zyprexa) is an antipsychotic used in the management of anorexia nervosa to enhance compliance with treatment and decrease agitation. Sertraline (Zoloft) is a selective serotonin reuptake inhibitor used to decrease binge episodes in clients with a binge-eating disorder (obesity). Fluoxetine (Prozac) is a selective serotonin reuptake inhibitor used to improve weight gain in the client with anorexia nervosa. Quetiapine (Seroquel) is an antipsychotic used in the treatment of schizophrenia.

7. 3. A client who has bulimia and is able to verbalize eating a variety of foods is showing success with treatment. Eating a variety of foods indicates that the client does not consider some foods as "forbidden foods" and understands that the key to success is proportion. A client should not take prescribed medicine only when responding to an urge to binge; medicine must be taken regularly until the therapist deems it is no longer necessary. Trying to do other things when feeling the urge to binge is a positive step, but it does not indicate success. A client cannot merely try to do other things when feeling the desire to eat. Success would be measured in being successful doing other tasks instead of eating. It is not a positive step for a client to say there is no longer a need to see the therapist. Seeing the therapist should be a regular commitment and not a capricious phenomenon.

8. 4. Routine serum laboratory tests are performed on all clients with eating disorders. Routine tests include calcium, magnesium, potassium, and sodium tests. Normal serum calcium is 9.0 to 10.5 mg/dl. Normal serum magnesium is 1.3 to 2.1 mEq/L. Normal serum potassium is 3.0 to 5.5 mEq/L. Normal serum sodium is 136 to 145 mEq/L.

9. 3. A client with anorexia nervosa generally will exhibit hypothermia, bradycardia, lanugo, and amenorrhea. However, an 11-year-old client with anorexia nervosa may have not started

menses and certainly has not had menses long enough to establish a pattern.

10. 3. Clients who have a history of anorexia frequently complain of feeling cold all the time that is unrelated to weather and clothing. Hypothermia is the result of dehydration or a loss of subcutaneous tissue.

11. 1. 3. 5. 6. Binge eating, also know as obesity, is an eating disorder not otherwise specified. A client with this disorder does not use compensatory mechanisms such as laxatives or diuretics or resort to purging. A client with a binge disorder is overweight and does not need to gain weight. The client should be instructed to avoid fasting because fasting leads to binging. The client should be informed on well-balanced nutrition and that there are no "forbidden foods." Avoiding the concept of "forbidden foods" eliminates the trigger to binge. The client should be instructed that the key to weight maintenance is a balance in the proportion of food and exercise. The client should be encouraged to plan for structured meals.

12. 3. Although a client with a binge-eating disorder needs to stop binging and eat a well-balanced diet, the best chance for recovery from a binge-eating disorder is cognitive behavioral therapy. Sertraline (Zoloft) is a selective reuptake inhibitor used in binge-eating disorders for the purpose of decreasing the binge episodes.

13. 4. It would be acceptable to delegate monitoring a client with an eating disorder after meals. Only a registered nurse can develop, create, and instruct a client.

14. 3. The priority action to take with any client who is threatening suicide is to assess the client for a detailed suicide plan. After assessing whether the client is serious and has developed a plan, it would be appropriate to assess how long the client has felt this way and whether the client has a support system. As with any disorder, the chance of recovery is greater with treatment.

15. 3. The priority action for the nurse to take when signing a client in from a pass at home is to search the client's belongings for laxatives, diuretics, or ipecac that the client can hide and use while in the hospital. Asking what the client did on pass, what was eaten, or if there was any difficulty with binging and purging behavior is relevant, but not the priority.

16. 3. Although a father who works a lot and is away from home, a sibling with food issues, and a friend with a body image problem all may be important factors in the well-being of a client with an eating disorder, the priority is the mother–daughter connection. Theory exists questioning a possible mother–daughter connection as having the greatest impact on the client's relationship with food.

17. 3. Although eating disorders are generally the domain of females, the incidence in males is increasing.

18. 4. 5. 6. A highly structured mealtime with scheduled meals is important to include in the plan of care for a client with anorexia nervosa. Mealtime should be limited to 30 minutes. The client should be monitored for up to 1 hour after meals to prevent hoarding of food or purging. Exercise is limited if the target weight is not maintained. The client is generally weighed two to three times a week at a regularly scheduled time and while wearing similar clothing. A weight gain of 3 to 5 pounds a week is the goal.

19. 3. 4. 6. Criteria for admission to the hospital for a client with anorexia nervosa include a rapid loss of weight equivalent to 30% of body weight in over 6 months, a failure to gain weight in an outpatient setting, a temperature of less than 36°C (96.8°F), a serum potassium level of less than 3 mEq/L, a systolic blood pressure of less than 70 mm Hg, a pulse of less than 40 beats per minute, and dysrhythmias.

20. 4. An appropriate nursing diagnosis for a client with a binge disorder is anxiety. A client with a binge disorder feels a great deal of distress over the binge behavior. Ineffective thermoregulation and risk for health maintenance are nursing diagnoses appropriate for bulimia.

21. 1. Selective serotonin reuptake inhibitors, such as sertraline (Zoloft), are used to decrease the binge episodes in a client with a binge-eating disorder. Olanzapine (Zyprexa) is an antipsychotic that may be used to increase cooperation with treatment and promote weight gain in a client with anorexia nervosa.

Amitriptyline (Elavil) and imipramine (Tofranil) are tricyclic antidepressants used in the treatment of depression.

22. 3. Telling the client with anorexia nervosa who is emaciated not to look in the mirror serves no purpose, because it is most likely an unrealistic goal. The client is obsessed with body image and frequently checks the mirror. Asking another person for his or her opinion also serves no purpose, because the client is obsessed with body size and most likely won't trust another person's opinion. The most effective intervention is for the nurse to be supportive of the client's self-image and to encourage the client to verbalize a fear of being fat.

23. 4. Tetany is a neuromuscular excitability associated with a critical decrease in the body's calcium level. An unpleasant tingling of the hands and around the mouth and muscular spasms are characteristic of tetany. If emergency treatment is not begun, laryngospasms may develop.

24. 4. It is essential that the nurse report a client with bulimia who has a serum calcium level of 8.6 mg/dl. Normal serum calcium is 9.0 to 10.5 mg/dl. A client with a low calcium level is at risk for developing tetany, which can be a life-threatening condition. Although a client with anorexia nervosa who has a pulse of 55 beats per minute and a systolic blood pressure of 90 mm Hg has bradycardia and hypotension, reporting these is not as critical as impending tetany. A serum potassium of 3.5 mEq/L is within the normal range.

25. 1. 2. 6. Clinical manifestations of hypokalemia include hypotension; a weak, thready pulse; constipation; hyporeflexia; increased urinary output; and shallow respirations.

REFERENCES

Antai-Otong, D. (2008). *Psychiatric nursing, biological and behavioral concepts* (2nd ed.). Clifton Park, NY: Delmar Cengage Learning.

Frisch, N. C., & Frisch, L. E. (2011). *Psychiatric mental health nursing* (4th ed.). Clifton Park, NY: Delmar Cengage Learning.

Sobel, S. (2004). *Eating disorders.* Sacramento, CA: CME Resource.

GERONTOLOGIC NURSING

CHAPTER 58

HEALTH ISSUES OF THE OLDER ADULT

I. THEORIES OF AGING

A. BIOLOGICAL THEORIES
1. AGING IS DIFFERENT AMONG HUMANS.
2. AGING IS DIFFERENT AMONG BODY SYSTEMS.
3. AGING AND DISEASE ARE NOT SYNONYMOUS.
4. OLDER ADULTS SHOULD BE ENCOURAGED TO CONTINUE THEIR DAILY ACTIVITIES.
5. GENETIC FACTORS
   a. Genetic program or biological clock predetermines life
   b. Senescence under genetic control at cellular level
   c. Mutations tend to cause organ decline.
6. CROSS-LINKING
   a. Cellular division is altered by chemical reactions.
   b. Cross-linking agents obstruct intracellular transport, leading to failure of body organs.
7. FREE RADICALS
   a. Free radicals replace useful biological information within molecules with faulty information, causing genetic disorders.
   b. As molecules accumulate, there is a physical decline.
   c. The effects of free radicals are counteracted by natural body oxidants.
8. AUTOIMMUNE REACTIONS
   a. Thyroid, bone marrow, and immune system are affected by the aging process.
   b. Decrease in thymus and a deterioration in the immune response
   c. Decrease in production of T-cell differentiation
   d. An increase in infections and cancers results in changes.
9. WEAR AND TEAR
   a. Cells wear out over an individual's life.
   b. Repeated injuries, trauma, or stress may hasten the process of aging.

B. PSYCHOLOGICAL THEORIES
1. INFLUENCED BY BIOLOGY AND SOCIOLOGY
2. INCLUDES BEHAVIORAL AND DEVELOPMENTAL ASPECTS OF LIFE
3. ADAPTIVE PROCESSES SUCH AS MEMORY, LEARNING CAPACITY, FEELINGS, INTELLECTUAL FUNCTIONING, AND MOTIVATIONS GUIDE THE OLDER ADULT TO MAKE SOME BIOLOGICAL CHANGES.
4. PAST ACCOMPLISHMENTS ARE INCORPORATED INTO LIFE TO PROMOTE SELF-ESTEEM.
5. INTELLECTUAL FUNCTIONING REMAINS INTACT FOR THE MAJORITY OF ADULTS.
6. MASLOW'S HIERARCHY OF HUMAN NEEDS
7. ERICKSON'S THEORY
   a. Ego integrity versus despair
   b. Older adult is concerned with guiding the next generation.
   c. Unsuccessful resolution may result in despair.

C. SOCIOLOGIC THEORIES
1. FOCUS ON ROLES AND RELATIONSHIP
2. SOCIETAL VALUES MAY DEFINE THE VIEW OF SELF.
3. OLDER ADULTS ARE INDIVIDUALS.
4. RESPONSES OF OLDER ADULTS SHOULD BE RESPECTED.
5. REALISTIC ACTIVITIES SHOULD BE PLANNED TO INCREASE SELF-CONFIDENCE.
6. OLDER ADULTS SHOULD BE ASSISTED IN THEIR ADAPTATION TO THEIR LIMITATIONS.
7. DISENGAGEMENT
   a. Mutual agreement between the older adult and society resulting in a withdrawal from society

b. Instead of interacting with society, older adults may become self-centered.

8. ACTIVITY

   a. A positive self-concept is necessary to maintain life satisfaction.

   b. The older adult should not withdraw from society.

9. CONTINUITY

   a. The older adult should be encouraged to continue with the same lifestyle.

   b. Maintain values, beliefs, and commitments that contribute to personalities

II. NURSING DIAGNOSES

   A. RISK FOR CONSTIPATION

   B. RISK FOR FALLS

   C. URINARY INCONTINENCE

   D. IMPAIRED PHYSICAL MOBILITY

   E. INEFFECTIVE SELF-HELP MANAGEMENT

   F. DISTURBED SLEEP PATTERN

Nursing Diagnoses: Definitions and Classification 2012–2014. Copyright © 2012, 1994–2012 by NANDA International. Used by arrangement with John Wiley & Sons Limited.

III. EFFECTS OF AGING ON THE BODY SYSTEMS

   A. DESCRIPTION

      1. THE OLDER ADULT'S PHYSICAL, PSYCHOLOGICAL, AND SOCIETAL WELL-BEING MAY ADVERSELY AFFECT ANY BODY SYSTEM, RESULTING IN ANY POSSIBLE NURSING DIAGNOSIS, SUCH AS IMPAIRED PHYSICAL MOBILITY, IMPAIRED MEMORY, IMBALANCED NUTRITION LESS THAN BODY REQUIREMENTS, SELF-CARE DEFICIT, AND SOCIAL ISOLATION.

   B. RESPIRATORY SYSTEM

      1. ALTERATIONS IN ANATOMY AND PHYSIOLOGY

         a. The lungs of an older adult are less flexible and compliant.

         b. Inspiratory and tidal volume decrease with age.

         c. Aging decreases the flexibility of the ribs and weakens chest wall muscles so that inspiration is not as deep.

         d. Atrophy of cilia

         e. Decreased and thickened alveoli

      2. ASSESSMENT

         a. Barrel chest

         b. Decreased cough reflex

         c. Increased infection

         d. Difficulty deep breathing

         e. Decreased sensitivity to hypoxia and hypercapnia

         f. Comorbidity may adversely affect gas exchange and airway clearance, resulting in chronic obstructive pulmonary disease (COPD), emphysema with a decrease in tidal volume, asthma, chronic bronchitis, pulmonary fibrosis, tuberculosis, and rarer conditions such as pneumocystis pneumonia.

      3. DIAGNOSTIC TESTS

         a. Chest x-ray

         b. Oxygen saturation

         c. Biopsy

         d. Sputum culture and sensitivity

         e. Computerized tomography (CT) scan

         f. Sleep evaluation to identify sleep apnea

      4. NURSING INTERVENTIONS

         a. Auscultate all lung fields anteriorly and posteriorly.

         b. Observe for color and capillary refill.

         c. Utilize pulse oximetry to measure O_2 saturation (expected saturation is 90–100% on room air).

            1) The O_2 saturation may be lower at higher altitudes in the older adult.

            2) Oxygen therapy is necessary only if the client is symptomatic, such as having shortness of breath or increased respiratory and heart rates.

         d. Assess for shortness of breath and dyspnea on exertion.

         e. Ask the client, "What is the hardest thing you do every day?" to assess for fatigue and quality of life.

         f. Monitor arterial blood gases, if indicated, evaluating for a decreased PaO_2 and increased $PaCO_2$ (the closer together they become, the more serious the client's condition).

         g. Observe sputum for color and presence of blood.

         h. Observe how fatigue and shortness of breath affect nutritional intake.

         i. Schedule activities to prevent extreme fatigue.

         j. Administer oxygen generally by nasal cannula at 2–3 L/min to the client with chronic lung conditions. A higher flow rate will depress the respiratory drive.

         k. Sequence activities to promote quality of life, such as a shower in a shower chair at night, so that the oxygen requirements for bathing will not interfere with food digestion as they would earlier in the day.

         l. Provide for comfort, such as oxygen administration and elevation of the head of the bed (client may prefer to sleep in a reclining chair or with an electric fan blowing to increase air circulation).

         m. Provide small, frequent, nutrient-dense feedings. If the client's CO_2 level is high, then the intake of carbohydrates may be decreased (carbohydrates are metabolized to produce CO_2 and water).

  n. Offer fluid intake to 2000–3000 ml a day unless contraindicated.

  o. Schedule medications such as nonsteroidal bronchodilators so that they do not interfere with rest periods because they have an adverse reaction of insomnia. These also increase heart and respiratory rate as well as blood pressure.

  p. Monitor the client for infection if taking steroids such as anti-inflammatory medications.

  q. Provide for immunizations for diseases that could be fatal for the client with a compromised respiratory system, such as influenza and pneumonia.

  r. Instruct the client about smoking cessation and avoidance of inhaled pollutants, such as wood smoke from a fireplace or aerosol sprays.

  s. Instruct the client's family member on how to perform postural drainage and clapping if prescribed.

    1) It is difficult for the older adult to assume the necessary positions.

    2) The family member may also be an older adult who does not have the strength to perform the treatment due to arthritis or chronic conditions.

C. CIRCULATION

  1. ALTERATIONS IN ANATOMY AND PHYSIOLOGY

    a. Decreased strength of ventricular contraction

    b. Decreased ejection fraction

    c. Arteries become less pliable.

    d. Less sensitive baroreceptors

    e. Thick and rigid heart valves such as aortic and mitral values

    f. Decline in pacemaker cells

  2. ASSESSMENT

    a. Varicose veins

    b. Hypertension

    c. Stenosis or insufficiency of heart valves

    d. Orthostatic hypotension

    e. Increased edema in dependent body parts

    f. Heart murmurs

    g. Dysrhythmias

    h. Comorbid conditions may cause serious cardiovascular problems such as diabetes mellitus, hypercholesterolemia, anemia, coronary artery disease, peripheral vascular disorders, congestive heart failure, conduction disorders, and dysrhythmias.

3. DIAGNOSTIC TESTS

  a. C reactive protein

  b. Complete blood count (CBC)

  c. Cholesterol (high-density lipoprotein [HDL] and low-density lipoprotein [LDL]) and triglyceride levels

  d. Echocardiogram (external and esophageal)

  e. Electrocardiogram

4. NURSING INTERVENTIONS

  a. Monitor blood pressure, heart rate and rhythm, cholesterol and triglyceride levels, oxygen saturation percentages, peripheral circulation, and renal function.

  b. Monitor skin color, temperature, and any discolorations.

  c. Monitor the client for changes in mental status such as confusion, which may be the result of an alteration in oxygenation. (Pneumonia or a myocardial infarction may present with confusion in the older adult.)

  d. Palpate the radial and pedal pulses.

  e. Auscultate pedal, apical, abdominal aorta, and carotid pulses by Doppler if appropriate.

  f. Assess blood pressure while lying, sitting, and standing.

  g. Instruct the client to stay warm with socks, gloves, and blankets rather than the use of external heat such as heating pads or heat lamps, which may cause burns.

  h. Assess for changes in mental status or cognition. An older adult experiencing a myocardial infarction may become agitated or nauseated because of the decreased perfusion without chest pain.

  i. Instruct the client or family member of any specific assessments needed related to medication administration such as taking a pulse for 1 full minute before administering digitalis preparations and notifying the physician if the pulse is less than 60 or over 100.

  j. Instruct the client's family member how to take, record, and report a blood pressure, and how to inspect the client's feet for alterations in circulation.

D. ELIMINATION

  1. ALTERATIONS IN ANATOMY AND PHYSIOLOGY

    a. Slowed gastrointestinal peristalsis

    b. Decreased absorption of nutrients from the gastrointestinal tract

    c. Decreased smooth muscle tone

    d. Weakened muscles used in swallowing

    e. Decrease in gastric enzymes

    f. Decreased sphincter tone

2. ASSESSMENT

    a. Decreased gastrointestinal motility

    b. Difficulty swallowing

    c. Heartburn

    d. Constipation

    e. Loss of teeth

    f. Decreased saliva

    g. Decreased taste

    h. Malabsorption

    i. Comorbid conditions that affect elimination patterns are those that primarily decrease mobility, such as arthritis or a cerebral vascular accident (CVA), or that decrease fluid intake, such as dementia or renal failure.

3. DIAGNOSTIC TESTS

    a. Urinalysis with culture and sensitivity

    b. Stool specimen for ova, parasites, and fecal fat

    c. Stool specimen for occult blood

    d. Colonoscopy

    e. Barium swallow or barium enema, or both

4. NURSING INTERVENTIONS

    a. Assess for an increased urinary output if the client is taking diuretics.

    b. Assess for diarrhea if the client is taking antibiotics.

    c. Monitor a male client who has benign prostatic hypertrophy for urinary frequency of small amounts of urine and nocturia.

    d. Monitor a female client for urinary incontinence that may occur as a result of having had many vaginal deliveries or cystocele.

    e. Assess for types of incontinence such as urge, stress, and neurogenic.

    f. Assess for constipation or perceived constipation. These may result in self-medications with over-the-counter (OTC) preparations. Laxative abuse can occur when the client's expectations for bowel movement regularity are not met.

    g. Monitor the client's urine for color, clarity, amount, and any inclusions. An older adult may not have the ability or the visual clarity to be an accurate reporter.

    h. Evaluate the client's daily fluid intake. The client may intentionally limit fluids in order to decrease trips to the toilet, especially if taking a diuretic.

    i. Evaluate the client's bowel elimination. Determine the client's definition of what are "normal" bowel movements. Identify OTC medications and methods used for regularity.

    j. Monitor bowel movements for color, consistency, amount, and frequency.

    k. Administer stool softeners, prune juice, fiber, and increased fluid intake for constipation.

    l. Administer laxatives if other methods for regularity fail, using enemas infrequently.

    m. Provide for regular toileting usually after breakfast.

    n. Implement a toileting schedule to prevent urinary incontinence. Incontinence may be not only embarrassing for the client but also a cause of social isolation, depression, and falls after hurrying to the toilet or slipping on a wet floor.

    o. Instruct the client to avoid caffeine and alcohol in the presence of urinary incontinence.

    p. Instruct the client on the importance of adequate (2000–3000 ml per day) intake of oral fluids and a diet rich in fiber.

    q. Assess a client with a urinary tract infection for confusion, incontinence, and anorexia rather than a fever, frequency, and urgency.

E. MOBILITY

1. ALTERATIONS IN ANATOMY AND PHYSIOLOGY

    a. Without use, muscles decrease in size and strength.

    b. Decreased bone density

    c. Tendons and ligaments lose elasticity.

    d. Narrowed intervertebral disks

2. ASSESSMENT

    a. Weak

    b. Reduced range of motion

    c. Unsteady balance, which may be compounded by inner ear problems, electrolyte imbalances, dehydration, anemia, and muscle weakness

    d. Osteoporosis results from inadequate calcium intake, inadequate vitamin D synthesis or ingestion, lack of weight-bearing activity or exercise, medications (such as corticosteroids), or smoking. As the bones weaken, the older adult is at risk for falls, fractures, kyphosis, and compression of vertebrae.

    e. Slowed gait because of chronic and degenerative conditions such as osteoarthritis, bunions, or obesity

3. DIAGNOSTIC TESTS

    a. Creatinine phosphokinase (CPK) to identify muscle activity

    b. Serum electrolytes

    c. X-rays, bone scans, and CT scans for skeletal anomalies

    d. Assessment of balance and gait

4. NURSING INTERVENTIONS
  a. Monitor electrolytes, fluid balance, blood counts, and ability to perform activities of daily living (ADLs).
  b. Assess muscle strength, gait, and balance.
  c. Complete a functional assessment profile.
  d. Identify the client's fall risk.
    1) Determine if shoes fit adequately.
    2) The presence of hazards in the home such as pets on the floor, throw rugs, clutter, electrical cords, and oxygen administration tubing
  e. Assess for consequences of immobility and institute preventive measures.
    1) Adequate hydration and leg exercises to prevent deep vein thrombosis and pulmonary embolism
    2) Range-of-motion (ROM) exercises to maintain muscle tone and prevent weakness
    3) Adequate exercise to prevent insomnia
    4) Diversional activities and social stimulation to prevent loneliness and depression
    5) Weight bearing as appropriate and calcium (1200–1500 mg/day) to prevent osteoporosis
    6) Adequate fluid intake (2000–3000 ml/day) to prevent hemoconcentration, urinary tract infection, constipation, and urinary lithiasis
    7) Adequate pain control so that the client is able to be mobile
    8) Monitor bowel movements and ensure adequate intake of fiber and fluids to prevent constipation.
    9) Observe skin frequently and prevent breakdown by providing position changes every 2 hours, adequate protein intake, and adequate fluid intake.

F. NEUROLOGICAL FUNCTION
  1. ALTERATIONS IN ANATOMY AND PHYSIOLOGY
    a. Decreased reflexes
    b. Decreased blood flow to the brain
    c. Deterioration of the myelin sheath
    d. The actual size of the brain in the normal older adult will decrease in size and weight by up to one-third.
  2. ASSESSMENT
    a. Sluggish reflexes
    b. Short-term memory problems
    c. Confusion
    d. Decreased ability to learn

3. DIAGNOSTIC TESTS
  a. Myelogram
  b. CT scan or other noninvasive scans
  c. Spinal tap
  d. Carotid or cerebral arteriogram
4. NURSING INTERVENTIONS
  a. Caution the older adult that she may have a slowed response while operating a motor vehicle.
  b. Monitor the client for short-term memory problems.
  c. Assess the client for atherosclerosis, hypertension, or transient ischemic attacks.
  d. Monitor cognition, level of consciousness, pupils, cranial nerves, and peripheral nerve function.
  e. Assess sensation and motor function.
  f. Evaluate the effect of medications on neurological function, such as an impairment in self-care.

G. SENSORY FUNCTION
  1. ALTERATION IN ANATOMY AND PHYSIOLOGY
    a. Vision changes from nearsightedness (myopia) to farsightedness (presbyopia) occur in most adults.
    b. Decreased blood supply to the ear
    c. Slowed pupil accommodation
    d. Atrophied olfactory fibers
    e. Decreased lacrimal secretions
    f. Larger, discolored, and more rigid lens
  2. ASSESSMENT
    a. Decreased taste and smell
    b. Decreased ability to distinguish item in the hands or on the feet
    c. Decreased hearing
    d. Increased sensitivity to glare
    e. Dry eyes
    f. Decreased ability to focus on objects
    g. Decreased ability to distinguish between sounds
    h. Decreased depth perception
    i. Excess wax production
  3. DIAGNOSTIC TESTS
    a. Tympanography
    b. Evaluation of cranial nerves
    c. Vision evaluation with measurement of intraocular pressure, optic nerve, and retina
    d. Evaluation of visual fields
  4. NURSING INTERVENTIONS
    a. Question the client related to loud prolonged noises earlier in life, such as rock music or machinery in the workplace.
    b. Assess the pupils and inform the client to avoid night driving because pupil accommodation slows.

c. Inform the client that food may not taste as good.

d. Assess the client for comorbid conditions that may pose serious safety risks for the older adult.

    1) Glaucoma—increase in intraocular pressure and decrease in peripheral vision leading to total loss of vision if untreated

    2) Macular degeneration—loss of central vision

    3) Cataracts—opacity of the lens that is so gradual that the client may be unaware of decreasing vision; leads to blindness but the lens can be replaced surgically and vision restored.

    4) Diabetes mellitus—retinopathy that leads to blindness; the loss of vision can be prevented by maintaining blood glucose levels within normal range.

e. Evaluate ability to hear, and inspect the ear canal for excess wax buildup.

f. Assess vision and ability to read printed instructions, and inspect the eye and lids.

g. Evaluate the range of odors that the client can recognize, focusing on the priority, which is the ability to recognize smoke in the environment.

h. Identify risks posed by sensory limitations.

i. Instruct the client on information vital to preventing further deterioration of eyesight, such as prescribed eyedrops for glaucoma that constrict the pupils and must be used for the rest of her life, and to maintain blood sugar within the normal limits.

H. INTEGUMENTARY SYSTEM

  1. ALTERATION IN ANATOMY AND PHYSIOLOGY

    a. Decreased sweat glands

    b. Decreased production of melanin and hair follicles

    c. Decreased blood supply to the nail beds

    d. Decreased subcutaneous fat

  2. ASSESSMENT

    a. Decreased ability to determine the differences between hot and cold

    b. Lack of skin turgor

    c. Dry hair, grayness, alopecia

    d. Brittle and dull fingernails and toenails

    e. Delayed wound healing

  3. DIAGNOSTIC TESTS

    a. Blanching sign

    b. Measurement of skin circumference

    c. Measurement of body weight

  4. NURSING INTERVENTIONS

    a. Instruct the client that she may be unable to distinguish between hot and cold temperatures, provide gloves and blankets for warmth, and use extreme caution when using a heating pad.

    b. Encourage an adequate intake of fluids to enhance skin turgor.

    c. Encourage an adequate intake of protein to enhance wound healing.

    d. Instruct the client to lubricate the skin daily.

    e. Instruct the client to bathe less frequently.

    f. Inform the client to provide adequate humidity in the environment.

I. GENITOURINARY SYSTEM

  1. ALTERATIONS IN ANATOMY AND PHYSIOLOGY

    a. Decreased size of the kidney

    b. Decreased renal blood flow

    c. Weak bladder and pelvic muscles

    d. Decreased number of nephrons

    e. Decreased glomerular filtration rate

  2. ASSESSMENT

    a. Inability to concentrate urine, resulting in dilute urine

    b. Urinary frequency, urgency, and retention; nocturia and incontinence

    c. Enlarged prostate in male clients

    d. Increased incidence of urinary tract infection

  3. DIAGNOSTIC TESTS

    a. Genitourinary examination

    b. Renal scan

    c. Kidney, ureter, and bladder x-ray

  4. NURSING INTERVENTIONS

    a. Instruct the client on an adequate oral intake.

    b. Maintain an accurate intake and output.

    c. Encourage the client to go to the bathroom every 2–3 hours.

    d. Avoid catheterization because that increases the incidence of urinary infections.

    e. Instruct the client to avoid fluids and caffeine at bedtime.

J. REPRODUCTIVE SYSTEM

  1. ALTERATIONS IN ANATOMY AND PHYSIOLOGY

    a. Decreased levels of estrogen in the female client

    b. Sclerotic penile veins and arteries

  2. ASSESSMENT

    a. Decreased production of vaginal secretions

    b. Painful intercourse

    c. Decreased ability to produce an erection

    d. Less frequency of ejaculations

3. DIAGNOSTIC TESTS: EXAMINATION OF THE GENITAL SYSTEM

4. NURSING INTERVENTIONS

   a. Instruct the client on good perineal care.

   b. Instruct the client to use vaginal lubricant for vaginal dryness and painful intercourse.

   c. Explore alterations to sexual activity such as rest before and after sexual activity.

IV. RELATED ISSUES OCCURRING WITH AGING

A. SLEEP AND REST

   1. ALTERATIONS IN SLEEP AND REST

      a. Older adults spend less time in rapid eye movement (REM) and Stage 4 sleep.

      b. Older adults may need only 6–7 hours of sleep a night and a nap in the afternoon, or they may stay up much later than they did when younger and sleep later in the morning.

      c. The ability to have quality sleep and rest is contingent on getting enough exercise and activity during waking hours.

   2. ASSESSMENT

      a. The presence of comorbid conditions may influence the quality and quantity of rest and sleep such as:

         1) Pain

         2) Depression

         3) Immobility

         4) Medications that cause insomnia such as bronchodilators (theophylline, aminophylline), stimulants (caffeine, atropine), or selective serotonin reuptake inhibitors (SSRIs) if taken at night

         5) Medications that interfere with REM sleep, such as some sleeping preparations

         6) Illicit drugs (amphetamines) and alcohol consumption

         7) Dementia with agitation and wandering

         8) Sleep apnea

         9) Anxiety

         10) Incontinence

   3. DIAGNOSTIC TESTS

      a. Sleep studies

      b. Levels of stimulants such as theophylline

      c. Evaluation of thyroid function

   4. NURSING INTERVENTIONS

      a. Observe the client's rest and sleep periods.

      b. Monitor oxygen saturation during sleep periods.

      c. Assess pain and client satisfaction with pain management.

      d. Evaluate the effects and adverse reactions of prescribed and OTC drugs.

      e. Question the client if she self-medicates with alcohol or drugs, attempting to increase sleep or rest.

      f. Formulate a schedule for rest and sleep periods with the client.

      g. Implement methods of promoting sleep and rest, such as adequate daytime activity, developing a bedtime routine, a fan or white noise machine to overcome background noises, toileting before bedtime, a warm bath in the evening, massage, bedtime snack or warm milk, decreased fluids after 6 p.m. to prevent awakening to go to the toilet, and no caffeine after 4 p.m.

      h. Instruct the client to use a night-light. In addition to providing a lighted path when the client gets out of bed, a night-light will also prevent shadows in the room, which may be confused for people or objects.

      i. Avoid using side rails. Use a very low bed with a bedside floor pad if the client has nighttime confusion to prevent falls or injury.

      j. Encourage the client to continue with previous nighttime routines such as using small amounts of alcoholic beverages to promote sleep if not contraindicated.

      k. Monitor the client for paradoxical effects of prescribed or OTC sleeping medications that may lead to agitation, confusion, and insomnia. If REM sleep is interrupted or decreased, the client may be confused or delirious. This may be mistaken for dementia.

B. IMMUNITY

   1. ALTERATIONS IN IMMUNITY

      a. Immunity in the older adult decreases with a decreased protein and is a major factor.

      b. Lymphocyte production is directly related to protein intake.

      c. If serum albumin is low, the lymphocyte count will be correspondingly low.

   2. ASSESSMENT

      a. Malnutrition

      b. Delayed wound healing

      c. Comorbid conditions or medications may also contribute to impaired immunity such as:

         1) Prednisone or prednisolone administration

         2) Diabetes mellitus

         3) Stress (such as from compounded losses—spouse, job, health, home)

         4) Human immunodeficiency virus (HIV)

3. DIAGNOSTIC TESTS
   a. Complete white count with differential
   b. Serum antibody levels
4. NURSING INTERVENTIONS
   a. Assess the amount of protein the client eats, understanding that older adults often do not eat enough protein because of cost, lack of interest in cooking, or inability to chew food.
   b. Assess the client for infections such as fungus in the mouth, vagina, or perianal area; virus such as herpes simplex 1 and 2; herpes zoster as shingles; respiratory infections; bacteria such as in pneumonia, bladder, and wound infections.
   c. Monitor vital signs.
   d. Inspect the skin frequently.
   e. Assess the client for confusion because this may be the first indication of infection, especially in the lungs or bladder.
   f. Monitor lung sounds.
   g. Monitor laboratory data related to immune function such as white count (without enough ingested protein, the white count may not be elevated in the presence of a bacterial infection).
   h. Administer supplemental dietary protein to alleviate low serum albumin.
   i. Prevent infection with adequate nutrition and appropriate immunizations for age, such as influenza, pneumonia, tetanus, and diphtheria.
   j. Encourage the client to eat adequate protein, change positions frequently, exercise, and increase fluids to prevent skin breakdown and promote healthy skin.
C. NUTRITION
   1. ALTERATIONS IN NUTRITION
      a. Significant changes in the gastrointestinal tract
      b. Dentition may change with the loss of teeth and the presence of gingivitis.
      c. Gastrointestinal motility and stomach emptying may slow.
      d. Gastric acidity and reflux may increase.
      e. Intestinal motility and absorption of nutrients may decrease.
      f. Metabolism is slower.
      g. Changes in taste and smell may decrease appetite.
   2. ASSESSMENT
      a. Decreased appetite
      b. Difficulty chewing

   c. There may be comorbid conditions that affect nutrition, such as:
      1) Diabetes mellitus
      2) Pernicious anemia
      3) Difficulty swallowing
      4) Dementia
      5) Decreased activity and mobility
      6) Polypharmacy that may decrease appetite; drug interactions, drug–food interactions
      7) Hyper- or hypothyroidism
      8) Malignancy
3. DIAGNOSTIC TESTS
   a. Upper and lower GI studies
   b. Dental examination
   c. Swallowing study
   d. Serum levels of vitamin B_{12}, iron, folic acid, and ferritin
4. NURSING INTERVENTIONS
   a. Obtain a written 24-hour dietary recall by the client.
   b. Perform a physical assessment of the mouth, hair, GI function, skin, and elimination patterns.
   c. Obtain an accurate weight.
   d. Assess the basal metabolic rate.
   e. Assess the client's ability to chew.
   f. Assess mental status, access to food, ability to prepare food, ability to purchase food, home arrangement, and safety with food storage and preparation.
   g. Identify all prescribed medications, OTC, herbal supplements, home remedies, vitamins, and dietary enhancements the client uses. Generally, fiber, medications, and alcohol will decrease appetite. The one exception is marijuana, which will increase the appetite.
   h. Monitor the older adult to determine:
      1) Carbohydrate intake: should be 50–60% of daily calories
      2) Protein intake: should be 10–20% of daily calories
      3) Fat intake: should be less than 30% of daily calories unless prescribed otherwise
      4) Water-soluble vitamins: vitamins B and C will be lost in the urine if the client is taking a diuretic or is losing excessive water in the urine from hyperglycemia.
      5) Fat-soluble vitamins: vitamins A, D, E, K will not be absorbed from the GI tract if the client is taking oil-containing laxatives, such as mineral oil, or is on a very-low-fat diet.
   i. Assess the client's appetite (small amounts of beer or red wine with or

before meals may stimulate the appetite of the older adult).

j. Assess for possible older adult abuse or neglect in regard to withholding funds or nutrition.

k. Plan exercise daily within the client's limitations and abilities (walking for 30 minutes per day is often the best exercise).

l. Provide nutrient-dense foods that can be chewed and swallowed easily. If dysphagia is present, liquids will need to be thickened to facilitate safe swallowing and prevent aspiration.

m. Provide a social atmosphere where the older adult does not have to eat alone and will not be rushed.

n. Provide utensils that the client can easily use, such as straws or large-handled silverware.

o. Feed the client only if she cannot feed herself so that autonomy, rather than learned helplessness, can be fostered.

p. Promote adequate nutrition by providing balanced meals with fiber (such as bran and psyllium), vitamins, and minerals (including calcium with vitamins because the older adult often is not in the sunshine enough to make her own vitamin D).

q. Offer finger foods that are easily chewed and swallowed for the client with dementia and agitation.

r. Offer frequent nutritious snacks. Older adults tend not to eat adequate meals.

s. Instruct the client how to increase the most often decreased nutrients (protein and calcium).

  1) Increase protein in the diet by including ground meats and dairy products, and adding nonfat dry milk to foods such as milkshakes, meatloaf, and scrambled eggs. Add egg whites to meatballs, hamburgers, casseroles, and baked goods.

  2) Increase calcium intake to 1200–1500 mg a day through OTC supplements with vitamin D and dairy products.

t. Increase fluids to 2000 ml a day. Older adults often do not drink enough fluids to avoid frequent trips to the toilet.

u. Evaluate appropriateness of restricted diets. Does not adding table salt to food decrease the taste so that the client does not eat? Does decreasing the percentage of ingested calories from fat to below 30% affect the absorption of fat-soluble vitamins (vitamins A, D, E, K) as well as the taste of foods? Does decreasing fat lead to decreasing protein intake?

D. PAIN
  1. ALTERATIONS IN PAIN
   a. Older adults often are unwilling to "complain" and talk about their pain.
   b. Older adults may think that pain is an inevitable part of aging, which it is not.
   c. Older adults may not want to ask for pain medication because they do not want to "bother" the caregiver.
   d. Older adults may decline pain medications because they are afraid of becoming addicted.
   e. Pain may be viewed as a part of life that must be tolerated or as a punishment for transgressions in life.
  2. ASSESSMENT
   a. Crying
   b. Rubbing a body part
   c. Moaning
   d. Depression
  3. NURSING INTERVENTIONS
   a. Assess the client's behavior and activity. Watch for decreased activity, insomnia, and restlessness.
   b. Utilize a visual pain scale that the older adult can see and understand easily.
   c. Administer the lowest possible dose of a drug, titrating the drug upward until the level of pain control is acceptable to the client.
   d. Administer drugs to the older adult in the IV or oral routes. The absorption of IM medications is unpredictable in the older adult.
   e. Assess the level of sedation and respiratory rate frequently.
     1) Respiratory depression is more likely with the first dose of an opioid, rather than later doses.
     2) Use adjuvant drugs such as nonsteroidal anti-inflammatory drugs (NSAIDs) and tricyclic antidepressants to support opioids.
     3) Round-the-clock dosing is the method of choice.
     4) Morphine is the opioid of choice for severe pain.
     5) Assess for GI distress or bleeding, or both, if the older adult is using NSAIDs for pain relief.
     6) Chronic pain may result in depression and spiritual distress.
     7) Every older adult who is taking opioids for pain must be on a bowel regimen, including dietary fiber, stool softener, adequate fluid intake, and a laxative, if needed.
   f. Identify what nonpharmacologic methods provide pain relief for the client, such as massage, heat or cold application (with caution),

hydrotherapy, meditation, guided imagery, relaxation therapy, or prayer.

E. POLYPHARMACY

1. OLDER ADULTS OFTEN TAKE MANY PRESCRIBED AND OTC MEDICATIONS.

2. PRESCRIBED MEDICATIONS AND OTC MEDICATIONS MAY INTERACT WITH EACH OTHER AND WITH FOOD.

3. OLDER ADULTS MAY NOT BE ABLE TO AFFORD ALL OF THE PRESCRIBED MEDICATIONS.

4. OLDER ADULTS MAY NOT BE ABLE TO MANAGE THE COMPLEXITIES OF MULTIPLE DRUGS AT DIFFERENT TIMES OF THE DAY.

5. VISUAL IMPAIRMENTS MAY AFFECT THE SAFETY OF SELF-ADMINISTRATIONS OF THE MANY MEDICATIONS.

6. OLDER ADULTS METABOLIZE MEDICATIONS MORE SLOWLY BECAUSE OF CHANGES IN LIVER AND KIDNEY FUNCTION ASSOCIATED WITH AGING AND COMORBID CONDITIONS.

7. MALABSORPTION IN THE GI TRACT WILL SLOW THE ABSORPTION OF DRUGS.

8. THE SYSTEMIC EFFECTS OF DRUGS WILL BE AFFECTED BY ALTERATIONS IN CIRCULATION.

9. DIAGNOSTIC TESTS
    a. Peaks and troughs of medications
    b. Serum levels of medications

10. NURSING INTERVENTIONS
    a. Determine the safety of the client's storage and self-administration of medications.
    b. Identify interactions among prescribed medications, OTC drugs, herbal preparations, and the client's diet.
    c. Inform all of the client's physicians of all drugs taken.
    d. Determine if the client actually takes all prescribed medications as directed by counting pills in prescription bottles.
    e. Set up a week's medications in a safety container as prescribed.
    f. Identify interactions and side effects of medications.
        1) Do any medications, such as antidepressants, adversely affect the client's appetite?
        2) Does the sheer size and number of medications such as large calcium, fiber, or potassium pills present a safety risk or decrease appetite?
        3) Is the client's quality of life affected by the medication schedule or financial burden?
        4) Instruct the client and family on all medications, interactions, and potential adverse reactions.

g. Determine the safest way to administer medications, such as crushing, thickening liquids, or a routine schedule.

F. COMMUNICATION

1. SPEAK CLEARLY AND IN A NORMAL TONE OF VOICE UNTIL THE OLDER ADULT'S HEARING ABILITY IS DETERMINED.

2. STAND IN THE CLIENT'S DIRECT LINE OF VISION. DO NOT APPROACH FROM BEHIND.

3. ASK PERMISSION TO SIT NEAR THE CLIENT OR STAND CLOSE BY AND TOUCH THE CLIENT AS APPROPRIATE.

4. IDENTIFY THE CLIENT'S LEVEL OF SCHOOLING AND ABILITY TO READ. WHAT LANGUAGE DOES THE CLIENT SPEAK AND READ? PROVIDE AN INTERPRETER AS NEEDED.

5. KEEP INSTRUCTIONS SIMPLE. PROVIDE INSTRUCTIONS IN WRITING AS WELL AS VERBALLY.

6. SPEAK TO THE OLDER ADULT AND NOT "OVER" OR AROUND HER.

7. WHEN INTERVIEWING THE OLDER ADULT, KEEP QUESTIONS SIMPLE. ALLOW TIME FOR A REPLY. IT MAY TAKE THE OLDER ADULT LONGER TO FORMULATE AN ANSWER.

8. ENCOURAGE THE FAMILY TO ALLOW THE OLDER ADULT TO TALK.

9. WHEN INSTRUCTING THE OLDER ADULT ABOUT HER CARE OR CONDITION, PROVIDE INFORMATION SIMPLY, VERBALLY, AND IN WRITING, WITH SCHEDULES AND DIRECTIONS CLEARLY DESCRIBED.

10. ACKNOWLEDGE THE WHOLE PERSON, INCLUDING HER CULTURE, ETHNICITY, AND RELIGION.

11. THE OLDER ADULT HAS A CULTURAL AND AN EXPERIENTIAL BACKGROUND THAT INFLUENCES WHO SHE IS TODAY AND HOW SHE WILL RESPOND TO HEALTH PROBLEMS.

12. THE COHORT OR EXPERIENTIAL GROUP TO WHICH THE CLIENT BELONGS MAY IDENTIFY HOW SHE HANDLES PROBLEMS—SUCH AS BEING A WORLD WAR II VETERAN, A VIETNAM VETERAN, OR A BABY BOOMER.

13. OLDER ADULTS ARE MORE DIFFERENT FROM EACH OTHER THAN ALIKE.

14. OLDER ADULTS SHOULD BE TREATED AS UNIQUE INDIVIDUALS.

15. AVOID DISCRIMINATION BASED ON AGE, INCOME, CULTURE, RACE, ETHNICITY, RELIGION, OR CHOICE OF LIFESTYLE.

PRACTICE QUESTIONS

1. A 92-year-old client with emphysema is experiencing chest pain. The nurse determines with pulse oximetry that the oxygen saturation is 83%. The nurse understands that it is essential that oxygen be administered by nasal cannula at which of the following rates?
   1. 8 L/minute
   2. 2 L/minute
   3. 5 L/minute
   4. 12 L/minute

2. An 86-year-old client has sustained a fractured femur and has had surgery to repair the fracture. The client is rubbing the surgical site and moaning. Which of the following is the priority nursing intervention?
   1. Administer the prescribed pain medication
   2. Assess the client's pain level
   3. Determine when the client last had pain medication
   4. Inspect the surgical site

3. Which of the following is the appropriate assessment for respiratory depression in the older adult after the administration of an opioid for analgesia? Respiratory depression is
   1. more likely after several doses of the same drug.
   2. most likely after the first dose.
   3. unlikely because the opioid is not prescribed for the older adult in large doses.
   4. unlikely if the drug is given orally.

4. A 73-year-old client has just undergone a colostomy for cancer of the colon. The client tells the nurse the pain is "8" on a scale of 0 to 10. Which of the following is the expected outcome of the nursing care for this client?
   1. The client does not ask for pain medication
   2. The client self-medicates with an over-the-counter medication
   3. The client verbalizes satisfaction with the level of pain and pain control
   4. The client states the pain is "4" on a scale of 0 to 10

5. The nurse assesses which of the following physiological manifestations as indicating that the client is experiencing acute pain? Select all that apply:
   [ ] 1. Verbalization of pain
   [ ] 2. Crying
   [ ] 3. Hypertension
   [ ] 4. Flushing
   [ ] 5. Tachycardia
   [ ] 6. Moist skin

6. The nurse assesses a 67-year-old client suspected of having a cataract for which of the following clinical manifestations? Select all that apply:
   [ ] 1. Halos around lights
   [ ] 2. Decrease in vision
   [ ] 3. Eye pain
   [ ] 4. Abnormal color perception
   [ ] 5. Glare
   [ ] 6. Headache

7. Which of the following principles should the nurse include in a class on biological theories? Select all that apply:
   [ ] 1. Behavioral and developmental aspects of life
   [ ] 2. Cellular division is altered by chemical reactions
   [ ] 3. The thyroid, bone marrow, and immune system are affected by the aging process
   [ ] 4. Focus on roles and relationship
   [ ] 5. Genetic program or biological clock predetermines life
   [ ] 6. Past accomplishments are incorporated into life to promote self-esteem

8. The nurse assesses a 92-year-old client who has experienced a recent cerebral vascular accident (CVA) with a cranial nerve VII dysfunction to be exhibiting which of the following manifestations?
   1. Loss of sense of smell
   2. Ptosis
   3. Difficulty in swallowing
   4. Asymmetry of facial features

9. Which of the following assessment findings should the nurse monitor for in an older adult with altered nutrition? Select all that apply:
   [ ] 1. Depression
   [ ] 2. Dementia
   [ ] 3. Decreased activity
   [ ] 4. Lack of skin turgor
   [ ] 5. Dysrhythmias
   [ ] 6. Polypharmacy

10. The nurse should include which of the following foods that has the most potassium per serving when instructing a 72-year-old client about foods that are high in potassium?
    1. Milk
    2. Oranges
    3. Colas
    4. Chicken

11. Which of the following is a priority for the nurse to assess when evaluating the hydration of an 87-year-old client?
    1. Height and weight
    2. Previous 24-hour intake
    3. Skin turgor on the back of the hand
    4. Blood pressure

12. During physical assessment of an older adult, the nurse should report which of the following cardiovascular changes that has occurred as a result of dehydration?
    1. Widened pulse pressure
    2. Tachycardia
    3. Hypertension
    4. Decreased respiratory rate

13. The nurse evaluates which of the following nursing assessment findings to be consistent with overhydration in a 72-year-old client admitted with congestive heart failure?
    1. Periorbital edema
    2. Edema of the hands
    3. Projectile vomiting
    4. Moist rales

14. The nurse monitors an older adult for which of the following clinical manifestations of a disturbed sleep pattern?
    Select all that apply:
    [ ] 1. Malnutrition
    [ ] 2. Increased infection
    [ ] 3. Pain
    [ ] 4. Immobility
    [ ] 5. Delayed wound healing
    [ ] 6. Taking theophylline

15. A 93-year-old client has been functioning independently in the home but has suddenly become confused. A family member asks the nurse, "Does this mean Dad has Alzheimer's disease?" Which of the following is the most appropriate response?
    1. "It is very likely your father has Alzheimer's disease."
    2. "Why do you think your father has dementia?"
    3. "Confusion can be a sign of an infection in an older adult."
    4. "Your father will have to be monitored over time."

16. A member of an older client's family asks the nurse why medications are ordered at half of the usual dose. Which of the following is the most appropriate response?
    1. "Medications for the older adult are prescribed at a pediatric dose."
    2. "The metabolism of the older adult is much like that of a child of the same weight."
    3. "Medications for the older adult may be at lower doses initially until responses are evaluated."

    4. "Older adults generally take a lower dose of a medication because of the cost."

17. When the nurse is taking a nursing history on a client, the client mentions, "I slipped on a wet spot on the way to the bathroom." Which of the following is a priority for the nurse to ask?
    1. "Have you started on any new medications?"
    2. "Do you drink caffeinated beverages?"
    3. "Have you experienced any incontinent episodes?"
    4. "Have you been feeling excessively weak recently?"

18. Which of the following should the nurse include in the medication instructions for an older adult who has back pain and for whom a mild opioid with codeine has been prescribed?
    1. Assess respirations three times a day
    2. Increase daily fiber and fluids
    3. Limit the administration of the medication to times of severe pain
    4. Avoid taking the medication more than two times a day

19. A hospice nurse caring for a terminally ill client should titrate the dose of morphine sulfate given to an older adult based on which of the following assessments?
    1. Blood pressure
    2. Level of consciousness
    3. Level of pain
    4. Request of family

20. An older adult asks the nurse why a daily bath is necessary. The nurse should respond that daily bathing
    1. stimulates circulation, provides relaxation, and mobilizes joints.
    2. adds hydration and prevents dry skin.
    3. including combing and brushing of the hair helps to remove excess oil from the scalp.
    4. is necessary to comply with agency policy.

21. Which of the following should the nurse include in the instructions given to an older adult about self-care and hygiene to achieve a positive outcome?
    1. A detailed description of the procedures
    2. A written description of the outcomes
    3. A description of the care center's routines
    4. An article on the importance of hygiene

22. The nurse evaluates which factor as a priority that will adversely affect mobility and self-care in the older adult?
    1. Weakness
    2. Level of consciousness
    3. Disease
    4. Family assistance

23. Older clients have individual preferences in carrying out activities of daily living (ADLs).

The nurse should include which intervention as a priority for encouraging independence in ADLs?
1. Allow the client to decide when to have a bath
2. Ask the client what ADLs are acceptable to perform
3. Provide total care for a client who is handicapped
4. Assess the client's abilities and preferences

24. The nurse finds an 88-year-old client lying on the floor unresponsive. The priority action for the nurse to take is
   1. start cardiopulmonary resuscitation (CPR).
   2. notify the physician.
   3. place the client back in bed.
   4. assess the respirations and pulse.

25. When planning to interview an older adult for a health history, the nurse should consider which of the following as a priority?

1. The purpose of the interview is to obtain pertinent historical data from the client
2. The interview is directed toward offering solutions to the client's problems
3. The interview should be conducted in the client's room
4. The goals of the interview vary

26. The registered nurse is planning clinical assignments for a geriatric nursing unit. Which of the following assignments should the nurse delegate to a licensed practical nurse?
   1. Assess a 67-year-old client after cataract surgery
   2. Monitor the serum electrolytes in an 87-year-old client with renal failure
   3. Take the vital signs of a 71-year-old client following a hip arthroplasty
   4. Perform a physical assessment on a 62-year-old client admitted for abdominal pain

ANSWERS AND RATIONALES

1. 2. In emphysema, the drive to breathe will be decreased or eliminated if oxygen is administered at a high rate. The best and safest initial rate of oxygen flow is 2 L to 3 L/minute. If higher flow rates are administered, the client may need artificial ventilation.

2. 2. Older adults may rub or pat a painful area rather than verbalize the pain. The priority intervention is to assess the client's pain level by asking the client. Administering pain medications, determining when the client had the last pain medication, and inspecting the surgical site are all appropriate interventions, but only after the current level of pain is assessed.

3. 2. Depending on the pain level, large doses may be prescribed for older adults. If a client is very sensitive to an opioid, the resulting respiratory depression is most likely to occur after the first dose. The route of administration will not decrease the likelihood of respiratory depression.

4. 3. An older adult in severe pain may not ask for pain medication because of a reluctance to "complain." The nurse cannot determine for the client what is an acceptable level of pain. A good outcome is achieved when the client can verbalize satisfaction with the level of pain and pain control.

5. 3. 5. Hypertension and tachycardia are physiological manifestations of acute pain.

Crying and verbalizing pain are psychological or emotional manifestations of pain. When a client is in acute pain, the skin is more likely to be cool and pale.

6. 2. 4. 5. A decrease in vision, abnormal color perception, and glare are clinical manifestations with cataracts. Halos around lights are common in glaucoma. Eye pain and headaches may be present in a variety of other eye disorders.

7. 2. 3. 5. Principles of biological theories include the following: cellular division is altered by chemical reactions; the thyroid, bone marrow, and immune system are affected by the aging process; and a genetic program or biological clock predetermines life. Principles of psychological theories include behavioral and developmental aspects of life and past accomplishments are incorporated into life to promote self-esteem. Focusing on roles and relationships is a principle in sociologic theories.

8. 4. An asymmetry of facial features is specific to cranial nerve VII, the facial nerve. A difficulty in swallowing is associated with cranial nerve IX, the glossopharyngeal nerve. Loss of smell is common with injury to cranial nerve I, the olfactory nerve. Ptosis occurs with damage to cranial nerve III, the oculomotor nerve.

9. 2. 3. 6. Assessment findings in altered nutrition for an older adult include dementia, decreased activity, and polypharmacy. Depression is an assessment finding for alterations in sleep and rest. Lack of skin turgor is an assessment finding in an altered integumentary system for an older adult. Dysrhythmia is an assessment finding with altered circulation.

10. 2. Citrus fruits, such as oranges, have the highest concentrations of potassium.

11. 4. Although weight and previous intake are important in evaluating hydration, blood pressure will give a more accurate indication of current hydration. Skin turgor should be checked in the older adult on the clavicle or forehead. A 24-hour intake of fluids may provide the nurse with additional information about the client's hydration status, but it is not the priority.

12. 2. A narrowed pulse pressure and hypotension indicate dehydration and decreased circulating blood volume. Tachycardia and an increased respiratory rate indicate the body is attempting to increase the circulation of oxygen in the blood.

13. 4. Periorbital edema and edema of the hands are related to kidney failure and overhydration. Projectile vomiting in the older adult may be related to increased intracranial pressure. Moist rales indicate left-sided heart failure in a client with congestive heart failure.

14. 3. 4. 6. Clinical manifestations in the assessment findings of altered sleep and rest include pain, immobility, and theophylline. Malnutrition and delayed wound healing are clinical manifestations in immunity. Increased infection is a clinical manifestation for an altered respiratory system.

15. 3. An older adult client who suddenly becomes confused may have developed an infection, generally of the lungs and bladder, or may be dehydrated. Confusion that occurs in delirium, Alzheimer's disease, and other forms of dementia develops slowly and over time. Telling a client's family that the client may have dementia and will have to be monitored over time shuts down communication. Telling the family that the acute confusion may be a sign of infection keeps communication open and offers information. Rather than a "why" question, the nurse could ask for more recent history on the client, such as whether the client has experienced a fall or head injury.

16. 3. Older adults do not metabolize medications at the same rates as children and younger adults do. The liver and kidneys may have impaired function. Even though a thin older adult may have a body weight similar to that of a child,

the dosage of medications must allow for age and comorbid conditions.

17. 3. Although asking clients if they have started on any new medications, drink caffeinated beverages, or are excessively weak is relevant when taking a health history, the possibility of incontinence is significant because the client stated that the fall was the result of "slipping on a wet spot."

18. 2. It is difficult for clients to count their own respirations accurately, and that measure is not necessary when taking codeine. The dosing of the medication should be "round the clock" to prevent severe pain. Older adult clients are more prone to constipation than younger clients, and fiber and fluids should be increased in the diet.

19. 3. The level of pain acceptable to the client determines the dose of pain medication given to a hospice client. The pain medication is then titrated.

20. 1. Daily bathing may damage fragile skin in the older adult. Daily combing and brushing of the hair helps stimulate the scalp and distribute the oil. Reasons for daily bathing include stimulating circulation, providing relaxation, and mobilizing joints.

21. 2. By giving the client a written description of the expected outcomes and then explaining the procedures and demonstrating the techniques, the nurse will facilitate learning and mutual goal setting.

22. 1. Older adults may have many chronic conditions that do not affect mobility or self-care. Weakness from any cause often means that older adults cannot be mobile and care for themselves.

23. 4. It is not advised to ask older clients when they want to take a bath because they may refuse activities of daily living (ADLs). Even clients who are handicapped are capable of autonomy and self-care. Asking the client what ADLs are acceptable to perform promotes dependency. Assessing the client's abilities, setting mutual goals, and planning care accordingly promote independence in the client.

24. 4. When finding a client unresponsive on the floor, the priority is to assess the respirations and pulse before notifying the physician or starting cardiopulmonary resuscitation (CPR).

25. 4. The interview for a health history should identify past and present problems. It should be conducted in a private environment, and the client's room may not be private. The interview is not for the purpose of offering solutions to the problems. Depending on the

setting and the reasons why the nurse is conducting the interview (such as to assess an acutely ill client or to evaluate a client still living at home who has a chronic condition), the goals may vary.

26. 3. A licensed practical nurse may take the vital signs on a client following a hip arthroplasty. Assessing, monitoring, and performing a physical assessment are all skills that require a registered nurse.

REFERENCES

Estes, M. (2010). *Health assessment and physical examination* (4th ed.). Clifton Park, NY: Delmar Cengage Learning.

Holfman Wold, G. (2012). *Basic geriatric nursing* (5th ed.). St. Louis, MO: Elsevier Mosby.

Touhy, T. A., & Jett, K. F. (2010). *Ebersole and Hess' gerontonological nursing & healthy aging* (3rd ed.). St. Louis, MO: Elsevier Mosby.

CHAPTER 59

DELIRIUM AND DEMENTIA

I. DEPRESSION

A. DESCRIPTION
1. DEPRESSION IS NOT A NORMAL PART OF AGING AND CAN BE INITIALLY CONFUSED WITH DELIRIUM OR DEMENTIA.
2. UP TO 30% OF OLDER WOMEN AND 20% OF OLDER MEN MAY HAVE CLINICAL DEPRESSION.
3. DEPRESSION IS UNDERTREATED IN THE OLDER ADULT AND CAN LEAD TO A DIMINISHED QUALITY OF LIFE AND INCREASED RISK OF SUICIDE.
4. THE DEPRESSION MAY BE LINKED TO A SIGNIFICANT LOSS OR LIFE CHANGE.
5. OLDER ADULTS WHO ARE AT GREAT RISK FOR SUICIDE ARE SINGLE MEN WITHOUT A CLOSE SUPPORT SYSTEM WHO HAVE CHRONIC ILLNESSES, CHRONIC PAIN, OR A TERMINAL ILLNESS.
6. THE CLIENT MAY SELF-MEDICATE WITH ALCOHOL OR OTHER DRUGS FOR THE DEPRESSION.
7. DENIAL, RATIONALIZATION, AND PROJECTION ARE OFTEN THE COPING MECHANISMS THAT PREVENT THE CLIENT AND FAMILY FROM SEEKING PROFESSIONAL HELP.
8. DEPRESSION IS GENERALLY DIURNAL, WITH CLINICAL MANIFESTATIONS WORSE IN THE MORNING.
9. GENERALLY, DEPRESSION HAS PERSISTED LONGER THAN 2 WEEKS AND MAY LAST FOR YEARS.

B. ASSESSMENT
1. CLINICAL MANIFESTATIONS OF DEPRESSION IN THE OLDER ADULT MAY BE TYPICAL OR ATYPICAL.
2. ANOREXIA OR OVEREATING, ESPECIALLY SWEETS AND STARCHES
3. ANGRY OUTBURSTS
4. FORGETFULNESS OR DECREASED ATTENTION SPAN
5. INSOMNIA OR SLEEPING TOO MUCH
6. LOSS OF INTEREST IN HYGIENE, PREVIOUS ACTIVITIES, OR THE FUTURE
7. DELUSIONS AND PARANOIA
8. SUBSTANCE ABUSE (ALCOHOL AND DRUGS)
9. PSYCHOMOTOR RETARDATION OR AGITATION
10. APATHY
11. RESTLESS SLEEP WITH EARLY MORNING AWAKENING
12. MAY BE AT RISK FOR SUICIDE

C. NURSING DIAGNOSES
1. ADULT FAILURE TO THRIVE
2. CHRONIC CONFUSION
3. DISTURBED THOUGHT PROCESSES

D. DIAGNOSTIC TESTS
1. GERIATRIC DEPRESSION SCALE (GDS)
2. BECK DEPRESSION INVENTORY (BDI)
3. CENTER FOR EPIDEMIOLOGICAL STUDIES DEPRESSION SCALE (CES-D)
4. MEDICAL EXAMINATION WITH LABORATORY TESTING TO RULE OUT CENTRAL NERVOUS SYSTEM (CNS) INFECTION SUCH AS SYPHILIS OR HUMAN IMMUNODEFICIENCY VIRUS (HIV)

E. NURSING INTERVENTIONS
1. ASSESS FOR CLINICAL MANIFESTATION OF DEPRESSION AFTER SIGNIFICANT LIFE EVENTS SUCH AS A LOSS OF A SPOUSE OR CLOSE RELATIVE, LOSS OF A JOB, CHANGE IN HEALTH STATUS, OR A MOVE.
2. ASSESS CHANGES IN APPEARANCE, WEIGHT, SLEEP PATTERNS, AFFECT, AND ABILITY TO FUNCTION.
3. MONITOR THE CLIENT FOR VERBALIZATION OF HOPELESSNESS,

FEAR OF THE FUTURE, CRYING, LOSS OF INTEREST IN PRIZED POSSESSIONS, RELATIONSHIPS, AND SELF-CARE.

4. DISCUSS DEPRESSION AND THE CLIENT'S FEELINGS.

5. REFER FOR NEUROPSYCHIATRIC EVALUATION, MEDICATION, AND PSYCHOTHERAPY AS APPROPRIATE.

6. MONITOR A CLIENT TAKING ANTIDEPRESSANTS FOR ADVERSE REACTIONS SUCH AS AGITATION, INSOMNIA, ANOREXIA, AND WEIGHT LOSS. (SEE CHAPTER 51.)

7. ENCOURAGE THE CLIENT TO WRITE FEELINGS IN A JOURNAL.

8. UTILIZE PLANNED REMINISCENCE THERAPY TO EMPHASIZE LIFE ACCOMPLISHMENTS, WHETHER IN A GROUP OR INDIVIDUALLY.

9. MONITOR FOR POSSIBLE SELF-DIRECTED HARM: REPORT AND REFER AS WARRANTED; REMOVE ITEMS THAT COULD BE USED FOR SELF-HARM SUCH AS CORDS, PLASTIC BAGS, FIREARMS, KNIVES, OR DRUGS; AND INSTITUTE SUICIDE PRECAUTIONS.

10. CONTRACT WITH THE CLIENT THAT HE WILL NOT HARM HIMSELF OR OTHERS.

11. IDENTIFY CONTRIBUTION OF LOSSES TO DEPRESSION AND HELP THE CLIENT HANDLE THESE LOSSES.

II. DELIRIUM

A. DESCRIPTION

1. A DECREASE IN COGNITIVE FUNCTION AND POSSIBLE ALTERATION IN CONSCIOUSNESS, WHICH IS REVERSIBLE

2. THE COGNITIVE CHANGES OCCUR RAPIDLY, SUCH AS IN A FEW HOURS OR WITHIN THE DAY, AND A CAUSE CAN USUALLY BE DETERMINED AND OFTEN CORRECTED.

3. COMMON CAUSES:
   a. Hypernatremia
   b. Hyponatremia
   c. Dehydration
   d. Fever greater than 104°F or 40°C
   e. Medication adverse reactions or interactions
   f. Low blood glucose
   g. Ketoacidosis
   h. Hypoxia
   i. Concussion
   j. Increased intracranial pressure from traumatic brain injury
   k. Subdural hematoma
   l. Drug or alcohol abuse
   m. Sensory overload or deprivation
   n. Sleep deprivation

4. RAPID ONSET, OFTEN BEING WORSE AT NIGHT

B. ASSESSMENT

1. FLUCTUATIONS IN AWARENESS AND ORIENTATION

2. DISORGANIZED THINKING

3. MAY EXPERIENCE ILLUSIONS, DELUSIONS, OR HALLUCINATIONS

4. HYPOKINETIC OR HYPERKINETIC

5. SLEEPLESSNESS, WITH THE CYCLE OFTEN REVERSED

6. CLINICAL MANIFESTATIONS, OFTEN WORSE AT NIGHT

C. NURSING DIAGNOSES

1. ADULT FAILURE TO THRIVE

2. ACUTE CONFUSION

3. DISORGANIZED THOUGHT PROCESSES

Nursing Diagnoses: Definitions and Classification 2012–2014. Copyright © 2012, 1994–2012 by NANDA International. Used by arrangement with John Wiley & Sons Limited.

D. DIAGNOSTIC TESTS

1. DIAGNOSTIC TESTING MAY BE USED TO CONFIRM A CAUSE OF THE DELIRIUM OR TO RULE OUT A CAUSE, SUCH AS A COMPUTERIZED TOMOGRAPHY (CT) SCAN OF THE HEAD TO RULE OUT TRAUMA OR BLEEDING.

2. SERUM ELECTROLYTE, COMPLETE BLOOD COUNT (CBC), BLOOD SUGAR, AND DRUG SCREENS

3. URINALYSIS AND CHEST X-RAY ARE NECESSARY TO INDICATE THE PRESENCE OF INFECTION.

4. AN ELECTROCARDIOGRAM (ECG) AND SERIAL ENZYME LEVELS MAY BE USED TO DETERMINE CARDIAC CAUSES.

5. OXYGENATION SATURATION LEVELS

E. NURSING INTERVENTIONS

1. ASSESS AND CAREFULLY DOCUMENT LEVEL OF CONSCIOUSNESS AND CHANGES IN MENTAL STATUS.

2. MONITOR OXYGEN SATURATION AND LABORATORY TESTS.

3. PROTECT FROM INJURY. INSTITUTE SAFE MEASURES SUCH AS SIDE RAILS UP, NOT LEAVING THE CLIENT ALONE, AND SEIZURE PRECAUTIONS.

4. CORRECT THE UNDERLYING CAUSE OF DELIRIUM, SUCH AS ADMINISTERING OXYGEN, FEEDING THE CLIENT IF LOW BLOOD SUGAR, REHYDRATING IF THERE IS DEHYDRATION, PROMOTING RESTFUL SLEEP, OR ADMINISTERING ANTIBIOTICS.

5. REORIENT TO PERSON, PLACE, AND TIME AS INDICATED.

6. MAKE SURE A CLIENT WHO WEARS EYEGLASSES OR USES A HEARING AID HAS THEM ON.

7. AVOID THE USE OF RESTRAINTS.

8. MONITOR THE CLIENT FOR COMPLICATIONS OF IMMOBILITY, AND IMPLEMENT ACTIVITIES SUCH AS ROM TO PREVENT SKIN BREAKDOWN.
9. OFFER SUPPORT TO THE CLIENT AND FAMILY.
10. ADMINISTER ANTIPSYCHOTICS SUCH AS HALOPERIDOL (HALDOL), ISPERIDONE (RISPERDAL), QUETIAPINE (SEROQUEL), AND OLANZAPINE (ZYPREXA). SEE CHAPTER 28 ON ANTIPSYCHOTICS.

III. **DEMENTIA/ALZHEIMER'S DISEASE**
   A. DESCRIPTION
      1. A SLOW LOSS OF COGNITIVE FUNCTION, WITH THE MAJOR SIGN INITIALLY BEING SHORT-TERM MEMORY LOSS
      2. PROGRESSES TO DEATH, OFTEN WITHOUT A DEFINITIVE CAUSE BEING DIAGNOSED
      3. OCCURS MOST OFTEN IN THE OLDER ADULT BUT CAN OCCUR IN A YOUNGER CLIENT WITH BRAIN INJURY OR DOWN SYNDROME
      4. THERE ARE MANY KNOWN CAUSES OF DEMENTIA, SUCH AS NEURODEGENERATIVE, VASCULAR, METABOLIC, IMMUNOLOGIC, SYSTEMIC, TRAUMA, OR DRUGS.
      5. MANY DEMENTIAS ARE OFTEN MISTAKENLY CALLED "ALZHEIMER'S."
      6. IF ALL OTHER POSSIBLE CAUSES OF DEMENTIA HAVE BEEN RULED OUT, A CLIENT WILL BE DIAGNOSED WITH ALZHEIMER'S-LIKE DEMENTIA (ALD).
      7. TYPES OF DEMENTIA INCLUDE ALZHEIMER'S (PLAQUES AND TANGLES IN THE BRAIN), VASCULAR OR MULTI-INFARCT DEMENTIA (DIMINISHED CIRCULATION TO MULTIPLE SMALL AREAS OF THE BRAIN), AND BRAIN DAMAGE FROM TRAUMA OR INFECTION.
      8. ALZHEIMER'S AND ALZHEIMER'S-LIKE DEMENTIA HAVE A PREDICTABLE DOWNWARD TRAJECTORY AND EXPECTED STAGES (SEE TABLE 59-1).
   B. ASSESSMENT
      1. ONSET IS GENERALLY INSIDIOUS.
      2. PROGRESSIVE CLINICAL MANIFESTATIONS THAT MAY BE STABLE OVER A PERIOD OF TIME SUCH AS MONTHS OR YEARS
      3. DISORIENTED TO PERSON, PLACE, AND TIME
      4. IMPAIRED JUDGMENT AND ABSTRACT REASONING
      5. MAY HAVE ILLUSIONS, DELUSIONS, OR HALLUCINATIONS

Table 59-1 Stages of Alzheimer's Disease

Stage	Clinical Manifestations
Stage 1: Early	Forgetfulness, often subtle and masked by the client
	Indecisiveness
	Increasing self-centeredness; decreasing interest in others, environment, and social activities
	Difficulty in learning new information
	Slowed reaction time
	Beginnings of compromised performance at home and at work
Stage 2: Middle	Progressing forgetfulness, inability to remember names of family members or close friends
	Tendency to lose things
	Confusion
	Fearfulness
	Easily induced frustration and irritability; sometimes, angry outbursts
	Repetitive storytelling
	Beginnings of communication problems (inability to remember words, apparent aphasia)
	Inability to follow simple directions
	Difficulty in calculating numbers
	Beginnings of getting lost in familiar places
	Evasive or anxious interactions with others
	Physical activity (pacing, wandering)
	Changes in sleep–rest cycle (with frequent activity at night)
	Changes in eating patterns (possible constant hunger or none at all)
	Neglect of activities of daily living (ADLs) and personal hygiene; changes in bowel and bladder continence; and dressing difficulties
	Inability to maintain safety without supervision
	Losses of social behaviors
	Paranoia
Stage 3: Late	Inability to communicate
	Inability to eat
	Incontinence (urine and feces)
	Inability to recognize family or friends
	Confinement to bed
	Total dependence relative to care

© Cengage Learning 2015

6. SLEEPLESSNESS WITH FREQUENT AWAKENINGS
7. DIFFICULTY IN CARRYING ON A CONVERSATION WITH A DIFFICULTY IN FINDING THE WORDS
   C. NURSING DIAGNOSES
      1. DISTURBED THOUGHT PROCESSES
      2. SELF-CARE DEFICIT
      3. INEFFECTIVE COPING
      4. WANDERING
      5. SOCIAL ISOLATION
      6. INEFFECTIVE THERAPEUTIC REGIMEN MANAGEMENT

7. INEFFECTIVE HEALTH MAINTENANCE
8. ANXIETY
9. CAREGIVER ROLE STRAIN

Nursing Diagnoses: Definitions and Classification 2012–2014. Copyright © 2012, 1994–2012 by NANDA International. Used by arrangement with John Wiley & Sons Limited.

D. DIAGNOSTIC TESTS
1. ALZHEIMER'S DISEASE CAN ONLY BE CONFIRMED ON AUTOPSY WHEN PLAQUES AND TANGLES ARE FOUND IN THE BRAIN.
2. CT SCAN AND MAGNETIC RESONANCE IMAGING (MRI) MAY DEMONSTRATE BRAIN ATROPHY, ENLARGED VENTRICLES IN LATE STAGE, OR A DECREASED SIZE OF THE BRAIN.
3. SINGLE-PHOTON EMISSION COMPUTED TOMOGRAPHY (SPECT), MAGNETIC RESONANCE SPECTROSCOPY (MRS), AND POSITRON EMISSION TOMOGRAPHY (PET) MAY DETECT CHANGES EARLY IN THE DISEASE AND MONITOR TREATMENT RESPONSE. APOLIPOPROTEIN E4 (APOE4) IS A GENE PRESENT ON CHROMOSOME 19 THAT CORRELATES WITH AND INCREASES THE RISK OF DEVELOPING ALZHEIMER'S DISEASE.
5. MINI-MENTAL STATE EXAM ASSESSES THE DEGREE OF COGNITIVE IMPAIRMENT. THE CLIENT MUST BE ABLE TO READ, WRITE, AND SEE TO COMPLETE THE EXAM.

6. A URINE TEST MEASURING ISOPROSTANES (BY-PRODUCTS OF FAT METABOLISM ASSOCIATED WITH FREE RADICALS) MAY MEASURE THE RISK OF DEVELOPING ALZHEIMER'S.

E. NURSING INTERVENTIONS
1. MAINTAIN A SAFE AND SECURE ENVIRONMENT AT ALL TIMES.
2. WITH EARLY COGNITIVE LOSS, INSTRUCT THE CLIENT AND FAMILY ON MEMORY TIPS SUCH AS A DAILY SCHEDULE AND ROUTINE, STICKY NOTES AS REMINDERS, AND LABELING OF HOUSEHOLD ITEMS, SUCH AS "BOB'S BATHROOM" OR "BOB'S CLOTHES."
3. MINIMIZE CHANGE IN THE ENVIRONMENT.
4. CLIENT SHOULD CARRY PERSONAL IDENTIFICATION AT ALL TIMES, INCLUDING NAME, ADDRESS, PHONE NUMBER, STATEMENT OF MEDICAL CONDITION, AND HOW TO CONTACT A FAMILY MEMBER.
5. INFORM THE FAMILY ABOUT DEMENTIA AND THE EXPECTED DOWNWARD COURSE OF THE ILLNESS.
6. PROVIDE SUPPORT FOR PLANNING LONG-TERM CARE AND HEALTH CARE DIRECTIVES.
7. ADMINISTER PRESCRIBED MEDICATIONS (SEE TABLE 59-2).

Table 59-2 Drugs Used to Treat Decreased Memory and Cognition in Alzheimer's Disease

Name	Classification	Action	Adverse Reactions	Nursing Interventions
Donepezil (Aricept)	Autonomic nervous system agent: cholinesterase inhibitor	Thought to increase acetylcholine in cerebral cortex	Headache, insomnia, fatigue, nausea, vomiting, diarrhea, bradycardia	Monitor for improvement of cognition. Monitor for signs and symptoms of GI upset or bleeding. Monitor asthma or chronic obstructive pulmonary disease (COPD) carefully. Monitor for bradycardia and fainting.
Rivastigmine (Exelon)	Autonomic nervous system agent: cholinesterase inhibitor	Inhibits acetylcholinesterase in the brain	Asthenia, sweating, syncope, fatigue, malaise, flulike symptoms, nausea, vomiting, diarrhea, anorexia, abdominal pain, dizziness, headache, hyperglycemia	Monitor cognitive function, dizziness, lab test results, weight, and anorexia.
Galantamine (Razadyne)	Autonomic nervous system agent: cholinergic; cholinesterase inhibitor	Acetylcholinesterase inhibitor	Weight loss, bradycardia, syncope, depression, insomnia, nausea, vomiting, diarrhea	Monitor all systems for significant changes.
Tacrine (Cognex)	Autonomic nervous system agent: cholinesterase inhibitor	Increases acetylcholine in the cerebral cortex	Diaphoresis, agitation, dizziness, confusion, nausea, vomiting, diarrhea, purpura	Monitor all systems for significant changes.

8. INSTRUCT THE CLIENT AND FAMILY AS APPROPRIATE ABOUT DEMENTIA AND HOW TO COPE WITH DECLINING COGNITIVE FUNCTION.

9. PREVENT FAMILY ROLE STRAIN AND BURNOUT AS MUCH AS POSSIBLE THROUGH RESPITE CARE, SUPPORT GROUPS, AND LONG-TERM CARE WHEN NEEDED.

10. BE ALERT FOR SIGNS OF OLDER ADULT CLIENT ABUSE OF CAREGIVERS OR CAREGIVER ABUSE OF THE VULNERABLE CLIENT.

11. AVOID ASKING "DON'T YOU REMEMBER WHEN . . .?"

12. FREQUENT AND INSISTENT REMINDERS ABOUT THE DATE OR CURRENT SITUATION SUCH AS THE DEATH OF A SPOUSE MAY INCREASE THE CLIENT'S AGITATION.

13. REDIRECT THE CLIENT AS THE BEST WAY TO HANDLE AGITATION.

14. PERMIT WANDERING WITHIN A SAFE ENVIRONMENT.

15. PROVIDE FINGER FOODS AND DRINKS TO PREVENT WEIGHT LOSS FROM THE ENERGY EXPENDITURE.

16. IMPLEMENT STOP SIGNS ON EXTERIOR DOORS OR PATHS ON THE FLOOR MARKED WITH WIDE TAPE THAT MAY PREVENT THE CLIENT FROM GOING OUTSIDE.

17. USE CHEMICAL RESTRAINT WITH DRUGS SUCH AS HALOPERIDOL (HALDOL) OR SEDATIVES AFTER OTHER INTERVENTIONS HAVE FAILED.

18. ASSESS THE CLIENT'S MENTAL STATUS BY ASKING THE CLIENT TO DRAW A CLOCK. THIS BRIEF EXAM OF MENTAL STATUS MAY INDICATE THE ABILITY TO FOLLOW DIRECTIONS AND THE MEMORY OF WHAT A CLOCK LOOKS LIKE.

19. ASSESS WEIGHT AND CHANGES IN WEIGHT, APPETITE, PRESENCE OF AGITATION, SAFETY CONCERNS SUCH AS WANDERING, SLEEPING PATTERNS, AND COPING BY THE CLIENT AND FAMILY, AND IMPLEMENT INTERVENTIONS AS APPROPRIATE.

20. PROVIDE A QUIET, CALM ENVIRONMENT FOR THE PHYSICAL AND MENTAL STATUS EXAM. IF THE CLIENT IS AGITATED OR ANXIOUS, A TRUSTED SIGNIFICANT OTHER SHOULD BE PRESENT. INSTRUCT THE FAMILY MEMBER NOT TO ANSWER FOR OR COACH THE CLIENT.

21. SPEAK SLOWLY AND IN SHORT SENTENCES. EXPRESS ONLY ONE IDEA OR QUESTION AT A TIME.

22. APPROACH THE CLIENT FROM THE FRONT AND NEVER FROM BEHIND. TOUCH THE CLIENT BY PERMISSION ONLY UNLESS IT IS AN EMERGENCY.

23. DO NOT CONTRADICT OR ARGUE WITH THE CLIENT OR ALLOW THE FAMILY TO DO SO. NEVER UTILIZE QUESTIONS THAT BEGIN WITH "DO YOU REMEMBER WHEN . . .?"

24. ENCOURAGE THE CLIENT TO PARTICIPATE IN A POSITIVE MANNER. KEEP INSTRUCTIONS SIMPLE.

25. UTILIZE AN ADULT DAY CARE CENTER AS APPROPRIATE

PRACTICE QUESTIONS

1. The nurse has determined that a confused older adult client who keeps pulling out the intravenous line and indwelling catheter is in need of soft wrist restraints. Which of the following should the nurse include in this client's plan of care?
   1. Obtain a p.r.n. restraint order
   2. Assess the placement of the wrist restraints, skin, and circulation every hour and document
   3. Place the client in a supine position after applying the restraints and secure the wrist restraints to the side rails when the client is in bed
   4. Remove the restraints once every 4 hours to perform activities of daily living

2. A family expresses concern to the nurse when their 96-year-old mother with dementia living in a long-term care facility seems more confused and does not remember the activities of daily living. Which of the following is the most appropriate response?
   1. "Don't worry; your mother is safe in the long-term care facility."
   2. "You need to remind your mother how to perform her basic needs."
   3. "Your mother will get worse as time goes on and the dementia progresses."
   4. "This must be frustrating for you."

3. A 77-year-old client expresses concern to a nurse in a walk-in psychiatric clinic of "going crazy or of having Alzheimer's disease" because

of feelings of being overwhelmed and sad all of the time, and misplacing things. Which of the following is the priority for the nurse to include in this client's plan of care?
1. Assist the client to develop areas of strength in coping
2. Make a psychosocial assessment
3. Explore the available supports for the client
4. Assure the client and dispel the idea of "going crazy"

4. Upon admission to a long-term care facility, an 83-year-old client is withdrawn, sitting quietly in a chair with the back to the door of the room. When the nurse speaks to the client, the client says, "Go away and leave me alone. Spend your time on someone who can use it. I just don't want to live if I have to stay here." Which of the following is the priority nursing action?
1. Create a welcoming and cheerful atmosphere
2. Encourage the client to discuss the feelings of hopelessness
3. Allow the client to have periods of solitude as asked for
4. Assess for depression and suicide potential

5. An 86-year-old client suddenly becomes confused about time, place, and person. After evaluating the oxygen saturation to be 98%, which of the following should the nurse assess first?
1. What medications the client is taking
2. Vital signs
3. Possibility of a recent fall
4. The client's pain level

6. A 56-year-old client diagnosed with Stage I (early-onset) Alzheimer's disease lives at home with family. A daughter asks the nurse, "How long will Dad be like this before his memory returns?" The best initial response the nurse can make is which of the following?
1. "He may never get better."
2. "This is just the beginning of a predicted decline."
3. "Tell me what you know about Alzheimer's disease."
4. "Is he taking his medicine for Alzheimer's disease?"

7. An older adult is picking at clothing and muttering, "Butterflies are all over me." The nurse does not see any butterflies. Which of the following is the priority for the nurse to perform?
1. Identify any risk for injury related to altered thought processes
2. Call for help
3. Provide a nonstimulating environment
4. Inform the client there are no butterflies in the room

8. An older adult's cognitive function has declined over the last 2 years. The family is concerned by the loss of short-term memory and the safety issues posed by the forgetfulness. A complete medical workup including a computerized tomography (CT) scan of the head has shown no medical cause for the cognitive changes. The nurse explains to the client and family that the medical diagnosis of Alzheimer's disease is based on
1. the information that no other cause can be found for the changes.
2. a blood test for C-reactive protein that was positive.
3. a loss of function seen on the Mini-Mental State Exam.
4. the results of an x-ray of the skull showing a decrease in the size of the brain.

9. When assessing an older adult, the nurse should be alert to the clinical manifestations of depression that may be masked by other chronic conditions. The cardinal and primary behavior exhibited in the depressed older adult is
1. a loss of interest in previously pleasurable activities.
2. inactivity.
3. drinking alcohol.
4. crying.

10. Donepezil hydrochloride (Aricept) has been prescribed for a client with Alzheimer's disease. Which of the following adverse reactions should the nurse include in the medication instructions given to the family?
Select all that apply:
[ ] 1. Headache
[ ] 2. Tachycardia
[ ] 3. Insomnia
[ ] 4. Hypotension
[ ] 5. Constipation
[ ] 6. Anorexia

11. Before preparing to use the Mini-Mental State Exam for cognitive function in an older adult, the nurse should consider which of the following limitations of the exam?
1. The test takes 1 hour to administer
2. The client must be able to see and write
3. The exam must take place in a dimly lit room
4. The exam is valid only with English-speaking clients

12. The nurse should consider which of the following medical etiologies in an older adult who has been healthy until recently but has developed dementia?
1. Sexually transmitted diseases
2. Electrolyte imbalances
3. Arthritis
4. Liver disease

13. Which of the following four older adult clients that the nurse is caring for does the nurse evaluate as most at risk for self-directed violence?
    1. A 76-year-old single man who lives in a retirement center and engages in community activities
    2. A widowed man who is 88 years old, lives alone, and has multiple chronic illnesses
    3. An 83-year-old woman who has type 2 diabetes mellitus and lives with her daughter
    4. A recently widowed woman with multiple chronic illnesses who lives near family

14. An older adult client with chronic depression tells the nurse, "Don't worry about me. I can manage the pain of my arthritis. The way I mix up my medications helps." The best initial response by the nurse is which of the following?
    1. "Don't mix your medications yourself. Take them only as prescribed."
    2. "That's dangerous. I'll have to take your narcotics from you."
    3. "That's dangerous. I'll have to call your daughter and have her give you your medications."
    4. "Tell me what you take and how you mix them."

15. The nurse is caring for an older adult with situational depression following the death of a spouse. What is the most important outcome for the nurse to plan for?
    1. The client will discuss the spouse and the meaning of the loss
    2. The client will not cry
    3. The client will speak of the spouse only positively
    4. The client will avoid talking about the spouse and engage in social activities

16. Which of the following is the priority nursing intervention for the nurse to include in the plan of care for a client with behavior problems related to dementia?
    1. Inform the client why the nursing interventions are necessary
    2. Instruct the caregivers on the process of dementia and care to be given
    3. Be consistent by repeating the same intervention as the client's dementia progresses
    4. Assist the client to perform difficult tasks

17. A nurse observes a family member continually reminding a client in late Stage II Alzheimer's disease of the date and place. The client is adamant that it is 1922 and the North Pole.

The nurse informs the family member that continually reminding the client of the date and place will result in
    1. a return of memory.
    2. increased retention of the information.
    3. a catastrophic reaction.
    4. an interest in having a calendar.

18. An 80-year-old client is admitted to the intensive care unit because of hemorrhaging after a stent is placed in her left femoral artery to improve circulation to the leg. The client is confused, not following instructions, and pulling at the intravenous tubing and indwelling catheter. The client's adult son tells the nurse, "My mom was never like this before. What have you done to her?" The best initial response the nurse can make is which of the following?
    1. "We've done nothing to her. She must have dementia."
    2. "Older adults will become confused after a bleed to the brain from decreased oxygen."
    3. "Your mother is acting like she is in alcohol withdrawal. Does she drink?"
    4. "You will need to talk to your mother's physician to get information about her condition."

19. An older client in a nursing facility suddenly becomes confused, paranoid, and verbally abusive to the staff. Which of the following is the priority nursing action?
    1. Ask the family members if they had a recent disagreement with the client
    2. Assess the vital signs and obtain a urine specimen
    3. Reorient the client to person, place, and time
    4. Ask whether the client is hearing voices

20. The nurse assesses which of the following behaviors in a client in early Stage I Alzheimer's disease?
    Select all that apply:
    [ ] 1. Masks forgetful behavior
    [ ] 2. Has a slow reaction time
    [ ] 3. Repetitive storytelling
    [ ] 4. Inability to follow simple directions
    [ ] 5. Becomes angry when challenged
    [ ] 6. Change in eating patterns

21. An older adult client with dementia becomes increasingly confused and wanders away from a long-term facility. The appropriate nursing action is to
    1. call law enforcement officials.
    2. restrain the client.
    3. follow the client and redirect from a safe distance.
    4. offer the client a ride back to the facility.

22. Which of the following should the nurse include in the education provided to a new graduate nurse to protect the nurse from injury when a client with dementia or delirium becomes aggressive?
    1. Gently place a hand on the client's shoulder to promote trust
    2. Lead the client to the activity area where there are others to distract the client
    3. Provide a quiet, calm atmosphere and offer simple directions
    4. Offer the client a meal

23. Donepezil hydrochloride (Aricept) is prescribed for an older adult with early dementia, Alzheimer's-like disease (ALD). When reviewing the client's medical conditions and medications, the nurse notifies the physician that there might be a serious interaction because the client has
    1. osteoarthritis.
    2. cancer of the pancreas.
    3. not had a yearly influenza immunization.
    4. bradycardia.

24. Rivastigmine (Exelon) is prescribed for a client with dementia. Which of the following would be an appropriate outcome of nursing care specific to this drug?
    1. The client will sleep 6 hours without waking during the night
    2. The client will eat 50% of all meals and snacks
    3. The client will maintain a weight within the normal range
    4. The client will maintain the serum potassium within normal range

25. The nurse monitors an older adult with Alzheimer's disease for which of the following adverse reactions to galantamine (Razadyne)?
    Select all that apply:
    [ ] 1. Anxiety
    [ ] 2. Bradycardia
    [ ] 3. Diarrhea
    [ ] 4. Increased appetite
    [ ] 5. Weight gain
    [ ] 6. Anemia

26. The registered nurse is planning the clinical assignments for a geriatric mental health unit. Which of the following assignments should the nurse delegate to a licensed practical nurse?
    1. Develop a plan of care for a client with dementia
    2. Perform a physical assessment on a client with Alzheimer's disease
    3. Administer donepezil hydrochloride (Aricept) to a client newly diagnosed with Alzheimer's disease
    4. Provide education to the family of a client with dementia

ANSWERS AND RATIONALES

1. 2. The standard of care for restraints is that they can be applied only with a written order from a health care provider. The order must be renewed every 24 hours. A p.r.n. order for restraints is not acceptable. Restraints should be removed once every 2 hours to perform activities of daily living. The client with wrist restraints should be placed in a lateral position to prevent aspiration. The condition of the skin, circulation, and placement of restraints must be assessed every hour. The assessment must also be documented.

2. 4. When a family expresses concern over their mother's confusion and decreased ability to perform her activities of daily living, the most appropriate response to the family is to acknowledge how frustrating it must be for the family. The nurse should not minimize family members' feelings or tell them how to feel. Reminding a client with short-term memory loss may increase agitation. Although the dementia will progress over time, reinforcing

that with the family is a negative response and may shut down communication.

3. 2. The first step of the nursing process is assessment. Before helping the client deal with a problem or exploring available resources, the nurse should determine if a problem is really present. Assuring the client and dispelling the idea of "going crazy" are negative interventions, and the nature of this client's condition is not yet known.

4. 4. Although creating a cheerful environment is important in a long-term care facility, the priority intervention is safety. Older adults who express not wanting to live if they have to stay there may be clinically depressed and at risk for self-harm. Encouraging clients to discuss feelings of hopelessness and allowing for periods of solitude may be appropriate interventions, but are not the priorities.

5. 2. In the case of delirium and a sudden change in mental status, the nurse should always assess for physiological causes—airway, breathing, and circulation—first. Although medications the client is taking, a recent fall, or the client's pain level may be possible causes of the delirium, the vital signs should be assessed first.

6. 3. The best response when the family of a client diagnosed with Stage I (early-onset) Alzheimer's disease asks when the family member will get better would be to ask family members how much they know about Alzheimer's. This is the best response because it facilitates open communication. Although the disease has a progressive course, telling the family that will close communication. Asking the family member if the client is taking medication for Alzheimer's disease is an inappropriate response, because it changes the subject.

7. 1. The first nursing action should be to identify any risks to the client or others because of the alteration in thought processes that the client is experiencing. It may be appropriate to provide a nonstimulating environment, but that is not the priority. Informing the client that there are no butterflies might precipitate a catastrophic reaction.

8. 1. The definitive diagnosis for Alzheimer's disease is only found on autopsy. When all other possible causes of cognitive decline are ruled out, the medical diagnosis of Alzheimer's disease (or Alzheimer's-like disease) is made. The Mini-Mental State Exam is one of many short tests to measure cognitive function, but it does not actually diagnose dementia. The older adult will show a decrease in the mass of the brain but may not have a corresponding loss of cognitive function. A blood test for C-reactive protein would not be positive for Alzheimer's disease.

9. 1. Loss of interest in previously enjoyable activities and withdrawal are indicators to the nurse that the client may be clinically depressed and in need of further assessment. Inactivity, drinking alcohol, and crying may be indicative of depression or other chronic conditions, not just depression.

10. 1. 3. 6. Donepezil hydrochloride (Aricept) is used in the treatment of mild to moderate Alzheimer's disease. Adverse reactions of Aricept include headache, bradycardia, insomnia, hypertension, diarrhea, and anorexia.

11. 2. The Mini-Mental State Exam does not require a specially trained individual and requires only 20 to 30 minutes to administer. The client must be able to see and write because the client will be asked to write a sentence as well as to copy a drawn figure.

12. 1. The first indication that a client has a sexually transmitted disease such as tertiary syphilis or HIV may be cognitive function changes and dementia.

13. 2. Older women, even if depressed, tend to be less likely to harm themselves, because they have social support and other interests. Older men without social support who have multiple chronic illnesses and live alone are more likely to commit suicide than older women.

14. 4. Clients with chronic illnesses and pain often adjust their own medications or add over-the-counter medications. A client's depression could be a result of the drugs or it could be the reason the client mixes medications. The nurse needs further information to identify risks for injury.

15. 1. It is most appropriate for the nurse to encourage clients who are experiencing situational depression over the loss of a spouse to verbalize their feelings. Crying is a normal and healthy expression of loss. The relationship with the spouse may not always have been positive, or the client may feel angry about the death. Setting an outcome that the client will speak positively describes how the client should feel and is not necessarily true.

16. 2. Educating the caregivers, whether family members or others, is always the priority when caring for a client with dementia. The caregivers must understand the disease and expected behaviors as well as the interventions for problem behaviors. The same interventions may not be effective as the condition changes. This should be part of the continued evaluation and part of the replanning.

17. 3. In late Stage II Alzheimer's disease there is no hope for memory return. Repeating reality orientation for the client whose reality is different may cause anxiety, anger, agitation, and a catastrophic reaction, such as running away or violence.

18. 2. Older adult clients may become confused after a bleed to the brain from decreased oxygen. Telling the family that the medical team has done nothing to the client is a defensive statement and would cut off communication. Dementia is a medical diagnosis, which the nurse does not make. The best initial response by the nurse is to answer the son's question. The nurse may need to know if the client has an alcohol abuse problem, but not until the son's concerns are answered. Passing the son off to the physician at this point would shut down communication with the son.

19. 2. Assessing the vital signs and obtaining a urine specimen is the priority in an older client who suddenly becomes confused and develops psychotic behavior. A urinary tract infection would be evident from an elevated temperature and bacteria in the urine specimen.

20. 1. 2. 5.   A client attempts to mask forgetful behavior, has a slow reaction time, and may become angry when challenged in early Stage I Alzheimer's disease. Repetitive storytelling, an inability to follow simple directions, and a change in eating patterns are behaviors exhibited in Stage II Alzheimer's.

21. 3.   When a client with dementia wanders away from a long-term care facility, the nurse should see if the client will return willingly with persuasion and redirection. If the client will not return, notifying law enforcement may be necessary, but the presence of law enforcement officials may also agitate and frighten the client. At no time should the nurse physically restrain the client alone or transport a client.

22. 3.   Touching an agitated client may increase aggression and precipitate violence against the nurse. The client should be in a quiet, calm atmosphere away from others and simple directions should be offered. Offering a meal may work as a temporary distraction, but the client at this point will be unable to sit and follow instructions about eating.

23. 4.   Aricept is a cholinesterase inhibitor used in the treatment of Alzheimer's disease, which may cause bradycardia with fainting.

24. 3.   Rivastigmine tartrate is used in the treatment of mild to moderate Alzheimer's disease. Nausea, vomiting, anorexia, and abdominal pain are adverse reactions to Exelon. The nurse should monitor weight weekly. Eating 50% of the food offered may not be sufficient to maintain body weight.

25. 2. 3. 6.   Adverse reactions of galantamine (Razadyne) include bradycardia, diarrhea, and anemia. Other adverse reactions include nausea, vomiting, and weight loss.

26. 3.   A licensed practical nurse may administer donepezil hydrochloride (Aricept) to a client with Alzheimer's disease. Developing a plan of care, performing a physical assessment, and providing education to a client's family on dementia are tasks that should be performed by a registered nurse.

REFERENCES

Daniels, R., & Nicoll, L. (2012). *Medical-surgical nursing.* Clifton Park, N.Y: Delmar Cengage Learning.

Estes, M. (2010). *Health assessment and physical examination* (4th ed.). Clifton Park, NY: Delmar Cengage Learning.

Holfman Wold, G. (2012). *Basic geriatric nursing* (5th ed.). St. Louis, MO: Elsevier Mosby.

Spratto, G. R., & Woods, A. L. (2012). *PDR nurse's drug handbook 2012.* Clifton Park, NY: Delmar Cengage Learning.

Touhy, T. A., & Jett, K. F. (2010). *Ebersole and Hess' gerontonological nursing & healthy aging* (3rd ed.). St. Louis, MO: Elsevier Mosby.

COMMUNITY HEALTH NURSING

CHAPTER 60

CASE MANAGEMENT

I. CASE MANAGEMENT

A. DESCRIPTION
1. A PROCESS IN WHICH A CLIENT'S HEALTH CARE ISSUES ARE MANAGED BY A PHYSICIAN OR NURSE
2. ASSISTS A CLIENT WITH COMPLEX, ACUTE, OR CHRONIC HEALTH CARE NEEDS
3. COORDINATES CARE FROM MULTIPLE SERVICES OR MULTIPLE PROVIDERS
4. STIMULATES THE CREATION OF NEW SERVICES WHERE NEEDED
5. ASSISTS THE CLIENT TO MEET IDENTIFIED HEALTH NEEDS WHEN THE CLIENT IS UNABLE TO MEET HER OWN NEEDS OR WORK HER WAY THROUGH THE HEALTH CARE SYSTEM
6. STRIVES TO PROMOTE SELF-CARE WHENEVER POSSIBLE
7. DECREASES FRAGMENTATION OF SERVICES AND PROMOTES CONTINUITY OF CARE
8. PROMOTES QUALITY, COST-EFFECTIVE OUTCOMES
9. INVOLVES ASSESSMENT, PLANNING, IMPLEMENTATION, COORDINATION, MONITORING, AND EVALUATION IN THE PROCESS OF PROVIDING CARE

B. THEORIES BEHIND THE DEVELOPMENT OF CASE MANAGEMENT
1. THE CURRENT HEALTH SYSTEM IS COMPLEX.
2. IT IS DIFFICULT FOR A CLIENT TO UNDERSTAND AND MANEUVER THROUGH THE SYSTEM ALONE.
3. TODAY A CLIENT LEAVES THE HOSPITAL "SICKER AND QUICKER" AND NEEDS HELP ONCE HOME.
4. A CLIENT NEEDS HELP TO FIND HEALTH CARE RESOURCES AND USE THEM APPROPRIATELY.
5. THE RESULTING FRAGMENTATION OF CARE MEANS GAPS IN SERVICES, INAPPROPRIATE USE OF SERVICES, AND POOR CONTINUITY OF CARE.
6. HEALTH CARE RESOURCES ARE SCARCE, AND VALUABLE RESOURCES MUST NOT BE WASTED.
7. INCREASED COST OF HEALTH CARE FORCES THIRD-PARTY PAYERS TO EXAMINE THE APPROPRIATE USE OF SERVICES, SUCH AS DIAGNOSTIC TESTS, LABORATORY COSTS, LENGTH OF HOSPITAL STAYS, AND LENGTH OF HOME HEALTH VISITS.
8. THE RESULT OF THE INCREASED COST OF HEALTH CARE NECESSITATES A CLIENT CARE COORDINATION PROGRAM IN HOSPITAL AND COMMUNITY SETTINGS TO MONITOR THE QUALITY OF CARE, IMPROVE EFFICIENCY IN THE SERVICES PROVIDED, AND REDUCE THE COST OF CARE.

C. CONCEPTS IN CASE MANAGEMENT
1. OFTEN BEGINS ON ADMISSION TO AN ACUTE CARE FACILITY, OR SHORTLY THEREAFTER
2. INVOLVES WORKING WITH THE CLIENT TO OVERSEE THE TRANSITION FROM THE ACUTE CARE SETTING BACK INTO THE COMMUNITY
3. CONTINUES AFTER DISCHARGE UNTIL THE CLIENT NO LONGER NEEDS THE SERVICES
4. OFTEN INVOLVES WORK WITH A HIGH-RISK POPULATION, SUCH AS CLIENTS WHO HAVE HAD CARDIAC SURGERY

D. LOCATION OF CASE MANAGEMENT SERVICES
1. SOME PROGRAMS ARE BASED IN HOSPITALS AND PROVIDE SHORT-TERM, ACUTE CARE FOCUS.
2. SOME PROGRAMS ARE BASED IN THE COMMUNITY TO PROVIDE MORE LONG-TERM, CHRONIC CARE FOCUS.

3. SERVICES MAY BE TRANSFERRED FROM THE HOSPITAL-BASED PROGRAMS TO MORE LONG-TERM, COMMUNITY-BASED SERVICES TO IMPROVE CONTINUITY OF CARE.

II. **THE CASE MANAGEMENT TEAM**
   A. MEMBERS OF THE CASE MANAGEMENT "TEAM"
      1. CLIENT
      2. CASE MANAGER (USUALLY A NURSE WITH A BACCALAUREATE OR MASTER'S DEGREE OR A SOCIAL WORKER)
      3. FAMILY MEMBERS
      4. PRIMARY HEALTH CARE PROVIDERS
      5. MEDICAL EQUIPMENT SUPPLIERS
      6. HEALTH MAINTENANCE ORGANIZATION (HMO) MANAGEMENT (WHEN APPLICABLE)
      7. OTHER HEALTH CARE PROVIDERS
      8. COMMUNITY RESOURCES (SUCH AS POLICE, PHARMACY, AND WELLNESS CENTER)
   B. CHARACTERISTICS OF THE CASE MANAGER
      1. CLINICAL KNOWLEDGE, SKILLS, AND EXPERIENCE
      2. KNOWLEDGE AND IDENTIFICATION OF APPROPRIATE COMMUNITY RESOURCES
      3. KNOWLEDGE OF FINANCING FOR DIFFERENT LEVELS OF HEALTH CARE, AN UNDERSTANDING OF THE ELIGIBILITY AND BENEFITS OF THIRD-PARTY PAYERS, AND THE ABILITY TO DETERMINE COST–BENEFIT RATIOS ARE ESSENTIAL.
      4. MANAGEMENT SKILLS AND EXPERIENCE TO DIRECT AND COORDINATE THE SERVICES FROM MULTIPLE PROVIDERS ARE NEEDED, AS WELL AS SPECIFIC SKILLS SUCH AS CONFLICT MANAGEMENT AND COLLABORATION.
      5. EXCELLENT COMMUNICATION SKILLS, BOTH ORALLY AND IN WRITING, FOR INTERACTION WITH CLIENTS AND PROVIDERS
      6. ABILITY TO MEET THE EDUCATIONAL AND COUNSELING NEEDS OF THE CLIENT
      7. CRITICAL THINKING AND PROBLEM-SOLVING SKILLS AND CREATIVITY AND FLEXIBILITY IN USING THESE SKILLS
      8. AN UNDERSTANDING OF THE ADVOCACY PROCESS AND A WILLINGNESS TO EMPOWER A CLIENT TO PARTICIPATE IN DECISIONS ABOUT HER OWN HEALTH CARE
      9. AN ABILITY TO USE TECHNOLOGY TO ENHANCE COORDINATION OF SERVICES
      10. AN UNDERSTANDING OF THE LEGAL AND ETHICAL ISSUES INVOLVED IN CASE MANAGEMENT
      11. A WILLINGNESS AND AN ABILITY TO WORK AUTONOMOUSLY, AND YET BE ABLE TO COLLABORATE WITH A LARGE NUMBER OF PROVIDERS IN COORDINATING SERVICES TO THE CLIENT

III. **CASE MANAGEMENT AND THE NURSING PROCESS**
   A. CASE MANAGEMENT PARALLELS THE NURSING PROCESS
      1. ASSESSMENT OF THE CLIENT'S CONDITION AND ENVIRONMENT IS CRITICAL IN IDENTIFYING NEEDS.
      2. PLANNING SHOULD INCLUDE SETTING GOALS, IDENTIFYING RESOURCES NEEDED, AND PLANNING OF ACTIVITIES.
      3. IMPLEMENTATION INCLUDES COORDINATION AND DELIVERY OF SERVICES, PLUS MAKING REFERRALS AS NEEDED.
      4. EVALUATION INVOLVES MONITORING THE CLIENT'S CONDITION, DETERMINING IF SERVICES ARE MEETING THE CLIENT'S NEEDS, CHANGING SERVICES IF NEW OR DIFFERENT SERVICES ARE NEEDED, AND CRISIS MANAGEMENT.
   B. TOOLS USED BY THE CASE MANAGER
      1. CRITICAL PATHWAYS, CAREMAPS, AND MULTIDISICPLINARY CARE PLANS ARE USED TO PLAN AND COORDINATE CARE.
      2. THE TOOLS SERVE AS GUIDELINES TO DIRECT SERVICES FROM ALL PROVIDERS UNDER THE GUIDANCE OF THE CASE MANAGER.
   C. FUNCTIONS IN CASE MANAGEMENT
      1. CASE FINDING
         a. The process of identifying clients who would benefit most from the services that case management can provide
      2. ASSESSMENT
         a. Comprehensive assessment of the client's needs, including physical, emotional, and social assessment and assessment of the availability of family support
      3. CARE PLANNING
         a. The main function of the case management process
         b. Development of a service plan, including the client's preferences, type, amount, and source of services;

family roles; and the case manager's role

c. The client becomes committed to the agency after the development of the service plan.

4. IMPLEMENTATION
   a. The process of carrying out the service plan in an efficient and cost-effective manner

5. REASSESSMENT AND EVALUATION
   a. The process of reassessing and reevaluating the service plan and making adjustments as needed
   b. Done at times when changes occur for the client, such as admission to the hospital, family crisis, admission to a nursing home, or any other event that affects any aspect of the client's health

D. CASE MANAGEMENT FOR INDIVIDUAL CLIENTS
   1. THE CASE MANAGER MUST INDIVIDUALIZE EACH PLAN OF CARE TO MEET THE NEEDS OF THE CLIENT USING CREATIVITY AND FLEXIBILITY, WHICH ARE THE KEYS TO A SUCCESSFUL PLAN.
   2. THE CASE MANAGER MUST WORK IN COLLABORATION WITH ALL MEMBERS OF THE HEALTH CARE TEAM.
   3. CASE MANAGEMENT FOR AN INDIVIDUAL MAY INCLUDE HELPING THE INDIVIDUAL AND FAMILY MEMBERS WITH THE FOLLOWING ARRANGEMENTS. (THESE ARE PROVIDED ONLY AS EXAMPLES AND ARE NOT MEANT TO BE AN INCLUSIVE LIST.)
      a. Appointments with the health care provider
      b. Obtaining the necessary equipment to be used at home
      c. Delivery of meals, groceries, and pharmacy supplies
   4. ARRANGEMENTS FOR HOME HEALTH NURSING VISITS OR VISITS FROM A HOME HEALTH CARE AIDE
   5. ARRANGEMENTS FOR TRANSPORTATION TO AND FROM MEDICAL APPOINTMENTS

6. CONTACTS WITH INSURANCE PROVIDERS
7. ARRANGEMENT OF PHYSICAL THERAPY, OCCUPATIONAL THERAPY, OR SPEECH THERAPY APPOINTMENTS IN THE HOME OR IN THE MEDICAL FACILITY
8. COORDINATION OF VOLUNTEERS THROUGH A LOCAL CHURCH OR SUPPORT GROUP
9. CONTACT WITH LOCAL POLICE AND FIRE DEPARTMENTS FOR SAFETY EDUCATION AND PLANS FOR EMERGENCY EVACUATION
10. CONTACT WITH LOCAL ELECTRICAL COMPANY TO ARRANGE EMERGENCY GENERATOR POWER IF OXYGEN OR OTHER ELECTRICAL EQUIPMENT IS REQUIRED IN THE CLIENT'S HOME

E. CASE MANAGEMENT IN THE COMMUNITY
   1. CASE MANAGEMENT IS OFTEN USED TO HELP AN INDIVIDUAL BUT CAN ALSO BE USED FOR GENERAL POPULATIONS WITHIN A COMMUNITY.
   2. CASE MANAGEMENT IS ESPECIALLY HELPFUL FOR POPULATIONS AT RISK.
   3. A CASE MANAGER COULD ASSIST GROUPS OF CLIENTS BY:
      a. Helping an older client to attain a healthier lifestyle
      b. Early identification, diagnosis, and treatment of children with physical disabilities
      c. Educating and monitoring school-aged children regarding early interventions for prevention of emergency hospitalizations for asthma
      d. Monitoring community services for clients with human immunodeficiency virus (HIV) or acquired immunodeficiency syndrome (AIDS)
      e. Providing occupational health services for multiple industries in a community
      f. Providing case finding, referral, and follow-up for high school substance abusers

PRACTICE QUESTIONS

1. The nurse working as a case manager understands that case management is often needed when the client
   1. cannot afford to stay in the hospital.
   2. has no one at home to help with the client's care.
   3. has complex acute or chronic health care needs.
   4. is too sick to care for oneself.

2. A client's family asks the nurse what the case manager's primary goal is. The most appropriate response of the nurse is to
   1. save the client money with cheaper care options.
   2. eliminate the need for multiple care providers.
   3. direct the care provided by speech and physical therapists.
   4. promote self-care of the client whenever possible.

3. A nurse has just accepted the position as a case manager at a local hospital. According to the definitions of various professional organizations that work with case managers, case management is a(n)
   1. position in the hospital's social service department.
   2. cost-effective way to provide direct nursing care.
   3. collaborative process between various health care providers.
   4. independent role of the nurse to provide cost-effective care.

4. A nurse is teaching a class about the history and development of case management. The nurse includes the information that case management developed as the result of many factors, such as which of the following?
   1. The current health system is complex but easily understood.
   2. Clients often stay in the hospital until they can care for themselves at home.
   3. Health care resources are scarce, so valuable resources must not be wasted.
   4. Third-party payers wanted to decrease the costs of hospital stays.

5. The nurse who has always used the nursing process when planning client care has just taken a position utilizing case management. Based on an understanding of the nursing process and the case management concept, the nurse understands that case management
   1. follows a more complex step-by-step model.
   2. uses care maps, not nursing care plans, for documentation.
   3. follows a process very similar to the nursing process.
   4. is a physician-directed process.

6. When planning a client's care, the nurse uses case management skills to help the client
   1. understand the variety of resources in the community.
   2. understand the importance of keeping appointment times.
   3. save money by always finding the least expensive options.
   4. save time by making phone calls for the client.

7. A nurse applied for a case manager position at the local hospital because the job description of the case manager is to
   1. decide what treatment will be provided.
   2. help clients determine the best care for the least cost.
   3. eliminate the competition from other providers.
   4. provide a service that costs very little to offer.

8. Which of the following would a school nurse perform when functioning as a case manager?
   1. Meet with the newspaper office to run an article on school nursing
   2. Team teach a class on healthy after-school snacks
   3. Contact the school board about the lack of computers in the school
   4. Discipline children in sports who do not adhere to weight-maintenance guidelines

9. In evaluating the nurse's role as a case manager, the nurse would determine which of the following skills as most beneficial in caring for clients?
   1. An ability to solve complex problems in a creative way
   2. A legal background, due to an increased atmosphere of lawsuits
   3. Extensive clinical experience as an intensive care nurse
   4. An ability to work according to established protocols and procedures

10. The case manager nurse should be assigned to provide services to which of the following clients?
    1. A mother experiencing her first pregnancy
    2. A client with newly diagnosed diabetes mellitus
    3. A client with a broken arm following a bicycle accident
    4. A group of teenagers who are members of SADD (Students against Drunk Driving)

11. Which of the following should the case manager nurse include in the plan of care for a client injured on the job who is now recovering from a broken leg?
    1. Assist the client with daily exercises to prevent muscle loss
    2. Prevent skin breakdown from limited mobility
    3. Coordinate visits with physical therapy in the home
    4. Provide transportation for the client to medical appointments when needed

12. The nurse is coordinating a case management system of care for which of the following purposes?
Select all that apply:
[ ] 1. Provides continuity of services
[ ] 2. Assists the client with method of payment
[ ] 3. Coordinates designated components of health care
[ ] 4. Avoids fragmented services
[ ] 5. Encourages the client to direct the decision making of the care
[ ] 6. Matches the intensity of the services with the client's needs over time

13. Which of the following is the priority for the nurse case manager planning the discharge of a client who is hospitalized for bone cancer?
1. Establish all physical therapy appointments for the next 3 months
2. Communicate primarily with the client's family instead of the client
3. Obtain all laboratory records to order the correct medications
4. Transfer the client's care to another case manager in the community setting

14. In caring for a client with a terminal condition, the nurse understands that the case management role in the hospital
1. begins when the client receives the diagnosis of cancer.
2. ends when the client is discharged to a home health service.
3. is not appropriate because a diagnosis of a terminal condition has been made.
4. begins when the order is written to begin chemotherapy.

15. A client has recently been hospitalized for open heart surgery and is going to be transferred to a skilled care facility for additional recovery. Which of the following is the role of the nurse case manager in the hospital?
1. Arrange transportation to the new facility
2. Obtain the necessary equipment to be used in the home
3. Deliver pharmaceutical supplies to the skilled care facility
4. Coordinate volunteers to help the client's spouse at home

ANSWERS AND RATIONALES

1. 3. Case management is a process used to assist individuals with complex health care problems by providing quality care with a cost-effective outcome. It organizes client care through a health care problem meeting, so that specific clinical and financial outcomes are achieved within a designated time period.

2. 4. The goal of case management is to help the client care for him- or herself. The case manager is responsible for coordinating care and establishing goals, from the admission phase through to discharge. The case manager works with all disciplines to facilitate care.

3. 3. Case managers do not usually work alone, but instead work with various health care team members to provide care for the client. Case management promotes collaboration, communication, and teamwork to provide the best possible care for the client in the most cost-effective manner possible. Case management also promotes timely discharge.

4. 3. Although health care resources are limited, case managers work to use these resources to provide quality care cost-effectively and to promote timely discharge.

5. 3. Case management follows a process very similar to the nursing process and includes assessment, planning, implementation, and evaluation.

6. 1. With a variety of resources available in the community, the client often needs help to find and use the most appropriate care for personal needs. The nurse may use case management to help the client understand available resources. The case manager usually does not make phone calls for the client and does not make sure the client gets to appointments on time.

7. 2. Hospitals needed a mechanism to find high-quality, cost-effective care to meet client needs. Case managers can assist the hospital and the clients to reduce the costs of care and ensure that a high quality of care will be provided.

8. 2. The focus of case managers in schools is to provide services for the enrolled students that improve health care. Teaching a class on healthy after-school snacks would provide such a service. Meeting with the newspaper office or contacting the school board does not focus directly on improving the health of the students. Disciplining children in sports who do not adhere to weight-maintenance guidelines is a punitive action and would not be performed by the nurse.

9. 1. Because the case manager must solve problems for clients in unique situations usually outside of the hospital setting, protocols may not be well established or in written form. The case manager must be flexible and creative in order to solve these problems. Having worked in an environment where established protocols and procedures were closely followed will also help the nurse now working as a case manager.

10. 2. Case managers usually work with clients who have complex or newly diagnosed conditions, such as a client newly diagnosed with diabetes mellitus.

11. 3. The case manager coordinates other members of the health care team to provide the multiple services needed by a client, but does not necessarily provide the care directly.

12. 1. 3. 4. 6. Case management is a type of delivery of care in which the health care needs of the client are managed by a nurse or physician. The purpose of case management is to ensure continuity of care and avoid fragmented services. It also coordinates all designated components of health care and matches the intensity of the services with the client's needs over time.

13. 4. Continuity of care is important in the care of clients. Because the hospital case manager may not be able to follow the client at home, it is a priority that the care of the client be transferred to a community case manager upon discharge.

14. 1. The case manager should be involved from the time that admission of the client and the process of case management are implemented, shortly after the diagnosis has been made. This ensures that multiple services are provided in an efficient and cost-effective manner.

15. 1. As a case manager, the nurse should help arrange the transition to the new facility, including transportation, transferring orders for medications and activities, and encouraging family involvement in the transfer. Equipment and volunteers needed in the home would not be arranged at the time of transfer. The new facility would be responsible for obtaining any pharmaceutical supplies.

REFERENCES

Daniels, R., & Nicoll, L. (2012). *Contemporary medical-surgical nursing.* Clifton Park, NY: Delmar Cengage Learning.

DeLaune, S. C., & Ladner, P. K. (2006). *Fundamentals of nursing: Standard and practice* (3rd ed.). Clifton Park, NY: Delmar Cengage Learning.

Hitchcock, J. E., Schubert, P. E., & Thomas, S. A. (2003). *Community health nursing: Caring in action* (2nd ed.). Clifton Park, NY: Delmar Cengage Learning.

CHAPTER 61

LONG-TERM CARE

I. LONG-TERM CARE

A. DESCRIPTION

1. WIDE RANGE OF SERVICES ADDRESSING THE PHYSICAL, PERSONAL, AND SOCIAL NEEDS PROVIDED TO THE OLDER CLIENT OR THE CLIENT WITH A FUNCTIONAL IMPAIRMENT WHO CAN NO LONGER CARE FOR SELF WITHOUT SUPERVISION OR ASSISTANCE

2. REQUIRED WHEN THE CLIENT NEEDS ASSISTANCE FOR GREATER THAN 30 DAYS

3. PROVIDED NOT ONLY TO THE OLDER CLIENT WHO HAS LOST THE ABILITY TO CARE FOR SELF IN THE HOME ENVIRONMENT BUT ALSO TO THE CLIENT WHO IS DEVELOPMENTALLY DISABLED OR MENTALLY IMPAIRED

4. INCREASING NEED FOR LONG-TERM CARE BECAUSE OF IMPROVED HEALTH CARE AND TECHNOLOGY, ALLOWING CLIENTS TO LIVE LONGER LIVES

5. PROVIDED ON A CONTINUUM, RANGING FROM THE MOST STRUCTURED CARE (NURSING FACILITY) TO THE LEAST STRUCTURED, SUCH AS A COMMUNITY-BASED PROGRAM

6. MOST COMMON SETTING IS THE SKILLED NURSING FACILITY (FORMERLY CALLED NURSING HOME OR CONVALESCENT CENTER), WHERE CLIENTS ARE CALLED RESIDENTS

7. MEDICAID OR OUT OF POCKET IS THE PRIMARY METHOD OF PAYMENT FOR LONG-TERM CARE.

8. APPROXIMATELY TWO OUT OF EVERY FIVE INDIVIDUALS IN THE UNITED STATES WILL REQUIRE SOME TYPE OF LONG-TERM CARE IN THEIR LIFETIME.

II. TYPES OF LONG-TERM FACILITIES

A. ASSISTED LIVING

1. SMALL CONGREGATE LIVING FACILITY DESIGNED FOR CLIENTS WHO CAN NO LONGER STAY IN THE HOME BUT DO NOT NEED SKILLED CARE

2. GENERALLY PRIVATE PAY UNLESS THE CLIENT QUALIFIES FOR MEDICAID REIMBURSEMENT

3. MINIMAL ASSISTANCE WITH ACTIVITIES OF DAILY LIVING AND MEDICATION MONITORING

4. MAY HAVE MEMORY CARE UNIT THAT IS LOCKED FOR CLIENTS WITH MILD DEMENTIA

5. PROMOTES SOCIALIZATION, ACTIVITIES, AND SMALL-GROUP OUTINGS SUCH AS LUNCH OR SHOPPING

6. COSTS RANGE FROM $2500 TO $5000 A MONTH, COVERING RENT, UTILITIES, HOUSEKEEPING, AND ACTIVITIES

7. FACILITIES ARE LICENSED BY THE STATE.

B. SUBACUTE CARE

1. TWENTY-FOUR-HOUR A DAY SKILLED NURSING CARE FOR A SHORT DURATION (GENERALLY SEVERAL MONTHS)

2. CLIENTS ARE MEDICALLY STABLE BUT REQUIRE SEVERAL COMPLEX MEDICAL TREATMENTS SUCH AS INTRAVENOUS THERAPY, VENTILATOR, TRACHEOSTOMY, OR WOUND CARE.

3. THE GOAL IS FOR THE CLIENT TO RETURN TO THE PREVIOUS LIVING ARRANGEMENT OR A LOWER LEVEL OF CARE.

4. UNITS GENERALLY ARE LOCATED IN SPECIFICALLY DESIGNATED AREAS OF LONG-TERM CARE FACILITIES.

C. SPECIAL CARE UNITS
1. SPECIAL UNITS IN LONG-TERM CARE FACILITIES DESIGNED TO PROVIDE CARE TO:
    a. Children and young adults with long-term disabilities
    b. Clients who have acquired immunodeficiency syndrome (AIDS)
    c. Clients with a cognitive impairment such as Alzheimer's disease and other forms of dementia
    d. Clients who have a chronic disabling mental illness or episodic acute life crisis
2. STAFF ON THESE UNITS GENERALLY HAVE IN-SERVICE TRAINING TO FACILITATE AN UNDERSTANDING OF THE SPECIAL CARE NECESSARY FOR THESE CLIENTS.
D. REHABILITATION UNIT
1. SPECIALIZED UNIT THAT PROVIDES SPEECH OR PHYSICAL THERAPY TO CLIENTS WITH A NEUROLOGICAL IMPAIRMENT
2. UNIT MAY BE EITHER A SPECIAL DESIGNATED UNIT IN A HOSPITAL OR A SEPARATE FACILITY
3. GOAL OF THERAPY IS TO RETURN THE CLIENT TO THE MAXIMAL LEVEL OF FUNCTIONING AND RETURN THE CLIENT TO THE PREVIOUS LIVING SITUATION
4. DURATION OF STAY IS GENERALLY WEEKS TO MONTHS
E. SKILLED NURSING CARE FACILITY
1. PROVIDES 24-HOUR A DAY CARE TO CLIENTS WHO ARE NOT ACUTELY ILL BUT ARE NOT ABLE TO BE REHABILITATED OR FUNCTION IN MINIMAL ASSISTED CARE UNITS
2. CLIENTS ARE CALLED RESIDENTS.
3. FORMERLY CALLED NURSING HOME OR CONVALESCENT CENTER
4. MANY FACILITIES UTILIZE A HOLISTIC APPROACH AND INCLUDE THE FAMILY AS MEMBERS OF THE HEALTH CARE TEAM.
5. THE GOAL OF THE FACILITY IS TO RESTORE THE RESIDENT TO THE HIGHEST LEVEL OF PHYSICAL, MENTAL, AND PSYCHOSOCIAL FUNCTION.
6. FACILITIES ARE ELIGIBLE TO APPLY FOR MEDICARE AND MEDICAID REIMBURSEMENT BUT MANY FACILITIES MAY CHOOSE NOT TO APPLY FOR CERTIFICATION.
7. SOME FACILITIES MAY HAVE UNITS DESIGNATED TO CARE FOR RESIDENTS WITH SPECIAL NEEDS SUCH AS ALZHEIMER'S DISEASE.

III. **ADMISSION TO LONG-TERM CARE FACILITY**
A. MAY BE TRANSFERRED FROM A HOSPITAL OR BE A DIRECT ADMISSION FROM THE CLIENT'S HOME
B. A HISTORY AND PHYSICAL MUST BE COMPLETED WITHIN 48 HOURS OF ADMISSION.
C. RESIDENTS MUST RECEIVE A COPY OF THE RESIDENT BILL OF RIGHTS, PART OF THE OMNIBUS BUDGET RECONCILIATION ACT (OBRA) OF 1987, WHICH MANDATES THE QUALITY OF CARE AT NURSING FACILITIES.
D. RESIDENTS MUST BE INFORMED ABOUT LIVING WILLS AND MEDICAL POWER OF ATTORNEY.
E. A GUARDIAN OR CONSERVATOR MAY BE APPOINTED BY THE COURT TO MANAGE A RESIDENT'S FINANCIAL DECISIONS WHEN HE HAS BEEN DECLARED "INCAPACITATED" OR HAS LOST DECISION-MAKING ABILITIES.
F. ESSENTIAL TO A POSITIVE ADJUSTMENT TO THE FACILITY IS AN ORIENTATION AND TOUR OF THE FACILITY AND INFORMATION ON ITS POLICIES AND PROCEDURES.
G. DEPENDING ON THE TYPE OF LONG-TERM CARE FACILITY, THE ANNUAL COST MAY BE IN EXCESS OF $40,000.

IV. **STAFFING OF LONG-TERM CARE FACILITIES**
A. DIRECTOR OF NURSING IS GENERALLY A REGISTERED NURSE WHO IS RESPONSIBLE TO BE ON DUTY 8 HOURS A DAY, 7 DAYS A WEEK AND ON CALL 24 HOURS A DAY TO ENSURE THE QUALITY OF CARE.
B. LICENSED PRACTICAL (LP) OR VOCATIONAL NURSES (VN): MORE JOB OPPORTUNITIES IN LONG-TERM CARE FACILITIES THAN HOSPITALS.
1. LP/VN MAY CHOOSE TO TAKE THE CERTIFICATION EXAMINATION FOR PRACTICAL AND VOCATIONAL NURSES IN LONG-TERM CARE (CEPN-LTC) OFFERED BY THE NATIONAL COUNCIL OF STATE BOARDS OF NURSING (NCSBN) AND USE THE ESSENTIAL "CLTC" WHEN WRITING A SIGNATURE.
2. AN LP/VN MUST BE IN A FACILITY 24 HOURS A DAY, 7 DAYS A WEEK.
C. CERTIFIED NURSE AIDES (CNAS): PERFORM BASIC NURSING CARE SUCH AS PERSONAL CARE OR ACTIVITIES OF DAILY LIVING ONLY UNDER THE SUPERVISION OF A LICENSED NURSE
D. CERTIFIED MEDICATION AIDES (CMAS): MAY BE PERMITTED IN SOME STATES TO ADMINISTER MEDICATIONS UNDER THE SUPERVISION OF A LICENSED NURSE BUT ONLY AFTER COMPLETING CNA

TRAINING AND A COURSE ON ADMINISTERING MEDICATIONS

E. THE LIMITED FUNDS AVAILABLE TO LONG-TERM CARE FACILITIES OFTEN PREVENT GERONTOLOGICAL CLINICAL NURSE SPECIALISTS (ADVANCED PRACTICE NURSES CERTIFIED BY THE BOARD OF NURSING EXAMINERS TO ASSESS AND PLAN RESIDENTS' CARE) OR GERIATRIC PSYCHIATRISTS FROM BEING EMPLOYED.

F. EACH FACILITY IS REQUIRED TO HAVE A DENTIST, PODIATRIST, AND MEDICAL DIRECTOR TO PROVIDE CARE TO RESIDENTS WITHOUT PERSONAL PHYSICIANS.

G. A SOCIAL WORKER MUST BE PRESENT IN LONG-TERM CARE FACILITIES WITH MORE THAN 120 BEDS.

V. ORIENTATION AND EDUCATION OF LONG-TERM CARE PERSONNEL

A. ORIENTATION
1. ORIENTATION TO LONG-TERM CARE FACILITY SHOULD START FROM DAY 1 OF EMPLOYMENT.
2. CONTINUING EDUCATION IS NOT A SUBSTITUTE FOR A COMPREHENSIVE ORIENTATION.
3. EXPERIENCED CNAS SHOULD PRECEPTOR NEW CNAS.
4. NEW CNAS SHOULD HAVE A REDUCED WORKLOAD DURING THE ORIENTATION PROCESS.

B. EDUCATION
1. WITHIN 4 MONTHS OF EMPLOYMENT, OBRA REQUIRES 75 HOURS OF TRAINING FOR A CERTIFIED AIDE.
2. FORMAL IN-SERVICE EDUCATION SHOULD BE PROVIDED TO EACH EMPLOYEE INSTEAD OF ON-THE-JOB TRAINING.
3. ESSENTIAL THAT INFORMATION ON AGING AND OLDER ADULT ABUSE BE INCLUDED
4. SIMULATING THE EXPERIENCES OF AGING ALLOWS NEW EMPLOYEES TO ROLE PLAY AND DEVELOP AN UNDERSTANDING OF LIFE AS AN OLDER CLIENT.

VI. PAYMENT IN LONG-TERM CARE FACILITIES

A. MEDICARE
1. HEALTH CARE INSURANCE PLAN ADMINISTERED BY THE FEDERAL GOVERNMENT TO OLDER ADULTS OVER THE AGE OF 65 YEARS
2. CONTAIN TWO PARTS
   a. Medicare Part A
      1) Primary payment for hospitalization
      2) Limited coverage for long-term care facility
      3) Covers a maximum of 100 days in a skilled nursing facility within 30 days of a hospitalization lasting a minimum of 3 days
   b. Medicare Part B
      1) Primarily covers physician and outpatient services

B. MEDICAID
1. FEDERALLY AND STATE-FUNDED HEALTH CARE PROVIDED TO LOW-INCOME CLIENTS
2. OLDER CLIENTS WHO RECEIVE A SOCIAL SECURITY BENEFIT AND QUALIFY FOR MEDICAID BASED ON FINANCIAL ASSETS WILL RECEIVE A PAYMENT TO BE USED FOR THE NURSING FACILITY.
3. ONLY CLIENTS WHO RESIDE IN MEDICAID-APPROVED FACILITIES ARE ELIGIBLE FOR PAYMENT.
4. EYE CARE, DENTAL CARE, PRESCRIPTIONS, HOSPITALIZATION, PHYSICIAN, AND PREVENTIVE SERVICES ARE COVERED.

C. LONG-TERM CARE INSURANCE
1. PROVIDED BY SOME EMPLOYERS
2. PREMIUMS CAN BE COSTLY.
3. COSTS AND BENEFITS SHOULD BE ANALYZED PRIOR TO PURCHASING COVERAGE.
4. DESIRABLE COVERAGE INCLUDES:
   a. $100 minimum daily coverage
   b. Home care and skilled nursing care facilities
   c. Guaranteed ability to renew for life
   d. Guaranteed lifetime premium
   e. Alzheimer's disease and other forms of dementia

D. VETERANS' AFFAIRS
1. PROVIDES LIMITED SERVICES
2. CHRONIC HEALTH PROBLEMS FOR SHORT-TERM REHABILITATION ARE COVERED.
3. SERVICE-RELATED DISEASES AND DISABILITIES ARE COVERED IN LONG-TERM FACILITIES.

E. PRIVATE PAY
1. SOME OLDER CLIENTS ARE FINANCIALLY CAPABLE OF PAYING FOR LONG-TERM CARE EITHER ON A TEMPORARY OR PERMANENT BASIS.
2. CLIENTS ADMITTED TO A LONG-TERM CARE FACILITY WHO EXHAUST PRIVATE FUNDS BECOME ELIGIBLE FOR MEDICAID.
3. UNFORTUNATELY, SOME LONG-TERM CARE FACILITIES ONLY RECEIVE PRIVATE PAYMENT FOR SERVICES.

VII. ETHNIC CONSIDERATIONS IN LONG-TERM CARE

A. DESCRIPTION

1. ETHNICITY IS A PRIORITY CONSIDERATION IN LONG-TERM CARE.
2. AN ATTEMPT TO UNDERSTAND THE CLIENT'S ETHNIC ORIGIN MUST BE INCLUDED WHEN CARING FOR AN OLDER ADULT CLIENT WHO IS HOSPITALIZED AND LONG-TERM CARE IS A CONSIDERATION.
3. FEW LONG-TERM CARE FACILITIES DEVOTED TO ONE ETHNIC ORIGIN EXIST.
4. SOME CULTURES, SUCH AS THE CHINESE, VIEW AGING AS A BLESSING AND TAKE CARE OF THE OLDER CLIENT IN THE HOME.
5. IT IS IMPOSSIBLE TO BE KNOWLEDGEABLE ON ALL CULTURES AND THEIR BELIEFS, SO ALL CLIENTS SHOULD BE TREATED HOLISTICALLY AND WITH RESPECT.

PRACTICE QUESTIONS

1. The nurse is screening a client with mild dementia who is unsafe in the home and needs minimal assistance with activities of daily living. The nurse should recommend which of the following facilities as the most appropriate placement for this client?
   1. Subacute care
   2. Skilled nursing care
   3. Rehabilitation unit
   4. Assisted living

2. An older client is considering purchasing long-term care insurance and asks the nurse how to select a good policy. The nurse should instruct a client that which of the following are characteristics to consider and are indicative of a good long-term care policy?
   Select all that apply:
   [ ] 1. The policy is expensive
   [ ] 2. Annual renewal guaranteed with stable medical condition
   [ ] 3. $100 daily coverage
   [ ] 4. Guaranteed lifetime premium
   [ ] 5. Excludes certain forms of dementia
   [ ] 6. Includes home care

3. Discharge plans are being made for a 74-year-old client who is widowed, lives alone, and had a left hip arthroplasty after a fall on the ice when volunteering in a day care. Which of the following facilities should the nurse discharge this client to?
   1. Assisted living
   2. Special care unit
   3. Rehabilitation unit
   4. Skilled nursing care facility

4. The registered nurse is preparing the work schedule at a skilled nursing care facility. Which of the following work assignments would be appropriate for the registered nurse to include?
   1. Unlicensed assistive personnel will administer drugs to residents
   2. A certified medication aide will perform uncomplicated dressing changes
   3. A licensed practical nurse will be on duty on all three shifts daily
   4. Unlicensed assistive personnel will cut the toenails of residents

5. The nurse assesses an older client in an assisted living facility who is crying uncontrollably and who tells the nurse, "I am going to be evicted because I ran out of money to live here." Which of the following is the priority response by the nurse?
   1. "I am sure something will work out for you."
   2. "Can you ask any of your family for money?"
   3. "You will qualify for Medicaid now that you have no money."
   4. "There are other financial options available to you."

6. Which of the following should receive priority when the nurse is developing the plan of care for an older client in a skilled nursing care facility?
   1. The client's age
   2. The client's financial resources
   3. The client's ethnic origin
   4. The client's physical and mental status

7. The nurse is teaching a class on long-term care. Which of the following should the nurse include in the lecture?
   1. A client has to be financially capable of privately paying to live in an assisted living facility
   2. The cost of assisted living facilities ranges from $500 to $900 per month

3. The annual cost of a long-term care facility for one client can be $40,000
4. A client has to be medically and psychologically stable to continue coverage under a long-term care insurance policy

8. A client being discharged from the hospital to an assisted living facility asks the nurse what the average cost is, in dollars per month. The most appropriate response by the nurse is what average cost? _____

9. The nurse is planning the new employee orientation and education for an unlicensed assistive personnel aide at a skilled nursing care facility. Which of the following should the nurse include in the orientation and education program? Select all that apply:
   [ ] 1. On-the-job training is better than formal in-service education
   [ ] 2. Seventy-five hours of training and education is required within 4 months of employment

   [ ] 3. New unlicensed assistive personnel can only work on a part-time basis for the first 6 months
   [ ] 4. The needs of an older client are no different from the needs of a younger client
   [ ] 5. Information on elder abuse
   [ ] 6. Simulated experiences on aging

10. An older adult client asks the nurse about the difference between Medicare Part A, Medicare Part B, and Medicaid. The appropriate response by the nurse is which of the following?
    1. "Medicare Part A covers physician and outpatient services."
    2. "Medicare Part B covers hospitalization."
    3. "Medicaid is granted for low-income clients who receive a Social Security benefit."
    4. "Medicaid fails to cover preventive services or hospitalization."

ANSWERS AND RATIONALES

1. 4. An assisted living facility is designed for a client who can no longer stay in the home and who needs only minimal assistance with activities of daily living or medication monitoring. A subacute care unit provides skilled nursing care 24 hours a day for a client with advanced dementia and who needs maximum assistance with activities of daily living. A rehabilitation unit provides specialized therapies, such as speech or physical therapy, for clients with neurological impairments who can return to the home environment after a period of rehabilitation lasting several weeks to months. Skilled nursing care would be necessary if a client needs care 24 hours a day in a structured environment, such as a nursing home facility.

2. 3. 4. 6. A comprehensive long-term care insurance policy would include coverage for Alzheimer's disease and other forms of dementia, home care, and a skilled nursing care facility; would have a guaranteed premium and renewal for life; and would allow a minimum of $100 a day coverage.

3. 3. It is most appropriate to discharge an older client who had a hip arthroplasty and was independent, living alone, and still working as a volunteer to a rehabilitation unit. The goal of a rehabilitation unit is to return the client to the

maximal level of functioning possible and to the home environment.

4. 3. A licensed practical or vocational nurse (LP/VN) should be on duty 24 hours a day, 7 days a week in a skilled nursing facility. Unlicensed assistive personnel cannot administer drugs. A certified medication aide (CMA) is a certified nurse aide who has taken an additional course on medication administration and may administer medications in some states. It is essential that the nurse making assignments know the law in the resident state. A certified medication aide cannot perform dressing changes and is not allowed to perform nursing care beyond personal care and activities of living.

5. 4. The priority response for the nurse to make to a client who has exhausted all personal financial resources in an assisted living facility is that there are other options available. Those other options may include family support or Medicaid. The nurse is not in a position to discuss or advise the client about financial matters. A financial advisor would be the best person to advise the client.

6. 3. Although the client's age, ethnic origin, financial resources, and physical and mental status are all important to consider when developing a plan of care for an older client in a long-term care facility, the priority is to consider the client's ethnic origin. Admission to a long-term care facility is viewed differently by people from different cultures, and the client's acceptance and perception of the long term will have a direct impact on the plan of care.

7. 3.   The annual expense for long-term care is very costly and may be in excess of $40,000. Approximately two out of every five individuals will need some kind of long-term care at some point in life. Medicaid and out-of-pocket payments are the primary methods of paying for long-term care. A client does not have to remain medically or psychologically stable to keep long-term care insurance. When choosing a long-term care insurance policy, it is essential that the policy include coverage for Alzheimer's disease and other forms of dementia.

8. $2500–$5000 per month. The cost of placement in an assisted living facility may range from $2500 to $5000 per month depending on the part of the country. This covers rent, utilities, housekeeping, and activities.

9. 2. 5. 6.   Information on aging and elder abuse should be included in the new employee orientation and education for unlicensed assistive personnel. Simulating the experiences of aging will assist the new employee in understanding aging. Seventy-five hours of training and education is required by the Omnibus Budget Reconciliation Act (OBRA) of 1987 within 4 months of employment. In-service education is more important than on-the-job training.

10. 3.   Medicare Part A covers hospitalization. Medicare Part B covers outpatient and physician services. Medicaid is a federally and state-funded health care program for low-income clients. Physician services, eye and dental care, prescriptions, and preventive services are covered under Medicaid.

REFERENCES

Daniels, R., & Nicoll, L. (2012). *Contemporary medical-surgical nursing.* Clifton Park, NY: Delmar Cengage Learning.

DeLaune, S. C., & Ladner, P. K. (2006). *Fundamentals of nursing: Standard and practice* (3rd ed.). Clifton Park, NY: Thomson Delmar Learning.

Hitchcock, J. E., Schubert, P. E., & Thomas, S. A. (2003). *Community health nursing: Caring in action* (2nd ed.). Clifton Park, NY: Thomas Delmar Learning.

CHAPTER 62

HOME HEALTH CARE

I. HOME HEALTH CARE

   A. EVOLUTION OF HOME HEALTH CARE
1. HOME CARE WAS THE PRIMARY SOURCE OF CARE FOR MANY YEARS.
2. HOME CARE WAS THE PRIMARY MODE OF HEALTH CARE IN THE 1800S.
3. CHARITIES WERE OFTEN A SOURCE OF HOME HEALTH CARE.
4. PUBLIC HEALTH NURSING BEGAN IN 1893 WITH THE DEVELOPMENT OF THE HENRY STREET SETTLEMENT.
5. THE AMERICAN RED CROSS ESTABLISHED A VISITING NURSE SERVICE FOR RURAL COMMUNITIES IN 1912.

   B. CHANGES IN HOME HEALTH CARE IN THE MID-TWENTIETH CENTURY
1. MANY HOME CARE AGENCIES WERE FORCED TO CLOSE WITH HEALTH CARE CHANGES THAT OCCURRED IN THE MID-TWENTIETH CENTURY.
2. HOSPITALS WERE BUILT TO CENTRALIZE CARE.
3. BY THE 1950S, MOST CARE WAS DELIVERED IN HOSPITALS AND HOME HEALTH CARE ALMOST DISAPPEARED.

   C. A REBIRTH OF HOME HEALTH CARE
1. DEVELOPMENT OF VOLUNTARY VISITING NURSES ASSOCIATIONS IN 1960 BEGAN THE DELIVERY OF CARE.
2. MEDICARE PROVIDED A SOURCE OF FUNDING FOR HOME CARE IN 1965.
3. MEDICARE INITIALLY COVERED HOME HEALTH CARE FOR THE OLDER ADULT AND LATER WAS EXPANDED TO INCLUDE YOUNGER, DISABLED INDIVIDUALS AND HOSPICE CARE.
4. THE FOCUS OF HOME CARE SHIFTED FROM HEALTH PROMOTION AND DISEASE PREVENTION TO CARE OF THE SICK AT HOME.
5. HOME HEALTH WAS VIEWED AS A COST-EFFECTIVE WAY TO PROVIDE CARE IN THE 1970S.

   D. HOME CARE TODAY
1. HOME CARE IS CONSIDERED THE FASTEST-GROWING SEGMENT OF HEALTH CARE.
2. THE FOCUS OF HEALTH CARE IS MOVING BACK TOWARD HEALTH PROMOTION AND DISEASE PREVENTION.

   E. WHY HOME HEALTH CARE GREW RAPIDLY
1. IT OFFERED A COST-EFFECTIVE WAY OF MEETING CLIENT NEEDS.
2. CLIENTS PREFERRED TO RECEIVE CARE IN THE COMFORT OF THEIR OWN HOMES; GREATER CLIENT SATISFACTION.
3. AS THE POPULATION AGED, MORE INDIVIDUALS NEEDED CARE AT HOME.
4. ADVANCES IN TECHNOLOGY ALLOWED CARE TO BE DELIVERED OUTSIDE OF INSTITUTIONS.
5. SHORTER HOSPITAL STAYS—PEOPLE WERE DISCHARGED "SICKER AND QUICKER."
6. MORE CARE WAS AVAILABLE AND OFFERED ON AN OUTPATIENT BASIS.
7. IT OFFERED A UNIQUE FORM OF HEALTH CARE DELIVERY.

   F. DESCRIPTION OF HOME HEALTH CARE
1. THE PROVISION OF HEALTH SERVICES IN THE HOME SETTING TO PROMOTE, MAINTAIN, OR RESTORE THE HEALTH OF THE INDIVIDUAL AND THE FAMILY
2. REQUIRES SKILLS IN ASSESSMENT, INTERVENTION, AND EVALUATION
3. ENCOURAGES CLIENTS TO FUNCTION AT THE HIGHEST LEVEL OF INDEPENDENCE POSSIBLE
4. PROVIDES A HOLISTIC VIEW OF THE CLIENT, INCLUDING ENVIRONMENTAL AND SOCIAL FACTORS, LIFESTYLE CHOICES, AND FAMILY RELATIONSHIPS THAT INFLUENCE HEALTH

5. REDUCES BARRIERS TO CARE SUCH AS TRANSPORTATION AND THE HIGH COSTS OF INSTITUTIONALIZATION
6. PROVIDES AN OPPORTUNITY FOR THE CLIENT TO EXERCISE MORE AUTONOMY AND CONTROL OVER HER CARE AND GREATER EMPOWERMENT
7. ADVANCES IN TECHNOLOGY HAVE ALLOWED MORE CARE TO BE PROVIDED IN THE HOME THAT USED TO BE AVAILABLE ONLY IN THE HOSPITAL.
8. PROVIDES CONTINUITY OF CARE OVER A LONG PERIOD OF TIME

G. TYPES OF HOME HEALTH AGENCIES
   1. OFFICIAL AGENCIES
      a. Publicly funded units in state or local health departments
      b. Supported by tax dollars
      c. Governed by local boards of health
   2. NONPROFIT AGENCIES
      a. Voluntary agencies supported by charities such as the United Way
      b. Privately owned, nongovernmental agencies
      c. Exempt from federal income tax
         1) Governed by a board of directors
         2) May partner with an official agency to avoid duplication of services
   3. PROPRIETARY AGENCIES
      a. Private, profit-making agencies
      b. Reimbursed for care through third-party payers
      c. Often part of national health care organizational chains managed by corporations
   4. INSTITUTION-BASED AGENCIES
      a. Usually part of a hospital
      b. Inpatient population is the greatest source of referrals
      c. Serves as a source of revenue for the hospital
      d. Governed by the same board that directs its parent company

H. FINANCING OF HOME HEALTH SERVICES
   1. MEDICARE IS THE LARGEST SINGLE PAYER OF HOME HEALTH CARE.
   2. MEDICARE PAYS FOR SKILLED NURSING VISITS (SNVS) FOR ALL PERSONS OLDER THAN 65.
   3. MEDICARE ALSO PAYS FOR COVERAGE OF INDIVIDUALS WHO ARE DISABLED AND HOSPICE CARE.
   4. HOME CARE IS COVERED UNDER PART B OF MEDICARE (SUPPLEMENTAL MEDICAL INSURANCE).

I. QUALIFICATIONS FOR FINANCING
   1. HOME CARE AGENCIES MUST QUALIFY UNDER THE CONDITIONS OF PARTICIPATION.
   2. COSTS ARE REIMBURSED ONLY FOR ALLOWABLE EXPENSES THAT OCCUR IN CARING FOR CLIENTS.
   3. DOCUMENTATION IS CRITICAL TO ACCURATELY REFLECT THE CARE GIVEN.
   4. PHYSICIANS MUST CERTIFY THAT CLIENTS ARE HOMEBOUND AND REQUIRE SKILLED NURSING CARE IN ORDER FOR SERVICES TO QUALIFY FOR MEDICARE REIMBURSEMENT.
   5. INDIVIDUAL PLANS OF CARE MUST BE COMPLETED AND UPDATED EVERY 60 DAYS FOR CARE TO BE REIMBURSED.
   6. MEASUREMENT AND REPORTING OF CLIENT OUTCOME DATA ARE USED TO DETERMINE REIMBURSEMENT TO AGENCIES (OUTCOMES AND ASSESSMENT INFORMATION SET—OASIS—IS REQUIRED BY ALL MEDICARE CERTIFIED AGENCIES).

J. OTHER SOURCES OF FINANCING
   1. MEDICAID—FOR LOW-INCOME CLIENTS OR CLIENTS WITH DISABILITIES
   2. PRIVATE INSURANCE
   3. PRIVATE PAY ("OUT OF POCKET")

K. THE NURSE'S ROLE IN HOME HEALTH CARE
   1. CASE FINDING AND FOLLOW-UP
      a. Identification of chronic health conditions
      b. Follow-up on communicable diseases and other risks to public health
      c. Abuse and neglect
      d. School health issues
   2. HEALTH PROMOTION AND ILLNESS IDENTIFICATION
      a. Prenatal and well-baby care
      b. Developmental assessment
      c. Healthy older adult services
   3. CARE OF THE SICK
      a. Chronic conditions
      b. Hospital follow-up for surgery, accidents, illnesses
      c. Terminal care and hospice

L. DIFFERENTIATING PUBLIC HEALTH AND HOME HEALTH
   1. PUBLIC HEALTH FOCUSES ON HEALTH PROMOTION AND PREVENTION.
   2. HOME HEALTH FOCUSES ON ILLNESS CARE AND POST-HOSPITAL FOLLOW-UP.
   3. SERVICES PROVIDED THROUGH HOME HEALTH CARE ARE OFTEN MULTIDISCIPLINARY AND MAY INCLUDE:
      a. Skilled nursing
      b. Physical therapy
      c. Occupational therapy

d. Speech therapy

e. Medical social services

f. Homemaker and home health aide, which is a service directly supervised by the nurse

M. QUALITY OF CARE

1. THE AMERICAN NURSES ASSOCIATION HAS ENDORSED THE STANDARDS OF HOME HEALTH NURSING AS THE BASIS FOR NURSING PRACTICE IN THE HOME.

N. DIFFERENTIATION OF NURSES' ROLES

1. THE GENERALIST ROLE INCLUDES:

a. Assessment of needs and planning of care

b. Provision of skilled nursing care

c. Documentation of services

d. Coordination and collaboration with other caregivers

e. Supervision by ancillary personnel involved in the care

f. Client advocacy

2. CERTIFICATION FOR A NURSE AS A HOME HEALTH GENERALIST REQUIRES A BACCALAUREATE OR HIGHER DEGREE AND EXPERIENCE IN HOME HEALTH NURSING.

3. THE SPECIALIST ROLE IS PREPARED FOR ADVANCED PRACTICE AND OFTEN SERVES AS:

a. Consultant

b. Administrator

c. Researcher

d. Clinical specialist and nurse practitioner

e. Educator

4. THE NURSE WHO FUNCTIONS AS A SPECIALIST IS USUALLY PREPARED WITH A MASTER'S DEGREE.

O. CAREGIVER ROLE

1. FAMILY CAREGIVERS

a. Are an integral part of the care provided in the home

b. Provide most of the essential, direct care to the client in the home

c. Provide care under the guidance and support of home health care professionals

d. Often assume the caregiver role out of necessity, not choice

e. Often experience role stress and strain for added responsibilities

f. Need support from the professional as well as the client

P. RESPITE CARE

1. FAMILY CAREGIVERS NEED RELIEF FROM RESPONSIBILITIES IN ORDER TO MAINTAIN THEIR OWN HEALTH.

2. FRIENDS MAY OFFER RELIEF IN THE FORM OF RESPITE CARE.

3. ADULT DAY CARE MAY BE PROVIDED IN THE COMMUNITY.

4. IN-HOME CARE MAY BE PROVIDED BY LOCAL AGENCIES.

Q. LEGAL AND ETHICAL ISSUES IN HOME HEALTH CARE

1. QUALIFICATIONS OF THE AGENCY

a. Licensing is usually required by state health departments.

b. Medicare certification is required for Medicare reimbursement.

c. Accreditation demonstrates commitment to provide quality care.

2. HOME CARE BILL OF RIGHTS

a. Written consent should be obtained at the start of care.

b. Details what can be expected from home care

c. Informs the client of rights while under services

1) Details quality-of-care issues

2) Right to participate in planning and continuity of care

3) Informed of advanced medical directives

4) Privacy issues

5) Financial information

R. ISSUES FOR THE TWENTY-FIRST CENTURY

1. CLIENTS HAVE NO LEGAL RIGHT TO HEALTH CARE IN THE UNITED STATES.

2. MANY PEOPLE ARE UNINSURED OR UNDERINSURED.

3. CONSUMERS ARE MORE EDUCATED AND CONCERNED ABOUT HEALTH CARE—THEY DEMAND A GREATER SATISFACTION WITH THE CARE THEY RECEIVE.

4. COST-CONTAINMENT PRESSURES BY GOVERNMENT AND THIRD-PARTY PAYERS CONTINUE TO PRESSURE HEALTH CARE INDUSTRY TO BECOME MORE EFFICIENT.

5. TECHNOLOGY IS CHANGING WHERE AND HOW HEALTH CARE IS DELIVERED.

6. TELEHEALTH IS CHANGING THE DELIVERY OF HEALTH CARE SERVICES.

7. NATIONAL STANDARDS AND GUIDELINES ARE ESSENTIAL TO MEASURE THE QUALITY OF CARE PROVIDED AND THE VIABILITY OF AGENCIES.

8. RESEARCH IS ESSENTIAL TO ENSURE THE QUALITY AND EFFICIENCY OF NURSING CARE PROVIDED IN THE HOME.

PRACTICE QUESTIONS

1. A nurse has been asked to teach a class about home health care to a local church group. Which of the following points should the nurse include in a class on home health care? Home health care
   1. is a relatively new phenomenon that began with Medicare.
   2. dates back to the beginning of the Red Cross in 1912.
   3. is only provided by charities and churches.
   4. was formally organized by visiting nurses in the late 1800s.

2. The nurse is establishing a home health care agency and knows it is important to understand the influence Medicare has had on the development of home health care because
   1. Medicare provided a regular source of funding for home health care.
   2. Medicare promoted the care of the disabled and the chronically ill.
   3. the cost of hospital care before Medicare was getting too high.
   4. clients were dissatisfied with the standards of home health care prior to Medicare.

3. When meeting with a client for the first time, the nurse working in home health care should include which of the following when describing the services that will be provided for the client?
   1. Care of the acute and chronically ill at home
   2. Health promotion activities for individual families in their homes
   3. Disease prevention in nursing homes in the community
   4. Care of clients who receive Medicare funding

4. Which of the following should the home health nurse include when providing home health care for a client?
   1. Custodial care for the client
   2. Charge for each service provided
   3. Receive direct payments from the client
   4. Plan visits based on client needs

5. Which of the following factors should the home health care nurse consider when planning care for a client in the home?
   1. The client is the only one designated to receive services
   2. The family should be included in all care rendered in the home
   3. The nurse will perform physical therapy exercises if needed

   4. All care should be completed in a designated period of time

6. A home health care nurse should include which of the following when informing a client about home care service?
   1. A dependency on the home care nurse will develop
   2. Greater autonomy and control over self-care are fostered
   3. Home care will cost more than staying in the hospital
   4. There are limits to advances in technology

7. When meeting with a client to explain the role of the nurse in home care, which of the following advantages of home care should be explained to the client? Home care
   1. allows the nurse to have primary control over the environment where the client will recover.
   2. saves the client money because the care is provided in a one-to-one situation and is always covered by insurance.
   3. provides a holistic view of the client that helps the nurse to establish appropriate goals and to plan appropriate care.
   4. encourages a dependent relationship between the nurse and the client.

8. The nurse should consider which of the following when interviewing for a position as a home health care nurse at an official agency? The care is
   1. funded by tax dollars at the state or local level.
   2. governed by a board of directors at the federal level.
   3. based in the local community hospital.
   4. certified by Medicare as long as the client is older.

9. When a client calls a nurse who has established a private nonprofit home care agency in the community, the nurse should explain that nurses at the agency
   1. are paid a salary exempt from federal income tax.
   2. work for an agency that is governed by the local board of health.
   3. are concerned about saving money for the stockholders of the corporation.
   4. may receive funding from voluntary agencies, such as the United Way.

10. A nurse working in a hospital-based home care agency is presenting the annual report to the

hospital board. The nurse states, "In order for the hospital to operate this home care agency,
1. the hospital must be a nonprofit agency."
2. third-party payers will reimburse all costs."
3. the primary source of referrals comes from the inpatient population."
4. funding is determined by the state board of health."

11. The home care nurse is assigned to change the dressing of a 78-year-old client following an emergency gallbladder surgery. The client asks the nurse if the home services will be covered by Medicare reimbursement. The most appropriate response by the nurse is which of the following?
1. "Reimbursement of services is based on the financial need of each client."
2. "Your home care will be covered because your physician certified you as homebound."
3. "I will update your plan of care every 6 months to maintain your coverage."
4. "Your care will be covered as a nonskilled nursing service."

12. The local hospital has contacted a new home health agency in the community to identify what services the agency can provide. Which of the following services would be appropriate for the nurse to include in the examples given to the hospital of care that is available?
1. Follow-up on three cases of tuberculosis in the local community
2. Teaching prenatal classes in the local hospital

3. Screening older people at a meal site for nutritional problems
4. Running a hospice at the local hospital

13. A public health nurse and a home health care nurse are meeting to discuss their roles in the community. The home health care nurse states that the nurse's role in home health care focuses on
1. health promotion in the home.
2. disease prevention in the home.
3. illness care in the hospital.
4. illness care in the home.

14. When planning the home care for a client who has returned home after suffering a stroke, the home health nurse should plan to supervise which of the following?
1. The speech therapist who works with the client
2. The discharge planner who works with the client and family
3. The home care aide who assists the client with personal cares
4. The physical therapist who helps the client regain mobility

15. During an initial home visit to assess the client's needs, the nurse should inform the client
1. about the physician's orders that mandate care.
2. about the client's rights at the start of care.
3. what must be paid by the client directly to Medicare.
4. that advanced medical directives do not apply in the home setting.

ANSWERS AND RATIONALES

1. 4. Home care was the primary source of care for many years. It began with charities, but was formally organized by visiting nurses in 1877 in New York. Medicare has helped provide a regular source of funding since Medicare began in 1965.

2. 1. Medicare is made up of two parts: Part A, or the hospital insurance, and Part B, or the supplemental medical insurance. Prior to Medicare, most home care was provided by voluntary agencies. In 1965, Medicare legislation was passed and provided a source of funding for home care.

3. 1. People are often discharged from the hospital before they are well enough to take care of themselves. Home health care is considered a cost-effective way to provide care to clients with acute or chronic illnesses in their own homes.

4. 4. The care for each client is planned by the nurse and based on an assessment of each client's individual needs. The home care agency is responsible for billing the client and paying the nurse. The nurse provides skilled nursing care, not custodial care.

5. 2. When in the home, the client and family members must all be included in any care provided. Working in the home assists the nurse to see how the client functions within the family setting and the home environment.

6. 2. Home care is a cost-effective way of meeting the client's needs in the comfort of the client's home, including the adaptation of high-tech equipment to the home environment. Clients are usually more satisfied with and have more control over the care given in their homes than the care given in institutions.

7. 3. Home care provides a holistic view of the client that influences the client's health. Being in the home environment provides an opportunity for the client to exercise more autonomy and control over personal care and encourages the client to function at the highest level of independence possible.

8. 1. Official agencies are publicly funded by taxes and operate in state or local health departments that fall under the control of local health departments. Being an official agency does not guarantee certification by Medicare. The agency must still qualify for Medicare certification.

9. 4. Private nonprofit agencies are governed by a board of directors and often receive funding from voluntary agencies. The agency, not the employees, has a tax exempt status. Proprietary agencies have stockholders who are concerned about making a profit.

10. 3. Most institutional-based agencies are operated and funded by hospitals and are governed by the hospital's board of directors. The hospital expects the home care agency to serve as a source of revenue by providing home care for inpatients after discharge.

11. 2. In order to qualify for reimbursement of home health care, the physician must certify that the client is homebound and requires skilled nursing care. Medicare only covers a client over the age of 65 years or a client who is permanently disabled. Outcome and Assessment Information Set (OASIS) is a mandated federal requirement for all home health agencies. Its purpose is to measure outcomes for outcome-based quality improvement. Data must be collected at admission and every 60 days until discharge.

12. 1. The home health nurse might be involved in case finding and follow-up that may impact the health in the community. The home health nurse is usually not involved in screening, teaching, or managing in specific organizations.

13. 4. Home health care focuses on illness care in the home and post-hospital follow-up. Public health focuses on health promotion and prevention in the community.

14. 3. Although the home health nurse may coordinate and collaborate with the discharge planner and the speech and physical therapists, the only supervisory responsibility will be with the home care aide.

15. 2. The Home Care Bill of Rights expects the nurse to obtain informed consent at the start of care, to detail what can be expected from the home care services, and to explain the rights of the client under those services, including the option for advanced medical directives.

REFERENCES

Daniels, R., & Nicoll, L. (2012). *Contemporary medical-surgical nursing.* Clifton Park, NY: Delmar Cengage Learning.

DeLaune, S. C., & Ladner, P. K. (2006). *Fundamentals of nursing: Standard and practice* (3rd ed.). Clifton Park, NY: Thomson Delmar Learning.

Hitchcock, J. E., Schubert, P. E., & Thomas, S. A. (2003). *Community health nursing: Caring in action* (2nd ed.). Clifton Park, NY: Thomson Delmar Learning.

CHAPTER 63

HOSPICE

I. HOSPICE

  A. DESCRIPTION

    1. HOSPICE IS PALLIATIVE RATHER THAN CURATIVE CARE OF THE DYING.

    2. THE FOCUS IS ON THE QUALITY OF LIFE, NOT ON EXTENDING LIFE.

    3. THE GOAL IS TO CREATE A BEAUTIFUL LIFE EVEN AS THE FAMILY REALIZES THAT LIFE EXPECTANCY IS SHORTENED.

    4. CLIENT AUTONOMY IS RESPECTED.

    5. CLIENT SELF-CARE CHOICES ARE RESPECTED EVEN WHEN THEY DISAGREE WITH THE NURSE'S.

    6. WRITTEN CONSENT IS REQUIRED TO ENTER A HOSPICE PROGRAM.

    7. A DO-NOT-RESUSCITATE (DNR) ORDER IS RECOMMENDED.

    8. THE INSURANCE BENEFIT CALLED HOSPICE IS NOT THE SAME AS THE HOSPICE CONCEPT.

      a. Many insurance companies pay for hospice care.

      b. Medicare has strict rules indicating that the life expectancy must be less than 6 months.

      c. Because death is hard to diagnose, most referrals are made during the last 3 weeks of life.

  B. THE CLIENT IS THE FAMILY

    1. THE FAMILY HAS SEVERAL DEVELOPMENTAL CHALLENGES TO FACE, SUCH AS RESOLVING RELATIONSHIPS, REVIEWING LIFE, FINDING MEANING IN LIFE, RESOLVING FINANCIAL AND SPIRITUAL ISSUES, GRIEVING FOR LOSSES, AND CONTROLLING CLINICAL MANIFESTATIONS.

    2. COMMON CLINICAL MANIFESTATIONS THE HOSPICE NURSE DEALS WITH ARE INDEPENDENCY ISSUES, SAFETY, GRIEF, PREPARING FINANCIALLY, HEALING RELATIONSHIPS, PAIN, RESPIRATORY CARE, SKIN CARE, BOWEL, SPIRITUAL ISSUES, ANXIETY, AND OTHER ISSUES RELATED TO HOSPICE.

    3. CAREGIVERS ARE GIVEN AS MUCH ATTENTION AS CLIENTS.

  C. EVOLUTION OF HOSPICE

    1. EVOLUTION IS BUILT ON THE IDEA OF A PLACE TO REST FROM THE TIMES OF THE CRUSADES.

    2. THE MEDICAL IDEA STARTED IN ENGLAND.

    3. HOSPICE HOUSES CELEBRATED THE JOURNEY TO THE END OF LIFE WITH HONEST, LOVING, INTENSE, AND PALLIATIVE CARE.

    4. VOLUNTEER ORGANIZATIONS BEGAN IN THE 1960S IN THE UNITED STATES.

    5. MEDICARE BENEFIT BEGAN IN 1985, CERTIFIED BY THE HOME CARE FINANCING ADMINISTRATION.

  D. HOSPICE PHILOSOPHY

    1. GRIEF SUPPORT IS GIVEN BEFORE AND AFTER THE DEATH OF A LOVED ONE.

    2. CARE IS PROVIDED BY AN INTERDISCIPLINARY TEAM.

      a. The team consists of family members, social workers, pastoral care leaders, home health aides, physicians, volunteers, bereavement counselors, registered nurses, and team coordinators.

      b. Other disciplines are often called in to aid the client's care, such as physical therapy, occupational therapy, music therapy, dietician, and recreational therapy.

      c. Team members meet weekly to discuss care needs and coordinate efforts.

3. CARE BEGINS WHEN FAMILIES AND THEIR PRIMARY CARE PROVIDERS DECIDE TO SWITCH THEIR FOCUS FROM CURE TO CARE COMFORT AND MANAGE CLINICAL MANIFESTATIONS.
4. HOSPICE IS AN IDEA, NOT A PLACE.
   a. Care is provided in the home, nursing home, hospital, hospice house, and so forth.
   b. The Medicare hospice benefit pays for caregivers, drugs, equipment, supplies, hospitalizations for terminal care, respite, and transfusions.
   c. Diagnostic treatments are not ordered or paid for.
   d. Bereavement care is provided for up to 1 year after death.
   e. Volunteers may provide family visits, caregiver respite, professional services, consultation, pastoral care, bereavement counseling, education, and comfort. Others serve only to raise funds for the hospice. Often the volunteer is the most vital member of the team for the family.

E. THE NURSE'S ROLE IN HOSPICE
   1. INSURANCE CASE MANAGERS COORDINATE CARE.
      a. May occur in hospitals, rehabilitation facilities, nursing homes, home health, outpatient clinics, office visits, life care, and hospice care
   2. HOSPICE NURSE
      a. Communicating, negotiating, providing flexible care hours, providing honest reports, working as a team with others involved in the care, providing a care management plan, and educating on the outcomes and goals
      b. Aggressively manage clinical manifestation
         1) The dying client suffers many discomforts, with the most common being nausea and vomiting, severe constipation, respiratory distress, insomnia, and pain.
         2) Psychological and neurological clinical manifestations such as depression, confusion, anxiety, agitation, and hallucinations.
         3) Care for caregivers and families through assessment, referral, support and intervention, education, respite, assistance,

and resource referrals; provide end-of-life care.
         4) Remain flexible as family members quickly go through painful adjustments.
      c. Educate both clients and physicians about the benefit of hospice in the acute care setting.

F. TYPES OF HOSPICE PROGRAMS
   1. PUBLIC AGENCIES
   2. HOSPITALS
   3. HOME HEALTH AGENCIES
   4. EXTENDED-CARE FACILITIES
   5. INDEPENDENT ORGANIZATIONS
   6. MAY BE FOR PROFIT OR NONPROFIT
   7. MAY BE IN AN INPATIENT OR FREESTANDING AGENCY

G. MEMBERS OF THE HOSPICE PROGRAM
   1. PHYSICIAN SERVICES
   2. REGISTERED NURSES
   3. VARIOUS THERAPY SERVICES
   4. SPIRITUAL AND BEREAVEMENT COUNSELING
   5. HOME HEALTH SERVICE AIDES
   6. HOMEMAKER SERVICES
   7. MEDICAL SUPPLIERS

H. PAIN MANAGEMENT
   1. DESCRIPTION
      a. An unpleasant sensation and emotional experience arising from actual or potential tissue damage
      b. There is acute pain and chronic pain.
   2. THERE ARE TWO TYPES OF PAIN MEDICATION: OPIOIDS AND NONOPIOIDS.
      a. Opioids are used for severe central nervous system (CNS) pain.
      b. Nonopioids are used for peripheral pain.
      c. Opioids cross the blood–brain barrier, causing CNS clinical manifestations such as drowsiness to sleep to unconsciousness, decreased mental and physical activity, headache, dizziness, confusion, dysphoria, unusual dreams, hallucinations, and delirium.
      d. Other opioid adverse reactions include respiratory depression, direct dilation of peripheral blood vessels, diminished peristaltic contractions, ureteral spasm, nausea and vomiting, papillary constriction, itching, and constipation.
      e. Opioid use is not recommended with certain conditions, including respiratory depression, liver or kidney disease, previous sensitivity to opioids, intracranial pressure, adrenal insufficiency, Addison's disease, alcoholism, urethral stricture, and

prostatic hypertrophy. Caution must be used during labor and delivery.

f. Nonsteroidal anti-inflammatory drugs (NSAIDs) are used in conjunction with opioids because they do not cause similar clinical manifestations.

g. Opioids are given either by demand dosing with a fixed dose or by constant-rate infusion plus demand dosing (see Table 63-1).

h. Do not give fentanyl until client is stabilized on an opioid.

i. Families are encouraged to use a pain medication as needed.

j. Taking opioids for pain relief is not addiction no matter the dose, duration, or frequency.

k. Agonists and nonagonists are the two types of opioids available.

3. EDUCATION IS THE PRIMARY NURSE ROLE IN PAIN MANAGEMENT.

4. CLIENT REPORT IS THE BEST ASSESSMENT TOOL.

5. IT IS A MYTH THAT PEOPLE ACT AS IF THEY ARE IN PAIN WHEN IN PAIN; THIS IS NOT TRUE BECAUSE THE CLIENT MAY LAUGH, SLEEP, OR TALK WHEN IN SEVERE PAIN.

6. HOSPICE NURSES ENCOURAGE COMBINING NONPHARMACOLOGICAL PAIN RELIEVERS WITH MEDICATION FOR PAIN MANAGEMENT.

a. Heat or cold, distraction, and relaxation are the common categories.

b. Distraction interventions include television, music, movies, reading, hobbies, and humor.

c. Relaxation methods include breathing, imagery, progressive muscle relaxation, and meditation.

d. Aroma therapy, herbs, and pressure and touch therapy may be helpful for some clients.

I. EDUCATION ISSUES

1. EDUCATION IS A CENTRAL ROLE FOR HOSPICE NURSES.

2. THE NURSE NEEDS TO KNOW HOW TO ASSESS LEARNER READINESS, PLAN AND PROVIDE EDUCATION, AND EVALUATE THE INTERVENTION.

3. SEVERAL THINGS AFFECT THE LEARNER'S READINESS TO LEARN, SUCH AS THE MEDICAL DIAGNOSIS, LEVEL OF CONSCIOUSNESS, DESIRE TO CHANGE, LIFESTYLE, RESOURCES, MEDICATIONS, HEALTH BELIEFS, AND FAMILY SUPPORT.

Table 63-1 Use and Dose Ranges of Opioids

Pain Medication	Use	Adult Dose	Route	Action Onset	Peak	Duration
Morphine	Moderate to severe, pulmonary edema, myocardial infarction (MI)	Adult > 50 kg: 30 mg every 3–4 hr, PO; 10 mg every 3–4 hr, IM, IV, or subcut; 0.8–1 mg/hr by bolus or 15 mg for continuous infusion	PO, IM, IV, subcut, EP	PO: 10–30 min IM: 10–30 min IV: 5–10 min Subcut: 10–30 min EP: 15–60 min	PO: 60–120 min IM: 30–60 min IV: 20 min Subcut: 50–90 min 60 min	4–5 hr
Meperidine (Demerol)	Moderate to severe	50–150 mg every 3–4 hr PO, IM, subcut 15–35 mg/hr IV infusion	PO, IM, IV, subcut	PO: 15 min IM: 10–15 min IV: 1 min Subcut: 10–15 min	PO: 60–90 min IM: 30–50 min IV: 5–7 min Subcut: 30–50 min	2–4 hr
Codeine	Mild to moderate	15–60 mg every 3–6 hr PO or 15–60 mg every 4–6 hr PO	PO	PO: 10–30 min	PO: 30–60 min	4–6 hr
Hydrocodone	Moderate to severe	5–10 mg every 4–6 hr PO	PO	10–30 min	30–60 min	4–6 hr
Fentanyl	Chronic	25 mcg/hr after assessment	TD (patch)	Slow	12–24 hr	24–48 hr
Hydromorphone (Diluadid)	Moderate to severe	2 mg every 3–4 hr PO to 4 mg every 4–6 hr PO	PO, IM, IV, subcut	PO: 30 min IM: 15 min IV: 10–15 min Subcut: 15 min	PO: 90–120 min IM: 30–60 min IV: 15–30 min Subcut: 30–90 min	PO: 4 hr IM: 4–5 hr IV: 2–3 hr Subcut: 4 hr

4. ASSESSMENT IS DONE DURING THE FIRST VISIT.
   a. The nurse needs to know the client's and family's knowledge, motivation, anxiety level, acceptance or denial of situations, and what level of change needs to occur.
5. THE ENVIRONMENT MAY AFFECT HOW FAST AND EFFECTIVE THE LEARNING CAN OCCUR—A BRIGHT, CLEAN, AND COMFORTABLE ENVIRONMENT WILL ENHANCE A POSITIVE OUTCOME.
6. LEARNING STYLES AFFECT EDUCATIONAL STRATEGIES.
   a. Start with a cultural assessment.
   b. Inform the client that performing a demo and return demo is a common strategy.
   c. Listening, negotiating, and contracting allow client control.
   d. Monitoring and evaluation are main roles once goals are set.
   e. Written materials may help decrease the client's high levels of anxiety and stress and also will inform the client on medication adverse reactions.
   f. Group supports are often more effective than nurse–client relationships.
   g. Telephone- and Internet-based groups may help the homebound.
   h. Clients with disabilities need aids.
      1) Verbal materials and assessments are helpful with the visually impaired.
      2) Visual aids prove beneficial with the hearing impaired.

J. DELIVERY OF THE EDUCATION
   1. PLANNING THE LESSON
      a. Learning goals are set by the family, client, and nurse together.
      b. Learning contracts or lesson plans are used to make the goals, strategies, and resources tangible.
         1) A lesson plan consists of the client's name, the learning goal, objectives, methods of teaching, resources available, time to teach, and method of evaluation.
         2) The educational contract begins with a simple statement of the learning goal after listing the client's name, diagnosis, and medications.
         3) The rest of the lesson plan is a statement of what the nurse will do.
   2. GIVING THE LESSON
      a. Give the lesson when the client and family are in the least pain.
      b. Provide materials for concept review.
      c. Give short and pointed lessons.
      d. Provide lots of repetition.

e. Provide methods for family control of personal progress.
f. Provide resources other than health care providers.

II. **NURSING DIAGNOSES SEEN IN HOSPICE**
   A. ACTIVITY INTOLERANCE
   B. ANXIETY
   C. CONSTIPATION
   D. DIARRHEA
   E. INEFFECTIVE BREATHING PATTERN
   F. DECREASED CARDIAC OUTPUT
   G. PAIN
   H. IMPAIRED VERBAL COMMUNICATION
   I. INEFFECTIVE COPING
   J. EXCESS FLUID VOLUME
   K. IMPAIRED GAS EXCHANGE
   L. GRIEVING
   M. RISK FOR INFECTION
   N. RISK FOR INJURY
   O. INEFFECTIVE HEALTH MAINTENANCE
   P. IMPAIRED PHYSICAL MOBILITY
   Q. IMBALANCED NUTRITION: LESS THAN BODY REQUIREMENTS
   R. IMPAIRED ORAL MUCOUS MEMBRANE
   S. POWERLESSNESS
   T. SELF-CARE DEFICIT: FEEDING, BATHING/ HYGIENE, DRESSING/GROOMING, AND TOILETING
   U. READINESS FOR ENHANCED SELF-CONCEPT
   V. DISTURBED SENSORY PERCEPTION: AUDITORY, VISUAL
   W. SEXUAL DYSFUNCTION
   X. IMPAIRED SKIN INTEGRITY
   Y. SOCIAL ISOLATION

Nursing Diagnoses: Definitions and Classification 2012–2014. Copyright © 2012, 1994–2012 by NANDA International. Used by arrangement with John Wiley & Sons Limited.

III. **CARING FOR THE MORIBUND CLIENT**
   A. THE MORIBUND PERIOD
      1. THE DYING PROCESS IS CALLED MORIBUND.
      2. CLIENTS APPROACH THE PERIOD DIFFERENTLY.
         a. Some quietly wait for family to leave the room.
         b. Others wait for a special family member to come.
         c. Some anticipate relief, whereas others fear what will happen.
         d. Other clients may exhibit hostile or angry behavior.
      3. DEVELOPMENTAL STAGES OF THE MORIBUND PERIOD INCLUDE DENIAL, ANGER, BARGAINING, DEPRESSION, AND ACCEPTANCE.
   B. THE NURSE'S ROLE
      1. PERFORM FREQUENT ASSESSMENTS OF THE CLIENT AND FAMILY MEMBERS.
      2. CONTACT THE CLIENT FREQUENTLY.

3. INCREASE THE CONTACT AS DEATH APPROACHES AND BRING THE CONTACT FROM DISTAL PORTIONS OF THE BODY CLOSER TO THE HEAD BECAUSE THE BODY LOSES SENSATION DISTALLY FIRST.
4. CHANGE THE POSITION FREQUENTLY.
5. PROVIDE PROPER MOUTH CARE.
6. MOISTEN THE LIPS.
7. MEET BASIC PHYSICAL NEEDS.
8. MONITOR VITAL SIGNS.
9. KEEP THE ROOM QUIET AND COMFORTABLY LIGHTED.

C. SIGNS OF APPROACHING DEATH
1. THE BODY RELAXES AND THE JAW DROPS.
2. BREATHING GROWS MORE LABORED.
3. THE BOWELS AND THE BLADDER LET GO.
4. CIRCULATION SLOWS AND BLOOD POOLS.
5. BLOOD PRESSURE DROPS.
6. EXTREMITIES COOL.
7. PROFUSE PERSPIRATION IS COMMON.
8. CHEYNE-STOKES RESPIRATIONS OCCUR.
9. THE PULSE BECOMES MORE RAPID AND WEAKER.
10. THE SKIN MOTTLES.
11. THE EYES NO LONGER RESPOND TO LIGHT.
12. HEARING IS THE LAST SENSE TO GO.

PRACTICE QUESTIONS

1. The daughter of a client asks the nurse how her mother can become a hospice client. Which of the following is the appropriate response by the nurse?
   1. "Anyone can make a hospice referral."
   2. "Your mother's physician must refer your mother."
   3. "The hospital discharge planner must make the referral from the hospital."
   4. "Your mother must start with home health first and then move to hospice."

2. The nurse assesses a hospice client to be unresponsive and incontinent, with limbs that are cool and mottling, and with a blood pressure of 80/48. The nurse evaluates this client as which of the following?
   1. Experiencing a drug overdose
   2. In need of transport to the hospital
   3. Moribund
   4. In need of a home health aide

3. When preparing for stabilization of a client with end-stage breast cancer who develops a gastrointestinal bleed, it would be essential for the nurse to explain which of the following?
   1. Stabilization at home because there is no hospitalization or hospice
   2. Stabilization at home because the client is terminal
   3. Hospitalization for stabilization paid by the client
   4. Hospitalization for stabilization paid by hospice

4. A nurse in the pediatric infectious disease unit should give which of the following information about hospice to the family of a child with acquired immunodeficiency syndrome (AIDS)?
   1. Hospice will pay for all the child's drugs
   2. Hospice provides an interdisciplinary team to support families
   3. Hospice means that the physician has given up on caring for the child
   4. Hospice means there is no longer hope for the child

5. A hospice nurse is caring for a client in the hospital with congestive heart failure who has problems of impaired mobility, skin alteration, impaired breathing, alteration in oral mucous membranes, and impaired nutrition. The client develops new-onset abdominal pain. The nurse should prepare the client for which of the following treatment modalities?
   1. Hospitalization to determine the etiology of the abdominal pain
   2. Laparoscopy to diagnose the etiology for the abdominal pain
   3. Aggressive relief of the clinical manifestations
   4. No change in the treatment for the abdominal pain

6. The nurse should inform the family of a client in hospice that which of the following services are available for Medicare coverage?
   Select all that apply:
   [ ] 1. Diagnostic services
   [ ] 2. Surgery
   [ ] 3. Medications
   [ ] 4. Curative radiation
   [ ] 5. Durable medical equipment
   [ ] 6. Psychiatrist

7. The nurse should include which of the following priority considerations to determine a client's readiness to learn?
Select all that apply:
[ ] 1. The client's medications
[ ] 2. The nurse's teaching ability
[ ] 3. The client's stress level
[ ] 4. The client's level of wellness
[ ] 5. The lesson plan
[ ] 6. The client's medical diagnosis

8. A dying client's family asks the nurse what is the life expectancy in months for the Medicare criteria for hospice. The most appropriate response by the nurse is how many months? _____

9. After receiving a terminal diagnosis of congestive heart failure, a client is hostile to family members and hospice staff. The family is very upset by this and asks the nurse why the client is so hostile. The most appropriate response by the nurse is which of the following?
1. "A terminal disease causes a sudden change in personality."
2. "The lack of oxygen to the brain causes the client to act angry."
3. "Drugs like digoxin (Lanoxin) can cause sudden mood shifts."
4. "This is a temporary stage, as the client prepares for an imminent death."

10. The hospice team has not been able to relieve the client's pain after repeated tries. One caregiver expresses concern to another caregiver that the pain is not real. The nurse tells the caregiver that pain is
1. an unpleasant sensory and emotional experience arising from tissue damage.
2. a cry for attention when clients do not cope with their mortality.

3. the result of an emotional reaction.
4. associated with all physical and mental illnesses.

11. A student nurse caring for a hospice client who is moribund and has not had a bowel movement for 5 days asks the nurse about giving the client an enema. Which of the following is the priority response by the nurse?
1. "Mineral oil is more effective than an enema."
2. "Maintaining a bowel program is essential to avoid pain and impactions."
3. "A stool softener may be administered."
4. "The body is slowing down and constipation is expected."

12. The nurse should prepare to administer which of the following drugs to a hospice client experiencing mild pain?
1. Codeine
2. Meperidine (Demerol)
3. Hydromorphone (Dilaudid)
4. Morphine

13. Which of the following drugs would be most appropriate for the nurse to administer to a client with end-stage carcinoma who has a recent diagnosis of uncontrollable pain?
1. Loratab with nonsteroidal anti-inflammatory drugs
2. Codeine with nonsteroidal anti-inflammatory drugs
3. Fentanyl
4. Morphine

14. Which of the following clients should the nurse refer to a hospice program?
1. A client recently diagnosed with breast cancer
2. A client scheduled for a bone marrow transplant
3. A client who has terminal ovarian cancer
4. A client who has pancreatic cancer

ANSWERS AND RATIONALES

1. 1. Hospice is a palliative program of coordinated care designed to deliver care to terminally ill clients and their families. Hospice relieves pain and other clinical manifestations without the intention of curing the client. Anyone can refer clients to hospice.

2. 3. Although drug overdose may produce some of the clinical manifestations, a client who is moribund, or nearing death, will exhibit cool mottled limbs, be unresponsive and incontinent, and have a low blood pressure.

3. 4. Medicare hospice will pay for the hospitalization to stabilize the client's clinical manifestations for respite, long-term, and short-term care.

4. 2. Medicare is the only insurance that guarantees medication payment. Medicare does not cover children. A decision to choose hospice care means that the family and caregivers switch from trying to cure to intensive caring, which includes control of the clinical manifestations. Trying to improve the family's quality of life becomes the goal.

5. 3. Hospice provides for aggressive relief of the clinical manifestations even within the hospital setting. It does not provide for surgery of other ailments, or for diagnosis of new conditions.

6. 3. 5. Hospice expenses covered under Medicare include medications and durable medical equipment. Diagnosis, curative treatments, and curative medications are not part of the hospice benefit.

7. 1. 3. 4. 6. Learning readiness is defined as how prepared the client is to learn when the educator first addresses learning. Medications, level of wellness, medical diagnosis, stress, desire to change, and many other conditions affect learning readiness. The nurse's teaching ability and the lesson plan both focus on the nurse and not the client's readiness.

8. 6 months. Medicare has strict rules indicating that the life expectancy must be less than 6 months.

9. 4. Hostility can be a reaction to the realization that one will soon die. The period is usually a short one, as the person generally adjusts to the facts and moves on to completing life's cycle.

10. 1. Pain is defined as an unpleasant sensory and emotional experience arising from tissue damage.

11. 4. The body slows down just before death and constipation is a common condition. Giving an enema or a stool softener would stress the body further. The caregiver can be directed to care in other ways that meet the client's needs during the last few hours before death.

12. 1. Codeine is the drug commonly given to ease the mild discomfort of a hospice client. Morphine, meperidine (Demerol), and hydromorphone (Dilaudid) are drugs used to treat moderate to severe pain.

13. 4. Morphine is appropriate for severe pain. Fentanyl is administered after a client has been on morphine sulfate for an extended time period.

14. 3. Although diagnoses of breast and pancreatic cancers and a client who is to have a bone marrow transplant all carry uncertain courses of treatment and prognoses, the client must already be determined to be terminal before a referral to hospice can be made.

REFERENCES

Daniels, R., & Nicoll, L. (2012). *Contemporary medical-surgical nursing.* Clifton Park, NY: Delmar Cengage Learning.

DeLaune, S. C., & Ladner, P. K. (2006). *Fundamentals of nursing: Standard and practice* (3rd ed.). Clifton Park, NY: Thomson Delmar Learning.

Hitchcock, J. E., Schubert, P. E., & Thomas, S. A. (2003). *Community health nursing: Caring in action* (2nd ed.). Clifton Park, NY: Thomson Delmar Learning.

LEGAL AND ETHICAL ISSUES IN NURSING

CHAPTER 64

CULTURAL DIVERSITY

I. **GUIDELINES FOR CULTURALLY SENSITIVE PRACTICE**
   A. SELF-EXAMINATION—DO NOT SAY AN UNDERSTANDING HAS TAKEN PLACE IF IT HAS NOT.
   B. USE OF LANGUAGE—ASK OTHERS HOW THEY WISH TO BE ADDRESSED.
   C. BODY LANGUAGE—FIND OUT WHAT IS APPROPRIATE, EYE CONTACT, TOUCHING, AND DISTANCE.
   D. DON'T ASSUME—FIND OUT WHO IS INVOLVED AND INCLUDE THEM.
   E. LISTEN—WHAT DOES THE CLIENT KNOW?

II. **KEY TERMS**
   A. ACCULTURATION: THE PROCESS OF LEARNING NORMS, BELIEFS, AND BEHAVIORAL EXPECTATIONS OF A GROUP; TO ACQUIRE THE MAJORITY GROUP'S CULTURE
   B. ANCESTRY: REFERS TO A PERSON'S NATIONALITY GROUP, LINEAGE, OR THE COUNTRY IN WHICH THE PERSON OR THE PERSON'S PARENTS OR RELATIVES WERE BORN BEFORE THEY CAME TO THE UNITED STATES
   C. ASSIMILATION: TO BECOME ABSORBED INTO ANOTHER CULTURE AND TO ADOPT ITS CHARACTERISTICS; TO DEVELOP A NEW CULTURAL IDENTITY
   D. BELIEF: BASIC ASSUMPTIONS OR PERSONAL CONVICTIONS THAT THE INDIVIDUAL BELIEVES ARE TRUE
   E. CULTURAL COMPETENCE: HAVING THE KNOWLEDGE, UNDERSTANDING, AND SKILLS REGARDING A DIVERSE CULTURE THAT ALLOW ONE TO PROVIDE ACCEPTABLE CARE
   F. CULTURAL DIVERSITY: THE DIFFERENCES IN VALUES, BELIEFS, NORMS, AND PRACTICES BETWEEN CULTURES
   G. CULTURE: VALUES, BELIEFS, NORMS, AND PRACTICES OF A PARTICULAR GROUP THAT ARE LEARNED AND SHARED AND GUIDE THINKING, DECISION, AND ACTION IN A PATTERNED WAY
   H. EMIC: PERSON'S WAY OF DESCRIBING AN ACTION OR EVENT, AN INSIDE VIEW
   I. ETHNICITY: A CULTURAL GROUP'S PERCEPTION OF THEMSELVES
   J. ETIC: THE INTERPRETATION OF AN EVENT BY SOMEONE WHO IS NOT EXPERIENCING THAT EVENT, AN OUTSIDE VIEW
   K. ETHNOCENTRISM: THE BELIEF THAT ONE'S OWN CULTURE IS SUPERIOR TO ALL OTHERS
   L. GENERALIZATIONS: BROAD INFORMATION ABOUT A CULTURE
   M. HERITAGE CONSISTENCY: OBSERVANCE OF THE BELIEFS AND PRACTICES OF ONE'S TRADITIONAL CULTURAL BELIEF SYSTEM
   N. HERITAGE INCONSISTENCY: OBSERVANCE OF THE BELIEFS AND PRACTICES OF ONE'S ACCULTURATED BELIEF SYSTEM
   O. SOCIALIZATION: PROCESS OF BEING RAISED WITHIN A CULTURE AND ACQUIRING THE CHARACTERISTICS OF THE GIVEN GROUP
   P. STEREOTYPE: FIXED NOTION OR CONCEPTION OF A PERSON OR GROUP WITH NO ALLOWANCE FOR INDIVIDUALITY
   Q. VALUES: PRINCIPLES THAT HAVE MEANING AND WORTH TO AN INDIVIDUAL, FAMILY, GROUP, OR COMMUNITY

III. **AFRICAN AMERICAN**
   A. COMMUNICATION
      1. ENGLISH SPEAKING
      2. NONVERBAL COMMUNICATION
         a. May be affectionate: affection is shown by hugging or touching, but touching in another's view may be viewed as offensive.

    b. Direct eye contact may be viewed as rude.
    c. Silence may indicate lack of trust for the caregiver.
    d. Head-nodding does not necessarily mean agreement.
    e. Nonverbal communication is very important.
    f. It may be viewed as intrusive to ask personal questions of someone whom an individual has just met.

B. TIME ORIENTATION
    1. FLEXIBLE TIME FRAME
    2. LIFE ISSUES MAY TAKE PRIORITY OVER KEEPING APPOINTMENTS.
    3. PRIMARILY PRESENT ORIENTED
    4. HAS A CLOSE PERSONAL SPACE

C. FAMILY STRUCTURE
    1. EXTENDED, MATRIARCHAL, AND MAY INCLUDE CLOSE FRIENDS IN KIN SUPPORT SYSTEM
    2. LARGE AND EXTENDED FAMILIES ARE IMPORTANT.
    3. FATHER OR ELDEST FAMILY MEMBER IS USUALLY THE SPOKESPERSON.
    4. ELDERS ARE TYPICALLY A SOURCE OF WISDOM AND DEMAND RESPECT.
    5. SINGLE-PARENT FAMILIES MAY BE FEMALE-HEADED HOUSEHOLDS SERVING AS BOTH CARETAKERS AND BREADWINNER.

D. RELIGION AND SPIRITUALITY
    1. RELIGION IS MAINLY PROTESTANT SUCH AS BAPTIST; HOWEVER, SOME ARE FOLLOWERS OF ISLAM OR OTHER FAITHS.
    2. PRAYER AND VISITS FROM A MINISTER ARE COMMON.
    3. AFFILIATION TO CHURCH COMMUNITY IS IMPORTANT.
    4. FAITH OR HERBALIST, OR BOTH MAY BE USED IN CONJUNCTION WITH BIOMEDICAL THERAPY.

E. DIETARY PRACTICE
    1. THREE MEALS DAILY, INCLUDING A LARGE MEAL IN LATE AFTERNOON, WHICH IS GENERALLY SUPPER.
    2. PREFER COOKED FOODS FOR RELIGIOUS REASONS.
    3. USUAL DIET INCLUDES MEAT, FISH, GREENS, RICE, POTATOES, CORN, AND YAMS.
    4. FOODS ARE GENERALLY SLOW-COOKED IN ADDED FAT.
    5. SOME PREGNANT CLIENTS MAY PARTICIPATE IN PICA OR THE INGESTION OF FOOD ITEMS SUCH AS STARCH USED IN LAUNDRY.

F. HEALTH AND ILLNESS BELIEFS
    1. A BELIEF THAT GOD, HEALTH, AND ILLNESS ARE CLOSELY CONNECTED.
    2. A HIGHER POWER EXTENDS TO EVERY FACET OF LIFE, INCLUDING HEALTH.
    3. ILLNESS CAN BE CLASSIFIED AS NATURAL AND UNNATURAL.
       a. Natural illness has natural causes and is caused by such things as exposure to cold air, rain, heat, impurities in the air, and bad food or water, such as in arthritis pain.
       b. An unnatural illness is caused by evil influences on the person.
       c. Professional health care workers can work to treat or cure the natural illnesses.
       d. Generic or traditional healers work to treat unnatural illnesses.
    4. PROPER DIET, PROPER BEHAVIOR, CLEANLINESS, AND EXERCISE IN FRESH AIR MAINTAIN HEALTH.

G. COMMON ILLNESSES
    1. HYPERTENSION
    2. CARDIOVASCULAR DISEASE
    3. STOMACH AND ESOPHAGEAL CANCER
    4. LACTOSE INTOLERANCE
    5. SICKLE CELL ANEMIA

H. NURSING INTERVENTIONS
    1. ENCOURAGE THE PARTICIPATION OF THE FAMILY.
    2. BE AWARE THAT A FOLK HEALER OR HERBALIST MAY BE CONSULTED BEFORE THE CLIENT SEEKS TREATMENT.
    3. EXPLORE WITH THE CLIENT THE MEANING OF HER NONVERBAL BEHAVIOR TO VALIDATE ITS MEANING.
    4. BE FLEXIBLE WITH THE USE OF TIME AND AVOID RIGIDITY IN THE SCHEDULING OF THE CLIENT'S CARE ACTIVITIES.
    5. VERIFY THE MEANING AND INTENT OF THE CLIENT'S WORDS.

IV. **ASIAN AMERICANS**
A. COMMUNICATION
    1. LANGUAGES INCLUDE CHINESE (ESPECIALLY MANDARIN), JAPANESE, KOREAN, VIETNAMESE, AND ENGLISH.
    2. NONVERBAL COMMUNICATION
       a. Quiet, polite, and tend not to disagree
       b. Eye contact may be considered rude and is avoided with authority figures.

    c. Keeping a respectful distance is recommended.

    d. Silence is valued.

    e. Head nodding does not generally mean agreement.

    f. The head is considered sacred and should not be touched.

    g. Usually do not touch others; unacceptable to touch members of the opposite sex

    h. An upturned palm may be viewed as offensive.

B. TIME ORIENTATION

    1. PROMPTNESS IS IMPORTANT; UNDERSTAND THE IMPORTANCE OF KEEPING APPOINTMENTS.

    2. ORIENTED MORE TO THE PRESENT

C. FAMILY STRUCTURE

    1. EXTENDED FAMILIES ARE COMMON; TWO OR THREE GENERATIONS OFTEN LIVE IN THE SAME HOUSEHOLD.

    2. A CLAN IS ANOTHER FORM OF FAMILY STRUCTURE. A CLAN IS A RECOGNIZED GROUPING OF FAMILIES WITH THE SAME LAST NAME AND LINE OF ANCESTORS.

    3. FAMILY UNIT IS VERY STRUCTURED AND HIERARCHICAL.

    4. MEN HAVE POWER AND AUTHORITY AND WOMEN ARE OBEDIENT, BUT WOMEN HAVE STRONG INFLUENCE IN THE HOME.

    5. OLDER ADULTS ARE VERY RESPECTED AND HONORED.

    6. EDUCATION IS HIGHLY VALUED.

D. RELIGION AND SPIRITUALITY

    1. RELIGIONS INCLUDE BUDDHISM, ISLAM, CATHOLICISM, PROTESTANT, AND TAOISM.

    2. BUDDHISTS PRACTICE ACT OF DANA (GENEROSITY), BELIEVED TO RETURN TO THEM IN THE FUTURE AS KARMA.

    3. CATHOLICS PRAY, RECITE THE ROSARY, AND MAY CONSULT THE CHAPLAIN.

    4. SOME PRACTICE ANCESTOR VENERATION, BELIEVING THE DECEASED GO TO A PLACE NEAR THE LIVING AND ARE ABLE TO HELP OR HINDER THE LIVING RELATIVES.

    5. MAY HAVE AN ALTAR FOR ANCESTOR WORSHIP

    6. SOME CHINESE USE HERBALISTS AND ACUPUNCTURISTS IN CONJUNCTION WITH WESTERN MEDICINE.

    7. MAY BELIEVE IN REINCARNATION

E. DIETARY PRACTICE

    1. USUALLY EAT THREE MEALS A DAY

    2. DIET IS USUALLY LOW IN FAT, ANIMAL PROTEIN, CHOLESTEROL, AND SUGAR.

    3. FISH, SOYBEANS, VEGETABLES, RICE, NOODLES, AND SOY SAUCE

    4. GENERALLY PREFER TEA, COFFEE, AND WATER BECAUSE MANY ASIANS ARE LACTOSE INTOLERANT

    5. FOR THE CHINESE, FOOD IS VIEWED AS IMPORTANT IN MAINTAINING THE BALANCE OF *YIN* (COLD) AND *YANG* (HOT) IN THE BODY. FOOD IS USED TO TREAT ILLNESS AND DISEASE.

    6. *YIN* FOODS, WHICH HAVE A POSITIVE ENERGY FORCE, INCLUDE FRUITS, VEGETABLES, AND COLD LIQUIDS.

    7. *YANG* FOODS, WHICH HAVE A NEGATIVE ENERGY FORCE, INCLUDE MEAT, EGGS, HOT SOUP AND LIQUIDS, AND OILY AND FRIED FOODS.

F. HEALTH AND ILLNESS BELIEFS

    1. HEALTH IS A STATE OF PHYSICAL AND SPIRITUAL HARMONY WITH NATURE.

    2. HEALTH IS ALSO MAINTAINING BALANCE BETWEEN *YIN* AND *YANG* INFLUENCES, NOT ONLY IN THE BODY BUT ALSO IN THE ENVIRONMENT.

    3. MOST PHYSICAL ILLNESSES ARE CAUSED BY AN IMBALANCE OF *YIN* AND *YANG*.

    4. CHRONIC ILLNESS MAY BE ATTRIBUTED TO KARMA AND MAY RESULT FROM BAD BEHAVIOR IN THIS LIFE OR IN PAST LIFE.

    5. HERBAL REMEDIES SUCH AS GINSENG ARE COMMONLY USED FOR ANEMIA, COLIC, DEPRESSION, OR INDIGESTION.

    6. TO PREVENT ILLNESS AND PROMOTE HEALTH, ONE SHOULD EAT A DIET BALANCED WITH *YIN* AND *YANG* FOODS.

    7. PRACTICES SUCH AS PINCHING, COINING (RUBBING A COIN OVER THE SKIN, CAUSING A MARK), AND CUPPING (APPLYING A GLASS OVER THE SKIN, SUCTION CREATED, CAUSES THE SKIN TO RISE UP AND TURN BLUE) ARE BELIEVED TO LET THE UNHEALTHY AIR CURRENTS OUT OF THE BODY.

    8. A BODY THAT IS HEALTHY MAY BE VIEWED AS A GIFT FROM THE ANCESTORS.

G. COMMON ILLNESSES

    1. HYPERTENSION

    2. LACTOSE INTOLERANCE

    3. STOMACH AND LIVER CANCER

H. NURSING INTERVENTIONS

    1. AVOID DIRECT EYE CONTACT AND GESTURING WITH THE HANDS.

    2. AVOID EXCESSIVE TOUCHING, AND BEFORE TOUCHING THE CLIENT'S HEAD EXPLAIN WHY IT IS NECESSARY TO DO SO.

3. BE AWARE THAT THE CLIENT MAY CONSULT A TRADITIONAL HEALER BEFORE CONSULTING MODERN MEDICINE.
4. EXPLORE RESPONSES TO QUESTIONS WITH THE CLIENT.
5. BE FLEXIBLE WITH THE USE OF TIME AND AVOID EXTREME RIGIDITY WHEN SCHEDULING CARES.

V. **HISPANIC AMERICANS**
  A. COMMUNICATION
    1. LANGUAGES INCLUDE SPANISH OR PORTUGUESE WITH MANY DIALECTS PRESENT.
    2. DIRECT CONFRONTATION IS CONSIDERED DISRESPECTFUL.
    3. IMPOLITE TO HAVE AN EXPRESSION OF NEGATIVE FEELINGS
    4. CONFIDENTIALITY IS IMPORTANT.
    5. VERY TACTILE, AND A HANDSHAKE OR EMBRACE IS OFTEN USED.
    6. POLITENESS AND MODESTY ARE VALUED.
    7. NONVERBAL COMMUNICATION
      a. Gestures are often used.
      b. Eye contact with authority figures is avoided typically and indicates respect and attentiveness.
      c. Touch, especially by strangers, is unappreciated.
      d. Silence may indicate lack of agreement; individuals tend to be verbally expressive.
      e. Emotion or pain is expressed through dramatic body gestures or facial expressions.
  B. TIME ORIENTATION
    1. PRESENT ORIENTED
    2. FLEXIBLE TIME FRAME
    3. COMFORTABLE WITH A CLOSENESS TO OTHER INDIVIDUALS
  C. FAMILY STRUCTURE
    1. GENERALLY PATRIARCHAL, WITH MALES MAKING THE DECISIONS AND MONEY AND FEMALES MANAGING THE HOUSEHOLD
    2. FAMILIES ARE TYPICALLY LARGE AND INCLUDE EXTENDED RELATIVES.
    3. LOYALTY AND OBLIGATION TO FAMILY ARE IMPORTANT.
    4. OLDER ADULTS ARE RESPECTED AND CHILDREN ARE EXPECTED TO OBEY THEIR PARENTS.
    5. TAKING CARE OF OLDER PARENTS IS SEEN AS A PRIVILEGE, NOT AN OBLIGATION.
  D. RELIGION AND SPIRITUALITY
    1. ROMAN CATHOLIC IS THE PREDOMINANT RELIGION.
    2. HOLD A WORLDVIEW THAT ONE MUST ACCEPT WHAT GOD GIVES AND A COMMON BELIEF THAT WHATEVER HAPPENS IS GOD'S WILL.
    3. RELIGIOUS CEREMONIES SUCH AS BAPTISM AND MARRIAGE ARE IMPORTANT.
    4. PRAYERS ARE COMMON, AND STATUES, CROSSES, AND CANDLES ARE EVIDENT IN MANY HOMES.
    5. HEALTH MAY RESULT FROM A STATE OF BALANCE BETWEEN "HOT" AND "COLD" FORCES OR "WET" AND "DRY" FORCES.
    6. ILLNESS MAY BE VIEWED AS A PUNISHMENT FOR THEIR SINS.
  E. DIETARY PRACTICES
    1. THE MAIN MEAL IS USUALLY AT NOON.
    2. RICE, BEANS, CORN, AND CHILIES ARE STAPLE FOODS.
    3. FRIED AND SPICY FOODS ARE CONSUMED.
  F. HEALTH AND ILLNESS BELIEFS
    1. IN TIME OF ILLNESS, INDIVIDUALS MAY UTILIZE BIOMEDICAL AND FOLK HEALTH SYSTEMS.
    2. SELF-MEDICATION AND USE OF "CURANDERA" (FOLK HEALER) ARE COMMON.
    3. OTHER TRADITIONAL HEALERS INCLUDE YERBEROS (HERBALISTS) AND SOBADORES (MASSEUSES).
    4. TRADITIONAL DISEASES INCLUDE:
      a. Empacho—stomach upset caused by eating the wrong foods at the wrong time of day or eating undercooked foods
      b. Caida de mollera—sunken fontanel caused by pulling the baby away from the breast or bottle too quickly, carrying the baby incorrectly, or from the baby falling
      c. Susto—fright sickness caused by a traumatic or frightening experience
    5. MANY INDIVIDUALS WILL NOT DISCUSS THEIR FOLK-HEALING REMEDIES WITH THE PROFESSIONAL HEALTH CARE PROVIDER OUT OF RESPECT.
  G. COMMON ILLNESSES
    1. PARASITE INFESTATION
    2. LACTOSE INTOLERANCE
    3. DIABETES
  H. NURSING INTERVENTIONS
    1. DISPLAY A NONJUDGMENTAL ATTITUDE REGARDING THE FOLK-HEALING THERAPIES, AND OBTAIN AS MUCH INFORMATION REGARDING HERBS AND SUPPLEMENTS USED.
    2. OFFER TO CALL A PRIEST WHEN THE CLIENT IS ILL.
    3. MAINTAIN PRIVACY AND CONFIDENTIALITY.

4. COMMUNICATION IS GENERALLY THROUGH THE HEAD OF THE FAMILY.
5. USE A GESTURE OF TOUCH WHEN EXAMINING A CHILD.
6. BE FLEXIBLE WHEN SCHEDULING CARE AND AVOID EXTREME RIGIDITY.

VI. **NATIVE AMERICANS**
A. COMMUNICATION—DEPENDS ON TRIBAL GROUP AND BAND, SUCH AS NAVAJOS, LAKOTA, SIOUX, AND OJIBWA
   1. LANGUAGES
      a. There are over 150 spoken Native American languages, although most speak English.
      b. Many of the languages involve a tonal speech in which the pitch is of great importance.
      c. Frequently use metaphors or anecdotes when speaking, and many times the Indian language does not have an equivalent single English word for translation.
      d. Typical speech pattern is slow with low tone of voice.
   2. NONVERBAL COMMUNICATION
      a. Maintain little eye contact—eye contact is considered a sign of disrespect.
      b. Silence is acceptable, viewed as positive, and a sign of respect for the speaker.
      c. It is very important to remain attentive during conversations and it is considered rude to indicate the person was not heard or to interrupt the speaker.
      d. Note taking during conversations or interviews is generally not acceptable.
      e. Lightly touching the hand when meeting or greeting a person is acceptable.
      f. Body language is an important mode of communication.
B. TIME ORIENTATION
   1. PRESENT TIME ORIENTATION
   2. TIME MAY BE VIEWED AS BEING ON A CONTINUUM, WITH NO BEGINNING AND NO END.
C. FAMILY STRUCTURE
   1. EXTREMELY FAMILY ORIENTED— THE TERM *FAMILY* TYPICALLY INVOLVES ALL MEMBERS OF THE EXTENDED FAMILY, SUCH AS FIRST COUSINS, BEING TREATED AS BROTHERS OR SISTERS.
   2. USUALLY A MALE FAMILY MEMBER WITH THE GREATEST AMOUNT OF PRESTIGE WILL RISE AS "LEADER" FOR THE EXTENDED FAMILY AND PROVIDE DIRECTION.
   3. OLDER ADULTS ARE HIGHLY RESPECTED AND PASS MANY OF THE TRADITIONS DOWN TO YOUNGER MEMBERS.
   4. CHILDREN ARE TAUGHT TO RESPECT TRADITIONS AND TO HONOR WISDOM.
   5. MOTHER IS TYPICALLY RESPONSIBLE FOR DOMESTIC DUTIES.
   6. IT IS COMMON FOR LARGE EXTENDED FAMILY TO VISIT A CLIENT IN THE HOSPITAL.
   7. PERSONAL SPACE IS VERY IMPORTANT, WITH SPACE HAVING NO BOUNDARIES.
   8. MASSAGE IS USED TO PROMOTE BONDING BETWEEN A MOTHER AND THE INFANT.
   9. COMMUNITY SOCIAL ORGANIZATIONS ARE VIEWED AS IMPORTANT.
D. RELIGION AND SPIRITUALITY
   1. RELIGIOUS AFFILIATION AND PRACTICES ARE AN INDIVIDUAL DECISION.
   2. BOTH TRADITIONAL AND A VARIETY OF CHRISTIAN RELIGIONS ARE PRACTICED.
   3. SACRED MYTHS AND LEGENDS ARE OFTEN VALUED.
   4. RELIGION AND PRACTICES IN HEALING GO TOGETHER.
E. DIETARY PRACTICE
   1. INFLUENCED BY TRIBAL BELIEFS, GEOGRAPHICAL AREA, AND AVAILABILITY
   2. TRADITIONAL DIETS IN THE PAST CONSISTED OF LOW-FAT FOODS, SUCH AS FRUITS, BERRIES, ROOTS, FISH, GAME, AND WILD GREENS.
   3. THE TRADITIONAL DIET HAS TRANSFORMED DUE TO THE SCARCITY OF THESE FOODS IN FEDERALLY DEFINED INDIAN GEOGRAPHICAL REGIONS.
   4. MODERN, PROCESSED FOODS, HIGH IN FAT AND SUGAR, ARE MORE COMMON NOW.
   5. LACTOSE INTOLERANCE IS COMMON BECAUSE MANY PEOPLE DO NOT DRINK MILK.
   6. CORN IS AN IMPORTANT STAPLE IN THE DIET.
F. HEALTH AND ILLNESS BELIEFS
   1. HEALTH IS BELIEVED TO REFLECT HARMONY WITH THE SURROUNDING ENVIRONMENT AND FAMILY.
   2. TRADITIONAL HEALTH BELIEFS FOCUS ON WELLNESS AND WHOLENESS.

3. TRADITIONAL REMEDIES MAY INCLUDE AN ACT OF PURIFICATION SUCH AS IMMERSION IN WATER, SWEAT LODGES, HERBAL MEDICINES, AND SPECIAL RITUALS.
4. HERBS AND ROOTS ARE CONSIDERED AGENTS OF NATURE OR SPIRITUAL HELPERS AND ARE USED MEDICINALLY.
5. MEDICINE MAN MAY BE CONSULTED AND IS CONSIDERED AN IMPORTANT PART OF TREATMENT.
6. SYMBOLIC OR SACRED ITEMS SUCH AS FEATHERS, STONES, ARROWHEADS, AND CORN POLLEN MAY BE USED FOR HEALING AND BLESSING.
7. BOTH TRADITIONAL AND WESTERN MEDICINE MAY BE UTILIZED.
8. IT IS FORBIDDEN TO TOUCH A DEAD BODY.

G. COMMON ILLNESSES
1. CARDIOVASCULAR DISEASE
2. DIABETES
3. ARTHRITIS
4. GLAUCOMA
5. TUBERCULOSIS

H. NURSING INTERVENTIONS
1. ENCOURAGE THE PARTICIPATION OF FAMILY MEMBERS.
2. ENCOURAGE THE CLIENT TO BRING PERSONAL ITEMS INTO THE HOSPITAL TO PERSONALIZE THE SPACE.
3. EXPLORE MESSAGES FOR CLARIFICATION.
4. UNDERSTAND THAT ALTHOUGH EYE CONTACT MAY BE ABSENT, THE CLIENT IS ATTENTIVE.

VII. **ARAB AMERICAN**
A. COMMUNICATION
1. LANGUAGES INCLUDE ARABIC (VARIATIONS EXIST IN DIALECTS) AND ENGLISH.
2. NONVERBAL COMMUNICATION
   a. Warm, shy, and modest
   b. When individuals feel accepted and trusted, they tend to be more expressive.
   c. Prefer closeness in space and with the same sex
   d. Typically very polite and may respond in ways to make others happy
   e. When men greet, hugging and kissing is common.

B. TIME ORIENTATION
1. PAST AND PRESENT ORIENTED
2. TYPICALLY "ON TIME" FOR BUSINESS ISSUES, MORE CASUAL AND SPONTANEOUS FOR INFORMAL GATHERINGS

C. FAMILY STRUCTURE
1. THE FAMILY IS THE STRONGEST SOCIAL UNIT IN ARAB CULTURE.
2. TYPICALLY THE ARAB-AMERICAN FAMILY IS PATRILINEAL, CONSISTING OF THE FATHER'S BROTHER'S FAMILIES, GRANDPARENTS ON THE FATHER'S SIDE, AND CHILDREN.
3. AT TIMES OF CRISES, FAMILY MEMBERS SHOW SUPPORT FINANCIALLY AND THROUGH THEIR PRESENCE.
4. THE CONCEPTS OF HONOR AND SHAME STRONGLY INFLUENCE THE FAMILY.
5. MOTHERS, SISTERS, DAUGHTERS, AND GRANDMOTHERS PROVIDE THE CARING FUNCTIONS.
6. THE FATHER, ELDEST SON, OR UNCLE USUALLY IS THE FAMILY SPOKESPERSON.
7. OLDER ADULTS ARE RESPECTED.
8. CHILDREN ARE SACRED AND EXPECTED TO BE OBEDIENT. ELDERS ARE MORE STRICT WITH GIRLS THAN BOYS.

D. RELIGION AND SPIRITUALITY
1. THE MAJORITY OF ARAB AMERICANS ARE MUSLIMS.
2. MUSLIM RELIGION (FOLLOWERS OF ISLAM) GREATLY AFFECTS THE LIVES OF ARAB AMERICANS.
3. THE ISLAMIC HOLY BOOK IS THE QURAN.
4. ISLAM IS BASED ON FIVE RELIGIOUS DUTIES REFERRED TO AS PILLARS:
   a. Profession of faith
   b. Prayer five times daily facing Mecca
   c. Fasting during Ramadan—Muslims do not eat, drink, or smoke from sunrise to sunset. Meals are served at night.
   d. Almsgiving (usually 2.5% of a person's total net worth)
   e. Pilgrimage to the Holy City of Mecca

E. DIETARY PRACTICE
1. A HEALTHY, HEARTY DIET IS IMPORTANT.
2. FRUITS, VEGETABLES, AND BREADS ARE COMMON.
3. MEATS USUALLY CONSIST OF CHICKEN AND LAMB SERVED WITH RICE OR SOUP.
4. AT HOME THE MEAL IS SERVED WITH PEOPLE TYPICALLY SITTING ON THE FLOOR.
5. THE MEAL IS OFTEN EATEN QUICKLY AND IN SILENCE.
6. UNDER ISLAMIC LAW, THE CONSUMPTION OF ALCOHOL AND IMPROPERLY SLAUGHTERED MEAT IS FORBIDDEN.

F. HEALTH AND ILLNESS BELIEFS
1. THE STRONG RELIGIOUS FOUNDATION OF ARAB AMERICANS IS IMPORTANT TO UNDERSTAND BECAUSE THIS GUIDES THEIR HEALTH AND ILLNESS BELIEF SYSTEM.
2. ARAB AMERICANS BELIEVE THAT GOD OR THE PROPHET MUHAMMAD IS OMNIPOTENT AND CAUSE FOR ALL HEALTH AND ILLNESS.
3. IF ONE LOSES FAITH IN GOD, THEN ILLNESS MAY BEFALL THAT PERSON.
4. A PERSON IS HEALTHY IF IN HARMONY WITH GOD.
5. FAMILY MEMBERS AND CLOSE FRIENDS ACCOMPANY CLIENTS TO THE HOSPITAL AND EXPECT TO PARTICIPATE IN CARE OR TAKE AN OVERSEEING ROLE.
6. ARAB AMERICANS SOMETIMES HAVE DIFFICULTY QUESTIONING MEDICAL AUTHORITIES AND BEING ACTIVELY INVOLVED IN MEDICAL DECISION MAKING AND OFTEN EXPECT THE PHYSICIAN TO MAKE MEDICAL DECISIONS.
7. HIGHLY TECHNICAL, INVASIVE THERAPIES ARE SEEN AS SUPERIOR TO NONINVASIVE TREATMENTS.
8. IMMEDIATE PAIN RELIEF IS EXPECTED AND MAY BE PERSISTENTLY REQUESTED.
9. THE BELIEF IN CONSERVING ENERGY FOR RECOVERY IS IN CONFLICT WITH THERAPIES THAT REQUIRE EXERTION.
10. HOME REMEDIES INCLUDE SWEATING RITUALS, RELIGIOUS VERSES, PRAYERS, AND A WELL-BALANCED DIET.
11. FOLK REMEDIES INCLUDE HERBS, OINTMENTS, FOODS, AND ENEMAS.

G. COMMON ILLNESSES
1. HYPERTENSION
2. CANCER

H. NURSING INTERVENTIONS
1. BE AWARE THAT THE CLIENT WILL BE PERSISTENT IN THE REQUEST FOR PAIN MEDICATION.
2. BE AWARE THAT THE CLIENT MAY RESORT TO HOME REMEDIES BEFORE SEEKING MEDICAL TREATMENT.
3. BE SUPPORTIVE OF THE CLIENT'S RELIGIOUS PREFERENCES.
4. ENCOURAGE THE CLIENT TO BE A PARTICIPANT IN THE HEALTH CARE.

VIII. EUROPEAN AMERICANS
A. COMMUNICATION
1. LANGUAGE—SPEAK THEIR NATIONAL DIALECTS AND ENGLISH

2. NONVERBAL COMMUNICATION
   a. Avoid close physical contact
   b. Direct eye contact is used and indicates trustworthiness.
   c. Handshake for greeting is appreciated and develops trust.
   d. Nodding is a gesture of approval.
   e. Silence may be used for either a sign of respect or disdain, depending on the circumstances.

B. TIME ORIENTATION
1. MOST ARE FUTURE ORIENTED, LOOKING TO THE FUTURE.

C. FAMILY STRUCTURE
1. FAMILY ORIENTED; EXTENDED FAMILY MEMBERS OFTEN LIVE TOGETHER, RELYING ON EACH OTHER FOR FINANCIAL AND EMOTIONAL SUPPORT, CHILD CARE, AND HOUSEHOLD TASKS.
2. THE FATHER TENDS TO HAVE THE GREATEST INFLUENCE AND MAKES DECISIONS.
3. CHILDREN PRIMARILY ARE CARED FOR BY THE MOTHER OR GRANDMOTHER.
4. EDUCATION, FAMILY, AND CULTURAL ACTIVITIES ARE HIGHLY VALUED.
5. THE INDIVIDUAL IS TYPICALLY HARD WORKING, SELF-RELIANT, AND INDEPENDENT.
6. OLDER ADULTS ARE HIGHLY RESPECTED.

D. RELIGION AND SPIRITUALITY
1. MAINLY JUDEO-CHRISTIAN

E. DIETARY PRACTICE
1. DIET IS HIGH IN CARBOHYDRATES, WITH BREAD BEING A STAPLE.
2. HIGH INTAKE OF RED MEAT

F. HEALTH AND ILLNESS BELIEFS
1. VIEW HEALTH AS THE ABSENCE OF DISEASE
2. MAY USE HOME REMEDIES BEFORE CONSULTING MODERN MEDICINE
3. MAY VIEW ILLNESS AS A NEGATIVE FORCE IN THEIR LIFE AND A RESULT OF THEIR SINS
4. MAY BE STOIC WHEN PRESENTING WITH PHYSICAL COMPLAINTS

G. COMMON ILLNESSES
1. CARDIOVASCULAR DISEASE
2. DIABETES
3. THALASSEMIA
4. BREAST CANCER

H. NURSING INTERVENTIONS
1. PAY PARTICULAR ATTENTION TO THE CLIENT'S BODY LANGUAGE.
2. OFFER SUPPORT TO THE CLIENT WHILE ATTEMPTING TO DECREASE THE NEGATIVE VIEW OF ILLNESS.
3. ENCOURAGE THE CLIENT TO CONSULT MODERN MEDICINE.

PRACTICE QUESTIONS

1. The outpatient care nurse is discussing postoperative dismissal teaching with an Asian-American client. During the discussion, the client looks at the floor, smiles at times, and nods his head. The nurse interprets this nonverbal behavior as a(n)
   1. acceptance of the dismissal instructions.
   2. understanding of the material taught.
   3. reflection of cultural values.
   4. ability to follow through with instructions.

2. The nurse in the emergency room is evaluating a head laceration on an 8-year-old Asian-American client. Prior to the physical assessment, the nurse should
   1. ask the parents to step out of the room.
   2. ask for permission to examine the head.
   3. touch the child gently, explaining the procedure.
   4. discuss the dismissal care of a laceration.

3. The admission nurse is gathering family information on an Asian-American client. The client mentions the term "clan." The nurse understands this term to mean
   1. a group of friends and relatives that accompanied the client.
   2. the client's spouse.
   3. a sacred symbol the client wishes to keep nearby at all times.
   4. a recognized group of families with the same last name and line of ancestors.

4. The nursing instructor is describing the Chinese-American philosophy of *yin* and *yang* to a group of nursing students. The instructor describes how foods are classified using this belief system. Which of the following statements should the nursing instructor include that correctly describes the *yin* and *yang* food correlation?
   1. *Yin* foods are hot
   2. *Yin* and *yang* deals with energy, not food
   3. *Yang* foods are cold
   4. Cold foods are consumed when a hot illness is present

5. The nurse in the urgent care center is assessing an Asian-American adolescent with complaints of a sore throat. When auscultating lung sounds, the nurse notices round bluish marks along each side of the client's back. The nurse reports this as which of the following?
   1. A potential skin infection
   2. A sign of abuse
   3. The practice of cupping
   4. An allergy to a medication

6. During a care conference involving the nurse, physician, social worker, Asian-American client, and Asian-American family members, some suggestions for further care are being discussed. The client is sitting in a chair at the edge of the room. The client looks only at the family and does not speak during the conference. The nurse assesses the client's behavior as
   1. withdrawal from the situation.
   2. a sign of denial regarding the condition.
   3. a lack of understanding of the discussion.
   4. a sign of respect for members of the health care team.

7. The nurse is reviewing follow-up instructions with an African-American client. The nurse notices that the client has missed two follow-up appointments in the last week. The client states "something else came up." The nurse interprets this as
   1. a lack of understanding of the follow-up routine.
   2. uncertainty of the willingness of the client to pursue further care.
   3. a sense of noncommitment toward the plan of care.
   4. a cultural value of a flexible time frame.

8. An African-American client with hypertension is attending a class on ways to take control of hypertension. The nurse explains dietary measures that can be used to help control blood pressure. Which of the following indicates the client has understood the material presented?
   1. "I love fried chicken, but will choose broiled skinless chicken as my entrée."
   2. "It is okay to use table salt, just not too much."
   3. "I can still drink wine or beer with my dinner; these fluids don't interfere with blood pressure."
   4. "I've never been a big vegetable eater; I don't suppose I need to start now."

9. An older adult African-American client has just received a diagnosis of prostate cancer. During a discussion with the family and nurse, the client states, "This is all in God's hands now; there's not much more I can do." The nurse interprets this statement as the client
   1. accepting the diagnosis.
   2. giving up on a possible cure.
   3. expressing feelings of loss of control.
   4. expressing a cultural belief in the connectedness of God, health, and illness.

10. The nurse is caring for an African-American client who recently had a hysterectomy. The client requests certain herbs from the dietician to be included with meals. When the meals arrive, the client and the faith healer perform a ritual over the herbs. The nurse assesses this as a(n)
    1. unacceptable event and reports it to the charge nurse.
    2. common practice to combine herbs, faith healing, and Western medicine.
    3. way for the client to think she has control.
    4. way for the client to individualize her own care.

11. The nurse in the diagnostic imaging center is preparing an African-American client with a history of headaches for a computerized tomography (CT) scan. Which of the following questions should the nurse avoid asking during the initial assessment?
    1. "Do you experience vision changes?"
    2. "Do you experience shortness of breath?"
    3. "Do you have a close relationship with your family?"
    4. "Do you typically experience headaches daily?"

12. The nurse is involved in discharge planning for an older Hispanic-American client with a terminal illness. The nurse offers services, such as Meals on Wheels, nursing care, and hospice. The client's family insists on providing all the care. The nurse identifies this situation as a(n)
    1. unrealistic expectation for members of the family.
    2. inability to accept other forms of help.
    3. common practice, as it is often seen as a privilege when family members care for older adults.
    4. way for family to stay in control of the older adult client.

13. A home health nurse is visiting a Hispanic-American client who does not speak English. A translator is not available at the time of the visit. The best approach for the nurse to overcome the language barrier is to
    1. discuss one issue at a time.
    2. write the medical terms down.
    3. offer to return at a different time.
    4. use simple words, gestures, and pictures.

14. A Hispanic-American client arrived at the emergency room complaining of severe stomach pains and cramps. Upon evaluation, the client described to the nurse a home remedy that included massage, prayer, rubbing, and gently pinching the spine. The nurse interpreted this behavior as a(n)

1. extreme attempt to avoid visiting a physician.
2. example of traditional folk remedies accepted by the Hispanic-American culture.
3. denial of the seriousness of the medical condition.
4. alternative approach with no scientific basis.

15. The nurse informs another nurse that which of the following statements best describes American Indians' beliefs about health?
    1. "The earth gives food, shelter, and medicine to humankind, and all things of the earth belong to human beings and nature."
    2. "Health is believed to reflect internal harmony."
    3. "Traditional health beliefs focus on illness and achieving health through nature."
    4. "The human body is viewed as several parts working together to attain health."

16. The nurse is explaining preoperative information to an American Indian client. The nurse observes the client to be quiet, looking at the picture on the wall, and not readily responding to the nurse's questions. This behavior would indicate the client
    1. is not accepting the information.
    2. has a hearing impairment.
    3. is listening to the nurse.
    4. is focusing on the environment.

17. The nurse admitting an American Indian client is working on the admission forms. The nurse has asked the client to speak louder and to repeat several comments. The client gets frustrated and won't continue the interview. Which of the following best describes this interaction?
    1. The nurse was unaware of acceptable forms of communication with Indian clients
    2. The client was feeling rushed during the interview process
    3. The nurse was seeking clarification during the interview
    4. The client was uncertain about the interview process

18. A nurse teaching a class on the characteristics of an Arab-American family unit uses the term "patrilineal." The nurse should include which of the following statements to best describe patrilineal?
    1. A concept of honor or shame in the family
    2. A philosophy of time orientation specific to the Arab culture
    3. A special bond evident in most Arab families
    4. A family group consisting of family members on the father's side

19. A nurse is reviewing a diet with an Arab-American client. The nurse understands that which of the following foods are typical in the Arab diet?
Select all that apply:
[ ] 1. Fried foods
[ ] 2. Rice
[ ] 3. Canned processed foods
[ ] 4. Soup
[ ] 5. Chicken
[ ] 6. Lamb

20. The nurse is teaching a class on the cultural aspects of the Arab-American client. Which of the following should the nurse include in this class?
   1. Friends are the strongest social unit in the Arab-American culture
   2. The majority of Arabs immigrating to the United States are Muslims
   3. Following Islam has no effect on the lifestyles of Arab Americans
   4. Mealtime is a social time of long duration

21. An Arab-American client is referred for continuing care related to dizziness and vision changes. The nurse understands that an Arab-American client would prefer which of the following therapies as a treatment of the condition?
   1. Continued monitoring of the clinical manifestations
   2. Computerized tomography (CT) scan of the head
   3. Blood work to check electrolytes
   4. Vision screening

22. A nurse caring for an Arab-American client is assessing the client's pain following angiography. The client is lying in bed, eyes tightly closed, and continually asks for more pain medication. The client states, "I asked for pain medication right away and I need it now!" Which of the following nursing actions would be most appropriate at this time?

   1. Check to see when the pain medication was last given
   2. Explain to the client that the nurse was not aware of the discomfort
   3. Try to obtain more information regarding the pain
   4. Inform the client that the pain medication will be administered after assisting another client

23. Which of the following should the nurse include in a class on the health belief system associated with clients of the Russian-American culture?
   1. A belief that man has little control over nature
   2. A belief that God's will is the only will
   3. A belief that nature, environment, and man are directly linked to health and wellness
   4. A belief that eating right will maintain health

24. A nurse educator is working with staff on cultural diversity issues related to nonverbal communication. The educator explains to another nurse that appropriate nonverbal communication in the Russian-American culture includes which of the following?
   1. Nodding is a gesture of approval
   2. Handshakes are avoided
   3. Direct eye contact is avoided
   4. Touch is considered an invasion of privacy

25. A care conference is scheduled to discuss the prognosis of a terminally ill Russian-American client. The family members insist that the client not be told the diagnosis. The nurse interprets this behavior as
   1. unacceptable because every client has a right to personal medical information.
   2. an ethical violation on the part of the family.
   3. a typical response in Russian-American cultural tradition to dealing with terminal illness.
   4. a dishonest way of communicating.

ANSWERS AND RATIONALES

1. 3. In the Asian-American culture, eye contact with authority figures is avoided. Head nodding does not necessarily reflect agreement. Direct eye contact is frequently viewed as rude. The Asian-American culture typically avoids confrontation. The word "no" is avoided because it would show disrespect.

2. 2. In the Asian-American culture, the head is considered sacred. Touching the head is seen as disrespectful. Permission must be sought to

touch the client. The parents should remain with the child to offer comfort and support.

3. 4. In the Asian-American culture, a clan is a family structure that includes a group of individuals considered ancestors and who have the same last name.

4. 4. In the Chinese-American culture, foods are classified as hot or cold and are transformed into *yin* and *yang* energy when metabolized by the body. *Yin* and *yang* represent a balance

between positive and negative forces. *Yin* foods are cold and *yang* foods are hot. Cold foods are eaten when a hot illness is present. Hot foods are eaten when a cold illness is present.

5. 3. In the Asian-American culture, cupping involves applying a glass over the skin to create a suction that causes the skin to swell and turn bluish. This practice is believed to let the unhealthy air currents out of the body. If an allergy to a medication existed, the rash typically would be located in more areas than just the back. Further investigation and discussion would be necessary before abuse could be suspected.

6. 4. The Asian-American culture is typically viewed as quiet, polite, and avoiding direct eye contact. Silence is valued and maintaining a distance is respected. Nonverbal communication is very important.

7. 4. A characteristic of African-American culture is the concept of time as flexible. The present takes precedent over the future. Members of the cultural group avoid rigidly scheduled appointments.

8. 1. In the African-American culture, clients typically enjoy fried, fatty foods and slow-cook foods in added fat. The client has made an appropriate alteration to this food choice by choosing broiled skinless chicken over fried chicken. Salt and alcohol should be avoided. Encouraging fresh fruits and vegetables is also appropriate.

9. 4. In the African-American culture, there is a strong belief in God and the view that God, health, and illness are interconnected.

10. 2. It is common in the African-American culture to combine Western medicine with other traditions. An herbalist or folk healer may be consulted before an individual seeks traditional medicine. Certainly the patient has a right to request herbs and a faith healer. This activity would not warrant the charge nurse being notified.

11. 3. In the African-American culture, it is considered intrusive to ask personal questions during the initial assessment. Asking a client about having vision changes, shortness of breath, or headaches is physiologically based; these questions take priority during the admission process.

12. 3. In the Hispanic-American culture, older adults are respected and honored. Extended families typically live together and provide care as necessary. This is seen as a privilege, not an obligation. Family members encourage involvement of the extended family.

13. 4. If a translator is not present with a client who does not speak English, communication will take more time. The nurse must be creative and patient. Using simple words, gestures, and pictures may prove helpful. Written medical terms will not be effective if the client doesn't understand English. Discussion of one issue at a time does not overcome the language barrier. Rescheduling home visits is not generally acceptable.

14. 2. Folk remedies are widely accepted practices in the Hispanic-American culture. At times, a combination of folk remedies and Western medicine is utilized. Many Hispanic-American clients will not discuss folk remedies with the physician.

15. 1. Traditional American Indian health beliefs reflect a bond between person and nature. Health is believed to reflect harmony with the surrounding environment and family. Traditional beliefs focus on wellness, not illness. The body is divided into two halves that are seen as plus and minus or two energy poles, one positive and one negative.

16. 3. Typical nonverbal behavior of American Indians is quiet listening. Silence is respected and eye contact is considered disrespectful. Communication style is often slow with a low tone of voice and reflection between statements.

17. 1. During an interview, asking an American Indian to speak louder and repeat responses is seen as rude and disrespectful.

18. 4. Patrilineal descent is typical of Arab-American families and means a family group consisting of family members on the father's side.

19. 2. 4. 5. 6. The Arab diet is rich in rice, soup, chicken, and lamb. Fried and canned foods are usually avoided. Pork is prohibited and meat is slaughtered in a specific fashion.

20. 2. The majority of Arab Americans immigrating to the United States are Muslims. Family members, not friends, are the strongest social unit. Following Islam is the pillar of the Arab-American lifestyle. Meals are often consumed very quickly and in silence.

21. 2. Generally, Arab-American clients prefer highly technical, even invasive, procedures over noninvasive treatment modalities.

22. 1. It is typical of the Arab-American culture that immediate pain relief is expected and may be persistently requested. Trying to obtain more information or explaining that the nurse was unaware of the discomfort is not appropriate at this time. Assisting another client should be delegated to another staff member.

23. 1. Russian-American cultural belief regarding health is very much the idea that one has little or no control over health and illness. Nature, environment, God's will, and eating right have no part in the belief system.

24. 1. Direct eye contact is used and appreciated in the Russian-American culture. Eye contact indicates trustworthiness and honesty. Touch and handshaking are used for formal greetings. Nodding is a gesture of approval.

25. 3. In the case of a terminal illness, a common Russian-American cultural practice is to only disclose the medical condition to nearest relatives. It is believed the client will do better if the client continues to have hope for recovery.

REFERENCES

Burkhardt, M. A., & Nathaniel, A. K. (2008). *Ethics and issues in contemporary nursing* (3rd ed.). Clifton Park, NY: Delmar Cengage Learning.

Kelly, P. (2012). *Nursing leadership and management.* Clifton Park, NY: Delmar Cengage Learning.

CHAPTER 65

LEADERSHIP AND MANAGEMENT

I. ISSUES IN HEALTH CARE DELIVERY

A. QUALITY HEALTH CARE ISSUES

1. **TYPES OF HEALTH CARE SERVICES**
   a. Primary health care is the level of services devoted to health promotion and the prevention of illness and disability.
   b. Secondary health care is the level of services focused on detection and early intervention in order to prevent further illness and disability.
   c. Tertiary health care services are devoted to restorative and rehabilitative services for clients who have chronic or irreversible conditions.

2. **POPULATION-BASED HEALTH CARE (SEE TABLE 65-1)**
   a. Description: Population-based health care focuses on the health care needs of a population of clients rather than individual clients.
   b. Management of care is the organized collection of activities designed to meet the needs of the client within a quality and efficient delivery system.

Table 65-1 Features of the New Role of Health Care Management in a Population-Based Health System

Emphasis on the continuum of care
Emphasis on maintaining and promoting wellness
Accountability for the health of defined populations
Differentiation based on ability to add value
Success achieved by increasing the number of covered individuals and keeping people healthy
Goal is to provide care at the most appropriate level
Integrated health delivery system
Managers oversee a market
Managers operate service areas across organizational borders
Managers actively pursue quality and continuous improvement

© Cengage Learning 2015

c. Evidence-based practice is the delivery of care for clients that is based not only on the clinical expertise of the nurse caregiver but also the recent research findings relative to the client's care needs.

3. **LEGAL AND ETHICAL ISSUES**
   a. Nurse practice acts guide the scope of practice for the professional nurse in each state. State boards of nursing monitor the legal practice of professional nurses in each state, and nurses must know the state law and use the nurse practice act for guidance and applicable action.
   b. *Negligence* and *malpractice* are terms that describe a lack of appropriate care as described by the nurse practice act and standards of care.
      1) Negligence is a deviation from the standard of care or carelessness in providing appropriate care that a person of ordinary prudence would exercise in the same circumstances.
      2) Malpractice is the failure of a licensed professional to act in a reasonable and prudent manner with respect to client care needs.
   c. Protective and reporting laws are those laws in each state that require a professional to report incompetent practice, client abuse situations, and professional impairment.
   d. Ethical practice and principles concern the process of making decisions relative to client care and professional practice that is based on distinction of right and wrong concerning knowledge and not just on opinion. Ethical decisions require knowledge, facts, and rules of the situation, options and courses of action that are appropriate, possible consequences, values, and desired goals and outcomes.

B. LEADERSHIP IN PROFESSIONAL NURSING

1. DESCRIPTION: A PROCESS IN WHICH THE LEADER INFLUENCES OTHER INDIVIDUALS OR GROUPS TOWARD GOAL ACHIEVEMENT. LEADERSHIP CAN BE DEMONSTRATED IN FORMAL OR INFORMAL ROLES.

2. LEADERSHIP CHARACTERISTICS
   a. Those attributes and personal characteristics demonstrated by individuals in leadership roles
   b. Vision: effective leaders focus on the professional, institutional, and purposeful vision that will provide direction toward goal achievement.
   c. Passion: the ability to motivate and guide people toward the goal
   d. Integrity: the knowledge of self that demonstrates the values of honesty and maturity and promotes trust among others

3. LEADERSHIP IN ACTION
   a. The traits demonstrated by a leader, such as intelligence, self-confidence, determination, integrity, and sociability; leadership effectiveness is usually demonstrated using one of the following leadership styles:
      1) Autocratic leadership: decisions are made by the leader and given directly to others through command and control of others.
      2) Democratic leadership: decisions are made by a participatory between the leader and others by delegation of authority to others in the system.
      3) Laissez-faire leadership: decision making is deferred to others by a passive and permissive approach.
      4) Transactional leadership: decisions may be implicitly defined using the power and formal authority of the organizational position to reward and punish performance.
      5) Transformational leadership: decisions are explicitly defined through collaboration, consultation, and consensus building among others.

C. MANAGEMENT IN PROFESSIONAL NURSING

1. DESCRIPTION: A PROCESS IN WHICH THE MANAGER COORDINATES ACTIONS AND RESOURCES TO ACHIEVE GOALS AND OUTCOMES FOR THE ORGANIZATION

2. MANAGEMENT PROCESS: THE ACTIVITIES OF PLANNING, ORGANIZING, COORDINATING, AND CONTROLLING HUMAN AND PHYSICAL RESOURCES IN ORDER TO ACHIEVE A GOAL
   a. POCC: Acronym describing the role function of the manager involving planning, organizing, coordinating, and controlling
   b. POSD-CORB: Acronym describing the role function of the manager involving planning, organizing, staffing, directing, coordinating, reporting, and budgeting
   c. Managerial roles and functions of the nurse
      1) Information processing roles: activities used to provide informational needs to others, such as monitor, disseminator, director, and spokesperson
      2) Interpersonal: behavioral activities used to motivate and communicate with others, such as director, leader, liaison, encourager, and spokesperson
      3) Decision-making roles: activities used to guide and direct goals, plans, and evaluative outcomes such as collaborator, entrepreneur, negotiator, delegator, and communicator

D. MANAGING CHANGE

1. CHANGE PROCESS: PROCESS OF ASSESSMENT, PLANNING, IMPLEMENTATION, EVALUATION, AND STABILIZATION EMPLOYED BY A LEADER OR MANAGER AS A FRAMEWORK TO GUIDE PLANNED CHANGE IN THE ORGANIZATION (SEE TABLE 65-2)

2. ROLE OF THE CHANGE AGENT (SEE TABLE 65-3): AN INDIVIDUAL WHO IS RESPONSIBLE FOR IMPLEMENTING A CHANGE PROJECT, ACTIVITY, OR PROCESS

3. RESPONSE TO CHANGE: BEHAVIORAL RESPONSE TO THE PROCESS AND OUTCOME OF PLANNED CHANGE EXHIBITED BY THOSE INVOLVED IN THE CHANGE PROJECT
   a. Innovators: those who embrace change and enjoy the challenge
   b. Early adopters: open and receptive to change but not obsessed with the need to change
   c. Early majority: those who really prefer the status quo but do not want to be left behind by the change event
   d. Late majority: those who adapt to change only after expressing negative feelings and skeptical ideas

Table 65-2 Comparison of Change Theories and Their Uses

Theorist and Year	Lewin (1951)	Lippitt (1958)	Havelock (1973)	Rogers (1983)
Title of Model	Force-Field Model	Phases of Change	Six-Step Change Model	Diffusion of Innovations Theory
Steps in Model (The steps in the models are spaced to indicate their correlation to Lewin's model.)	Unfreeze	Diagnose problem Assess motivation and capacity for change Assess change agent's motivation and resources	Build relationship Diagnose problem Acquire resources	Awareness
	Move	Select progressive change objective Choose appropriate role of change agent	Choose solution Gain acceptance	Interest Evaluation Trial
	Refreeze	Maintain change Terminate helping relationship	Stabilization and self-renewal	Adoption

Adapted from Swansburg, R. C., & Swansburg, R. J. (1998). Introductory management and leadership for nurses (2nd ed., p. 327). Boston: Jones & Bartlett.

Table 65-3 Roles and Characteristics of the Change Agent

Leader of change process
Manages process and group dynamics
Understands feelings of group experiencing the change
Maintains momentum and enthusiasm
Maintains vision of change
Communicates change, progress, and feelings
Knowledgeable about the organization
Trustworthy
Respected
Intuitive

© Cengage Learning 2015

e. Laggards: those who prefer tradition and stability; suspicious of the change
f. Rejectors: those who openly oppose and reject the change project and may hinder the outcome to the point of sabotage

E. CLIENT-CARE MANAGEMENT
  1. MODELS OF CLIENT CARE DELIVERY: ORGANIZATIONAL MODELS FOR STAFFING OR THE WORK OF DELIVERY OF CARE TO CLIENTS
    a. Total client care: the registered nurse is responsible for the total care of clients assigned for the shift with or without assistance from a licensed practical nurse (LPN) or an unlicensed assistant personnel (UAP).
    b. Functional nursing: nursing care is divided into functional units that are assigned to one of the staff members whose specific duties are compatible with the work to be done.
    c. Team nursing: nursing care assignments are given to a team of staff with the responsibility for the entire care of a group of clients. A team leader coordinates and supervises all the care provided by others on the team.
    d. Primary nursing: the registered nurse is the designated primary care provider for clients with responsibility and accountability for the quality care of the clients assigned on a 24-hour basis.
    e. Client-centered or client-focused care: care-delivery model where assignment of care is based on client needs rather than staff needs. Care teams are usually interdisciplinary and assigned to a group of clients.
    f. Differentiated nursing practice: roles, functions, and work of the registered nurse are established according to a set of criteria such as education, clinical experience, competence, and certification.
  2. EFFECTIVE STAFFING PATTERNS
    a. Client classification and needs: a system of measurement for describing the nursing workload requirements for a specific client or group of clients based on client care needs
    b. Nurse staffing: the process of evaluating the quantity and quality of nursing staff patterns necessary to meet standards of care for clients and to ensure quality client outcomes
    c. Client care outcomes: the process of measuring the effectiveness of client care results based on diagnosis, standards of care, and length of hospital stay and staffing patterns

Table 65-4 Delegation Suggestions for RNs

1. Include all personnel in the delegation process when making assignments.

2. Assess what is to be delegated and identify who would best complete the assignment.

3. Communicate the duty to be performed and identify the time frame for completion. The expectations for personnel should be clear and concise.

4. Avoid removing duties once assigned. This should be considered only when the duty is above the level of the personnel, as when the client's care is in jeopardy because client status has changed.

5. Evaluate the effectiveness of the delegation of duties, check in frequently, and ask for a feedback report on the outcomes of care delivery.

6. Accept minor variations in the style in which the duties are performed. Individual styles are acceptable as long as the duty is performed correctly within the scope of practice.

© Cengage Learning 2015

3. ISSUES IN MANAGING CLIENT CARE
   a. Delegation: the transferring of authority to perform selected nursing tasks to a competent individual (see Table 65-4)
   b. Accountability and responsibility: accountability is the legal liability for overall nursing care of clients assumed by the nurse. Responsibility includes each nurse's personal obligation, reliability, and dependability to perform client care at an acceptable level based on standards of care.
   c. Appropriate team delegation: the assignment of client care tasks and duties to personnel who are educated or licensed to perform specific quality care tasks. Delegation considerations include potential harm to the client, complexity of care needed, skill at problem solving, predictability of client care outcomes, and need for appropriate therapeutic interaction (see Figure 65-1).
   d. Conflict resolution: the ability to resolve conflict or disagreements between other individuals. Sources of conflict include differences of opinion about resources, values, personalities, cultural, and threats to personal self-esteem or organizational position.
   e. Conflict resolution techniques (see Table 65-5): strategies used to resolve the conflict process

II. **LEADING AND MANAGING CLIENT CARE**
   A. EFFECTIVE TEAM BUILDING
      1. DEFINITION OF TEAMS: A SMALL GROUP OF INDIVIDUALS WITH A SET OF SKILLS THAT COMPLEMENT EACH OTHER AND WHO ARE COMMITTED TO A COMMON PURPOSE, ATTAINMENT OF GOALS, DESIRED OUTCOMES, AND PERFORMANCE ACCOUNTABILITY
      2. ROLES WITHIN TEAMS ARE DESIGNATED OR EMERGE AS THE PURPOSE AND GOALS OF THE TEAM BECOME CLEAR. SOME INDIVIDUALS TAKE ON INFORMAL ROLES TO FACILITATE GROUP EFFECTIVENESS.
         a. Team leaders usually take on the leadership and management planning, organizing, and creation of the team process.
         b. Coordinators are similar to leaders in that they are aware of the team goals and direction and assist in keeping the team moving in the right direction.
         c. The mobilizer assists the leader and coordinator in keeping the team energized and interested in goal attainment.
         d. The team questioner is the person who asks the questions, even the ones that others want to ask but avoid, in order to keep the project goals and outcomes clear and concise.
         e. The antagonist is the team member who looks at the situation in the opposite manner as other team members and provides a "devil's advocate" approach to the team process.
         f. The team recorder is the person who records the details of team meetings, process, outcomes, and evaluation.
      3. ROLES OF DYSFUNCTIONAL TEAM MEMBERS INCLUDE THOSE ROLES AND ACTIVITIES THAT HINDER THE TEAM PROGRESS AND GOAL ATTAINMENT.
         a. Criticizers are characterized by resistance to all activities, plans, and goals of the team. If the process is not implemented in a way that they agree with, every action and comment is negative.
         b. Passive team members rarely have input for the team and remain in a quiet, noncontributing mode for fear of rebuttal from other team members.
         c. Detailers are those who get so saturated with the details of the team that it is difficult for them to focus on the goal and to see the bigger issues of the team.
         d. Controllers are those team members who try to monopolize the team process by constantly sharing their personal opinions.
         e. Team pleasers are those who avoid negative comments and unfavorable decisions in order to please the leader or other group members.

Figure 65-1 Considerations in delegation

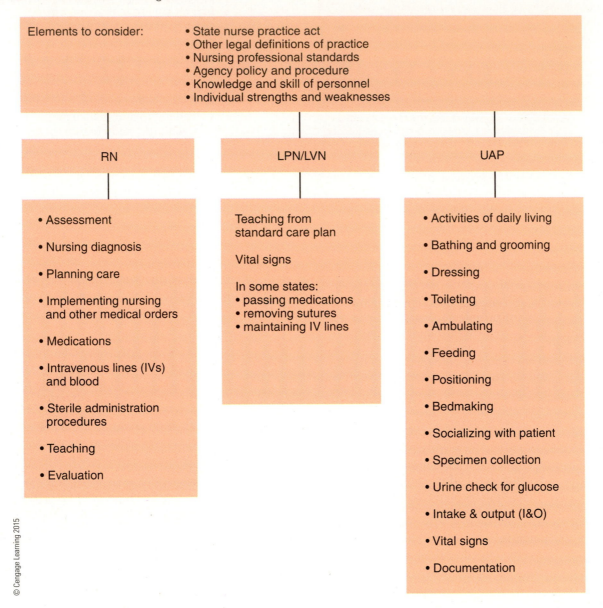

© Cengage Learning 2015

4. TEAM EVALUATION IS IMPORTANT IN ORDER TO ASSESS ACCOMPLISHMENT OF GOALS AND OUTCOMES. EVALUATION OF THE PURPOSE, GOALS, IMPLEMENTATION, OUTCOMES, AND TEAM MEMBER PARTICIPATION ARE IMPORTANT TO ENSURE FUTURE SUCCESS AND OUTCOMES.

B. EFFECTIVE COMMUNICATION STRATEGIES

1. ELEMENTS OF THE COMMUNICATION PROCESS (SEE FIGURE 65-2)

a. Communication is the exchange of information, often an interactive process that is influenced by the context.

b. Modes of communication include verbal, nonverbal, and electronic.

2. NURSES MUST BE EFFECTIVE COMMUNICATORS AND LEARN VARIOUS TECHNIQUES FOR ENHANCING INTERACTIONS WITH OTHER NURSES, THE INTERDISCIPLINARY HEALTH CARE TEAM, AND CLIENTS AND FAMILIES. COMMUNICATION SKILLS INCLUDE ATTENDING, RESPONDING, CLARIFYING, AND CONFRONTING (SEE TABLE 65-6).

3. BECAUSE NURSES COMMUNICATE WITH MANY DIVERSE INDIVIDUALS AND GROUPS IN THE WORK SETTING, SKILL SHOULD ALSO BE DEVELOPED RELATED TO THE IDENTIFICATION OF BARRIERS TO THE

Table 65-5 Summary of Conflict Resolution Techniques

Conflict Resolution Technique	Advantages	Disadvantages
Avoiding—ignoring the conflict	Does not make a big deal out of nothing; conflict may be minor in comparison to other priorities	Conflict can become bigger than anticipated; source of conflict might be more important to one person or group than others
Accommodating—smoothing or cooperating; one side gives in to the other side	One side is more concerned with an issue than the other side; stakes not high enough for one group and that side is willing to give in	One side holds more power and can force the other side to give in; the importance of the stakes are not as apparent to one side as the other; can lead to parties feeling "used" if they are always pressured to give in
Competing—forcing; the two or three sides are forced to compete for the goal	Produces a winner; good when time is short and stakes are high	Produces a loser; leaves anger and resentment on losing sides
Compromising—each side gives up something and gains something	No one should win or lose but both should gain something; good for disagreements between individuals	May cause a return to the conflict if what is given up becomes more important than the original goal
Negotiating—high-level discussion that seeks agreement but not necessarily consensus	Stakes are very high and solution is rather permanent; often involves powerful groups	Agreements are permanent, even though each side has gains and losses
Collaborating—both sides work together to develop optimal outcome	Best solution for the conflict and encompasses all goals important to each side	Takes a lot of time; requires commitment to success
Confronting—immediate and obvious movement to stop conflict at the very start	Does not allow conflict to take root; very powerful	May leave impression that conflict is not tolerated; may make something big out of nothing

© Cengage Learning 2015

Figure 65-2 Basic communication model

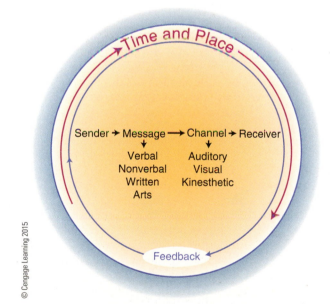

Time and Place

Sender → Message —→ Channel → Receiver

Verbal   Auditory
Nonverbal   Visual
Written   Kinesthetic
Arts

Feedback

© Cengage Learning 2015

Table 65-6 Additional Communication Skills

Skill	Description
Supporting	Siding with another person or backing up another person: "I can see that you would feel that way."
Focusing	Centers on the main point: "So your main concern is . . ."
Open-ended questioning	Allows for patient-directed responses: "How did that make you feel?"
Providing information	Supplies one with knowledge he did not previously have: "It's common for people with pneumonia to be tired."
Using silence	Allows for intrapersonal communication
Reassuring	Restores confidence or removes fear: "I can assure you that tomorrow . . ."
Expressing appreciation	Shows gratitude: "Thank you" or "You are thoughtful."
Using humor	Provides relief and gains perspective; may also cause harm so use carefully
Conveying acceptance	Makes known that one is capable or worthy: "It's okay to cry."
Asking related questions	Expands the listener's understanding: "How painful was it?"

© Cengage Learning 2015

COMMUNICATION PROCESS. BARRIERS TO EFFECTIVE COMMUNICATION INCLUDE GENDER AND CULTURAL DIFFERENCES, EMOTIONAL ISSUES SUCH AS STRESS AND ANGER, INCONGRUENT INTERACTIVE RESPONSES, AND CONFLICT (SEE TABLE 65-7).

C. INFLUENCE OF POWER
   1. DEFINITION OF *POWER*: THE ABILITY TO INFLUENCE OTHERS TOWARD GOAL ATTAINMENT; POWER INCLUDES THE ABILITY TO INFLUENCE ANOTHER INDIVIDUAL'S THINKING OR BEHAVIOR OR BOTH.

Table 65-7 Additional Barriers to Communication

Barrier	Description
Offering false reassurances	Promising something that cannot be delivered
Being defensive	Acting as though one has been attacked
Stereotyping	Unfairly categorizing someone based on his traits
Interrupting	Speaking before the other has completed his message
Inattention	Not paying attention
Stress	A state of tension that gets in the way of reasoning
Unclear expectations	Ill-defined tasks or duties that make successful completion unlikely

© Cengage Learning 2015

FOR EXAMPLE, THE NURSE INFLUENCES THE BEHAVIOR OF THE CLIENT AND FAMILY DURING HEALTH TEACHING SESSIONS.

2. SOURCES OF POWER RELATE TO FACTORS THAT ALLOW AN INDIVIDUAL TO INFLUENCE ANOTHER AND MAY BE FORMAL OR INFORMAL AND CONSCIOUS OR UNCONSCIOUS.

   a. Expert power: results from the knowledge and skill that a person possesses
   b. Legitimate power: derived from a position or role that a person holds personally or professionally; associated with some degree of authority as a result of the position
   c. Referent power: result of how much others like the individual, respect held for the individual, and trustworthiness of the person.
   d. Reward or coercive power: derived by the ability a person has to offer reward, punishment, or fear over another individual
   e. Connection power: the ability of an individual to connect to others and increase his influence by the number of people in the group with whom he is associated
   f. Information power: derived from a person's ability or position to influence others by the amount and kind of information possessed
   g. Empowerment versus disempowerment in managing client care

   1) Empowerment: the process of facilitating the participation of others in decision making or a specific activity through instilling the belief that the others have power that needs to be activated
   2) Disempowerment: the process of disabling or diminishing power in an individual or group by influencing the perceived power of that individual or group based on image, opinion, or actions

D. TIME MANAGEMENT IN NURSING
   1. DESCRIPTION
      a. The process or skill of decision making and priority setting that maximizes the most effective and productive use of time
      b. Nurse managers, nursing staff, and individuals connected to the health care delivery team must understand the larger organizational picture of the unit or institution in order to develop achievable goals and use time effectively.
      c. Time management strategies such as knowledge of the overall situation, planning and achieving quality outcomes, and priority setting are important in the overall achievement of client care outcomes. The following order of priority for client care is one example of an approach to time management on a given shift:
         1) Life-threatening or potentially life-threatening conditions
         2) Activities that ensure safety for clients, families, and coworkers
         3) Activities essential to the plan of care and achievement of optimal client outcomes
      d. Proper time management is important in decreasing the stress and burnout felt by nurses who are spending numerous hours in the work of managing client care. Strategies to enhance personal time management include scheduling personal time for self using periods of downtime efficiently, controlling distractions that interfere with personal time, and setting attainable personal goals such as exercise, rest, and education.

PRACTICE QUESTIONS

1. A family has recently moved to a new metropolitan area and is looking for a health care delivery system that will serve the needs of all family members, including a father who is an older adult and recently had a stroke and is in need of rehabilitative services. The nurse informs the family that which of the following agencies would be the best health care choice?
   1. A home health care service
   2. A university medical center and outpatient services
   3. A suburban community hospital
   4. Health promotion services for the entire family

2. A family selected population-based health care practice of America. The nurse manager teaching this family about the health care services available would include which of the following statements?
   1. "We have an asthma clinic specifically for clients of all ages."
   2. "The major initiative of our care delivery system is restorative care."
   3. "The main advantage to families is that palliative care is the main priority."
   4. "If specialty care is needed, the health care provider will make a referral to a tertiary care system."

3. Based on an understanding of evidence-based client care, the nurse manager should include which of the following instructions for the staff on how to address the home-care needs of a group of clients who have had knee replacements?
   1. "I know from experience that these clients will need a concrete exercise plan."
   2. "Most clients exhibit anxiety when describing the stairs within their homes."
   3. "Knee replacement care is complex because of the age of these clients."
   4. "Dietary instructions at home are based on common standards of practice and the most recent research for promoting healing."

4. A new graduate nurse is interviewing for a staff position in a health care delivery system that has agencies in five different states. Which of the following statements indicates that the new nurse understands the legalities of nursing practice, if hired by this company?

   1. "Standards of practice are established by the governing agency, so practice issues will be covered at each agency site."
   2. "A registered nurse license is acknowledged in all of the 50 states without additional paperwork."
   3. "The nurse practice act in each state will provide the legal guidelines for professional nursing practice."
   4. "The nurse will practice nursing at any of the five agencies based on the nurse practice act in the nurse's home state."

5. After reviewing incident reports for 1 month, a nurse working in the risk management department at a local health care facility determines which of the following violations of client care is most common?
   1. Physical abuse
   2. Substance abuse
   3. Malpractice actions
   4. Negligence of care

6. Which of the following laws require a nurse to report a peer who is keeping a portion of narcotics ordered for a client?
   1. Reporting laws
   2. Malpractice laws
   3. Jurisdiction laws
   4. Civil court laws

7. Which of the following should the nurse manager include in staff development classes related to ethical decision making?
   1. The practice of ethics is the philosophy of individual opinion and values
   2. Ethical decisions made in client care are based on the opinion of the client and family
   3. Ethical decision making is based on knowledge, facts, and a strong commitment to right and wrong
   4. Ethical decision making in client care can only be made by an interdisciplinary team

8. The nursing manager on the orthopedic unit evaluates a new staff nurse on the night shift as a born "leader," based on which of the following true leadership qualities?
   1. Having incomplete intake and output records on the night shift was a problem; records have been consistently complete since the new staff nurse arrived
   2. The new staff nurse has scheduled staff journal club discussions once a month to increase current knowledge about client care issues

3. The new staff nurse always works overtime when asked by the nurse manager
4. Incomplete shift counts for medications was first noticed by the new staff nurse

9. The astute nurse manager who wishes to empower the nurses on the unit recognizes that strategies must be found to promote their leadership ability. Which of the following supports the nurse manager's knowledge of leadership?
   1. Leadership qualities are demonstrated by those in formal and informal management positions
   2. Nurses at all levels of the organizational chart are not responsible for leadership traits
   3. Leadership characteristics are not measurable on performance appraisals
   4. Only top-level managers have the vision, passion, and integrity to demonstrate leadership

10. The nurse leader who empowers the staff to participate in decision-making activities is exhibiting which of the following leadership styles?
    1. Laissez-faire
    2. Situational
    3. Autocratic
    4. Democratic

11. The nurse describes which of the following leadership models as an integral part of the democratic leadership style?
    1. Transactional
    2. Transformational
    3. Transdepartmental
    4. Transprofessional

12. The management process is incorporated in many job descriptions, such as head nurse, staff nurse, nutritionist, and therapist. Which of the following managerial activities are common to all health care positions?
    Select all that apply:
    [ ] 1. Budgeting
    [ ] 2. Planning
    [ ] 3. Organizing
    [ ] 4. Liaison
    [ ] 5. Coordinating
    [ ] 6. Spokesperson

13. Which of the following are priorities for the nurse manager to incorporate into the nurse manager role of guiding and directing goal achievement?
    Select all that apply:
    [ ] 1. Collaborator
    [ ] 2. Caregiver
    [ ] 3. Negotiator
    [ ] 4. Delegator
    [ ] 5. Communicator
    [ ] 6. Liaison

14. The nurse manager introduces to the staff the new organizational policy and procedural changes for administering blood products. According to Lewin's model for implementing change, which of the following steps of the change process is the nurse manager addressing?
    1. Unfreeze
    2. Move
    3. Refreeze
    4. Evaluate

15. A staff nurse has been assigned to the Standards of Care Committee in which the standard of care for wound care and dressing changes is going to be refined. As an effective change agent, the staff nurse will need to exhibit which of the following characteristics?
    1. Quality interpersonal skills
    2. Respect from clients and families
    3. Expertise in clinical therapeutics
    4. High ethical decision making

16. The nurse manager and staff of a 25-bed surgical unit have decided to change the client care delivery model from primary nursing to team nursing. The nurse manager prepares which of the following statements for the administration that is most appropriate to support this change?
    1. "No transition period will be necessary because all staff have experience working in teams."
    2. "The staffing goal is to have four teams, with a total of three to four RNs, two to three LPNs, and two nursing assistants for each shift."
    3. "The nursing assistants, who are also senior nursing students, have the knowledge and skill to lead a staffing team."
    4. "The registered nurses on the unit will be assigned 24 hours of responsibility for client care planning."

17. Based on an understanding of the differentiated nursing practice model, nurses on the burn and trauma unit have decided to assign certain client care activities because
    1. nurses have client care rounds and discuss differences in client outcomes.
    2. there is a pay differential for registered nurses who work overtime.
    3. all unit staff are accountable for annual validation of cardiopulmonary resuscitation (CPR), safety precautions, and client confidentiality guidelines.
    4. Bachelor of science nurses (BSNs) and master of science nurses (MSNs) are expected to plan and implement education and research-based staff development sessions.

18. Based on an understanding of the nurse manager role, the nurse manager was notified at home of a staffing issue for the night shift because the
    1. nurse manager must be an autocratic leader.
    2. nurse manager has 24-hour, 7-day-a-week accountability for nursing care.
    3. regular staff members do not have managerial responsibility for problem-solving outcomes of staffing issues.
    4. nurse manager is responsible for all staff decisions, including staffing changes.

19. Which of the following roles is the charge nurse applying when assigning unlicensed assistive personnel (UAP) to tasks of custodial care, vital sign monitoring, and intake and output measurement for all the clients on the unit?
    1. Delegation
    2. Accountability
    3. Responsibility
    4. Outcome measurement

20. The nurse manager incorporates which of the following functional roles of the team members when planning to conduct a class on effective team building and group process?
    1. There will always be one person who wants to dominate the discussion using personal examples
    2. Every group needs a person in the role of creator, coordinator, and record keeper
    3. An effective team always rallies around the leadership traits demonstrated by the group or team spokesperson
    4. Some teams are motivated to get the job done in spite of dysfunctional behavior of a few team members

21. The communication process is essential to the leader or manager role and to the role of the manager of client care. It is essential for all managers, including the manager of client care, to be effective communicators. The nurse who effectively analyzes the communication process understands that messages are
    1. synchronous and asynchronous.
    2. coded and encoded.
    3. verbal and nonverbal.
    4. native and foreign.

22. Which of the following communication skills should the nurse include when planning to manage client care?
    Select all that apply:
    [ ] 1. Observation
    [ ] 2. Attending
    [ ] 3. Teaching
    [ ] 4. Responding
    [ ] 5. Clarifying
    [ ] 6. Focusing

23. The nurse should consider which of the following sources of power to be most effective within an organization?
    1. Expert
    2. Referent
    3. Connection
    4. Legitimate

24. The nurse should include which of the following in the discharge instructions given to a client who was recently diagnosed with diabetes mellitus to promote dietary compliance?
    1. Empowerment
    2. Authority
    3. Connectedness
    4. Charisma

25. The nurse manager called a meeting with one of the unit team leaders because clients have complained that they are not receiving their medication on time. The nurse manager should include which of the following good time management strategies during the meeting with the unit team leader?
    1. The nurse manager wants all team leaders to take the first hour of each shift to set client care priorities
    2. The nurse manager realizes that time management strategies are unrealistic when staffing is too low
    3. All team leaders must look at the overall work to be done and set appropriate priorities
    4. Optimal outcomes can only be achieved by implementing essential physical tasks

26. The charge nurse must transfer a client from a medical-surgical unit to a maternity unit in order to make a bed available. It would be most appropriate for the charge nurse to transfer which client?
    1. A 55-year-old client with tonic-clonic seizures
    2. A 22-year-old client with a gastrointestinal bleed on a vasopressin (Pitressin) drip
    3. A 40-year-old client who had a knee replacement with a continuous motion device
    4. A 30-year-old mastectomy client who will be discharged

ANSWERS AND RATIONALES

1. 2. Tertiary health care services include restorative and rehabilitative services for clients of all ages. A university medical center with outpatient services is best equipped to deliver care across the continuum for this family. A home health care service, suburban community, and health promotion services for the entire family are limited to a specific level of care.

2. 1. Population-based health care practice is the development, provision, and evaluation of multidisciplinary health care services to population groups experiencing an increased risk in partnership with consumers of health care and the community, in order to improve the health of the community and its diverse population groups. Population-based care is a managed care approach for a specific group of clients, not just individuals. The goal of care in a population-based system is to maintain and promote wellness, not restorative care. Specialty care and palliative care can be a part of the services, but may not be the priority; referral to a larger system is not necessary.

3. 4. Evidenced-based practice is a combination of knowledge and expertise in clinical practice, as well as the most recent research findings, used with each specific client. Although clients usually understand the exercise plan needed to strengthen overall muscle and joints, anxiety can be minimized with teaching and practice dealing with steps. Knee replacement care is complex, but the age of the client is not relevant. Dietary instructions, such as increase in protein, are important for healing following a knee replacement.

4. 3. Nurse practice acts may differ from state to state. The state board of nursing for each state monitors the legal practice of nursing in each state. Although standards of care may be policy at each agency, they do not override the standards outlined in the nurse practice act for each agency's state. Once an RN license has been obtained, reciprocity to practice in other states must be granted by each state board.

5. 4. Negligence is the most common violation of client care in health care facilities. Negligence is a deviation from the appropriate standard of care, usually due to carelessness. Physical abuse, substance abuse, and malpractice actions are all criminal acts and occur less frequently.

6. 1. Reporting laws in each state require a professional to report incompetent practice, client abuse, and professional impairment. Malpractice laws, jurisdiction laws, and civil court laws may vary from state to state.

7. 3. Making ethical decisions requires skill in analyzing knowledge, facts, rules of care, and a strong personal distinction between what is right and wrong in a specific client situation. Opinion is not the driving force in decision making. Ethical decision making in client care made by an interdisciplinary team is ultimately possible when ethics committees meet to discuss individual client cases. It is important to remember that every nurse practices as an individual professional and incorporates ethical decision making into everyday practice.

8. 2. Knowing the importance of keeping up-to-date on practice issues and having the confidence to implement a strategy to discuss client care issues as a new staff member both demonstrate leadership quality in this staff nurse.

9. 1. Leadership qualities and an ability to influence others to achieve goals can be exhibited by any employee in an organization. Individuals with good management skills may not demonstrate leadership ability.

10. 4. Democratic leaders seek participation in decision-making activities by all levels of staff affected at the unit level. Laissez-faire leadership is a passive and permissive style of leadership that defers decision making. An autocratic leadership style involves decision making that is centralized, with the leader making decisions and using power to command and control others. Situational leadership confirms that there is not one best leadership style, but rather that effective leadership is matched to the group's level of task-relevant readiness.

11. 2. Transformational leadership theory includes explicitly seeking collaboration, consultation, and consensus building among team members. Transactional leadership model is aligned with transactional leadership. Transdepartmental and transprofessional are strategies, not leadership models, for gathering information across departments within an organization or within the profession as a whole.

12. 2. 3. 5. Managers of human resources, client care, and other health-related disciplines include role functions of planning, organizing, and coordinating client care activities. Not all personnel have the responsibilities of budgeting, department liaison, or director and spokesperson.

13. 1. 3. 4. 5. Although functioning as a caregiver and liaison is possible, the functions that are the priority for the nurse manager are collaborator, negotiator, delegator, and communicator. Nurse managers may have to assume the duties of caregiver in certain circumstances, but usually they do not have a client care assignment. The liaison role is usually carried out by the nursing staff, on behalf of the client. The nurse manager would function as spokesperson to speak on behalf of the staff of a department.

14. 1. The first step for implementing change, or unfreezing, is to assist others to understand the need for change and the steps necessary to implement the change. Communication and information sharing are essential in this step. Actual implementation of the change and accepting the change as the standard of care are activities that occur with moving and refreezing. Evaluating is necessary for overall quality management, but is not a part of the change process as described by Lewin's change theory.

15. 1. Although respect from clients and families, expertise in clinical therapeutics, and high ethical decision making are admirable for the staff nurse, the change process related to procedure of wound care and dressing changes will need to be discussed hospital-wide, unit by unit, utilizing quality interpersonal skills. Teaching and information sharing are essential when a change affects so many people, and these require quality interpersonal skills.

16. 2. A staffing goal of having four teams with a total of three to four RNs, two to three LPNs, and two nursing assistants is the best staffing option for implementing care based on flexibility and acuity of client care for a 25-bed unit. Transition in staffing and operational issues will be necessary even if all staff members have previously worked using a team nursing model. Assuming that all nursing assistants are senior nursing students is not a legally sound staffing assignment. Assigning a registered nurse to be responsible for 24-hour client care is indicative of a primary nursing model.

17. 4. Expectations to plan and implement education and research-based staff development sessions by bachelor of science nurses (BSNs) and master of science nurses (MSNs) are best, considering that the assignment of educational sessions is based on the education level of the nursing staff. Differentiated practice includes the assignment of duties based on education level, competence, and certification. Nurses who have client care rounds, staff nurses who work overtime, and unit staff members who are held accountable for violation of unit requirements all require nurses to do similar activities regardless of education, clinical expertise, and competence levels.

18. 2. The nurse manager has 24-hour, 7-day-a-week accountability for nursing care. Nursing staff members are participative decision makers because of their position in the organization.

Staff members should have input into the overall decision-making process.

19. 1. Delegation is the assignment of tasks to others who are competent and skilled to perform them. Accountability and responsibility are qualities that all caregivers must demonstrate, regardless of level of position. Although the unlicensed assistive personnel (UAP) may collect data to carry out a nursing task, a nurse at a higher education level would be responsible for the overall evaluation and reporting.

20. 2. Every group needs a person in the role of creator and coordinator as well as a record keeper. This description contains the functional roles of members of a team. A dominator is a person who wants to dominate. Some teams always rally around the leadership traits of a member of the group or team, but it takes all team members working together collaboratively to be an effective team. Some teams are motivated to get the job done in spite of the dysfunctional behavior of a few team members, but to be a more effective group all team members need to work together.

21. 3. The most effective communication process includes both verbal and nonverbal cues. The terms synchronous and asynchronous and coded and encoded describe communication concepts within computer technology. Native and foreign describe language as being one's first, or native, language or a language learned later, that is, a foreign language.

22. 2. 4. 5. 6. Facilitating communication requires more than verbal and nonverbal cues. Strategies to enhance understanding of the message communicated by the client and others will assist the nurse to provide quality, accurate feedback. Communication skills that should be used to manage client care include attending, responding, clarifying, and focusing. Observation and teaching are skills needed by the nurse in planning client care, but are not necessarily strategies for accurate and effective communication.

23. 4. Legitimate power is the minimum source of power, derived by merely holding a position of authority. Expert, referent, and connection are all sources of power that are derived in ways other than by holding a position. Expert power is power derived from the knowledge and skills the nurse possesses. Referent power, also known as charismatic power, is power conferred by others, based on their respect and liking for an individual, group or organization. Connection power is the connection between nurses having power, such as networking between positions of authority.

24. 1. Empowerment involves the ability to facilitate the participation of others to action and appropriate decision making. In the case of a client with diabetes mellitus and the need for dietary compliance, the nurse facilitates empowerment and compliance by teaching the client what the correct choices are. Authority and charisma do not ensure compliance. For some older clients, these traits of authority and charisma might be negative influences. Connectedness is a possible influence on the client, but because it would require that the nurse connect often with the client to assess compliance, it would not be a realistic motivator.

25. 3. All team leaders must look at the overall work to be done and set appropriate priorities. Time management can be accomplished by knowing the overall needs of the clients and then setting appropriate priorities. Team leaders who take the first half hour of every shift to set priorities are lacking time management skills; the tasks could be handled by efficient shift reporting. During a nursing shortage, time management skills are essential and should be realistic.

26. 1. Obstetrical nurses would have the appropriate knowledge and skills to care for a client having seizures because they routinely care for pregnant women who have hypertension and experience eclampsia (seizures).

REFERENCE

Kelly, P. (2012). *Nursing leadership and management* (3rd ed.). Clifton Park, NY: Delmar Cengage Learning.

CHAPTER 66

ETHICAL ISSUES

I. **ETHICS**
   A. DESCRIPTION
      1. ETHICS IS A WAY OF EXAMINING, UNDERSTANDING, AND MAKING DECISIONS ABOUT WHAT ACTIONS ARE RIGHT OR WRONG ACCORDING TO SOCIETAL NORMS AND ACCEPTED MORALITY.
      2. IT IS THE RESPONSIBILITY OF ALL NURSES TO RECOGNIZE ETHICAL ISSUES AND APPLY ETHICAL PRINCIPLES AND METHODS OF ETHICAL DECISION MAKING ON A DAILY BASIS.
      3. AN ETHICAL ISSUE OR DILEMMA ARISES WHEN THERE IS A DECISION TO BE MADE BUT IT IS NOT CLEAR WHAT MAY BE RIGHT OR WRONG DUE TO REASONABLE ARGUMENTS AND CONFLICTING MORAL PRINCIPLES OR RULES FOR EITHER ACTION.
      4. ETHICAL THEORIES GUIDE THE WAY A NURSE EXAMINES A SITUATION.
      5. PROFESSIONS SUCH AS NURSING DEVELOP CODES OF CONDUCT TO COMMUNICATE THE VALUES OF THE PROFESSION AND REINFORCE AND GUIDE ETHICAL BEHAVIOR AMONG ITS MEMBERS IN ORDER TO DEMONSTRATE ITS COMMITMENT TO THE TRUST GRANTED IT BY SOCIETY.
      6. ETHICS COMMITTEES EXIST TO PROVIDE CONSULTATION AND GUIDANCE TO HEALTH CARE PROFESSIONALS FACED WITH COMPLEX ETHICAL DILEMMAS; HOWEVER, THEIR PURPOSE IS NOT TO RESOLVE THE DILEMMA.
   B. PHYSIOLOGICAL BASIS ON WHICH TO ESTABLISH ETHICAL THEORIES
      1. NATURALISM
         a. View of moral judgment that sees ethics as dependent on human nature and psychology
         b. Explains differences in moral codes to social conditions and at the same time suggesting a basic congruence to the possession by underlying psychological tendencies, suggesting there is a universality in moral judgment
         c. Individuals or a group of individuals make judgments based on feelings about certain actions in certain situations, resulting in most individuals' judgments being much the same in situations that are the same.
      2. RATIONALISM
         a. Opposite view of naturalism
         b. Belief that feelings, although viewed as similar in people, may not be similar at all
         c. The foundation of this belief is based on absolute truth that is not dependent on human nature.
         d. Belief that values in ethics have an origin in the nature of the universe or God that may become known through the process of reasoning
         e. Belief that there are truths about the world that are not only true but universal and superior to the information received by the senses
         f. Perceive moral rules as true

II. **ETHICAL THEORIES**
   A. DESCRIPTION: A FRAMEWORK THAT GUIDES A NURSE'S REFLECTION ON THE DILEMMA
   B. TYPES
      1. UTILITARIANISM
         a. The right action is that which yields the greatest good for the greatest number of people.
         b. Gives equal weight to all parties involved in the dilemma
         c. Based on the principle of utility or achieving the maximum value out of the action

      d. "Act utilitarianism"—moral rules can be suspended in some circumstances if they do not maximize the greatest good for the greatest number.

      e. "Rule utilitarianism"—moral rules may not be suspended because doing so does not lead to the greatest good in the long run.

  2. KANTIANISM

      a. Categorical imperative—the action is right if such an action is willed to become a universal law.

      b. Persons must be treated as ends and never as only a means to an end.

      c. Correct actions are based on one's obligations to others.

      d. May be called deontology or formalism

  3. VIRTUE OR CHARACTER ETHICS

      a. Believes an individual is capable of learning and practicing through the repetition of acts

      b. The virtue is habituated.

      c. May be used to nurture or predict character in individuals

III. ETHICAL PRINCIPLES

  A. DESCRIPTION

    1. MAKE UP PRINCIPLE-BASED OR COMMON-MORALITY THEORY

    2. INCORPORATE CONCEPTS FROM OTHER THEORIES

    3. MUST BE BALANCED AGAINST EACH OTHER WHEN MAKING AN ETHICAL DECISION

  B. AUTONOMY

    1. SELF-RULE AND FREEDOM TO ACT

    2. OPPOSITE OF PATERNALISM

    3. NURSES MUST SAFEGUARD THE CLIENTS' AUTONOMY BY PROVIDING INFORMATION AND PROTECTING CLIENTS FROM CONTROLLING CONSTRAINTS SO THEY MAY USE THEIR FREEDOM EFFECTIVELY.

    4. A CLIENT'S AUTONOMY SHOULD BE RESPECTED AS LONG AS IN SO DOING IT DOES NOT POSE A GREATER HARM TO OTHERS.

    5. MAY BE SUSPENDED IF A CLIENT IS INCAPABLE OF SELF-RULE, SUCH AS INFANTS OR SUICIDAL CLIENTS

    6. LIMITED AUTONOMY TO MAKE DECISIONS ABOUT MEALS AND SOME CARE SHOULD BE GRANTED EVEN TO CLIENTS WHO ARE NOT DEEMED COMPETENT TO MAKE LEGAL OR OTHER TYPES OF DECISIONS

    7. INFORMED CONSENT—PROVIDING SUFFICIENT INFORMATION AND GUIDANCE TO THE CLIENT SO THAT SHE MAY ACCEPT OR DECLINE A PROCEDURE OR PARTICIPATION IN RESEARCH IS BASED ON THIS PRINCIPLE.

  C. BENEFICENCE

    1. DOING GOOD OR TO BENEFIT OTHERS

    2. WHAT ONE OUGHT TO DO, SUCH AS PREVENTING OR REMOVING HARM OR PROMOTING GOOD

    3. REQUIRED TO DO GOOD BASED ON THE RELATIONSHIP BETWEEN PARTIES, SUCH AS THE NURSE–CLIENT RELATIONSHIP

    4. USUALLY OVERRIDDEN BY RESPECT FOR AUTONOMY, SUCH AS THE NURSE RESPECTING THE CLIENT'S RIGHT TO AUTONOMY TO CHOOSE OVER THE NURSE'S OBLIGATION TO DO GOOD

  D. NONMALEFICENCE

    1. OBLIGATION NOT TO CAUSE INTENTIONAL HARM

    2. MUST BE OBEYED REGARDLESS OF RELATIONSHIP

    3. PROVIDE REASONS FOR LEGAL PROHIBITION OF CERTAIN ACTIVITIES

  E. JUSTICE

    1. FAIRNESS AND APPROPRIATE DISTRIBUTION OF RESOURCES

    2. THESE CONCEPTS RELATE TO HEALTH CARE POLICY AND SOCIAL PROGRAMS.

  F. CONFIDENTIALITY

    1. REQUIRES NONDISCLOSURE OF PRIVATE OR SECRET INFORMATION THAT ONE IS ENTRUSTED WITH

    2. THIS PRINCIPLE IS BASED ON THE OATHS OF NURSING.

    3. NOT DIVULGING INFORMATION SHARED IN CONFIDENCE

    4. CLIENTS HAVE A RIGHT TO EXPECT THAT THEIR PRIVATE MEDICAL INFORMATION WILL NOT BE SHARED WITH ANYONE OTHER THAN THOSE NEEDING IT TO PROVIDE THEIR CARE.

  G. FIDELITY

    1. RELATES TO THE CONCEPT OF FAITHFULNESS AND THE PRACTICE OF KEEPING PROMISES AND LOYALTY WITHIN THE NURSE–CLIENT RELATIONSHIP

    2. PROMISE KEEPING AND TRUST

    3. LOYALTY TO THE CLIENT

    4. CLIENT ABANDONMENT IS AN EXAMPLE OF BREACHING THIS RULE.

  H. VERACITY

    1. TRUTH TELLING

    2. THE OBLIGATION TO TELL THE TRUTH IS BASED ON RESPECT FOR OTHERS.

    3. VITAL TO MAINTENANCE OF THE THERAPEUTIC RELATIONSHIP

IV. ETHICAL DECISION MAKING

A. DESCRIPTION

1. MULTIPLE FRAMEWORKS EXIST BY WHICH TO SYSTEMATICALLY EVALUATE THE ETHICAL THEORIES AND PRINCIPLES RELEVANT AND IN CONFLICT IN A GIVEN ETHICAL DILEMMA.
2. NURSES SHOULD CHOOSE AND USE ETHICAL DECISION-MAKING TOOLS TO GUIDE THEM IN THEIR ACTIONS.
3. HOSPITAL ETHICS COMMITTEES SHOULD BE UTILIZED BY NURSES WHENEVER THERE IS CONFLICT OVER RESOLUTION OF AN ETHICAL DILEMMA.

V. RELATIONSHIP BETWEEN ETHICS AND THE LAW

A. DESCRIPTION

1. ETHICS IS THE FOUNDATION OF THE LAW.
2. LAW IS THE SYSTEM OF RULES OF ACTION OR CONDUCT THAT DETERMINES THE BEHAVIOR OF INDIVIDUALS IN RESPECT TO RELATIONSHIPS WITH OTHERS AND THE GOVERNMENT.
3. BECAUSE LAWS ARE CREATED BY INDIVIDUALS, ETHICS AND LAW ARE NOT ALWAYS CONGRUENT.
4. LAWS FALL INTO PUBLIC OR PRIVATE REALMS AND ARE CONSTITUTIONAL, STATUTORY, OR ADMINISTRATIVE.
   a. Constitutional law is based on the Constitution and takes precedence over all other laws.
   b. Legislative law, also known as statutory law, is developed at the state or federal legislatures.
   c. Administrative law consists of legal powers given to administrative agencies by legislative bodies and the rules the agencies implement to carry out those policies such as the state boards of nursing.
   d. Common law, also known as case law, is a type of law based on previous court decisions.

B. TYPES OF LAW

1. PUBLIC LAW IS THE RELATIONSHIP BETWEEN INDIVIDUALS AND THE GOVERNMENT.
2. PRIVATE LAW IS THE RELATIONSHIP BETWEEN INDIVIDUALS.
3. CONTRACT LAW DEALS WITH THE OBLIGATIONS AND RIGHTS OF INDIVIDUALS WHO MAKE CONTRACTS, SUCH AS AN IMPLIED CONTRACT BETWEEN THE NURSE AND THE CLIENT TO DELIVER SAFE AND COMPETENT CARE.
4. TORT LAW IS AN INJURY OR WRONGFUL ACT THAT AN INDIVIDUAL SUFFERS BECAUSE OF ANOTHER INDIVIDUAL'S INTENTIONAL OR UNINTENTIONAL ACTIONS INVOLVING THE CONCEPTS OF MALPRACTICE AND NEGLIGENCE, MAKING IT THE DIVISION OF LAW THE NURSE IS MOST FAMILIAR WITH.
   a. Negligence is the omission of an act that another reasonable individual would do in the same situation, such as a nurse who fails to wipe up a water spill on the floor that the client had spilled.
   b. Malpractice is a type of negligence in which there is a professional misconduct due to a lack of professional skill that results in harm to the client, such as a medication error.

VI. LEGAL ISSUES

A. INFORMED CONSENT

1. PROVIDES LEGAL PROTECTION TO A CLIENT'S RIGHT TO PERSONAL AUTONOMY, SUCH AS A CLIENT WHO MAY CHOOSE A COURSE OF ACTION REGARDING THE PLAN FOR HER HEALTH CARE
2. INCLUDES DISCLOSURE AND ESSENTIAL INFORMATION THAT WILL ALLOW A CLIENT TO MAKE AN INFORMED DECISION ABOUT THE CARE RECEIVED (SEE TABLE 66-1)
3. THE CLIENT HAS THE OPPORTUNITY TO ACCEPT OR REFUSE THE PROPOSED TREATMENT.
4. ALTHOUGH TREATMENT RECOMMENDATIONS MAY BE GIVEN, THE CLIENT'S CONSENT MUST BE FREE OF COERCION OR MANIPULATION BY THE HEALTH CARE PROVIDER.
5. BEFORE WITNESSING A CONSENT, THE NURSE SHOULD ASSESS IF THE CLIENT HAS A CLEAR

Table 66-1 Content of Informed Consent

The nature of the health concern and prognosis if nothing is done
Description of all treatment options, even those that the health care provider does not favor or cannot provide
The benefits, risks, and consequences of the various treatment alternatives, including noninterventions

UNDERSTANDING OF A PROPOSED PROCEDURE OR NEEDS FURTHER EXPLANATION, SUCH AS EXPLAINING THE BENEFITS AND RISKS OF SURGERY.

B. ADVANCE DIRECTIVES

   1. DIRECTIONS THAT ARE IMPLEMENTED OR WITHHELD OR A DESIGNATION OF SOMEONE WHO WILL ACT AS A SURROGATE IN MAKING DECISIONS FOR AN INDIVIDUAL WHO LOSES THE CAPABILITY TO MAKE DECISIONS

   2. MAY BE CONSIDERED A FORM OF WRITTEN CONSENT FOR FUTURE INTERVENTIONS, SUCH AS LIFE AND DEATH ISSUES WHEN THE CLIENT IS UNABLE TO MAKE THOSE DECISIONS

   3. THE PATIENT SELF-DETERMINATION ACT REQUIRES HOSPITALS, NURSING HOMES, HEALTH MAINTENANCE ORGANIZATIONS, AND HOME CARE AGENCIES TO PROVIDE WRITTEN INFORMATION TO ADULT CLIENTS REGARDING THEIR RIGHTS TO MAKE DECISIONS ABOUT THEIR HEALTH CARE DECISIONS.

   4. NURSES HAVE THE RESPONSIBILITY TO MAKE SURE CLIENTS HAVE THE RIGHT TO COMPLETE ADVANCE DIRECTIVES AND TO ENSURE THAT THEIR WISHES ARE CARRIED THROUGH WHEN THE TIME COMES.

   5. NURSES NEED TO KNOW THEIR STATE'S STATUTES THAT GUIDE ADVANCE DIRECTIVES.

   6. THE NURSE HAS THE RESPONSIBILITY TO UNDERSTAND THE CLIENT'S WISHES FOR ADVANCE DIRECTIVES AND TO COMMUNICATE THOSE WISHES TO OTHER MEMBERS OF THE HEALTH CARE TEAM.

   7. A CLIENT WHO IS ADMITTED WITH AN ADVANCE DIRECTIVE DOES NOT NECESSARILY MEAN THAT THE CLIENT HAS A DO-NOT-RESUSCITATE (DNR) ORDER.

C. DO NOT RESUSCITATE ORDERS

   1. DIRECTIONS TO WITHHOLD CARDIOPULMONARY RESUSCITATION (CPR) THAT MUST BE WRITTEN AND PLACED IN A CLIENT'S MEDICAL RECORD

   2. WHETHER TO INITIATE CPR REQUIRES PROFESSIONAL, ETHICAL, LEGAL, AND INSTITUTIONAL CONSIDERATIONS.

   3. THE GENERAL PRINCIPLE FOR WHEN TO IMPLEMENT CPR IS THAT IT SHOULD BE INITIATED UNLESS IT WOULD BE FUTILE TO DO SO OR UNLESS THE PHYSICIAN HAS SPECIFIC ORDERS NOT TO DO SO.

   4. THE DNR ORDER SHOULD BE IMMEDIATELY DOCUMENTED IN A CLIENT'S MEDICAL RECORD, STATING WHY THE ORDER WAS WRITTEN, WHO GAVE THE CONSENT, WHO WAS PRESENT FOR THE DISCUSSION, IF THE CLIENT WAS COMPETENT TO GIVE CONSENT, AND THE TIME FRAME FOR THE DNR ORDER.

   5. PRIOR TO MAKING AN INFORMED CONSENT, THE CLIENT AND THE FAMILY SHOULD BE INFORMED ABOUT THE CLIENT'S CONDITION AND PROGNOSIS.

   6. A DNR ORDER REQUIRES THE NURSE TO BE FOCUSED ON COMFORT INTERVENTIONS AND TO SERVE AS A SUPPORT SYSTEM.

   7. THE NURSE NEEDS TO BE INFORMED OF EACH CLIENT'S ORDERS.

PRACTICE QUESTIONS

1. A student nurse asks the nurse, "Why did my advisor recommend an ethics class for me?" Which of the following is the best response by the nurse?
   1. "It is the responsibility of nurses to recognize ethical dilemmas in clinical situations."
   2. "Ethics must be learned in order to obey the law."
   3. "You must have misunderstood because nurses do not have to study ethics."
   4. "You may find studying ethics interesting."

2. The nurse tells another nurse that which of the following best describes the purpose of the American Nurses Association Code for Nurses?
   1. To communicate the values of the profession
   2. To defend the actions of nurses in lawsuits
   3. To develop the good character of nurses
   4. To help recognize nurses for their ethical behavior

3. Which of the following is the best example of an ethical dilemma faced by the nurse?
   1. Deciding whether or not to place a client in a private room
   2. Deciding whether or not to tell a client about the client's diagnosis
   3. Deciding the order in which staff members should take their breaks
   4. Deciding whether or not to ask another nurse to care for a very complex patient

4. A nurse is asked to keep the client's cancer progression from family members until after a daughter's wedding next week, so as not to distract from this important day. This will require the nurse to withhold information from the client's spouse and daughter who accompanied the client to the clinic. Which of the following actions by the nurse best demonstrates the theory of utilitarianism?
   1. The nurse tells the client that truth telling is an ethical rule that nurses must uphold and asks the client to reconsider this request
   2. The nurse tells the client's spouse about the disease progression in secret, making the spouse promise not to tell the client
   3. The nurse does as the client wishes and keeps the diagnosis from the family until after the wedding
   4. The nurse informs the client that sharing the diagnosis will facilitate coping and that the family must be told today in the clinic

5. A nurse is asked to keep the client's cancer progression from family members indefinitely. This will require the nurse to withhold information from the client's spouse, who frequently accompanies the client to the clinic. Which of the following actions by the nurse best demonstrates the theory of Kantianism?
   1. The nurse persuades the client to tell the family because it is the right thing to do
   2. The nurse considers multiple ethical principles and supports the client in telling the family, as should be done universally in such a situation
   3. The nurse remembers the ethical rule of truth telling and decides to tell the client's spouse in secret
   4. The nurse considers multiple ethical principles and does not tell the family, because client confidentiality is of primary importance

6. After the physician explains the surgery to the client, the nurse provides the client with information about surgery, answers the client's questions, and allows the client to agree or refuse to have surgery. Which of the following ethical principles is best described by the nurse's actions?
   1. Nonmaleficence
   2. Beneficence
   3. Truth telling
   4. Autonomy

7. The nurse informs a young, healthy client that the scarce amount of flu vaccine will be given to older clients and those with immunosuppressed responses first. Which of the following ethical principles is best described by the nurse's statement?
   1. Beneficence
   2. Autonomy
   3. Justice
   4. Nonmaleficence

8. The nurse chooses to delay taking a break so that pain medication could be administered on time rather than making the client wait until the nurse's break is complete. Which of the following ethical principles is best described by the nurse's action?
   1. Beneficence
   2. Justice
   3. Nonmaleficence
   4. Autonomy

9. A mentally ill client with an order for a general diet requests a vegetarian meal. Which of the following actions by the nurse best demonstrates the nurse's understanding of the principle of autonomy?
   1. Tell the client that a vegetarian meal cannot be substituted for a general diet
   2. If necessary, obtain an order from the physician for a vegetarian meal; otherwise, provide a vegetarian meal per the client's request
   3. Contact the client's family and obtain their consent to provide a vegetarian meal to the client
   4. Contact the client's medical power of attorney for permission to make a diet change

10. The nurse returns to the client's room in exactly four hours to administer the next dose of pain medication as promised. Which of the following ethical rules is best demonstrated by the nurse?
    1. Justice
    2. Nonmaleficence
    3. Fidelity
    4. Confidentiality

ANSWERS AND RATIONALES

1. 2. 1. Recognizing ethical dilemmas is the responsibility of all nurses, as well as physicians. Ethical behavior is a component of both law and religion, but knowledge of these areas does not render studying ethics unnecessary.

2. 1. The ethical codes of professions, such as nursing, are developed to communicate the values of the profession and to guide ethical behavior among its members. The code cannot make nurses behave ethically, nor is its purpose to defend nursing to other professionals or in legal matters.

3. 2. An ethical dilemma exists when the nurse must make a decision about what is right or wrong, but there are conflicting moral principles or rules with any action taken. While deciding on room assignments and breaks are decisions nurses make daily, these are not ethical dilemmas. Nurses should use good judgment and refuse being assigned to clients whose care is too complex for their training. Withholding information about a diagnosis potentially brings up conflicting issues of veracity, fidelity, and beneficence and is therefore an ethical dilemma.

4. 3. Utilitarianism is a moral theory that holds an action is judged as good or bad in relation to the consequences. It attempts to maximize the greatest good for the greatest number, giving equal weight to all parties involved. The nurse must consider the feelings of the client, family members, and all others potentially affected by the sharing of the diagnosis. According to the theory of utilitarianism, the nurse must suspend the principle of veracity in order to fulfill the wishes of the client and sustain the happiness that is sure to come to the family members through the wedding celebration. Although obtaining support from one's family does support coping, there is no indication that the client is not coping well at this time, and there will be time for coping after the wedding. The nurse must also consider the obligation to uphold the client's confidentiality.

5. 2. Kantianism, also called deontology, is based on the rationalist view that the rightness or wrongness of an act depends on the nature of the act. The theory of Kantianism uses the categorical imperative to test actions. This imperative states that a person should act as

one would wish everyone to act (as if it were a universal law) in that situation. It also says that persons should be treated as ends rather than as means to an end. Pressuring the client treats the client as a means to the end, with which the nurse feels more comfortable and avoids conflict. Keeping the disease progression secret supports the client in treating the spouse as a means to an end by being dishonest. Neither truth telling nor confidentiality alone always applies under this theory, but what is important is a consideration of how one ought to behave if one's actions were to become a universal law. Because sharing the cancer diagnosis with the family is known to support coping of the client and family, it would be generally accepted to support this behavior in most situations in order to uphold principles of beneficence, autonomy, and rule of veracity. Therefore, the nurse should not take the responsibility of telling, but should provide guidance, education, and support to the client's behavior of telling.

6. 4. The principle of autonomy is upheld when sufficient information and guidance are provided by the nurse so that the client may freely give informed consent. Beneficence is doing good, whereas nonmaleficence is not doing harm. Truth telling is an ethical rule rather than a principle, and relates to the nurse's obligation to be truthful out of respect for the client.

7. 3. Equitable distribution of resources is described by the principle of justice. Beneficence is doing good, and nonmaleficence is not doing harm. Autonomy is providing the freedom to act.

8. 1. Beneficence is described as doing what one ought to do to promote good. Nonmaleficence is not causing intentional harm. Justice is the equitable distribution of resources. Autonomy is upholding a client's right to make informed choices.

9. 2. Limited autonomy, such as what type of meal to eat, may be granted to those clients who are not deemed competent for other medical decisions. Neither the client's family nor the power of attorney needs to be contacted to make a diet change, even if they make other types of medical decisions for the client.

10. 3. Justice and nonmaleficence are ethical principles dealing with fair distribution of

services and doing no harm. These are
principles, not rules. Confidentiality is
an ethical rule emphasizing the importance
of respecting the client's right to privacy

of information. Fidelity is the rule
demonstrated by this nurse by keeping
the promise made and returning with the
pain medication.

REFERENCES

Burkhardt, M. A., & Nathaniel, A. K. (2008). *Ethics and issues in contemporary nursing* (3rd ed.). Clifton Park, NY: Delmar Cengage Learning.

Kelly, P. (2012). *Nursing leadership and management.* Clifton Park, NY: Delmar Cengage Learning.

CHAPTER 67

LEGAL ISSUES FOR OLDER ADULTS

I. **LEGAL ISSUES OF THE OLDER ADULT**
   A. DESCRIPTION
      1. REGISTERED NURSES PRACTICING WITH OLDER ADULTS AND THEIR FAMILIES NEED KNOWLEDGE OF BASIC LAWS AND MUST BE SURE THEIR PRACTICE FALLS WITHIN LEGAL BOUNDARIES.
      2. CLIENTS AND FAMILIES MAY ASK FOR ADVICE ABOUT WILLS AND ADVANCE DIRECTIVES.
      3. NURSES MUST BE ADVOCATES FOR OLDER ADULTS AND PROTECT THEIR RIGHTS.
   B. LEGAL RISKS FOR NURSING PRACTICE WITH THE OLDER ADULT
      1. SITUATIONS THAT INCREASE THE RISK OF LIABILITY FOR A NURSE INCLUDE:
         a. Working with insufficient resources
         b. Failing to follow policies and procedures
         c. Taking shortcuts
         d. Working when physically or emotionally exhausted
      2. WHEN THE STANDARD OF CARE FOR A GIVEN GROUP, SUCH AS OLDER ADULTS, OR SITUATION IS NOT FOLLOWED BY THE NURSE, NEGLIGENCE OR MALPRACTICE MAY BE CHARGED.
         a. Administering the incorrect dosage of a medication and the client suffers harm
         b. Identifying a serious client behavior such as respiratory distress and not informing the physician in a timely manner
         c. Not providing for the safety of a client, such as pouring liquid soap for wound cleansing into a medicine cup and leaving it at the bedside of a client who is confused and the client drinks it
         d. Failing to turn an immobile client for an entire shift and the client gets a pressure ulcer
         e. Placing a food tray outside the reach of a client who is unable to self-feed
      3. THE FOLLOWING CONDITIONS MUST BE PRESENT FOR MALPRACTICE TO EXIST:
         a. There was a failure to perform at the level of the standard of care.
         b. Physical or mental injury resulted to the client or a violation of the client's right resulted from the nurse's negligence.
      4. ACTS THAT COULD RESULT IN LEGAL LIABILITY INCLUDE:
         a. Assault: a deliberate threat or attempt to harm another person that the person believes could be carried through, such as telling a client that if breakfast is not eaten, lunch will not be provided.
         b. Battery: unconsented touching of the client in a socially impermissible way or carrying through an assault, such as performing a procedure without consent
         c. Defamation of character: an oral or written communication to a third party that damages a person's reputation, such as when transferring a client from one facility to another and writing on the transfer papers "He's a dirty old man. Watch out!"
         d. False imprisonment: unlawful restraint or detention of a person, such as physically preventing a client who is competent from leaving a facility or even telling a client that she will be tied to the bed or locked up when trying to leave
         e. Fraud: willful and intentional misrepresentation intended to produce an unlawful gain, such as overcharging a client for services; older adults tend to be trusting and easy prey for fraud from strangers, acquaintances, or unscrupulous family members.

f. Invasion of privacy: invading the right of a client to personal privacy, for example, an unwanted publicity such as putting a picture of the client in the paper without permission, releasing a medical record to unauthorized persons, giving client information to an inappropriate person or agency (allowing a student nurse who is not assigned to a client to look at that client's chart), or having one's private affairs made public (discussing a client in a public place where the discussion can be heard). Federal regulations, as well as the state, govern the client's privacy.

g. Larceny: unlawful taking of a client's possession, such as taking the client's personal items including candy, jewelry, or monies from a nursing home resident or clothing that is given to another resident to wear

h. Negligence: omission or commission of an act that departs from acceptable and reasonable standards of practice, such as failing to monitor a client's bowel movement pattern and the client develops an impaction

i. Malfeasance: committing an unlawful or improper act, such as a nurse performing surgery on a client's leg ulcer

j. Misfeasance: performing an act improperly, such as a nurse starting a prescribed intravenous infusion in the foot of a client with impaired circulation

k. Nonfeasance: failure to take proper action, such as not notifying the physician of a serious change in the client's status

l. Malpractice: failure to abide by the standards of practice of the nursing profession, such as not checking if the nasogastric tube is in the stomach before administering the tube feeding

m. Criminal negligence: to disregard protecting the safety of another person, such as allowing a client who is confused and receiving oxygen to have access to cigarettes and a lighter in an unsupervised situation

C. INFORMED CONSENT
   1. DESCRIPTION
      a. Consent is a voluntary act by which a person agrees to have something done to the person by someone else.
      b. Informed consent is a process by which a client knows the reason for the proposed treatment as well as its benefits and risks and is implied by signing a consent form.
      c. Clients have the right to know the full implications of procedures and make an independent decision as to whether or not the procedure should be performed. Obtaining an informed consent in the older adult may be difficult if the client has been declared legally incompetent and has a guardian. Clients who have a fluctuating level of mental function or who are not fully able to comprehend are incapable of giving legal consent. Consent must be obtained from the legal guardian.
      d. Protects the client's right to self-determination
      e. If in doubt about whether written consent is necessary in a given situation, it is best to err on the side of safety by obtaining witnessed consent from the client if the client is competent or from the legal guardian.
      f. If the client or guardian refuses a prescribed procedure it is useful to have the responsible party sign a release stating that consent is denied and that the risks associated with refusing consent are understood such as refusing to receive a prescribed influenza vaccination.

D. COMPETENCY
   1. DESCRIPTION
      a. Competency is the client's ability to make rational decisions regarding care
      b. The client must be able to make decisions voluntarily.
      c. The client has access to information relevant to the health problem and to related decisions.
      d. The client must be legally declared incompetent before a designated guardian has the right to make health care decisions.
      e. Advance directives signed by a client who is competent and witnessed provides for a surrogate to make health care decisions if the client is no longer able to do so.

E. SUPERVISION OF OTHER HEALTH CARE TEAM MEMBERS
   1. DESCRIPTION
      a. The registered nurse has the responsibility to supervise the care delegated to other licensed and unlicensed personnel.
      b. This supervision may be direct or indirect as identified in the nurse practice laws of the legal jurisdiction.

F. MEDICATION ADMINISTRATION
  1. EACH LEGAL JURISDICTION IDENTIFIES WHO MAY ADMINISTER MEDICATIONS TO NOT ONLY ALL CLIENTS BUT ALSO TO VULNERABLE OLDER ADULTS.
    a. The registered nurse caring for older adults has the responsibility to know the prescribed medications, adverse reactions, interactions, and contraindications even if a licensed or unlicensed personnel, such as a medication aide a family member, administers the medications in the nursing home or in the client's home.

G. RESTRAINTS
  1. DESCRIPTION
    a. The Omnibus Budget Reconciliation Act (OBRA) designates the rights of the client and the responsibilities of the providers of health care regarding the use of either physical or chemical restraint, or both.
    b. The older adult has a right to the safest and least restrictive environment.
    c. Other methods to avoid restraints should be used, such as looking in on the client whenever passing the client's room or keeping the bed in the lowest possible position.
    d. Restraints are legal only if they are used to protect the client or others from harm.
    e. If the nurse applied restraints in an emergency situation to a client who is combative or unruly, the nurse must obtain an order immediately.
    f. A legal order from a licensed prescriber, such as a physician or nurse practitioner, is necessary for physical restraints of a client. This includes the use of side rails, a lap belt restraint, or a chest restraint.
    g. The use of a chemical agent, such as a sedative, for restraint of the client must also require a legal order.
    h. A restraint such as bed rails should be agreed to in writing by a client who is competent or by the legal guardian.
    i. Documentation of the client behavior, need for the restraint for safety, monitoring the client frequently, and removal of the restraint must be performed frequently and according to agency policy.

H. TELEPHONE ORDERS
  1. DESCRIPTION
    a. Medical orders from a physician are frequent in the care of the older adult whether in home health or long-term care.
    b. The possibility of error is great with a verbal order. Repetition and clarification of the order is necessary to prevent errors.
    c. Agency policy will identify if a registered nurse may take a verbal order from the physician's office personnel.

I. "NO-CODE" ORDERS
  1. DESCRIPTION
    a. Each legal jurisdiction will identify the scope of medical orders that indicate "no-code" status for a client.
    b. In general, if the client does not have advance directives all measures will be used to resuscitate a client and prolong life. Kinship laws vary with legal jurisdiction, and next of kin may be able to identify for a client who is unable to make his wishes known what measures should be taken.

J. ADVANCE DIRECTIVES
  1. DESCRIPTION
    a. Clients who are competent have the right to complete advance directives for health care, which could be followed in the event that they are unable at some time to make their own decisions.
    b. In many legal jurisdictions, next of kin may request additional medical measures to prolong life.

K. ISSUES RELATED TO DEATH AND DYING
  1. DESCRIPTION
    a. An older adult may have an advance directive with which family members disagree.
    b. Older adults may delegate important decisions to family members who do not understand the ramifications of health care choices they may make, such as putting a client with end-stage congestive heart failure on a ventilator.

L. ABUSE AND NEGLECT OF VULNERABLE OLDER ADULTS
  1. DESCRIPTION
    a. Older adults may be the victims of emotional, physical, and sexual abuse.
    b. The registered nurse must be alert to the signs of abuse and neglect, possibly from caregivers.
    c. Signs of abuse include unexplained bruises or welts; multiples bruises; unexplained fractures, abrasions, and lacerations; multiple injuries; withdrawal or passivity; fear; depression; and hopelessness.
    d. Signs of neglect include dehydration; malnourishment; overmedication or undermedication; desertion or abandonment; inappropriate or soiled clothes; lack of glasses, dentures, or

other aids if usually worn; and being left unattended.

   e. Exploitation of the vulnerable older adult includes disappearance of possessions, being forced to sell possessions or change a will, being overcharged for home repairs,

inadequate living environment, inability to afford social activities, being forced to sign over control of finances, and having no money for food or clothes.

   f. The registered nurse must report abuse, neglect, and exploitation to the proper authorities.

PRACTICE QUESTIONS

1. A nurse admitted an older adult with a history of alcohol abuse. The client asked for assurance that leather restraints would not be used under any circumstances during alcohol withdrawal after surgery. The nurse promised that no restraints would be used. After surgery, the client was very agitated, delirious, and combative. Although restraints were indicated to preserve the client's safety, the nurse opposed using them because of the promise made. This action by the nurse was
   1. appropriate because of the nurse's promise.
   2. inappropriate because the promise was not safe.
   3. a violation of the American Nurses Association Code of Ethics for Nurses.
   4. a violation of the American Nurses Association Nursing Standards.

2. A staff member observes a nurse assigned to a postoperative nursing unit reading the chart of a friend's grandmother who is a client on the unit. The nurse is not assigned to this client and does not have a responsibility for this client's care. The client was just diagnosed with terminal cancer and the family does not know. The staff member evaluates the action by the nurse as
   1. appropriate because the nurse is a health care worker and assigned to the unit.
   2. inappropriate because the grandmother is not assigned to the nurse.
   3. not being a violation of the client's privacy because the nurse does not tell anyone what is in the chart.
   4. gaining information to assist a friend through a difficult time.

3. The nurse is concerned about the medical care a long-term care resident is receiving. The nurse asks an opinion about the medical care from a physician who is not responsible for the client. The nurse has
   1. violated the principle of confidentiality.

   2. acted appropriately to gain information on the client's behalf.
   3. gone to the appropriate chain of command.
   4. followed institutional policy.

4. A nursing home resident is offered the opportunity to participate in research on a new drug therapy to treat pressure ulcers. The resident decides after signing the consent form not to participate in the research project. Based on an understanding of the legal issues related to nursing homes, which of the following is appropriate in this situation? The client
   1. cannot withdraw from the study after the consent is signed.
   2. can withdraw at any time from the study.
   3. cannot participate in a study because of being incompetent.
   4. can withdraw only if the family requests withdrawal.

5. The nurse is eating lunch in a nursing home cafeteria. Two nurse aides can be heard at the next table talking about a resident by name. Which of the following is the priority nursing action?
   1. Talk to the nurse aides privately later about this inappropriate behavior
   2. Tell the nurse aides they are being overheard and should talk quietly
   3. Report them to their supervisor
   4. Tell the nurse aides that they are breaching confidentiality

6. The nurse is working in an outpatient same-day surgery unit. An 86-year-old client signs the surgical consent form and asks the nurse, "What did I just sign? My wife always takes care of the paperwork." Which of the following is the priority nursing action?
   1. Assess what the client understands about the surgery
   2. Notify the surgeon that the client does not understand the surgery

3. Ask the client's wife to explain the consent for surgery

4. Ask the client's wife to sign the consent form because the client is not competent

7. Which of the following is the appropriate nursing action when a nursing student assigned to the surgery suite for observation asks the nurse for permission to photocopy the surgical record from a client's chart for an assignment the student must write?
   1. Photocopy the pages for the student
   2. Allow the student to photocopy the pages without the client's name
   3. Allow the student to write down pertinent but no identifying information
   4. Ask the physician for permission to photocopy the pages

8. The nurse working in a long-term care facility is orientating a new nurse to the facility. The nurse should tell the new nurse that which of the following is the priority reason that health care issues of older adults become an ethical dilemma?
   1. The choices for health care options do not seem to be clearly right or wrong
   2. Decisions are made based on value systems
   3. Decisions are made quickly
   4. The legal rights of the client coexist with the health professional's obligation to provide care for the client

9. A nurse is accused of which of the following when writing on an older adult's transfer papers to a long-term care facility that "he is a dirty old man"?
   1. Defamation of character
   2. Negligence
   3. Malfeasance
   4. Invasion of privacy

10. The temporary nurse from a registry is working on the night shift in a long-term care facility. This nurse has had little experience working with the older adult. Which of the following is an appropriate assignment for the charge nurse to give the nurse from the registry?
    1. An 83-year-old hospice client who is expected to die soon
    2. Administration of medication to 18 clients
    3. Six clients who are stable
    4. Two clients with fevers of unknown origin

11. The nurse is planning care for a group of older adult clients. Which of the following clients is a priority for the nurse to care for first?
    1. An 87-year-old client in need of a dressing change
    2. An 83-year-old client with an infected total knee replacement incision

3. A 92-year-old client who has a temperature of 38.3°C, or 101°F
4. A 90-year-old client who has potassium of 6.7 mEq/L

12. A nurse is teaching a class of new graduate nurses on negligence. Which of the following situations is a priority for the nurse to include in the class as an example of negligence?
    1. Not giving a prescribed medication to an older adult
    2. Not turning off the oxygen at the bedside when a client at home wants to smoke in bed
    3. Not allowing a family member to awaken an older adult client who is sleeping
    4. Talking about a client outside of the long-term care facility

13. One of the unlicensed assistive personnel (UAPs) caring for an older adult with fragile skin report to the nurse a red, painful, and swollen IV site in the hand. Which of the following requests by the nurse does the UAP interpret as inappropriate and illegal?
    1. "Tell the client I'll be there as soon as I can."
    2. "Carefully take the IV out."
    3. "Put a cool washcloth on the IV site."
    4. "Elevate the client's hand on a pillow."

14. After reviewing the records of four older clients in a long-term care facility, which of the following situations does the nurse recognize as violating the client's right to privacy?
    1. Administering a medication to a client in the presence of other clients
    2. Placing the client's name on the client's bed
    3. Placing a photograph of the client in the medication administration record
    4. Placing a photograph of the client in the medical record

15. A 66-year-old client is admitted to a long-term care facility for rehabilitation following a total hip replacement. The client refuses to stay in the facility and tells the nurse, "I am going to walk home." Which of the following is the appropriate action by the nurse?
    1. Tell the client that rehabilitation is necessary and leaving is not possible
    2. Restrain the client to prevent the client from leaving
    3. Call security to restrain the client
    4. Do not prohibit the client from leaving

16. The older adult client in a long-term care facility is soiled with feces. The client calls out, "Stop, don't hurt me. Help!" while being bathed by the nurse. Because the nurse did not have the client or the client's guardian's expressed

permission to bathe the client, the nurse is at risk for being accused of
1. assault.
2. battery.
3. malpractice.
4. negligence.

17. A 66-year-old client with developmental disabilities and schizophrenia living in a long-term care facility develops pneumonia and is seriously ill. There are no advance directives and no legal guardian. Which of the following is the appropriate nursing intervention as the client's condition worsens?
    1. Do not resuscitate because of the impairment of the client
    2. Do not resuscitate because of the age of the client
    3. Provide all possible medical treatment including resuscitation
    4. Call the client's physician for a do not resuscitate order

18. A nurse observes a staff member telling an older adult client that if the client does not take prescribed oral medications, dessert will be withheld. The nurse reports the behavior of the staff member as
    1. assault.
    2. battery.
    3. malpractice.
    4. negligence.

19. A new employee to a long-term care facility asks the nurse if pictures of the residents may be taken. The appropriate response is, "Pictures
    1. cannot be published without the resident's or guardian's permission."
    2. may only be taken by the family."
    3. can be published if the residents are not identified."
    4. will not violate the right to privacy when taken discreetly."

20. An older adult client receives a gift of boxed chocolate candy. The client has dementia and does not understand that the candy is the client's and what it is. The nurse should
    1. tell the client the candy is the client's and offer a piece.
    2. offer the candy to the other clients.
    3. send the candy home with the client's family.
    4. throw the candy away, as the client is unable to eat it.

21. Based on an understanding of the legal liability in health care, a nurse who fails to monitor the bowel movement pattern of an older adult client, which leads to an impaction, has committed which of the following?

1. Misfeasance
2. Malpractice
3. Assault
4. Negligence

22. A nurse allowed an older adult who is confused to hold onto her purse. Later, the client was receiving oxygen by nasal prongs and attempted to light a cigarette with a cigarette lighter from the purse. An explosion, fire, and injury subsequently resulted. The case goes to court and the nurse is charged with which of the following?
    1. Negligence
    2. Battery
    3. Criminal negligence
    4. Malfeasance

23. An older adult client tells the nurse that the client has human immunodeficiency virus (HIV). The nurse should
    1. document this information in the client's chart.
    2. tell the client's physician.
    3. inform the health care team who will come in contact with the client.
    4. encourage the client to disclose this information to the client's physician.

24. The nurse caring for an older adult tears the skin of the client while removing a piece of tape. The skin is attached to the upper arm and to the tape. The nurse cuts the attached part of the skin with a scissors in order to remove the tape. The nurse fails to understand that if harm comes to the client during the act of cutting the skin with the scissors, which of the following could the nurse be charged with?
    1. Malpractice
    2. Negligence
    3. Acceptable practice
    4. Assault

25. The nurse caring for an older adult client soiled with feces fails to clean and bathe the client, leaving the client for another staff member to care for. Another nurse reports this nurse as guilty of
    1. nonmaleficence.
    2. negligence.
    3. malpractice.
    4. assault.

26. Which of the following should the nurse include when teaching a class on restraint application in the older adult?
    1. Restraints should be removed and reapplied every 4 hours
    2. Place a client with extremity restraints in a prone position to ensure safety

3. A physician must evaluate a client within one hour after restraints are applied in an emergency situation
4. A client should have a belt restraint on at all times as a safety precaution

27. The nurse should include which of the following in the plan of care for a client who is confused, combative, bedridden, and has a vest restraint?
   1. Securely tie the straps of the vest restraint to the side rails of the bed
   2. Crisscross the vest in the front and tie the vest with a quick-release knot
   3. Remove the client's gown before applying the vest to ensure a snug fit
   4. Provide hygienic care around the vest, taking care not to untie or remove the vest

28. The nurse is caring for an older adult client who is very combative and is constantly hitting the staff at a long-term care facility. The decision was made that extremity restraints are temporarily necessary. Which of the following is most appropriate to include in this client's plan of care?
   1. Place the client in a lateral position
   2. Insert one finger between the restraint and the client's extremity
   3. Secure the restraint to the nonmovable part of the bed
   4. Remove the restraint after four hours to assess the skin

29. The nurse appropriately applies a mummy restraint to which of the following clients?
   1. An older adult client who is confused
   2. A screaming child prior to an eye irrigation
   3. An adolescent who is having a drug reaction
   4. An older adult client who is combative and scratching the staff

30. The registered nurse is preparing to delegate nursing tasks. Which of the following should the nurse delegate to unlicensed assistive personnel?
   1. Perform a neurovascular assessment on an older adult client who has a jacket restraint
   2. Assess the skin integrity of an older adult client with a belt restraint
   3. Perform range-of-motion exercises on an older adult client with an extremity restraint
   4. Assess the oxygenation status of an older adult client with a vest restraint

31. The registered nurse is preparing the client assignments for the day in a long-term care facility. Which of the following client assignments would be appropriate for the registered nurse to delegate to unlicensed personnel?
   1. Application of a prescribed restraint
   2. Administration of medications through a nasogastric tube
   3. Assessment of a postoperative stoma
   4. Irrigation of a Foley catheter

ANSWERS AND RATIONALES

1. 2. The nurse should not have made a promise that would possibly compromise the client's safety. The client could also receive some medication for the agitation, delirium, or combative behavior.

2. 2. Nurses only have the right to health care information that involves the clients for whom they are responsible and to whom the nurses have a duty.

3. 1. A resident of a long-term facility, as other clients, has the right to confidentiality about personal health care information. If the nurse has a concern, the matter should be discussed with the primary physician.

4. 2. Even though living in a long-term care facility, the older adult is considered competent unless legally declared otherwise. A client can withdraw from a research study at any time.

5. 4. Residents of a nursing home, as all clients, have the right to confidentiality. The priority action

is to deal with this inappropriate behavior as soon as it occurs. The nurse has the responsibility to protect the resident's privacy.

6. 1. Assessment of the client's understanding of the surgery is essential. If a client has signed a surgical consent form then questions what was signed, it is a priority to assess what the client understands. After assessing what the client understands, or if the client is incompetent, then it would be appropriate to notify the physician.

7. 3. When a nursing student wants to photocopy a client's medical record, nonidentifying information may be written down. The client has the right to confidentiality and any information that could be linked to the client, such as names or addresses, cannot be shared.

8. 4. Although health care options do not seem clearly right or wrong and decisions in a long-term care facility are made quickly, the priority reason health care issues in older adults become highly charged ethical dilemmas is that the client's rights to care and for a dignified death are managed in the context of the health professional's obligations to provide care.

9. 1. Defamation of character is an oral or written communication to a third party that damages a person's reputation, such as transferring a client from one facility to another and writing on the discharge papers that "he is a dirty old man."

10. 3. A nurse who is not familiar with the agency or the clients should be assigned to the most stable clients. Assigning a nurse to a hospice client, to clients with fevers of unknown etiology, or to administering medication to clients all require knowledge of the particular clients.

11. 4. Although a client with an infected knee replacement, a temperature of 38.3°C, or 101°F, and a client in need of a dressing change all need an assessment by the nurse, the client with a potassium level of 6.7 mEq/L is the most acute and at risk.

12. 2. Negligence is the result of either omitting to do something that another reasonable person, guided by those ordinary considerations that ordinarily regulate human affairs, would do, or of doing something another reasonable or prudent person would not do. If there is imminent danger to a client, the nurse must take every measure to protect the client. It may be appropriate for the nurse such as in the case of a client with a sudden rash and the nurse withholds a prescribed antibiotic, which may contribute to the development of the rash. It is inappropriate to talk about a client outside of a long-term care facility because it violates the client's right to privacy, but it is not negligence.

13. 2. Unlicensed assistive personnel cannot legally perform a nursing function such as removing an IV. This would be interpreted as inappropriate and illegal.

14. 1. The medications that a client receives are private. The medications should not be administered where someone else, such as another client, can see what the client is receiving. Placing the client's name on the client's bed, and placing a photograph in the client's medical record or medication administration record are for the client's safety and do not violate the right to privacy. Only authorized personnel have access to that information.

15. 4. A client who is in a long-term care facility for rehabilitation and who wants to go home is competent and able to make decisions, even if those decisions may endanger the client's health. It would be inappropriate to prevent the client from leaving, because the client can make health care decisions unless incompetence has been declared. Restraining the client would be false imprisonment or battery.

16. 2. Because the client is protesting the bathing, the nurse could be accused of battery without the permission of the guardian. Battery is the unlawful touching of another person. Assault is an unjustifiable attempt or a threat to touch a person without consent that results in fear of immediate harm. The touching may not actually occur. Malpractice is a type of negligence in which any unreasonable act or professional misconduct results in injury to the client. Negligence is the failure to do something that a reasonable person, led by those ordinary considerations that ordinarily regulate human affairs, would do, or the doing of something another reasonable person would not do.

17. 3. In the absence of advance directives by the client or a guardian, the nurse must provide all appropriate care.

18. 1. Assault is a deliberate threat that the client believes could be carried through, or an unjustifiable attempt or threat to touch a person without consent that results in fear of immediate harm. Battery is unlawful touching of another person. Malpractice is a type of negligence in which any unreasonable act or professional misconduct results in injury to the client. Negligence is the omission of doing something that a reasonable person, led by those ordinary considerations that ordinarily regulate human affairs, would do or doing something another reasonable person would not do.

19. 1. The right to privacy includes the publishing of pictures or any other information about a client without the client's or guardian's permission. The nurse has the responsibility to advocate for and protect the client's privacy. Pictures may be taken in a long-term care facility for the purpose of placing the photograph in the client's medical record or on the medication administration record.

20. 1. When a client with dementia does not recognize that the candy gift belongs to the client, the nurse should take every opportunity to get the client to enjoy it. The candy is a gift and the personal property of the client. The nurse cannot take the candy. This could constitute larceny.

21. 4. Negligence is the omission or commission of an act that departs from the acceptable and reasonable standards of practice. The nurse is expected to monitor the elimination patterns of clients. A nurse that fails to monitor a client's bowel movement pattern and the client develops an impaction is accused of negligence.

22. 3. Criminal negligence is the disregard of protecting the safety of another person. The nurse has the responsibility to protect the client. In this case, the nurse failed to protect the client with oxygen from lighting cigarettes with a lighter and sustaining injury.

23. 4. The nurse must protect the client's right to privacy of health care information. Documenting a client's HIV status in the client's chart, telling the client's physician, and informing the health care team who will come in contact with the client all violate the client's right to privacy.

24. 1. Cutting the skin of a client with a scissors could be considered a medical procedure and not within the scope of nursing practice. A charge of malpractice could result. Malpractice is a type of negligence in which any unreasonable act or professional misconduct results in injury to the client. Negligence is the omission or commission of an act that departs from the acceptable and reasonable standards of practice. Assault is an unjustifiable attempt or threat to touch a person without consent that results in fear of immediate harm. The touching may not actually occur.

25. 2. The nurse is failing to perform an expected action, keeping the client clean and safe from harm. This is negligence. Negligence is the omission or commission of an act that departs from the acceptable and reasonable standards of practice. Malpractice is a type of negligence in which any unreasonable act or professional misconduct results in injury to the client. Assault is an unjustifiable attempt or threat to touch a person without consent that results in fear of immediate harm. The touching may not actually occur. Nonmaleficence is a principle that requires the nurse to act in such a way as to prevent harm to a client.

26. 3. The least restrictive type of restraint should be used. If restraints are used in an emergency situation, a physician must evaluate the client within one hour after the restraint is applied. Restraints should be reassessed every hour and removed every two hours. Wrist and ankle restraints should not be applied with the client in a prone position because there is an increased risk for aspiration. The client should be placed in a supine position. A belt restraint should not be used just because the client is an older adult and without justification. This is considered false imprisonment.

27. 2. A vest restraint should be crisscrossed in the front and tied with a quick-release knot. The restraint should be applied over the client's clothes to prevent friction on the skin. A restraint should never be tied to the side rails of the bed. This poses the risk of strangulation.

28. 1. A client who has an extremity restraint should be placed in the lateral position. Placing this client in a supine position would place the client at risk for aspiration. Two fingers should be inserted under a restraint to prevent it from being too tight. The restraint should never be applied to the nonmovable part of the bed, to avoid the restraint from becoming too tight when the bed is raised or lowered. The skin under a restraint must be assessed every hour and the restraint must be removed every 2 hours.

29. 2. A mummy restraint is most generally used with a small child during some kind of short-term examination or treatment. Older adult clients should never be restrained because they are confused or combative. An adolescent would never be restrained just because of a drug reaction.

30. 3. Performing specific assessments, such as a neurovascular or an oxygenation assessment, or checking for skin integrity should not be delegated to unlicensed assistive personnel. These tasks require the skills of a nurse. Unlicensed assistive personnel may perform range-of-motion exercises on a client who has a restraint.

31. 1. Although unlicensed assistive personnel should not perform any assessments on a client with a restraint, they have been trained to apply the restraint. Administration of medications through a nasogastric tube, assessment of a postoperative stoma, and irrigation of a Foley catheter should be performed by a nurse.

REFERENCE

Burkhardt, M. A., & Nathaniel, A. K. (2008). *Ethics and issues in contemporary nursing* (3rd ed.). Clifton Park, NY: Delmar Cengage Learning.

SYMBOLS AND ABBREVIATIONS

Symbol	Meaning		Symbol	Meaning
~	similar		<	less than
≅	approximately		%	percent
@	at		+	positive
√	check		−	negative
Δ	change		♀	female
↑	increased		♂	male
↓	decreased		△△△	trimester of pregnancy
=	equals			(one triangle for
#	pounds			each trimester)
>	greater than			

2,3-DPG	2,3-diphosphoglycerate		ATSDR	Agency for Toxic Substances and Disease Registry
AACN	American Association of Colleges of Nursing		BCR	bulbocavernosus reflex
AAOHN	American Association of Occupational Health Nurses		BMI	body mass index
			BMR	basal metabolic rate
AARP	American Association of Retired Persons		BN	bachelor in nursing
ABG	arterial blood gases		BP	blood pressure
A/C	alternative/complementary		BScN	bachelor of science in nursing (in Canada)
acetyl-CoA	acetyl coenzyme A		BSE	breast self-examination
ADA	Americans with Disabilities Act		BSN	bachelor of science in nursing
ADAMHA	Alcohol, Drug Abuse, and Mental Health Administration		BUN	blood urea nitrogen
			C	Celsius; also called centigrade
ADH	antidiuretic hormone		CAI	computer-assisted instruction
ADL	activities of daily living		CAM	complementary and alternative medicine
ADP	adenosine diphosphate		CAT	computerized adaptive testing
ADR	adverse drug reactions		CAUSN	Canadian Association of University Schools of Nursing
AEB	as evidenced by			
AGF	angiogenesis factor		CBC	complete blood count
AGS	American Geriatric Society		CBE	charting by exception
AHA	American Hospital Association		CDC	Centers for Disease Control and Prevention
AHNA	American Holistic Nurses Association		CEUs	continuing education units
AHRQ	Agency for Healthcare Research and Quality		CHD	coronary heart disease
AIDS	acquired immunodeficiency syndrome		CLIA	Clinical Laboratory Improvement Act
AJN	American Journal of Nursing		cm	centimeter
AMB	as manifested by		CNA	Canadian Nurse Association
ANA	American Nurses Association		CNATS	Canadian Nurses Association Testing Service
ANS	autonomic nervous system		CNM	certified nurse midwife
AONE	Association of Nurse Executives		CNO	community nursing organization
AORN	Association of Perioperative Registered Nurses		CNP	chronic nonmalignant pain
APN	advanced practice nurse		CNS	central nervous system; clinical nurse specialist
APRN	advanced practice registered nurse			
APS	American Pain Society		CO_2	carbon dioxide
APTT	activated partial thromboplastin time		COBRA	Consolidated Omnibus Budget Reconciliation Act
ASCN	Association of Collegiate Schools of Nursing			
AST	aspartate aminotransferase		COPD	chronic obstructive pulmonary disease
AT	axillary temperature		CPK	creatine phosphokinase
ATP	adenosine triphosphate		CPM	continuous passive motion

CPN	central parenteral nutrition	IV	intravenous
CPR	cardiopulmonary resuscitation	IVP	intravenous pyelogram
CPT	chest physiotherapy	JCAHO	Joint Commission on Accreditation of Healthcare Organizations
CQI	continuous quality improvement	kcal	kilocalorie
CRNA	certified registered nurse anesthetist	kg	kilogram
CSF	cerebrospinal fluid	l or L	liter
CST	computerized clinical simulation testing	LAS	localized adaptation syndrome
CT	computed tomography	lb	pound
CVA	cerebral vascular accident	LDH	lactic dehydrogenase
DDS	doctor of dental science	LDL	low-density lipoprotein
DHHS	Department of Health and Human Services	LLQ	left lower quadrant
dl	deciliter; also abbreviated dL	LMP	last menstrual period
DNR	do not resuscitate	LOC	level of consciousness
DNSc	doctorate of nursing in science	LPN	licensed practical nurse
DRGs	diagnostic-related groups	LUQ	left upper quadrant
DSN	doctorate of science in nursing	LVN	licensed vocational nurse
DUS	Doppler ultrasound stethoscope	m	meter
DVT	deep vein thrombosis	MA	master of arts
EBP	evidence-based practice	MAC	mid-upper-arm circumference
ECG	electrocardiogram (also known as an EKG)	MAR	medication administration record
ED	emergency department	MD	doctor of medicine
EEG	electroencephalogram	MDRO	multiple-drug-resistant organism
EN	enteral nutrition	mEq	milliequilvalent
EOL	end of life	mEq/L	milliequivalent per liter
EPA	Environmental Protection Agency	mg	milligram
EPO	exclusive provider organization	MH	malignant hyperthermia
EPR	electronic patient record	MI	myocardial infarction
ESR	erythrocyte sedimentation rate	ml	milliliter; also abbreviated mL
ET	ear canal temperature; enterostomal therapist	mm	millimeter
F	Fahrenheit	mm Hg	millimeters of mercury
FAF	fibroblast activating factor	MN	master in nursing
FAS	fetal alcohol syndrome	mOsm	milliosmole; also spelled milliosmol
FDA	Food and Drug Administration	mOsm/L	milliosmole per liter
FiO$_2$	fraction of inspired oxygen	MRI	magnetic resonance imaging
ft	feet	MRSA	methicillin-resistant *Staphylococcus aureus*
g	gram	MSN	master of science in nursing
GAS	general adaptation syndrome	NACGN	National Association of Colored Graduate Nurses
GCS	Glasgow Coma Scale	NANDA	North American Nursing Diagnosis Association
GI	gastrointestinal tract	NCCAM	National Center for Complementary and Alternative Medicine
GNP	gross national product	NCEP	National Cholesterol Education Program
GST	general systems theory	NCLEX	National Council Licensing Examination
gtt	drop	NCLEX-PN	National Council Licensure Examination for Practical Nurses
HBD	alpha-hydroxybutyrate dehydrogenase	NCLEX-RN	National Council Licensure Examination for Registered Nurses
HBV	hepatitis B virus	NCSBN	National Council of State Boards of Nursing
Hct	hematocrit	NCVHS	National Committee on Vital and Health Statistics
HDL	high-density lipoprotein	NIC	Nursing Interventions Classification
HEPA	high-efficiency particulate air	NIH	National Institutes of Health
Hgb	hemoglobin	NINR	National Institute of Nursing Research
HIPDB	Healthcare Integrity and Protection Data Bank	NLN	National League for Nursing
HIS	hospital information system	NMDS	Nursing Minimum Data Set
HIV	human immunodeficiency virus	NOC	Nursing Outcomes Classification
HMO	health maintenance organization	NP	nurse practitioner
HPN	home parenteral nutrition	NPDB	National Practitioner Data Bank
HPNA	Hospital and Palliative Nurses Association	NPO	*(non per os)* nothing by mouth (to eat or drink)
HQIA	Healthcare Quality Improvement Act	NS	nutrition support
HRSA	Health Resources and Services Administration	NSNA	National Student Nurses Association
HSV-2	herpes simplex virus 2	NST	nutritional support team
HT	healing touch	OBRA	Omnibus Budget Reconciliation Act
ICN	International Council of Nurses	OOB	out of bed
IHS	Indian Health Service	OR	operative room
IM	intramuscular	OSHA	Occupational Safety and Health Administration
in	inch		
I&O	intake and output		
IOM	Institute of Medicine		
IPPB	intermittent positive-pressure breathing		
IRA	individual retirement account		
ISMP	Institute of Safe Medication Practices		

OT	occupational therapist; oral temperature
OTC	over-the-counter drugs
oz	ounce
P	pulse
PA	physician assistant
PaO$_2$ (PAO$_2$)	partial pressure of oxygen dissolved in arterial blood plasma
Pap	Papanicolaou test
PAT	pulmonary artery temperature
PC	potential complication
PCA	patient-controlled analgesia
PCO$_2$	partial pressure of carbon dioxide dissolved in arterial blood plasma
PCP	primary care provider
PEG	percutaneous endoscopic gastrostomy
PERRLA	pupils equal, round, reactive to light, and accommodation
pH	hydrogen ion concentration of a solution
PID	pelvic inflammatory disease
PIE	problem, intervention, evaluation
PIEE	pulsed irrigation enhanced evacuation
PKU	phenylketonuria
PMR	progressive muscle relaxation
PMS	premenstrual syndrome
PN	parenteral nutrition
PNI	psychoneuroimmunology
PNS	peripheral nervous system
PO	*(per os)* by mouth
PO$_2$	partial pressure of oxygen in a mixture of gases, or in solution
POCT	point-of-care testing
POMR	problem-oriented medical record
POR	problem-oriented record
PPN	peripheral parenteral nutrition
PPO	preferred provider organization
PPS	prospective payment system
prn	*(pro re nata)* as needed
PRO	peer review organization
PSRO	professional standards review organization
PT	physical therapist; prothrombin; prothrombin time
PTSD	post-traumatic stress disorder
PTT	partial thromboplastin
PURT	prompted urge response toileting
q	every
QA	quality assurance
R	respiration
RAS	reticular activating system
RBC	red blood cell
RD	registered dietitian
RDA	recommended dietary allowance
RDDA	recommended daily dietary allowances
REM	rapid eye movement

RHC	rural health clinic
RLQ	right lower quadrant
RN	registered nurse
RNA	registered nurse's assistant
ROM	range of motion
RPCH	rural primary care hospital
RPh	registered pharmacist
RT	rectal temperature; related to respiratory therapist
RUQ	right upper quadrant
SA	sinoatrial node
SAECG	signal-averaged electrocardiography
SaO$_2$	percent saturation of arterial blood (hemoglobin) with oxygen
SBC	school-based clinic
S-CDTN	self-care deficit theory of nursing
SI	*le Systeme International d'Unites* (the international system of units)
SL	sublingual
SLT	social learning theory
SMDA	Safe Medical Devices Act
SMI	sustained maximum inspiration
SO	source-oriented charting
SOAP	subjective data, objective data, assessment, plan
SOAPIE	subjective data, objective data, assessment, plan, implementation, evaluation
STD	sexually transmitted disease
STG	short-term goal
SUI	stress urinary incontinence
SW	social worker
T	temperature
TCM	traditional Chinese medicine
TEFRA	Tax Equity Fiscal Responsibility Act
TENS	transcutaneous electrical nerve stimulation
TMJ	temporomandibular joint
TNA	total nutrient admixture
TPN	total parenteral nutrition
TQM	total quality management
TSE	testicular self-examination
TT	therapeutic touch
UAP	unlicensed assistive personnel
UHDDS	uniform hospital discharge data set
UNL	unified nursing language
USPHS	United States Public Health Service
VA	Veterans Affairs
VLDL	very low density lipoprotein
V/Q	ventilation/perfusion mismatch
VRE	vancomycin-resistant enterococci
WBC	white blood cell
WIC	Women, Infants, and Children
WNL	within normal limits

INDEX

Page numbers in italics reference figures, and those followed by "t" reference tables.